Biomedical Ethics

Biomedical Ethics

FOURTH EDITION

Thomas A. Mappes
Frostburg State University

David DeGrazia
George Washington University

McGRAW-HILL, INC.

New York   St. Louis   San Francisco
Auckland   Bogotá   Caracas   Lisbon   London
Madrid   Mexico City   Milan   Montreal
New Delhi   San Juan   Singapore   Sydney
Tokyo   Toronto

Biomedical Ethics

Copyright © 1996, 1991, 1986, 1981 by McGraw-Hill, Inc. All rights reserved.
Printed in the United States of America. Except as permitted under the United
States Copyright Act of 1976, no part of this publication may be reproduced or
distributed in any form or by any means, or stored in a data base or retrieval
system, without the prior written permission of the publisher.

This book is printed on acid-free paper.

2 3 4 5 6 7 8 9 0 FGR FGR 9 0 9 8 7 6

ISBN 0-07-040141-1

This book was set in Plantin by ComCom, Inc.
The editors were Judith R. Cornwell and Tom Holton;
the production supervisor was Louise Karam.
The cover was designed by Rafael Hernandez.
Quebecor Printing/Fairfield was printer and binder.

Library of Congress Cataloging-in-Publication Data
Biomedical ethics / [edited by] Thomas A. Mappes, David DeGrazia.—
    4th ed.
        p.   cm.
    Reprinted from various sources.
    Includes bibliographical references.
    ISBN 0-07-040141-1
    1. Medical ethics.   2. Bioethics.   I. Mappes, Thomas A.
    II. DeGrazia, David.
        [DNLM: 1. Ethics, Medical—collected works.   2. Bioethics—
    collected works.   W 50 B6153 1996]
R724.B49   1996
174' .2—dc20
DNLM/DLC
for Library of Congress   95-9348

ABOUT THE AUTHORS

Thomas A. Mappes holds a B.S. in chemistry from the University of Dayton and a Ph.D. in philosophy from Georgetown University. He is professor of philosophy at Frostburg State University, where he has taught since 1973. He is the coeditor (with Jane S. Zembaty) of *Social Ethics: Morality and Social Policy* (McGraw-Hill, 4th ed., 1992) and his published work appears in journals such as *American Philosophical Quarterly* and *Kennedy Institute of Ethics Journal*. In 1985, the Frostburg State University Foundation presented him with the Faculty Achievement Award for Teaching.

David DeGrazia earned a B.A. from the University of Chicago, an M.St. from Oxford University, and a Ph.D. from Georgetown University, each in philosophy. He has been teaching philosophy and biomedical ethics at George Washington University since 1989. He is the author of *Taking Animals Seriously* (forthcoming, Cambridge University Press) and of articles published in such journals as *Journal of Medicine and Philosophy, Public Affairs Quarterly, History of Philosophy Quarterly,* and *Southern Journal of Philosophy.*

CONTENTS

PREFACE

This fourth edition of *Biomedical Ethics,* like its predecessors, is designed to provide an effective teaching instrument for courses in biomedical ethics. Although the basic character of the book remains unchanged, it has been substantially revised and updated. More than 50 percent of the book's readings are new to the fourth edition, and a number of new chapter sections have been developed. For example, there are now sections on such topics as determinations of competence (Chapter 2), managing mental illness and dementia (Chapter 5), advance directives (Chapter 6), genetic engineering and the Human Genome Project (Chapter 9), and health-care-delivery systems (Chapter 10); there is also an expanded section on animal experimentation (Chapter 4). Moreover, the General Introduction (Chapter 1) has been extensively revised. For example, it now includes sections on virtue ethics, the ethics of care and feminist ethics, and casuistry.

In this fourth edition we have retained all the structural features that made earlier editions of the book effective teaching instruments. We have maintained the comprehensive character of the text, once again organized the subject matter so that it unfolds in an efficient and natural fashion, and retained a number of helpful editorial features, such as the headnotes that precede each selection and the annotated bibliographies at the end of each chapter. We have also retained (and updated) the appendix of case studies. Finally, inasmuch as the value of any textbook anthology is largely dependent upon the quality of its readings, we have once again assembled a set of readings characterized by high-quality analysis and, to the greatest extent possible, clarity of writing style. As in the past, we have also taken care to choose readings that reflect diverse viewpoints with regard to the leading issues in biomedical ethics.

The introductions to each chapter of this book provide one of its most important editorial features. In the introductions we explicitly identify the central issues in each chapter and scan the various positions on these issues together with their supporting argumentation. Whenever possible, we draw out the relationship between the arguments that appear in a certain chapter and the ethical concepts and approaches discussed in the General Introduction. Whenever necessary, we also provide background conceptual clarification and factual information. In this vein, as a matter of course, we explicate the meaning of technical biomedical terms and introduce relevant biomedical information. The purpose of the chapter introductions is to enhance the effectiveness of the book as a teaching instrument. This same central purpose is shared by the book's other editorial features, which include biographical as well as argument sketches preceding each selection and annotated bibliographies at the end of each chapter. The annotated bibliographies provide substantial guidance for further reading and research. The various entries in the bibliographies, like the various readings in each chapter, reflect diverse viewpoints.

The first three editions of *Biomedical Ethics* were developed through the joint efforts of Thomas A. Mappes and Jane S. Zembaty. This fourth edition was developed through the joint efforts of Thomas A. Mappes and David DeGrazia. One of the present editors (T.A.M.) would like to express his gratitude to Jane Zembaty for two decades of friendship and professional collaboration (which is ongoing in connection with other projects). Both of the present editors (T.A.M. and D.D.) want to acknowledge their extensive indebtedness to her for numerous passages, analyses, organizational structures, and insights originally embodied in earlier editions and carried over to the fourth.

We wish to thank Frostburg State University and George Washington University for their support of this project. In particular, gratitude is expressed to President Catherine Gira of Frostburg State University for her support of a sabbatical leave in the Fall of 1993. We are indebted to the Kennedy Institute, Georgetown University, whose bioethics library has been a significant ally in our research efforts. We greatly appreciate the helpful assistance of the library staff, especially Pat Milmoe McCarrick and Mary Carrington Coutts. We are also indebted to the reference librarians at Frostburg State University, and to the following professors who provided McGraw-Hill with useful review information: Arthur L. Caplan, University of Minnesota; Joseph W. Devlin, LaSalle University; Frank W. Derringh, CUNY–New York City Technical College; Patricia Fauser, Illinois Benedictine College; Jack Glickman, SUNY-Brockport; Sharon Gold, Rensselaer Polytechnic Institute; Melanie McLeod, University of Michigan, Flint; Heather Hull Mara, Albuquerque TVI Community College; William May, University of Southern California; John Messerly, Ursuline College; Michael J. Meyer, Santa Clara University; Betty Odello, Los Angeles Pierce College; Anthony Preus, Binghamton University; Ed Sherline, University of Wyoming; Anita M. Superson, University of Kentucky; Ronald M. Uritus, Barry University; Gregory L. Weiss, Roanoke College; and Thomas Young, Mansfield University. We are especially grateful to Judy Cornwell, our editor at McGraw-Hill, for her consistent responsiveness to our needs and concerns, to Joy Kroeger-Mappes, Frostburg State University, for her valuable criticisms and advice, and to Lawrence P. Ulrich, University of Dayton, for providing some of the case-study material in the Appendix. Finally, we must express our thanks to Sara Chant for her exemplary work as a research assistant, to Shelley Drees for her valuable help with manuscript preparation, and to Fergus Laughland for his assistance in proofreading.

Thomas A. Mappes
David DeGrazia

Biomedical Ethics

CHAPTER 1

GENERAL INTRODUCTION

A number of ethical issues (or problem areas) can be identified as associated with the practice of medicine and/or the pursuit of biomedical research. This set of ethical issues constitutes the subject matter of biomedical ethics. The proper task of biomedical ethics is to advance reasoned analysis in an effort to clarify and resolve such issues. What we term "biomedical ethics" is also commonly termed "bioethics." Although both terms are very well established and can be used interchangeably, *biomedical ethics* has the virtue of making more explicit the concern with issues associated with the practice of medicine. In any case, it is necessary in this context to understand *the practice of medicine* in an inclusive way, as referring not only to the professional activities of physicians but also to the distinctive activities of other health-care professionals.

THE NATURE OF BIOMEDICAL ETHICS

In order to situate biomedical ethics properly as a subdiscipline within the more general discipline of ethics, it is necessary to consider the nature of ethics as a philosophical discipline. *Ethics,* understood as a philosophical discipline, can be conveniently defined as the *"philosophical* study of morality." As such, it must be immediately distinguished from the *scientific* study of morality, often called "descriptive ethics." The goal of descriptive ethics is to attain empirical knowledge about morality. The practitioner of descriptive ethics is dedicated to describing existing moral views and, subsequently, explaining such views by advancing an account of their causal origin. Moral views, no less than other aspects of human experience, provide behavioral and social scientists a range of phenomena that stand in need of explanation. For example, why does a certain individual have such a Victorian view of sexual morality? A Freudian psychologist might attempt an explanation in terms of basic Freudian categories and early childhood experience. Why does a particular group of people manifest such a high incidence of moral advocacy for physician-assisted suicide? A sociologist might study the group in question and ultimately suggest an explanation based on factors such as the following: Many members of the group have seen loved ones die only after extensive suffering. Many members of the group identify themselves as nonreligious.

Ethics as a philosophical discipline stands in contrast to descriptive ethics. (Hereafter, the expression *ethics* is used to designate the philosophical discipline, as distinct from descrip-

1

tive ethics.) Philosophers commonly subdivide ethics into (1) normative ethics and (2) metaethics, although the precise relationship of these two branches is a matter of some dispute. In normative ethics, philosophers attempt to determine what is morally right and what is morally wrong with regard to human action.[1] In metaethics, philosophers are concerned with tasks such as analyzing the nature of moral judgments and specifying appropriate methods for the justification of particular moral judgments and theoretical systems. It seems plausible to maintain that deliberations in normative ethics are to some extent dependent upon and cannot be completely detached from metaethical considerations. Whatever the precise relationship between normative ethics and metaethics, it is important to see that *normative ethics* is logically distinct from *descriptive ethics*. Whereas descriptive ethics attempts to describe (and explain) those moral views that in fact *are accepted,* normative ethics attempts to establish which moral views are *justifiable* and thus *ought to be accepted.* In *general* normative ethics, the task is to advance and provide a reasoned justification of an overall theory of moral obligation, thereby establishing an ethical theory that provides a general answer to the question: What is morally right and what is morally wrong? In *applied* normative ethics, as opposed to general normative ethics, the task is to resolve particular moral problems—for example: Can abortion be morally justified, and, if so, under what conditions?

In light of the distinctions just made, it is now possible to identify biomedical ethics as one branch of applied (normative) ethics.[2] The task of biomedical ethics is to resolve ethical problems associated with the practice of medicine and/or the pursuit of biomedical research. Clearly, since there are ethical problems associated with other aspects of life, there are other branches of applied ethics. Business ethics, for example, is concerned with the ethical problems associated with the transaction of business. Importantly, in all branches of applied ethics, the particular issues under discussion are *normative* in character. Is this particular practice right or wrong? Is it morally justifiable? In applied ethics, the concern is not to establish which moral views people do in fact have. That is a descriptive matter. The concern in applied ethics, as in general normative ethics, is to establish which moral views are justifiable.

The following questions are typically raised in biomedical ethics: Is a physician morally obligated to tell a terminally ill patient that he or she is dying? Are breaches of medical confidentiality ever morally defensible? Can euthanasia be morally justified? Is surrogate motherhood morally justified? Normative ethical questions such as these are concerned with the morality of certain acts and practices. Other questions in biomedical ethics focus on the ethical justifiability of laws. For example, is society justified in having laws that restrict the availability of abortion? Should we have laws that prohibit physician-assisted suicide? Should we have laws that allow others to commit an individual, against his or her will, to a mental institution? The appearance of questions of this latter type shows that deliberations in biomedical ethics are intertwined not only with deliberations in general normative ethics but also with deliberations in social-political philosophy and the philosophy of law. In these latter disciplines, a central theoretical question concerns the justifiable limits of law. Strictly speaking, if biomedical ethics is a type of applied ethics, ethics must be broadly understood as overlapping with social-political philosophy and the philosophy of law.

Although many of the ethical issues falling within the scope of biomedical ethics have historical roots, especially insofar as they are related to various codes of medical ethics, biomedical ethics did not crystallize into a full-fledged discipline until very recently. Only since about 1970 have the various trappings of a relatively autonomous discipline become manifest. Numerous centers for research in biomedical ethics now exist. Two of the most prominent are The Hastings Center (now located in Briarcliff Manor, New York) and the Kennedy Institute of Ethics, Georgetown University (Washington, D.C.). New journals continue to appear, conferences abound, and the field has its own encyclopedia, *The Encyclopedia of Bioethics,* first published in 1978. An increasing number of philosophers, theologians, and other professionals now identify biomedical ethics as an area of specialization.

If, as is clear, many of the ethical issues falling within the scope of biomedical ethics have historical precedents, why has the field emerged as a vigorous and highly visible discipline only recently? Two cultural developments are at the root of the contemporary prominence of biomedical ethics: (1) the awesome advance of biomedical research as attended by the resultant development of biomedical technology and (2) the practice of medicine in an increasingly complicated institutional setting.

Consider first the impact of recent biomedical research. It has been responsible not only for the creation of historically unprecedented ethical problems but also for adding new dimensions to old problems and making the solution of those old problems a matter of greater urgency. Some developments—for example, those associated with reproductive technologies such as in vitro fertilization—seem to present us with ethical problems that are genuinely unprecedented. More commonly, however, the advance of biomedical research has simply added complexity to old problems and created a sense of urgency with regard to their solution. Euthanasia is not a new problem; however, our ability to save the lives of severely impaired newborns who would have died in the past and our ability to sustain the biological processes of irreversibly comatose individuals have added new dimensions and, surely, a new urgency. Abortion is not a new problem, but the development of various techniques of prenatal diagnosis has created the new possibility of genetic abortion. Indeed, the many successes of biomedical research in our own time, as manifested in the associated technological developments, call attention to the value of systematic biomedical research on human subjects and thus occasion reexamination of ethical limitations with regard to human experimentation.

The practice of medicine in an increasingly complicated institutional setting is, along with the advance of biomedical research, largely responsible for the contemporary prominence of biomedical ethics. In the past, the practice of medicine was largely confined within the bounds of the physician-patient relationship. Now, however, hospitals and other health-care institutions are intimately intertwined with physicians and allied personnel in the delivery of medical care. We have also witnessed an extension of the consumer rights movement into the health-care arena, a heightened emphasis on the legal requirements of informed consent, and an accompanying escalation of concern within the health-care community about legal liability. As a result, health-care professionals and institutions now find it necessary to pay closer attention to the interplay among medical, legal, and ethical considerations. Moreover, as a society we have become increasingly conscious of issues of social justice. We hear talk of a right to health care and are confronted with numerous problems of allocation.

It is frequently said that biomedical ethics is an interdisciplinary field, and some explication of its interdisciplinary character might prove helpful. First, there is a sense in which biomedical ethics is interdisciplinary within philosophy itself, that is, inasmuch as deliberations in biomedical ethics are intertwined not only with deliberations in general normative ethics but also with deliberations in social-political philosophy and the philosophy of law. Second, there is a sense in which biomedical ethics is interdisciplinary precisely because the issues under discussion are frequently approached not only from the vantage point of moral philosophy (the principal vantage point in the collection of readings in this text) but also from the vantage point of moral theology. Whereas philosophical arguments are constructed without presupposing the truth of any religious claims, that is, without reliance on religious *faith*, theological arguments are constructed within a faith framework. There is yet a third sense in which biomedical ethics is said to be interdisciplinary. In this sense, the most prominent one, biomedical ethics is interdisciplinary by reference to the disciplines of medicine and biology. Medical judgments and the findings of biology often play a crucial role in ethical deliberations. (The findings of the social sciences can be relevant as well.) It is also important to recognize that the *experience* of health-care professionals and biomedical researchers is often essential to ensure that ethical discussions retain firm contact with the concrete realities that permeate the practice of medicine and the pursuit of biomedical research.

Although the issues of biomedical ethics are essentially normative, they are intertwined with both conceptual issues and factual (i.e., empirical) issues. For example, suppose we are concerned with the ethical acceptability of intervention for the sake of preventing a person from committing suicide. Our basic concern is with a normative question; however, we must face the problem of clarifying the nature of suicide, a conceptual issue. For example, if a Jehovah's Witness, on the basis of religious principle, refuses a lifesaving blood transfusion, is the resultant death to be classified as a suicide? In addition to facing conceptual perplexities, we are also faced with an important factual question: Do those who typically attempt suicide really want to die? Presumably psychologists and sociologists have important things to tell us on this score. In the end, of course, we want to reach an ethical conclusion. However, ethical deliberations must proceed in the light of conceptual structures and factual beliefs. In the case of some issues in biomedical ethics, underlying factual issues are especially prominent. For example, in addressing the normative question of whether it is ever morally permissible to use children as research subjects, it is important to consider a factual question: To what extent can therapeutic techniques be developed for children in the absence of research employing children as research subjects? In the case of other issues in biomedical ethics, associated conceptual issues command special attention. For example, one could hardly discuss the normative issue of whether it is appropriate to transplant vital organs from brain-dead patients without closely examining the concept of death.

It is helpful to approach the literature of biomedical ethics with an eye toward distinguishing conceptual, factual, and normative issues. Furthermore, with regard to normative issues, which are the central issues of biomedical ethics, one cannot hope to situate argumentation in biomedical ethics properly without some awareness of the various types of ethical theory developed in general normative ethics. Such theories provide the frameworks within which many of the arguments in biomedical ethics are formulated.

ETHICAL THEORIES

As discussed in this section, an ethical theory provides an ordered set of moral standards (in some cases, simply one *ultimate* moral principle) that is to be used in assessing what is morally right and what is morally wrong regarding human action in general. A proponent of any such theory puts it forth as a framework within which a person can correctly determine, on any given occasion, what he or she (morally) ought to do.

The Critical Assessment of Competing Ethical Theories

Since a number of competing ethical theories may be identified, the question that immediately arises is what criteria are relevant to an assessment of these competing theories? There is no easy way to answer this very fundamental and very controversial question, but let us start with those considerations whose relevance is unlikely to be disputed. Any theory in any field is rightly expected to be internally consistent. Thus a theory can be faulted on the basis of inconsistency. In a similar vein, any theory is surely flawed to the extent that it is either unclear and/or incomplete. It might also be claimed that lack of simplicity should count against a theory, but the relevance of this consideration is somewhat problematic. Perhaps simplicity should be understood as a subsidiary criterion, one whose relevance is limited to the case of deciding between two theories otherwise judged to be equally defensible. Surely a theory that exhibits simplicity is more elegant, more aesthetically pleasing, than one that does not. However, if the latter theory is otherwise more adequate, it would seem to retain a superiority over the former.

If the above considerations are relevant to a critical assessment of theories in any field, we must yet identify considerations relevant to our particular concern, the critical assessment of (normative) ethical theories. Responsive to this task, it is suggested that the following criteria should be identified as embodying the two most important considerations. (1) The implications of an ethical theory must be largely reconcilable with our experience of the moral life. (2) An ethical theory must provide effective guidance where it is most needed, that is, in those situations where substantive moral considerations can be advanced on both sides of an issue. Although many philosophers would endorse the relevance of these two criteria, perhaps not so many would be willing to assign them the exclusive prominence suggested here. Nevertheless, in support of identifying them as the principal criteria relevant to a critical assessment of competing ethical theories, it can be pointed out that analogous considerations are clearly relevant (and prominent) in the critical assessment of empirical (i.e., scientific) theories. When competing empirical theories are under critical examination, it is surely relevant to ask which of the competitors gives a better account of the facts. It is also relevant to ask which of the competitors is superior in terms of heuristic value, that is, which can function to guide future research most effectively. In embracing the priority of criteria 1 and 2 we are saying that an adequate ethical theory must achieve two major goals, analogous to the goals that must be achieved by an adequate empirical theory. An adequate ethical theory must accord with the "facts" of the moral life as we experience it, and it must function heuristically by guiding us when we are confronted with moral perplexity. An ethical theory should, on the one hand, make sense out of the moral life by exhibiting the structures underlying our ordinary moral thinking. On the other hand, it should illuminate our moral judgment precisely where it is experienced to falter—in the face of moral dilemmas.

There is certainly no suggestion here that the standards embodied in criteria 1 and 2 can be applied in some mechanical-like fashion to assess the relative adequacy of a proposed ethical theory. Intellectual judgments on these matters are necessarily complex and subtle. In saying, for example, that an adequate ethical theory must accord with our experience of the moral life, we certainly do not want to insist that each and every divergence from the verdict of "commonsense morality" must be interpreted as counting against an ethical theory. Perhaps we would be better advised to revise our moral judgment in light of the theory. (In empirical science, fact-theory mismatches are sometimes resolved not by modifying the theory but by reinterpreting the facts in the light of the theory.) In embracing criterion 1 we undoubtedly commit ourselves to a point of view incompatible with the acceptance of an ethical theory that is revisionary in some wholesale sense, but we do not commit ourselves to the view that "commonsense morality" is sacrosanct. If an ethical theory successfully captures the underlying structures of our ordinary moral thinking, it will of course be true that its implications in large measure accord with our ordinary moral thinking. If the theory, however, cannot be reconciled with a relatively smaller range of our ordinary moral judgments, we may decide to interpret this disharmony as the product of some inadequacy in "commonsense morality" rather than as an inadequacy in the proposed theory.

Teleological versus Deontological Theories

With the introduction of criteria 1 and 2, we are now prepared to undertake a survey of alternative ethical theories. Our immediate concern is the identification, articulation, and critical consideration of those ethical theories that are at once both prominent in general normative ethics and frequently reflected in argumentation advanced in biomedical ethics. In a later section, under the heading of "Alternative Directions and Methods," some additional theoretical perspectives are presented.

In contemporary discussions, ethical theories are frequently grouped into two basic, and mutually exclusive, classes—*teleological* and *deontological*. Any ethical theory that claims the rightness and wrongness of human action is *exclusively* a function of the goodness and badness of the consequences resulting directly or indirectly from that action is a teleological theory. Consequences are all-important here. A deontological theory maintains, in contrast, that the rightness and wrongness of human action is *not exclusively* (in the extreme case, not at all) a function of the goodness and badness of consequences. In accordance with this specification, a theory is deontological (rather than teleological) if it places limits on the relevance of teleological considerations. Thus, an ethical theory in which the moral rightness and wrongness of human action is construed as totally independent of the goodness and badness of consequences would be only one kind, albeit the strongest or most extreme kind, of deontological theory.

The most prominent teleological ethical theory is the theory known as "utilitarianism." The adequacy of utilitarianism and the issue of its proper explication continue to be dominant concerns in contemporary discussions of ethical theory. For this reason, and especially because much argumentation in biomedical ethics is based on utilitarian reasoning, utilitarianism warrants our detailed attention. However, it should first be noted that utilitarianism is not the only ethical theory that is correctly categorized as teleological. One other notable teleological theory is the theory known as "ethical egoism." The basic principle of ethical egoism can be phrased as follows: *A person ought to act so as to promote his or her own self-interest.* An action is morally right if, when compared to possible alternatives, its consequences are such as to generate the greatest balance of good over evil *for the agent*. (The impact of action on other people is irrelevant except as it may indirectly affect the agent.) Ethical egoism is a teleological theory precisely because, by the terms of the theory, the rightness and wrongness of human action is exclusively a function of the goodness and badness of consequences.

Ethical egoism is an enormously problematic theory, one whose implications seem to be intensely at odds with our ordinary moral thinking. Under certain conditions, ethical egoism leads us to the conclusion that it is a person's moral obligation to perform an action that is flagrantly antisocial in nature. Consider this example. Mr. A loves to set buildings on fire; nothing makes him happier than watching a building burn. He recognizes that arson destroys property and subjects human life to serious risk, but he happens to be a thoroughly unsympathetic person, one whose well-being is not negatively affected by the misfortune of others. Of course, it would not be in A's best self-interest (and thus would not be A's moral obligation) to burn down a building if there is a good chance that he will be caught. (The punishment for arson is severe.) However, if A is very clever and if it is virtually certain that he will not be caught, ethical egoism seems to imply that arson is the morally right thing for him to do.

Another problematic feature of ethical egoism is that it cannot be publicly advocated without inconsistency. Suppose that Ms. B embraces ethical egoism. Accordingly, she considers it her moral obligation always to act in such a way as to promote her individual self-interest. Can she now publicly advocate ethical egoism, that is, encourage others to adopt the view that each person's moral obligation is to act in such a way as to promote his or her individual self-interest? No. Since it is to *her* advantage that others *not* act egoistically, it follows that it would be immoral for her to publicly advocate ethical egoism.

In reducing morality to considerations of personal prudence, it can be argued, ethical egoism destroys the very sense behind morality. Morality, it would seem, functions (at least in part) to restrict the pursuit of personal self-interest. It is not that morality prohibits the pursuit of personal self-interest; rather it functions to place limits on this pursuit. In "collapsing" morality into prudence, ethical egoism does not accord with a commonly experienced phenomenon of the moral life, the tension between self-interest and morality, between "what would be best for me" and "what is the morally right thing."

In fairness to ethical egoism, it must be noted that its proponents have sometimes devised ingenious arguments in an attempt to minimize the sort of difficulties just discussed. However, ethical egoism is not widely defended in contemporary discussions of ethical theory, and it surely plays an insignificant role in discussions of biomedical ethics. It has been introduced primarily as a notable instance of a teleological yet nonutilitarian theory. Attention will now be focused on utilitarianism.

In its classical formulation, utilitarianism is found most prominently in the works of two English philosophers, Jeremy Bentham (1748–1832) and John Stuart Mill (1806–1873). In contemporary discussions, a distinction is made between two kinds of utilitarianism—*act-utilitarianism* and *rule-utilitarianism*. Although it is somewhat controversial whether a significant distinction can be maintained between these two versions of utilitarianism, it is presumed for the sake of exposition that two distinct utilitarian ethical theories can indeed be articulated.[3]

Act-Utilitarianism

Human action typically takes place within the fabric of our social existence. Thus, an action performed by one person often affects not only the agent but also the lives of many others. Consider a man who refuses to stop smoking even though he suffers from emphysema. He will not be the only one to suffer the consequences; certainly those who care about him will also. His refusal to give up smoking, since it has the effect of further damaging his health, also produces a higher level of anxiety among the members of his family. Among the other detrimental consequences of his continuing to smoke is the negative impact, although small, on the productivity of those around him when he smokes. However, the various consequences of a single action are seldom uniformly good or uniformly bad. In addition to the bad consequences already indicated, there are also a number of good consequences that result from the refusal to stop smoking. Most notably, the emphysema patient continues to derive the satisfaction associated with cigarette smoking. In addition, it is likely that his continuing to smoke will make him less irritable around others. When the various consequences of a single action are fully analyzed, more often than not we find ourselves confronted with a mixture of good and bad. For example, if a person throws a late-night party, it is true that those in attendance may have a very good time, but it is also true that the neighbors may lose out on some much needed sleep.

The basic principle of act-utilitarianism can be stated as follows: *A person ought to act so as to produce the greatest balance of good over evil, everyone considered.* Act-utilitarianism stands in vivid contrast to ethical egoism, which directs a person always to act so as to produce the greatest balance of good over evil *for oneself* (i.e., the agent). The act-utilitarian is committed to the proposition that the interests of everyone affected by an action are to be weighed in the balance along with the interests of the agent. Everyone's interests are entitled to an impartial consideration. According to the act-utilitarian, an action is morally right if, when compared to possible alternatives, its likely consequences are such as to generate the greatest balance of good over evil, everyone considered. If we refer to the net balance of good over evil (everyone considered) that is likely to be produced by a certain action as its (overall) *utility*, then we can say that act-utilitarianism directs a person always to choose that alternative that has the greatest utility. Thus we can express the basic principle of act-utilitarianism as follows: A person ought to act so as to maximize utility.

For the act-utilitarian, calculation is a paramount element in the moral assessment of action. The question is always this: What is the utility of each of my alternatives in this particular set of circumstances? However, any system of utilitarian calculation must ultimately be anchored in some conception of intrinsic value (i.e., that which is good or desirable in and of itself). The act that will maximize utility (by our definition) is the act that is likely to produce the greatest balance of good over evil, everyone considered. However, what is to count as "good" and what as "evil" in our calculations? The answers provided within the framework of classical utilitarianism reflect a so-called hedonistic theory of intrinsic value. According to Bentham, only pleasure (understood broadly to include any type of satisfaction or enjoyment) has intrinsic value; only pain (understood broadly to include any dissatisfaction, frustration, or displeasure) has intrinsic disvalue. According to Mill, only happiness has intrinsic value; only unhappiness has intrinsic disvalue. To what extent there is substantive disagreement between Bentham and Mill on this matter is a complex question that cannot be dealt with here. It should be mentioned, however, that many contemporary utilitarian thinkers have embraced more elaborate and nonhedonistic theories of intrinsic value.[4] Nevertheless, for the sake of exposition, we shall presume that a hedonistic theory of intrinsic value, in the spirit of Bentham and Mill, underlies utilitarian calculation.

In the spirit of act-utilitarianism, in order to determine what I should do in a certain situation, I must first attempt to delineate alternative paths of action. Next, I attempt to foresee the consequences (sometimes numerous and far-reaching) of each alternative action. Then I attempt, in each case, to evaluate the consequences and to weigh the good against the bad, considering the impact of my action on everyone whom it is likely to affect. Such a reckoning will reveal the act that is likely to produce the greatest balance of good over evil, and this act is the morally right act for me in my particular circumstances. (If it appears likely that two competing actions would produce the same balance of good over evil, then either action will qualify as the morally correct action.) In some situations, it is true, no matter what I do, more evil (pain or unhappiness) will come into the world than good (pleasure or happiness). In such unfortunate situations, according to the act-utilitarian, the morally right act is the one that will bring the least amount of evil into the world.

Act-utilitarianism can rightly be understood as a form of "situation ethics." The act-utilitarian has no sympathy for the notion that certain kinds of actions are intrinsically wrong, that is, wrong by their very nature. Rather, a certain kind of action (e.g., lying) may be wrong in one set of circumstances yet right in another. The circumstances in which an action is to be performed are relevant to its morality (i.e., its rightness or wrongness) because the consequences of the action will vary depending on the circumstances. Thus, the morality of action is a function of the situation confronting the agent—"situation ethics."

The situational character of act-utilitarianism is reflected in the act-utilitarian attitude toward moral rules. Among the "commonsense rules of morality" are the following: "do not kill," "do not injure," "do not steal," "do not lie," "do not break promises," and so forth. According to the act-utilitarian, these rules are to be understood merely as rules of thumb. They are, for the most part, reliable guides for human action, especially relevant when time constraints undermine the possibility of careful calculation. In most circumstances, acting in accordance with a moral rule is the way to maximize utility, but in some cases this is not so. In these latter cases, whenever there is good reason to believe that breaking a moral rule will produce a greater balance of good over evil (everyone considered), the right thing to do is to break it. In such a case, it would be wrong to follow the rule. Lying is usually wrong, breaking promises is usually wrong, killing is usually wrong, but whenever circumstances are such that there is good reason to believe that breaking a certain moral rule will maximize utility, the rule should be broken. Of course, the act-utilitarian insists, one must be cautious in concluding that any given exception to a moral rule is indeed justified. One must be wary of rationalization and not allow one's own interests to weigh more heavily than the interests of others in the utilitarian calculation. Most importantly, one must not be simpleminded in a consideration of the likely consequences of breaking a moral rule. Indirect and long-term consequences must be considered as well as direct and short-term consequences. Lying on a certain occasion may seem to promote most effectively the interests of those immediately involved, but perhaps the lie will provide a bad example for less reflective people, or perhaps it will contribute to a general breakdown of trust among human beings. In this same vein, one prominent contemporary act-utilitarian emphasizes the significance of the long-term, indirect consequences of promise breaking, while at the same time exhibiting the underlying act-utilitarian attitude toward moral rules:

> The rightness or wrongness of keeping a promise on a particular occasion depends only on the goodness or badness of the consequences of keeping or of breaking the promise on that particular occasion. Of course part of the consequences of breaking the promise, and a part to which we will normally ascribe decisive importance, will be the weakening of faith in the institution of promising. However, if the goodness of the consequences of breaking the rule is *in toto* greater than the goodness of the consequences of keeping it, then we must break the rule. . . .[5]

Act-utilitarianism has often been criticized on the grounds that, due to the extensive sort of calculations it seems to demand, it cannot function as a useful guide for human action. In the spirit of this criticism, the following questions are asked: How can I possibly predict all the consequences of my actions? How am I to assign weights to the various kinds of human satisfactions—for example, the pleasure of eating a cheeseburger versus the aesthetic enjoyment of the ballet? How am I to weigh the anxiety of one person against the inconvenience of another? Besides, how am I supposed to have time to do these extensive calculations? Act-utilitarians, in response to such questions, usually appeal rather directly to "commonsense." They say, typically: There is no escape from a consideration of probabilities in rational decision making; predict as best you can and weigh as best you can, considering the time you have available for deliberation. All that can be expected is that you come to grips with the likely consequences of your alternatives in a serious-minded, sensible way, and then act accordingly.

Examples of Act-Utilitarian Reasoning in a Biomedical Context   The following examples are provided in an effort to exhibit act-utilitarian reasoning as it might arise in a biomedical context. It is not claimed that an act-utilitarian must necessarily reach the conclusion suggested in each case. It is only claimed that an act-utilitarian might plausibly reach the stated conclusion.

(1) A severely impaired newborn, believed to have no realistic chance of surviving more than a few weeks, has contracted pneumonia. (The treatment of impaired newborns is discussed in Chapter 7.) A physician, in conjunction with the parents of the infant, must decide whether to fight off the pneumonia with antibiotics, thereby prolonging the life of the infant. The alternative is simply to allow the infant to die. It seems clear that the interests of all those immediately involved are best served by deciding not to treat the pneumonia. Surely the infant has nothing to gain, and something to lose, by a slight extension of a pain-filled life. The parents, whose suffering cannot be eradicated whatever action is taken, nevertheless will find some relief knowing that their child's suffering has ended. In addition, hospital resources can be better utilized than to prolong the dying process of an infant who cannot benefit from further treatment. However, there may be decisive consequences of allowing death to occur that are indirect and long-term in nature. Perhaps allowing this infant to die will contribute to a breakdown of protective attitudes toward infants in general. No, the risk of this untoward consequence seems minimal. Withholding antibiotics, thereby allowing the infant to die, is the right thing to do in this particular case.

(2) A biomedical researcher, on the basis of animal studies she has conducted, believes that a certain drug therapy has great promise for the treatment of a particular kind of cancer in human beings. At present, however, her primary concern is to establish an appropriate

dosage level for human beings; there have been several troublesome side effects exhibited by the animals who received large doses of the drug. Over the years, the researcher has found that students at her university are very willing to volunteer themselves as research subjects in experiments that can be identified as presenting only minimal risks to themselves. They are, however, understandably reluctant to volunteer for experiments that seem to present more substantial risks. The researcher in this particular case cannot honestly say that there are no substantial risks for research subjects. She expects, in particular, that perhaps 30 to 40 percent of the research subjects will have to contend with very prolonged nausea. However, if she is honest in conveying this information to potential research subjects, it is unlikely that they will volunteer in sufficient numbers. (The ethics of experimentation on human subjects is discussed in Chapter 4.) Perhaps, she reasons, it is justifiable in this particular case to withhold information about the risk of very prolonged nausea. After all, it is very likely that numerous people will eventually derive great benefit from the therapeutic technique under study. Surely this likely benefit far outweighs the short-term discomfort of a much smaller number. Suppose, however, the deception comes to light. If those who routinely volunteer as research subjects are given a reason to distrust those conducting the experiments, the overall research effort on campus will be negatively affected. This seems to be a decisive consideration. In this particular case, then, deception would be wrong. (If there were no realistic chance of the deception being discovered, it seems that the conclusion would be different.)

(3) In the 1960s when kidney dialysis machines were scarce, it was not possible for all who needed them to be accorded access. A hospital administrator or perhaps a committee has been charged with the responsibility of deciding, in essence, whose lives will be saved. (Such decisions are often referred to as "microallocation decisions") On a particular occasion, when there is room for one more patient, there are two candidates in great need. One of the candidates, a civic-minded woman of 40, is married and the mother of four children. The other candidate, an unmarried man of the same age, is known to be a drifter and an alcoholic. It seems clear, at first glance, that the consequences of saving the woman's life are far superior to those of saving the man's life. Her husband, her children, and the community in general would be negatively affected in very substantial ways by her death. However, is it not problematic to accord a person access to a scarce medical resource on the basis of his or her social role? If a precedent of this sort is set, will not those whose lives are less "socially useful" become somewhat anxious and fearful? On the other hand, perhaps this negative consequence will be balanced by a positive consequence; that is, people will be more inclined to become "socially useful." It still seems clear that the woman in this case should have priority over the man.

Critical Assessment of Act-Utilitarianism   Act-utilitarianism arguably fares poorly when measured against a previously identified standard: The implications of an ethical theory must be largely reconcilable with our experience of the moral life. In a number of ways, it can be argued, act-utilitarianism clashes with our experience of the moral life. This perceived failure to accord with our ordinary moral thinking is reflected in the following well-known objections to act-utilitarianism.

(1) Act-Utilitarianism Confronts Individuals with an Overly Demanding Moral Standard. We are accustomed to thinking that at least some of our decisions are matters of "mere prudence," rightly decided on the basis of "what is best for me." Which major a college student should choose is a good example of a choice that we are inclined to consider essentially a nonmoral matter, a matter of "mere prudence." According to the act-utilitarian, however, a person is continually under a moral obligation to produce the greatest balance of good over evil, everyone considered. Whereas ethical egoism seems to wrongly "collapse" morality into prudence, it would seem that act-utilitarianism "expands" morality so as to destroy the realm of prudence. No aspect of a person's life can be considered merely a matter of prudence.

Every decision is a moral decision, to be made on the basis of utilitarian calculation. However, no matter how noble it might be for a college student to decide his or her major on the basis of a utilitarian calculation, it would seem that one is certainly not under an obligation to proceed in this manner. Doing so, we would ordinarily say, is not one's duty but, rather, is something "above and beyond the call of duty." Act-utilitarianism, in directing a person always to act so as to maximize utility, seems problematically to imply that it is one's duty to act in a way that we ordinarily consider "above and beyond the call of duty."

(2) Act-Utilitarianism Does Not Accord with Our Experience of Particular, Morally Significant Relationships. In our experience of the moral life, we are continually aware of highly particular, morally significant relationships that exist between ourselves and others. We are related to particular individuals in a host of morally significant ways, such as spouse to spouse, parent to child, creditor to debtor, promisor to promisee, employer to employee, teacher to student, physician or nurse to patient. In view of such relationships, it is ordinarily thought, we have special obligations—obligations that function to restrict the effort to maximize utility. Parents, we are strongly inclined to say, are obligated to care for their children even if there is good reason to think that the time and energy necessary for this task would maximize utility if redirected to some other task. In the same way, by virtue of the special relationship that exists between a physician and a patient, would it not be wrong for a physician to make decisions regarding a patient's treatment in the manner of an act-utilitarian? For a physician to damage the interests of an individual patient in an effort to maximize utility surely seems wrong. W. D. Ross, who has vigorously pressed this overall line of criticism against act-utilitarianism, asserts that the "essential defect of the . . . theory is that it ignores, or at least does not do full justice to, the highly personal character of duty."[6]

(3) Act-Utilitarianism Does Not Accord with Our Conviction That Individuals Have Rights. The notion of rights plays an important part in our ordinary moral thinking, but act-utilitarianism seems incapable of accommodating this notion. Moreover, in certain circumstances, the action that would maximize utility (and thus the right action according to the act-utilitarian) is one that we are inclined to consider seriously immoral precisely because it entails the violation of some person's right. For example, it seems that act-utilitarianism would allow an innocent person to be unjustly punished, as long as circumstances were such as to make this line of action the one that would generate the greatest balance of good over evil. Suppose extreme social unrest has been created by a wave of unsolved crimes. The enraged crowd will violently erupt, bringing massive evil into the world, unless the authorities punish someone (anyone) in an effort to appease the appetite for vengeance. So act-utilitarianism seems to allow the unjust treatment of a person as a scapegoat, as a mere means to a social end. But surely an innocent person has a right not to be punished, and it is by reference to this right that the wrongness of scapegoating is most naturally understood. Similarly, "the common moral opinion that painless undetected murders of old unhappy people are wicked, no matter what benefits result"[7] can be thought to rest on the contention that people, however old and unhappy, nevertheless have a *right* to life. It is often asserted against act-utilitarianism that it is a defective theory because it allows "the end to justify the means." At least part of the sense behind this charge can be made out in reference to the notion of rights. Certain means of achieving a desirable social end are simply wrongful because they entail the violation of a person's right. Contra act-utilitarianism, such means cannot be justified by the end.

Act-utilitarians have responded in two different ways to the overall claim that the theory cannot be reconciled with our ordinary moral thinking. Some say, in essence, "so much the worse for our ordinary moral thinking." In their view, we must simply overhaul our collective moral consciousness and embrace the mind-set of the act-utilitarian. Most act-utilitarians, however, do not adopt this revisionary stance. Rather, they seek to demonstrate that the clash between act-utilitarianism and our ordinary moral thinking is not nearly so severe as the above criticisms suggest. They argue that, when act-utilitarianism is properly applied, when all the significant long-term, indirect consequences are taken into account, the theory does not give rise to conclusions that seem so patently objectionable. It is very doubtful, however, that this strategy of argument can completely rescue act-utilitarianism from its difficulties.

Perhaps act-utilitarianism fares better when measured against the second of our previously identified standards: An ethical theory must provide effective guidance where it is most needed. At the very least, it must be said in favor of act-utilitarianism that it provides a reasonably clear decision procedure, a sense of direction, for the resolution of moral dilemmas. In the face of moral considerations that incline our judgment in conflicting ways, act-utilitarianism counsels us to analyze the likely consequences of alternative actions in order to determine the alternative that will maximize utility. Still, however well act-utilitarianism might be thought to fare with regard to our second standard, it seems to encounter significant problems when measured against our first standard. Indeed, in contemporary times, most utilitarian thinkers have rejected act-utilitarianism in favor of a theory known as rule-utilitarianism.[8]

Rule-Utilitarianism

The basic principle of act-utilitarianism has previously been formulated as follows: A person ought to act so as to produce the greatest balance of good over evil, everyone considered. In contrast, the basic principle of rule-utilitarianism can be formulated as follows: *A person ought to act in accordance with the rule that, if generally followed, would produce the greatest balance of good over evil, everyone considered.* If the demand to produce the greatest balance of good over evil, everyone considered, is referred to as the principle (standard) of utility, then the principle of utility is the basic ethical principle in both the act-utilitarian and the rule-utilitarian systems. However, in the act-utilitarian system, determining the morally correct action is a matter of assessing alternative actions directly against the standard of utility; whereas in the rule-utilitarian system, determining the morally correct action involves an *indirect* appeal to the principle of utility. In the spirit of rule-utilitarianism, a moral code is first established by reference to the principle of utility. That is, a set of valid moral rules is established by determining which rules (as opposed to conceivable alternatives), if generally followed, would produce the greatest balance of good over evil. In rule-utilitarianism, individual actions are morally right if they are in accord with those rules.

The difference between act-utilitarian reasoning and rule-utilitarian reasoning can be represented schematically as follows:

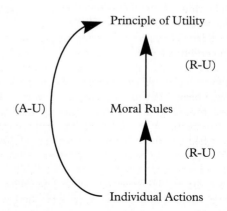

Principle of Utility

(R-U)

(A-U)   Moral Rules

(R-U)

Individual Actions

Act-utilitarian reasoning embodies a single-stage procedure; rule-utilitarian reasoning, a two-stage procedure. Because the act-utilitarian is committed to assessing individual actions strictly on the basis of utilitarian considerations, act-utilitarianism is often referred to as "extreme" or "unrestricted" utilitarianism. Because the rule-utilitarian is committed to developing a moral code (a set of moral rules) on the basis of utilitarian considerations and then assessing individual actions not on the basis of utilitarian considerations but on the basis of accordance with the moral rules that have been established, rule-utilitarianism is often referred to as "restricted" utilitarianism.

For the act-utilitarian, moral rules have a very subordinate status. They are merely "rules of thumb," providing some measure of practical guidance. For the rule-utilitarian, moral rules assume a much more fundamental status, indeed a theoretical primacy. Only in reference to established moral rules can the moral assessment of individual actions be carried out. Thus the first and most crucial step for the rule-utilitarian is the articulation of a set of moral rules, themselves justified on the basis of utilitarian considerations. Underlying this task is the question of which rules (as opposed to conceivable alternatives), if generally followed, would produce the greatest balance of good over evil, everyone considered. That is, which rules, if adopted or recognized in our moral code, would maximize utility?

As a first approximation of a set of moral rules that could be justified on the basis of utilitarian considerations, consider the "commonsense rules of morality," such as "do not kill," "do not steal," "do not lie," "do not break promises." It is not difficult to think of such rules as resting upon a utilitarian foundation. Surely the consequences of the adoption of the rule "do not kill" are dramatically better than the consequences of the adoption of the rule "kill whenever you want." If the latter rule were generally followed, society would be reduced to a profoundly uncivilized level. Similarly, the consequences of the adoption of the rule "do not steal" are dramatically better than the consequences of the adoption of the rule "steal whenever you want." If the former rule is generally followed, individuals will enjoy an important measure of personal security. If the latter rule were adopted by a society, anxiety and tension would dominate social existence. As for lying and promise breaking, if people felt free to engage in such behavior, the numerous advantages that derive from human trust and cooperation would evaporate. However, the rules thus far exhibited as having a utilitarian foundation are essentially prohibitions. Are there not also rules of a more positive sort that could also be justified on the basis of utilitarian considerations? It would seem so. Consider rules such as "come to the aid of people in distress" and "prevent innocent people from being harmed." It surely seems that human welfare would be enhanced by the adoption of such rules as part of the overall fabric of our moral code.

According to the rule-utilitarian, an individual action is morally right when it accords with the rules or moral code established on a utilitarian basis. However, the account of moral rules thus far presented is too simplistic. In order to be plausible, the rules that constitute the moral code must be understood as incorporating certain exceptions. The need to recognize justified exceptions is perhaps most apparent when we remember that moral rules, if stated unconditionally, can easily come into conflict with each other. When an obviously agitated person waves a gun and inquires as to the whereabouts of a third party, it may not be possible to act in accordance with both the rule "do not lie" and the rule "prevent innocent people from being harmed." Indeed, it is precisely this sort of situation that inclines us to consider incorporating an exception into our rule against lying. Suppose we say, "Do not lie *except* when necessary to prevent an innocent person from being harmed." When the possibility of a justified exception is raised, the rule-utilitarian employs the following decision procedure. The question is posed, Would the adoption of the rule with the exception have better consequences than the adoption of the rule without the exception? If so, the exception is a justified one; the rule incorporating the exception has greater utility than the rule without the exception. In the face of our proposed exception to the rule against lying, the rule-utilitarian would probably conclude that it does constitute a justified exception. The adoption of the rule "do not lie *except* when necessary to protect an innocent person from being harmed" would seem to preserve essentially all the social benefits provided by the adoption of the rule "do not lie," while at the same time bringing about an additional social benefit, an increased measure of personal security for potential victims of assault.

Examples of Rule-Utilitarian Reasoning in a Biomedical Context   (1) A substantive problem in biomedical ethics (discussed in Chapter 2) has to do with the morality of a physician's lying to a patient, in particular, whether it is right for a physician to lie to a patient, saying that the patient's illness is not terminal when it is believed to be so. The rule-utilitarian would conceptualize this issue as raising the possibility of a justified exception to the rule against lying. (Notice that an act-utilitarian, in contrast, would insist on assessing every individual case on its own utilitarian merits.) Suppose we consider incorporating into the rule against lying an exception to this effect: *"except* when in the judgment of a physician it would be better for a patient that he or she not know that his or her illness is believed to be terminal." Would the adoption of the rule incorporating this exception have better consequences than the adoption of the rule without the exception? The correct answer to this question is perhaps arguable, but it would seem that the rule-utilitarian would conclude that the proposed exception is an unjustified one. It is perhaps true that adoption of a rule incorporating the proposed exception would result in many patients being spared (at least temporarily) the distress that accompanies knowledge of one's impending death. On the other hand, it seems that this gain would be dwarfed by the distress and anxiety that would emerge from the erosion of trust within the confines of the physician-patient relationship. Whether a more limited exception could be formulated to a rule-utilitarian's satisfaction remains an open question.

(2) Another substantive problem in biomedical ethics (discussed in Chapter 7) has to do with the morality of mercy killing. Suppose a terminally ill patient, in great pain, requests that a physician terminate his or her life by administering a lethal dose of a drug. Such a case can be said to raise the issue of voluntary (active) euthanasia. The rule-utilitarian would conceptualize this issue (and other issues such as suicide and abortion) as raising the possibility of a justified exception to our rule against killing. Notice that at least one exception to our rule against killing is relatively uncontroversial. Killing in self-defense is justifiable, according to the rule-utilitarian, because although the adoption of the rule "do not kill" has dramatically better consequences than the adoption of the rule "kill whenever you want," adoption of the rule "do not kill *except* in self-defense" has still better consequences. As for voluntary (active) euthanasia, perhaps we should say that strong rule-utilitarian arguments can be advanced on both sides of the issue. Rule-utilitarian proponents of voluntary (active) euthanasia emphasize that social acceptance of this practice would result in great benefits—the primary one being that many dying people would be able to escape an extension of an anguished dying process. On the other side of the issue, however, we find, among a number of important concerns, insistence that availability of the lethal dose would create a climate of fear and anxiety among the elderly. Will dying people not come to feel that their families, to whom they have become a burden, expect them to ask for the lethal dose?

(3) A final illustration of rule-utilitarian reasoning in a biomedical context can be presented in reference to the principle of medical confidentiality (discussed in Chapter 3). This principle, which has an obvious basis in a rule-utilitarian structure, demands that information revealed within the context of a therapeutic relationship be held confidential. If patients could not rely on this expectation, they would be reluctant to communicate information that is essential to their proper treatment. Still, are there not justifiable exceptions to the principle of medical confidentiality? Suppose, for example, a patient reveals to his or her therapist an intention to kill or injure a third party. Is it not incumbent upon the therapist to break medical confidentiality in an effort to ensure protection for the third party? The situation just

described is the basis of the *Tarasoff* case considered in Chapter 3, and rule-utilitarian arguments on both sides of the issue can be found in the judicial opinions presented. There is an obvious benefit associated with the recognition of an exception to medical confidentiality based on the interests of innocent third parties; namely, threatened people will sometimes be saved from injury and death. On the other hand, it is argued, emotionally disturbed patients are likely to become more inhibited in communicating with therapists; thus their cures will be inhibited, and a greater incidence of violence against innocent people will result.

Critical Assessment of Rule-Utilitarianism   Rule-utilitarianism, it would seem, goes a long way toward alleviating the perceived difficulties of act-utilitarianism. Although act-utilitarians have charged rule-utilitarians with "superstitious rule-worship,"[9] it is act-utilitarianism rather than rule-utilitarianism that seems to clash with our ordinary moral thinking on this score. Indeed, rule-utilitarianism, in somewhat vivid contrast to act-utilitarianism, seems to fare reasonably well when measured against the standard that the implications of an ethical theory must be largely reconcilable with our experience of the moral life.

Whereas act-utilitarianism seems to confront individuals with an overly demanding moral standard, placing each of us under a continuing obligation to maximize utility with each of our actions, rule-utilitarianism is far less demanding of individuals. It requires only that individuals conform their actions to the rules that constitute a utilitarian-based moral code, and this requirement accords well with our ordinary moral thinking. Rule-utilitarianism also seems to accord reasonably well with our experience of particular, morally significant relationships. We commonly perceive ourselves as having special obligations arising out of our various morally significant relationships, and we think of these obligations as incompatible with functioning in the manner of an act-utilitarian. For example, parents have a special obligation to care for their children, physicians have a special obligation to act in the interests of their patients, and so forth. Such special obligations can be understood as having a rule-utilitarian foundation, as deriving from rules that, if generally followed, would maximize utility. Thus rule-utilitarianism seems to remedy another perceived difficulty of act-utilitarianism.

It is less clear that rule-utilitarianism is capable of providing a complete remedy for another perceived difficulty of act-utilitarianism, that is, its inability to provide an adequate theoretical foundation for individual rights. Surely rule-utilitarianism does not lead us so easily as does act-utilitarianism to conclusions that are incompatible with our ordinary moral thinking about the rights of individuals. For example, in suggesting that the painless murder of an old, unhappy (but not suicidal) person is the right thing as long as it can be done in complete secrecy, act-utilitarianism seems to clash violently with our conviction that such an action is patently objectionable, inasmuch as it constitutes a violation of a person's right to life. Rule-utilitarianism, in contrast, would never lead us to the conclusion that this sort of killing is morally legitimate. Surely the consequences of adopting the rule "do not kill *except* in the case of old, unhappy people who can be killed in complete secrecy" are dramatically worse than the consequences of adopting the rule without such an exception. If the rule with the exception were adopted, the lives of elderly people would be filled with anxiety and fear. In addition to rescuing utilitarian thinking from such obvious clashes with our ordinary moral thinking, rule-utilitarianism suggests a way of accommodating the notion of individual rights. Just as our special obligations can be understood as deriving from rules in a utilitarian-based moral code, so too can an individual's rights be understood in this fashion. A person's right to life, for example, can be understood as a correlate of our utilitarian-based rule against killing. Of course, whatever exceptions are properly incorporated into our rule against killing will factor out as limitations on a person's right to life. Whether rule-utilitarianism in this manner can provide an adequate theoretical foundation for individual rights is a very controversial matter. Its critics charge that it cannot.

Closely related to the claim that rule-utilitarianism does not provide an adequate theoretical foundation for individual rights is the somewhat broader claim that rule-utilitarianism fails to provide an adequate theoretical grounding for what we take to be the obligations of justice. This broader criticism, which is also vigorously advanced against act-utilitarianism, is perhaps the principal residual difficulty confronting rule-utilitarianism. Critics of rule-utilitarianism allege, for example, that the theory is compatible with the blatant injustice of enslaving one segment of a society's population or at least discriminating against this segment. The idea is that social rules discriminating against an explicitly identified minority group might function to maximize utility by bringing about more happiness in the advantaged majority than unhappiness in the disadvantaged minority. Rule-utilitarians are inclined to argue in response to this line of criticism that when the consequences of adopting "unjust rules" are completely analyzed, it is never true that their adoption can be justified on utilitarian grounds. Rather, the rule-utilitarian contends, "the rules of justice" rest on a secure utilitarian foundation. Whether rule-utilitarianism, in this manner, can adequately be reconciled with the perceived obligations of justice is a matter of contemporary debate.

Rule-utilitarianism also seems to fare reasonably well when measured against the second of our suggested standards: An ethical theory must provide effective guidance where it is most needed. In the dilemma situation, where one moral rule, or principle, inclines us one way and another moral rule, or principle, inclines us another way, the rule-utilitarian instructs us to establish relative priority by considering the consequences of incorporating appropriate exceptions into the rules that are in conflict. The dilemma is to be resolved by adoption of a rule that will maximize utility. Although this decision procedure sometimes entails very complex factual analysis and deliberation, it does seem to provide us a substantial measure of explicit guidance. Since rule-utilitarianism also seems to be reasonably harmonious with our ordinary moral thinking, it is an ethical theory that cannot easily be dismissed.

Kantian Deontology

The most prominent of the classical deontological theories is that developed by the German philosopher Immanuel Kant (1724–1804). Kantian deontology continues to command substantial attention in contemporary discussions of ethical theory and, importantly, is the underlying framework of much argumentation in biomedical ethics. In both of these respects, Kantian deontology is similar to utilitarianism and, like utilitarianism, warrants our detailed attention.

Kant sees utilitarianism as embodying a radically wrong approach in ethical theory. He emphasizes the need to avoid the "serpent-windings" of utilitarian thinking and refers to the principle of utility as "a wavering and uncertain standard." There is indeed a single, fundamental principle that is the basis of all moral obligation, but this fundamental principle is *not* the principle of utility. The "supreme principle of morality," the principle from which all of our various duties derive, Kant calls the "categorical imperative."

Although our present objective is an exposition of Kantian deontology, the enormous complexity of Kant's moral philosophy is a formidable obstacle to any concise exposition of the structure of Kant's ethical system. In particular, we are faced with the problem that Kant formulated the basic principle of his system, the categorical imperative, in a number of different ways. Although Kant insists that his various formulations are all equivalent, this contention is explicitly denied by many of his expositors and critics. Thus, if we are to provide a coherent account of Kantian deontology, mindful of the need to provide an account that is especially useful in dealing with issues in biomedical ethics, it seems advisable to settle on a favored formulation of the categorical imperative. Since two of Kant's formulations of the categorical imperative are especially prominent, it will suffice for our purposes to choose a favored formulation from these two.

According to what we will call the "first formulation," the categorical imperative tells us: "Act only on that maxim through which you can at the same time will that it should become a universal law."[10] According to what we will call the "second formulation," the categorical imperative tells us: "Act in such a way that you always treat humanity, whether in your own person or in the person of any other, never simply as a means, but always at the same time as an end."[11] The first formulation of the categorical imperative has often been compared with the Golden Rule ("do unto others as you would have them do unto you"), and it may be true that both of these principles, when suitably interpreted, have roughly the same implications. At any rate, it is apparently the case that Kant considered the first formulation to be the most basic of all his formulations. Yet, despite this fact, and despite the fact that ethical theorists have tended to pay more attention to the first formulation than the second, it is the second formulation that we take to have greater promise for the task at hand. Two major reasons can be advanced for choosing to exhibit the structure of Kant's ethical system in reference to the second formulation of the categorical imperative. First, the second formulation embodies a central notion—respect for persons—that is somewhat easier to grasp and apply than the more formalistic notion of universalizability, which is the core element of the first formulation. Second, when argumentation in biomedical ethics reflects a Kantian viewpoint, it is almost always couched in terms of the second formulation rather than the first.

Kantian deontology is an ethics of respect for persons. In Kant's view, every person, by virtue of his or her humanity (i.e., rational nature) has an inherent dignity. All persons, as rational creatures, are entitled to respect, not only from others but also from themselves as well. Thus the categorical imperative directs each of us to "act in such a way that you always treat humanity, whether in your own person or in the person of any other, never simply as a means, but always at the same time as an end." From this fundamental principle, according to Kant, a host of particular duties can be derived. The resultant system of duties includes duties to self as well as duties to others. In each of these cases, "perfect duties" must be distinguished from "imperfect duties," thus generating a fourfold classification of duties: (1) perfect duties to self, (2) imperfect duties to self, (3) perfect duties to others, and (4) imperfect duties to others. Although the distinction between perfect and imperfect duties is not a transparent one, its structural importance in the Kantian system is hard to overemphasize. Perfect duties require that we do or abstain from certain acts. *There are no legitimate exceptions to a perfect duty.* Such duties are binding in all circumstances, because certain kinds of action are simply incompatible with respect for persons, hence strictly impermissible. Imperfect duties, by contrast, require us to pursue or promote certain goals (e.g., the welfare of others). However, action in the name of these goals must never be at the expense of a perfect duty. One of Kant's most prominent commentators relates the distinction between perfect and imperfect duties to the categorical imperative in the following way: "We transgress perfect duties by treating any person *merely* as a means. We transgress imperfect duties by failing to treat a person as an end, even though we do not actively treat him as a means."[12]

Our discussion of Kant's fourfold classification of duties begins with a consideration of perfect duties to others. A transgression in this category of duty occurs whenever one person treats another person merely as a means. It is strictly impermissible for person A to treat person B merely as a means because such treatment is incompatible with respect for B as a person. Notice that Kant does not claim that it is morally wrong for one person to use another as a means. His claim is that it is morally wrong for one person to use another *merely* as a means. In the ordinary course of life, it is surely unavoidable (and morally unproblematic) that each of us in numerous ways uses others as means to achieve our various ends. A college teacher uses students as a means to achieve his or her livelihood. A college student uses instructors as a means of gaining knowledge and skills. Such human interactions, presumably based on the voluntary participation of the respective parties, are quite compatible with a principle of respect for persons. However, respect for persons entails that each of us recognize the rightful authority of other persons (as rational beings) to conduct their individual lives as they see fit. We may legitimately recruit others to participate in the satisfaction of our personal ends, but they are used merely as a means whenever we undermine the voluntary or informed character of their consent to interact with us in some desired way. Person A coerces person B at knifepoint to hand over $200. A uses B merely as a means. If A had requested of B a gift of $200, leaving B free to determine whether or not to make the gift, A would have proceeded in a manner compatible with respect for B as a person. Person C deceptively rolls back the odometer of a car and thereby manipulates person D's decision to buy the car. C uses D merely as a means. C has acted in a way that is strictly incompatible with respect for D as a person.

In the Kantian system, among the most notable of our perfect duties to others are: (1) the duty not to kill an innocent person, (2) the duty not to lie, and (3) the duty to keep promises. Murder (the killing of an innocent person), lying, and promise breaking are actions that are intrinsically wrong. However beneficial the consequences of such an action might be in a given circumstance, the action is strictly impermissible. (Notice the antiutilitarian character of Kant's thinking.) The murderer exhibits obvious disrespect for the person of the victim. The liar, in misinforming another person, violates the respect due to that person as a rational creature with a fundamental interest in the truth. A person who makes a promise issues a guarantee upon which the recipient of the promise is entitled to rely in his or her future planning. The person who breaks a promise shows disrespect for another by undermining the effort to conduct the affairs of one's life. By murdering, lying, or breaking a promise, an agent uses another person merely as a means to the agent's own ends.

According to Kant, each person has not only perfect duties to others but also perfect duties to self. The categorical imperative demands that no person (including oneself) be treated merely as a means. It is no more permissible to manifest disrespect for one's own person than to do so for the person of another. Kant insists, for example, that each person has a perfect duty to self to avoid drunkenness. Since drunkenness undermines a person's rational capacities, it is incompatible with respect for oneself as a rational creature. Kant believes that individuals debase themselves in the effort to achieve pleasure via inebriation. Inebriates treat themselves merely as a means (to the end of pleasure). But surely the foremost example of a perfect duty to self in the Kantian system is the duty not to commit suicide. To terminate one's own life, Kant insists, is strictly incompatible with respect for oneself as a person. In eradicating one's very existence as a rational creature, a person treats oneself merely as a means (ordinarily to the end of avoiding discomfort or distress). Suicide is an action that is intrinsically wrong, and there are no circumstances in which it is morally permissible.

In addition to the notion of perfect duties (both to self and others), the Kantian system also incorporates the notion of imperfect duties. Whereas perfect duties require, in essence, strict abstention from those actions that involve using a person merely as a means, imperfect duties have a very different underlying sense. Imperfect duties require the promotion of certain goals. In broad terms, there are two such goals—an agent's personal perfection (i.e., development) and the happiness or welfare of others. Respect for oneself as a person requires commitment to the development of one's capacities as a rational being. Thus Kant spoke of an imperfect duty to self to develop one's talents. The sense of this duty is that, by and large, it is up to each individual to decide which talents to cultivate and which to deemphasize. But a person is not free to abandon the goal of personal development. Although the duty to develop one's talents requires no *specific* actions, it does require each individual to formulate a plan of life that embodies a commitment to the goal of personal development.

Before discussing Kant's final category of duty, imperfect duty to others, it will prove helpful to introduce the notion of *beneficence*.[13] If one acts in such a way as to further the happiness or welfare of another, then one acts beneficently. (A benevolent person is one who is inclined to act beneficently.) Beneficence may be contrasted with *nonmaleficence,* which is ordinarily understood as the noninfliction of harm on others. One who harms ("does evil" to) another acts in a maleficent fashion. One who *refrains* from harming others acts in a nonmaleficent fashion. One who acts, in a more positive way, to contribute to the welfare of others acts in a beneficent fashion. Beneficence is a generic notion that can best be understood as including the following types of activity: (1) preventing evil or harm from befalling someone, (2) removing an evil that is presently afflicting someone, and (3) providing benefits ("doing good") for someone. Although it is sometimes difficult to decide which of these categories is the most appropriate classification for a particular beneficent action, the following examples seem relatively straightforward. Pushing someone out of the path of an oncoming car is an example of the first type of activity. Curing a patient's disease is an example of the second. Giving someone a $100 gift is an example of the third.

According to Kant, respect for other persons requires not only that we avoid using them merely as a means (by the observance of our perfect duties to others) but also that we commit ourselves in some general way to furthering their happiness or welfare. Thus Kant considers what we will call the "duty of beneficence" to be an imperfect duty to others. As with the duty to develop our talents, an imperfect duty to self, the duty of beneficence requires no *specific* actions. One does not violate the duty of beneficence by refusing to act beneficently in any individual case where the opportunity arises. What is required instead of specific actions is that each person incorporate in his or her life plan a commitment to promote the well-being of others. Individuals are free to choose the sorts of actions they will embrace in an effort to further the well-being of others (e.g., contributing to the relief of famine victims); they are not free to abandon the general goal of furthering the well-being of others.

Since the duty of beneficence is an imperfect duty in the Kantian system, action in the name of beneficence must never be taken at the expense of a perfect duty. For example, it is impermissible to lie or break a promise in an effort to save a third party from harm. The same is true with regard to the imperfect duty to develop one's talents. For example, if one has resolved (quite properly) to develop one's creative powers, it is nevertheless impermissible to do so by "creatively" defrauding others.

The Kantian Framework in a Biomedical Context   With our exposition of Kantian deontology now complete, we are in a position to exhibit some of the more important implications of this ethical theory in the realm of biomedical ethics. To begin with, the theory has an obvious relevance to the much-discussed problem of whether or not a physician may justifiably lie to a patient (an issue discussed in Chapter 2). Since every person has a perfect duty to others not to lie, a straightforward implication of Kantian deontology is that a physician may *never* lie to a patient. If a patient, diagnosed as terminally ill by a physician, inquires about his or her prognosis, the physician may be much inclined to lie, motivated by a desire to protect the patient from the psychological turmoil that would accompany knowledge of his or her true condition; but action in the name of beneficence (an imperfect duty) may never be at the expense of a perfect duty. This same analysis is relevant to the use of placebos by physicians. Sometimes a patient becomes psychologically dependent on a certain medication. When the medication is discontinued, because the physician is convinced it is no longer needed and because its continued use represents a threat to health, the patient complains of the reemergence of symptoms. If such a patient is given a placebo, that is, a therapeutically inert but harmless substance, misrepresented as a medication, the patient may feel fine. Nevertheless, despite the fact that placebos may be capable of enhancing patient welfare, their employment is morally impermissible, at least in cases involving an explicit lie.

Kantian deontology has some very important and very direct implications for the ethics of experimentation with human subjects (a topic discussed in Chapter 4). Since it is morally wrong for any person to use any other person merely as a means, it follows that it is morally wrong for a biomedical researcher to use a human research subject merely as a means. From this consideration it is but a short step to the requirement of voluntary informed consent as a basic principle of research ethics. If a researcher is engaged in a study that involves human subjects, we may presume that the immediate "end" being sought by the researcher is the successful completion of the study. But notice that the researcher may desire this particular end for any number of reasons: the speculative understanding it will provide; the technology it will make possible; the eventual benefit of humankind; personal recognition in the eyes of the scientific community; a raise in pay; and so forth. This mixture of self-centered and benevolent motivations may be considered the researcher's less immediate ends. If researchers are to avoid using their research subjects merely as means (to the ends of the researchers), surely they must refrain from coercing the participation of their subjects and, in addition, provide information about the research project (most notably, risks to the subjects) sufficient for the subjects to make a rational decision with regard to their personal participation. Thus respect for persons demands that researchers honor the requirement of voluntary informed consent.

Suppose a researcher explains to a potential research subject how important it is that he or she consent to participate. There is no question but that the research project at issue, if brought to a successful conclusion, will provide substantial benefit to humankind. Does the potential subject have a moral obligation to participate? Surely not. Within the framework of Kantian deontology, the duty of beneficence is an imperfect duty. A person must on occasion act beneficently, but there is no obligation to perform any *specific* beneficent action. Interestingly enough, the same line of thought would seem to apply to the question of whether a physician has a moral obligation to come to the aid of a seriously injured person (not by prior agreement the physician's patient) in an emergency situation.

Critical Assessment of Kantian Deontology   Are the implications of Kantian deontology largely reconcilable with our experience of the moral life? Can this theory function to provide effective guidance in the face of perceived moral dilemmas? These two questions reflect the criteria suggested earlier as most central to the assessment of the relative adequacy of an ethical theory.

Before indicating some of the ways in which Kantian deontology can be thought to be at odds with our ordinary moral thinking, it is important to emphasize that the theory does successfully account for crucial aspects of our experience of the moral life. To begin with, Kantian deontology provides an obvious foundation for the "commonsense rules of morality." The wrongfulness of actions that fly in the face of these rules—actions such as killing, injuring, stealing, lying, breaking promises—can very plausibly be understood as flowing from the categorical imperative. The Kantian deontologist maintains that these actions are wrong because they involve treating another person merely as a means, and there is something very compelling about the notion of respect for persons as the core notion of morality.

Kantian deontology also seems to provide a secure foundation for the notion of individual rights, a notion that is very prominent in our ordinary moral thinking. Individual rights, in the Kantian system, are to be understood as the correlates of our perfect duties to others. (Imperfect duties, in contrast, do not generate rights.) For example, each of us has a perfect *duty* not to kill an innocent person; thus every innocent person has a *right* not to be killed. More generally, every person has a right not to be used by another merely as a means. An innocent person has a right not to be punished, no matter how socially desirable the consequences might be in a certain set of circumstances. A potential research subject has a right not to be coerced or deceived into participation, even if the satisfactory completion of the study promises great benefit for humankind. In its insistence that individual rights cannot be overridden by "utilitarian" considerations, Kantian deontology achieves accord with our firmly entrenched (if somewhat vague) conviction that the end does not justify the means.

Yet, there are aspects of Kantian deontology that cannot be easily reconciled with our experience of the moral life. One very prominent difficulty has to do with the Kantian contention that keeping promises and not lying are both duties of perfect obligation. We are quite at home, in our ordinary moral thinking, with both a duty to keep promises and a duty not to lie, but it is the exceptionless character of these duties in the Kantian system that we find troublesome. Surely in extreme cases, we are inclined to say, these duties must yield to more weighty moral considerations. For example, if a person breaks a rather trivial promise (say, to return a book at a certain time) in order to respond to the needs of a person in serious distress, surely he or she has not acted immorally. Or again, if a person lies to a would-be murderer about the whereabouts of the intended victim, surely the liar has not (all things considered) acted immorally. The Kantian deontologist sees in such examples a clash between a perfect duty and the imperfect duty of beneficence, and the Kantian teaching is that the former may never yield to the latter. But it would seem that a theory with such implausible implications stands in need of revision. Perhaps the problem is not only that Kantian deontology overstates the significance of certain "perfect" duties but also that it understates the significance of the duty of beneficence, at least that aspect of beneficence that has to do with preventing serious harm from befalling another or alleviating the serious distress of another.

In our everyday existence as moral agents, we are accustomed to the idea that we have a number of important duties to others. It is less clear that the Kantian notion of duties to self can be reconciled with our experience of the moral life. This is difficult territory. For one thing, the issue of suicide (discussed in Chapter 7) seems to confound our moral "commonsense" in a way that blatant wrongs such as murder, rape, and slavery do not. Still, despite significant disagreement, suicide is considered by many to be morally wrong. But the issue is this: Do those who consider suicide morally wrong experience the duty not to commit suicide as a duty to self? It seems more likely that this duty is experienced as a duty to others (who may be negatively affected by one's suicide) or, in the case of religious believers, as a duty to God. A similar argument could be made with regard to the imperfect duty to develop one's talents.

It cannot be denied that Kantian deontology, to a substantial degree, is reconcilable with our experience of the moral life. On the other hand, it appears that the theory is attended with some significant and unresolved difficulties. How does Kantian deontology fare when measured against the second of our standards, the requirement that an ethical theory provide effective guidance in the face of moral dilemmas? Once again, it seems, the verdict is somewhat mixed.

It might be argued that Kantian deontology, by sorting our various duties into the categories of perfect and imperfect and assigning priority to perfect duties, provides us with a structure in terms of which moral dilemmas can be resolved. This is perhaps true to the extent that our perplexity can be analyzed in terms of perfect duties marshaled against imperfect duties, but even here it is difficult to overlook the fact that the priority of perfect over imperfect duties is itself a somewhat problematic feature of Kantian deontology. One is tempted to say that even if the theory provides reasonably *clear* guidance, it sometimes fails to provide *correct* guidance.

W. D. Ross's Theory of Prima Facie Duties

In a book entitled *The Right and the Good* (1930), the English philosopher W. D. Ross proposed a deontological theory that has received considerable attention among ethical theorists. The point of departure for the development of Ross's theory is his concern to provide a defensible account of "cases of conscience," that is, situations that confront us with a conflict of duties. One perceived line of obligation pulls us in one direction; another perceived line of obligation pulls us in a contrary direction. We find ourselves unsettled and uncertain but cannot avoid a choice. Which duty takes precedence over the other? The parent of a young child has promised to attend a community meeting, but the child seems to need special attention. Since our social existence is complex, conflict-of-duty situations are a recurrent feature of our daily life. In the biomedical context, such situations are pervasive.

For understandable reasons, Ross maintains that neither the Kantian nor the utilitarian can provide an account of conflict-of-duty situations that harmonizes with what he calls "ordinary moral consciousness." We have just considered the relevant deficiency in the Kantian approach. It is implausible to maintain that the duty of beneficence can never take precedence over the duty to keep promises or the duty not to lie. As for the utilitarian approach (and here it is clear that Ross has act-utilitarianism in mind), this theory's insistence that in reality we have only the one duty of maximizing utility clashes with our conviction that we have distinct lines of obligation to distinct people. In order to provide an adequate account of conflict-of-duty situations, Ross maintains, it is essential to introduce the notion of "prima facie duty." The Latin phrase *prima facie,* now commonplace in moral philosophy, literally means "at first glance." But the word *conditional* best expresses the sense of the phrase as Ross intends it. A prima facie duty is a conditional duty. A prima facie duty (as opposed to an absolute duty) can be overridden by a more stringent duty.

According to Ross, there are no absolute, or unconditional, duties, only prima facie duties. But what is the basis of our prima facie duties? Both the utilitarian and the Kantian assert that our various duties have a unitary basis in a fundamental principle of morality. The utilitarian believes that our various duties can be derived from the principle of utility. The Kantian believes that our various duties can be derived from the categorical imperative. Ross, in vivid contrast, maintains that our various prima facie duties have no unitary basis. Rather, they emerge out of our numerous "morally significant relations," relations such as promisee to promiser, creditor to debtor, spouse to spouse, child to parent, friend to friend, citizen to the state, fellow human being to fellow human being. "Each of these relations is the foundation of a *prima facie* duty, which is more or less incumbent on me according to the circumstances of the case."[14]

In unproblematic circumstances, where we are bound by only one prima facie duty, this particular prima facie duty is our *actual* duty. In conflict-of-duty situations, where two (or more) prima facie duties compete for priority, only one of these duties, the more stringent one in the circumstances, can be our actual duty. We have, for example, both a prima facie duty to keep promises and a prima facie duty to assist those who are in need. According to Ross, when these two duties come into conflict, it is clear (in terms of our "ordinary moral consciousness") that the duty to keep promises is usually more incumbent upon us than the duty to assist those who are in need. However, if the promise is relatively trivial and the need of another is compelling—a matter of serious distress—then it is equally clear that the priority is reversed. In the difficult cases, Ross maintains, there is in principle no hard-and-fast rule to apply. In his view, the best anyone can do is to make a reflective, "considered decision" as to which of the competing prima facie duties has the priority in any given situation.

According to Ross, "there is nothing arbitrary about [our] *prima facie* duties. Each rests on a definite circumstance which cannot seriously be held to be without moral significance."[15] Accordingly, he proposes the following division of our prima facie duties.

(1) *Duties of fidelity* include keeping promises, honoring contracts and agreements, and telling the truth. Duties in this class rest on a person's previous acts. In giving one's word to do something, a person creates the duty to do so. (Ross thinks that by entering a conversation, a person implicitly agrees to tell the truth.) Notice that a person's so-called role responsibilities can be identified as an important subclass of duties of fidelity. For example, a teacher has certain responsibilities as a teacher, a physician certain responsibilities as a physician, and

a nurse certain responsibilities as a nurse. In taking on a certain social role, a person brings into existence various duties of fidelity. In addition, further duties of fidelity arise out of agreements (both explicit and implicit) that a person enters into while functioning in a professional capacity.

(2) *Duties of reparation* also rest on a person's previous acts. Any person, by wrongfully treating someone else, creates the duty to rectify the wrong that has been perpetrated. For example, if A steals a certain amount of money from B, A thereby brings into existence the duty to repay this amount. (3) *Duties of gratitude* rest on previous acts of other persons, that is, beneficial services provided by them. If A has provided a good service for B when B was in need, B thereby stands under a duty to provide a good service for A when A is in need.

(4) *Duties of beneficence* "rest on the mere fact that there are other beings in the world whose condition we can make better."[16] (5) *Duties of nonmaleficence* rest on the complementary fact that we can also make the condition of other beings worse. The duties in this category, which Ross recognizes as especially stringent, can be summed up under the heading of "not injuring others." The duty not to kill is an obvious example.

(6) *Duties of justice* "rest on the fact or possibility of a distribution of pleasure or happiness (or of the means thereto) which is not in accordance with the merit of the persons concerned."[17] Benefits are to be distributed in accordance with personal merit, and existing unjust patterns of distribution are to be rectified. (7) *Duties of self-improvement* "rest on the fact that we can improve our own condition."[18]

Prima Facie Duties in a Biomedical Context   Ross's framework of prima facie duties is helpful for conceptualizing many of the moral dilemmas that arise in a biomedical context. In analyzing such dilemmas as they arise from the point of view of health-care professionals, the category of duties of fidelity is especially important. Consider, for example, the physician-patient relationship (a topic discussed in Chapter 2). The social understanding or implicit agreement that underlies this relationship undoubtedly includes a number of important provisions. Among these are the provision that the physician is to act in the best medical interest of the patient and the provision that the physician is to keep confidential any personal information that comes to light within the context of the physician-patient relationship. In the very act of accepting a patient for treatment, a physician thereby incurs a number of important prima facie duties of fidelity.

Suppose a physician is convinced that lying to a patient is in the best medical interest of the patient. In Ross's scheme, the prima facie duty not to lie, itself a duty of fidelity, comes into conflict with another duty of fidelity, the prima facie duty to act in the best medical interest of the patient. Since neither duty is unconditional, in one case the duty not to lie might be more incumbent upon the physician, whereas in another case the duty to act in the best interest of the patient might be the more stringent duty. Suppose, in a different case, a physician is treating a patient suffering from a condition that renders the patient in his or her occupation a danger to others. In addition, suppose that the patient is a bus driver subject to blackouts. The patient is desperate to keep his or her job and refuses to divulge the problem to his or her employer. Should the physician break medical confidentiality and notify the patient's employer in an effort to ensure the public safety? In this case, the prima facie duty of beneficence comes into conflict with a duty of fidelity, the prima facie duty to keep medical confidentiality. (Justifiable exceptions to the duty to keep medical confidentiality are discussed in Chapter 3.)

Among the explicit role responsibilities of a typical hospital nurse is the obligation to follow a physician's orders in the treatment of patients. By the simple act of accepting employment in the hospital setting, a nurse thereby incurs, among other numerous duties of fidelity, the prima facie duty to obey a physician's orders. An important moral dilemma for the hospital nurse arises when, in the judgment of the nurse, following a physician's order would be detrimental to the patient. (This dilemma is discussed in Chapter 3.) Thinking in terms of Ross's theory, we can structure the dilemma as follows. The prima facie duty to follow a physician's orders comes into conflict with two other prima facie duties. First there is a relevant duty of nonmaleficence. A nurse should not act in a way that would, in effect, injure another person. Second, there is another relevant duty of fidelity, deriving from the fact that a nurse has an implicit contract or agreement with the patient to act in his or her best medical interest. Is the collective force of these two prima facie duties more incumbent upon the nurse than the prima facie duty to follow a physician's orders? Since the duty of nonmaleficence is recognized by Ross (and "ordinary moral consciousness") as especially stringent, it seems that in most cases, at least where the potential harm to patients is significant, the nurse must conclude that it would be wrong to follow the physician's order.

Abstracting from any relevant role responsibilities on the part of health-care professionals, the issue of the moral justifiability of mercy killing (discussed in Chapter 7) might be conceptualized, in accordance with Ross's scheme, as a moral dilemma involving the conflict between a duty of beneficence and a duty of nonmaleficence. A terminally ill person suffering unbearable pain could be understood to benefit from an immediate and painless death. Thus we have on one hand a duty of beneficence—the prima facie duty to come to the assistance of a person in serious distress—and on the other hand a duty of nonmaleficence—the prima facie duty not to kill.

Critical Assessment of Ross's Theory   Since Ross developed his theory of prima facie duties explicitly in reference to the promptings of "ordinary moral consciousness," it would be surprising if his theory could not be reconciled with our experience of the moral life. Indeed, let us put aside whatever worries might be expressed on this score, for there is a much more obvious deficiency in Ross's theory. Recall that we have asked not only that an ethical theory be largely reconcilable with our experience of the moral life but also that it provide us with effective guidance where it is most needed, in the face of moral dilemmas. And despite the fact that Ross's theory provides us with a helpful framework for conceptualizing our moral dilemmas, it provides us with virtually no substantive guidance for resolving them.

In the difficult cases, where two prima facie duties come into strong conflict, Ross holds that there are no principles we can appeal to in an effort to make an appropriate decision. The most we can do, in his view, is render a "considered decision" as to which duty is more incumbent upon us in a certain situation. Although it is fine to be told to make a considered decision, what exactly is worthy of consideration in reaching a decision? At this point, there is a strong argument for moving beyond Ross's theory. One plausible approach would identify *considerations of coherence* (within our overall system of moral convictions) as the relevant standard. (See the discussion of "Reflective Equilibrium and Appeals to Coherence" later in this chapter.) If Ross's theory were supplemented with a coherence-based decision procedure, the advantages of thinking in terms of prima facie duties could be combined with a plausible methodology for mediating among conflicting duties.

RELEVANT CONCEPTS AND PRINCIPLES

The concepts of autonomy and paternalism are of fundamental importance in biomedical ethics. Closely associated with these concepts is a set of principles, called "liberty-limiting principles," which are often invoked in order to justify limitations on individual liberty. This section provides an examination of these relevant concepts and principles. It also provides a brief exposition of a set of principles under the heading of "The Principles of Biomedical Ethics."

Autonomy

Many discussions in biomedical ethics presume the importance of individual autonomy, stressing the right of autonomous decision makers to determine for themselves what will be done to their bodies. This "right of self-determination" is said to limit what physicians, nurses, and other health-care professionals can justifiably do to patients. In fact, this right is often taken so seriously that professionals who act against their patients' wishes, even to save their patients' lives, are condemned as morally blameworthy and leave themselves open to charges of battery. In view of all this, it is useful to discuss the following questions, the first a conceptual question and the second an ethical one. (1) What sense of autonomy is operative in the widespread presumption that individual autonomy is an important value? (2) What is the ethical basis for the value accorded to individual autonomy?

The Concept of Autonomy   Autonomy is typically defined as self-governance or self-determination. Individuals are said to act autonomously when they, and not others, make the decisions that affect their lives and act on the basis of their decisions. This general characterization needs to be explicated, however, since autonomy is a complex notion. Writers in biomedical ethics often conceptually distinguish several senses of autonomy in order to clarify some of the issues raised when questions are asked about justified infringements or limitations of individual autonomy: (1) autonomy as liberty of action; (2) autonomy as freedom of choice; and (3) autonomy as effective deliberation.[19] A brief consideration of these three senses of autonomy will also serve to emphasize the various ways in which an individual's action, thought, or choice may be less than fully autonomous.

1 Autonomy as Liberty of Action   Think of a would-be physician, Mark, who sits under a tree waiting for medical knowledge to permeate his being. No one is forcing Mark to sit under the tree. He is free to leave anytime he chooses. His action results from his conscious intention to sit under the tree. (He does not mistakenly believe, for example, that he is sitting in medical school.) His action is also voluntary in the sense that it is not the result of coercion or duress. If autonomy is treated simply as a synonym for "liberty of action," then Mark is acting autonomously insofar as his action is intentional and voluntary. Mark's autonomy would be violated, however, if he were physically forced to sit under the tree or if someone were to coerce him into sitting there by threatening him with harm.

When autonomy is identified with liberty of action, the primary contrast drawn is between autonomy and coercion. Coercion involves the deliberate use of force or the threat of harm. The coercer's purpose is to get the person being coerced to do something he or she would not otherwise be willing to do. "Occurrent" coercion involves the use of physical force. "Dispositional" coercion involves the threat of harm.[20] An unscrupulous medical researcher, for example, might literally force individuals to participate as research subjects, as was done in Nazi Germany. This is occurrent coercion. The researcher might also bring about the desired participation by threatening reluctant patients with some harm, such as the withdrawal of care essential for the patient's recovery. This is dispositional coercion. Moreover, with regard to the threat of harm, human beings can coerce other human beings either directly or by enacting laws that threaten them with harm. Laws as well as individuals can be coercive. For example, a physician is constrained from actively killing patients by laws that threaten harm (in the form of punishment) to those who do so.

2 Autonomy as Freedom of Choice   Suppose that a 26-year-old, recently divorced man is the father of three children. He decides that it would be a good idea for him to have a vasectomy, which is a sterilization procedure involving minor surgery. However, there is only one physician (a urologist) who performs the procedure in the rural area where the young man lives, and finances prohibit his traveling to obtain the vasectomy elsewhere. If the urologist refuses to perform the procedure (perhaps based on the conviction that vasectomy is an unwise choice for a man so young), the 26-year-old man is not free to act on his decision. Note that his lack of freedom is not due to coercion. Nevertheless, his autonomy is limited in the sense that his range of choice is narrowed. Consider as well a patient who does not want to go through the process of choosing between alternative forms of treatment (surgery versus chemotherapy, for example) and asks the physician to make the choice without giving the patient any details about the risks and benefits of each. If the physician does not accede to the request and insists upon giving the patient the requisite information, the patient's liberty of action is not being constrained by coercion. Nonetheless, the patient's range of choice is narrowed insofar as the way he or she is treated is not in accordance with the preferred choice.

The following example illustrates how a change at the level of policy might effectively function to limit autonomy understood as freedom of choice. Suppose that Medicaid funding for abortion has been widely available in a certain state, but then new legislation results in a dramatic cutback of such funding. Because there will now be a number of poor women who are no longer effectively free to act on the decision to procure an abortion, it is plausible to say that the new legislation has resulted in limitations on the autonomy of these women.

3 Autonomy as Effective Deliberation   The accounts of limitations on autonomy provided in the discussions of autonomy as liberty of action and autonomy as freedom of choice focus on factors external to the agent that limit his or her autonomy. The first focuses on the coercion exerted on the agent by others, either directly or indirectly. The second focuses on the unavailability of options that the agent might have chosen. By contrast, autonomy as effective deliberation focuses on the agent's internal states and on related internal constraints.

In many discussions in biomedical ethics, autonomy is closely allied with rationality. An autonomous individual is characterized as one who is capable of making *rational* and *unconstrained* decisions and acting accordingly. Thus an individual *exercises* autonomy only to the extent that he or she acts without constraint on the basis of rational and unconstrained decisions. The criteria of rationality and constraint are central here. Under what conditions are individuals and their decisions and actions unconstrained? We have already discussed some of the constraints on an individual's actions. Our present discussion focuses on autonomy and constraints in relation to the agent's decision-making process. This requires distinguishing between two senses of rationality.

According to the first sense of rationality, individuals are properly described as rational when they are capable of choosing the best means to some chosen end. In this sense of rationality, someone who wants to be a physician and attends medical school in order to attain this end is acting rationally. Someone with the same desire who, like Mark in our earlier example, sits under a tree and meditates for 12 hours a day, waiting for medical knowledge to "permeate his being," is acting irrationally. To be rational in this sense entails being capable of reasoning well on the basis of good evidence about the best means to achieve some end. Someone in our society, for example, who does not use contraceptives during intercourse because she believes that an amulet she wears will keep her from getting pregnant is acting irrationally. To be rational in this sense also entails being able to postpone immediate gratification when such postponement is necessary to achieve chosen goals. Would-be physicians in medical school who party every night because they enjoy doing so, even though this seriously jeopardizes their chances of succeeding in school, are acting irrationally.

A second sense of rationality involves choosing ends rather than means to those ends. All thinking beings have goals or ends they believe are in their interest to pursue. Being able to select and identify appropriate goals or interests is an important aspect of rationality. In this sense of rationality, an individual is properly described as rational if he or she is capable of choosing appropriate ends, although what counts as an appropriate end is a notorious matter of dispute. One who chooses unprofitable or self-destructive ends, for example, may be characterized as irrational. Would-be suicides are often described as irrational in this sense, as are masochists. Would-be suicides might sometimes be rational in the first sense, that is, capable of choosing the most efficient and painless way to end their lives. However, those who hold that the choice of death as an end is always inappropriate would consider all would-be suicides irrational in the second sense.

If rational acts must be based on decisions concerning the best means to maximize appropriately chosen ends, a fully rational person will have to have a number of abilities:

1. The ability to formulate appropriate goals, especially long-term goals.

2. The ability to establish priorities among these goals.

3. The ability to determine the best means to achieve chosen goals.

4. The ability to act effectively to realize these goals.

5. The ability to either abandon the chosen goals or modify them if the consequences of using the available means are undesirable or if the means are inadequate.

To sum up the discussion of autonomy as effective deliberation thus far, an individual is autonomous in this sense only to the extent that he or she possesses the abilities requisite for effective reasoning and the disposition to exercise those abilities. These abilities can be limited in many ways. When they are, decisions and actions may be less than fully rational. First, some individuals may not have sufficiently developed the necessary abilities or may even be incapable of sufficiently developing them. Second, even individuals who have the requisite abilities may be unable to *exercise* them on a particular occasion due to various internal factors. For example, emotions such as fear may make the impartial weighing of information impossible. Laziness may keep an individual from learning all the pertinent information. The presence of pain or the use of drugs may also affect the exercise of reasoning abilities. It may be best, therefore, to speak of *degrees* of rationality and irrationality since many factors can make decisions and actions less than fully rational without pushing them to the irrational end of the spectrum.

Furthermore, autonomy as effective deliberation may be constrained in ways that do not affect the "rationality" of the decision. Lies, deception, and a lack of appropriate information can all limit the effective exercise of the abilities required for rational deliberation. Physicians, for example, can constrain their patients' decision-making processes by deliberately withholding information. A patient who is told about only one possible kind of therapy and lacks information about alternatives cannot weigh the relative risks and benefits of all possible therapies in relation to long-term ends. In that situation a patient's "choice" of the therapy recommended by the physician is much less than fully autonomous. Yet the choice might be rational both because the patient's deliberative process has been logical and because it may actually be in the latter's best interests in light of long-term goals. However, to the extent that the patient's decision-making processes are constrained by the lack of information, the patient cannot effectively exercise his or her autonomy.

In summary, an individual is autonomous or self-determining only to the extent that he or she possesses the abilities necessary for effective deliberation, is free of internal constraints in the exercise of those abilities, and is neither coerced by others nor has his or her range of options narrowed by them. A person's autonomy can be infringed upon, limited, or usurped by others in many ways including coercion, deception, lying, failing to supply necessary information, and narrowing the individual's range of options, for example, by refusing to act in accordance with his or her expressed desires. It can also be diminished by internal factors, such as strong emotions, the lack of appropriate capacities, fever, compulsion, and severe pain. To respect others' autonomy or right of self-determination is to treat them as individuals having the abilities required to be rational decision makers, capable of identifying their own interests and making their own reflective choices about the best means to advance them. Individual A fails to respect individual B's autonomy if A imposes constraints on B's deliberative process or liberty of action or if A narrows B's range of choices. In each of these cases, A interferes in some way with the effective exercise of B's autonomy, and this is incompatible with the principle of respect for autonomy.

The Value of Autonomy   What is the basis for the moral value accorded to individual autonomy? The strongest claims regarding its moral primacy come from Kant and from certain other deontologists. In Kant's view, persons, unlike things, must always be accorded respect as self-determining subjects. They must be treated as ends in themselves and never merely as objects. For Kant, the fundamental principle of morality, respect for persons as moral agents, entails respect for personal autonomy. Such respect is due them as a right—autonomous agents are entitled to respect. If persons were not taken to be autonomous agents, there would be no basis for the moral responsibility we have toward other human beings, which precludes our using them, as we do cattle, chickens, rocks, land, and trees, simply to serve our own ends. But how does Kant understand autonomy?

Kant's primary focus is on the autonomy of the will. For Kant, "Autonomy of the will is the property the will has of being a law to itself."[21] What Kant calls the "dignity of man as a rational creature" is due to human beings possessing just that property that enables them to govern their own actions in accordance with rules of their own choosing. Putting aside many complexities in Kant's own thinking, a Kantian position central in biomedical ethics describes autonomy in terms of self-control, self-direction, or self-governance. The individual capable of acting on the basis of effective deliberation, guided by reason, and neither driven by emotions or compulsions nor manipulated or coerced by others, is, on a Kantian position, the model of autonomy.

For utilitarians, autonomy is an important value. John Stuart Mill, who speaks of individuality rather than autonomy, argues, for example, that liberty of action and thought is essential in developing both the intellectual and character traits necessary for truly human happiness:

> The human faculties of perception, judgment, discriminative feeling, mental activity, and even moral preference, are exercised only in making a choice. He who does anything because it is the custom makes no choice. He gains no practice either in discerning or in desiring what is best. The mental and moral, like the muscular powers, are improved by being used. . . .
>
> He who lets the world, or his own portion of it, choose his plan of life for him, has no need of any other faculty than the ape-like one of imitation. He who chooses his plan for himself employs all his faculties. He must use observation to see, reasoning and judgment to foresee, activity to gather materials for decision, discrimination to decide, and when he has decided, firmness and self-control to hold to his deliberate decision. . . .
>
> Where, not the person's own character, but the traditions or customs of other people are the rule of conduct, there is wanting one of the principal ingredients of human happiness.[22]

For Mill, persons possessing "individuality" are autonomous in a very strong sense, reflectively choosing their own plans of life, making their own decisions without manipulation by others, and exercising firmness and self-control in acting on their decisions.

Despite the high value placed on autonomy by utilitarians, their interest in autonomy differs from the Kantian one. On a Kantian view, respect for the autonomy of rational agents is entailed by the fundamental principle of morality, which serves as a limiting criterion for all moral conduct. That is, it places limits on what one individual can do to another human being without acting immorally. As noted earlier, one person can never use another as a subject in a medical experiment without his or her consent, no matter what potential good consequences for society as a whole might result. For a utilitarian such as Mill, respect for individual autonomy has utility value. A society that fosters respect for persons as autonomous agents will be a more progressive and, on balance, a happier society because its citizens will have the opportunities to develop their capacities to act as rational, responsible moral agents. If it could be shown that respect for individual autonomy does not have sufficient utility value, the utilitarian might have no good grounds for objecting to practices that infringe upon that autonomy.

Liberty-Limiting Principles

Since autonomy is accorded such great moral value, a moral justification must be given for any infringement on or limitation or usurpation of autonomy. Many of the discussions in biomedical ethics explore such *proposed* justifications. The following exposition centers on the most general kinds of reasons advanced in these discussions.

Six suggested general reasons, most frequently considered when limitations of liberty (one aspect of autonomy) are at issue, are embodied in six principles, often called "liberty-limiting principles," stated below.[23] It is important to note at the outset that while some writers advance these principles as legitimate liberty-limiting principles, others argue against the legitimacy of many, or even most, of them.

1. A person's liberty is justifiably restricted to prevent that person from harming others (the harm principle).

2. A person's liberty is justifiably restricted to prevent that person from offending others (the offense principle).

3. A person's liberty is justifiably restricted to prevent that person from harming himself or herself (the principle of paternalism).

4. A person's liberty is justifiably restricted to benefit that person (the principle of extreme paternalism).

5. A person's liberty is justifiably restricted to prevent that person from acting immorally (the principle of legal moralism).

6. A person's liberty is justifiably restricted to benefit others (the social welfare principle).

These liberty-limiting principles are most frequently discussed when questions are raised about the justification of coercive laws, such as laws limiting access to hallucinogenic drugs. But the considerations they embody are also pertinent when applied to individual acts and practices that infringe upon or limit others' *autonomy*. It should also be noted that more than one of these principles might be advanced to justify a proposed limitation or infringement.

The harm principle is the most widely accepted liberty-limiting principle. Few will dispute that the law is within its proper bounds when it constrains individuals from performing acts that will seriously harm other persons or will seriously impair important institutional practices. Laws that threaten thieves, murderers, and the like with punishment, for example, are usually perceived as a necessary part of any social system. Individual acts of coercion whose intent is to prevent individuals from harming others are also usually considered morally permissible. A bystander, for example, who prevents a terrorist from killing or wounding someone, is praised and not blamed for interfering with the terrorist's action. Aside from the harm principle, however, the moral legitimacy of the liberty-limiting principles under discussion here is a matter of dispute.

According to the offense principle, the law may justifiably be invoked to prevent offensive behavior in public. "Offensive" behavior may be understood as behavior that causes shame, embarrassment, or discomfort to onlookers. In the leading example of the relevance of the offense principle to biomedical ethics, individuals who behave offensively in public have sometimes been involuntarily committed to mental institutions, even though their behavior did not pose a serious threat of harm to themselves or others. If individuals are committed to mental institutions simply because their behavior is considered offensively eccentric, then the offense principle is being invoked, at least implicitly. Attacks on the use of such grounds to deprive individuals of much of their autonomy are attacks on the legitimacy of the offense principle.

According to the principle of legal moralism, liberty may justifiably be limited to prevent immoral behavior or, as it is often expressed, to "enforce morals." Acts such as kidnapping, murder, and fraud are undoubtedly immoral, but the principle of legal moralism does not have to be invoked to justify laws against them. An appeal to the harm principle already provides a widely accepted independent justification. The principle of legal moralism usually comes to the fore only when so-called victimless crimes are at issue. Is it justifiable to legislate against homosexual acts, gambling, or prostitution simply on the grounds that such activities are thought to be morally unacceptable? In biomedical ethics, the principle of legal moralism is sometimes invoked, at least implicitly, when it is argued that suicide is an immoral act and that, therefore, it is justifiable to act to prevent suicide, even if the decision to take one's own life is the result of careful deliberation. Many do not accept the principle of legal moralism as a legitimate liberty-limiting principle, however. Mill holds, for example, that to accept the principle is tantamount to permitting a "tyranny of the majority."

The social welfare principle also has some relevance in biomedical ethics. According to this principle, in a version that employs the concept of autonomy rather than the concept of liberty, individual autonomy can justifiably be restricted to benefit others. Such justifications are sometimes attempted in discussions of biomedical and behavioral research. It is argued, for example, that using human beings as research subjects without informing them (thus bypassing their consent) is morally justified if the research project promises some potentially great benefit to others in society. Those who find such justifications questionable may be wary about accepting the social welfare principle as a legitimate principle.

The liberty-limiting principles that are most prominent in the literature of biomedical ethics are the paternalistic principles. Disagreements about the legitimacy of paternalistic justifications affect the resolution of a number of important issues in biomedical ethics. Physicians or nurses, for example, who lie to patients in order to spare them pain are often accused of acting on questionable (i.e., paternalistic) grounds. The paternalistic justifications offered for certain laws that are of special concern in biomedical ethics are also frequently attacked. Among such laws are those that allow courts to commit individuals to mental institutions either in order to keep them from harming themselves or in order to force them to receive treatment. Because of the centrality of paternalism in biomedical ethics, it is essential to examine the concept of paternalism as well as some of the arguments offered both for and against paternalistic actions and practices.

Paternalism

The definition of *paternalism* most widely cited is Gerald Dworkin's: "[Paternalism is] the interference with a person's liberty of action justified by reasons referring exclusively to the welfare, good, happiness, needs, interests, or values of the person being coerced."[24] When paternalism in the legal system is at issue, this definition is acceptable since laws, backed by force or the threat of harm, are by nature coercive. However, many of the actions considered paternalistic in biomedical ethics do not fit this definition. Consider the following examples:

1. A patient has frequently asserted that he would immediately commit suicide if he were ever diagnosed with Alzheimer's disease, and his physician believes he is serious. The patient says that Alzheimer's disease is antithetical to everything he values in life. The physician has now arrived at a diagnosis of Alzheimer's disease, but she lies to the patient about the diagnosis. She does so because she believes that a deliberate premature death is incompatible with the patient's best interests.

2. A physician believes that surgery is the best available treatment for a patient's cancer. The physician does not disclose significant information about nonsurgical alternatives because he believes that the patient would be inclined to choose one of these alternatives, and he wants to ensure that the patient consents to the treatment that the physician believes to be in the patient's best interests.

3. A physician refuses to perform an abortion for a woman who lives in a small, isolated town with no other physicians. They both know that the woman cannot afford to travel elsewhere to have the abortion. The physician refuses to perform the abortion because she believes that the woman will eventually regret the decision and become seriously depressed about it.

Note that none of these cases involves coercion; yet each can be correctly described as involving paternalism. In each of the cases, a physician has in one way or another infringed upon or limited a patient's autonomy. In the third case, the physician has narrowed a patient's range of choice to exclude the preferred choice, ostensibly for the patient's own good. In the first two cases, a physician has denied a patient information vital to effective deliberation, again for the patient's own good. In all three cases, physicians have treated patients as individuals incapable of making the correct judgments about their own best interests. In all three cases, a physician has effectively usurped a patient's decision-making power, substituting his or her judgment for the patient's. While it is difficult to capture this sense of paternalism in a precise definition, a rough definition can be given as follows: *Paternalism* is the interference with, limitation of, or usurpation of individual autonomy justified by reasons referring exclusively to the welfare or needs of the person whose autonomy is being interfered with, limited, or usurped.

Is such paternalistic behavior ever morally justified? If the answer is yes, under what conditions do paternalistic grounds constitute good reasons, either for coercion or for effectively taking decisions out of individuals' hands for their own good? In considering the justifiability of paternalistic actions, keep in mind the difference between the principle of paternalism and the principle of extreme paternalism. The latter would apply to paternalistic actions whose intent is to benefit individuals, whereas the former would apply to paternalistic actions whose intent is to keep individuals from harm.

In the framework of Kantian ethical theory, the moral fundamentality of individual autonomy seems to prohibit any paternalistic actions when the individuals affected are capable of self-governance or self-determination. It would always be morally wrong, for example, for physicians to withhold information about surgical procedures from patients simply because the physicians believed that their patients would refuse to undergo potentially beneficial procedures if informed of all the risks. Charles Fried, a contemporary ethicist who adopts a Kantian approach to paternalism in the medical context, maintains that patients must never be denied relevant information. By withholding it, physicians fail to treat patients as ends in themselves. In Fried's view, patients can never be treated simply as means to ends, even when the ends in question are their own ends (e.g., their restored health).[25]

John Stuart Mill provides the classical utilitarian statement on the illegitimacy of paternalistic actions. This statement is sometimes cited in court opinions concerning the right of self-determination in medical matters. Mill argues:

> [O]ne very simple principle [is] entitled to govern absolutely the dealings of society with the individual in the way of compulsion and control, whether the means used be physical force in the form of legal penalties, or the moral coercion of public opinion. That principle is, that the sole end for which mankind are warranted, individually or collectively, in interfering with the liberty of action of any of their number, is self-protection. That the only purpose for which power can be rightfully exercised over any member of a civilized community, against his will, is to prevent harm to others. His own good, either physical or moral, is not sufficient warrant. He cannot rightfully be compelled to do or forbear because it will be better for him to do so, because it will make him happier, because, in the opinions of others, to do so would be wise, or even right.[26]

In this statement, Mill asserts that while prevention of harm to others is sometimes sufficient justification for interfering with another's autonomy, the individual's own good never is. Mill rejects paternalistic interventions because of the high utility value that he assigns to individual autonomy. In assigning it this value, he assumes that individuals are, on the whole, better judges of their own interests than anyone else, so that minimizing paternalistic interventions will maximize human happiness. However, Mill himself qualifies his rejection of paternalism in the following way:

> [T]his doctrine is meant to apply only to human beings in the maturity of their faculties. We are not speaking of children, or of young persons below the age which the law may fix as that of manhood or womanhood. Those who are still in a state to require being taken care of by others, must be protected against their own actions as well as external injury.[27]

In the kinds of cases he cites, Mill assumes that people are justified in acting paternalistically because they are better judges of an individual's interests than the individual himself or herself. Arguing in this way, Mill seems to open the door for the justification of paternalism in the case of individuals who may not be able to identify and advance their own interests correctly because they lack the required level of ability for effective deliberation. Such individuals, often described as having "diminished autonomy" insofar as they lack the necessary abilities or capacities for self-determination, include infants, young children, and the severely mentally retarded. It is important to see that the paternalistic restrictions Mill allows would limit autonomy as liberty of action to the extent that they involve coercion. They would also limit autonomy as freedom of choice to the extent that they narrow the range of available choices. However, they do not limit autonomy in the sense central to Mill's, as well as Kant's, moral position since those with diminished autonomy lack what is essential for an appropriate level of effective rational deliberation.

Many contemporary attempts to justify *some* paternalistic actions adopt an approach similar to Mill's, stressing the apparently diminished autonomy of those who are treated paternalistically. If their autonomy were not so compromised, the argument runs, they would want the benefits involved and would want to avoid the harms. Those who argue in this way must deal with an underlying conceptual issue. They must identify the criteria that should be used in determining whether a person's autonomy is sufficiently diminished to justify paternalism. In light of our earlier discussion of rationality, constraint, and autonomy, it seems plausible to hold the following view regarding diminished autonomy. When a person's autonomy (in the third sense) is significantly constrained by intellectual lacks (e.g., lack of reasoning ability or ignorance of relevant facts), it is sufficiently impaired to justify paternalistic acts, especially when necessary to prevent serious, irrevocable harm. Two examples may be helpful here. People under the influence of hallucinogenic drugs who decide to leap from twentieth-floor windows in order to get home more quickly, believing that they (like Superman) can fly, are hardly acting in an autonomous manner. Their decisions are grossly inconsistent with the best inductive evidence we possess regarding what happens to human beings who leap out of windows. Severely retarded individuals who decide to go out alone in a busy city but are incapable of understanding traffic signals would also seem to be acting in a significantly nonautonomous way. They are unaware of the kind of risk they would be running by going out alone. In both cases, there is good reason to assume that the individuals are incapable, whether temporarily or permanently, of the level of reasoning required for sufficiently autonomous decision making. Thus, paternalistic interventions seem to be justified.

Does the fact that a decision will result in death or some other serious, irrevocable harm *always* provide sufficient grounds for the claim that autonomy is so severely diminished that paternalism is justified? Some especially problematic cases involve decisions to commit suicide. Many suicide attempts are the result of temporary disorientation associated with drugs, alcohol, or extreme, but reversible, depression. In accordance with our earlier discussion of rationality and autonomy, decisions to commit suicide in these cases can be considered significantly irrational and thus nonautonomous. Indeed, cases involving individuals who are so constrained in their reasoning that they are temporarily or permanently incapable of correctly assessing the probable severely harmful results of their acts would seem to provide clear instances of autonomy that is sufficiently diminished to justify paternalism. However, some decisions to end or risk life may be based on carefully thought-out reasons and may be either consistent with the person's own long-term conception of a satisfying or meaningful life or the result of a new but reflective reassessment of ultimate values and goals. It would beg the question to call these latter decisions irrational and, therefore, nonautonomous, in order to justify paternalistic interventions, simply on the grounds that the person's intended act will probably result in serious self-harm. It may be that in the case of those ends that are usually considered highly undesirable (e.g., death or the possibility of severe injury), it should be presumed that the individual's choice is not rational and, therefore, not an autonomous one. This presumption would justify, at best, temporarily constraining someone from certain acts in order to establish the rationality of the choice.

In summary, it can plausibly be maintained that paternalistic interventions can be justified either (1) when intervention is responsive to the welfare of an individual whose autonomy is significantly diminished or (2) when temporary constraint is necessary to prevent a person from acting to bring about *presumably* irrational self-harming outcomes until it can be determined that the individual is acting autonomously. Paternalism in accordance with these two conditions is often called "weak paternalism," and it is entirely consistent with Mill's criticism of paternalism (which is essentially a rejection of so-called "strong paternalism"). The interventions that are characteristic of weak paternalism do not show a lack of respect for individual autonomy. In the first case, an individual is simply incapable of acting in a significantly autonomous manner. In the second, the point of the intervention is to ensure that an individual will not harm himself or herself while acting nonautonomously. Thus the legitimacy of weak paternalism is widely accepted. In contrast, the legitimacy of strong paternalism is a hotly disputed issue. Strong paternalism is characterized by interventions that go beyond the limits set by conditions 1 and 2. Advocates of strong paternalism maintain that paternalistic interference with autonomous actions and choices can sometimes be justified.

Note that the distinction between weak and strong paternalism is not the same as the distinction between paternalism and extreme paternalism (as reflected in the statement of liberty-limiting principles). Discussions of the distinction between weak and strong paternalism often focus on actions and practices whose intention is to prevent harm and thus on the principle of paternalism rather than the principle of extreme paternalism. However, a similar distinction can be made in regard to extreme paternalism. A weak form of extreme paternalism would allow paternalistic interferences intended to benefit those whose autonomy is significantly diminished. This would stand in contrast to a strong form of extreme paternalism, which would allow beneficial paternalistic interferences even in the case of persons whose autonomy is not significantly diminished.

The mildly mentally retarded may pose special problems when questions of justified paternalism are raised, precisely because they *may* lack the abilities necessary for autonomy as effective deliberation. Whether the mildly retarded lack such abilities is a matter of dispute, however. Many people classified as mildly mentally retarded are capable of effective deliberation if they are given appropriate training and information. In the case of mentally retarded individuals who are capable of effective deliberation, paternalistic treatment would seem to be justified only if strong paternalism is justified. However, if strong paternalism is not justified in the case of the nonmentally retarded, then it would also not be justified in the case of mildly mentally retarded individuals capable of effective deliberation. On the other hand, in the case of mentally retarded individuals whose autonomy is diminished to the point that paternalistic interferences in their lives would be instances of weak paternalism, paternalistic actions whose intent is to benefit these individuals could be as justifiable as those whose intent is to keep them from harm.

Is strong paternalism ever justified? One defense of strong paternalism rests on a prudential argument that itself appeals to the importance of autonomy. We are aware that we often act in ignorance and that we are often tempted to act in ways incompatible with what we see as our long-term interests. Acting in ignorance, or too weak-willed to resist temptation, we may do ourselves serious irreversible harm of a sort that would severely diminish our autonomy. We are also aware that accidents, illnesses, diseases, and emotional pressures may diminish our rational capacities and thus our autonomy. We should be willing, therefore, to accept those paternalistic acts, laws, and practices whose intent is either to protect individual autonomy from being severely diminished or, if it has already been diminished, to restore it. This argument is advanced in order to justify the following kinds of laws: (1) laws, such as those against the sale of laetrile (a "cure" for cancer that researchers believe has no merit), that protect us against our own ignorance; (2) laws, such as those against the sale of hallucinogenic drugs (without prescription), that protect us against our own weaknesses of the will and/or ignorance; and (3) laws that allow courts and psychiatrists to commit the "mentally ill" to institutions against their will in order to cure them (restore their autonomy) or to keep them from the kind of self-harm that might further reduce their autonomy. The same sort of prudential argument is sometimes invoked to justify paternalistic acts by physicians when these acts are performed to prevent some serious deterioration of the patient's autonomy. However, some of the constraining interventions that would seem to be justified by this line of argument are very problematic. Some individuals, for example, might prefer to give in to temptations, weighing the pleasures of using hallucinogenic drugs more highly than its dangers or risks. Others might want to have access to laetrile, hoping that it will help and willing to risk the possibility that it might not. The involuntary civil commitment of the mentally ill for their own good is perhaps even more questionable, as some of the readings in Chapter 5 bring out.

A radically different defense of paternalism on the part of the state is offered by critics of the liberal individualist tradition, which is associated with both natural right theorists such as John Locke and utilitarians such as Mill. These critics question the need to justify laws and government practices whose intent is to benefit or keep from self-harm the members of society being constrained. In this view, a need to justify the state's interference with individual autonomy arises from a social-political theory that misunderstands the relationship between the state and the individual and mistakenly stresses the primacy of individual interests rather than the interests of the social whole. The ideal of the liberal-individualist tradition in social-political theory is a society with a minimal amount of state interference with individual autonomy. Critics of this social-political ideal reject the justifications that are offered in defense of the primacy accorded individual autonomy as simply expressions of an ideological commitment to "Western liberal thought." The ideology of the critics stresses the primacy of the interests of society as a whole. A social-political system committed to the latter ideal perceives all individual acts as significant for society at large and government regulation of any of those acts as part of the state's legitimate role. Any final assessment of such a defense of state paternalism, of course, is intimately intertwined with the resolution of fundamental questions about the relationship between the individual and the state.

In a totally different vein, indirect support for opposition to paternalism comes from certain sociologists, psychologists, and other social theorists who offer analyses to explain the recent emphasis on antipaternalism in American society. They attribute much of the recent stress on antipaternalism to a growing awareness of both the class differences in our society and the fact that those who perform paternalistic acts (e.g., psychiatrists, judges, physicians, and the administrators and staffs of mental institutions) are usually members of the upper-middle class, while those who are treated paternalistically are usually members of the poorer, less-privileged classes. An awareness of this class difference, and of the related differences in interests and values, gives rise to serious doubts about both the ability and the willingness of those wielding paternalistic authority to act in the interests of those whom they typically constrain. On this analysis, it is not the moral legitimacy of the principle of paternalism that is really at issue when paternalistic acts and practices are increasingly rejected. Rather, what is at issue are the abuses resulting from so-called paternalistic acts that do not in fact serve to benefit (or keep from harm) the individuals constrained but do serve the ends of the members of the professions wielding paternalistic authority. This line of argument is intended to point out that the current antipaternalistic stress is probably not the result of conscious deliberation about the legitimacy of central ethical principles but a rejection of what passes as justified paternalism in a class society in which the "constrainers" are neither knowledgeable nor altruistic enough to perceive correctly the interests of those they constrain. However, the factual claims, if correct, tend to support a Mill-like claim that unless the interests and values of constrainers and constrainees coincide, individual self-interest is better served in the long run if paternalism is rejected rather than accepted.

The Principles of Biomedical Ethics

One prominent approach to problems in biomedical ethics has been articulated by Tom L. Beauchamp and James F. Childress in *Principles of Biomedical Ethics,* originally published in 1979. The basic idea is that problems can be appropriately identified, analyzed, and resolved by reference to a set of four principles, each of which corresponds to a prima facie (i.e., conditional) obligation. The four principles, tailored specifically to be relevant in the field of biomedical ethics, are as follows: the principle of respect for autonomy, the principle of nonmaleficence, the principle of beneficence, and the principle of justice.

This distinctive principle-based approach has much in common with W. D. Ross's theory of prima facie duties, which can also be understood as a principle-based approach. In each case, we are dealing with several prima facie principles of obligation. So in each case, it is common for the principles of the system to conflict, thus requiring a judgment as to which principle has overriding weight or significance. As expressed by Beauchamp and Childress in their third edition, "Which principle overrides in a case of conflict will depend on the particular context. . . ."[28]

Frequent references to "the principles of biomedical ethics," both individually and collectively, can be found in the literature of biomedical ethics (including the readings collected in this textbook). As presented by Beauchamp and Childress, each of the principles must ultimately be understood by reference to numerous distinctions and clarifications. For our purposes, however, it is useful to identify a central (if less than complete) meaning for each principle. The *principle of respect for autonomy* requires that health-care professionals not interfere with the effective exercise of patient autonomy. The *principle of nonmaleficence* requires that health-care professionals not act in ways that entail harm or injury to patients. The *principle of beneficence* requires that health-care professionals act in ways that promote patient welfare. (The closely related concepts of beneficence and nonmaleficence are briefly explicated in our earlier discussion of Kantian deontology.) The *principle of justice* requires that social benefits (e.g., health-care services) and social burdens (e.g., taxes) be distributed in accordance with the demands of justice. Although this articulation of the principle of justice is somewhat uninformative, it is impossible to give the principle any clearer content without considering questions that are at issue in competing theories of distributive justice. These theories are discussed in the introduction to Chapter 10.

ALTERNATIVE DIRECTIONS AND METHODS

There is presently emerging a growing challenge both to recently dominant ethical theories, such as those previously discussed, and to the idea that these theories can simply be *applied* to generate satisfactory solutions to concrete problems. In biomedical ethics, criticisms have increasingly been directed at two broad approaches to ethical reasoning. These approaches are known as *deductivism* and *principle-based ethics* (also called "principlism"). A deductivist theory, such as utilitarianism or Kantianism, features a single foundational principle that supposedly provides a basis for all ethical justification.[29] According to this approach, correct ethical judgments can, in principle, be derived from the foundation, given relevant factual information (e.g., concerning the consequences of possible actions, in utilitarianism). As we saw in the previous section, principle-based ethics features a framework of several principles, rules, or duties, none of which takes absolute priority over any other. In principle-based ethics, as it is commonly understood,[30] one considers whatever principles, rules, or duties are relevant in the circumstances, settling conflicts by determining which seems more weighty.[31] Specific criticisms of deductivism and principle-based ethics will emerge in the discussions of leading alternative approaches.

Virtue Ethics

An emphasis on the moral evaluation of *actions* is common both to deductivist theories and to principle-based ethics. These approaches offer principles or rules of conduct as their main source of moral guidance. One is directed to maximize utility, never to treat persons as mere means to one's ends, or the like. Sometimes principles or rules are expressed in the language of rights and duties. For example, it is said that competent adults have a right to refuse medical treatment and health-care professionals have a duty to respect the decision making of competent adults. In contrast, virtue ethics, the tradition of Plato and Aristotle, gives *virtuous character* a preeminent place. For our purposes, virtues may be understood as character traits that are morally valued, such as truthfulness, courage, compassion, and sincerity. In virtue ethics, agents—those performing the actions—are the focus. Whereas the principal concern in an action-based approach to ethics is with the right thing to do, the principal concern in a virtue-based approach is with what kind of person to be.

In recent years there has been a significant revival of virtue ethics, a development affecting bioethics. Some theorists have argued that mainstream theories have overemphasized action-guides to the neglect of issues of character. What is needed, they maintain, is a *supplementation* of action-based ethics with virtue ethics. Other theorists have defended the more radical thesis that the neglect of virtue has caused action-based ethical theories to be *importantly misconceived* (so that merely supplementing them is insufficient). Among these theorists, some have argued for a robust *integration* of action-based ethics and virtue ethics (without giving priority to either), while others have gone further, calling for the *replacement* of action-based ethics by virtue ethics.

What arguments can be advanced in favor of virtue ethics? One difficulty with theories that are solely action based is that they seem to neglect the fact that we often morally judge people's motivations and character, not just their actions. For example, in praising someone's kindness or criticizing a person's meanness, our evaluation makes no explicit reference to actions. Sometimes we even fault a person who acts rightly but with questionable motivation or attitude. For example, consider a person who gives to charities only when seeking public office, or a surgeon who only begrudgingly solicits a patient's informed consent to surgery. Conversely, sometimes we temper our blame of a person who has acted wrongly if, in doing so, admirable motives and character traits were displayed. For example, we might moderate our criticism of someone who lied to assuage another's feelings, even if we think lying was the wrong choice.

Another argument addresses what is most useful in guiding moral choice. It is claimed that principles, rules, and codes are of little use in actual decision making (e.g., in biomedical contexts). Such action-guides are too abstract to provide practical guidance. Moreover, they often conflict. (The suggestion that conflicts can be effectively resolved by appeal to an ethical theory immediately confronts the problem that there is such extensive disagreement on which theory is most adequate.) A more effective approach, according to this argument, is to cultivate enduring traits (such as competence, attentiveness, honesty, compassion, and loyalty) through education, the influence of role models, and habitual exercise of those traits. Such virtues, it is claimed, are a more reliable basis, in practice, for morally correct action than is knowledge of principles, rules, or codes.

The arguments surveyed so far are compatible with the program of supplementing action-based theories with virtue ethics. Even the idea that virtues are more useful in practice is consistent with these claims. (1) Ethics is more centrally concerned with what people should do (virtues being generally reliable means for doing the right thing). (2) Right action, in principle, can be characterized without reference to virtue. However, the following arguments are more radical. They suggest that virtue is often at least as morally important or fundamental as right action and that sometimes the latter cannot even be characterized independently of virtue.

First, several philosophers have argued that in many cases right action cannot be described in an illuminating way without referring to virtue. Consider the idea that we should help those who are suffering. (This idea expresses a principle of action.) Truly helping someone often requires keen attention to the subtleties of the situation at hand to determine whether, and what sort of, intervention is called for. Would calling a particular student aside, telling him or her an anecdote, and offering advice be helpful, or would it be intrusive and condescending? One cannot reliably perform acts that are helpful (as opposed to intrusive or condescending) without exercising a capacity for discernment, which involves such virtues as emotional attunement and sympathetic insightfulness.[32] Since being helpful in such circumstances involves being virtuous, the proper conclusion is that virtue partly constitutes right action.

Second, the manner in which we act—what we express in our action—can matter as much as, or more than, what we do. (We might even say that our manner of acting is part of what we do.) Suppose Earl borrows money from his brother, Jake, and promises to repay him within a month. Four weeks later Jake gently reminds Earl of his promise. If Earl then storms into his brother's house, slams down the money, and marches off in resentment and anger, he has fulfilled his duty to keep a promise, but he has not acted well. A full account of how Earl should have conducted himself would include a description of the manner in which he should have acted (perhaps courteously). Here, again, the conclusion is that virtue partly constitutes right action.

Moreover, sometimes emotional responses, which can reveal a person's character, are of paramount moral importance (a point suggested in the last example). This is especially evident in situations in which no particular action is morally called for. For example, a social worker might be deeply affected by another social worker's detailed account of a patient who lost his job and committed suicide. If the two work at different hospitals, there is probably nothing the first social worker can do about the tragedy. However, her pain at a stranger's plight reveals virtue; complete indifference arguably would reveal a moral deficiency.[33]

While the above arguments probably succeed in showing the need to integrate virtue ethics and action-based ethics (and perhaps undermine the claim that action has priority), there are compelling reasons to resist the stronger thesis that virtue ethics should *replace* action-based approaches. First, while action-guides such as principles and rules are not exhaustive of what is important in the moral life, neither is virtue. One can be well motivated and have a good character yet act wrongly; conversely, acting without virtue does not *always* mean doing the wrong thing. (This is consistent with the view that virtue sometimes partly constitutes right action.) Morally, we are concerned with both action and character, doing and being.

Second, the specificity of such action-guides as rules, codes, and rights-claims often provides an attractive form of bottom-line moral protection. Rules such as those requiring informed consent for medical interventions and prohibiting therapists from having sexual relations with psychiatric patients provide an important bedrock of action requirements. In fact, such rules can often help professionals establish relationships with patients in which certain virtues can more naturally be exercised.

Similarly, it seems unlikely that any specification of virtues would be sufficient to guide conduct. In bioethics we are interested in such questions as, Is it ever right for a therapist to violate patient confidentiality, and, if so, when? Such a question probably cannot be answered by appeal to virtue alone. In conclusion, it would seem that an adequate portrait of the moral life would include action-guides such as principles, rules, and rights-claims—not just virtues. The question we are left with, then, is not whether both virtues and action-guides have important places in ethical theory and bioethics, but rather how to understand in greater detail their roles and relationship to one another.

How might virtues play a role in biomedical ethics? Here is one example. A physician has just received test results strongly suggesting that her 30-year-old patient has inoperable ovarian cancer. Neither of them expected such a calamity. The physician knows that she has an obligation to inform her patient of the results. However, in reflecting on how to broach and discuss this matter with her, the physician finds such principles as beneficence and non-maleficence too general to be useful; no helpful rules of conduct come to mind, either. The physician keeps coming back to such ideas as *compassion, sensitivity,* and *honesty.* Although these words describe virtues, we could say that "Be compassionate," "Be sensitive," and "Be honest" are rules of action. Nevertheless, such instructions do not really tell the physician how to handle her delicate predicament. To handle it well, she will have to *be* compassionate, sensitive, and honest (and no set of rules can explain how to be that way). The physician, in other words, will have to be virtuous. She might find it useful to model her behavior on that of a mentor or colleague whom she identifies as having the desired qualities.

The Ethics of Care and Feminist Ethics

The ethics of care and feminist ethics represent further challenges to recently dominant ethical theories, to deductivism, and to principle-based ethics. While the ethics of care and feminist ethics both stem importantly from the moral experience of women, they represent overlapping—but certainly not identical—sets of concerns.

Like virtue ethics, the ethics of care pays considerable attention to affective components of the moral life, but with special emphasis on empathy and concern for the needs of others—that is, on caring. Like casuistry (an approach discussed in the next section), it emphasizes the particularities and context of moral judgment and rejects impartiality as an essential feature of morality. The ethics of care also underscores the moral importance of relationships and the responsibilities to which they give rise.

Perhaps more than any other work, Carol Gilligan's study of gender differences in ethical thinking has brought the ethics of care into the mainstream of philosophical discussion.[34] In a study of responses to moral conflicts, Gilligan finds that females tend to focus on details about the relationships among the persons involved and to seek innovative solutions that protect everyone's interests. In contrast, males typically try to identify and apply a relevant principle or rule (which they take to be universal or valid from an impartial perspective), even if doing so means sacrificing someone's interests. Gilligan calls the former approach an *ethic of care* (or responsibility) and the latter (which includes recently dominant ethical theories) an *ethic of justice*. She notes in her study that the empirical correlations were imperfect; males sometimes work from the care perspective and women sometimes use the justice approach. In any event, the tendencies she notes are striking, for they suggest that traditional approaches to ethics have been more responsive to the moral experience of males than to that of females. Gilligan concludes that there is no reason to consider the care perspective inferior and that an ideal ethics would incorporate both approaches.

As originally characterized by Gilligan and now generally understood, the ethics of care downplays rights and allegedly universal principles and rules in favor of an emphasis on caring, interpersonal relationships, and context. Numerous specific criticisms of recently dominant ethical theories have been developed in the ethics of care literature. A summary of several critical arguments follows.

To begin with, there is a problematic presumption underlying theories such as utilitarianism and Kantianism. The presumption is that impartiality is a fundamental aspect of moral thinking. In reality, impartiality is a demand reflective of male thinking; the partiality that comes with caring relationships is no less legitimate. Indeed, certain relationships merit special weight. For example, in many contexts, a father should favor his own children's interests over those of other children. Moreover, the abstract principles of traditional theories have very limited practical use; contextualization and attention to detail are needed for problem solving in ethics. In many complex situations involving ethical conflicts, such principles as "Respect all persons as ends in themselves" and "Maximize utility" simply provide inadequate guidance.

Furthermore, ethical theories featuring abstract principles tend to neglect affective components of the moral life. Caring responsiveness to others' needs is often morally preferable to detached, dispassionate moral evaluation. For example, the ethics of care would strongly affirm a health-care professional's heartfelt dedication to a patient, without conditioning its value on good consequences or respect for persons. The abstract nature of recently dominant theories also tends to cover up certain morally salient experiences—such as being a woman, a parent, a minority, or a professional who has particular working relationships with other professionals.

A health-care professional working within the spirit of the ethics of care would bear in mind (or internalize) considerations such as these: (1) the individualized needs, both physical and psychological, of the patient; (2) how to respond in a caring, personalized manner to those needs; (3) the likely impact of various options on the quality of the relationships among the involved persons, including the patient and professional, but also other members of the health-care team and any involved family members; and (4) how to attain or maintain the best possible relationships among those persons. Suppose a nurse faces a conflict between loyalty to a patient and loyalty to the attending physician, who refuses to disclose certain medical options to the patient. The "justice" approach might view the dilemma in terms of overall utility, conflicting rights, or the like. In contrast, the ethics of care would emphasize the lived relationships and the responsibilities inherent in them, the impact of possible responses on those relationships, and the prospects for conflict resolution.

The relationship between *feminist ethics* and the ethics of care is a complex one, and this complexity is reflected in the different ways that various feminists have responded to the emergence and widespread discussion of the ethics of care. Some feminists have celebrated the reception accorded the ethics of care and feel validated by the recognition of a distinctly female moral perspective. Others, however, have reacted negatively to at least certain aspects of the ethics of care.

Feminist ethics can be initially characterized in the following ways: (1) As with the ethics of care, it is firmly committed to the view that the moral experience of women must be taken seriously (but often with a critical eye to the role that the subordination of women may play in shaping that experience). (2) It is deeply committed to the overriding moral importance of ending oppression—with special emphasis on the subordination of women.

These features of feminist ethics together motivate a redirection of focus to women (and, to an important extent, minorities and other historically disadvantaged groups). This focus includes both an emphasis on the importance of women's interests and special attention to issues that especially concern or affect women. Thus, in bioethics, feminist ethics urges careful examination of the interests of women as decision makers in maternal-fetal conflicts and as the almost exclusive participants in the profession of nursing. Special attention is also given, for example, to the distinctive needs of women in the area of medical research, to the moral complexities of surrogate motherhood, and to arguably sexist undercurrents in the promotion of in vitro fertilization and in various medical practices surrounding childbirth.

In feminist ethics, a critical eye is turned toward practices and institutions that may perpetuate and legitimate forms of oppression. Some of these practices and institutions, feminists argue, are so deeply embedded in our culture that they go unnoticed. Susan Sherwin states:

> In pursuing feminist ethics, we must continually raise the question, What does it mean for women? When, for example, feminists consider medical research, confidentiality, or the new reproductive technologies, they need to ask not only most of the standard moral questions but also the general questions of how the issue under consideration relates to the oppression of women and what the implications of a proposed policy would be for the political status of women. Unless such questions are explicitly asked, the role of practices in the oppression of women (or others) is unlikely to be apparent, and offensive practices may well be morally defended.[35]

Some feminists have charged proponents of the ethics of care with naïveté for accepting women's moral experiences at face value—without questioning the oppressive practices and attitudes that may have helped make certain experiences and ways of thinking typical for women. Sherwin, for example, argues:

> Because gender differences are central to the structures that support dominance relations, it is likely that women's proficiency at caring is somehow related to women's subordinate status.[36]

Nurturing, caring, and the disposition to preserve relationships at almost any cost may simply be the survival skills of an oppressed group; Sherwin notes that such dispositions are also found among formerly colonized persons of both genders. Some feminists also argue that the value of mothering, so affirmed in the ethics of care, may be tied to the norm of the nuclear family—a norm that can be seen as discounting the perspectives of homosexuals, persons in single-parent families, and others who remain legally unmarried. They point out that caring has led some women to direct nearly all of their energies to others' needs, without adequately attending to their own. While caring is an admirable trait in many circumstances, these feminists maintain, it is sometimes better withheld when a focus on rights and autonomy is necessary. In general, they conclude, we must not valorize the traits that tend to perpetuate women's subordinate status.[37]

How might we assess the ethics of care and feminist ethics as alternatives to recently dominant theories and to the idea that these theories can simply be applied in order to resolve concrete problems? The care perspective's emphasis on relationships and the affective components of the moral life merits careful attention; arguably, the traditional theories greatly understate their significance. (Ross's theory, which highlights morally significant relationships, is a partial exception.) The critical-minded attention of feminist ethics to oppression, inequalities, and issues pertaining to women and other disadvantaged groups is surely valuable. In addition, the feminist caution about gender stereotyping is well-taken. Uncritical acceptance of traditionally feminine and masculine qualities may lead too easily to the assignment of people to "appropriate" roles (such as women to midnight infant feedings and men to aggressive professional pursuits).

However, the distance between these alternative perspectives, on the one hand, and recently dominant theories, on the other, can easily be overdrawn. Utilitarians, for example, should be firmly dedicated to the eradication of oppression (given all of its bad consequences). Kantian respect for persons, while perhaps vague and abstract, is at least compatible with caring and special relationships (the validity of which could be impartially recognized). Caring attention to particularities might even provide a useful way of specifying or supplementing abstract but worthy principles.

In the end, Gilligan argues that "care" and "justice" are both only parts of a broader ethics, and few proponents of the care perspective propose that it monopolize ethics. In a pluralistic spirit, one might adopt a similar attitude toward feminist ethics, concentrating on whatever insight and illumination this perspective brings to ethics. Here is a concluding suggestion from Sherwin:

> I do not envision feminist ethics to be a comprehensive . . . theory that can be expected to resolve every moral question with which it is confronted. It is a theoretical perspective that must be combined with other considerations to address the multitude of moral dilemmas that confront human beings. . . . Although very little of the literature in ethics addresses the issue of sexism or any other form of systematic oppression, surely the responsibility to do so in one's moral evaluations is implicit. Feminist ethics has assumed leadership in pursuing such analysis.[38]

Casuistry: Case-Based Reasoning in Historical Context

Casuistry, which has received a great deal of attention in recent years, is a method of moral reasoning that was reawakened from three centuries of slumber with the publication of *The Abuse of Casuistry,* by Albert Jonsen and Stephen Toulmin.[39] Following Aristotle and other philosophers as well as theologians throughout the ages, the authors contend that the "top-down" reasoning inherent in deductivism and principle-based ethics (as they understand it) is entirely inadequate for the resolution of concrete problems, such as those that arise in bioethics. (Jonsen and Toulmin never clearly distinguish deductivism and principle-based ethics. While some of their criticisms concern both approaches, others concern only deductivism.)

First, according to the casuists, no simple, unified ethical theory can capture the great diversity of our moral ideas, a consideration that helps to account for the fact that there is such extensive disagreement about ethical theories. Second, our actual moral thinking does not typically consist of straightforward deductive reasoning (deriving an ethical judgment from a supreme principle). *Practical wisdom* is required to determine which of various norms (principles or rules) applies in a complicated or ambiguous case. For example, if a patient awaiting admission to a fully occupied intensive care unit better fulfills admission criteria than someone already admitted, would it ever be right to admit the waiting patient if doing so would be detrimental to the one who would be displaced? Casuists doubt that the answers to such questions can be derived from a traditional ethical theory, such as utilitarianism or Kantianism, or from a set of abstract principles. Third, such approaches miss the fact that moral certainty, where it exists, concerns particular cases. For example, that a particular person acts wrongly in torturing for sadistic pleasure is far more certain than any full-blown ethical theory could be.

The alternative of casuistry is a form of case-based reasoning. It begins with clear "paradigm" cases in which some norm is clearly relevant and indicates the right action or judgment. For example, if we learn that a man stole a car just for a thrill, we know he acted wrongly. From this and similar cases we can extract a *maxim,* "Stealing is wrong," which holds in the absence of unusual circumstances. The paradigm cases serve to illuminate other cases by way of analogy. Maxims are refined as new cases are confronted in which the norms apply ambiguously (for example, if someone finds an expensive watch in a classroom and does not attempt to locate its owner) or in conflict (for example, if someone believes that temporarily appropriating a bicycle is the only way to save an innocent person's life). Often, the refinements involve stating exceptions.

In order to reach a defensible moral judgment in any particular case, we must first determine which paradigms are relevant. Difficulties arise, of course, when paradigms fit only ambiguously or when two or more paradigms fit in conflicting ways. Jonsen and Toulmin see the history of moral practice as revealing an ongoing clarification of the use of paradigms and of admitted exceptions. This brings us to an important point.

Moral reasoning about cases cannot proceed without reference to actual moral traditions. Casuists assert the priority of *practice* over theory. Moral norms are to be found in practice; practice is not to be justified (or condemned) by absolute moral principles, because there are none. In rejecting the idea of a timeless, rationally required ethical theory, the casuists have important allies in such American pragmatists as William James (1842–1910) and John Dewey (1859–1952). But the emphasis on practice is not simply a broad historicism, grounding our understanding of morality in the developing Western moral tradition. Also crucial are the specific institutions and practices (such as those of American medicine) that provide the context for any set of ethical problems. To illustrate their method, casuists point to case law—including, in bioethics, classic cases such as *Quinlan, Conroy,* and *Cruzan,* which have greatly illuminated the ethics of terminating life-sustaining treatment.

For an example of casuistry in action, consider the question of whether Jehovah's Witness parents have the right to refuse a blood transfusion for their young child who will die without one. Rather than appealing to an ethical theory or to general principles such as beneficence or respect for autonomy, a casuist would try to reason by analogy from cases about which we have relatively settled opinions. The casuist would cite various cases that support (1) the right of competent adults to refuse medical treatment for themselves, and (2) the right of parents to make decisions for their children. Regarding the second right, we let parents send their children to private religious schools, for example. On the other hand, society tends to limit parental discretion if choices amount to serious neglect. Thus, while parents have much discretion over where to send their children to school, they may not keep them out of school (unless comparable tutoring is provided); that choice is regarded as seriously detrimental to a child's well-being. Similarly, a casuist might argue that, because refusing a blood transfusion would ensure the child's death, such a choice would be seriously neglectful and therefore beyond the bounds of parental discretion. Unlike the parents, the child has not autonomously chosen to be a Jehovah's Witness. If and when he or she becomes an adult, he or she may choose or reject this value system and make medical and other decisions accordingly.

How viable is casuistry as an alternative to recently dominant theories and top-down methods of ethical reasoning? It certainly avoids the remoteness from concrete problems that arguably plagues utilitarianism and Kantianism. Indeed, it seems to capture the way much of our ethical reasoning actually proceeds. Moreover, casuistry is capable of producing consensus even when people disagree about ethical theories. Furthermore, the casuists are surely right that at least some specific moral judgments are more certain than any ethical theory.

At the same time, a number of problems confront casuistry. Some concern the work of the currently leading proponents, Jonsen and Toulmin. For example, while they identify casuistry as an alternative to top-down approaches represented in the theories already described, they never clearly distinguish their primary targets: deductivism and principle-based ethics. This omission is significant, because some of their criticisms can be validly made against at most one of these approaches. For instance, while some specific moral judgments are more certain than any *complete ethical theory,* it is far from clear that such judgments are more certain than any *principle.* Since principle-based ethics involves the use of principles (as opposed to the use of a complete ethical theory), the casuists' point about the locus of ethical certainty may only constitute an advantage over deductivism.

One might therefore wonder whether casuistry is so different from principle-based ethics. Casuists claim that moral certainty is to be found in particular cases. However, giving priority to the particular over the general may be undermined by the following possibility: *grasping the ethical significance of a case is indistinguishable from grasping a prima facie principle or rule that applies to that case.* We can grasp that a man's slapping a child without special cause is wrong. However, in order to make this judgment, we must also grasp the prima facie wrongness of some kind of action, such as harming the innocent or hurting children. For it is something about the man's action that is understood to make it wrong. There seems to be no reason to claim that judgments about particular cases are more certain than judgments about prima facie principles or rules relevant to such cases. Indeed, it is not clear that the two kinds of judgments can be completely separated.

Another possible charge against casuistry is that it is overly "intuitionistic" in resolving difficult cases. Suppose we start with the established view that a competent adult patient may refuse medical treatment. May such a patient also refuse all nutrition and hydration? If so, what makes this second kind of case *relevantly similar* to the first, such that the maxim guiding the first (respecting competent adult patients' refusals) applies also to the second? Where matters are debatable, how does one *justify* particular judgments? At this point, the casuist is likely to vest decision-making authority in community judgment. Such a judgment becomes incorporated into the community's evolving traditions and practices. For example, our society has judged that food and water can be thought of, in medical settings, as similar to medical care. So a competent adult patient may refuse them.

While casuistry can respond to the charge of being overly intuitionistic by appealing to traditions and practices, it must then confront the charge of being too *accepting* of the latter. Why take at face value the ethical convictions woven into our cultural traditions and professional practices? American medical practice, for instance, may embody a vision of the physician-nurse relationship that is elitist and sexist. Therefore, is it not unsound, as contemporary feminists would insist, to appeal to established medical practice in considering issues concerning the interactions of physicians and nurses? To take another example, arguably neither broad cultural traditions nor the professional practice of researchers has sufficient critical "edge" to confront squarely the question of whether animals should be used in biomedical research and, if so, with what restrictions.

Finally, by focusing so exclusively on cases, casuistry risks (1) being unable to make progress with especially controversial issues and (2) missing very general and fundamental issues, the resolution of which may be relevant to specific cases. As an example of problem (1), case analysis is almost certainly insufficient to illuminate the moral status of animals. In our society today there is fundamental disagreement about animals' moral status, so people are likely to have widely varying responses to individual cases. Regarding (2), fundamental issues can be missed because of excessive faith in precedents (previous cases). How do we know our precedents are right? For example, the fact that Medicare covers renal dialysis and kidney transplants, open-heart surgery, and certain other treatments may seem to weigh in favor of funding heart transplants. But perhaps we never should have funded those other treatments in the first place.[40]

In conclusion, while casuistry embodies important insights about ethical reasoning, it faces significant challenges. Contrary to the claims of recent defenders, casuistry may be compatible with principle-based ethics. Further reflection on its strengths and weaknesses may suggest that casuistry is best regarded as part of a more comprehensive model of ethical reasoning.

Reflective Equilibrium and Appeals to Coherence

Recently dominant approaches (whether deductivist or principle-based) are sometimes criticized for viewing ethical justification as essentially "downward"; that is, *theories or principles,* assumed to be firmly established, are thought to justify our judgments about particular cases. On the other hand, casuistry may oversimplify the nature of ethical reasoning in the opposite direction. Casuists claim that ethical certainty lies in *cases,* the study of which allows us to identify maxims to be used and revised in exploring new cases. Arguably, each of these models is excessively rigid in giving priority to one level of ethical conviction: general norms (theories or principles) or particular cases. Perhaps our ethical insights and reasoning lack any such exclusive foundation.

According to the model of *reflective equilibrium,* formulated by John Rawls, no level of ethical conviction deserves such priority.[41] Justification occurs at all levels of generality: (1) theories, (2) principles and rules of differing degrees of specificity, and (3) judgments about cases. Judgments made at any level can be used to revise judgments at any other level.

The reflective-equilibrium model directs us to start with *considered judgments,* that is, those judgments about which we have a very high degree of certainty after careful and extensive consideration. These judgments differ in some ways from the paradigm cases of casuistry. First, considered judgments may be of any level of generality. Some may be specific case judgments (as in casuistry); others may be rules such as a prohibition of rape; still others may be principles, such as the principle of respect for autonomy. Second, a judgment counts as a considered judgment only if it is reasonably believed not to have resulted from bias. (Casuistry, again, ties its paradigm case judgments so closely to accepted practices that many such judgments may be suspected of bias.) From a set of considered judgments, one can begin a process of belief revision in an effort to achieve a more coherent overall set of beliefs. (What coherence involves is described below.)

For example, one might initially believe it appropriate to test drug addicts without their consent for HIV; requiring consent might make it difficult to gather data that would be useful for the future treatment of HIV-infected patients. But Kant's principle that we should never treat persons merely as means casts doubt on this initial judgment. Such patients are not treated as ends in themselves unless they are given the option to refuse testing. This revision of judgments moves "downward," but in the present model one may also revise "upward." For example, mindful of a case in which a psychiatric patient threatens to kill an identified third party, we might revise a principle of patient confidentiality to allow exceptions in this sort of case.

One point stressed by defenders of the reflective-equilibrium model is that revisions are never considered final; we must always admit the possibility that our ethical convictions (sometimes even considered judgments) will require modification in light of further considerations. Thus, while we strive, through continual reflection, for a state of equilibrium in our total set of ethical convictions (hence the model's name), we are never finished with moral inquiry. New problems arise, and fresh information and novel insights make us question old judgments. As in casuistry, moral reasoning is viewed as dynamic and is not expected to produce a final, rationally necessary theory.

But how do we know which judgments or norms should get revised when there is a conflict? In the cases above, why not (1) reject or revise the prohibition against treating persons merely as means or (2) retain confidentiality as an exceptionless principle, instead of the other way around in each case? How can we *justify* any particular resolution of conflicts? In brief, conflicts are to be settled by making revisions that seem to produce the greatest *coherence* in our overall system of ethical convictions.

Appeals to coherence may be understood, more specifically, to include requirements of logical consistency, argumentative support, and plausibility.[42] *Logical consistency* is simply the avoidance of outright contradiction. For example, it is logically inconsistent to hold that killing an innocent person is always wrong, yet it would be right to grant this particular person's request to be killed on grounds of mercy. *Argumentative support* is the giving of reasons for one's ethical views—reasons that must be consistent with one's reasoning about other ethical issues. Thus, if one favors paternalistically prohibiting the use of certain drugs but opposes paternalistic seat belt laws, one must provide argumentative support explaining why paternalism is justified in one case but not in the other. In the absence of any argument for a relevant distinction, the combination of claims appears incoherent. The third requirement for selecting among alternative viewpoints is *plausibility*. Suppose someone argues that no actions are ethically right or wrong (a logically consistent position) because all ethical judgments are just an expression of taste (argumentative support). This view is utterly implausible. It implies that it is not wrong to commit genocide out of sheer racial hatred. Thus, in the present model one seeks logically consistent judgments, backed by ethical reasons or arguments, that are largely plausible upon reflection.[43]

The reflective-equilibrium model, involving appeals to coherence, appears to be gaining support as more theorists and professionals question the adequacy of more traditional approaches. The model is especially favored by those contemporary philosophers who identify with the spirit of the early American pragmatists (who saw ethical reasoning as dynamic and rejected claims of an absolute foundation for morality). The model incorporates the case-based reasoning of casuistry, as well as the downward argumentation associated with principle-based ethics.[44] It concedes to deductivism that sometimes theoretical thinking is needed to check our particular judgments. Depending on how it is developed, the model can also include many insights and elements of virtue theory as well as the ethics of care and feminist ethics. Overall, it may seem to offer a flexible and balanced approach to moral reasoning.

Nevertheless, the model of reflective equilibrium has its difficulties. Arguably, it buys flexibility and freedom from dogmatism at the cost of vagueness and lack of structure. Utilitarianism and Kantianism, in contrast, provide a relatively clear framework to be applied in ethics. Casuistry, by focussing on concrete cases, may provide a clearer method for approaching some issues. A critic could argue that, in the reflective-equilibrium model, one might not know where to start or how to proceed. A defender of the model might respond as follows. Theoretically, we start with considered judgments; in practice, we often simply start wherever we have ethical concern, and we use various tools of reasoning as we work toward more coherent positions. While this model is receiving increasing attention in bioethics and appears to have many strengths, it may be premature to judge its overall adequacy as an alternative to casuistry and recently dominant approaches.

T.A.M. and D.D.

NOTES

1 Efforts to determine what is morally good and what is morally bad with regard to human character also fall under the heading of normative ethics. This aspect of normative ethics is of central importance in a school of thought known as *virtue ethics*. A discussion of virtue ethics is presented later in Chapter 1.

2 Some scholars prefer to identify biomedical ethics as a type of *practical* ethics, rather than *applied* ethics. Their underlying concern is to avoid any suggestion that particular moral problems can be effectively resolved simply by "applying" ethical theories or principles. We continue to employ the commonly used category of applied ethics, but in no way do we mean to imply the appropriateness of any mechanical-like "application" model. (See the section, "Alternative Directions and Methods.")

3 In what follows, the two versions of utilitarianism are articulated in ways intended to emphasize a contrast between them. There are alternative ways of articulating both act-utilitarianism and rule-utilitarianism, and some of these articulations bring the two versions of utilitarianism much closer than our account suggests.

4 Probably a majority of contemporary utilitarians take the satisfaction of preferences to constitute intrinsic value. See, for example, Jonathan Glover, *Utilitarianism and Its Critics* (New York: Macmillan, 1990), Part 2.

5 J. J. C. Smart, "Extreme and Restricted Utilitarianism," in Michael D. Bayles, ed., *Contemporary Utilitarianism* (New York: Doubleday, 1968), p. 100.

6 W. D. Ross, *The Right and the Good* (Oxford: The Clarendon Press, 1930), p. 22.

7 Alan Donagan, "Is There a Credible Form of Utilitarianism?" in *Contemporary Utilitarianism*, p. 189. Donagan's point is that act-utilitarianism is "monstrous" and "incredible" because it seems to recommend such murders.

8 The distinction between act-utilitarianism and rule-utilitarianism is a distinction that has become prominent only in contemporary times. Accordingly, the writings of Bentham and Mill are somewhat ambiguous with regard to these categories. Although Bentham is probably rightly understood as an act-utilitarian, a very strong case can be made for interpreting Mill as a rule-utilitarian. See, for example, J. O. Urmson, "The Interpretation of the Moral Philosophy of J. S. Mill," in *Contemporary Utilitarianism*, pp. 13–24.

9 Smart, "Extreme and Restricted Utilitarianism," p. 107.

10 Immanuel Kant, *Groundwork of the Metaphysic of Morals*, trans. H. J. Paton (New York: Harper & Row, 1964), p. 88.

11 *Ibid.*, p. 96.

12 H. J. Paton, *The Categorical Imperative: A Study in Kant's Moral Philosophy* (Chicago: University of Chicago Press, 1948), p. 172.

13 The account of beneficence suggested here reflects an analysis originally presented by Tom L. Beauchamp and James F. Childress in Chapters 4 and 5 of *Principles of Biomedical Ethics* (New York: Oxford University Press, 1979).

14 Ross, *The Right and the Good,* p. 19.

15 *Ibid.,* p. 20.

16 *Ibid.,* p. 21.

17 *Ibid.*

18 *Ibid.*

19 Writers in biomedical ethics and social philosophy characterize autonomy in various ways. Bruce L. Miller, for example, distinguishes four senses of autonomy: autonomy as liberty of action, autonomy as authenticity, autonomy as effective deliberation, and autonomy as moral reflection. (Our discussion follows Miller to some extent but diverges in important ways.) Gerald Dworkin prefers to distinguish between liberty and freedom on the one hand and autonomy on the other, using *autonomy* much more narrowly than Miller. See Bruce L. Miller, "Autonomy and the Refusal of Lifesaving Treatment," *Hastings Center Report* 11 (August 1981), pp. 25–28; and Gerald Dworkin, "Autonomy and Informed Consent," in President's Commission, *Making Health Care Decisions,* Appendix G (1982), pp. 63–81.

20 The distinction between occurrent and dispositional coercion is made by Michael D. Bayles in "A Concept of Coercion," in J. Roland Pennock and John D. Chapman, eds., *Coercion: Nomos XIV* (Chicago: Aldine-Atherton, 1972), pp. 16–29.

21 Kant, *Groundwork,* p. 108.

22 John Stuart Mill, *Utilitarianism, On Liberty, Essay on Bentham,* ed. Mary Warnock (New York: New American Library, 1962), pp. 187, 185. All quotations in this chapter are from this edition of *On Liberty.*

23 Joel Feinberg's discussion of such principles served as a guide for the formulations adopted here. See Joel Feinberg, *Social Philosophy* (Englewood Cliffs, NJ: Prentice-Hall, 1973), Chapter 2.

24 Gerald Dworkin, "Paternalism," *The Monist* 56 (1972), p. 65.

25 Charles Fried, *Medical Experimentation: Personal Integrity and Social Policy* (New York: American Elsevier, 1974), p. 101.

26 Mill, *On Liberty,* p. 135.

27 *Ibid.*

28 Beauchamp and Childress, *Principles of Biomedical Ethics,* 3d ed. (1989), p. 51.

29 Such a foundational principle might have a complex structure (unlike that of utilitarianism or Kantianism). For example, a foundational principle might consist of two or more simpler principles arranged in a strict hierarchy.

30 But see the section, "Reflective Equilibrium and Appeals to Coherence," later in the chapter.

31 Two influential works of principle-based ethics in biomedical ethics are Beauchamp and Childress, *Principles of Biomedical Ethics* (4th ed., 1994); and National Commission for the Protection of Human Subjects of Biomedical and Behavioral Research, *The Belmont Report: Ethical Principles and Guidelines for Research Involving Human Subjects* (Washington, DC: Government Printing Office, 1979).

32 Arguments of this sort can be found in, for example, Iris Murdoch, *The Sovereignty of Good* (London: Routledge and Kegan Paul, 1970); and Martha Nussbaum, *Love's Knowledge* (New York: Oxford University Press, 1990).

33 The last three paragraphs have benefitted from ideas in Alisa L. Carse, "Rules of Conduct and the Uncodifiability of Virtue" (unpublished manuscript).

34 Carol Gilligan, *In a Different Voice: Psychological Theory and Women's Moral Development* (Cambridge, MA: Harvard University Press, 1982).

35 Susan Sherwin, *No Longer Patient: Feminist Ethics and Health Care* (Philadelphia, PA: Temple University Press, 1992), p. 55.

36 *Ibid.,* p. 50.

37 See Sherwin, *No Longer Patient,* pp. 49–51. Cf. Sara Ruddick, "Remarks on the Sexual Politics of Reason," in Eva Feder Kittay and Diana T. Meyers, eds., *Women and Moral Theory* (Savage, MD: Rowman & Littlefield, 1987), p. 246; John M. Broughton, "Women's Rationality and Men's Virtues: A Critique of Gender Dualism in Gilligan's Theory of Moral Development," in Mary Jeanne Larrabee, ed., *An Ethic of Care: Feminist and Interdisciplinary Perspectives* (New York: Routledge, 1993), p. 134; and Zella Luria, "A Methodological Critique," in Larrabee, *An Ethic of Care,* pp. 202–203.

38 Sherwin, *No Longer Patient,* p. 57.

39 Albert R. Jonsen and Stephen Toulmin, *The Abuse of Casuistry: A History of Moral Reasoning* (Berkeley: University of California Press, 1988).

40 John D. Arras, "Getting Down to Cases: The Revival of Casuistry in Bioethics," *The Journal of Medicine and Philosophy* 16 (1991), p. 46.

41 See "Outline for a Decision Procedure for Ethics," *Philosophical Review* 60 (1951), pp. 177–197; and *A Theory of Justice* (Cambridge, MA: Harvard University Press, 1971).

42 Strictly speaking, coherence involves other theoretical virtues as well, such as simplicity and clarity. Moreover, any proponent of this model—in fact, of any model or theory—must seek not only coherence among ethical beliefs but also coherence between ethical beliefs and empirical facts. Thus the claim that surgery without anesthesia on dogs is morally appropriate because dogs are incapable of suffering is undermined by evidence showing that dogs, in fact, can suffer.

43 A commonly cited distinction pertaining to the present model is that between "narrow" and "wide" reflective equilibrium. See, for example, Norman Daniels, "Wide Reflective Equilibrium and Theory Acceptance in Ethics," *Journal of Philosophy* 76 (1979), pp. 256–282; and Margaret Holmgren, "The Wide and Narrow of Reflective Equilibrium," *Canadian Journal of Philosophy* 19 (1989), pp. 43–60.

44 Indeed, contrary to its reputation as an exclusively top-down form of reasoning, principle-based ethics may be best understood as a version of reflective equilibrium that emphasizes principles. See David DeGrazia, "Moving Forward in Bioethical Theory: Theories, Cases, and Specified Principlism," *Journal of Medicine and Philosophy* 17 (1992), pp. 511–539.

ANNOTATED BIBLIOGRAPHY: CHAPTER 1

Bayles, Michael D., ed.: *Contemporary Utilitarianism* (New York: Doubleday, 1968). This volume includes ten articles by contemporary philosophers. Various points of view on the nature and justifiability of utilitarian theory are represented.

Beauchamp, Tom L., and James F. Childress: *Principles of Biomedical Ethics,* 4th ed. (New York: Oxford University Press, 1994). The authors advocate a principle-based approach in bioethics. Chapters 3–6 provide an account of principles organized by reference to four headings: respect for autonomy, nonmaleficence, beneficence, and justice. Chapter 8 provides a discussion of "Virtues and Ideals in Professional Life."

Blustein, Jeffrey: *Care and Commitment: Taking the Personal Point of View* (New York: Oxford University Press, 1991). Blustein argues for a synthesis of insights from recently dominant ethical theories, the ethics of care, and recent philosophical work on personal integrity into a unified moral outlook.

Carse, Alisa L.: "The 'Voice of Care': Implications for Bioethical Education," *Journal of Medicine and Philosophy* 16 (February 1991), pp. 5–28. After elucidating contrasting features of recently dominant ethical theories and the ethics of care, Carse draws implications of the latter for bioethics education.

Childress, James F.: *Who Should Decide?: Paternalism in Health Care* (New York: Oxford University Press, 1982). In this extended discussion of paternalism, Childress examines the metaphors and principles underlying the disputes about professional paternalism in health care.

Christman, John, ed.: *The Inner Citadel: Essays on Individual Autonomy* (New York: Oxford University Press, 1989). This anthology provides a collection of articles on the nature and value of individual autonomy.

Donagan, Alan: *The Theory of Morality* (Chicago: University of Chicago, 1977). In this book, Donagan provides a theory of morality whose philosophical basis is Kant's "second formulation" of the categorical imperative.

Dworkin, Gerald: *The Theory and Practice of Autonomy* (Cambridge: Cambridge University Press, 1988). In Part 1, Dworkin examines the nature and value of autonomy. In Part 2, he applies the general framework developed in Part 1 to various moral questions.

Foot, Philippa: *Virtues and Vices* (Oxford: Blackwell, 1978). Foot argues that virtue is more central, morally, than obligation; the paradigm moral person is one who is disposed by character to be rightly motivated.

Glover, Jonathan, ed.: *Utilitarianism and Its Critics* (New York: Macmillan Publishing Company, 1990). The various selections in this anthology incorporate both objections to utilitarianism and attempts to defend utilitarianism against the objections.

Holmes, Helen Bequaert, and Laura M. Purdy, eds.: *Feminist Perspectives in Medical Ethics* (Bloomington: Indiana University Press, 1992). The aim of this anthology is to show how feminist ethics and the ethics of care can advance medical ethics. Most of the contributors focus on specific issues in medical ethics that especially affect the interests of women.

Jonsen, Albert R.: "Casuistry as Methodology in Clinical Ethics," *Theoretical Medicine* 12 (December 1991), pp. 295–307. Jonsen focuses on how casuistry can be a useful technique of practical reasoning for clinical ethicists and ethics consultants.

———, and Stephen Toulmin: *The Abuse of Casuistry: A History of Moral Reasoning* (Berkeley: University of California Press, 1988). After examining the history of casuistry and the criticism it has received, the authors argue for its revival.

Journal of Medicine and Philosophy 15 (April 1990). The articles included in this issue appear under the heading of "Philosophical Critique of Bioethics." Various methodological issues are considered, and several of the articles develop criticisms of the principle-based approach associated with Beauchamp and Childress in *Principles of Biomedical Ethics*.

Kant, Immanuel: *Groundwork of the Metaphysic of Morals,* translated and analyzed by H. J. Paton (New York: Harper & Row, 1964). In this work, a basic reference point, Kant offers an overall statement and defense of his ethical theory.

Kittay, Eva Feder, and Diana T. Meyers, eds.: *Women and Moral Theory* (Savage, MD: Rowman & Littlefield, 1987). Contributors to this anthology examine and debate (1) the empirical basis for asserted gender differences in moral problem solving, (2) specific aspects of moral deliberation, and (3) political and legal implications of the ethics of care and feminist ethics.

Larrabee, Mary Jeanne, ed.: *An Ethic of Care: Feminist and Interdisciplinary Perspectives* (New York: Routledge, 1993). This anthology focusses on Carol Gilligan's work and its implications. Special attention is given to debates in moral philosophy, empirical claims in psychology about alleged gender differences in moral reasoning, and challenges to Gilligan's work that claim it excludes African-American and other cultures.

Lindley, Richard: *Autonomy* (Atlantic Highlands, NJ: Humanities Press, 1986). After examining various conceptions of autonomy and some related principles, Lindley discusses several specific practical problems regarding autonomy, including social practices in regard to those who are mentally handicapped or mentally ill.

MacIntyre, Alasdair: *After Virtue: A Study in Moral Theory* (Notre Dame, IN: University of Notre Dame Press, 1981). Advancing the disquieting thesis that contemporary moral language consists of the fragmented remnants of a worldview no longer accepted in the secular West, MacIntyre advocates a return to Aristotelean virtue ethics.

Mill, John Stuart: *Utilitarianism, On Liberty, Essay on Bentham,* edited by Mary Warnock (New York: New American Library, 1962). In his famous essay *Utilitarianism,* Mill offers a classic statement of the utilitarian position. In his equally well-known essay *On Liberty,* he defends the classic liberal view regarding the limitation of individual liberty.

Rawls, John: *A Theory of Justice* (Cambridge, MA: Harvard University Press, 1971). In this classic work, Rawls presents and defends his theory of justice as an alternative to utilitarian theory. In doing so, he also argues for and uses the method of reflective equilibrium.

Sartorius, Rolf, ed.: *Paternalism* (Minneapolis: University of Minnesota Press, 1983). The various articles in this collection deal with the nature and justifiability of paternalism.

APPENDIX: SELECTED REFERENCE SOURCES IN BIOMEDICAL ETHICS

Lineback, Richard H., ed.: *The Philosopher's Index* (Bowling Green, OH: Philosophy Documentation Center, Bowling Green State University). This reference source, issued quarterly, is "an international index to philosophical periodicals and books." Both a subject index and an author index are provided, as are abstracts of articles. The subject index identifies useful material on virtually any topic of importance in biomedical ethics.

Reich, Warren T., ed. in chief: *Encyclopedia of Bioethics,* 2d ed. (New York: Macmillan, 1995). This five-volume set is a basic reference source in biomedical ethics. The set contains 460 original articles, and each article is followed by a selected bibliography.

Walters, LeRoy, and Tamar Joy Kahn, eds.: *Bibliography of Bioethics* (Washington, DC: Kennedy Institute of Ethics, Georgetown University). This bibliography, whose volumes are issued annually, is the most comprehensive source available. Its cumulated contents are also available from BIOETHICSLINE, an on-line database of the National Library of Medicine. (The database is updated bimonthly.)

CHAPTER 2

THE PHYSICIAN-PATIENT RELATIONSHIP

INTRODUCTION

What moral rules should govern physicians in dealing with patients? What qualities of character would a virtuous physician display? Are physicians ever morally justified in acting paternalistically toward their patients? Are they ever morally justified in withholding information from their patients, lying to them, or treating them without their consent? This chapter confronts such questions as it examines some of the fundamental moral issues associated with the physician-patient relationship and, consequently, with many of the other issues in this book.

Physicians' Obligations and Virtues

The Hippocratic Oath, reprinted in this chapter, reflects the traditional paternalism of the medical profession. The oath requires physicians to act so as to "benefit" the sick and "keep them from harm," but it says nothing about patients' rights. Most of the medical codes of ethics developed through the years by the American Medical Association reveal a similar approach. They articulate the standards and virtues that should guide physicians in their professional relationships with patients and others but remain silent on patients' rights. For example, physicians are expected to promote their patients' well-being, but nothing is said about a patient's right to define his or her own well-being—or to participate in decisions affecting it. In contrast, the discussions that have taken place over the past quarter of a century in biomedical ethics have frequently emphasized patients' rights, especially their right of self-determination. This emphasis reflects a growing change in lay attitudes toward physicians.

For a long time physicians were viewed as dedicated, hardworking, selfless individuals who could be expected to do everything in their power to benefit their patients. Patients, on the other hand, were viewed as dependent individuals having an obligation to trust their physicians. It was often taken for granted that doctors, because of their purported wisdom, objectivity, benevolence, and skill, were in the best position to decide what was in their patients' best interests. Professional codes of medical ethics reflected this view of the physician-patient relationship, affirming that physicians would act to benefit, and not exploit, the often vulnerable patients over whom they frequently held great influence and power.

Current attitudes toward physicians are very different, due to many factors including the following. First, the physician-patient relationship has become increasingly impersonal as the growth of medical knowledge and technology has made medicine more complex. Growing complexity has led to increased specialization and the growth of large, depersonalized medical institutions. Second, the rise of "iatrogenic illnesses," which are those resulting from medical interventions, has sometimes raised doubts about the skills and judgment of physicians. Third, there is a growing perception that many physicians engage in practices that sometimes compromise patients' interests for the sake of physicians' financial gain. In an article reprinted in this chapter, Edmund D. Pellegrino argues that a physician's virtue is of paramount importance in situations in which altruism and self-interest appear to conflict.

In keeping with such changing attitudes toward physicians, many recent discussions of medical ethics have attempted to expose and criticize the extensive paternalism embodied in traditional codes of medical ethics. Many authors have rejected as morally unacceptable professional codes that sanction paternalistic justifications for medical practices—such as lying for a patient's "own good"—that violate a patient's right to self-determination. However, in a 1990 statement, "Fundamental Elements of the Patient-Physician Relationship," reprinted in this chapter, the American Medical Association acknowledges numerous patient rights, including the right to receive information relevant to one's medical care.

Paternalism and Respect for Patient Autonomy

Is acting in accord with the traditional commitment to foster a patient's well-being always compatible with acting in accord with the principle of respect for patient autonomy? In their analysis of numerous models, or metaphors, of the physician-patient relationship, in an article reprinted here, James F. Childress and Mark Siegler suggest that these two goals are not always compatible. The paternalism model, which emphasizes the traditional medical commitment to serve patient well-being, is usually inadequate in today's world, according to the authors. Physicians and patients may disagree in their health-related values (for example, cases in which only the physician considers addiction to cigarettes a disease), or they may disagree about the relative value of health in comparison with other values (as when a Jehovah's Witness refuses a blood transfusion, knowing that death will inevitably result, while the patient's physician considers the transfusion necessary). As the authors put it, paternalism "tends to concentrate on care rather than respect, patients' needs rather than their rights, and physicians' discretion rather than patients' autonomy or self-determination."

That is not to say that paternalism is never justified, however. Childress and Siegler defend the commonly accepted form of paternalism (identified in Chapter 1 as weak paternalism) in which a patient is incompetent and at risk of harm. Moreover, the authors ultimately recommend, for many physician-patient interactions in which the patient is competent, the metaphor of *negotiation*. This metaphor illuminates two important aspects of medical relationships: (1) the autonomy of both parties (where autonomy is construed not as a goal that can be imposed on a patient, but as a constraint on permissible interactions between autonomous persons) and (2) the ongoing nature of the relationship. The metaphor of negotiation invites both patient and physician to determine what they consider acceptable terms for continuing the relationship. Those terms may involve one or more of the models Childress and Siegler discuss—even paternalism, because a patient might autonomously decide to turn the medical decision-making reins over to a physician willing to take them.

As presented in Chapter 1, paternalism is the interference with, limitation of, or usurpation of individual autonomy justified by reasons referring exclusively to the welfare or needs of the person whose autonomy is being interfered with, limited, or usurped. In acting paternalistically, physicians in effect act as if they, and not their patients, can best identify what is in their patients' best interests as well as the best means to advance those interests. Many commentators argue that paternalism and respect for patients' autonomy are incompatible. But Terrence F. Ackerman argues in this chapter that genuine respect for autonomy may require physicians to override patients' treatment-related preferences (suggesting at least weak paternalism) in order to help them regain some of the autonomy lost due to the constraining effects of illness. While affirming the importance of honesty and respect for patients' rights, Ackerman criticizes the interpretation of respect for autonomy that takes it to be essentially a principle of *noninterference*. To understand his concern, it is helpful to discuss two kinds of cases in which the values perceived as fundamental in physician-patient interactions—promotion of patient well-being and respect for patient autonomy—appear to conflict.

First, a patient's abilities for effective deliberation may be so severely constrained by illness (e.g., high fever, delirium) that autonomous decisions are virtually impossible and "apparent" decisions may be inconsistent with the patient's history of decisions and values. In such cases, the promotion of a patient's well-being may require acting against his or her expressed wishes. This would appear to violate the principle of respect for autonomy, but the conflict between the two values may not be real. If the patient's autonomy as effective deliberation is so severely diminished and the desires expressed are also inconsistent with the patient's history and values, the principle of respect for autonomy would not even seem to apply. When there are compelling reasons to believe that a patient's decisions are not autonomous and that as a result the patient cannot exercise the right of self-determination, no paternalistic usurpation of that right—no *strong* paternalism—is involved when decisions are made for the patient.

Second, a patient and physician may disagree about just what constitutes the patient's well-being (a point noted by Childress and Siegler). A physician, for example, might insist on continuing aggressive treatment in the case of a cancer patient, even though past treatment has brought no positive results. The patient might have a strong desire to discontinue the recommended therapy and let life end without the additional discomforts caused by the therapy. To foster the patient's well-being, then, the physician might think it necessary to resort to paternalistic practices intended to circumvent the patient's decision. In such a case the physician may see a conflict between two obligations—an obligation to promote the patient's well-being, as understood from an objective medical standpoint, and an obligation to respect the patient's right of self-determination. The physician may believe that any chance of prolonging life, no matter how slight, justifies continuing treatment. But while the prolongation of life is generally regarded as a good and its premature termination a harm, the paternalistic model itself does not commit one to the prolongation of life irrespective of the harms that might be incurred by the patient. Thus the physician's belief that this life must be prolonged, whatever the discomfort to the patient and no matter how brief the extension of life, may be due to the physician's own values rather than to some indisputably objective medical values. The patient, however, may believe that a few extra days or weeks of uncomfortable in-hospital life, with an extremely small chance of further prolonging life, are not worth the price. If the patient's decision is the result of reflection and in keeping with his or her history of decisions and values, respect for autonomy would seem to require acting in accord with the *patient's* perception of his or her well-being. If the patient's decision is not in accord with his or her history of decisions and values but *is* the result of a careful reflective reevaluation of those values, respect for autonomy would again seem to require acting in accord with the patient's choices. The conflict here is not between an obligation to respect autonomy and an obligation to promote patient well-being but between two different conceptions of *well-being*. The conflict arises because what constitutes a person's well-being is to some extent a subjective, or personal, judgment.

The problematic cases that concern Ackerman arise because of the constraining effects illness has on autonomy. In relation to the first kind of case, for example, it is sometimes difficult to judge to what extent a patient's capacity for effective deliberation is undermined. In the face of such uncertainty, does the physician's obligation to promote the patient's well-being entail an obligation to act so as to "restore the patient's autonomy" to the greatest extent possible, even if this involves some measure of paternalism? Ackerman holds that the physician's obligation is to act to restore autonomy. This suggests (in Childress and Siegler's terms) that autonomy is a goal to be sought when it is absent or diminished, not just a constraint on physician-patient interactions when the patient is already considered autonomous. Ackerman gives examples intended to show how psychological states (such as depression) or social factors (such as family influence) can constrain a patient's decision making. He argues that physicians have an obligation to act in ways that will offset the effects of these constraints in order to make the patient more autonomous. It is not clear that all of Ackerman's examples involve paternalism, since they do not all involve the usurpation of patients' decision making. In any event, physicians who act as Ackerman recommends run the danger exemplified by the second kind of case, when they fail to see that a disagreement with a patient about some course of treatment may be due, not to the constraining effects of illness on autonomy, but to a disagreement about values.

Truth-Telling

Traditional codes of medical ethics have little to say about deception, lying, or truth-telling. Yet some of the most widely disputed issues in biomedical ethics center on the physician's obligation to be truthful with the patient and on the patient's right to know the truth. Until recently, it was not unusual for physicians to lie to patients about their illnesses for paternalistic reasons. Nor was it unusual for physicians to prescribe alternating injections of sterilized water with injections of painkilling drugs for patients who were told that all the injections contained some opiate. In the first kind of case, physicians often argued that patients did not want to know the truth or that the truth would harm the patient. In the second kind of case, they often argued that the deceptive practices were justified because water does have a psychotherapeutic effect but is much less dangerous to the patient than too frequent injections of opiates. This latter view is succinctly expressed in a letter written to *The Lancet*:

> Whenever pain can be relieved with a ml of saline, why should we inject an opiate? Do anxieties or discomforts that are allayed with starch capsules require administration of a barbiturate, diazepam, or propoxyphene?[1]

Are physicians ever morally justified in paternalistic lies or deceptive practices? If so, under what conditions?

One way to approach these questions is to begin with more general questions. Is it always morally wrong to lie? Is it always right to tell the truth? In answering these questions, of course, we must give reasons to justify the position taken. If it is *always* wrong to lie or to deceive others intentionally, then it is wrong for anyone, including physicians, to do so. If lies and intentional deception are *sometimes* morally acceptable, then it is necessary to specify the conditions that make them acceptable. Once these conditions are determined, we can explore the particular physician-patient situation to see whether it satisfies them.

Rule-utilitarians, for example, faced with deciding under what conditions, if any, lies and deceptive practices are justified, would have to consider the possible consequences of adopting and following a particular rule. In the medical context, they would ask, "What would be the effect on the physician-patient relationship if physicians followed the rule, 'Lie to your patients whenever you believe that doing so is in the patient's best interests'?" In weighing the potential consequences of following such a rule, they would have to take account of the erosive effect that following it would have on patients' trust of physicians.

Suppose a physician argued as follows: Physicians ought to lie to patients because (1) it is extremely difficult to convey the technical facts and uncertainties inherent in a medical situation to persons who lack medical training, (2) most patients do not want to know the truth, and (3) the truth can harm patients. In responding to this argument, a rule-utilitarian would have to examine the three factual claims underpinning this view, a task carried out by Roger Higgs in this chapter (though without special reference to the theory of rule-utilitarianism). In response to the first argument, Higgs replies that (*a*) while communicating the patient's medical situation to the patient may be difficult, it is generally not impossible, and (*b*) the admission " 'I do not know' can be a major piece of honesty." In response to the second argument, Higgs cites studies suggesting that most patients *do* want the truth. In response to the third, Higgs contends the following: (*a*) While the truth can sometimes harm patients, such cases are less common than physicians have claimed; (*b*) the manner of disclosure is crucial to the likelihood of harm; and (*c*) lying can also be harmful by preventing a patient from being able to plan appropriately for the future and by weakening a patient's trust of physicians.

The rule-utilitarian who agreed with Higgs's findings would still be faced with determining whether exceptions should be built into a rule against lying to patients. These exceptions would probably be designed to cover cases in which there is very strong evidence to show that a patient does not want to know or would be seriously harmed by knowing. The rule-utilitarian would then have to determine whether the harm done to these patients would be outweighed by the overall good consequences of following a rule that prohibits all lying to patients.

Deontologists, of course, take a different approach. Immanuel Kant, whose deontological position is discussed in Chapter 1, is usually read as defending an absolutist position: All lies, including those done out of altruistic motives, are wrong. Not all deontologists agree with this absolutist position. As noted in Chapter 1, W. D. Ross maintains, for example, that there is a prima facie obligation not to lie or intentionally deceive but that this obligation can sometimes be overridden by some other prima facie obligation. In medicine, the overriding obligation might sometimes be the physician's obligation to promote the patient's medical well-being.

In the end, perhaps the kind of situation in which it is most plausible to argue that physicians may lie or deceive is one in which truthfulness seems likely to destroy a patient's hope. An example would be that of a critically ill patient who might be devastated by the disclosure that her cancer is inoperable; without hope, she might quickly succumb to her disease. In one of this chapter's readings, Howard Brody cautions against the hasty assumption that truthful disclosure would have this effect. He argues that physicians can seldom entirely dash a patient's hope, because hope is extraordinarily resilient. Moreover, in his view, disclosing the truth is usually compatible with inspiring hope, by responding to important patient concerns other than survival. Brody's examples include the patient's hope that death will be relatively painless, the hope that he or she will not be abandoned before death, and the hope that loved ones will maintain contact in the time remaining.

Informed Consent

Discussions about truth-telling and lying in medical ethics frequently arise in conjunction with discussions of the requirements of informed consent. It is now widely accepted that both law and morality require that competent adults not be subjected to interventions without their informed and voluntary consent. But lying to patients or even withholding information from them can seriously undermine their ability to make informed decisions and, therefore, to give informed consent. In order to be able to give such consent, and thereby exercise their right of self-determination, patients must have access to relevant information, and physicians are usually the only ones in a position to supply it. Judge Spotswood W. Robinson III affirms this point in a judicial opinion, reprinted in this chapter, in which he argues that physicians have a duty to "satisfy the vital informational needs of the patient."

The informed-consent requirement is a relatively recent addition to the ethical constraints governing the physician-patient relationship. Traditional codes of medical ethics recognize no physician obligation to inform patients about the risks and benefits of alternative diagnostic and treatment techniques. The doctrine of informed consent was introduced into case law in 1956. Since then, however, it has received a great deal of attention in biomedical ethics as both a legal and an ethical requirement. In 1982, for example, Congress assigned the task of determining the ethical and legal implications of the informed-consent requirement to the President's Commission for the Study of Ethical Problems in Medicine and Biomedical and Behavioral Research. In its report, the commission describes ethically valid consent "as an ethical obligation that involves a process of shared decisionmaking based upon the mutual respect and participation [of patients and health care professionals]"[2] and identifies two values as providing the ethical foundation of the requirement: respect for the patient's autonomy, or the right of self-determination, and the promotion of the patient's well-being.

Much of the literature on informed consent focuses on several difficulties that affect the application of the requirement. (1) Who is *competent* to give consent? (2) When is consent *informed*? That is, how much information must a patient receive and understand before his or her consent is informed rather than partially informed or uninformed? (3) When is consent *voluntary*? Each of these questions is briefly examined in order to show some of the difficulties that affect the application of the requirement. It is important to note that the problems here are both conceptual and empirical. The meaning of the concepts *informed, competent,* and *voluntary* must be explicated so that it can be determined just what counts as voluntary and informed consent. Then, in a particular case, it must be determined whether the individual in question is capable of giving voluntary and informed consent.

(1) Who is competent to give consent? The patient who is sick enough to be in a hospital or institution may not be functioning normally enough to be a rational decision maker. Patients who are under great emotional stress, who are frightened, or who are in severe pain are often considered less than competent decision makers. In a burn center in California, for example, the following procedure has been used when a patient with burns over 60 percent or more of his or her body is admitted. During the first two hours after the patient is severely burned, there is no pain since the nerve endings are anesthetized. Patients during this time are given a choice. They can opt either to start a course of treatment, which will be prolonged and excruciatingly painful but may save their lives, or to receive painkilling medication and care until they die. Can a patient in such circumstances, even if free from pain, be considered clear-minded enough to weigh these alternatives?

Recent work on competence stresses that it is not "all or nothing." Still, for practical purposes in medical decision making, some threshold must be used to determine who is considered competent and who is not. The commission's report maintains that individuals should be judged to be incapable of decision making only when they lack the ability to make decisions that promote their well-being in keeping with their own previously expressed values and preferences. Allen E. Buchanan and Dan W. Brock in this chapter defend a "sliding-scale" model of competence, according to which different standards of competence apply depending on the kinds of medical decisions being made. However, in a reading reprinted here, Tom Tomlinson replies that what should vary from case to case is not standards of competence itself but standards of *evidence* for determining competence.

(2) How much information must patients be given before their consent is informed? Suppose a patient suffering from breast cancer agrees to have a radical mastectomy. She is not told that studies indicate that this radical surgery is not more effective than much less radical surgery. Has the patient been given sufficient information for her decision to count as an informed one? What criteria must the physician use in determining when sufficient information has been given? Is more information better than less? Studies have shown that patients receiving long, detailed explanations of the risks and purposes of a procedure may comprehend and retain very little of the significant information. In contrast, those who are given less detailed information may be able to comprehend and retain more of the important facts.[3]

(3) When is consent really voluntary? It is often argued that it is very easy to manipulate even highly competent patients into giving consent when the request is made by someone in a position of authority. For example, it has been shown that physicians, whose patients sometimes see them as "god" figures, and therapists, whose judgments patients generally trust, find it very easy to get the consent they request. When patients are influenced in this way, is their consent sufficiently voluntary?

Recent work on informed consent, such as that of the president's commission, stresses the importance of the process of communication and of the patient's cognitive-information processing. Studies have been undertaken both to understand and to improve the procedures used to get "informed consent."[4] If the goal is informed consent, it may be insufficient simply to transmit information to patients via a form or a short conversation listing possible risks and alternatives; it is necessary to determine how much the patient has understood and perhaps even some of the other factors that may affect the patient's decision, such as concern about a physician's reaction to a refusal.

Consider the example of a terminally ill, diabetic, cancer-ridden patient who, after repeatedly rejecting amputation of his gangrenous left foot, suddenly assented. His consent appeared to be both voluntary and informed. However, given his history and the staff's knowledge of his values, a decision was made to call in an ethics consultant to determine the reasons for the patient's change of mind. After a long conversation with the patient, the consultant learned that the patient had consented to the amputation only because he erroneously believed that without his consent the physician and the hospital would refuse to continue their care. Once he understood that this belief was incorrect, he withdrew his assent to the amputation. The staff members' knowledge of this patient's character and values as well as their concern that the consent be truly informed and voluntary may not be the norm, but this case illustrates that informed consent requires more than forms and cursory rituals. It also shows the need for medical professionals to have insight into the communication processes they use to achieve informed consent.

What extent, or quality, of communication can be reasonably expected—legally and morally—as a standard of informed consent? Whatever the answer, is it compatible with good medical practice? In one of this chapter's readings, Howard Brody criticizes the prevailing legal standards of informed consent for encouraging the impression that informed consent is separate from, and even interferes with, sound medical care. In his view, part of the problem stems from the fact that most physician-patient encounters occur in the context of primary care, whereas the courts and many commentators appear to take surgery and other risky procedures as the paradigm of such encounters. Brody discusses the advantages of a "conversation" standard of informed consent (which is illustrated in the case of the diabetic patient just described), but he argues that this demanding standard is probably not feasible legally. As a compromise, Brody recommends a "transparency" standard, under which a physician can be said to have provided adequate disclosure when his or her essential thinking about the medical situation has been made transparent to the patient.

Some Other Issues Related to the Physician-Patient Relationship

One cluster of issues related to the physician-patient relationship concerns various types of conflicts of interest. (1) One type of conflict of interest pits *patients' interests against the health-related interests of physicians.* Do physicians have an obligation, stemming from their professional roles, to provide health care when doing so puts them at risk? For example, do physicians have an obligation to care for individuals who have AIDS or who are infected with the human immunodeficiency virus (HIV)? In two of this chapter's readings, Edmund D. Pellegrino and John D. Arras address both the general question of physicians' obligations to provide care even when doing so puts them at personal risk and questions dealing specifically with physicians' obligations toward those with AIDS or HIV. (2) A second type of conflict of interest pits *patients' interests against the financial interests of physicians.* In an article reprinted in this chapter, Ronald M. Green examines ethical arguments for and against the practice of medical joint-venturing, which involves physicians' referring their patients to facilities in which the physicians have a financial interest. (3) A final type of conflict of interest pits *patients' interests against society's financial interests.* Marcia Angell, in one of this chapter's readings, examines the current American expectation that doctors act as "double agents." Such a conflict comes about because in addition to the traditional expectation that doctors ally themselves with patients in addressing their medical needs, doctors today are also pressured to respond to society's need to curtail medical costs. What is at stake in this tension, she argues, is the patient-centered ethic that forms the very moral core of medicine.

In the concluding reading of this chapter, Michael J. Meyer explores the relatively unexamined topic of patients' duties. Meyer contends that certain patient duties are grounded in the nature of the patient-professional relationship. He presents several examples of what he takes to be such duties.

D.D.

NOTES

1 J. Sice, "Letter to the Editor," *The Lancet* 2 (1972), p. 651.
2 President's Commission for the Study of Ethical Problems in Medicine and Biomedical and Behavioral Research, *Making Health Care Decisions: The Ethical and Legal Implications of Informed Consent in the Patient-Practitioner Relationship,* Vol. 1: *Report* (Washington, DC: U.S. Government Printing Office, 1982), p. 2.
3 On this point, see Ralph J. Alfidi, "Controversy, Alternatives, and Decisions in Complying with the Legal Doctrine of Informed Consent," *Radiology* 114 (January 1975), pp. 231–234.
4 Barrie R. Cassileth et al., "Informed Consent—Why Are Its Goals Imperfectly Realized?" *New England Journal of Medicine* 302 (1980), pp. 896–900; and T. M. Grundner, "On the Readability of Surgical Consent Forms," *ibid.*, pp. 900–902.

Physicians' Obligations and Virtues

The Hippocratic Oath

Little is known about the life of Hippocrates, a Greek physician born about 460 B.C. We know that he was a widely sought, well-known, and influential healer who is said to have lived 85, 90, 104, or 109 years. A collection of documents known as the *Hippocratic Writings* (largely written from the fifth to the fourth century B.C.) is believed to represent the remains of the Hippocratic school of medicine. Some of the works in this collection are credited to Hippocrates. The oath reprinted here, however, is believed to have been written by a philosophical sect known as the Pythagoreans in the latter part of the fourth century B.C.

For the Middle Ages and later centuries, the Hippocratic Oath embodied the highest aspirations of the physician. It sets forth two sets of duties: (1) duties to the patient and (2) duties to the other members of the guild (profession) of medicine. In regard to the patient, it includes a set of absolute prohibitions (e.g., against abortion and euthanasia) as well as a statement of the physician's obligation to help and not to harm the patient.

I swear by Apollo Physician and Asclepius and Hygieia and Panaceia and all the gods and goddesses, making them my witnesses, that I will fulfill according to my ability and judgment this oath and this covenant:

To hold him who has taught me this art as equal to my parents and to live my life in partnership with him, and if he is in need of money to give him a share of mine, and to regard his offspring as equal to my brothers in male lineage and to teach them this art—if they desire to learn it—without fee and covenant; to give a share of precepts and oral instruction and all the other learning to my sons and to the sons of him who has instructed me and to pupils who have signed the covenant and have taken an oath according to the medical law, but to no one else.

I will apply dietetic measures for the benefit of the sick according to my ability and judgment; I will keep them from harm and injustice.

Reprinted with permission of the publisher from *Ancient Medicine: Selected Papers of Ludwig Edelstein,* edited by Owsei Temkin and C. Lilian Temkin, p. 6. Copyright © 1967 by the Johns Hopkins Press: Baltimore.

I will neither give a deadly drug to anybody if asked for it, nor will I make a suggestion to this effect. Similarly I will not give to a woman an abortive remedy. In purity and holiness I will guard my life and my art.

I will not use the knife, not even on sufferers from stone, but will withdraw in favor of such men as are engaged in this work.

Whatever houses I may visit, I will come for the benefit of the sick, remaining free of all intentional injustice, of all mischief and in particular of sexual relations with both female and male persons, be they free or slaves.

What I may see or hear in the course of the treatment or even outside of the treatment in regard to the life of men, which on no account one must spread abroad, I will keep to myself holding such things shameful to be spoken about.

If I fulfill this oath and do not violate it, may it be granted to me to enjoy life and art, being honored with fame among all men for all time to come; if I transgress it and swear falsely, may the opposite of all this be my lot.

Fundamental Elements of the Patient-Physician Relationship
Council on Ethical and Judicial Affairs, American Medical Association

This 1990 statement asserts (1) the collaborative nature of the patient-physician relationship and (2) a set of patient rights. Regarding the collaborative relationship, patients are said to have a responsibility to work cooperatively with physicians in addressing health-related needs. Patients' rights include the right to accept or refuse recommended medical treatments, the right to confidentiality, and the right to "have available adequate health care."

From ancient times, physicians have recognized that the health and well-being of patients depends on a collaborative effort between physician and patient. Patients share with physicians the responsibility for their own health care. The patient-physician relationship is of greatest benefit to patients when they bring medical problems to the attention of their physicians in a timely fashion, provide information about their medical condition to the best of their ability, and work with their physicians in a mutually respectful alliance. Physicians can best contribute to this alliance by serving as their patients' advocate and by fostering the following rights:

1. The patient has the right to receive information from physicians and to discuss the benefits, risks, and costs of appropriate treatment alternatives. Patients should receive guidance from their physicians as to the optimal course of action. Patients are also entitled to obtain copies or summaries of their medical records, to have their questions answered, to be advised of potential conflicts of interest that their physicians might have, and to receive independent professional opinions.

2. The patient has the right to make decisions regarding the health care that is recommended by his or her physician. Accordingly, patients

Reprinted with permission of the publisher from *JAMA*, vol. 264 (December 26, 1990), p. 3133. Copyright © 1990, American Medical Association.

may accept or refuse any recommended medical treatment.

3. The patient has the right to courtesy, respect, dignity, responsiveness, and timely attention to his or her needs.

4. The patient has the right to confidentiality. The physician should not reveal confidential communications or information without the consent of the patient, unless provided for by law or by the need to protect the welfare of the individual or the public interest.

5. The patient has the right to continuity of health care. The physician has an obligation to cooperate in the coordination of medically indicated care with other health care providers treating the patient. The physician may not discontinue treatment of a patient as long as further treatment is medically indicated, without giving the patient sufficient opportunity to make alternative arrangements for care.

6. The patient has a basic right to have available adequate health care. Physicians, along with the rest of society, should continue to work toward this goal. Fulfillment of this right is dependent on society providing resources so that no patient is deprived of necessary care because of an inability to pay for the care. Physicians should continue their traditional assumption of a part of the responsibility for the medical care of those who cannot afford essential health care.

The Virtuous Physician and the Ethics of Medicine
Edmund D. Pellegrino

Edmund D. Pellegrino is director of the Center for Clinical Bioethics, Georgetown University, as well as John Carroll Professor of Medicine and Medical Humanities and professor of community and family medicine at Georgetown Medical School. Widely published in medical ethics, he is coauthor of *A Philosophical Basis of Medical Practice* (1981) and *For the Patient's Good* (1988). He is also coeditor of *Catholic Perspectives on Medical Morals* (1989).

Pellegrino defends a vision of medical ethics in which virtue ethics and duty-based ethics are each essential components. Citing several important codes of medical ethics, including the Hippocratic Oath, Pellegrino argues for a three-tiered system of obligations incumbent upon physicians. In "ascending order of ethical sensitivity," they are (1) obedience to the law, (2) observance of moral rights and fulfillment of moral duties, and (3) the practice of virtue. According to Pellegrino, physicians' practice of virtue distinguishes itself less in the avoidance of clearly unethical actions than in the avoidance of actions at the ambiguous margin of moral responsibility, where altruism is pitted against self-interest. Examples of practices at this moral margin include investing in for-profit hospitals, selling services for whatever the market will bear, and making referrals on the basis of friendship and reciprocity rather than skill.

. . . In most professional ethical codes, virtue and duty-based ethics are intermingled. The Hippocratic Oath, for example, imposes certain duties like protection of confidentiality, avoiding abortion, not harming the patient. But the Hippocratic physician also pledges: ". . . in purity and holiness I will guard my life and my art." This is an exhortation to be a good person and a virtuous physician, in order to serve patients in an ethically responsible way.

Likewise, in one of the most humanistic statements in medical literature, the first century A.D. writer, Scribonius Largus, made *humanitas* (compassion) an essential virtue. It is thus really a role-specific duty. In doing so he was applying the Stoic doctrine of virtue to medicine [1, 5].

The latest version (1980) of the AMA 'Principles of Medical Ethics' similarly intermingles duties, rights, and exhortations to virtue. It speaks of 'standards of behavior', 'essentials of honorable behavior', dealing 'honestly' with patients and colleagues and exposing colleagues 'deficient in character'. The *Declaration of*

From *Virtue and Medicine: Explorations in the Character of Medicine,* edited by Earl E. Shelp, pp. 248–253. © 1985 by D. Reidel Publishing Company. Reprinted by permission of Kluwer Academic Publishers.

Geneva, which must meet the challenge of the widest array of value systems, nonetheless calls for practice 'with conscience and dignity' in keeping with 'the honor and noble traditions of the profession'. Though their first allegiance must be to the Communist ethos, even the Soviet physician is urged to preserve 'the high title of physician', 'to keep and develop the beneficial traditions of medicine' and to 'dedicate' all his 'knowledge and strength to the care of the sick'.

Those who are cynical of any protestation of virtue on the part of physicians will interpret these excerpts as the last remnants of a dying tradition of altruistic benevolence. But at the very least, they attest to the recognition that the good of the patient cannot be fully protected by rights and duties alone. Some degree of supererogation is built into the nature of the relationship of those who are ill and those who profess to help them.

This too may be why many graduating classes, still idealistic about their calling, choose the Prayer of Maimonides (not by Maimonides at all) over the more deontological Oath of Hippocrates. In that 'prayer' the physician asks: ". . . may neither avarice nor miserliness, nor thirst for glory or for a great reputation engage my mind; for the enemies of truth and philanthropy may easily deceive me and make me forgetful of my lofty aim of doing good to thy children." This is an unequivocal call to virtue and it is hard to imagine even the most cynical graduate failing to comprehend its message.

All professional medical codes, then, are built of a three-tiered system of obligations related to the special roles of physicians in society. In the ascending order of ethical sensitivity they are: observance of the laws of the land, then observance of rights and fulfillment of duties, and finally the practice of virtue.

A legally based ethic concentrates on the minimum requirements—the duties imposed by human laws which protect against the grosser aberrations of personal rights. Licensure, the laws of torts and contracts, prohibitions against discrimination, good Samaritan laws, definitions of death, and the protection of human subjects of experimentation are elements of a legalistic ethic.

At the next level is the ethics of rights and duties which spells out obligations beyond what law defines. Here, benevolence and beneficence take on more than their legal meaning. The ideal of service, of responsiveness to the special needs of those who are ill, some degree of compassion, kindliness, promise-keeping, truth-telling, and non-maleficence and specific obligations like confidentiality and autonomy, are included. How these principles are applied, and conflicts among them resolved in the patient's best interests, are subjects of widely varying interpretation. How sensitively these issues are confronted depends more on the physician's character than his capability at ethical discourse or moral casuistry.

Virtue-based ethics goes beyond these first two levels. We expect the virtuous person to do the right and the good even at the expense of personal sacrifice and legitimate self-interest. Virtue ethics expands the notions of benevolence, beneficence, conscientiousness, compassion, and fidelity well beyond what strict duty might require. It makes some degree of supererogation mandatory because it calls for standards of ethical performance that exceed those prevalent in the rest of society [6].

At each of these three levels there are certain dangers from over-zealous or misguided observance. Legalistic ethical systems tend toward a justification for minimalistic ethics, a narrow definition of benevolence or beneficence, and a contract-minded physician-patient relationship. Duty- and rights-based ethics may be distorted by too strict adherence to the letter of ethical principles without the modulations and nuances the spirit of those principles implies. Virtue-based ethics, being the least specific, can more easily lapse into self-

righteous paternalism or an unwelcome over-involvement in the personal life of the patient. Misapplication of any moral system even with good intent converts benevolence into maleficence. The virtuous person might be expected to be more sensitive to these aberrations than someone whose ethics is more deontologically or legally flavored.

The more we yearn for ethical sensitivity the less we lean on rights, duties, rules, and principles, and the more we lean on the character traits of the moral agent. Paradoxically, without rules, rights, and duties specifically spelled out, we cannot predict what form a particular person's expression of virtue will take. In a pluralistic society, we need laws, rules, and principles to assure a dependable minimum level of moral conduct. But that minimal level is insufficient in the complex and often unpredictable circumstances of decision-making, where technical and value desiderata intersect so inextricably.

The virtuous physician does not act from unreasoned, uncritical intuitions about what feels good. His dispositions are ordered in accord with that 'right reason' which both Aristotle and Aquinas considered essential to virtue. Medicine is itself ultimately an exercise of practical wisdom—a right way of acting in difficult and uncertain circumstances for a specific end, i.e., the good of a particular person who is ill. It is when the choice of a right and good action becomes more difficult, when the temptations to self-interest are most insistent, when unexpected nuances of good and evil arise and no one is looking, that the differences between an ethics based in virtue and an ethics based in law and/or duty can most clearly be distinguished.

Virtue-based professional ethics distinguishes itself, therefore, less in the avoidance of overtly immoral practices than in avoidance of those at the margin of moral responsibility. Physicians are confronted, in today's morally relaxed climate, with an increasing number of new practices that pit altruism against self-interest. Most are not illegal, or, strictly speaking, immoral in a rights- or duty-based ethic. But they are not consistent with the higher levels of moral sensitivity that a virtue-ethics demands. These practices usually involve opportunities for profit from the illness of others, narrowing the concept of service for personal convenience, taking a proprietary attitude with respect to medical knowledge, and placing loyalty to the profession above loyalty to patients.

Under the first heading, we might include such things as investment in and ownership of for-profit hospitals, hospital chains, nursing homes, dialysis units, tie-in arrangements with radiological or laboratory services, escalation of fees for repetitive, high-volume procedures, and lax indications for their use, especially when third party payers 'allow' such charges.

The second heading might include the ever decreasing availability and accessibility of physicians, the diffusion of individual patient responsibility in group practice so that the patient never knows whom he will see or who is on call, the itinerant emergency room physician who works two days and skips three with little commitment to hospital or community, and the growing over-indulgence of physicians in vacations, recreation, and 'self-development'.

The third category might include such things as 'selling one's services' for whatever the market will bear, providing what the market demands and not necessarily what the community needs, patenting new procedures or keeping them secret from potential competitor-colleagues, looking at the investment of time, effort, and capital in a medical education as justification for 'making it back', or forgetting that medical knowledge is drawn from the cumulative experience of a multitude of patients, clinicians, and investigators.

Under the last category might be included referrals on the basis of friendship and reciprocity rather than skill, resisting consultations and second opinions as affronts to one's competence, placing the interest of the referring physician above those of the patients, looking the other way in the face of incompetence or even dishonesty in one's professional colleagues.

These and many other practices are defended today by sincere physicians and even encouraged in this era of competition, legalism, and self-indulgence. Some can be rationalized even in a deontological ethic. But it would be impossible to envision the physician committed to the virtues assenting to these practices. A virtue-based ethics simply does not fluctuate with what the dominant social mores will tolerate. It must interpret benevolence, beneficence, and responsibility in a way that reduces self interest and enhances altruism. It is the only convincing answer the profession can give to the growing perception clearly manifest in the legal commentaries in the FTC ruling that medicine is nothing more than business and should be regulated as such.

A virtue-based ethic is inherently elitist, in the best sense, because its adherents demand more of themselves than the prevailing morality. It calls forth that extra measure of dedication that has made the best physicians in every era exemplars of what the human spirit can achieve. No matter to what depths a society may fall, virtuous persons will always be the beacons that light the way back to moral sensitivity; virtuous physicians are

the beacons that show the way back to moral credibility for the whole profession.

Albert Jonsen, rightly I believe, diagnoses the central paradox in medicine as the tension between self-interest and altruism [4]. No amount of deft juggling of rights, duties, or principles will suffice to resolve that tension. We are all too good at rationalizing what we want to do so that personal gain can be converted from vice to virtue. Only a character formed by the virtues can feel the nausea of such intellectual hypocrisy.

To be sure, the twin themes of self-interest and altruism have been inextricably joined in the history of medicine. There have always been physicians who reject the virtues or, more often, claim them falsely. But, in addition, there have been physicians, more often than the critics of medicine would allow, who have been truly virtuous both in intent and act. They have been, and remain, the leaven of the profession and the hope of all who are ill. They form the sea-wall that will not be eroded even by the powerful forces of commercialization, bureaucratization, and mechanization inevitable in modern medicine.

We cannot, need not, and indeed must not, wait for a medical analogue of MacIntyre's 'new St. Benedict' to show us the way. There is no new concept of virtue waiting to be discovered that is peculiarly suited to the dilemmas of our own dark age. We must recapture the courage to speak of character, virtue, and perfection in living a good life. We must encourage those who are willing to dedicate themselves to a "higher standard of self effacement" [2].

We need the courage, too, to accept the obvious split in the profession between those who see and feel the altruistic imperatives in medicine, and those who do not. Those who at heart believe that the pursuit of private self-interest serves the public good are very different from those who believe in the restraint of self-interest. We forget that physicians since the beginnings of the profession have subscribed to different values and virtues. We need only recall that the Hippocratic Oath was the Oath of physicians of the Pythagorean school at a time when most Greek physicians followed essentially a craft ethic [3]. A perusal of the Hippocratic Corpus itself, which intersperses ethics and etiquette, will show how differently its treatises deal with fees, the care of incurable patients, and the business aspects of the craft.

The illusion that all physicians share a common devotion to a high-flown set of ethical principles has done damage to medicine by raising expectations some members of the profession could not, or will not, fulfill.

Today, we must be more forthright about the differences in value commitment among physicians. Professional codes must be more explicit about the relationships between duties, rights, and virtues. Such explicitness encourages a more honest relationship between physicians and patients and removes the hypocrisy of verbal assent to a general code, to which an individual physician may not really subscribe. Explicitness enables patients to choose among physicians on the basis of their ethical commitments as well as their reputations for technical expertise.

Conceptual clarity will not assure virtuous behavior. Indeed, virtues are usually distorted if they are the subject of too conscious a design. But conceptual clarity will distinguish between motives and provide criteria for judging the moral commitment one can expect from the profession and from its individual members. It can also inspire those whose virtuous inclinations need re-enforcement in the current climate of commercialization of the healing relationship.

To this end the current resurgence of interest in virtue-based ethics is altogether salubrious. Linked to a theory of patient good and a theory of rights and duties, it could provide the needed groundwork for a reconstruction of professional medical ethics as that work

matures. Perhaps even more progress can be made if we take Shakespeare's advice in *Hamlet:* "Assume the virtue if you have it not. . . . For use almost can change the stamp of nature."

BIBLIOGRAPHY

[1] Cicero: 1967, *Moral Obligations,* J. Higginbotham (trans.), University of California Press, Berkeley and Los Angeles.
[2] Cushing, H.: 1929, *Consecratio Medici and Other Papers,* Little, Brown and Co., Boston.
[3] Edelstein, L.: 1967, 'The Professional Ethics of the Greek Physician', in O. Temkin (ed.), *Ancient Medicine: Selected Papers of Ludwig Edelstein,* Johns Hopkins University Press, Baltimore.
[4] Jonsen, A.: 1983, 'Watching the Doctor', *New England Journal of Medicine* 308: 25, 1531–1535.
[5] Pellegrino, E.: 1983, '*Scribonius Largus* and the Origins of Medical Humanism', address to the American Osler Society.
[6] Reader, J.: 1982, 'Beneficence, Supererogation, and Role Duty', in E. Shelp (ed.), *Beneficence and Health Care,* D. Reidel, Dordrecht, Holland, pp. 83–108.

Physician-Patient Models and Patient Autonomy

Metaphors and Models of Doctor-Patient Relationships: Their Implications for Autonomy

James F. Childress and Mark Siegler

James F. Childress is Kyle Professor of Religious Studies and professor of medical education at the University of Virginia. Widely published in biomedical ethics, he is the author of *Who Should Decide?: Paternalism in Health Care* (1982) and coauthor of *Principles of Biomedical Ethics* (4th ed., 1994). Mark Siegler is professor of medicine and director of the Center for Clinical Medical Ethics at the University of Chicago. His many articles include "Therapeutic Research Protocol: Should Patients Pay?" and "Confidentiality in Medicine—A Decrepit Concept," and he is coauthor of *Clinical Ethics* (3d ed., 1992).

Childress and Siegler examine five models, or metaphors, for the physician-patient relationship: (1) *paternalism* (the physician as caring parent, the patient as child); (2) *partnership* (both parties as collaborating in pursuit of the shared goal of the patient's health); (3) *contract* (physician and patient as related to each other by specific contracts, detailing their obliga-

Theoretical Medicine, vol. 5 (1984), pp. 17–30. © 1984 by D. Reidel Publishing Company. Reprinted by permission of Kluwer Academic Publishers.

tions and rights); (4) *friendship* (physician and patient as intimately related due to the highly personal nature of health); and (5) *technical assistance* (the physician as technician, the patient as customer). The authors then explore the relative advantages and disadvantages of regarding the physician-patient relationship as a relationship between *intimates* or as one between *strangers,* before examining the implications of each for patient autonomy. They conclude by developing the metaphor of *negotiations* as a way to understand many interactions between physicians and patients.

INTRODUCTION

Many metaphors and models have been applied to relationships between patients and physicians. One example is an interpretation of physician-patient relationships as paternalistic. In this case, the physician is regarded as a parent and the patient is regarded as a child. Opponents of such a paternalistic view of medicine rarely reject the use of metaphors to interpret medical relationships; rather, they simply offer alternative metaphors, for example, the physician as partner or the patient as rational contractor. Metaphors may operate even when patients and physicians are unaware of them. Physician-patient conflicts may arise if each party brings to their encounter a different image of medicine, as, for example, when the physician regards a paternalistic model of medicine as appropriate, but the patient prefers a contractual model.

As these examples suggest, metaphors involve seeing something as something else, for example, seeing a lover as a red rose, human beings as wolves, or medical therapy as warfare. Metaphors highlight some features and hide other features of their principal subject.[1] Thus, thinking about a physician as a parent highlights the physician's care for dependent others and his or her control over them, but it conceals the patient's payment of fees to the physician. Metaphors and models may be used to describe relationships as they exist, or to indicate what those relationships ought to be. In either the descriptive or the prescriptive use of metaphors, this highlighting and hiding occurs, and it must be considered in determining the adequacy of various metaphors. When metaphors are used to describe roles, they can be criticized if they distort more features than they illuminate. And when they are used to direct roles, they can be criticized if they highlight one moral consideration, such as care, while neglecting others, such as autonomy.

Since there is no single physician-patient relationship, it is probable that no single metaphor can adequately describe or direct the whole range of relationships in health care, such as open heart surgery, clinical research, and psychoanalysis. Some of the most important metaphors that have shaped health care in recent years include: parent-child, partners, rational contractors, friends, and technician-client. We want to determine the adequacy of these metaphors to describe and to direct doctor-patient relationships in the real world. In particular, we will assess them in relation to patient and physician autonomy.

METAPHORS AND MODELS OF RELATIONSHIPS IN HEALTH CARE

(1) The first metaphor is *paternal* or *parental,* and the model is paternalism. For this model, the locus of decision-making is the health care professional, particularly the physician, who has 'moral authority' within an asymmetrical and hierarchical relationship. (A variation on these themes appear in a model that was especially significant earlier—the priest-penitent relationship.)

Following Thomas Szasz and Marc Hollender, we can distinguish two different versions of paternalism, based on two different prototypes.[2] If we take the *parent-infant relationship* as the prototype, the physician's role is active, while the patient's role is passive. The patient, like the infant, is primarily a dependent recipient of care. This model is applied easily to such clinical situations as anesthesia and to the care of patients with acute trauma, coma, or delirium. A second version takes the *parent-adolescent child* relationship as the prototype. Within this version, the physician guides the patient by telling him or her what to expect and what to do, and the patient co-operates to the extent of obeying. This model applies to such clinical situations as the outpatient treatment of acute infectious diseases. The physician instructs the patient on a course of treatment (such as antibiotics and rest), but the patient can either obey or refuse to comply.

The paternalist model assigns moral authority and discretion to the physician because good health is assumed to be a value shared by the patient and the physician and because the physician's competence, skills, and ability place him or her in a position to help the patient regain good health. Even if it was once the dominant model in health care and even if many patients and physicians still prefer it, the paternalist model is no longer adequate to describe or to direct all relationships in health care. Too many changes have occurred. In a pluralistic society such as ours, the assumption that the physician and patient have common values about health may be mistaken. They may disagree about the *meaning* of health and disease (for example, when the physician insists that cigarette smoking is a disease, but the patient claims that it is merely a nasty habit) or about the *value* of health relative to other values (for example, when the physician wants to administer a blood transfusion to save the life of a Jehovah's Witness, but the patient rejects the blood in order to have a chance of heavenly salvation).

As a normative model, paternalism tends to concentrate on care rather than respect, patients' needs rather than their rights, and physicians' discretion rather than patients' autonomy or self-determination. Even though paternalistic actions can sometimes be justified, for example, when a patient is not competent to make a decision and is at risk of harm, not all paternalistic actions can be justified.[3]

(2) A second model is one of *partnership,* which can be seen in Eric Cassell's statement: "Autonomy for the sick patient cannot exist outside of a good and properly functioning doctor-patient relation. And the relation between them is inherently a *partnership*".[4] The language of collegiality, collaboration, association, co-adventureship, and covenant is also used. This model stresses that health care professionals and their patients are partners or colleagues in the pursuit of the shared value of health. It is similar to the paternalist model in that it emphasizes the shared general values of the enterprise in which the participants are involved. But what makes this model distinctive and significant is its emphasis on the equality of the participants' interpretations of shared values such as health, along with respect for the personal autonomy of all the participants.[5] The theme of equality does not, however, cancel a division of competence and responsibility along functional lines within the relationship.

Szasz and Hollender suggest that the prototype of the model of 'mutual participation' or partnership is the adult-adult relationship. Within this model the physician helps the patient to help himself, while the patient uses expert help to realize his (and the physician's) ends. Some clinical applications of this model appear in the care of chronic diseases and psychoanalysis. It presupposes that "the participants (1) have approximately equal power, (2) be mutually interdependent (i.e., need each other), and (3) engage in activity that will be in some ways satisfying to both". Furthermore, "the physician does not know what is best for the patient. The search for this becomes the essence of the therapeutic interaction. The patient's own experiences furnish indispensable information for eventual agreement, under otherwise favorable circumstances, as to what 'health' might be for him".[6]

Although this model describes a few practices, it is most often offered as a normative model, indicating the morally desirable and even obligatory direction of practice and research.[7] As a normative model, it stresses the equality of value contributions and the autonomy of both professionals and other participants, whether sick persons or volunteers for research.

(3) A third model is that of *rational contractors.* Health care professionals and their patients are related or should be related to each other by a series of specific contracts. The prototype of this model is the specific contract by which individuals agree to exchange goods and services, and the enforcement of such contracts by governmental sanctions. According to Robert Veatch, one of the strongest proponents of the contractual model in health care, this model is the best compromise between the *ideal of partnership,* with its emphasis on both equality and autonomy, and the *reality* of medical care, where mutual trust cannot be presupposed. If we could realize mutual trust, we could develop partnerships. In the light of a realistic assessment of our situation, however, we can only hope for contracts. The model of rational contracts, according to Veatch, is the only realistic way to share responsibility, to preserve both equality and autonomy under less than ideal circumstances, and to protect the integrity of various parties in health care (e.g., physicians are free not to enter contracts that would violate their consciences and to withdraw from them when they give proper notice).[8]

Such a model is valuable but problematic both descriptively and normatively. It neglects the fact that sick persons do not view health care needs as comparable to other wants and desires, that they do not have sufficient information to make rational contracts with the best providers of health services, and that current structure of medicine obstructs the free operation of the marketplace and of contracts.[9] This model may also neglect the virtues of benevolence, care, and compassion that are stressed in other models such as paternalism and friendship.

(4) A fourth attempt to understand and direct the relationships between health care professionals and patients stresses *friendship*. According to P. Lain Entralgo,

> Insofar as man is a part of nature, and health an aspect of this nature and therefore a natural and objective good, the *medical relation* develops into comradeship, or association for the purpose of securing this good by technical means. Insofar as man is an individual and his illness a state affecting his personality, the medical relation ought to be more than mere comradeship—in fact it should be a friendship. All dogma apart, a good doctor has always been a friend to his patient, to all his patients.[10]

For this version of 'medical philia', the patient expresses trust and confidence in the physician while the doctor's "friendship for the patient should consist above all in a desire to give effective technical help—benevolence conceived and realised in technical terms".[11] Technical help and generalized benevolence are 'made friendly' by explicit reference to the patient's personality.

Charles Fried's version of 'medical philia' holds that physicians are *limited, special-purpose friends* in relation to their patients. In medicine as well as in other professional activities such as law, the client may have a relationship with the professional that is analogous to friendship. In friendship and in these relationships, one person assumes the interests of another. Claims in both sets of relationships are intense and demanding, but medical friendship is more limited in scope.[12]

Of course, this friendship analogy is somewhat strained, as Fried recognizes, because needs (real and felt) give rise to medical relationships, even if professionals are free not to meet them unless they are emergencies, because patients pay professionals for their 'personal care', and because patients do not have reciprocal loyalties. Nevertheless, Fried's analysis of the medical relationship highlights the equality, the autonomy, and the rights of both parties—the 'friend' and the 'befriended'. Because friendship, as Kant suggested, is "the union of two persons through equal and mutual love and respect", the model of friendship has some ingredients of both paternalism (love or care) and anti-paternalism (equality and respect).[13] It applies especially well to the same medical relationships that fit partnership; indeed, medical friendship is very close to medical partnership, except that the former stresses the intensity of the relationship, while the latter stresses the emotional reserve as well as the limited scope of the relationship.

(5) A fifth and final model views the health care professional as a *technician*. Some commentators have referred to this model as plumber, others as engineer; for example, it has been suggested that with the rise of scientific medicine the physician was viewed as "the expert engineer of the body as a machine".[14] Within this model, the physician 'provides' or 'delivers' technical service to patients who are 'consumers'. Exchange relations provide images for this interpretation of medical relations.

This model does not appear to be possible or even desirable. It is difficult to imagine that the health care professional as technician can simply present the 'facts' unadorned by values, in part because the major terms such as health and disease are not value-free and objective. Whether the 'technician' is in an organization or in direct relation to clients, he or she serves some values. Thus, this model may collapse into the contractual model or a bureaucratic model (which will not be discussed in this essay). The professional may be thought to have only technical authority, not moral authority. But he or she remains a moral agent and thus should choose to participate or not in terms of his or her own commitments, loyalties, and integrity. One shortcoming of the paternalist and priestly models, as Robert Veatch notes, is the patient's "moral abdication", while one shortcoming of the technician model is the physician's "moral abdication".[15] The technician model offers autonomy to the patient, whose values dominate (at least in some settings) at the expense of the professional's moral agency and integrity. In other models such as contract, partnership, and friendship, moral responsibility is shared by all the parties in part because they are recognized, in some sense, as equals.

RELATIONS BETWEEN INTIMATES AND BETWEEN STRANGERS

The above models of relationships between physicians and patients move between two poles: intimates and strangers.[16] In relations of intimacy, all the parties know each other very well and often share values, or at least know which values they do not share. In such relations, formal rules and procedures, backed by sanctions, may not be necessary; they may even be detrimental to the relationships. In relations of intimacy, trust rather than control is dominant. Examples include relationships between parents and children and between friends. Partnerships also share some features of such relationships, but their intimacy and shared values may be limited to a specific set of activities.

By contrast, in relations among strangers, rules and procedures become very important, and control rather than trust is dominant.[17] Of course, in most relations there are mixtures of trust and control. Each is present to some degree. Nevertheless, it is proper to speak about relations between strangers as structured by rules and procedures because the parties do not know each other well enough to have mutual trust. Trust means confidence in and reliance upon the other to act in accord with moral principles and rules or at least in accord with his or her publicly manifested principles and rules, whatever they might be. But if the other is a stranger, we do not know whether he or she accepts what we would count as moral principles and rules. We do not know whether he or she is worthy of trust. In the absence of intimate knowledge, or of shared values, strangers resort to rules and procedures in order to establish some control. Contracts between strangers, for example, to supply certain goods, represent instances of attempted control. But contractual relations do not only depend on legal sanctions; they also presuppose confidence in a shared structure of rules and procedures. As Talcott Parsons has noted, "transactions are actually entered into in accordance with a body of binding rules which are not part of the ad hoc agreement of the parties".[18]

Whether medicine is now only a series of encounters between strangers rather than intimates, medicine is increasingly regarded by patients and doctors, and by analysts of the profession—such as philosophers, lawyers, and sociologists—as a practice that is best understood and regulated *as if it were* a practice among strangers rather than among intimates. Numerous causes can be identified: First, the pluralistic nature of our society; second, the decline of close, intimate contact over time among professionals and patients and their families; third, the decline of contact with the 'whole person', who is now parcelled out to various specialists; fourth, the growth of large, impersonal, bureaucratically structured institutions of care, in which there is discontinuity of care (the patient may not see the same professionals on subsequent visits).[19]

In this situation, Alasdair MacIntyre contends, the modern patient "usually approaches the physician as stranger to stranger: and the very proper fear and suspicion that we have of strangers extends equally properly to our encounters with physicians. We do not and cannot know what to expect of them. . . ".[20] He suggests that one possible response to this situation is to develop a rule-based bureaucracy in which "we can confront *any* individual who fills a given role with exactly the same expectation of exactly the same outcomes. . . ". Our encounters with physicians and other health care professionals are encounters between strangers precisely because of our pluralistic society: several value systems are in operation, and we do not know whether the physicians we encounter share our value systems. In such a situation, patient autonomy is "a solution of last resort" rather than "a central moral good". Finally patients have to decide for themselves what will be done to them or simply delegate such decisions to others, such as physicians.

Just as MacIntyre recognizes the value of patient autonomy in our pluralistic society, so John Ladd recognizes the value of the concept of rights among strangers.[21] He notes that a legalistic, rights-based approach to medicine has several important advantages because rules and rights "serve to define our relationships with strangers as well as with people whom we know . . . In the medical context . . . we may find ourselves in a hospital bed in a strange place, with strange company, and confronted by a strange physician and staff. The strangeness of the situation makes the concept of rights, both legal and moral, a very useful tool for defining our relationship to those with whom we have to deal".

Rules and rights that can be enforced obviously serve as ways to control the conduct of others when we do not know them well enough to be able to trust them. But all of the models of health care relationships identified above depend on some degree of trust. It is too simplistic to suppose that contracts, which can be legally enforced, do away with trust totally. Indeed, as we have argued, a society based on contracts depends to a very great extent on trust, precisely because not everything is enforceable at manageable cost. Thus, the issue is not simply whether trust or control is dominant, but, in part, the basis and extent of trust. Trust, at least limited trust, may be possible even among strangers. There may be a presumption of trust, unless the society is in turmoil. And there may be an intermediate notion of 'friendly strangers'. People may be strangers because of differences regarding values or uncertainty regarding the other's values; they may be friendly because they accept certain rules and procedures, which may ensure that different values are respected. If consensus exists in a pluralistic society, it is primarily about rules and procedures, some of which protect the autonomy of agents, their freedom to negotiate their own relationships.

PHYSICIAN-PATIENT INTERACTIONS AS NEGOTIATIONS

It is illuminating, both descriptively and prescriptively, to view some encounters and interactions between physicians and patients as negotiations. The metaphor of negotiation has its home in discussions to settle matters by mutual agreement of the concerned parties. While it frequently appears in disputes between management and labor and between nations, it does not necessarily presuppose a conflict of interests between the parties. The metaphor of negotiation may also illuminate processes of reaching agreement regarding the terms of continuing interaction even when the issue is mainly the determination of one party's interests and the means to realize those interests. This metaphor captures two important characteristics of medical relationships: (1) it accents the autonomy of both patient and physician, and (2) it suggests a process that occurs over time rather than an event which occurs at a particular moment.

The model of negotiation can both explain what frequently occurs and identify what ought to occur in physician-patient interactions. An example can make this point: A twenty-eight-year-old ballet dancer suffered from moderately severe asthma. When she moved from New York to Chicago, she changed physicians and placed herself in the hands of a famed asthma specialist. He initiated aggressive steroid therapy to control her asthma, and within several months he had managed to control her wheezing. But she was distressed because her dancing had deteriorated. She suspected that she was experiencing muscle weakness and fluid accumulation because of the steroid treatment. When she attempted to discuss her concerns with the physician, he maintained that "bringing the disease under complete control—achieving a complete remission of wheezes—will be the best thing for you in the long run". After several months of unhappiness and failure to convince the physician of the importance of her personal goals as well as her medical goals, she sought another physician, insisting that she didn't live just to breathe, but breathed so that she could dance.[22]

As in this case—and despite the claims of several commentators—people with medical needs generally do not confront physicians as strangers and as adversaries in contemporary health care. As we suggested earlier, even if they can be viewed as strangers in that they often do not know each other prior to the encounter, both parties may well proceed with a presumption of trust. Patients may approach physicians with some trust and confidence in the medical profession, even though they do not know the physicians before them. Indeed, codes of medical ethics have been designed in part to foster this trust by indicating where the medical profession stands and by creating a climate of trust. Thus, even if patients approach individual physicians as strangers, they may have some confidence in these physicians as members of the profession as they negotiate the particular terms of their relationship. At the other extreme, some patients may approach physicians as adversaries or opponents. But for negotiation to proceed, some trust must be present, even if it is combined with some degree of control, for example, through legal requirements and the threat of legal sanctions.

The general public trust in the medical profession's values and skills provides the presumptive basis for trust in particular physicians and can facilitate the process of negotiation. But, as we noted earlier, in a pluralistic society, even people who are strangers, i.e., who share very few substantive values, may be 'friendly' if they share procedural values. Certain procedural values may provide the most important basis for the trust that is necessary for negotiation; indeed, procedural principles and rules should structure the negotiation in order to ensure equal respect for the autonomy of all the parties.

First, the negotiation should involve adequate disclosure by both parties. In this process of communication—much broader and richer than most doctrines of informed consent recognize—both parties should indicate their values as well as other matters of relevance. Without this information, the negotiation cannot be open and fair. Second, the negotiation should be voluntary, i.e., uncoerced. Insofar as critical illness can be viewed as 'coercing' individuals through the creation of fear, etc., it may be difficult to realize this condition for patients with certain problems. However, for the majority of patients this condition is achievable. Third, the accommodation reached through the negotiation should be mutually acceptable.[23]

What can we say about the case of the ballet dancer in the light of these procedural requirements for negotiation? It appears that the relationship foundered not because of inadequate disclosure at the outset, or along the way, but because of the patient's change in or clarification of her values and the physician's inability to accommodate these other values. The accommodation reached at the outset was mutually acceptable for a time. Initially their values and their metaphors for their relationship were the same. The physician regarded himself as a masterful scientist who was capable technically of controlling a patient's symptoms of wheezing. In fact, he remarked on several occasions: "I have never met a case of asthma I couldn't help". The patient, for her part, selected the physician initially for the same reasons. She was unhappy that her wheezing persisted, and she was becoming discouraged by her chronic health problem. Because she wanted a therapeutic success, she selected an expert who would help her achieve that goal. Both the patient and the physician made several voluntary choices. The patient chose to see *this* physician and to see him for several months, and the physician chose to treat asthma aggressively with steroids.

In a short time, the patient reconsidered or clarified her values, discovering that her dancing was even more important to her than the complete remission of wheezing, and she wanted to renegotiate her relationship so that it could be more mutual and participatory. But her new metaphor for the relationship was incompatible with the physician's nonnegotiable commitment to his metaphor—which the patient had also accepted at the outset. Thus, the relationship collapsed. This case illustrates both the possibilities and the limitations of the model of negotiation. Even when the procedural requirements are met, the negotiation may not result in a satisfactory accommodation over time, and the negotiation itself may proceed in terms of the physician's and the patient's metaphors and models of the relationships, as well as the values they affirm.

Autonomy constrains and limits the negotiations and the activities of both parties: Neither party may violate the autonomy of the other or use the other merely as a means to an end. But respecting autonomy as a constraint and a limit does not imply seeking it as a *goal* or praising it as an *ideal*.[24] This point has several implications. It means, for example, that patients may exercise their autonomy to turn their medical affairs completely over to physicians. A patient may instruct the physician to do whatever he or she deems appropriate: "You're the doctor; whatever you decide is fine". This relationship has been characterized as "paternalism with permission",[25] and it is not ruled out by autonomy as a constraint or a limit. It might, however, be ruled out by a commitment to autonomy as an ideal. Indeed, commitment to autonomy as an ideal can even be paternalistic in a negative sense; it can lead the health care professional to try to force the patient to be free and to live up to the ideal of autonomy. But our conception of autonomy as a constraint and a limit prevents such actions toward competent patients who are choosing and acting voluntarily. Likewise, maintenance, restoration, or promotion of the patient's autonomy may be, and usually is, one important goal of medical relationships. But its importance can only be determined by negotiation between the physician and the patient. The patient may even subordinate the goal of autonomy to various other goals, just as the ballet dancer subordinated freedom from wheezing to the power to dance.

This view of autonomy as a limit or a constraint, rather than an ideal or a goal, permits individuals to define the terms of their relationship. Just as it permits the patient to acquiesce in the physician's recommendations, it permits the physician to enter a contract as a mere technician to provide certain medical services, as requested by the patient. In such an arrangement, the physician does *not* become a mere means or a mere instrument to the patient's ends. Rather, the physician exercises his or her autonomy to enter into the relationship to provide technical services. Such actions are an expression of autonomy, not a denial of autonomy. If, however, the physician believes that an action requested by the patient—for example, a specific mode of therapy for cancer or a sterilization procedure—is not medically indicated, or professionally acceptable, or in the patient's best interests, he or she is not obligated to sacrifice autonomy and comply. In such a case, the professional refuses to be an instrument of or to carry out the patient's wishes. When the physician cannot morally or professionally perform an action (not legally prohibited by the society) he or she may have a duty to inform the patient of other physicians who might be willing to carry out the patient's wishes. A refusal to be an instrument of another's wishes is very different from trying to prevent another from realizing his or her goals.

Negotiation is not always possible or desirable. It is impossible, or possible only to a limited extent, in certain clinical settings in which the conditions for a fair, informed, and voluntary negotiation are severely limited, often because one party lacks some of the conditions for autonomous choices. First, negotiation may be difficult if not impossible with some types of patients, such as the mentally incompetent. Sometimes paternalism may be morally legitimate or even morally obligatory when the patient is not competent to negotiate and is at risk. In such cases, parents, family members, or others may undertake negotiation with the physician, for example, regarding defective newborns or comatose adults. But health care professionals and the state may have to intervene in order to protect the interests of the patient who cannot negotiate directly. Second, the model of negotiation does not fit situations in which patients are forced by law to accept medical interventions such as compulsory vaccination, involuntary commitment, and involuntary psychiatric treatment. In such situations, the state authorizes or requires treatment against the wishes of the patient; the patient and the physician do not negotiate their relationship. Third, in some situations physicians have dual or multiple allegiances, some of which may take priority over loyalty to the patient. Examples include military medicine, industrial medicine, prison medicine, and university health service. The physician is not free in such settings to negotiate in good faith with the patient, and the patient's interests and rights may have to be protected by other substantive and procedural standards and by external control. Fourth, negotiation may not be possible in some emergencies in which people desperately need medical treatment because of the risk of death or serious bodily harm. In such cases, the physician may *presume* consent, apart from a process of negotiation, if the patient is unable to consent because of his/her condition or if the process of disclosing information and securing consent would consume too much time and thus endanger the patient. Finally, procedural standards are important for certain types of patients, such as the poor, the uneducated, or those with 'unattractive medical problems' (e.g., drug addiction, obesity, and hypochondriasis). In such cases, there is a tendency— surely not a universal one—to limit the degree of negotiation with the patient because of social stigmatization. A patient advocate may even be appropriate.

In addition to the procedural requirements identified earlier, there are societal constraints and limits on negotiation. Some actions may not be negotiable. For example, the society may prohibit 'mercy killing', even when the patient requests it and the physician is willing to carry it out.[26] Such societal rules clearly limit the autonomy of both physicians and patients, but some of these rules may be necessary in order to protect important societal values. However, despite such notable exceptions as 'mercy killing', current societal rules provide physicians and patients with considerable latitude to negotiate their own relationship and actions within that relationship.

If negotiation is a process, its accommodations at various points can often be characterized in terms of the above models—parent-child, friends, partners, contractors, and technician-consumer. Whatever accommodation is reached through the process of negotiation is not final or irrevocable. Like other human interactions, medical relationships change over time. They are always developing or dissolving. For example, when a patient experiencing anginal chest pain negotiates a relationship with a cardiologist, he may not have given or even implied consent to undergo coronary angiography or cardiac surgery if the cardiologist subsequently believes that it is necessary. Medical conditions change, and people change, often clarifying or modifying their values over time. In medical relationships either the physician or the patient may reopen the negotiation as the relationship evolves over time and may even terminate the relationship. For example, the ballet dancer in the case discussed above elected to terminate the relationship with the specialist. That particular relationship had not been fully negotiated in the first place. But even if it had been fully negotiated, she could have changed her mind and terminated it. Such an option is essential if the autonomy of the patient is to be protected over time. Likewise, the physician should have the option to renegotiate or to withdraw from the relationship (except in emergencies), as long as he or she gives adequate notice so that the patient can find another physician.

NOTES

1 On metaphor, see George Lakoff and Mark Johnson, *Metaphors We Live By* (Chicago: University of Chicago Press, 1980).
2 See Thomas S. Szasz and Marc H. Hollender, 'A contribution to the philosophy of medicine: The basic models of the doctor-patient relationship', *Archives of Internal Medicine* 97, (1956) 585–92; see also, Thomas S. Szasz, William F. Knoff, and Marc H. Hollender, 'The doctor-patient relationship and its historical context', *American Journal of Psychiatry* 115, (1958) 522–28.
3 For a fuller analysis of paternalism and its justification, see James F. Childress, *Who Should Decide?: Paternalism in Health Care* (New York: Oxford University Press, 1982).
4 Eric Cassell, 'Autonomy and ethics in action', *New England Journal of Medicine* 297, (1977) 333–34. Italics added. Partnership is only one of several images and metaphors Cassell uses, and it may not be the best one to express his position, in part because he tends to view autonomy as a goal rather than as a constraint.
5 According to Robert Veatch, the main focus of this model is "an equality of dignity and respect, an equality of value contributions". Veatch, 'Models

for ethical medicine in a revolutionary age', *Hastings Center Report* 2, (June 1972) 7. Contrast Eric Cassell who disputes the relevance of notions of "equality" and "inequality". *The Healer's Art: A New Approach to the Doctor-Patient Relationship* (Philadelphia: J. B. Lippincott Company, 1976), pp. 193–94.

6 Thomas S. Szasz and Marc H. Hollender, 'A contribution to the philosophy of medicine: The basic models of the doctor-patient relationship', pp. 586–87. (See Note 2.)

7 See, for example, Paul Ramsey, 'The ethics of a cottage industry in an age of community and research medicine', *New England Journal of Medicine* 284, (1971) 700–706; *The Patient as Person: Explorations in Medical Ethics* (New Haven: Yale University Press, 1970), esp. Chap. 1; and Hans Jonas, 'Philosophical reflections on experimenting with human subjects', Ethical Aspects of Experimentation with Human Subjects, *Daedalus* 98, (1969) 219–47.

8 Robert Veatch, 'Models for ethical medicine in a revolutionary age', p. 7. (See Note 5.)

9 See Roger Masters, 'Is contract an adequate basis for medical ethics?', *Hastings Center Report* 5, (December 1975) 24–28. See also May, 'Code and covenant or philanthropy and contract?', in *Ethics in Medicine: Historical Perspectives and Contemporary Concerns,* ed. by Stanley Joel Reiser, Arthur J. Dyck, and William J. Curran (Cambridge, Mass.: The MIT Press, 1977), pp. 65–76.

10 P. Lain Entralgo, *Doctor and Patient,* trans. from the Spanish by Frances Partridge (New York: McGraw-Hill Book Co., World University Library, 1969), p. 242.

11 *Ibid.,* p. 197.

12 See Charles Fried, *Medical Experimentation: Personal Integrity and Social Policy* (New York: American Elsevier Publishing Co., Inc., 1974), p. 76. Our discussion of Fried's position is drawn from that work, *Right and Wrong* (Cambridge, Mass.: Harvard University Press, 1978), Chap. 7, and 'The lawyer as friend: The moral foundations of the lawyer-client relation', *The Yale Law Journal* 85, (1976) 1060–89.

13 Immanuel Kant, *The Doctrine of Virtue,* Part II of *The Metaphysic of Morals,* trans. by Mary J. Gregor (New York: Harper and Row, Harper Torchbook, 1964), p. 140.

14 Thomas S. Szasz, William F. Knoff, and Marc H.

Hollender, 'The doctor-patient relationship and its historical context', p. 525. See also Robert Veatch, 'Models for ethical medicine in a revolutionary age', p. 5, and Leon Kass, 'Ethical dilemmas in the care of the ill: I. What is the physician's service?', *Journal of the American Medical Association* 244, (1980) 1815 for criticisms of the technical model (from very different normative positions).

15 Veatch, 'Models for ethical medicine in a revolutionary age', p. 7.

16 See Stephen Toulmin, 'The tyranny of principles', *Hastings Center Report* 11, (December 1981) 31–39.

17 On trust and control, see James F. Childress, 'Nonviolent resistance: Trust and risk-taking', *Journal of Religious Ethics* 1, (1973) 87–112.

18 Talcott Parsons, *The Structure of Social Action* (New York: The Free Press, 1949), p. 311.

19 On the factors in the decline of trust, see Michael Jellinek, 'Erosion of patient trust in large medical centers', *Hastings Center Report* 6, (June 1976) 16–19.

20 Alasdair MacIntyre, 'Patients as agents', in *Philosophical Medical Ethics: Its Nature and Significance,* ed. by Stuart F. Spicker and H. Tristram Engelhardt, Jr. (Boston: D. Reidel Publishing Co., 1977).

21 John Ladd, 'Legalism and medical ethics', *The Journal of Medicine and Philosophy* 4, (March 1979) 73.

22 This case has been presented in Mark Siegler, 'Searching for moral certainty in medicine: A proposal for a new model of the doctor-patient encounter', *Bulletin of the New York Academy of Medicine* 57, (1981) 56–69.

23 See *ibid.* for a discussion of negotiation. Other proponents of a model of negotiation include Robert A. Burt, *Taking Care of Strangers: The Rule of Law in Doctor-Patient Relations* (New York: Free Press, 1979) and Robert J. Levine, *Ethics and Regulation of Clinical Research* (Baltimore: Urban and Schwarzenberg, 1981).

24 See the discussion in Childress, *Who Should Decide?,* Chap. 3.

25 Alan W. Cross and Larry R. Churchill, 'Ethical and cultural dimensions of informed consent', *Annals of Internal Medicine* 96, (1982) 110–13.

26 See Oscar Thorup, Mark Siegler, James Childress, and Ruth Roettinger, 'Voluntary exit: Is there a case of rational suicide?', *The Pharos* 45, (Fall 1982) 25–31.

Why Doctors Should Intervene
Terrence F. Ackerman

Terrence F. Ackerman is chair of the department of human values and ethics at the University of Tennessee and an adjunct member in medical ethics at St. Jude Children's Hospital. He is coeditor of *Clinical Medical Ethics: Exploration and Assessment* (1987) and coauthor of *A Casebook of Medical Ethics* (1989).

Ackerman criticizes the notion of respect for autonomy that identifies it with noninterference. He argues that noninterference fails to respect patient autonomy because it does not take account of the transforming effects of illness. Ackerman's major contention is that the autonomy of those who are ill is limited by all kinds of constraints—physical, cognitive, emotional, and social. Ackerman argues in favor of sometimes overriding patients' treatment-related preferences, maintaining that real respect for the autonomy of patients requires physicians actively to attempt to neutralize the impediments that interfere with patients' choices, helping them to restore control over their lives.

Patient autonomy has become a watchword of the medical profession. According to the revised 1980 AMA Principles of Medical Ethics,[1] no longer is it permissible for a doctor to withhold information from a patient, even on grounds that it may be harmful. Instead the physician is expected to "deal honestly with patients" at all times. Physicians also have a duty to respect the confidentiality of the doctor-patient relationship. Even when disclosure to a third party may be in the patient's interests, the doctor is instructed to release information only when required by law. Respect for the autonomy of patients has given rise to many specific patient rights—among them the right to refuse treatment, the right to give informed consent, the right to privacy, and the right to competent medical care provided with "respect for human dignity."

While requirements of honesty, confidentiality, and patients' rights are all important, the underlying moral vision that places exclusive emphasis upon these factors is more troublesome. The profession's notion of respect for autonomy makes noninterference its essential feature. As the Belmont Report has described it, there is an obligation to "give weight to autonomous persons' considered opinions and choices while refraining from obstructing their actions unless they are clearly detrimental to others."[2] Or, as Tom Beauchamp and James Childress have suggested, "To respect autonomous

Reprinted with permission of the author and the publisher from *Hastings Center Report*, vol. 12 (August 1982), pp. 14–17.

agents is to recognize with due appreciation their own considered value judgments and outlooks even when it is believed that their judgments are mistaken." They argue that people "are entitled to autonomous determination without limitation on their liberty being imposed by others."[3]

When respect for personal autonomy is understood as noninterference, the physician's role is dramatically simplified. The doctor need be only an honest and good technician, providing relevant information and dispensing professionally competent care. Does noninterference really respect patient autonomy? I maintain that it does not, because it fails to take account of the transforming effects of illness.

"Autonomy," typically defined as self-governance, has two key features. First, autonomous behavior is governed by plans of action that have been formulated through deliberation or reflection. This deliberative activity involves processes of both information gathering and priority setting. Second, autonomous behavior issues, intentionally and voluntarily, from choices people make based upon their own life plans.

But various kinds of constraints can impede autonomous behavior. There are physical constraints—confinement in prison is an example—where internal or external circumstances bodily prevent a person from deliberating adequately or acting on life plans. Cognitive constraints derive from either a lack of information or an inability to understand that information. A consumer's ignorance regarding the merits or defects of a particular product fits the description. Psychological constraints, such as anxiety or depression, also inhibit adequate deliberation. Finally, there are social constraints—such as institutionalized roles and expectations ("a woman's place is in the home," "the doctor knows best") that block considered choices.

Edmund Pellegrino suggests several ways in which autonomy is specifically compromised by illness:

> In illness, the body is interposed between us and reality—it impedes our choices and actions and is no longer fully responsive. . . . Illness forces a reappraisal and that poses a threat to the old image; it opens up all the old anxieties and imposes new ones—often including the real threat of death or drastic alterations in life-style. This ontological assault is aggravated by the loss of . . . freedoms we identify as peculiarly human. The patient . . . lacks the knowledge and skills necessary to cure himself or gain relief of pain and suffering. . . . The state of being ill is therefore a state of "wounded humanity," of a person compromised in his fundamental capacity to deal with his vulnerability.[4]

The most obvious impediment is that illness "interposes" the body or mind between the patient and reality, obstructing attempts to act upon cherished plans. An illness may not only temporarily obstruct long-range goals; it may necessitate permanent and drastic revision in the patient's major activities, such as working habits. Patients may also need to set limited goals regarding control of pain, alteration in diet and physical activity, and rehabilitation of functional impairments. They may face considerable difficulties in identifying realistic and productive aims.

The crisis is aggravated by a cognitive constraint—the lack of "knowledge and skills" to overcome their physical or mental impediment. Without adequate medical understanding, the patient cannot assess his or her condition accurately. Thus the choice of goals is seriously hampered and subsequent decisions by the patient are not well founded.

Pellegrino mentions the anxieties created by illness, but psychological constraints may also include denial, depression, guilt, and fear. I recently visited an eighteen-year-old boy who was dying of a cancer that had metastasized extensively throughout his abdomen. The doctor wanted to administer further chemotherapy that might extend the patient's life a few months. But the patient's nutritional status was poor, and he would need intravenous feedings prior to chemotherapy. Since the nutritional therapy might also encourage tumor growth, leading to a blockage of the gastrointestinal tract, the physician carefully explained the options and the risks and benefits several times, each time at greater length. But after each explanation, the young man would say only that he wished to do whatever was necessary to get better. Denial prevented him from exploring the alternatives.

Similarly, depression can lead patients to make choices that are not in harmony with their life plans. Recently, a middle-aged woman with a history of ovarian cancer in remission returned to the hospital for the biopsy of a possible pulmonary metastasis. Complications ensued and she required the use of an artificial respirator for several days. She became severely depressed and soon refused further treatment. The behavior was entirely out of character with her previous full commitment to treatment. Fully supporting her overt wishes might have robbed her of many months of relatively comfortable life in the midst of a very supportive family around which her activities centered. The medical staff stalled for time. Fortunately, her condition improved.

Fear may also cripple the ability of patients to choose. Another patient, diagnosed as having a cerebral tumor that was probably malignant, refused life-saving surgery because he feared the cosmetic effects of neurosurgery and the possibility of neurological damage. After he became comatose and new evidence suggested that the tumor might be benign, his family agreed to surgery and a benign tumor was removed. But he later died of complications related to the unfortunate delay in surgery. Although while competent he had agreed to chemotherapy, his fears (not uncommon among candidates for neurosurgery) prevented him from accepting the medical intervention that might have secured him the health he desired.

Social constraints may also prevent patients from acting upon their considered choices. A recent case involved a twelve-year-old boy whose rhabdomyosarcoma had metastasized extensively. Since all therapeutic interventions had failed, the only remaining option was to involve him in a phase 1 clinical trial. (A phase 1 clinical trial is the initial testing of a drug in human subjects. Its primary purpose is to identify toxicities rather than to evaluate therapeutic effectiveness.) The patient's course had been very stormy, and he privately expressed to the staff his desire to quit further therapy and return home. However, his parents denied the hopelessness of his condition, remaining steadfast in their belief that God would save their child. With deep regard for his parents' wishes, he refused to openly object to their desires and the therapy was administered. No antitumor effect occurred and the patient soon died.

Various social and cultural expectations also take their toll. According to Talcott Parsons, one feature of the sick role is that the ill person is obligated ". . . to seek *technically competent* help, namely, in the most usual case, that of a physician and to *cooperate* with him in the process of trying to get well."[5] Parsons does not describe in detail the elements of this cooperation. But clinical observation suggests that many patients relinquish their opportunity to deliberate and make choices regarding treatment in deference to the physician's superior educational achievement and social status ("Whatever you think, doctor!"). The physical and emotional demands of illness reinforce this behavior.

Moreover, this perception of the sick role has been socially taught from childhood—and it is not easily altered even by the physician who ardently tries to engage the patient in decision making. Indeed, when patients are initially asked to participate in the decision-making process, some exhibit considerable confusion and anxiety. Thus, for many persons, the institutional role of patient requires the physician to assume the responsibilities of making decisions.

Ethicists typically condemn paternalistic practices in the therapeutic relationship, but fail to investigate the features that incline physicians to be paternalistic. Such behavior may be one way to assist persons whose autonomous behavior has been impaired by illness. Of course, it is an open moral question whether the constraints imposed by illness ought to be addressed in such a way. But only by coming to grips with the psychological and social dimensions of illness can we discuss how physicians can best respect persons who are patients.

RETURNING CONTROL TO PATIENTS

In the usual interpretation of respect for personal autonomy, noninterference is fundamental. In the medical setting, this means providing adequate information and competent care that accords with the patient's wishes. But if serious constraints upon autonomous behavior are intrinsic to the state of being ill, then noninterference is not the best course, since the patient's choices will be seriously limited. Under these conditions, real respect for autonomy entails a more inclusive understanding of the relationship between patients and physicians. Rather than restraining themselves so that patients can exercise whatever autonomy they retain in illness, physicians should actively seek to neutralize the impediments that interfere with patients' choices.

In *The Healer's Art,* Eric Cassell underscored the essential feature of illness that demands a revision in our understanding of respect for autonomy:

> If I had to pick the aspect of illness that is most destructive to the sick, I would choose the loss of control. Maintaining control over oneself is so vital to all of us that one might see all the other phenomena of illness as doing harm not only in their own right but doubly so as they reinforce the sick person's perception that he is no longer in control.[6]

Cassell maintains, "The doctor's job is to return control to his patient." But what is involved in "returning control" to patients? Pellegrino identifies two elements that are preeminent duties of the physician: to provide technically competent care and to fully inform the patient. The noninterference approach emphasizes these factors, and their importance is clear. Loss of control in illness is precipitated by a physical or mental defect. If technically competent therapy can fully restore previous health, then the patient will again be in control. Consider a patient who is treated with antibiotics for a routine throat infection of streptococcal origin. Similarly, loss of control is fueled by lack of knowledge—not knowing what is the matter, what it portends for life and limb, and how it might be dealt with. Providing information that will enable the patient to make decisions and adjust goals enhances personal control.

If physical and cognitive constraints were the only impediments to autonomous behavior, then Pellegrino's suggestions might be adequate. But providing information and technically competent care will not do much to alter psychological or social impediments. Pellegrino does not adequately portray the physician's role in ameliorating these.

How can the doctor offset the acute denial that prevented the adolescent patient from assessing the benefits and risks of intravenous feedings prior to his additional chemotherapy? How can he deal with the candidate for neurosurgery who clearly desired that attempts be made to restore his health, but feared cosmetic and functional impairments? Here strategies must go beyond the mere provision of information. Crucial information may have to be repeatedly shared with patients. Features of the situation that the patient has brushed over (as in denial) or falsely emphasized (as with acute anxiety) must be discussed in more detail or set in their proper perspective. And the physician may have to alter the tone of discussions with the patient, emphasizing a positive attitude with the overly depressed or anxious patient, or a more realistic, cautious attitude with the denying patient, in order to neutralize psychological constraints.

The physician may also need to influence the beliefs or attitudes of other people, such as family members, that limit their awareness of the patient's perspective. Such a strategy might have helped the parents of the dying child to conform with the patient's wishes. On the other hand, physicians may need to modify the patient's own understanding of the sick role. For example, they may need to convey that the choice of treatment depends not merely upon the physician's technical assessment, but on the quality of life and personal goals that the patient desires.

Once we admit that psychological and social constraints impair patient autonomy, it follows that physicians must carefully assess the psychological and social profiles and needs of patients. Thus, Pedro Lain-Entralgo insists that adequate therapeutic interaction consists in a combination of "objectivity" and "cooperation." Cooperation "is shown by psychologically reproducing in the mind of the doctor, insofar as that is possible, the meaning the patient's illness has for him."[7] Without such knowledge, the physician cannot assist patients in restoring control over their lives. Ironically, some critics have insisted that physicians are not justified in acting for the well-being of patients because they possess no "expertise" in securing the requisite knowledge about the patient.[8] But knowledge of the patient's psychological and social situation is also necessary to help the patient to act as a fully autonomous person.

BEYOND LEGALISM

Current notions of respect for autonomy are undergirded by a legal model of doctor-patient interaction. The relationship is viewed as a typical commodity exchange—the provision of technically competent medical care in return for financial compensation. Moreover, physicians and patients are presumed to have an equal ability to work out the details of therapy, *provided that* certain moral rights of patients are recognized. But the compromising effects of illness, the superior knowledge of physicians, and various institutional arrangements are also viewed as giving the physician an unfair power advantage. Since the values and interests of patients may conflict with those of the physician, the emphasis is placed upon noninterference.[9]

This legal framework is insufficient for medical ethics because it fails to recognize the impact of illness upon autonomous behavior. Even if the rights to receive adequate information and to provide consent are secured, affective and social constraints impair the ability of patients to engage in contractual therapeutic relationships. When people are sick, the focus upon equality is temporally misplaced. The goal of the therapeutic relationship is the "development" of the patient—helping to resolve the underlying physical (or mental) defect, and to deal with cognitive, psychological, and social constraints in order to restore autonomous functioning. In this sense, the doctor-patient interaction is not unlike the parent-child or teacher-student relationship.

The legal model also falls short because the therapeutic relationship is not a typical commodity exchange in which the parties use each other to accomplish mutually compatible goals, without taking a direct interest in each other. Rather, the status of patients as persons whose autonomy is compromised constitutes the very stuff of therapeutic art. The physician is attempting to alter the fundamental ability of patients to carry through their life plans. To accomplish this delicate task requires a personal knowledge about and interest in the patient. If we accept these points, then we must reject the narrow focus of medical ethics upon noninterference and emphasize patterns of interaction that free patients from constraints upon autonomy.

I hasten to add that I am criticizing the legal model only as a *complete* moral framework for therapeutic interaction. As case studies in medical ethics suggest, physicians and patients *are* potential adversaries. Moreover, the disability of the patient and various institutional controls provide physicians with a distinct "power advantage" that can be abused. Thus, a legitimate function of medical ethics is to formulate conditions that assure noninterference in patient decision making. But various positive interventions must also be emphasized, since the central task in the therapeutic process is assisting patients to reestablish control over their own lives.

In the last analysis, the crucial matter is how we view the patient who enters into the therapeutic relationship. Cassell points out that in the typical view ". . . the sick person is seen simply as a well person with a disease, rather than as qualitatively different, not only physically but also socially, emotionally, and even cognitively." In this view, ". . . the physician's role in the care of the sick is primarily the application of technology . . . and health can be seen as a commodity."[10] But if, as I believe, illness renders sick persons "qualitatively different," then respect for personal autonomy requires a therapeutic interaction considerably more complex than the noninterference strategy.

Thus the current "Principles of Medical Ethics" simply exhort physicians to be honest. But the crucial requirement is that physicians tell the truth in a way, at a time, and in whatever increments are necessary to allow patients to effectively use the information in adjusting their life plans.[11] Similarly, respecting a patient's refusal of treatment maximizes autonomy only if a balanced and thorough deliberation precedes the decision. Again, the "Principles" suggest that physicians observe strict confidentiality. But the more complex moral challenge is to use confidential information in a way that will help to give the patient more freedom. Thus, the doctor can keep a patient's report on family dynamics private, and still use it to modify attitudes or actions of family members that inhibit the patient's control.

At its root, illness is an evil primarily because it compromises our efforts to control our lives. Thus, we must preserve an understanding of the physician's art that transcends noninterference and addresses this fundamental reality.

REFERENCES

1 American Medical Association, *Current Opinions of the Judicial Council of the American Medical Association* (Chicago, Illinois: American Medical Association, 1981), p. ix. Also see Robert Veatch, "Professional Ethics: New Principles for Physicians?," *Hastings Center Report* 10 (June 1980), 16–19.

2 The National Commission for the Protection of Human Subjects of Biomedical and Behavioral Research, *The Belmont Report: Ethical Principles and Guidelines for the Protection of Human Subjects of Research* (Washington, D.C.: U.S. Government Printing Office, 1978), p. 58.

3 Tom Beauchamp and James Childress, *Principles of Biomedical Ethics* (New York: Oxford University Press, 1980), p. 59.

4 Edmund Pellegrino, "Toward a Reconstruction of Medical Morality: The Primacy of the Act of Profession and the Fact of Illness," *The Journal of Medicine and Philosophy* 4 (1979), 44–45.

5 Talcott Parsons, *The Social System* (Glencoe, Illinois: The Free Press, 1951), p. 437.

6 Eric Cassell, *The Healer's Art* (New York: Lippincott, 1976), p. 44. Although Cassell aptly describes the goal of the healer's art, it is unclear whether he considers it to be based upon the obligation to respect the patient's autonomy or the duty to enhance the well-being of the patient. Some parts of his discussion clearly suggest the latter.

7 Pedro Lain-Entralgo, *Doctor and Patient* (New York: McGraw-Hill, 1969), p. 155.

8 See Allen Buchanan, "Medical Paternalism," *Philosophy and Public Affairs* 7 (1978), 370–90.

9 My formulation of the components of the legal model differs from, but is highly indebted to, John Ladd's stimulating analysis in "Legalism and Medical Ethics," in John Davis et al, editors, *Contemporary Issues in Biomedical Ethics* (Clifton, N.J.: The Humana Press, 1979), pp. 1–35. However, I would not endorse Ladd 's position that the moral principles that define our duties in the therapeutic setting are of a different logical type from those that define our duties to strangers.

10 Eric Cassell, "Therapeutic Relationship: Contemporary Medical Perspective," in Warren Reich, editor, *Encyclopedia of Bioethics* (New York: Macmillan, 1978), p. 1675.

11 Cf. Norman Cousins, "A Layman Looks at Truth-telling," *Journal of the American Medical Association* 244 (1980), 1929–30. Also see Howard Brody, "Hope," *Journal of the American Medical Association* 246 (1981), pp. 1411–12.

Truth-Telling

On Telling Patients the Truth
Roger Higgs

Roger Higgs is general practitioner at King's College School of Medicine and Dentistry in London, England. He is the author of "Child Autonomy" and "Not the Last Word on Euthanasia" and the coauthor of *Mental Health and Primary Care* (1993).

Higgs argues for the paramount importance of physicians' telling patients the truth, before taking on the complex issue of whether this rule has exceptions. He considers and rejects most of the arguments commonly offered to justify lying to patients or otherwise deceiving them. In the end, he maintains, "there are *some* circumstances in which the health professions are probably exempted from society's general requirement for truthfulness," but these are very rare circumstances in which there are clearly no acceptable alternatives.

. . . [T]hose with experience, either as patients or professionals, will immediately recognize the situation. Although openness is increasingly practised, there is still uncertainty in the minds of many doctors or nurses faced with communicating bad news; as for instance when a test shows up an unexpected and probably incurable cancer, or when meeting the gaze of a severely ill child, or answering the questions of a mother in mid-pregnancy whose unborn child is discovered to be badly handicapped. What should be said? There can be few who have not, on occasions such as these, told less than the truth. Certainly the issue is a regular preoccupation of nurses and doctors in training. Why destroy hope? Why create anxiety, or something worse? Isn't it 'First, do no harm'?[1]

The concerns of the patient are very different. For many, fear of the unknown is the worst disease of all, and yet direct information seems so hard to obtain. The ward round goes past quickly, unintelligible words are muttered—was I supposed to hear and understand? In the surgery the general practitioner signs his prescription pad and clearly it's time to be gone. Everybody is too busy saving lives to give explanations. It may come as a shock to learn that it is policy, not just pressure of work, that prevents a patient learning the truth about himself. If truth is the first casualty, trust must be the second. 'Of course they wouldn't say, especially if things were bad,' said the elderly woman just back from out-

patients, 'they've got that Oath, haven't they?' She had learned to expect from doctors, at the best, silence; at the worst, deception. It was part of the system, an essential ingredient, as old as Hippocrates. However honest a citizen, it was somehow part of the doctor's job not to tell the truth to his patient. . . .

[I]t is easier to decide what to do when the ultimate outcome is clear. It may be much more difficult to know what to say when the future is less certain, such as in the first episode of what is probably multiple sclerosis, or when a patient is about to undergo a mutilating operation. But even in work outside hospital, where such dramatic problems arise less commonly, whether to tell the truth and how much to tell can still be a regular issue. How much should this patient know about the side effects of his drugs? An elderly man sits weeping in an old people's home, and the healthy but exhausted daughter wants the doctor to tell her father that she's medically unfit to have him back. The single mother wants a certificate to say that she is unwell so that she can stay at home to look after her sick child. A colleague is often drunk on duty, and is making mistakes. A husband with venereal disease wants his wife to be treated without her knowledge. An outraged father demands to know if his teenage daughter has been put on the pill. A mother comes in with a child to have a boil lanced. 'Please tell him it won't hurt.' A former student writes from abroad needing to complete his professional experience and asks for a reference for a job he didn't do.[2] Whether the issue is large or small, the truth is at stake. What should the response be?

Discussion of the apparently more dramatic situa-

Reprinted from Michael Lockwood, ed., *Moral Dilemmas in Modern Medicine* (1985), pp. 187–191, 193–202, by permission of Oxford University Press. © Roger Higgs 1985.

tions may provide a good starting point. Recently a small group of medical students, new to clinical experience, were hotly debating what a patient with cancer should be told. One student maintained strongly that the less said to the patient the better. Others disagreed. When asked whether there was any group of patients they could agree should never be told the truth about a life-threatening illness, the students chose children, and agreed that they would not speak openly to children under six. When asked to try to remember what life was like when they were six, one student replied that he remembered how his mother had died when he was that age. Suddenly the student who had advocated non-disclosure became animated. 'That's extraordinary. My mother died when I was six too. My father said she'd gone away for a time, but would come back soon. One day he said she was coming home again. My younger sister and I were very excited. We waited at the window upstairs until we saw his car drive up. He got out and helped a woman out of the car. Then we saw. It wasn't mum. I suppose I never forgave him—or her, really.'[3]

It is hard to know with whom to sympathize in this sad tale. But its stark simplicity serves to highlight some essential points. First, somehow more clearly than in the examples involving patients, not telling the truth is seen for what it really is. It is, of course, quite possible, and very common in clinical practice, for doctors (or nurses) to engage in deliberate deceit without actually *saying* anything they believe to be false. But, given the special responsibilities of the doctor, and the relationship of trust that exists between him and his patient, one could hardly argue that this was morally any different from telling outright lies. Surely it is the *intention* that is all important. We may be silent, tactful, or reserved, but if we intend to deceive, what we are doing is tantamount to lying. The debate in ward or surgery is suddenly stood on its head. The question is no longer 'Should we tell the truth?' but 'What justification is there for telling a lie?' This relates to the second important point, that medical ethics are part of general morality, and not a separate field of their own with their own rules. Unless there are special justifications, health-care professionals are working within the same moral constraints as lay people. A lie is a lie wherever told and whoever tells it.

But do doctors have a special dispensation from the usual principles that guide the conduct of our society? It is widely felt that on occasion they do, and such a dispensation is as necessary to all doctors as freedom from the charge of assault is to a surgeon. But if it is impossible to look after ill patients and always be open and truthful, how can we balance this against the clear need for truthfulness on all other occasions? If deception is like a medicine to be given in certain doses in certain cases, what guidance exists about its administration?

. . . Although the writer of the 'Decorum' in the Hippocratic corpus advises physicians of the danger of telling patients about the nature of their illness '. . . for many patients through this cause have taken a turn for the worse',[4] the Oath itself is completely silent on this issue. This extraordinary omission is continued through all the more modern codes and declarations. The first mention of veracity as a principle is to be found in the American Medical Association's 'Principles of Ethics' of 1980, which states that the physician should 'deal honestly with patients and colleagues and strive to expose those physicians deficient in character or competence, or who engage in fraud and deception'.[5] Despite the difficulties of the latter injunction, which seems in some way to divert attention from the basic need for honest communication with the patient, here at last is a clear statement. This declaration signally fails, however, to provide the guidance that we might perhaps have expected for the professional facing his or her individual dilemma.

The reticence of these earlier codes is shared, with some important exceptions, by medical writing elsewhere. Until recently most of what had been usefully said could be summed up by the articles of medical writers such as Thomas Percival, Worthington Hooker, Richard Cabot, and Joseph Collins, which show a wide scatter of viewpoints but do at least confront the problems directly.[6] There is, however, one widely quoted statement by Lawrence Henderson, writing in the *New England Journal of Medicine* in 1955.[7] 'It is meaningless to speak of telling the truth, the whole truth and nothing but the truth to a patient . . . because it is . . . a sheer impossibility . . . Since telling the truth is impossible, there can be no sharp distinction between what is true and what is false.' . . .

But we must not allow ourselves to be confused, as Henderson was, and as so many others have been, by a failure to distinguish between truth, the abstract concept, of which we shall always have an imperfect grasp, and *telling* the truth, where the intention is all important. Whether or not we can ever fully grasp or express the whole picture, whether we know ultimately what the truth really is, we must speak truthfully, and intend to convey what we understand, or we shall lie. In Sissela Bok's words 'The moral question of whether you are lying or not is not *settled* by establishing the truth or falsity of what you say. In order to settle the question, we must know whether you *intend your statement to mislead.*'[8] . . .

Most modern thinkers in the field of medical ethics would hold that truthfulness is indeed a central principle of conduct, but that it is capable of coming into conflict with other principles, to which it must occasionally give way. On the other hand, the principle of veracity often receives support from other principles. For instance, it is hard to see how a patient can have autonomy, can make a free choice about matters concerning himself, without some measure of understanding of the facts as they influence the case; and that implies, under normal circumstances, some open, honest discussion with his advisers.[9] . . .

Once the central position of honesty has been established, we still need to examine whether doctors and nurses really do have, as has been suggested, special exemption from being truthful because of the nature of their work, and if so under what circumstances. . . . It may finally be decided that in a crisis there is no acceptable alternative, as when life is ebbing and truthfulness would bring certain disaster. Alternatively, the moral issue may appear so trivial as not to be worth considering (as, for example, when a doctor is called out at night by a patient who apologizes by saying, 'I hope you don't mind me calling you at this time, doctor', and the doctor replies, 'No, not at all.'). However, . . . occasions of these two types are few, fewer than those in which deliberate deceit would generally be regarded as acceptable in current medical practice, and should regularly be debated 'in public' if abuses are to be avoided.[10] To this end it is necessary now to examine critically the arguments commonly used to defend lying to patients.

First comes the argument that it is enormously difficult to put across a technical subject to those with little technical knowledge and understanding, in a situation where so little is predictable. A patient has bowel cancer. With surgery it might be cured, or it might recur. Can the patient understand the effects of treatment? The symptom she is now getting might be due to cancer, there might be secondaries, and they in turn might be suppressible for a long time, or not at all. What future symptoms might occur, how long will she live, how will she die—all these are desperately important questions for the patient, but even for her doctor the answers can only be informed guesses, in an area where uncertainty is so hard to bear.

Yet to say we do not know anything is a lie. As doctors we know a great deal, and *can* make informed guesses or offer likelihoods. The whole truth may be impossible to attain, but truthfulness is not. 'I do not

know' can be a major piece of honesty. To deprive the patient of honest communication because we cannot know everything is, as we have seen, not only confused thinking but immoral. Thus deprived, the patient cannot plan, he cannot choose. If choice is the crux of morality, it may also, as we have argued elsewhere, be central to health. If he cannot choose, the patient cannot ever be considered to be fully restored to health.[11]

This argument also raises another human failing—to confuse the difficult with the unimportant. Passing information to people who have more restricted background, whether through lack of experience or of understanding, can be extremely difficult and time-consuming, but this is no reason why it should be shunned. Quite the reverse. Like the difficult passages in a piece of music, these tasks should be practiced, studied, and techniques developed so that communication is efficient and effective. For the purposes of informed consent, the patient must be given the information he needs, as a reasonable person, to make a reasoned choice.

The second argument for telling lies to patients is that no patient likes hearing depressing or frightening news. That is certainly true. There must be few who do. But in other walks of life no professional would normally consider it his or her duty to suppress information simply in order to preserve happiness. No accountant, foreseeing bankruptcy in his client's affairs, would chat cheerfully about the Budget or a temporarily reassuring credit account. Yet such suppression of information occurs daily in wards or surgeries throughout the country. Is this what patients themselves want?

In order to find out, a number of studies have been conducted over the past thirty years.[12] In most studies there is a significant minority of patients, perhaps about a fifth, who, if given information, deny having been told. Sometimes this must be pure forgetfulness, sometimes it relates to the lack of skill of the informer, but sometimes with bad or unwelcome news there is an element of what is (perhaps not quite correctly) called 'denial'. The observer feels that at one level the news has been taken in, but at another its validity or reality has not been accepted. This process has been recognized as a buffer for the mind against the shock of unacceptable news, and often seems to be part of a process leading to its ultimate acceptance.[13] But once this group has been allowed for, most surveys find that, of those who have had or who could have had a diagnosis made of, say, cancer, between two-thirds and three-quarters of those questioned were either glad to have been told, or declared that they would wish to know. Indeed, surveys reveal that most *doctors* would themselves wish to be told the truth, even though (according to earlier studies at least) most of those same doctors said they would not speak openly to their patients—a curious double standard! Thus these surveys have unearthed, at least for the present, a common misunderstanding between doctors and patients, a general preference for openness among patients, and a significant but small group whose wish not to be informed must surely be respected. We return once more to the skill needed to detect such differences in the individual case, and the need for training in such skills.

Why doctors have for so long misunderstood their patients' wishes is perhaps related to the task itself. Doctors don't want to give bad news, just as patients don't want it in abstract, but doctors have the choice of withholding the information, and in so doing protecting themselves from the pain of telling, and from the blame of being the bearer of bad news. In addition it has been suggested that doctors are particularly fearful of death and illness. Montaigne suggested that men have to think about death and be prepared to accept it, and one would think that doctors would get used to death. Yet perhaps this very familiarity has created an obsession that amounts to fear. Just as the police seem over-concerned with violence, and firemen with fire, perhaps doctors have met death in their professional training only as the enemy, never as something to come to terms with, or even as a natural force to be respected and, when the time is ripe, accepted or even welcomed. . . .

. . . Paternalism may be justifiable in the short term, and to 'kid' someone, to treat him as a child because he is ill, and perhaps dying, may be very tempting. Yet true respect for that person (adult or child) can only be shown by allowing him allowable choices, by granting him whatever control is left, as weakness gradually undermines his hold on life. If respect is important then at the very least there must be no acceptable or effective alternative to lying in a particular situation if the lie is to be justified.

. . . However, a third argument for lying can be advanced, namely, that truthfulness can actually do harm. 'What you don't know can't hurt you' is a phrase in common parlance (though it hardly fits with concepts of presymptomatic screening for preventable disease!) However, it is undeniable that blunt and unfeeling communication of unpleasant truths can cause acute distress, and sometimes long-term disability. The fear that professionals often have of upsetting people, of causing a scene, of making fools of themselves by letting unpleasant emotions flourish, seems to have elevated this argument beyond its natural limits. It is not unusual to find that the fear of creating harm will deter a surgical

team from discussing a diagnosis gently with a patient, but not deter it from performing radical and mutilating surgery. Harm is a very personal concept. Most medical schools have, circulating in the refectory, a story about a patient who was informed that he had cancer and then leapt to his death. The intended moral for the medical student is, keep your mouth shut and do no harm. But that may not be the correct lesson to be learned from such cases (which I believe, in any case, to be less numerous than is commonly supposed). The style of telling could have been brutal, with no follow-up or support. It may have been the suggested treatment, not the basic illness, that led the patient to resort to such a desperate measure. Suicide in illness is remarkably rare, but, though tragic, could be seen as a logical response to an overwhelming challenge. No mention is usually made of suicide rates in other circumstances, or the isolation felt by ill and warded patients, or the feelings of anger uncovered when someone takes such precipitate and forbidden action against himself. What these cases do, surely, is argue, not for no telling, but for better telling, for sensitivity and care in determining how much the patient wants to know, explaining carefully in ways the patient can understand, and providing full support and 'after-care' as in other treatments.

But even if it is accepted that the short-term effect of telling the truth may sometimes be considerable psychological disturbance, in the long term the balance seems definitely to swing the other way. The effects of lying are dramatically illustrated in 'A Case of Obstructed Death?'[14] False information prevented a woman from returning to healthy living after a cancer operation, and robbed her of six months of active life. Also, the long-term effect of lies on the family and, perhaps most importantly, on society, is incalculable. If trust is gradually corroded, if the 'wells are poisoned', progress is hard. Mistrust creates lack of communication and increased fear, and this generation has seen just such a fearful myth created around cancer.[15] Just how much harm has been done by this 'demonizing' of cancer, preventing people coming to their doctors, or alternatively creating unnecessary attendances on doctors, will probably never be known.

There are doubtless many other reasons why doctors lie to their patients; but these can hardly be used to justify lies, even if we should acknowledge them in passing. Knowledge is power, and certainly doctors, though usually probably for reasons of work-load rather than anything more sinister, like to remain 'in control'. Health professionals may, like others, wish to protect themselves from confrontation, and may find it easier to coerce or manipulate than to gain permission. There may be a desire to avoid any pressure for change. And there is the constant problem of lack of time. . . .

If the importance of open communication with the patient is accepted, [however,] we need to know when to say what. If a patient is going for investigations, it may be possible at that time, before details are known, to have a discussion about whether he would like to know the details. A minor 'contract' can be made. 'I promise to tell you what I know, if you ask me.' Once that time is past, however, it requires skill and sensitivity to assess what a patient wants to know. Allowing the time and opportunity for the patient to ask questions is the most important thing, but one must realize that the patient's apparent question may conceal the one he really wants answered. 'Do I have cancer?' may contain the more important questions 'How or when will I die?' 'Will there be pain?' The doctor will not necessarily be helping by giving an extended pathology lesson. The informer may need to know more: 'I don't want to avoid your question, and I promise to answer as truthfully as I can, but first . . .' It has been pointed out that in many cases the terminal patient will tell the doctor, not vice versa, if the right opportunities are created and the style and timing is appropriate. Then it is a question of not telling but listening to the truth.[16]

If in spite of all this there still seems to be a need to tell lies, we must be able to justify them. That the person is a child, or 'not very bright', will not do. Given the two ends of the spectrum of crisis and triviality, the vast middle range of communication requires honesty, so that autonomy and choice can be maintained. If lies are to be told, there really must be no acceptable alternative. . . . If we break an important moral principle, that principle still retains its force, and its 'shadow' has to be acknowledged. As professionals we shall have to ensure that we follow up, that we work through the broken trust or the disillusionment that the lie will bring to the patient, just as we would follow up and work through bad news, a major operation, or a psychiatric 'sectioning'. This follow-up may also be called for in our relationship with our colleagues if there has been major disagreement about what should be done.

In summary, there are *some* circumstances in which the health professions are probably exempted from society's general requirement for truthfulness. But not telling the truth is usually the same as telling a lie, and a lie requires strong justification. Lying must be a last resort, and we should act as if we were to be called upon to defend the decision in public debate, even if our duty of confidentiality does not allow this in practice. We should always aim to respect the other impor-

tant principles governing interactions with patients, especially the preservation of the patient's autonomy. When all is said and done, many arguments for individual cases of lying do not hold water. Whether or not knowing the truth is essential to the patient's health, telling the truth is essential to the health of the doctor–patient relationship.

NOTES

1 *Primum non nocere*—this is a latinization of a statement which is not directly Hippocratic, but may be derived from the *Epidemics* Book 1 Chapter II: 'As to diseases, make a habit of two things—to help, or at least do no harm.' *Hippocrates*, 4 Vols. (London: William Heinemann, 1923–31), Vol. I. Translation W. H. S. Jones.

2 Cases collected by the author in his own practice.

3 Case collected by the author.

4 Quoted in Reiser, Dyck, and Curran (eds), *Ethics in Medicine, Historical Perspectives and Contemporary Concerns* (Cambridge, Mass.: MIT Press, 1977).

5 American Medical Association, 'Text of the American Medical Association New Principles of Medical Ethics' *American Medical News* (August 1–8, 1980), 9.

6 To be found in Reiser *et al.*, op. cit. (see n. 4 above).

7 Lawrence Henderson, 'Physician and Patient as a Social System', *New England Journal of Medicine*, 212 (1935).

8 Sissela Bok, *Lying: Moral Choice in Public and Private Life* (London: Quartet, 1980).

9 Alastair Campbell and Roger Higgs, *In That Case* (London: Darton, Longman and Todd, 1982).

10 John Rawls, *A Theory of Justice* (Cambridge, Mass.: Harvard University Press, Belknap Press, 1971).

11 Op. cit. (see n. 9 above).

12 Summarized well in Robert Veatch, 'Truth-telling I' in Warren T. Reich (ed.), *Encyclopaedia of Bioethics* (New York: Free Press, 1978).

13 The five stages of reacting to bad news, or news of dying, are described in *On Death and Dying* by Elizabeth Kübler-Ross (London: Tavistock, 1970). Not everyone agrees with her model. For another view see a very stimulating article 'Therapeutic Uses of Truth' by Michael Simpson in E. Wilkes (ed.), *The Dying Patient* (Lancaster: MTP Press, 1982). 'In my model there are only two stages—the stage when you believe in the Kübler-Ross five and the stage when you do not.'

14 Roger Higgs, 'Truth at the last—A Case of Obstructed Death?', *Journal of Medical Ethics*, 8 (1982), 48–50, and Roger Higgs, 'Obstructed Death Revisited', *Journal of Medical Ethics*, 8 (1982), pp. 154–56.

15 Susan Sontag, *Illness as Metaphor* (New York: Farrar, Straus and Giroux, 1978).

16 Cicely Saunders, 'Telling Patients', *District Nursing* (now *Queens Nursing Journal*) (September 1963), pp. 149–50, 154.

Hope
Howard Brody

Howard Brody, a medical doctor who is also trained in philosophy, is professor of family practice and philosophy at Michigan State University, where he is also director of the Center for Ethics and Humanities in the Life Sciences. He is the author of *Ethical Decisions in Medicine* (1976), *Stories of Sickness* (1988), and *The Healer's Power* (1992).

Brody considers the problem of how to observe the ethical requirement to tell patients the truth without destroying their hope. He argues that, because hope is much more resilient than physicians generally assume, it can in fact rarely be taken away. Moreover, he contends, "it is almost always possible to combine frank and accurate disclosure of the truth with an invigorating infusion of hope." Brody supports this claim with examples of forms of hope that are compatible with grim medical prognoses; one such example is patients' hope that they will not be abandoned by their physicians.

Those of us who talk about ethical issues in medicine have our spiel on "truth-telling" down pat. We talk about the historical background of the policy of benign deception[1]; about data that show that patients generally suspect the truth anyway[2]; about recent changes in physician behavior in the direction of complete disclosure of unwelcome diagnostic news[3]; and finally, about the important ethical principles of autonomy and individual self-determination.[4,5] But sooner or later comes the rejoinder, delivered with the air of laying down the trump card: "All of that sounds very good. But how can you possibly justify ever taking away the patient's hope?"

In debates on medical ethics, this question is all too often left unanswered. I believe that there is a satisfactory answer and that it has more to do, as Norman Cousins very correctly pointed out, with the "art of

medicine" rather than the ethics of medicine.[6] It is possible to tell the patient his true diagnosis in such a way as to leave him and his family emotionally devastated. It is also possible to prescribe the wrong dose of digoxin or to operate on the left knee for an arthropathy present on the right. We should not confuse botching our jobs with adhering to an erroneous ethical principle.

We know from placebo research how potent the patient's emotions and ideas can be in healing the body. We also know that the physician is placed in a pivotal role to influence the patient's ideas and emotions for better or for worse.[7] Since hope is such a powerful medicine, we ought to manage our therapeutic relationships so as to maximize its effects. But to do so, we ought to have a more precise idea of hope's psychopharmacological properties than is commonly gained from the truth-telling debate.

I would like to offer two rather rash observations about hope in this attempt to advance our understanding. The first is that, while we talk with great facility about the dangers of taking away the patient's hope, I

Reprinted with permission of the publisher from *JAMA*, vol. 246 (September 25, 1981), pp. 1411–1412. Copyright © 1981, American Medical Association.

am not sure that we really have the power to do so except in very rare instances.

One does not have to practice medicine for long before one becomes aware of the profound emotional impact that our most innocent, off-handed remarks can have on our patients. As most of us would not have become physicians if we did not have the desire, at some level, to wield power over our fellow creatures, these incidents tend to confirm our satisfying myths of omnipotence. We may forget the much greater numbers of our patients who go on smoking despite our dire warnings, or who always seem to have a few extra penicillin pills in the medicine cabinet despite our firm admonishment to "take the pills four times a day until the prescription is completely gone."

Anecdotes have been told of patients who die of their terminal cancer, firmly convinced that they are in perfect health and that the slides must have been mixed up in the laboratory. I have had an elderly man tell me with great gusto how ten years ago his physicians had told him that he had only six months to live with his prostatic carcinoma. Certainly, anecdotes can be offered to support the opposing view also; but I think that in general hope may be more resilient than we realize. The most callous pronouncement of doom may prompt not despair, but rather an intense commitment to proving that SOB wrong. And, if more sophisticated defense mechanisms fail, denial is not a bad thing to fall back on.

The second rash observation is that it is almost always possible to combine frank and accurate disclosure of the truth with an invigorating infusion of hope. For one thing, in many cases, the actual facts are not as grim as we think, if the patient is motivated to hear the good news along with the bad. We can truthfully tell the patient with terminal cancer, "Statistically I would say that your life span is more likely to be measured in months rather than years," along with the additional message, "Somehow a few lucky or highly motivated patients seem to beat the odds and live much longer than we expect." The patient, depending on his or her own needs at the time, can choose to hear that the glass is 95% empty or that it is 5% full.

But there is a more important reason why we can almost always give hope even along with the direst tidings. It is suggested in a poem by Emily Dickinson:

The heart asks pleasure first,
And then escape from pain,
And then those little anodynes
That deaden suffering,

And then to go to sleep,
And then if it should be
The will of its inquisitor
The privilege to die.

If we were as good at listening to our patients as we are at telling them things, we would learn that hope is not automatically equated with survival. Hope means different things to different people; and hope means different things to the same person as he moves through different stages of his illness and his emotional reaction to it. The man who last year hoped for a cure for his arthritis may now hope that, on a good day, he can get in nine holes of golf. And, for those unfortunates for whom those who would keep them alive have become truly the "inquisitor" instead of the savior, hope may mean a pain-free and oblivious death.

Giving hope, then, need not consist of, "You really don't have cancer after all," or, "We removed all the cancer surgically and your ten-year survival prognosis is excellent." Giving hope can be: "We will be able to give you medicines to keep you free of pain," or, "You will still be around this weekend to visit with your grandchildren when they come," or, "I will not abandon you." (Which in turn makes us wonder, when patients "lose hope" after being told the truth in a callous, brutal manner, if they are not responding to the unspoken message of the physician's detachment and abandonment rather than to the spoken words.) When we talk to patients and find out what is really worrying them, we can almost always give some realistic assurances.

If we understand the psychopharmacological features of hope in this way, we realize that setting hope-maintaining against truth-telling is to create a false dichotomy. There is no fundamental conflict between our moral duty to preserve hope—to heal our patients with our words and not just with our medicines—and our moral duty to respect our patients as adult human beings who should be given the information they need to make their own free choices about their lives. We as physicians can maintain the demeanor that calms and reassures our patients—the positive sense of "arrogance" described by Franz Ingelfinger[8]—and still take the initiative in disclosing truth. And once we realize that this is possible, we can turn our attention to the real question, which is how to learn and how to teach the skills necessary to do it as well as possible.

1 Reiser SJ: Words as scalpels: Transmitting evidence in the clinical encounter. *Ann Intern Med* 1980;92:837–842.

2 McIntosh J: Patients' awareness and desire for information about diagnosed but undisclosed malignant disease. *Lancet* 1976;2:300–303.

3 Novack DH, Plumer R, Smith RL, et al: Changes in physicians' attitudes toward telling the cancer patient. *JAMA* 1979;241:897–900.

4 Beauchamp TL, Childress JF: *Principles of Biomedical Ethics.* New York, Oxford University Press, 1979.

5 Brody H: *Ethical Decisions in Medicine,* ed 2. Boston, Little Brown & Co, 1981.

6 Cousins N: A layman looks at truth telling in medicine. *JAMA* 1980;244:1929–1930.

7 Brody H: *Placebos and the Philosophy of Medicine.* Chicago, University of Chicago Press, 1980.

8 Ingelfinger FJ: Arrogance. *N Engl J Med* 1980; 303:1507–1511.

Informed Consent

Opinion in *Canterbury v. Spence*
Judge Spotswood W. Robinson III

Spotswood W. Robinson III is senior circuit judge on the United States Court of Appeals, District of Columbia. Prior to his appointment to the bench, Judge Robinson served as associate professor of law at Howard University (1939–1949) and as the dean of the Law School (1960–1963).

A 19-year-old man, John W. Canterbury, developed paraplegia after a laminectomy (a surgical procedure). Prior to the surgery, his physician, William Thornton Spence, did not inform Canterbury that the operation involved the risk of paralysis. Canterbury brought an action against the physician and the hospital. In defending his decision to withhold the information from the patient, Dr. Spence testified that communicating the 1 percent risk "is not good medical practice because it might deter patients from undergoing needed surgery and might produce adverse psychological reactions which could preclude the success of the operation." In this selection, Judge Robinson argues that an adult patient of sound mind has the right to determine what should be done to his or her body. Because of this right, a physician has the duty to inform the patient about those dangers that "are material" to the patient's decision. The court allows two exceptions to this rule of disclosure. It holds, however, that a physician cannot remain silent simply because divulgence might prompt the patient to forgo therapy that the physician perceives as necessary.

Suits charging failure by a physician adequately to disclose the risks and alternatives of proposed treatment are not innovations in American law. They date back a good half-century, and in the last decade they have multiplied rapidly. There is, nonetheless, disagreement among the courts and the commentators on many major questions, and there is no precedent of our own directly in point. For the tools enabling resolution of the issues on this appeal, we are forced to begin at first principles.

U.S. Court of Appeals, District of Columbia Circuit; May 19, 1972. 464 Federal Reporter, 2nd Series, 772. Reprinted with permission of West Publishing Company.

The root premise is the concept, fundamental in American jurisprudence, that "[e]very human being of adult years and sound mind has a right to determine what shall be done with his own body. . . ." True consent to what happens to one's self is the informed exercise of a choice, and that entails an opportunity to evaluate knowledgeably the options available and the risks attendant upon each. The average patient has little or no understanding of the medical arts, and ordinarily has only his physician to whom he can look for enlightenment with which to reach an intelligent decision.[1] From these almost axiomatic considerations springs the need, and in turn the requirement, of a reasonable divulgence by physician to patient to make such a decision possible.[2]

A physician is under a duty to treat his patient skillfully, but proficiency in diagnosis and therapy is not the full measure of his responsibility. The cases demonstrate that the physician is under an obligation to communicate specific information to the patient when the exigencies of reasonable care call for it. Due care may require a physician perceiving symptoms of bodily abnormality to alert the patient to the condition. It may call upon the physician confronting an ailment which does not respond to his ministrations to inform the patient thereof. It may command the physician to instruct the patient as to any limitations to be presently observed for his own welfare, and as to any precautionary therapy he should seek in the future. It may oblige the physician to advise the patient of the need for or desirability of any alternative treatment promising greater benefit than that being pursued. Just as plainly, due care normally demands that the physician warn the patient of any risks to his well-being which contemplated therapy may involve.

The context in which the duty of risk-disclosure arises is invariably the occasion for decision as to whether a particular treatment procedure is to be undertaken. To the physician, whose training enables a self-satisfying evaluation, the answer may seem clear, but it is the prerogative of the patient, not the physician, to determine for himself the direction in which his interests seem to lie. To enable the patient to chart his course understandably, some familiarity with the therapeutic alternatives and their hazards becomes essential.

A reasonable revelation in these respects is not only a necessity but, as we see it, is as much a matter of the physician's duty. It is a duty to warn of the dangers lurking in the proposed treatment, and that is surely a facet of due care. It is, too, a duty to impart information which the patient has every right to expect.[3] The patient's reliance upon the physician is a trust of the kind which traditionally has exacted obligations beyond those associated with arms-length transactions. His dependence upon the physician for information affecting his well-being, in terms of contemplated treatment, is well-nigh abject. As earlier noted, long before the instant litigation arose, courts had recognized that the physician had the responsibility of satisfying the vital informational needs of the patient. More recently, we ourselves have found "in the fiducial qualities of [the physician-patient] relationship the physician's duty to reveal to the patient that which in his best interests it is important that he should know." We now find, as a part of the physician's overall obligation to the patient, a similar duty of reasonable disclosure of the choices with respect to proposed therapy and the dangers inherently and potentially involved. . . .

Once the circumstances give rise to a duty on the physician's part to inform his patient, the next inquiry is the scope of the disclosure the physician is legally obliged to make. The courts have frequently confronted this problem but no uniform standard defining the adequacy of the divulgence emerges from the decisions. Some have said "full" disclosure, a norm we are unwilling to adopt literally. It seems obviously prohibitive and unrealistic to expect physicians to discuss with their patients every risk of proposed treatment—no matter how small or remote—and generally unnecessary from the patient's viewpoint as well. Indeed, the cases speaking in terms of "full" disclosure appear to envision something less than total disclosure, leaving unanswered the question of just how much.

The larger number of courts, as might be expected, have applied tests framed with reference to prevailing fashion within the medical profession. Some have measured the disclosure by "good medical practice," others by what a reasonable practitioner would have bared under the circumstances, and still others by what medical custom in the community would demand. We have explored this rather considerable body of law but are unprepared to follow it. The duty to disclose, we have reasoned, arises from phenomena apart from medical custom and practice. The latter, we think, should no more establish the scope of the duty than its existence. Any definition of scope in terms purely of a professional standard is at odds with the patient's prerogative to decide on projected therapy himself. That prerogative, we have said, is at the very foundation of the duty to disclose, and both the patient's right to know and the physician's correlative obligation to tell him are diluted to the extent that its compass is dictated by the medical profession.[4]

In our view, the patient's right of self-decision shapes the boundaries of the duty to reveal. That right can be effectively exercised only if the patient possesses enough information to enable an intelligent choice. The scope of the physician's communications to the patient, then, must be measured by the patient's need, and that need is the information material to the decision. Thus the test for determining whether a particular peril must be divulged is its materiality to the patient's decision: all risks potentially affecting the decision must be unmasked. And to safeguard the patient's interest in achieving his own determination on treatment, the law must itself set the standard for adequate disclosure.

Optimally for the patient, exposure of a risk would be mandatory whenever the patient would deem it significant to his decision, either singly or in combination with other risks. Such a requirement, however, would summon the physician to second-guess the patient, whose ideas on materiality could hardly be known to the physician. That would make an undue demand upon medical practitioners, whose conduct, like that of others, is to be measured in terms of reasonableness. Consonantly with orthodox negligence doctrine, the physician's liability for nondisclosure is to be determined on the basis of foresight, not hindsight; no less than any other aspect of negligence, the issue on nondisclosure must be approached from the viewpoint of the reasonableness of the physician's divulgence in terms of what he knows or should know to be the patient's informational needs. If, but only if, the fact-finder can say that the physician's communication was unreasonably inadequate is an imposition of liability legally or morally justified.

Of necessity, the content of the disclosure rests in the first instance with the physician. Ordinarily it is only he who is in position to identify particular dangers; always he must make a judgment, in terms of materiality, as to whether and to what extent revelation to the patient is called for. He cannot know with complete exactitude what the patient would consider important to his decision, but on the basis of his medical training and experience he can sense how the average, reasonable patient expectably would react. Indeed, with knowledge of, or ability to learn, his patient's background and current condition, he is in a position superior to that of most others—attorneys, for example—who are called upon to make judgments on pain of liability in damages for unreasonable miscalculation.

From these considerations we derive the breadth of the disclosure of risks legally to be required. The scope of the standard is not subjective as to either the physician or the patient; it remains objective with due regard for the patient's informational needs and with suitable leeway for the physician's situation. In broad outline, we agree that "[a] risk is thus material when a reasonable person, in what the physician knows or should know to be the patient's position, would be likely to attach significance to the risk or cluster of risks in deciding whether or not to forgo the proposed therapy."

The topics importantly demanding a communication of information are the inherent and potential hazards of the proposed treatment, the alternatives to that treatment, if any, and the results likely if the patient remains untreated. The factors contributing significance to the dangerousness of a medical technique are, of course, the incidence of injury and the degree of the harm threatened. A very small chance of death or serious disablement may well be significant; a potential disability which dramatically outweighs the potential benefit of the therapy or the detriments of the existing malady may summon discussion with the patient.

There is no bright line separating the significant from the insignificant; the answer in any case must abide a rule of reason. Some dangers—infection, for example—are inherent in any operation; there is no obligation to communicate those of which persons of average sophistication are aware. Even more clearly, the physician bears no responsibility for discussion of hazards the patient has already discovered, or those having no apparent materiality to patients' decision on therapy. The disclosure doctrine, like others marking lines between permissible and impermissible behavior in medical practice, is in essence a requirement of conduct prudent under the circumstances. Whenever nondisclosure of particular risk information is open to debate by reasonable-minded men, the issue is for the finder of the facts.

Two exceptions to the general rule of disclosure have been noted by the courts. Each is in the nature of a physician's privilege not to disclose, and the reasoning underlying them is appealing. Each, indeed, is but a recognition that, as important as is the patient's right to know, it is greatly outweighed by the magnitudinous circumstances giving rise to the privilege. The first comes into play when the patient is unconscious or otherwise incapable of consenting, and harm from a failure to treat is imminent and outweighs any harm threatened by the proposed treatment. When a genuine emergency of that sort arises, it is settled that the impracticality of conferring with the patient dispenses with need for it. Even in situations of that character the physician should, as current law requires, attempt to secure a relative's consent if possible. But if time is too short to accommodate discussion, obviously the physician should proceed with the treatment.

The second exception obtains when risk-disclosure poses such a threat of detriment to the patient as to become unfeasible or contraindicated from a medical point of view. It is recognized that patients occasionally become so ill or emotionally distraught on disclosure as to foreclose a rational decision, or complicate or hinder the treatment, or perhaps even pose psychological damage to the patient. Where that is so, the cases have generally held that the physician is armed with a privilege to keep the information from the patient, and we think it clear that portents of that type may justify the physician in action he deems medically warranted. The critical inquiry is whether the physician responded to a sound medical judgment that communication of the risk information would present a threat to the patient's well-being.

The physician's privilege to withhold information for therapeutic reasons must be carefully circumscribed, however, for otherwise it might devour the disclosure rule itself. The privilege does not accept the paternalistic notion that the physician may remain silent simply because divulgence might prompt the patient to forgo therapy the physician feels the patient really needs. That attitude presumes instability or perversity for even the normal patient, and runs counter to the foundation principle that the patient should and ordinarily can make the choice for himself. Nor does the privilege contemplate operation save where the patient's reaction to risk information, as reasonably foreseen by the physician, is menacing. And even in a situation of that kind, disclosure to a close relative with a view to securing consent to the proposed treatment may be the only alternative open to the physician. . . .

NOTES

1 Patients ordinarily are persons unlearned in the medical sciences. Some few, of course, are schooled in branches of the medical profession or in related fields. But even within the latter group variations in degree of medical knowledge specifically referable to particular therapy may be broad, as for example, between a specialist and a general practitioner, or between a physician and a nurse. It may well be, then, that it is only in the unusual case that a court could safely assume that the patient's insights were on a parity with those of the treating physician.

2 The doctrine that a consent effective as authority to perform therapy can arise only from the patient's understanding of alternatives to and risks of the therapy is commonly denominated "informed consent." The same appellation is frequently assigned to the doctrine requiring physicians, as a matter of duty to patients, to communicate information as to such alternatives and risks. See, *e.g.,* Comment, Informed Consent in Medical Malpractice, 55 Calif. L. Rev. 1396 (1967). While we recognize the general utility of shorthand phrases in literary expositions, we caution that uncritical use of the "informed consent" label can be misleading. See, *e.g.,* Plante, An Analysis

of "Informed Consent," 36 Ford. L. Rev. 639, 671–72 (1968).

In duty-to-disclose cases, the focus of attention is more properly upon the nature and content of the physician's divulgence than the patient's understanding or consent. Adequate disclosure and informed consent are, of course, two sides of the same coin—the former a *sine qua non* of the latter. But the vital inquiry on duty to disclose relates to the physician's performance of an obligation, while one of the difficulties with analysis in terms of "informed consent" is its tendency to imply that what is decisive is the degree of the patient's comprehension. As we later emphasize, the physician discharges the duty when he makes a reasonable effort to convey sufficient information although the patient, without fault of the physician, may not fully grasp it. Even though the factfinder may have occasion to draw an inference on the state of the patient's enlightenment, the fact-finding process on performance of the duty ultimately reaches back to what the physician actually said or failed to say. And while the factual conclusion on adequacy of the revelation will vary as between patients—as, for example, between a lay patient and a physician-patient—the fluctuations are attributable to the kind of divulgence which may be reasonable under the circumstances.

3 Some doubt has been expressed as to the ability of physicians to suitably communicate their evaluations of risks and the advantages of optional treatment, and as to the lay patient's ability to understand what the physician tells him. Karchmer, Informed Consent: A Plaintiff's Medical Malpractice "Wonder Drug," 31 Mo. L. Rev. 29, 41 (1966). We do not share these apprehensions. The discussion need not be a disquisition, and surely the physician is not compelled to give his patient a short medical education; the disclosure rule summons the physician only to a reasonable explanation. That means generally informing the patient in non-technical terms as to what is at stake: the therapy alternatives open to him, the goals expectably to be achieved, and the risks that may ensue from particular treatment and no treatment. So informing the patient hardly taxes the physician, and it must be the exceptional patient who cannot comprehend such an explanation at least in a rough way.

4 For similar reasons, we reject the suggestion that disclosure should be discretionary with the physician.

The Values Underlying Informed Consent

President's Commission for the Study of Ethical Problems in Medicine and Biomedical and Behavioral Research

The President's Commission, created in 1978, began its deliberations early in 1980 and ended them in 1983. Its task was to consider several issues raised by the practice of medicine and the distribution of health care. The Commission issued reports on the informed-consent requirement, the definition of death, genetic screening and counseling, the compensation of research subjects, and the distribution of health care. During its life, the Commission included twenty-one commissioners. It was chaired by Morris B. Abraham; its executive director was Alexander Morgan Capron.

The Commission identifies and discusses two values that should guide decision making in the health-care provider-patient relationship: the promotion of a patient's well-being and respect for a patient's self-determination. The Commission locates the ethical foundation of informed consent in the promotion of these two values and makes recommendations intended to ensure that these values are respected and enhanced. In making its recommendations, the Commission rejects the idea that obtaining informed consent is simply a matter of reciting the contents of a form and getting a signature. It sees ethically valid consent as a *process* of shared decision making based on mutual respect and participation. Although stressing the importance of self-determination, the Commission recognizes that some people may be permanently incapable of making their own decisions and that others may be temporarily unable to exercise their right of self-determination. It, therefore, provides some recommendations about making decisions for those unable to do so.

What are the values that ought to guide decisionmaking in the provider-patient relationship or by which the success of a particular interaction can be judged? The Commission finds two to be central: promotion of a patient's well-being and respect for a patient's self-determination.

SERVING THE PATIENT'S WELL-BEING

Therapeutic interventions are intended first and foremost to improve a patient's health. In most circumstances, people agree in a general way on what "improved health" means. Restoration of normal functioning (such as the repair of a fractured limb) and avoidance of untimely death (such as might occur without the use of antibiotics to control life-threatening infections in otherwise healthy persons) are obvious

Reprinted from President's Commission for the Study of Ethical Problems in Medicine and Biomedical and Behavioral Research, *Making Health Care Decisions,* Volume One: Report (1982), pp. 41–46, 2–6.

examples. Health care is, in turn, usually a means of promoting patients' well-being. The connection between a particular health care decision and an individual's well-being is not perfect, however. First, the definition of health can be quite controversial: does wrinkled skin or uncommonly short stature constitute impaired health, such that surgical repair or growth hormone is appropriate? Even more substantial variation can be found in ranking the importance of health with other goals in an individual's life. For some, health is a paramount value; for others—citizens who volunteer in time of war, nurses who care for patients with contagious diseases, hang-glider enthusiasts who risk life and limb—a different goal sometimes has primacy.

Absence of Objective Medical Criteria   Even the most mundane case—in which there is little if any disagreement that some intervention will promote health—may well have no objective medical criteria that specify a single best way to achieve the goal. A fractured limb can be repaired in a number of ways; a life-threatening infection can be treated with a variety of antibiotics; mild diabetes is subject to control by diet, by injectable natural insulin, or by oral synthetic insulin substitutes. Health care professionals often reflect their own value preferences when they favor one alternative over another; many are matters of choice, dictated neither by biomedical principles or data nor by a single, agreed-upon professional standard.

In the Commission's survey it was clear that professionals recognize this fact: physicians maintained that decisional authority between them and their patients should depend on the nature of the decision at hand. Thus, for example, whether a pregnant woman over 35 should have amniocentesis was viewed as largely a patient's decision, whereas the decision of which antibiotic to use for strep throat was seen as primarily up to the doctor. Furthermore, on the question of whether to continue aggressive treatment for a cancer patient with metastases in whom such treatment had already failed, two-thirds of the physicians felt it was not a scientific, medical decision, but one that turned principally on personal values. And the same proportion felt the decision should be made jointly (which 64% of the doctors claimed it usually was).

Patients' Reasonable Subjective Preferences
Determining what constitutes health and how it is best promoted also requires knowledge of patients' subjective preferences. In pursuit of the other goals and interests besides health that society deems legitimate, patients may prefer one type of medical intervention to another, may opt for no treatment at all, or may even request some treatment when a practitioner would prefer to follow a more conservative course that involved, at least for the moment, no medical intervention. For example, a slipped disc may be treated surgically or with medications and bed rest. Which treatment is better can be unclear, even to a physician. A patient may prefer surgery because, despite its greater risks, in the past that individual has spent considerable time in bed and become demoralized and depressed. A person with an injured knee, when told that surgery has about a 30% chance of reducing pain but almost no chance of eliminating it entirely, may prefer to leave the condition untreated. And a baseball pitcher with persistent inflammation of the elbow may prefer to take cortisone on a continuing basis even though the doctor suggests that a new position on the team would eliminate the inflammation permanently. In each case the goals and interests of particular patients incline them in different directions not only as to how, but even as to whether, treatment should proceed.

Given these two considerations—the frequent

absence of objective medical criteria and the legitimate subjective preferences of patients—ascertaining whether a health care intervention will, if successful, promote a patient's well-being is a matter of individual judgment. Societies that respect personal freedom usually reach such decisions by leaving the judgment to the person involved.

The Boundaries of Health Care   This does not mean, however, that well-being and self-determination are really just two terms for the same value. For example, when an individual (such as a newborn baby) is unable to express a choice, the value that guides health care decisionmaking is the promotion of well-being—not necessarily an easy task but also certainly not merely a disguised form of self-determination.

Moreover, the promotion of well-being is an important value even in decisions about patients who can speak for themselves because the boundaries of the interventions that health professionals present for consideration are set by the concept of well-being. Through societal expectations and the traditions of the professions, health care providers are committed to helping patients and to avoiding harm. Thus, the well-being principle circumscribes the range of alternatives offered to patients: informed consent does not mean that patients can insist upon anything they might want. Rather, it is a choice among medically accepted and available options, all of which are believed to have some possibility of promoting the patient's welfare, including always the option of no further medical interventions, even when that would not be viewed as preferable by the health care providers.

In sum, promotion of patient well-being provides the primary warrant for health care. But, as indicated, well-being is not a concrete concept that has a single definition or that is solely within the competency of health care providers to define. Shared decisionmaking requires that a practitioner seek not only to understand each patient's needs and develop reasonable alternatives to meet those needs but also to present the alternatives in a way that enables patients to choose one they prefer. To participate in this process, patients must engage in a dialogue with the practitioner and make their views on well-being clear. The majority of physicians (56%) and the public (64%) surveyed by the Commission felt that increasing the patient's role in medical decisionmaking would improve the quality of health care.[1]

Since well-being can be defined only within each individual's experience, it is in most circumstances congruent to self-determination, to which the Report now turns.

RESPECTING SELF-DETERMINATION

Self-determination (sometimes termed "autonomy") is an individual's exercise of the capacity to form, revise, and pursue personal plans for life. Although it clearly has a much broader application, the relevance of self-determination in health care decisions seems undeniable. A basic reason to honor an individual's choices about health care has already emerged in this Report: under most circumstances the outcome that will best promote the person's well-being rests on a subjective judgment about the individual. This can be termed the instrumental value of self-determination.

More is involved in respect for self-determination than just the belief that each person knows what's best for him- or herself, however. Even if it could be shown that an expert (or a computer) could do the job better, the worth of the individual, as acknowledged in Western ethical traditions and especially in Anglo-American law, provides an independent—and more important—ground for recognizing self-determination as a basic principle in human relations, particularly when matters as important as those raised by health care are at stake. This noninstrumental aspect can be termed the intrinsic value of self-determination.

Intrinsic Value of Self-Determination   The value of self-determination readily emerges if one considers what is lost in its absence. If a physician selects a treatment alternative that satisfies a patient's individual values and goals rather than allowing the patient to choose, the absence of self-determination has not interfered with the promotion of the patient's well-being. But unless the patient has requested this course of conduct, the individual will not have been shown proper respect as a person nor provided with adequate protection against arbitrary, albeit often well-meaning, domination by others. Self-determination can thus be seen as both a shield and a sword.

Freedom from Interference   Self-determination as a shield is valued for the freedom from outside control it is intended to provide. It manifests the wish to be an instrument of one's own and "not of other men's acts of will."[2] In the context of health care, self-determination overrides practitioner-determination even

if providers were able to demonstrate that they could (generally or in a specific instance) accurately assess the treatment an informed patient would choose. To permit action on the basis of a professional's assessment rather than on a patient's choice would deprive the patient of the freedom not to be forced to do something—whether or not that person would agree with the choice. Moreover, denying self-determination in this way risks generating the frustration people feel when their desires are ignored or countermanded. . . .

SUMMARY OF CONCLUSIONS AND RECOMMENDATIONS

. . . The ethical foundation of informed consent can be traced to the promotion of two values: personal well-being and self-determination. To ensure that these values are respected and enhanced, the Commission finds that patients who have the capacity to make decisions about their care must be permitted to do so voluntarily and must have all relevant information regarding their condition and alternative treatments, including possible benefits, risks, costs, other consequences, and significant uncertainties surrounding any of this information. This conclusion has several specific implications:

1. Although the informed consent doctrine has substantial foundations in law, it is essentially an ethical imperative.

2. Ethically valid consent is a process of shared decisionmaking based upon mutual respect and participation, not a ritual to be equated with reciting the contents of a form that details the risks of particular treatments.

3. Much of the scholarly literature and legal commentary about informed consent portrays it as a highly rational means of decisionmaking about health care matters, thereby suggesting that it may only be suitable for and applicable to well-educated, articulate, self-aware individuals. Whether this is what the legal doctrine was intended to be or what it has inadvertently become, it is a view the Commission unequivocally rejects. Although subcultures within American society differ in their views about autonomy and individual choice and about the etiology of illness and the roles of healers and patients,[3] a survey conducted for the Commis-

sion found a universal desire for information, choice, and respectful communication about decisions.[4] Informed consent must remain flexible, yet the process, as the Commission envisions it throughout this Report, is ethically required of health care practitioners in their relationships with all patients, not a luxury for a few.

4. Informed consent is rooted in the fundamental recognition—reflected in the legal presumption of competency—that adults are entitled to accept or reject health care interventions on the basis of their own personal values and in furtherance of their own personal goals. Nonetheless, patient choice is not absolute.

• Patients are not entitled to insist that health care practitioners furnish them services when to do so would violate either the bounds of acceptable practice or a professional's own deeply held moral beliefs or would draw on a limited resource on which the patient has no binding claim.

• The fundamental values that informed consent is intended to promote—self-determination and patient well-being—both demand that alternative arrangements for health care decisionmaking be made for individuals who lack substantial capacity to make their own decisions. Respect for self-determination requires, however, that in the first instance individuals be deemed to have decisional capacity, which should not be treated as a hurdle to be surmounted in the vast majority of cases, and that incapacity be treated as a disqualifying factor in the small minority of cases.

• Decisionmaking capacity is specific to each particular decision. Although some people lack this capacity for all decisions, many are incapacitated in more limited ways and are capable of making some decisions but not others. The concept of capacity is best understood and applied in a functional manner. That is, the presence or absence of capacity does not depend on a person's status or on the decision reached, but on that individual's actual functioning in situations in which a decision about health care is to be made.

• Decisionmaking incapacity should be found to exist only when people lack the ability to make decisions that promote their well-being in con-

formity with their own previously expressed values and preferences.

• To the extent feasible people with no decisionmaking capacity should still be consulted about their own preferences out of respect for them as individuals.

5. Health care providers should not ordinarily withhold unpleasant information simply because it is unpleasant. The ethical foundations of informed consent allow the withholding of information from patients only when they request that it be withheld or when its disclosure per se would cause substantial detriment to their well-being. Furthermore, the Commission found that most members of the public do not wish to have "bad news" withheld from them.

6. Achieving the Commission's vision of shared decisionmaking based on mutual respect is ultimately the responsibility of individual health care professionals. However, health care institutions such as hospitals and professional schools have important roles to play in assisting health care professionals in this obligation. The manner in which health care is provided in institutional settings often results in a fragmentation of responsibility that may neglect the human side of health care. To assist in guarding against this, institutional health care providers should ensure that ultimately there is one readily identifiable practitioner responsible for providing information to a particular patient. Although pieces of information may be provided by various people, there should be one individual officially charged with responsibility for ensuring that all the necessary information is communicated and that the patient's wishes are known to the treatment team.

7. Patients should have access to the information they need to help them understand their conditions and make treatment decisions. To this end the Commission recommends that health care professionals and institutions not only provide information but also assist patients who request additional information to obtain it from relevant sources, including hospital and public libraries.

8. As cases arise and new legislation is contemplated, courts and legislatures should reflect

this view of ethically valid consent. Nevertheless, the Commission does not look to legal reforms as the primary means of bringing about changes in the relationship between health care professionals and patients.

9. The Commission finds that a number of relatively simple changes in practice could facilitate patient participation in health care decisionmaking. Several specific techniques—such as having patients express, orally or in writing, their understanding of the treatment consented to—deserve further study. Furthermore, additional societal resources need to be committed to improving the human side of health care, which has apparently deteriorated at the same time there have been substantial gains in health care technology. The Department of Health and Human Services, and especially the National Institutes of Health, is an appropriate agency for the development of initiatives and the evaluation of their efficacy in this area.

10. Because health care professionals are responsible for ensuring that patients can participate effectively in decisionmaking regarding their care, educators have a responsibility to prepare physicians and nurses to carry out this obligation. The Commission therefore concludes that:

- Curricular innovations aimed at preparing health professionals for a process of mutual decisionmaking with patients should be continued and strengthened, with careful attention being paid to the development of methods for evaluating the effectiveness of such innovations.
- Examinations and evaluations at the professional school and national levels should reflect the importance of these issues.
- Serious attention should be paid to preparing health professionals for team practice in order to enhance patient participation and well-being.

11. Family members are often of great assistance to patients in helping to understand information about their condition and in making decisions about treatment. The Commission recommends that health care institutions and professionals recognize this and judiciously attempt to involve family members in decisionmaking for patients, with due regard for the privacy of patients and for the possibilities for coercion that such a practice may entail.

12. The Commission recognizes that its vision of health care decisionmaking may involve greater commitments of time on the part of health professionals. Because of the importance of shared decisionmaking based on mutual trust, not only for the promotion of patient well-being and self-determination but also for the therapeutic gains that can be realized, the Commission recommends that all medical and surgical interventions be thought of as including appropriate discussion with patients. Reimbursement to the professional should therefore take account of time spent in discussion rather than regarding it as a separate item for which additional payment is made.

13. To protect the interests of patients who lack decisionmaking capacity and to ensure their well-being and self-determination, the Commission concludes that:

- Decisions made by others on patients' behalf should, when possible, attempt to replicate the ones patients would make if they were capable of doing so. When this is not feasible, decisions by surrogates on behalf of patients must protect the patients' best interests. Because such decisions are not instances of personal self-choice, limits may be placed on the range of acceptable decisions that surrogates make beyond those that apply when a person makes his or her own decisions.
- Health care institutions should adopt clear and explicit policies regarding how and by whom decisions are to be made for patients who cannot decide.
- Families, health care institutions, and professionals should work together to make health care decisions for patients who lack decisionmaking capacity. Recourse to courts should be reserved for the occasions when concerned parties are unable to resolve their disagreements over matters of substantial import, or when adjudication is clearly required by state law. Courts and legislatures should be cautious about requiring judicial review of routine health care decisions for patients who lack capacity.

- Health care institutions should explore and evaluate various informal administrative arrangements, such as "ethics committees," for review and consultation in nonroutine matters involving health care decisionmaking for those who cannot decide.
- As a means of preserving some self-determination for patients who no longer possess decisionmaking capacity, state courts and legislatures should consider making provision for advance directives through which people designate others to make health care decisions on their behalf and/or give instructions about their care.

The Commission acknowledges that the conclusions contained in this Report will not be simple to achieve. Even when patients and practitioners alike are sensitive to the goal of shared decisionmaking based on mutual respect, substantial barriers will still exist. Some of these obstacles, such as long-standing professional attitudes or difficulties in conveying medical information in ordinary language, are formidable but can be overcome if there is a will to do so. Others, such as the dependent condition of very sick patients or the ever-growing complexity and subspecialization of medicine, will have to be accommodated because they probably cannot be eliminated. Nonetheless, the Commission's vision of informed consent still has value as a measuring stick against which actual performance may be judged and as a goal toward which all participants in health care decisionmaking can strive. . . .

NOTES

1 Many physicians and patients said they believed an increased patient role would give the patient a better understanding of the medical condition and treatment, would improve physician performance in terms of the honesty and scope of discussion, and would generally improve the doctor-patient relationship. However, a number of physicians claimed that greater patient involvement would improve the quality of care because it would improve compliance and would make patients more cooperative and willing to accept the doctor's judgment.

2 Isaiah Berlin, "Two Concepts of Liberty," in *Four Essays on Liberty,* Clarendon Press, Oxford (1969) at 118–38.

3 Robert A. Hahn, *Culture and Informed Consent: An Anthropological Perspective* (1982), Appendix F, in Volume Three of this Report.

4 The Commission's survey of the public broke down these responses on the basis of variables such as age, gender, race, education, and income.

Transparency: Informed Consent in Primary Care
Howard Brody

A biographical sketch of Howard Brody is found on page 83.

Brody argues that accepted legal standards of informed consent, as commonly employed by the courts, give physicians the unhelpful message that informed consent is essentially a legalistic exercise intruding upon good medical care—an impression especially likely in the context of primary-care medicine. An alternative that would send physicians the right message, a "conversation" standard, is probably not legally workable, according to the author. Brody contends that a compromise, the "transparency" standard, sets reasonable obligations for physicians and permits courts to review appropriately. According to this standard, disclo-

Reprinted with permission of the author and the publisher from *Hastings Center Report*, vol. 19 (September–October 1989), pp. 5–9. © The Hastings Center.

sure is considered adequate when the physician's basic thinking has been made transparent to the patient.

While the patient's right to give informed consent to medical treatment is now well-established both in U.S. law and in biomedical ethics, evidence continues to suggest that the concept has been poorly integrated into American medical practice, and that in many instances the needs and desires of patients are not being well met by current policies.[1] It appears that the theory and the practice of informed consent are out of joint in some crucial ways. This is particularly true for primary care settings, a context typically ignored by medical ethics literature, but where the majority of doctor-patient encounters occur. Indeed, some have suggested that the concept of informed consent is virtually foreign to primary care medicine where benign paternalism appropriately reigns and where respect for patient autonomy is almost completely absent.[2]

It is worth asking whether current legal standards for informed consent tend to resolve the problem or to exacerbate it. I will maintain that accepted legal standards, at least in the form commonly employed by courts, send physicians the wrong message about what is expected of them. An alternative standard that would send physicians the correct message, a conversation standard, is probably unworkable legally. As an alternative, I will propose a transparency standard as a compromise that gives physicians a doable task and allows courts to review appropriately. I must begin, however, by briefly identifying some assumptions crucial to the development of this position even though space precludes complete argumentation and documentation.

CRUCIAL ASSUMPTIONS

Informed consent is a meaningful ethical concept only to the extent that it can be realized and promoted within the ongoing practice of good medicine. This need not imply diminished respect for patient autonomy, for there are excellent reasons to regard respect for patient autonomy as a central feature of good medical care. Informed consent, properly understood, must be considered an essential ingredient of good patient care, and a physician who lacks the skills to inform patients appropriately and obtain proper consent should be viewed as lacking essential medical skills necessary for practice. It

is not enough to see informed consent as a nonmedical, legalistic exercise designed to promote patient autonomy, one that interrupts the process of medical care.

However, available empirical evidence strongly suggests that this is precisely how physicians currently view informed consent practices. Informed consent is still seen as bureaucratic legalism rather than as part of patient care. Physicians often deny the existence of realistic treatment alternatives, thereby attenuating the perceived need to inform the patient of meaningful options. While patients may be informed, efforts are seldom made to assess accurately the patient's actual need or desire for information, or what the patient then proceeds to do with the information provided. Physicians typically underestimate patients' desire to be informed and overestimate their desire to be involved in decision-making. Physicians may also view informed consent as an empty charade, since they are confident in their abilities to manipulate consent by how they discuss or divulge information.[3]

A third assumption is that there are important differences between the practice of primary care medicine and the tertiary care settings that have been most frequently discussed in the literature on informed consent. The models of informed consent discussed below typically take as the paradigm case something like surgery for breast cancer or the performance of an invasive and risky radiologic procedure. It is assumed that the risks to the patient are significant, and the values placed on alternative forms of treatment are quite weighty. Moreover, it is assumed that the specialist physician performing the procedure probably does a fairly limited number of procedures and thus could be expected to know exhaustively the precise risks, benefits, and alternatives for each.

Primary care medicine, however, fails to fit this model. The primary care physician, instead of performing five or six complicated and risky procedures frequently, may engage in several hundred treatment modalities during an average week of practice. In many cases, risks to the patient are negligible and conflicts over patient values and the goals of treatment or nontreatment are of little consequence. Moreover, in contrast to the tertiary care patient, the typical ambulatory patient is much better able to exercise freedom of choice and somewhat less likely to be intimidated by either the severity of the disease or the expertise of the physician; the opportunities for changing one's mind once treatment has begun are also much greater. Indeed, in primary care, it is much more likely for the full process of informed consent to treatment (such as the beginning and the dose adjustment of an anti-hypertensive medication) to occur over several office visits rather than at one single point in time.

It might be argued that for all these reasons, the stakes are so low in primary care that it is fully appropriate for informed consent to be interpreted only with regard to the specialized or tertiary care setting. I believe that this is quite incorrect for three reasons. First, good primary care medicine ought to embrace respect for patient autonomy, and if patient autonomy is operationalized in informed consent, properly understood, then it ought to be part and parcel of good primary care. Second, the claim that the primary care physician cannot be expected to obtain the patient's informed consent seems to undermine the idea that informed consent could or ought to be part of the daily practice of medicine. Third, primary care encounters are statistically more common than the highly specialized encounters previously used as models for the concept of informed consent.[4]

ACCEPTED LEGAL STANDARDS

Most of the literature on legal approaches to informed consent addresses the tension between the community practice standard and the reasonable patient standard, with the latter seen as the more satisfactory, emerging legal standard.[5] However, neither standard sends the proper message to the physician about what is expected of her to promote patient autonomy effectively and to serve the informational needs of patients in daily practice.

The community practice standard sends the wrong message because it leaves the door open too wide for physician paternalism. The physician is instructed to behave as other physicians in that specialty behave, regardless of how well or how poorly that behavior serves patients' needs. Certainly, behaving the way other physicians behave is a task we might expect physicians to readily accomplish; unfortunately, the standard fails to inform them of the end toward which the task is aimed.

The reasonable patient standard does a much better job of indicating the centrality of respect for patient autonomy and the desired outcome of the informed consent process, which is revealing the information that a reasonable person would need to make an informed and rational decision. This standard is particularly valuable when modified to include the specific informational and decisional needs of a particular patient.

If certain things were true about the relationship between medicine and law in today's society, the reasonable patient standard would provide acceptable guidance to physicians. One feature would be that physicians esteem the law as a positive force in guiding their practice, rather than as a threat to their well-being that must be handled defensively. Another element would be a prospective consideration by the law of what the physician could reasonably have been expected to do in practice, rather than a retrospective review armed with the foreknowledge that some significant patient harm has already occurred.

Unfortunately, given the present legal climate, the physician is much more likely to get a mixed or an undesirable message from the reasonable patient standard. The message the physician hears from the reasonable patient standard is that one must exhaustively lay out all possible risks as well as benefits and alternatives of the proposed procedure. If one remembers to discuss fifty possible risks, and the patient in a particular case suffers the fifty-first, the physician might subsequently be found liable for incomplete disclosure. Since lawsuits are triggered when patients suffer harm, disclosure of risk becomes relatively more important than disclosure of benefits. Moreover, disclosure of information becomes much more critical than effective patient participation in decisionmaking. Physicians consider it more important to document what they said to the patient than to document how the patient used or thought about that information subsequently.

In specialty practice, many of these concerns can be nicely met by detailed written or videotaped consent documents, which can provide the depth of information required while still putting the benefits and alternatives in proper context. This is workable when one engages in a limited number of procedures and can have a complete document or videotape for each.[6] However, this approach is not feasible for primary care, when the number of procedures may be much more numerous and the time available with each patient may be considerably less. Moreover, it is simply not realistic to expect even the best educated of primary care physicians to rattle off at a moment's notice a detailed list of significant risks attached to any of the many drugs and therapeutic modalities they recommend.

This sets informed consent apart from all other aspects of medical practice in a way that I believe is widely perceived by nonpaternalistic primary care physicians, but which is almost never commented upon in the medical ethics literature. To the physician obtaining informed consent, *you never know when you are finished.* When a primary care physician is told to treat a patient for strep throat or to counsel a person suffering a normal grief reaction from the recent death of a relative, the physician has a good sense of what it means to complete the task at hand. When a physician is told to obtain the patient's informed consent for a medical intervention, the impression is quite different. A list of as many possible risks as can be thought of may still omit some significant ones. A list of all the risks that actually have occurred may still not have dealt with the patient's need to know risks in relation to benefits and alternatives. A description of all benefits, risks, and alternatives may not establish whether the patient has understood the information. If the patient says he understands, the physician has to wonder whether he really understands or whether he is simply saying this to be accommodating. As the law currently *appears* to operate (in the perception of the defensively minded physician), there never comes a point at which you can be certain that you have adequately completed your legal as well as your ethical task.

The point is not simply that physicians are paranoid about the law; more fundamentally, physicians are getting a message that informed consent is very different from any other task they are asked to perform in medicine. If physicians conclude that informed consent is therefore not properly part of medicine at all, but is rather a legalistic and bureaucratic hurdle they must overcome at their own peril, blame cannot be attributed to paternalistic attitudes or lack of respect for patient autonomy.

THE CONVERSATION MODEL

A metaphor employed by Jay Katz, informed consent as conversation, provides an approach to respect for patient autonomy that can be readily integrated within primary care practice.[7] Just as the specific needs of an individual patient for information, or the meaning that patient will attach to the information as it is presented, cannot be known in advance, one cannot always tell in advance how a conversation is going to turn out. One must follow the process along and take one's cues from the unfolding conversation itself. Despite the absence of any formal rules for carrying out or completing a conversation on a specific subject, most people have a good intuitive grasp of what it means for a conversation to be finished, what it means to change the subject in the middle of a conversation, and what it means to later reopen a conversation one had thought was completed when something new has just arisen. Thus, the metaphor suggests that informed consent consists not in a formal process carried out strictly by protocol but in a conversation designed to encourage patient participation in all medical decisions to the extent that the patient wishes to be included. The idea of informed consent as physician-patient conversation could, when properly developed, be a useful analytic tool for ethical issues in informed consent, and could also be a powerful educational tool for highlighting the skills and attitudes that a physician needs to successfully integrate this process within patient care.

If primary care physicians understand informed consent as this sort of conversation process, the idea that exact rules cannot be given for its successful management could cease to be a mystery. Physicians would instead be guided to rely on their own intuitions and communication skills, with careful attention to information received from the patient, to determine when an adequate job had been done in the informed consent process. Moreover, physicians would be encouraged to see informed consent as a genuinely mutual and participatory process, instead of being reduced to the one-way disclosure of information. In effect, informed consent could be demystified, and located within the context of the everyday relationships between physician and patient, albeit with a renewed emphasis on patient participation.[8]

Unfortunately, the conversation metaphor does not lend itself to ready translation into a legal standard for determining whether or not the physician has satisfied her basic responsibilities to the patient. There seems to be an inherently subjective element to conversation that makes it ill-suited as a legal standard for review of controversial cases. A conversation in which one participates is by its nature a very different thing from the same conversation described to an outsider. It is hard to imagine how a jury could be instructed to determine in retrospect whether or not a particular conversation was adequate for its purposes. However, without the possibility for legal review, the message that patient autonomy is an important value and that patients have important rights within primary care would seem to be severely undermined. The question then is whether some of the important strengths of the conversation model can be retained in another model that does allow better guidance.

THE TRANSPARENCY STANDARD

I propose the transparency standard as a means to operationalize the best features of the conversation model in medical practice. According to this standard, adequate informed consent is obtained when a reasonably informed patient is allowed to participate in the medical decision to the extent that patient wishes. In turn, "reasonably informed" consists of two features: (1) the physician discloses the basis on which the proposed treatment, or alternative possible treatments, have been chosen; and (2) the patient is allowed to ask questions suggested by the disclosure of the physician's reasoning, and those questions are answered to the patient's satisfaction.

According to the transparency model, the key to reasonable disclosure is not adherence to existing standards of other practitioners, nor is it adherence to a list of risks that a hypothetical reasonable patient would want to know. Instead, disclosure is adequate when the physician's basic thinking has been rendered transparent to the patient. If the physician arrives at a recommended therapeutic or diagnostic intervention only after carefully examining a list of risks and benefits, then rendering the physician's thinking transparent requires that those risks and benefits be detailed for the patient. If the physician's thinking has not followed that route but has reached its conclusion by other considerations, then what needs to be disclosed to the patient is accordingly different. Essentially, the transparency standard requires the physician to engage in the typical patient-management thought process, only to *do it out loud in language understandable to the patient.*[9]

To see how this might work in practice, consider the following as possible general decision-making strategies that might be used by a primary physician:

1. The intervention, in addition to being presumably low-risk, is also routine and automatic. The physician, faced with a case like that presented by the patient, almost always chooses this treatment.

2. The decision is not routine but seems to offer clear benefit with minimal risk.

3. The proposed procedure offers substantial chances for benefit, but also very substantial risks.

4. The proposed intervention offers substantial risks and extremely questionable benefits. Unfortunately, possible alternative courses of action also have high risk and uncertain benefit.

The exact risks entailed by treatment loom much larger in the physician's own thinking in cases 3 and 4 than in cases 1 and 2. The transparency standard would require that physicians at least mention the various risks to patients in scenarios 3 and 4, but would not necessarily require physicians exhaustively to describe risks, unless the patient asked, in scenarios 1 and 2.

The transparency standard seems to offer some considerable advantages for informing physicians what can legitimately be expected of them in the promotion of patient autonomy while carrying out the activities of primary care medicine. We would hope that the well-trained primary care physician generally thinks before acting. On that assumption, the physician can be told exactly when she is finished obtaining informed consent—first, she has to share her thinking with the patient; secondly, she has to encourage and answer questions; and third, she has to discover how participatory he wishes to be and facilitate that level of participation. This seems a much more reasonable task within primary care than an exhaustive listing of often irrelevant risk factors.

There are also considerable advantages for the patient in this approach. The patient retains the right to ask for an exhaustive recital of risks and alternatives. However, the vast majority of patients, in a primary care setting particularly, would wish to supplement a standardized recital of risks and benefits of treatment with some questions like, "Yes, doctor, but what does this really mean for me? What meaning am I supposed to attach to the information that you've just given?" For example, in scenarios 1 and 2, the precise and specific risk probabilities and possibilities are very small considerations in the thinking of the physician, and reciting an exhaustive list of risks would seriously misstate just what the physician was thinking. If the physician did detail a laundry list of risk factors, the patient might very well ask, "Well, doctor, just what should I think about what you have just told me?" and the thoughtful and concerned physician might well reply, "There's certainly a small possibility that one of these bad things will happen to you; but I think the chance is extremely remote and in my own practice I have never seen anything like that occur." The patient is very likely to give much more weight to that statement, putting the risks in perspective, than he is to the listing of risks. And that emphasis corresponds with an understanding of how the physician herself has reached the decision.

The transparency standard should further facilitate and encourage useful questions from patients. If a patient is given a routine list of risks and benefits and then is asked "Do you have any questions?" the response may well be perfunctory and automatic. If the patient is told precisely the grounds on which the physician has made her recommendation, and then asked the same question, the response is much more likely to be individualized and meaningful.

There certainly would be problems in applying the transparency standard in the courtroom, but these do not appear to be materially more difficult than those encountered in applying other standards; moreover, this standard could call attention to more important features in the ethical relationship between physician and patient. Consider the fairly typical case, in which a patient suffers harm from the occurrence of a rare but predictable complication of a procedure, and then claims that he would not have consented had he known about that risk. Under the present "enlightened" court standards, the jury would examine whether a reasonable patient would have needed to know about that risk factor prior to making a decision on the proposed intervention. Under the transparency standard, the question would instead be whether the physician thought about that risk factor as a relevant consideration prior to recommending the course of action to the patient. If the physician did seriously consider that risk factor, but failed to reveal that to the patient, he was in effect making up the patient's mind in advance about what risks were worth accepting. In that situation, the physician could easily be held liable. If, on the other hand, that risk was considered too insignificant to play a role in determining which intervention ought to be performed, the physician may still have rendered his thinking completely transparent to the patient even though that specific risk factor was not mentioned. In this circumstance, the physician would be held to have done an adequate job of disclosing information.[10] A question would still exist as to whether a competent physician ought to have known about that risk factor and ought to have considered it more carefully prior to doing the procedure. But that question raises the issue of negligence, which is where such considerations properly belong, and removes the problem from the context of informed consent. Obviously, the standard of informed consent is misapplied if it is intended by itself to prevent the practice of negligent medicine.

TRANSPARENCY IN MEDICAL PRACTICE

Will adopting a legal standard like transparency change medical practice for the better? Ultimately only empirical research will answer this question. We know almost nothing about the sorts of conversations primary care physicians now have with their patients, or what would happen if these physicians routinely tried harder to share their basic thinking about therapeutic choices. In this setting it is possible to argue that the transparency standard will have deleterious effects. Perhaps the physician's basic thinking will fail to include risk issues that patients, from their perspective, would regard as substantial. Perhaps how physicians think about therapeutic choice will prove to be too idiosyncratic and variable to serve as any sort of standard. Perhaps disclosing basic thinking processes will impede rather than promote optimal patient participation in decisions.

But the transparency standard must be judged, not only against ideal medical practice, but also against the present-day standard and the message it sends to practitioners. I have argued that that message is, "You can protect yourself legally only by guessing all bad outcomes that might occur and warning each patient explicitly that he might suffer any of them." The transparency standard is an attempt to send the message, "You can protect yourself legally by conversing with your patients in a way that promotes their participation in medical decisions, and more specifically by making sure that they see the basic reasoning you used to arrive at the recommended treatment." It seems at least plausible to me that the attempt is worth making.

The reasonable person standard may still be the best way to view informed consent in highly specialized settings where a relatively small number of discrete and potentially risky procedures are the daily order of business. In primary care settings, the best ethical advice we can give physicians is to view informed consent as an ongoing process of conversation designed to maximize patient participation after adequately revealing the key facts. Because the conversation metaphor does not by itself suggest measures for later judicial review, a transparency standard, or something like it, may be a reasonable way to operationalize that concept in primary care practice. Some positive side-effects of this might be more focus on good diagnostic and therapeutic decisionmaking on the physician's part, since it will be understood that the patient will be made aware of what the physician's reasoning process has been like, and better documentation of management decisions in the patient record. If these occur, then it will be clearer that the standard of informed consent has promoted rather than impeded high quality patient care.

ACKNOWLEDGMENTS

I plan to develop these ideas at somewhat greater length, with special emphasis on the duty to disclose remote risks, in a volume to be titled *The Healer's Power* (in preparation). I am grateful to Margaret Wallace and Stephen Wear for their insightful comments during the preparation of this manuscript.

REFERENCES

1 Charles W. Lidz *et al.*, "Barriers to Informed Consent," *Annals of Internal Medicine* 99:4 (1983), 539–43.
2 Tom L. Beauchamp and Laurence McCullough, *Medical Ethics: The Moral Responsibilities of Physicians* (Englewood Cliffs, NJ: Prentice-Hall, 1984).
3 For a concise overview of empirical data about contemporary informed consent practices see Ruth R. Faden and Tom L. Beauchamp, *A History and Theory of Informed Consent* (New York: Oxford University Press, 1986), 98–99 and associated footnotes.
4 For efforts to address ethical aspects of primary care practice, see Ronald J. Christie and Barry Hoffmaster, *Ethical Issues in Family Medicine* (New York: Oxford University Press, 1986); and Harmon L. Smith and Larry R. Churchill, *Professional Ethics and Primary Care Medicine* (Durham, NC: Duke University Press, 1986).
5 Faden and Beauchamp, *A History and Theory of Informed Consent,* 23–49 and 114–50. I have also greatly benefited from an unpublished paper by Margaret Wallace.
6 For a specialty opinion to the contrary, see W. H. Coles *et al.*, "Teaching Informed Consent," in *Further Developments in Assessing Clinical Competence,* Ian R. Hart and Ronald M. Harden, eds. (Montreal: Can-Heal Publications, 1987), 241–70. This paper is interesting in applying to specialty care a model very much like the one I propose for primary care.
7 Jay Katz, *The Silent World of Doctor and Patient* (New York: Free Press, 1984).
8 Howard Brody, *Stories of Sickness* (New Haven: Yale University Press, 1987), 171–81.
9 For an interesting study of physicians' practices on this point, see William C. Wu and Robert A. Pearlman, "Consent in Medical Decisionmaking: The Role of Communication," *Journal of General Internal Medicine* 3:1 (1988), 9–14.
10 A court case that might point the way toward this line of reasoning is *Precourt v. Frederick,* 395 Mass. 689 (1985). See William J. Curran, "Informed Consent in Malpractice Cases: A Turn Toward Reality," *New England Journal of Medicine* 314:7 (1986), 429–31.

Determinations of Competence

Standards of Competence

Allen E. Buchanan and Dan W. Brock

Allen E. Buchanan is professor of business, philosophy, and medical ethics at the University of Wisconsin, Madison. He is the author of *Marx and Justice: The Radical Critique of Liberalism* (1982) and *Ethics, Efficiency, and the Market* (1982). Dan W. Brock is professor of philosophy and biomedical ethics at Brown University, where he is also director of the Center for Biomedical Ethics. Many of his articles are collected in *Life and Death: Philosophical Essays in Biomedical Ethics* (1993). Buchanan and Brock both served on the staff of the President's

Reprinted with the permission of Cambridge University Press from *Deciding for Others: The Ethics of Surrogate Decision Making,* pp. 48–57. © 1989, Cambridge University Press.

Commission for the Study of Ethical Problems in Medicine and Biomedical and Behavioral Research. They are the coauthors of *Deciding for Others* (1989), from which this selection is reprinted.

Buchanan and Brock argue that an adequate standard for evaluating a patient's competence must focus on the process of reasoning leading up to a patient's medical decision, rather than on the decision itself. According to the authors, competence evaluations must strike a balance between the values of (1) patient self-determination and (2) patient well-being (specifically, protecting patients from harm that might result from their own choices). Because both the importance to the patient of self-determination and the degree of expected harm from an unfortunate choice can vary greatly from case to case, Buchanan and Brock argue that no single standard of competence is appropriate for all decisions. They offer several examples of how self-determination and well-being can be balanced in specific cases to set appropriate standards of competence.

[I.] DIFFERENT STANDARDS OF COMPETENCE

A number of different standards of competence have been identified and supported in the literature, although statutory and case law provide little help in articulating precise standards.[1] It is neither feasible nor necessary to discuss here all the alternatives that have been proposed. Instead, the range of alternatives will be delineated and the difficulties of the main standards will be examined in order to clarify and defend [our decision-relative analysis.] More or less stringent standards of competence in effect strike different balances between the values of patient well-being and self-determination.

A. A Minimal Standard of Competence

An example of a minimal standard of competence is that the patient merely be able to express a preference. This standard respects every expressed choice of a patient, and so is not in fact a criterion of *competent* choice at all.[2] It entirely disregards whether defects or mistakes are present in the reasoning process leading to the choice, whether the choice is in accord with the patient's own conception of his or her good, and whether the choice would be harmful to the patient. It thus fails to provide any protection for patient well-being, and it is insensitive to the way the value of self-determination itself varies both with the nature of the decision to be made and with differences in people's capacities to choose in accordance with their conceptions of their own good.

B. An Outcome Standard of Competence

At the other extreme are standards that look solely to the *content* or *outcome* of the decision—for example, the standard that the choice be a reasonable one, or be what other reasonable or rational persons would choose. On this view, failure of the patient's choice to match some such allegedly objective outcome standard of choice entails that it is an incompetent choice. Such a standard maximally protects patient well-being—although only according to the standard's conception of well-being—but fails adequately to respect patient self-determination.

At bottom, a person's interest in self-determination is his or her interest in defining, revising over time, and pursuing his or her own particular conception of the good life. [With so-called ideal or objective] theories of the good for persons, there are serious practical or fallibilist risks associated with any purportedly objective standard for the correct decision—the standard may ignore the patient's own distinctive conception of the good and may constitute enforcement of unjustified ideals or unjustifiably substitute another's conception of what is best for the patient. Moreover, even such a standard's theoretical claim to protect maximally a patient's well-being is only as strong as the objective account of a person's well-being on which the standard rests. Many proponents of ideal theories only assert the ideals and fail even to recognize the need for justifying them, much less proceed to do so.

Although ascertaining the correct or best theory of individual well-being or the good for persons is a complex and controversial task, . . . any standard of individual well-being that does not ultimately rest on an individual's own underlying and enduring aims and values is both problematic in theory and subject to intolerable abuse in practice. There may be room in some broad policy decisions or overall theories of justice for more "objective" and interpersonal measures of well-being that fail fully to reflect differences in individuals' own views of their well-being,[3] but we believe there is *much less room* for such purportedly objective measures in the kind of judgments of concern here—judgments about appropriate treatment for an individual patient. Thus, a standard that judges competence by comparing the content of a patient's decision to some objective standard for the correct decision may fail even to protect appropriately a patient's well-being.

C. A Process Standard of Decision-Making Competence

An adequate standard of competence will focus primarily not on the content of the patient's decision but on the *process* of the reasoning that leads up to that decision. There are two central questions for any process standard of competence. First, a process standard must set a level of reasoning required for the patient to be competent. In other words, how well must the patient understand and reason to be competent? How much can understanding be limited or reasoning be defective and still be compatible with competence? The second question often passes without explicit notice by those evaluating competence. How certain must those persons evaluating competence be about how well the patient has understood and reasoned in coming to a decision? This second question is important because it is common in cases of marginal or questionable competence for there to be a significant degree of uncertainty about the patient's reasoning and decision-making process that can never be eliminated.

[II.] RELATION OF THE PROCESS STANDARD OF COMPETENCE TO EXPECTED HARMS AND BENEFITS

Because the competence evaluation requires striking a balance between the two values of respecting patients' rights to decide for themselves and protecting them from the harmful consequences of their own choices, it should be clear that no single standard of competence— no single answer to the questions above—can be ade-

quate for all decisions. This is true because (1) the degree of expected harm from choices made at a given level of understanding and reasoning can vary from none to the most serious, including major disability or death, and because (2) the importance or value to the patient of self-determination can vary depending on the choice being made.

There is an important implication of this view that the standard of competence ought to vary in part with the expected harms or benefits to the patient of acting in accordance with the patient's choice—namely, that just because a patient is competent to consent to a treatment, it does *not* follow that the patient is competent to refuse it, and vice versa. For example, consent to a low-risk lifesaving procedure by an otherwise healthy individual should require only a minimal level of competence, but refusal of that same procedure by such an individual should require the highest level of competence.

Because the appropriate level of competence properly required for a particular decision must be adjusted to the consequences of acting on that decision, no single standard of decision-making competence is adequate. Instead, the level of competence appropriately required for decision making varies along a full range from low/minimal to high/maximal. Table 1 illustrates this variation, with the treatment choices listed used only as examples of any treatment choice with that relative risk/benefit assessment.

The net balance of expected benefits and risks of the patient's choice in comparison with other alternatives will usually be determined by the physician. This assessment should focus on the expected effects of a particular treatment option in forwarding the patient's underlying and enduring aims and values, to the extent that these are known. When the patient's aims and values are not known, the risk/benefit assessment will balance the expected effects of a particular treatment option in achieving the general goals of health care in prolonging life, preventing injury and disability, and relieving suffering as against its risks of harm. The table indicates that the relevant comparison is with other available alternatives, and the degree to which the net benefit/risk balance of the alternative chosen is better or worse than that for optimal alternative treatment options. It should be noted that a choice might properly require only low/minimal competence, even though its expected risks exceed its expected benefits or it is more generally a high-risk treatment, because all other available alternatives have substantially worse risk/benefit ratios.

Table 1 also indicates, for each level of competence, the relative importance of different *grounds* for believing that a patient's own choice best promotes his or her well-being. This brings out an important point. For *all* patient choices, other people responsible for deciding whether those choices should be respected should have grounds for believing that the choice, if it is to be honored, is reasonably in accord with the patient's well-being (although the choice need not, of course, *maximally* promote the patient's interests). When the patient's level of decision-making competence need be only at the low/minimal level, as in the agreement to a lumbar puncture for presumed meningitis, these grounds derive only minimally from the fact that the patient has chosen the option in question; they principally stem from others' positive assessment of the choice's expected effects on the patient's well-being.

At the other extreme, when the expected effects of the patient's choice for his or her well-being appear to be substantially worse than available alternatives, as in the refusal of a simple appendectomy, the requirement of a high/maximal level of competence provides grounds for relying on the patient's decision as itself establishing that the choice best fits the patient's good (his or her own underlying and enduring aims and values). The highest level of competence should assure that no significant mistakes in the patient's reasoning and decision making are present, and is required to rebut the presumption that the choice is not in fact reasonably related to the patient's interests.

When the expected effects for the patient's well-being of his or her choice are approximately comparable to those of alternatives, as in the choice of a lumpectomy for treatment of breast cancer, a moderate/median level of competence is sufficient to provide reasonable grounds that the choice promotes the patient's good and that her well-being is adequately protected. It is also reasonable to assume that as the level of competence required increases (from minimal to maximal), the instrumental value or importance of respecting the patient's self-determination increases as well, specifically the part of the value of self-determination that rests on the assumption that persons will secure their good when they choose for themselves. As competence increases, other things being equal, the likelihood of this happening increases.

Thus, according to the concept of competence endorsed here, a particular individual's decision-making

TABLE 1   Decision-Making Competence and Patient Well-Being

The patient's treatment choice	Others' risk/ benefit assessment of that choice in comparison with other alternatives	Level of decision-making competence required	Grounds for believing patient's choice best promotes/protects own well-being.
Patient consents to lumbar puncture for presumed meningitis	Net balance substantially better than for possible alternatives	Low/minimal	Principally the benefit/risk assessment made by others
Patient chooses lumpectomy for breast cancer	Net balance roughly comparable to that of other alternatives	Moderate/median	Roughly equally from the benefit/risk assessment made by others and from the patient's decision that the chosen alternative best fits own conception of own good
Patient refuses surgery for simple appendectomy	Net balance substantially worse than for another alternative or alternatives	High/maximal	Principally from patient's decision that the chosen alternative best fits own conception of own good

capacity at a given time may be sufficient for making a decision to refuse a diagnostic procedure when foregoing the procedure does not carry a significant risk, although it would not necessarily be sufficient for refusing a surgical procedure that would correct a life-threatening condition. The greater the risk relative to other alternatives—where risk is a function of the severity of the expected harm and the probability of its occurrence—the greater the level of communication, understanding, and reasoning skills required for competence to make that decision. It is not always true, however, that if a person is competent to make one decision, then he or she is competent to make another decision so long as it involves equal risk. Even if the risk is the same, one decision may be more complex, and hence require a higher level of capacity for understanding options and reasoning about consequences.

In the previous section, we rejected a standard of competence that looks to the content or outcome of the decision in favor of a standard that focuses on the process of the patient's reasoning. This may appear inconsistent with our insistence here that the appropriate level of decision-making capacity required for competence should depend in significant part on the effects for the patient's well-being of accepting his or her choice, since what those effects are clearly depends on the content or outcome of the patient's choice. However, there is no inconsistency. The competence evaluation addresses the process of the patient's reasoning, whereas the degree of defectiveness and limitation of, and uncertainty about, that process that is compatible with competence depends in significant part on the likely harm to the patient's well-being of accepting his or her choice. To the extent that they are known, the effects on the patient's well-being should be evaluated in terms of his or her own underlying and enduring aims and values, or, where these are not known, in terms of the effects on life and health. Thus in our approach there is no use of an "objective" standard for the best or correct decision that is known to be in conflict with the patient's own underlying and enduring aims and values, which was the objectionable feature of a content or outcome standard of competence.

The evaluation of the patient's decision making will seek to assess how well the patient has understood the nature of the proposed treatment and any significant alternatives, the expected benefits and risks and the likelihood of each, the reason for the recommendation, and then whether the patient has made a choice that reasonably conforms to his or her underlying and enduring aims and values. Two broad kinds of defect are then possible; first, "factual" misunderstanding about the nature and likelihood of an outcome, for example from limitations in cognitive understanding resulting from stroke or from impairment of short-term memory resulting from dementia; second, failure of the patient's choice to be based on his or her underlying and enduring aims and values, for example because depression has temporarily distorted them so that the patient "no longer cares" about restoration of the function he or she had valued before becoming depressed.[4]

A crude but perhaps helpful way of characterizing the proper aim of the evaluator of the competence of a seemingly harmful or "bad" patient choice is to think of him or her addressing the patient in this fashion: "Help me try to understand and make sense of your choice. Help me to see whether your choice is reasonable, not in the sense that it is what I or most people would choose, but that it is reasonable for you in light of your underlying and enduring aims and values." This is the proper focus of a *process* standard of competence.

Some may object that misguided paternalists will always be ready to assert that their interference with the patient's choice is "deep down" in accord with what we have called the patient's "underlying and enduring aims and values," or at least with what these would be except for unfortunate distortions. If there is no objective way to determine a person's underlying and enduring aims and values then the worry is that our view will lead to excessive paternalism. We acknowledge that this determination will often be difficult and uncertain, for example in cases like severe chronic depression, leading to genuine and justified uncertainty about the patient's "true" aims and values. But any claims that the aims and values actually expressed by the patient are not his underlying and enduring aims and values should be based on evidence of the distortion of the actual aims and values independent of their mere difference with some other, "better" aims and values. Just as the process standard of competence focuses on the process of the patient's reasoning, so also it requires evidence of a process of distortion of the patient's aims and values to justify evaluating choices by a standard other than the patient's actually expressed aims and values. . . .

NOTES

1 See especially Roth, L. H., Meisel, A., & Lidz, C. W. (1977). Tests of Competency to Consent to Treatment. *American Journal of Psychiatry,* 134, 279–84;

what they call "tests" are what we call "standards." An excellent discussion of competence generally, and of Roth, et al.'s tests for competence in particular, is Freedman, B. (1981). Competence, Marginal and Otherwise. *International Journal of Law and Psychiatry*, *4*, 53–72.

2 Cf. Freedman, *op. cit.*

3 For example, John Rawls makes such claims for an objective and interpersonal account of "primary goods" to be used in evaluating persons' well-being within a theory of justice; cf. Rawls, J. (1971). *A The-*

ory of Justice. Cambridge, MA: Harvard University Press. Cf. also Scanlon, T. (1975). Preference and Urgency. *Journal of Philosophy*, *72*, 655–69.

4 This second kind of decision-making defect illustrates the inadequacy of the tests that Roth, Meisel & Lidz call "the ability to understand" and "actual understanding" tests (cf. Roth, et al. (pp. 281–82), *op. cit.* The clinically depressed patient may evidence no failure to understand the harmful consequences of his choice, but instead evidence indifference to those consequences as a result of his depression.

Who Decides, and What?
Tom Tomlinson

Tom Tomlinson is associate professor of philosophy and assistant director of the Center for Ethics and Humanities in the Life Sciences, Michigan State University. He is the author of such articles as "Misunderstanding Death on a Respirator," "The Irreversibility of Death: Reply to Cole," and "Casuistry in Medical Ethics."

Tomlinson reviews and challenges Buchanan and Brock's "sliding-scale" conception of competence standards. One problematic implication of their view, he argues, is that a patient could simultaneously be competent to accept a treatment yet incompetent to refuse it (if, for example, the risks associated with refusing the treatment are very great). In Tomlinson's view, Buchanan and Brock confuse (1) the sound idea of a variable standard of *evidence* for competence (which is justified by the fact that the stakes of making correct competence assessments are higher in some cases than in others) and (2) the idea of a variable standard of *competence itself.*

. . . The concept of competence [advanced in Buchanan and Brock's book, *Deciding for Others,*] shares much with the view that has been dominant since the reports of the President's Commission for the Study of Ethical Problems in Medicine, which, as staff members, Buchanan and Brock helped to write. Competence is decision relative because decisions of different complexities may call on different mental capacities. Adult persons should be presumed competent. Because of the importance of self-determination, the burden of proving a person's incompetence rests on others.

The capacities necessary for making a competent

Reprinted with permission of the publisher from *Medical Humanities Review,* vol. 5 (July 1991), pp. 73–76.

decision start with the capacity for understanding the facts pertinent to the decision at hand, including not only an intellectual grasp of the facts, but the capacity to understand imaginatively what it would feel like to experience the outcomes of the various alternative choices. The capacity for communication is also required, both as a means for others to evaluate understanding and for the person to communicate the preferred choice. Competence also requires capacities for reasoning and deliberation—again, not in the abstract, but for inferring from the facts how the various choices will affect one's values and goals. The last capacity important for competence is the possession of a set of values that is "consistent, stable, and affirmed" as one's own.

Although all of these capacities are matters of

degree, competence itself is not a matter of degree, but of threshold. One is either competent to make a given decision at a given time, or one is not. The problem, then, is where to set the threshold.

Buchanan and Brock argue that the threshold is set by balancing the two values that are served by the process of informed consent: the patient's well-being and the patient's self-determination. Although they acknowledge that there are competing standards for defining well-being, they think that all the plausible standards are substantially subjective: that is, a person's well-being must be understood in terms of the hierarchy of values that the person himself or herself affirms. The value of self-determination is partly instrumental because it is more likely to result in choices that enhance well-being as defined in the individual's own terms; and it is partly intrinsic because we often prefer to decide for ourselves, even when we don't think we would make the best decision.

Setting the level of the threshold of competence requires balancing these two values in order to steer between two dangers. Setting the threshold too high will take decision-making authority away from a patient who was competent to exercise it and will compromise the value of self-determination. Setting the threshold too low will permit an incompetent patient to choose unwisely and will compromise the value of protecting the patient's well-being.

Buchanan and Brock observe that anyone who advocates, as they do, a "process standard" that assesses the process of reasoning by which the patient came to a decision, must answer two questions. First, how well must the patient understand and reason to be judged competent; and, second, how certain must the evaluators be that their assessment of the patient's understanding is accurate? When the patient would pay a high price if we are wrong about his or her competence, we will want to be very certain indeed.

They believe that these considerations argue for a sliding-scale standard of competence. When there is a low risk of harm in respecting the patient's choice, a minimal capacity for understanding is sufficient. When there is a high risk of harm, we should require the patient to demonstrate a maximal capacity for understanding.

[A] particular individual's decision-making capacity at a given time may be sufficient for making a decision to refuse a diagnostic procedure when forgoing the procedure does not carry a significant risk, although it would not necessarily be sufficient for refusing a surgical proce-

dure that would correct a life-threatening condition. The greater the risk relative to other alternatives . . . the greater the level of communication, understanding, and reasoning skills required for competence to make that decision.

One implication of this view is that assessing a patient's competence is perfectly defensible when the patient refuses treatment, even if the patient's competence would not have been questioned if treatment had been accepted. Refusal is never in itself sufficient evidence of incompetence.

Does this sliding-scale model provide the most defensible conception of competence? One important set of objections comes from Charles Culver and Bernard Gert, most recently in the *Milbank Quarterly* in 1990. Even though competence, in their view, remains relative to the kind of decision to be made, it is a characteristic of persons, not of any specific decision. This point is illustrated most vividly by considering a counterintuitive consequence of the sliding-scale model: that a patient could be competent to accept treatment, but not competent to reject the very same treatment. In Buchanan and Brock's view, the decision to accept life-saving and benign treatment is a low-risk decision that requires only a minimal level of understanding to be competent. The decision to reject that treatment, however, is a high-risk decision that requires a high level of understanding to be competent. Therefore, the status of the patient who decides to refuse treatment that he or she had previously accepted could change from competent to incompetent, even though nothing has changed about the patient's level of understanding, medical condition, treatment procedures, or any other fact except the choice itself. For Culver and Gert, competence is the capacity of the patient to understand and appreciate the facts pertaining to a specific kind of decision, a capacity that can be evaluated prior to and independently of the decision finally made and is the same for refusal as for acceptance of treatment. Culver and Gert agree with Buchanan and Brock that deciding whether the patient's choice will be respected requires consideration of the patient's well-being, but they argue that it is done by assessing the rationality of the decision rather than the competence of the decision maker. Even a competent patient's choice can be "seriously irrational"—can threaten serious harm for no good reason. When that is the case, the competent patient's choice should be overruled.

Buchanan and Brock reply at least to earlier versions of this argument by agreeing that competence, in our common-sense notion of it, is a characteristic of persons. But they reject Culver and Gert's conception because it allows a fully competent patient's choice to be overruled for paternalistic reasons. This is a position that breaks too sharply with our ethical and legal traditions, which accord almost absolute decisional authority to the competent patient. This criticism of Culver and Gert is aimed in the right direction but could be much stronger. For them, respect for autonomy drops out altogether as a moral consideration in decisions about respecting refusal of treatment. For Culver and Gert, only the rationality or irrationality of the refusal is relevant to any decision about respecting it, regardless of competence as they understand it. Since rationality is taken to be a characteristic of a decision and in no respect a characteristic of the patient, the rationality of the patient's choice is to be judged without reference to that person's individual values and goals, but instead from a social or more ideal perspective. Respect for the intrinsic worth of individual, idiosyncratic conceptions of the good no longer operates as a brake on paternalistic interventions.

Buchanan and Brock could have avoided Culver and Gert's objection entirely if they hadn't confused the need for a variable standard of *evidence* for competence with a variable standard of *capacity* for competence. Culver and Gert are right in arguing that competence is a characteristic of persons and that the capacities required for competence vary with the complexities of the decision that is pending, not with the risk to the patient's well-being that one decision or another poses. Contrary to Buchanan and Brock, competence itself is not a balancing concept that weighs self-determination against well-being. Nevertheless, the level of risk to the patient's well-being remains relevant to the assessment of competence because it determines what the stakes of an incorrect assessment are and, in turn, how certain we need to be that the patient's decision is in fact a com-

petent one. When the consent is to a lifesaving and benign procedure, it doesn't matter whether we are wrong to judge the patient competent; we will treat the patient in any case. When, however, that patient changes his or her mind and refuses the procedure, it matters a great deal whether we're wrong in judging the patient to be competent and, in the name of self-determination, we permit the refusal to stand. In this circumstance, we rightly demand a much higher degree of evidence for that person's competence, not because the capacities necessary for a competent decision about this treatment have changed, but because our need to be sure about the patient's possession of those capacities has escalated dramatically.

This approach is a third position that incorporates elements of the other two. Competence is a capacity of persons that is independent of consent and refusal and does not weigh self-determination against well-being; and yet the risks to a patient's well-being justify a different approach to evaluating competence when the patient is refusing treatment rather than consenting to it. The irrationality of the patient's choice, judged from a position external to the patient's own hierarchy of values and goals, is no more than a red flag that indicates the need to inquire into the patient's competence more closely; contrary to Culver and Gert, it is not, in itself, a consideration that can be weighed paternalistically against the competent patient's right to self-determination, a right that remains nearly absolute.

After all is said and done, this dispute may in some part be a philosophical tempest in a teapot. The ethically significant question is when an adult's refusal of treatment may be overruled, and on that question it is hard to distinguish between *when it is competent, but irrational* (Culver and Gert) and *when it is irrational, hence difficult to find competent* (Buchanan and Brock). As a practical matter, any of these conceptions would end up treating cases in much the same way. . . .

Altruism, Self-Interest, and Medical Ethics
Edmund D. Pellegrino

A biographical sketch of Edmund D. Pellegrino is found on page 61.

Pellegrino argues that there are two conceptions of medicine today and each has different implications regarding physicians' duty to treat AIDS patients. The first conception sees medicine as an occupation like any other and the physician as having the same "rights," including the right to refuse services, as any other individual engaged in a business or a craft. The second, advanced by the author, distinguishes between medicine and other careers or forms of livelihood on three grounds: (1) the nature of illness itself; (2) the fact that the physician's knowledge is not individually owned and ought not to be used primarily for personal benefit; and (3) the physician's public acknowledgment, in taking an oath on graduation, of a collective covenant to use the acquired competence in the interests of the sick. In Pellegrino's account, these grounds give rise to an obligation on the part of physicians to make their knowledge available to all who need it, even if that involves effacing their own self-interests.

Nothing more exposes a physician's true ethics than the way he or she balances his or her own interests against those of the patient. Whether the physician is refusing to care for patients with the acquired immunodeficiency syndrome . . . or withdrawing from emergency department service for fear of malpractice suits, striking for better pay or fees, or earning a gatekeeper's bonus by blocking access to medical care, the question raised is the same. Does medicine entail effacement of the physician's self-interests—even to the point of personal and financial risk? Is some degree of altruism a moral obligation, or is nonmaleficence the limit of the physician's mandatory beneficence? How far does physician advocacy go?[1] What does the concept of physician as advocate mean?[2]

. . . Although the question is not new, the historic and ethical precedents are inconsistent. Even now, with respect to caring for AIDS patients, the guidelines are confusing. Item VI of the current American Medical Association Principles affirms the physician's right to choose whom to treat. The Ethical and Judicial Council acknowledges the tradition to treat but permits "alternate arrangements" for physicians emotionally unable to comply. On the other hand, the American College of Physicians and the Infectious Disease Society of Amer-

ica are unequivocal about the physician's duty to treat.[3]

These inconsistencies cannot be resolved without a more explicit choice between two fundamentally opposed conceptions of medicine itself. One conception calls for self-effacement by the physician, while the other accommodates physician self-interest. Not to choose between these two is to reinforce the cynics, discourage the conscientious, and undermine the moral credibility of our whole enterprise. Some of us would argue that there is a right answer, but that a wrong answer is more honest than no answer at all.

The arguments of those who defend refusals to care for AIDS patients are several: AIDS was not in the social contract when they entered medicine, obligations to self and family override obligations to patients, physicians who contract AIDS are permanently lost to society and their patients, treating patients when one is fearful or hostile only compromises their care, some physicians are emotionally unable to cope, and house staff carry an unfair share of the risks.

Leaving aside the fact that the risks of contagion are disproportionate to the fear, these arguments are cogent only if we accept the conception of medicine that undergirds them, i.e., medicine is an occupation like any other, and the physician has the same "rights" as the businessman or the craftsman. Medical knowledge belongs to the physician to be dispensed in the marketplace on terms set by its owner. Being ill and in need of care is no different from needing any other service or commodity. Competence and avoidance of harm are all that can legitimately be demanded of physicians. . . .

There are at least three things specific to medicine that impose an obligation of effacement of self-interest on the physician and that distinguish medicine from business and most other careers or forms of livelihood.[4]

First is the nature of illness itself. The sick person is in a uniquely dependent, anxious, vulnerable, and exploitable state. Patients must bare their weakness, compromise their dignity, and reveal intimacies of body and mind. The predicament forces them to trust the physician in a relationship of relative powerlessness. Moreover, physicians invite that trust when offering to put knowledge at the service of the sick. A medical need in itself constitutes a moral claim on those equipped to help.

Second, the knowledge the physician offers is not proprietary. It is acquired through the privilege of a medical education. Society sanctions certain invasions of privacy such as dissecting the human body, participating in the care of the sick, or experimenting with human subjects. The student is permitted access to the world's medical knowledge, much of it gained by observation and experiment on generations of sick persons. All of this, and even financial subsidization for medical education, is permitted for one purpose—that society have an uninterrupted supply of trained medical personnel.

The physician's knowledge, therefore, is not individually owned and ought not be used primarily for personal gain, prestige, or power. Rather, the profession holds this knowledge in trust for the good of the sick. Those who enter the profession are automatically parties to a collective covenant—one that cannot be interpreted unilaterally.

Finally, this covenant is publicly acknowledged when the physician takes an oath at graduation. This—not the degree—is the graduate's formal entry into the profession. The oath—whichever one is taken—is a public promise that the new physician understands the gravity of this calling and promises to be competent and to use that competence in the interests of the sick. Some degree of effacement of self-interest is thus present in every medical oath. That is what makes medicine truly a profession.

These three things—the nature of illness, the nonproprietary character of medical knowledge, and the oath of fidelity to the patients' interests—generate strong moral obligations. To refuse to care for AIDS patients, even if the danger were much greater than it is, is to abnegate what is essential to being a physician. The physician is no more free to flee from danger in performance of his or her duties than the fireman, the policeman, or the soldier. To be sure, society and the profession have complementary obligations to reduce the risks and distribute the obligation fairly. However, physicians and other health professionals cannot avoid the obligation to make their knowledge available to all who need it.

Two divergent conceptions of medicine oppose each other in medical ethics today. One entails self-effacement, the other rejects it. What the AIDS epidemic and, in their own ways, the commercialization of medicine have done is to force an explicit choice. To make that choice, we need something we do not yet have—a moral philosophy of medicine, something that goes beyond professional codes, or the analysis of ethical puzzles. What is called for is a return to the normative quest of classic ethics—the quest for what it is to be a good physician and for what kind of person the physician should be. . . .

NOTES

1 Sade R: Medical care as a right: A refutation. *N Engl J Med* 1971;285:1288–1292.
2 Hotchkiss WS: Doctor as patient advocate. *JAMA* 1987;258:947–948.
3 Health and Public Policy Committee, American College of Physicians and the Infectious Disease Society of America: Acquired immune deficiency syndrome. *Ann Intern Med* 1986;104:575–581.
4 Pellegrino ED, Thomasma DC: *The Good of the Patient: The Restitution of Beneficence in Medical Ethics.* New York, Oxford University Press Inc., in press.

AIDS and the Duty to Treat
John D. Arras

John D. Arras is associate professor of bioethics, Albert Einstein College of Medicine and Montefiore Medical Center, and adjunct associate professor of bioethics at Barnard College. Arras is the coeditor of *Ethical Issues in Modern Medicine* (4th ed., 1995). His published articles include "Quality of Life in Neonatal Ethics: Beyond Denial and Evasion" and "Getting Down to Cases: The Revival of Casuistry in Bioethics."

As Pellegrino does, Arras raises this question: Do physicians have an obligation to place themselves at risk in the service of patients? Arras criticizes those who have stressed the voluntary nature of the physician-patient "contract," finding voluntarism an unacceptable basis for medical practice in the age of AIDS. He discusses and criticizes some attempts to establish a duty to provide care, including the attempt to use the notion of a social contract between society and the medical profession as a basis for the duty. Dissatisfied with the social contract approach, Arras focuses on a virtue-based approach to the problem. He briefly discusses the moral tradition found in the history of the medical profession and maintains that recent history reveals a very strong commitment on the part of physicians to place patients' needs first, even at the risk of their own health. Arras concludes by responding to the question, "Can or should the traditional duty to treat be extended to include HIV-infected patients?"

Do physicians, by virtue of their role as health care professionals, have a duty to treat HIV-infected patients? Must they subject themselves to the very small, but nonetheless terrifying, risk of becoming infected themselves in order to live up to the ethical demands of their calling? For most physicians toiling in the front lines against AIDS, this is a new and totally unanticipated moral question that has yet to receive a clear and satisfying answer.

The current generation of physicians has experienced very little exposure to serious occupational risk. Well protected by antiseptic techniques and antibiotics for a period of roughly thirty years, doctors in developed countries have come to believe (with some justification) that they are exempt from the riskier aspects of medicine that had claimed the lives of so many of their predecessors. Prior to this *pax antibiotica,* risk and fear accompanied physicians daily, especially during the all-too-frequent periods of plague and virulent infectious disease. For many, if not most, of these physicians, to be a doctor *meant* that one was willing to take personal risks for the benefit of patients. One entered the profes-

sion with a keen appreciation of the hazards. By abruptly dispelling this perception of relative safety, AIDS has compelled today's physicians to reopen the traditional inquiry into the moral relationship between hazard and professional duty.

AIDS has likewise highlighted the limits of most contemporary bioethical inquiries into the physician-patient relationship. In their singleminded campaign against the excesses of medical paternalism, most bioethicists have been content merely to refute physicians' claims to moral expertise and special prerogatives based upon their Hippocratic duty to benefit the patient. In undermining this claim, bioethicists have completely ignored the question of whether physicians might still have special *responsibilities* as healers.

Moreover, the bioethicists' favorite metaphor for describing the physician-patient relationship, the contract between free and equal moral agents, has further obscured the issue of physicians' obligations to place themselves at risk in the service of their patients. By stressing the voluntary nature of the physician-patient "contract," bioethicists have inadvertently reinforced the notion that physicians, as free moral agents, have a perfect right to choose whomever they wish to serve. This claim to contractual freedom, enshrined in the 1957 AMA Code of Ethics,[1] likewise fails to address the

Reprinted with permission of the author and the publisher from *Hastings Center Report,* vol. 18 (April/May 1988), Special Supplement, pp. 10–14, 16–18.

question of whether physicians have a special duty to enter into contracts with hazardous patients.

Although there are many ways in which physicians can fail to discharge their putative duty to care for HIV-infected patients, ranging from outright refusal to foot-dragging, I shall focus on the central problem of categorical refusal to treat due to fear of infection. Do all physicians have an ethical duty to treat HIV-infected patients in spite of the risk, or can physicians fully discharge their moral duty to such persons by referring them to other physicians who are willing and capable of treating them? In short, is voluntarism an ethically acceptable basis for medical practice in the age of AIDS?

PROTECTING THE VULNERABLE: INDIVIDUAL RIGHTS AND PROFESSIONAL OBLIGATIONS

One promising starting point for our inquiry is to focus on the medical need of HIV-infected patients. These persons harbor a potentially lethal virus and may already be manifesting symptoms of ARC (AIDS Related Complex) or AIDS. They may require treatment of AIDS related conditions—such as Kaposi's sarcoma and pneumocystis pneumonia—or they may incidentally have other health problems requiring attention, such as kidney failure, heart defects, or dental problems. Although the diagnosis of HIV disease renders their plight particularly poignant, these patients resemble all patients with serious illnesses insofar as they are sick, vulnerable, and needy.

One compelling, though still contested, response to such health needs is to claim that they establish either an individual right to health care or at least a social duty to provide it.[2] This approach holds that because of the pivotal importance of health needs, including those needs created by AIDS, each person either infected with the virus or manifesting symptoms has a claim, grounded in justice, to the provision of needed health care.

The obvious drawback of this approach for our purposes is that it entirely avoids the question of physicians' individual or collective responsibility for HIV-infected patients. Whether we accept the language of individual rights or the language of societal obligation, the duty to provide care could be interpreted to fall squarely upon society through the vehicle of government, not on physicians as individuals or as a profes-

sional group. A voluntaristic system, with special incentives for those willing to treat, is compatible with this kind of societal duty.

A closely related argument makes use of the notion of a social contract between society and the medical profession. In exchange for the performance of a vital public service—that is, ministering to the needs of the sick and vulnerable—physicians as a group are granted monopolistic privileges over the practice of medicine. By seeking and receiving such a benefit, physicians incur a corresponding obligation founded on the notion of reciprocity.[3] If physicians are granted a monopoly over medical practice and then refuse to treat certain patients who are perhaps the most vulnerable members of society, who else will treat them? Just as the police have a duty to protect defenseless citizens based on their monopoly over the legitimate use of force, so physicians have a duty to treat those in medical need, even in the face of some personal risk.

By establishing some sort of duty to treat, the social contract approach thus improves upon the right-to-health-care argument, but we must concede immediately that it locates the duty not on the shoulders of each and every physician, but rather at the level of the medical profession. Since the parties to this contract are society and the profession, the social contract cannot generate, at least in the first instance, the kind of responsibility that goes through the profession to each individual member. So long as society's vital interest in caring for the vulnerable is secured, the social contract is upheld, no matter what the response of individual physicians.

This is where the analogy between physicians and the police breaks down. Whereas both groups have a professional monopoly on providing a vital public service, as well as the corresponding professional duty to provide it, individual police officers are also expected to take risks in the course of their ordinary duties. Whether they like it or not, they have to go down that dark alley where danger lurks. The reason for this disparity in the terms of these two social contracts is that police officers cannot usually delegate their risky business to others. Except for medical emergencies and personnel at public hospitals—the two obvious exceptions to the social contract's inattention to individual performance—physicians can usually refer undesirable or especially hazardous cases to others.

The sort of duty to treat generated by the social contract strategy is thus clearly compatible, at least in theory, with a voluntaristic system. Indeed, some might argue that such a voluntaristic system provides an optimal solution to the problem of AIDS: the patients get respectful care from physicians who really wish to provide it; unwilling doctors are freed from professional or legal coercion; and willing physicians are rewarded either by their own virtue or by incentives. In theory, everyone's needs and interests are thus secured by the social contract under conditions of maximal freedom of choice.

In practice, however, there is reason to believe that such a voluntaristic system might prove to be either unstable or inadequate. In the first place, such systems might place unfair demands upon those physicians who are willing to treat HIV-infected patients. If the majority of hospital-based physicians exempt themselves from the care of such patients, thereby dumping the burden upon a willing few, the resulting division of labor might easily be perceived as being grossly unfair. Those who undertook the nearly exclusive care of AIDS patients would thereby expose themselves to higher risk of both psychological burnout and eventual infection. In response to this perception, recalcitrant physicians might well agree to treat their fair share of AIDS patients so that the burden might be more or less equally distributed among the staff. Even so, it must be conceded that this shift from voluntarism to egalitarianism would be attributable, not to any putative individual duty to patients, but rather to a perceived duty to treat one's *colleagues* fairly.

An individualized duty to treat HIV-infected patients might nevertheless be empirically derived from the social contract if we could demonstrate that a voluntaristic system failed to perform according to the terms of the contract. Indeed, if it could be shown that voluntaristic systems tended to harm HIV-infected patients or failed to meet their needs, then the social contract could consistently call for the imposition of a duty to treat upon each and every doctor.

Demonstrating likely harms to HIV-infected patients under a purely voluntaristic system is not difficult. First, refusing to treat a person because he or she has AIDS or HIV infection ordinarily constitutes an insult of monumental proportions. The prospective patient is stigmatized and made to feel like an outcast. In itself this amounts to a significant injury.[4]

Secondly, the delays inherent in any system of widespread referrals might themselves cause significant harms. If patients suffering from severe or painful maladies are refused care by a physician or clinic and referred elsewhere, their conditions may well be exacerbated by the time they find someone willing and able to treat them.[5]

But perhaps the most obvious and serious problem with any voluntaristic system is that it would in all probability lead to lack of access and to substandard care. The dental profession provides an interesting case in point. A recent informal poll of the 4,100 member Chicago Dental Society revealed only three dentists, all from the same clinic, who were willing to accept new AIDS referrals.[6]

Even if a voluntaristic system were able to produce enough willing physicians to solve the problem of access, the quality of the care received would remain an open question. Although it is possible (but not likely) that such a system could find the right incentives to achieve acceptable levels of quality, the history of our treatment of poor, stigmatized, and unpopular groups indicates that AIDS patients, like the insane and criminals, will most likely receive inadequate and substandard care. In either case, if the system were unable to secure either access or quality, the social contract through the conditions of licensure would justify the imposition of an individualized duty to treat.[7]

An individual duty to treat can thus be empirically derived from the collective duty ascribed to the profession, and this duty can justifiably be imposed by the state in conformity with the social contract. Perhaps this is enough to get the job done, and perhaps in the long run that is what matters most to AIDS patients; but it is certainly not the stuff on which legends of professional virtue are based. In order to ground the sort of individualized and unmediated duty to treat patients—despite substantial hazard—that we associate with the historical tradition of medicine, we have to shift our focus from the specific task of meeting social needs to understanding traditional conceptions of the virtuous physician.

CONCEPTIONS OF PROFESSIONAL VIRTUE

In general, virtue-based accounts of the physician-patient relationship depend upon both a specific conception of the goal or good of the medical art and an account of the virtues (for example, competence, courage, fidelity) necessary to attain that good.[8] In contrast to the more standard bioethical methodologies that attempt to marshall rules and principles toward the resolution of specific quandaries or dilemmas, virtue ethics is more concerned with articulating the character and role-specific duties of the good physician. There are two different approaches to virtue ethics that speak to the issue of physicians' duty to treat. One relies on a rather abstract end-means relationship; the other attempts to ground the notion of the virtuous physician in an analysis of the commitments endorsed by the profession historically. . . .

Moral Tradition and Medical Virtue

[The latter] virtue-based approach relies, not on the nature or essence of medicine *sub specie aeternitatis*, but rather on the notion of a moral tradition embedded in the on-going history of the profession. Proponents of this view would agree with Alasdair MacIntyre's claim that we cannot answer the question "What am I to do?" without first answering the prior question "Of what story or stories do I find myself a part?"[9] They would then proceed to tell a story, to relate a history, of a profession that has incorporated a willingness to take risks for the benefit of patients as a constitutive element in physicians' self-understanding. Over time, this account would explain, the profession elevated the ideal of steadfast devotion to the well being of patients to the status of a fundamental duty, a definitive element inherent in the very role of physician. According to this story, physicians, if queried about their commitment to accept risk in the line of duty, would simply respond, "This is who we are; this is what we do. Those who fail to treat are cowards and not true physicians."

1. The Problem of Evidence   Incredibly, however, this is a history that has yet to be written. Apart from two pertinent articles that adopt contradictory positions, there are no focused, comprehensive, historical studies of physicians' duty to treat.[10] This is obviously a major problem for the virtue-based approach, since it attempts to ground the duty to treat in the historical practice and traditional self-understandings of physicians. In the absence of a reliable historical record, the status of the virtue-based duty is problematical.

To be sure, there is some historical evidence attesting to the existence of a self-perceived duty. Darrel M. Amundsen notes, for example, that as early as the 14th century, flight in the face of plague was regarded, both by physicians and the public at large, as a dereliction of duty and a shameful thing.[11] Although many physicians did, in fact, flee the plague, Amundsen contends that a standard of behavior had emerged according to which their retreat would be harshly judged. In support of this view, he quotes Guy de Chauliac, the Pope's physician at Avignon, who ruefully declared, "And I, to avoid

infamy, dared not absent myself but with continual fear preserved myself as best I could."

Another important example of self-sacrificial behavior motivated by medical duty is provided by Benjamin Rush during the great yellow fever epidemic at Philadelphia in 1793.[12] Although Rush's extraordinary devotion to patients during the epidemic has become the stuff of legend—as opposed, sadly, to the efficacy of his violent treatments—it is crucial to note that his courage was perceived by himself and others as required by duty. His acts were courageous, not because they went beyond the call of duty, but rather because he did his duty when others might be sorely tempted to flee from it.[13]

In spite of this "oral tradition" attesting to a duty to treat, we still lack rigorous historical studies that would establish an unbroken chain of professional duty stretching from the advent of the Black Death in Europe to modern times. Moreover, it is noteworthy that the only medical historian who has attempted to focus on this vast stretch of time has come to a very different conclusion. According to Daniel Fox, the history of medicine is marked, not so much by an unbroken tradition of risk taking for patients, as by a tradition of negotiation between civic leaders and the medical profession to provide for the needs of patients during epidemics. In short, Fox claims that voluntarism, rather than any individualized professional duty to treat, has been the historical norm.[14]

2. The Burden of Proof   Notwithstanding the absence of hard historical data on the duty to treat throughout the past six centuries, two salient facts suggest that the burden of proof should lie with those who would deny the existence of this duty. First, the persistence of an oral tradition or "folk wisdom" among physicians attesting to a duty to take risks for patients tells us a good deal about how physicians have traditionally understood their professional role. This sort of narrative tradition can still speak powerfully to us even if it does not meet the exacting standards of contemporary historiography.

Second, even if historians eventually demonstrate that voluntarism, rather than individual duty, best describes the behavior and beliefs of most physicians from the Middle Ages to the 20th century, they will most likely have to concede that, from the latter half of the 19th century onwards, tales of heroism eclipse accounts of flight as a sense of individual duty became indisputably rooted in the medical conscience. Even Zuger and Miles, who eventually conclude that the duty to treat cannot be firmly grounded in the vast canvass of medical history, admit that from the 1850s onwards "it becomes far more difficult to find recorded instances of physicians' reluctance to accept the risks that epidemics entailed for them. The stories of the cholera pandemics of the 19th century, the plague in the Orient, the influenza pandemic of 1918, polio in the 1950s, are largely ones of medical heroism."[15]

This firm understanding of the physician's duty was explicitly recognized as early as 1847 in the first code of ethics of the American Medical Association, which stated that ". . . when pestilence prevails, it is their duty to face the danger, and to continue their labors for the alleviation of the suffering, even at the jeopardy of their own lives."[16] Language to this effect remained in the Code until 1957, when it was dropped on account of medicine's (ultimately provisional) conquest of pestilential diseases.[17] Following a prolonged period of indecision on the physician's duty to treat HIV-infected patients, the A.M.A. in November 1987 unambiguously reaffirmed the duty to treat in the face of risk.[18] Although such codes are by no means infallible guides to the moral sensibilities of physicians, they at least provide good evidence of a profession's considered ethical judgments and of its own sense of identity.

Thus, although the historical record is woefully incomplete and physicians' track record is markedly inconsistent, our recent history reveals a very strong professional commitment to place the needs of the patient first, even at the risk of one's own health or life. This historical understanding, based perhaps more on *story* than on *historiography,* is aptly captured in Arnold Relman's claim that "the risk of contracting the patient's disease is one of the risks that is inherent in the profession of medicine. Physicians who are not willing to accept that risk. . . . ought not to be in the practice of medicine."[19] . . .

AIDS AND THE DUTY TO TREAT

Can or should the traditional duty* to treat be extended to include HIV-infected patients? To answer this ques-

*_Editors' note:_ In a section not included in this excerpt from his article, Arras identifies six features of this duty to treat: (1) It is _a particularistic duty_—a duty based on a particular shared vision of the good animating a particular moral tradition. (2) It is a duty that may be grounded in several factors: (a) an empathetic response to patients' needs and medical vulnerability by those who, by virtue of their medical skills, possess an exclusive

tion, we must ask additional questions about the nature of the risks posed by AIDS to physicians. What exactly is the risk of transmission through occupational exposure? And, how should this risk be evaluated?

What Is the Risk?   Since physicians do not usually have sex or share needles with their patients, the most likely routes of transmission are needle-stick accidents and blood splashing. In contrast to the risk of acquiring hepatitis B through an errant needle stick, the risk of HIV infection from similar accidents is very small—probably no more than one per every 200 incidents.[20] Even this low level of risk can be essentially eliminated for many physicians by scrupulous attention to established infection-control recommendations.

This is not to say that there is no risk at all. By February 1988, at least eight health care workers had acquired HIV infection through occupational exposure, and those who go on to develop full-blown AIDS will almost certainly die. Moreover, some physicians may be at higher risk for HIV infection. Surgeons, obstetricians and emergency room personnel, for example, appear to be disproportionately vulnerable to needle sticks and exposure to blood. Significantly, however, existing studies do not indicate a higher rate of occupational HIV transmission among these "high blood profile" specialties.[21]

Evaluating the Risk of AIDS   In addition to the task of scientifically estimating their actual exposure to risk, physicians must also evaluate this risk. Is it worth running? At first glance, this would appear to be an easy question for a historically based virtue ethics, since the objective risk of death from occupational exposure to HIV simply pales in comparison with the risks run by

and awesome power; (b) physicians' indebtedness to society for the social contributions that enable physicians to acquire the necessary knowledge and skills; and (c) a shared ideal of medicine as a profession dedicated to the good of others. (3) It is _an individualized duty_—a duty that binds each and every physician to treat regardless of whether other physicians might be available. (4) In keeping with the previous feature, this duty to treat _rules out volunteerism._ Those who refuse to treat are bad physicians even if they succeed in referring all of their patients to others who satisfy all their medical needs. (5) It _has not been entirely self-imposed_ but forged in an ongoing dialogue with society at large and thus has been subject to _social reinforcement._ (6) It is a duty that has a limit, one set by the level of risk involved. The problem is to determine the threshold of "acceptable risk," which is the dividing line between duty and supererogation.

previous generations of physicians. But we must recall that the threshold separating duty from supererogation depends upon culturally relative definitions of reasonable or acceptable risks. What if risks that were acceptable thirty, sixty, or one hundred years ago are no longer deemed reasonable by physicians and the society at large?

Conditions certainly have changed, and these changes are responsible for much of our current perplexity regarding the limits of the duty to treat. Perhaps most importantly, the world (or at least the industrialized, affluent part of it) is now a much safer place. Prior to the development of antibiotics, antisepsis, and vaccines, the entire population of the world might be said to have constituted a gigantic "high risk group" for early death from pestilence and other killer diseases. Life for most people, including physicians, was on average much shorter than it is today.

Thus, to a 19th century physician, death from yellow fever would no doubt have seemed a tragic but not extraordinary possibility. By contrast, present day physicians fully expect to live a long life; they no longer believe that anyone, especially themselves, should die from an infectious disease.

Notwithstanding this displacement of the threshold of supererogation, today's medical profession appears to be extending its historical commitment to encompass those who suffer from HIV and AIDS. As the A.M.A. policy statement recently made clear, "that tradition must be maintained. . . . A physician may not ethically refuse to treat a patient whose condition is within the physician's current realm of competence solely because the patient is seropositive."[22] Although some physicians have privately or publicly engaged in categorical refusals to care for HIV-infected patients,[23] they appear to constitute, in the words of Surgeon General Koop, "a fearful and irrational minority."[24] To be sure, many physicians, especially the younger ones who bear most of the burden of caring for AIDS patients, tread a narrow path like Guy de Chauliac between fear of AIDS and fear of infamy; but very few are driven by fear to renounce the care of AIDS patients altogether.

Thus, while our altered perceptions of relative risk may help to account for resistance to treating AIDS patients, it appears that the medical profession has collectively decided, albeit with a significant amount of internal dissent, to view most occupational exposures to HIV disease as at least comparable to other risks inherent in the practice of medicine—that is, as "acceptable risks."

Notwithstanding this consensus on the basic issue, a significant number of physicians, especially those who are no longer subjected to the discipline of internship and residency programs, have come to the conclusion that for them the risk is not worth running, even if they concur with the CDC's low estimates. How can this be explained?

The answer lies, at least in part, in the way some of these physicians perceive those afflicted with HIV disease. In refusing to deal with such patients, many physicians seem not merely to be saying, "Why should I risk my life?" but rather, "Why should I risk my life for the likes of homosexuals and intravenous drug abusers?" In other words, these physicians want to know why they must incur even small risks of serious harm for the benefit of morally suspect groups. It is one thing, they say, to risk one's life for an "innocent" child afflicted with AIDS through no fault of his own, but it is quite another thing to expose oneself to risks for patients who have "brought it upon themselves" through behaviors that are either illegal, immoral, or both.[25]

This attempt to turn the HIV-infected person into a complete Other by means of distancing and devaluation is often supplemented by a simultaneous movement of imaginative identification. As he evelutes the risks, the physician places himself in the shoes of the AIDS patient, but instead of achieving sympathy, this act of identification often yields only horror. The physician must contemplate not only the risk of death, however small, but also the risk of dying as people often die of AIDS in our society—that is, as outcasts, as stigmatized objects of fascination and disgust.

The appropriate societal response to a reluctance to treat based on this kind of fear should be a renewed effort to extend compassion and humane services to *all* AIDS sufferers. The fear of stigmatization is real and a matter of legitimate concern. Although it does not justify categorical refusals to treat, such fear is not a shameful response to societal intolerance. If physicians are to be expected to put their lives on the line, the least society can do is to treat them and their families with gratitude and the utmost respect if they become infected.

But as for those physicians who refuse to treat because they do not deem the lives and health of homosexuals and drug addicts to be worth the slightest exposure to risk, it would seem that they violate an even more basic duty traditionally espoused by the medical profession: the duty to treat all patients with respect for their human dignity, irrespective of considerations of their personal attributes, their social or economic status, or the nature of their disease. . . .

ACKNOWLEDGMENTS

This paper accumulated numerous debts. I am grateful to Michael Alderman, Ronald Bayer, Nancy Dubler, Liz Emrey, Robert Klein, Dorothy Levenson, Tom Murray, Kathleen Nolan, Nancy Rhoden, David Willis, Peter Williams, and the members of The Hastings Center's project on "AIDS and Professional Responsibility," for many trenchant criticisms and helpful suggestions. I gratefully acknowledge the support of the New York Council for the Humanities.

REFERENCES

1 *Judicial Council of the American Medical Association: Current Opinions of the Judicial Council of the American Medical Association* (Chicago: American Medical Association, 1986), ix.

2 For a general discussion of the comparative merits of "rights-based" and "social duty" approaches to equity, see John Arras, "Retreat from the Right to Health Care," *Cardozo Law Review* 6:2 (Winter 1984), 321–45.

3 Compare John Rawls, *A Theory of Justice* (Cambridge, MA: Harvard University Press, 1971), 102–03.

4 Richard Goldstein, "AIDS and the Social Contract," *The Village Voice* 32:52 (December 29, 1987), 14ff.

5 See *Report on Discrimination Against People with AIDS* (January 1986–June 1987) and *AIDS and People of Color: The Discriminatory Impact* (August 1987).

6 "AIDS Clinic Being Weighed by Chicago Dental Society," *New York Times* (July 21, 1987), B4.

7 Since most state licensure laws do not address the issue of physicians' refusal to initiate treatment contracts, this imposition would most likely require fresh legislation.

8 Cf. Earl Shelp, ed., *Virtue and Medicine* (Boston: Reidel Publishing Company, 1985).

9 Alasdair MacIntyre, *After Virtue* (Notre Dame: Notre Dame University Press, 1981), 201.

10 Darrel M. Amundsen, "Medical Deontology and Pestilential Disease in the Late Middle Ages," *Journal of the History of Medicine and Allied Sciences* 32 (1977), 403–21; and Daniel M. Fox, "The Politics of Physicians' Responsibility in Epidemics: A Note on History," *Hastings Center Report* 18:2 (April/May 1988).

11 Amundsen, "Medical Deontology," 408.

12 See generally, J.H. Powell, *Bring Out Your Dead: The Great Plague of Yellow Fever in Philadelphia in 1793* (Philadelphia: University of Pennsylvania Press, 1949).

13 On the relationships between courage, duty, and supererogation, see Douglas N. Walton, *Courage: A Philosophical Investigation* (Berkeley: University of California Press, 1986).

14 Fox, "The Politics of Physicians' Responsibility in Epidemics."

15 Abigail Zuger and Steven H. Miles, "Physicians, AIDS, and Occupational Risk," *Journal of the American Medical Association* 258, No. 14 (October 9, 1987), 1924–1928.

16 *Code of Ethics of the American Medical Association, 1847.* Reprinted in Chauncey D. Leake, ed., *Percival's Medical Ethics* (Huntington, NY: Krieger Publishing Company, 1975).

17 This interpretation of the A.M.A.'s decision to drop this provision was recently confirmed by Nancy Dickey, M.D., a member of the A.M.A. Council on Ethical and Judicial Affairs, at a meeting of the Hastings Center's project on "AIDS and Professional Responsibilities."

18 American Medical Association Council on Ethical and Judicial Affairs, *Report on Ethical Issues Involved in the Growing AIDS Crisis* (November 1987).

19 *Cardiovascular News* (August 1987), 7.

20 James R. Allen, "Health Care Workers and the Risk of HIV Transmission," *Hastings Center Report* 18:2 (April 1988).

21 See M.D. Hagen, et al., "Routine Preoperative Screening for HIV," *JAMA* 259:9 (March 4, 1988), 1357–59.

22 AMA Council on Ethical and Judicial Affairs, "Issues Involved in the Growing AIDS Crisis," December 1987.

23 "AIDS Fear Spawns Ethics Debate as Some Doctors Withhold Care," *New York Times* (July 11, 1987), A1, 12.

24 "Doctors Who Shun AIDS Patients are Assaulted by Surgeon General," *New York Times* (September 10, 1987), A1.

25 As a family practitioner from Illinois put it, "I would not knowingly treat a homosexual patient with AIDS, but I would treat patients who got the disease by blood transfusion, and I would treat children with AIDS." "What Doctors Think About AIDS," *MD* (January 1987), 95.

Medical Joint-Venturing: An Ethical Perspective
Ronald M. Green

Ronald M. Green is John Phillips Professor of Religion and director of the Institute for the Study of Applied and Professional Ethics at Dartmouth College. His published works include "Method in Bioethics: A Troubled Assessment," *Religion and Moral Reason* (1988), and *The Ethical Manager: A New Method for Business Ethics* (1994). Green served on the National Institutes of Health Human Embryo Research Panel.

Green argues that the practice of medical joint-venturing—in which physicians refer patients to facilities (e.g., surgery centers) in which they have a financial interest—is ethically indefensible. This practice, he contends, fails even to meet ethical standards appropriate to business, which require an agent in a fiduciary relationship with another person to give undivided attention to the other's interests. Green considers and rejects two arguments in support of medical joint ventures: (1) that they are part of long-accepted business practices in medicine and raise no ethical questions that have not been settled; and (2) that the practice generates sufficient societal benefits to warrant an exception to the usual rules concerning conflicts of interest. He concludes by cautioning that medicine cannot afford to risk further loss of societal trust and respect by accepting joint-venturing.

In 1986 a national chain opened a new radiological facility in Philadelphia near the office of Dr. Robert Hochberg, a private radiologist. Within several months, Hochberg noticed a decline in his business. Two and a half years later, less than half as many patients were using his office. Some of this was attributable to the superior technology at the competing facility, which boasted a state-of-the-art magnetic resonance imaging (MRI) machine. But Hochberg also blames the decline on what he believes are the chain's unfair business practices. When the new center opened, Hochberg notes, it recruited local doctors as limited partners, many of whom previously referred patients to him. According to Hochberg, "A few of the guys just turned off the spigot."[1]

A year earlier, Dr. William Birnbaum, a radiologist in Irvine, California, was approached by a colleague demanding a share of his profit. Birnbaum says he was told that if he didn't comply with the request, this colleague and the other physicians would stop referring patients to Birnbaum. "He said he wanted a piece of the action," Birnbaum later commented. "He said since it was their patients, they deserved some of the income."[2]

Reprinted with permission of the author and the publisher from *Hastings Center Report*, vol. 20 (July–August 1990), pp. 22–26. © The Hastings Center.

Implicit in this request was the threat that the others might open a competing facility, which they eventually did.

These stories suggest that medicine is no longer immune to the hardball tactics and hostile takeovers reported in the business pages of the newspapers. Behind these anecdotes, however, lies a development with potentially major impact on the quality of health care in this country and the future of the medical profession: the enormous growth in the number of medical facilities owned in "limited partnerships" by physicians who refer their own patients to them. Radiological offices, with their expensive CAT-scan and MRI technologies, are probably at the forefront of this development, but physician-ownership also plays a major role in the growth of many new outpatient, nonhospital medical facilities. These include women's health centers, alcohol and drug abuse treatment facilities, home health care services, freestanding urgent/primary care offices, same-day surgery centers, cardiopulmonary testing services, sports medicine clinics, parenteral nutrition services, and diagnostic medical laboratories.[3] In some cases, new hospital-based facilities have been opened in collaboration with groups of physician-investors or existing facilities have been "privatized" to stimulate physician referral to them.[4]

Although accurate figures are hard to come by,

congressional analysts have estimated that tens of thousands of doctors already invest in limited partnerships,[5] and one independent health care analyst believes that physicians hold shares or are partners in medical facilities that generate tens of billions of dollars a year in medical services.[6] A 1988 survey by the American Medical Association indicated that 7 percent of physicians polled had an ownership interest in a health care facility to which they refer patients,[7] while a 1989 report by the Inspector General of the Department of Health and Human Services (HHS) indicates that physicians own or invest in at least 25 percent of the independent clinical labs to which they refer patients, 27 percent of independent physiological labs, including radiology and MRI centers, and 8 percent of durable medical equipment businesses.[8]

LEGAL CONTROVERSIES

Much of this activity involves what is called "joint-venturing" by physicians and their financial backers. Typically, a group of investors guided by a consulting firm will recruit physician-investors in a proposed facility. As "limited partnerships" these arrangements do not have to include other nonphysician investors and may exclude doctors who use or own competing facilities. Once a center is organized, partners are strongly encouraged to refer patients. The quarterly dividend statements mailed to each partner typically contain a record of his or her rate of usage along with reminders of each partner's responsibility to refer patients to the facility. These centers can be enormously profitable. In many cases, physicians have recovered their investment within several years and reports of annual rates of return in excess of 50 percent are not uncommon. In view of this, it is not hard to imagine how seriously the encouragements to refer patients are taken, especially if they contain an implicit threat of exclusion from the partnership for low rates of usage.

Such activities have not been free of controversy. Considerable attention has focused on the legal question of whether these joint ventures violate the Medicare and Medicaid antifraud and abuse law, which prohibits the offering or receiving of "any remuneration (including any kickback, bribe, or rebate)" in return for referring an individual for Medicare- and Medicaid-financed services.[9] At issue is whether profits in joint enterprises of this sort that are not directly keyed to individual referrals or rates of referral come within the statute's prohibitions. To this point, interpretations of this law have

permitted the distribution of profits in proportion to the ownership of the venture so long as no payments were made according to the amount of business generated through referrals.[10] Faced with uncertainties about the statutes, however, investors have repeatedly sought "safe harbor" rulings by HHS defining activities exempt from prosecution. This debate may eventually be cut short by congressional action. Legislation introduced last year by Representative Fortney H. "Pete" Stark (D-California) would forbid Medicare reimbursement for referrals by physicians to facilities in which they have an ownership interest or compensation arrangement with the provider.[11]

SETTING ETHICAL STANDARDS

Whichever direction legislation takes, the ethical issues raised by these practices are more fundamental and more enduring. In the future large areas of medical care not financed by federal or state government will be subject only to the ethical standards held to govern the conduct of the profession. These standards will also shape physicians' attitudes toward joint venture practices and their response to future legislative initiatives. But determining what these ethical standards should be is a complex matter involving not only the question of what constitutes a fair disbursement of health care dollars but more basic questions about the impact of these practices on the doctor-patient relationship and the quality of health care generally. Although joint-venturing has drawn far less attention from medical ethicists than areas of medical entrepreneurialism such as for-profit hospitals or HMOs, the ethical questions here are no less pressing. They include such matters as the nature of the fiduciary relationship between doctor and patient, the impact of these new arrangements on patients' trust in physicians' treatment recommendations, and the question of whether these arrangements do or do not create incentives for the costly (and possibly dangerous) overutilization of diagnostic and other medical procedures.

Medical organizations have begun to wrestle with professional standards of ethics in debates over proposed code provisions or amendments that would expressly forbid physicians from referring patients to facilities in which they have a significant ownership interest. Although the AMA has rejected such a provision—opting instead for a more limited rule requiring physicians merely to disclose ownership interests to patients[12]—the American College of Physicians and the

American College of Radiology have concluded that disclosure does not provide sufficient protection for patients' interests and have added outright prohibitions on self-referral to their codes.[13] The forums for scholarly discussion of the issue include medical journals and a substantial report by the Institute of Medicine's Committee on Implications of For-Profit Enterprise in Health Care. The editor of the *New England Journal of Medicine* and the IOM report both strongly recommend an outright ban on physician self-referral.[14]

AN INTOLERABLE CONFLICT OF INTEREST

Without reviewing all the arguments and responses to these practices, I want to add my voice to the side of those who favor an ethical ban on physicians' referral of patients to facilities in which they have an ownership interest. I believe such practices patently violate the most elemental ethical standards governing not only medicine but ordinary business conduct, especially the requirement that an agent standing in a fiduciary relationship to another person avoid "self-dealing" and give undivided attention to the interests of that person. I see no compelling reason to bend the standards in this case. Whatever positive objectives medical "joint-venturing" involves, such as physicians' development of new diagnostic or care alternatives, can be attained without permitting policies that introduce an intolerable conflict of interest into the heart of patient care.

The violation of basic medical and business ethics standards here is obvious. For generations, medical codes have prohibited fee-splitting among physicians, the practice of returning a percentage of the fees generated by referral for medical consultation.[15] Behind this ban lies a fear that fee-splitting encourages a "trafficking" in sick people and a view of patients as financial resources rather than persons. A further assumption is that even the appearance of such practices might seriously undermine patients' trust in physicians' decisions. Clearly, however, apart from the absence of an immediate *quid pro quo,* nothing ethically distinguishes the newer practices of self-referral from older forms of fee-splitting. In both cases, physicians profit from their referrals and powerful incentives work to encourage a trade in "warm bodies."

The mounting evidence that physicians significantly tend to "overutilize" medical facilities in which they have ownership interest suggests that these concerns are justified. Studies done in Michigan in 1981 and 1984, for example, showed that patients referred to a facility owned by their physician typically underwent 40 percent more tests than patients referred to a non-physician-owned facility.[16] A privately commissioned update of the 1984 study done in 1988 showed that physicians with financial ownerships in a lab ordered 64 percent more tests than doctors without an investment.[17] And the 1989 HHS report uncovered a pervasive pattern of overutilization. It indicated that patients of referring physicians who own or invest in independent clinical laboratories received 45 percent more clinical laboratory services than Medicare patients in general and that patients of those doctors who have a financial interest in physiological labs, for radiology, computer scanning and MRI, used 13 percent more testing services than Medicare patients generally. The report estimated that in 1987 the overutilization of clinical laboratory services cost the Medicare system $28 million nationally.[18]

Comparing self-referral in joint ventures with norms governing related business activity illustrates how basic the conflict of interest is here. Possibly the closest analogue to physicians in this respect are corporate purchasing managers. Like physicians, purchasing managers are legal and ethical fiduciaries of the principals they serve. But a recent draft of the "Standards and Guidelines" of the National Association of Purchasing Management expressly forbids purchasing managers from engaging in personal business with suppliers in ways that encroach on their primary duty of loyalty to the employer.[19] In view of this, the relevant question before physicians is how they can justify a less demanding standard for their own "purchasing" activities.

A number of arguments have been advanced in response to this question, but two merit explicit attention. One is that "joint ventures" of this sort are continuous with long-accepted business practices in medicine and hence raise no ethical questions that have not already been settled. A second argument moves in a different direction. It accepts the relative novelty of the practice of "joint-venturing" but maintains that it generates sufficient benefits to society to warrant an exception to prevailing rules dealing with conflict of interest. Each of these arguments, I believe, is unpersuasive.

CUSTOMARY BEHAVIOR

The first argument points out that physicians have long been in a position of potential financial conflict of interest with their patients. Physicians in traditional fee-for-service practices, for example, have always had an incentive to overrecommend or overutilize their own services to the financial detriment of their patients. Society has learned to rely on the professional judgment and integrity of doctors rather than imposing rigid norms or arbitrary social intervention to prevent abuses. The development of office-based medical laboratories or radiological facilities extended this pattern without requiring a change in ethics and the newer joint ventures represent only a further extension of what has become customary behavior. Why, then, should doctors be prohibited from sending patients across town for a laboratory report when they can now ethically and legally send them across the hall?[20]

There are several replies to this position. For one thing, it is not true that matters of conflict of interest in fee-for-service medicine have always been regarded as best left entirely to physicians' discretion. The increasing requirement of outside review in insurance payment procedures suggests that society recognizes the potential for conflicts of interest here. There have also recently been proposals for new procedures in the billing of office-based diagnostic or laboratory services (including de-coupling payment from levels of usage by establishing set charges to all patients to recover the costs of capital investment in facilities).[21] If these concerns apply in the office setting, however, they grow in proportion to the powerful incentives operating on physicians to refer patients to joint-venture facilities outside their office.

Indeed, the very externality of these joint ventures introduces a new and important set of differences from previous practice. Whatever entrepreneurial activities have transpired within the context of a physician's office have usually been immediately visible to patients and supporting staff. Excesses or abuses were subject to review by all parties and were constrained by the face-to-face relationship between doctor and patient. This changes when the patient is sent across town to a large facility, however: The physician's control and responsibility substantially diminish and the physician becomes subject to pressure by outside individuals with financial or professional concerns of their own.

In addition, the externalization of diagnosis and care opens the door to virtually unlimited financial exploitation of patients. Whatever incentive there may be to overutilize services in the medical office setting is significantly limited by the physician's own time and resources. Where the primary office (or offices) is converted into a referral facility for further physician-owned medical services, however, these limits vanish. It now

becomes possible to view one's practice as a lucrative industrial enterprise, in which the physician and his primary care associates serve only as initial screening agents for patients who become factors deliverable for value-added processing. These considerations suggest the need for ethical—and perhaps legal—restraints on joint-venturing that would neither be necessary nor appropriate in the office setting.

THE SOCIAL VALUE ARGUMENT

A second major argument admits the potential for enhanced conflict of interest created by these ventures, but stresses their overwhelming social value and the need for freedom from restraint for this value to be realized. Those who argue this way point out that many of the services financed by joint-venturing result from the effort to provide new and more efficient medical care outside the hospital setting. Some, like same-day ophthalmological surgery centers, utilize new technologies that greatly reduce patient costs and inconvenience. Others, like MRI facilities, have often been started to bypass slow-moving hospital and governmental boards, whose bureaucratic mentality makes them unresponsive to medical need. Defenders of joint-venturing contend as well that physicians in a community are often best qualified to identify useful medical innovations. To prohibit such activities by new ethical restraints, they argue, would slow progress and institutionalize the vested interests that oppose new procedures or approaches to health care delivery.

These are powerful arguments. They not only contain a great deal of truth, they are a warning against a return to older forms of medical ethical thinking (such as the traditional ban on advertising) whose primary aim was to restrain competition and medical initiative. But as impressive as these arguments are, they miss the point. To address the central problem of conflict of interest here we do not have to prohibit physicians from acting as medical entrepreneurs. Doctors can remain free to identify new medical needs and to band together as investors to meet them. Indeed, they may even decide to devote the bulk of their time to such activities. *All that needs to be prohibited is physicians' referral of patients to facilities they own or in which they invest.* With this simple ban on self-referral incorporated in the ethics of the profession, the troubling link between financial gain and a physician's care recommendations is broken and patients need not worry about their doctor's motives in treatment decisions.

Admittedly, this prohibition will not remove all problems. New and innovative technologies, for instance, may be available only through a physician-financed facility, and an outright ban on self-referral may either discourage physicians from taking a lead in developing these facilities or may seriously disadvantage a particular doctor's patients. But this problem is not insurmountable. Proposals for legal prohibitions on self-referral typically make exception for "sole rural providers." Surely something like this could be developed, even for densely populated urban areas, to permit physicians to introduce innovative technologies and facilities.

It might also be feared that because of the vast sums of money involved here, a ban on self-referral might stimulate forms of collusion between providers, with physicians covertly agreeing to refer patients to one another's facilities. It would be unfortunate if this occurred, but it is not a decisive argument against ethically prohibiting these activities. If a ban makes sense, the appropriate first response to the possibility of evasion is not easing of the restriction but better communication of the reasons for it and more effective procedures for enforcing it.

PATIENT TRUST, PROFESSIONAL ESTEEM

The stakes here are important. Physicians understandably feel buffeted by the events of the past two decades. New forms of corporate practice have threatened their traditional autonomy, while cost-containment efforts by government and insurers, the expense of malpractice insurance, and increased competition from a variety of sectors have eroded their income. Small wonder that many doctors look to entrepreneurialism and joint-venturing as a positive development for themselves and their profession.

They are right to do so as long as this new area grows in a way consistent with the central values of the profession. One of these values is patients' trust. If joint-venturing undermines this by giving patients reason to think they are nothing but currency in the hands of medical entrepreneurs it will weaken their cooperation with the medical system and more than offset any promised medical gains. This problem might become especially acute if financial considerations lead some physicians to overutilize potentially dangerous radiological examinations or other invasive medical procedures.

In that case, joint-venturing would lead to violations of the fundamental principal of medical ethics, "Above all, do no harm," with incalculable consequences for medicine as a whole.

Physicians must also consider the impact of joint-venturing on the respect traditionally accorded their profession. Medicine is in transition today and can well do without the images of cutthroat behavior contained in the stories mentioned at the outset. If these images proliferate, physicians will end by losing assets more valuable than any financial investment: their self-esteem and the esteem of the communities they serve.

REFERENCES

1 Robert P. Hey and Barbara Bradley, "Partnership Pays Off—For Some," *The Christian Science Monitor,* 8 December 1988, 5–6.
2 Michael Waldholz, "Warm Bodies: Doctor-Owned Labs Earn Lavish Profits in a Captive Market," *The Wall Street Journal,* 1 March 1989, A1, A6.
3 Joan B. Trauner, Harold S. Luft, and Joy O. Robinson, *Entrepreneurial Trends in Health Care Delivery: The Development of Retail Dentistry and Freestanding Ambulatory Services.* A Report by the Institute for Health Policy Studies, University of California, San Francisco for the Federal Trade Commission (Washington, DC: U.S. Federal Trade Commission, 1982).
4 Waldholz, "Warm Bodies," A6.
5 Barbara Bradley and Robert P. Hey, "MDs' Investments Reap Controversial Profits," *The Christian Science Monitor,* 8 December 1988, 1.
6 Waldholz, "Warm Bodies," A6.
7 American Medical Association, Center for Health Policy Research, *SMS Report,* 3:2 (Chicago: American Medical Association, 1989).
8 Richard P. Kusserow, *Financial Arrangements Between Physicians and Health Care Businesses. Report to Congress* (Washington, DC: Department of Health and Human Services, Office of Inspector General, Office of Analysis and Inspections, May 1989), Control #OAI-12-88-01410:iii.
9 Medicare-Medicaid Antifraud and Abuse Amendments, Social Security Act (PL 95-142, 25 October 1977). *United States Statutes at Large* 91:1182–83; Sections 1877(b),1909(b). Redesignated as: Section 1128B per PL 100–93 101 *Stat.* 689, 18 August 1987.
10 Bradford H. Gray, ed., *For-Profit Enterprise in Health*

Care (Washington, DC: National Academy Press, 1986), 161.

11 H.R. 939, "Ethics in Patient Referrals Act," was introduced in February 1989. It permits exceptions for group practices, sole rural providers and prepaid plans. Since its introduction it has been subject to extensive lobbying by the AMA and other professional societies opposing or supporting joint venturing. Among the amendments offered by opponents is a "grandfather" clause that would permit self-referral to joint ventures established before March 1, 1989.

12 American Medical Association, *Current Opinions of the Judicial Council of the American Medical Association—1984* (Chicago: American Medical Association, 1984); "Physician Referral—The AMA View," *Journal of the American Medical Association* 262:3 (21 July 1989), 395–96.

13 American College of Physicians, *Ethics Manual* (Philadelphia: American College of Physicians, 1984), 21; American College of Radiology, "Policy Statement: Ethics in Patient Referrals, 1988" (Reston, VA; American College of Radiology, 1988).

14 Arnold S. Relman, "Dealing with Conflicts of Interest," *The New England Journal of Medicine* 313 (1985), 749–51 and "Antitrust Law and the Physician Entrepreneur," *The New England Journal of Medicine* 313 (1985), 884–85; Gray, *For-Profit Enterprise*, esp. ch. 8.

15 See, for example, the Ad Hoc Committee on Medical Ethics, *American College of Physicians Ethics Manual*, "Part I: History of Medical Ethics, the Physician and the Patient, the Physician's Relationship to Other Physicians, the Physician and Society," *Annals of Internal Medicine* 101 (1984), 129–37.

16 State of Michigan, Department of Social Services, Medicaid Services Administration, Bureau of Health Services Review, Medicaid Monitoring Section, "Utilization of Medicaid Laboratory Services by Physicians With/Without Ownership Interest in Clinical Laboratories: A Comparative Analysis of Six Selected Laboratories" (Lansing, MI: July 9, 1981); Blue Cross and Blue Shield of Michigan, Medical Affairs Division, Charlotte J. Bartzack, ed., "A Comparison of Laboratory Utilization and Payout to Ownership" (Detroit, MI: Blue Cross and Blue Shield of Michigan, 1984).

17 This study was commissioned by Metpath, a laboratory that has been hurt by competition from limited partnerships. For a discussion of this and other more recent studies, see Robert P. Hey and Barbara Bradley, "Patient Care vs. Physicians' Investments," *The Christian Science Monitor*, 12 December 1988, 6.

18 Kusserow, *Financial Arrangements*, iii.

19 National Association of Purchasing Management, "Standards and Guidelines for Ethical Purchasing Practices" (Tempe, AZ: National Association of Purchasing Management, 1989), 3. This draft document does permit ownership of stock in a supplier "provided that the interest is solely of an investment nature" (3).

20 Hey and Bradley, "Partnership Pays Off," 6.

21 Gray, *For-Profit Enterprise*, 163.

The Doctor as Double Agent
Marcia Angell

Marcia Angell is executive editor of *The New England Journal of Medicine*. Her articles include "Patient Preferences in Randomized Clinical Trials," "How Much Will Health Care Reform Cost?" and "Breast Implants—Protection or Paternalism?"

Angell examines the contemporary expectation that American doctors should function as "double agents"—with conflicting allegiances to patients' medical needs and to society's financial interests. Because this situation is a result of rapidly increasing medical costs, them-

Reprinted with permission of the publisher from *Kennedy Institute of Ethics Journal*, vol. 3 (September 1993), pp. 279–286.

selves the result of an inherently inflationary health-care finance system, the solution, Angell argues, is to restructure the system to remove the inflationary pressures. Failure to do so, she concludes, is to endanger the patient-centered ethic at the moral core of medicine.

IN EARLIER TIMES—that is, before 1980—it was generally agreed that the doctor's sole obligation was to take care of each patient. The doctor was the patient's fiduciary or agent, and the doctor was to act only in the patient's interest. Now all that has changed. Many of us—economists, governmental officials, corporate executives, even ethicists, and yes, even many doctors themselves—now believe that doctors have other obligations that compete with their obligation to the patient. In particular, they believe that doctors have acquired an obligation to save resources for society. Doing so requires doctors to practice with one eye on costs, which may mean sometimes denying beneficial care that they would surely have provided in earlier times.

According to the new view, doctors are no longer simply agents for their patients. They are now agents for society's needs as well. They are, in short, *double agents,* expected to decide whether the benefits of treatment to their patients are worth the costs to society. Many distinguished ethicists have enthusiastically embraced this new ethic (Callahan 1990; Morreim 1991). To them, keeping an eye on the price tag means saving scarce resources for other, more important uses.

How did this extraordinary shift in our view of doctors' obligations come about? Is it just coincidence that it began with our first realization—roughly in the mid-1970s—that our seemingly endless resources were in fact finite? And is it just coincidence that it accorded with the wishes of the third-party payers—who discovered during the 1980s that they had severe and growing budgetary problems? In short, can it be that the ethical underpinnings of the practice of medicine have been scrapped in a single decade for financial reasons? Is economics driving ethics?

I'll begin with my conclusions. I believe that doctors *are* now asked to be double agents and that their dual obligation is a recent construct, which arose out of the economic difficulties of the large third-party payers. I will argue that we embrace this new ethic at our peril. Even if we as a society decide that health care should take a smaller piece of the national economic pie, there are ways to do this that do not entail rebuilding—and perhaps destroying—almost overnight, the ethical underpinnings of the profession.

HISTORICAL REVIEW

First, a quick review of how we got here. This requires an economic analysis, since my thesis is that economics is now driving ethics. The economic history of health care in the United States can be divided into three phases. First, there was the phase of the true market, lasting until roughly World War II. Patients paid doctors out-of-pocket for their medical care. If the price was too high, the doctor was confronted with an unhappy patient. Even after private insurance companies began to flourish in the 1930s, the premiums were still paid out-of-pocket and so patients continued to feel the costs, although the pain was blunted. Fortunately, medical care was fairly inexpensive. Unfortunately, it was also relatively ineffective, compared with the power of modern medicine.

The second phase was marked by the entry of big business into the health care picture. Big business began to offer health insurance as a fringe benefit in order to evade the wage and price controls in effect during World War II. Offering health insurance was tantamount to increasing wages, and furthermore, it was not taxed. The connection between employment and health insurance was thus an historical accident that haunts us still. But the important effect of this connection for the discussion here is that it insulates patients from the costs of medical care. Neither doctors nor patients had to worry any longer about the costs of medical care. With the enactment of Medicare and Medicaid in 1966, this insulation from costs spread to the poor and, most importantly, to the elderly—a politically powerful group. By the end of the 1960s, anything resembling a true market in health care had vanished. Nearly everyone was covered by third-party payers—government, business, and private insurance companies. And medical care was becoming both more expensive and more effective. Despite the increasing costs, the third parties happily paid the charges, with few questions asked.

The third phase began with the realization that health care costs were consistently rising far more rapidly than the GNP. Now that patients and doctors and hospitals were insulated from accountability, there were no limits on the expansion of the health care industry in this country. It was open-ended and nearly risk-free, absorbing an ever greater share of our domestic spending. While national expenditures for other social goods, such as education, stagnated or declined, expenditures for health care rose rapidly—from roughly 6 percent of the GNP in 1965 to nearly 10 percent in 1980 to 13 percent in 1991 (Stoline and Weiner 1993).

Not only was there nothing to stop the inflation, but there were features that virtually guaranteed it. These included the piecework, fee-for-service reimbursement system that is greatly skewed toward high-technology procedures and specialists. Doctors, of course, act as both providers and purchasing agents, so these highly paid specialists could easily generate their own business. For example, the cardiologist who recommends coronary angiography to a patient also bills for it.

COST CONTAINMENT

In the 1970s, the Arab oil embargo made Americans realize that our resources were finite. Health care costs began to occupy the attention of some experts and policymakers. By the 1980s, it became clear to nearly everyone that we could not indefinitely sustain rising health care costs, and for the first time, efforts were made to control them. "Cost containment" crept into the lexicon, and by the end of the 1980s the *New England Journal of Medicine* probably received more manuscripts about cost containment than about cancer. The efforts to control costs were spearheaded by the major third parties—government and big business. They were responding essentially to budgetary problems, not to moral problems. They went about cost containment in a number of ad hoc, uncoordinated ways, as briefly mentioned below. None of them was notably successful. In fact health care costs rose even faster—I believe, *because* of cost containment efforts, not despite them.

Regulation by third parties, including managed care, simply led to the growth of an expensive and intrusive new bureaucracy. Efforts to foster competition led to increased marketing, not to lower prices. And attempts to limit demand through higher deductibles and copayments simply shifted costs and limited care,

primarily to the most vulnerable. Efforts by insurers to avoid risks also shifted costs. In general, savings to one part of the system were costs to another. In fact, the dominant characteristic of the American health care system is that there is no system. There is just a hodgepodge of arrangements, existing independently, often working at cross purposes, and generating enormous administrative costs. Indeed, administrative costs—billing, marketing, underwriting, claims processing, utilization review—now consume more than 20 cents of the health care dollar (Woolhandler and Himmelstein 1991).

Why do I recapitulate this sorry history of the economics of the American health care system? I do so because it is important to understand the context in which doctors are being invited to act as double agents. They are invited to do so in an open-ended, inherently inflationary system (or, rather, nonsystem) that spends roughly 40 percent more per citizen on health care than the next most expensive health care system in the world and at least twice as much on administrative costs. Further, this system is embedded in a society that routinely spends billions and billions on such goods as tobacco, television ads, and cosmetics. Clearly, we as a society are not facing scarcity; instead we are facing the inefficient and frivolous use of vast resources.

SAVING FOR THIRD PARTIES

What precisely is the doctor supposed to do as double agent? In a nutshell, doctors are supposed to tailor their care of patients to save money for third parties. For example, under the DRG system of hospital reimbursement for Medicare patients, doctors are supposed to be agents for the hospital, discharging patients as rapidly as possible and keeping services to a minimum so that the hospital can game the system. In many HMOs doctors are expected to keep costs as low as possible, and some HMOs even directly reward doctors with bonuses when the HMO comes out ahead. They may also withhold a portion of doctors' salaries if they refer patients to specialists too often or use too many tests and procedures. Thus, doctors are agents for the HMO and have a direct incentive to undertreat their patients, just as in the fee-for-service system they have an incentive to overtreat them. Other forms of managed care also deter doctors from delivering care. Those that require utilization review often make it so complicated and difficult to get approval for hospitalization or procedures that the doctor is reluctant even to try. And it should be noted that nearly all medical care these days is managed in one way or another, by which I mean it is subject to efforts of insurers to limit care.

In essence, then, doctors are increasingly being asked, in one way or another, to save money for a third party—and sometimes for themselves—by scrimping on the medical care they deliver. But the pressure is seldom described in these terms. Instead, it is described as practicing "cost-effective" medicine. "Cost-effective" is the new watchword. It used to be a technical term that referred to the least expensive of two equally effective alternatives, or to the most effective of two equally costly ones. Now it is simply a shorthand for any attempt to save money. The word sounds fine, and who can object to it?

JUSTIFICATION FOR DOUBLE AGENTS

But how can we justify asking doctors to deprive their patients of care, including clearly beneficial care that in other circumstances they would not hesitate to provide? Just as the problem is new, so are the ethical justifications.

First, it is claimed that limiting care is what society wishes, and that the medical profession has an obligation not only to accept the will of society but to further it. Doctors are simply anticipating and delivering what is expected of them by the body politic, despite the fact that individual patients may want something else when they are sick.

Second, it is argued that because third parties now pay for nearly all medical care, they have gained a legitimate voice—indeed, the overriding voice—in how much medical care patients should receive. I find this a peculiarly American argument. Essentially the message is that whoever pays the piper calls the tune. The purest example of this view is the Oregon plan for rationing the care received by Medicaid patients. This is often described as a decision to allocate scarce resources rationally and justly, but it is, of course, nothing of the sort. It is instead a matter of taxpayers deciding to limit the care received by the poor, on the grounds that the taxpayers are funding it. Those who drew up the priority list of medical services are not those to whom it would apply. Even if we were to accept the idea that paying for medical care confers the right to limit it, we should remember that most patients do in fact still pay for their medical care, just as they always did. They simply pay in advance and indirectly, through their work or their taxes. The third parties are not using their own money.

The third justification for doctors to be double agents is the most compelling. It appeals to the doctor as good citizen or, more dramatically, to the doctor as

occupant of a metaphorical lifeboat with limited supplies. According to this view, resources saved in denying patients expensive medical care could be used to provide less expensive care to a larger number of patients. Or it could be used for even more important public purposes, such as education. This line of argument has been put forward most persuasively by Dan Callahan (1990) who contends that Americans have overvalued individual health care compared with other social goods.

ARGUMENTS AGAINST DOUBLE AGENTS

Despite these justifications, I see five serious problems with the view that doctors should act to contain costs, patient by patient. First and most simply, this view of the role of doctors is based on the premise that resources in our health care system are in fact scarce. But, of course, they aren't. The mere fact that we spend so much more on health care than all other advanced nations is proof that our health care resources are plentiful. Given that in 1990 we spent about $2,566 on every man, woman, and child in the United States, and Canada spent only $1,770, we can hardly claim inadequate resources (Schieber, Poullier, and Greenwald 1992). And since Americans and Canadians are subject to the same ailments and have roughly the same outcomes, we must assume that our system is grossly inefficient. Clearly, the answer to an inefficient system is not to stint on care, but rather to restructure the system to make it more efficient.

Second, enlisting doctors as ad hoc rationers presumes that resources saved by denying health care would be put to better use. But in our system there is absolutely no reason to think that it would. As Norman Daniels (1986) has pointed out, in the United Kingdom or Canada, resources saved by denying care would be used for presumably more valuable health care, but that is not the case here. In the U.S., we do not have a closed system in which funds taken from one form of health care are diverted to another that is deemed to be more important. Instead, funds not used for health care may find their way into any sector of the larger economy, to be used for anything—e.g., defense, education, farm subsidies, or personal savings. Furthermore, even funds that remain within the health care system might not be used for more effective care; instead, money saved on, say, heart transplantation may very well find its way to a hospital's public relations office or to higher salaries for administrators. Under these circumstances, it is very difficult to sustain an ethical argument for doctors acting as double agents. The only principled way to ration health care is to close the system and establish limits that apply to everyone—not just to the poor.

Third, asking doctors to be double agents overlooks an important symbolic function of health care. Our society was founded on the principle that individuals enjoy a set of basic rights that cannot be denied them. As medicine has become increasingly effective in preserving life, medical care has come to be counted among these rights. Thus, doctors are seen to preserve a basic human right, namely life, just as criminal lawyers are seen to preserve liberty by defending their clients. Lawyers do not decide part way through a trial to call it quits because it's just too expensive to go on with it. In both situations, there has been a consensus that the single-minded focus on the patient or the client serves the broader interests of society. This argument is particularly compelling in a society as unequal as ours. People will tolerate the vast inequities in income and privilege in this country only if they feel assured that their irreducible set of rights is truly protected. It has been suggested that high technology medicine may serve precisely such a reassuring function in our society. And public opinion polls tend to support this view (Blendon 1991). The public, in contrast to the third-party payers, does not feel that we are spending too much on health care, only that we are not getting our money's worth.

Fourth, when doctors act as double agents, they are merely acting on their own particular prejudices. They are deciding that this or that medical service costs too much. This is not a medical judgment, but a political or philosophical one. Another doctor (or a plumber or electrician) might make quite a different judgment. This is no way to allocate health care.

And fifth and perhaps most important, the doctor as double agent is not honest. Sick people need and expect their doctors' single purpose to be to heal them. The doctor-patient relationship would not survive a candid statement by the doctor that only care that seems to the doctor to be worth the money will be provided. Anything short of full efforts to heal the individual patient, then, must involve a hidden agenda—an ethically indefensible position.

CONCLUSION

In sum, we should be loath to abandon or modify the patient-centered ethic, and we should be wary of ethical justifications for doing so. Unfortunately, history shows us that ethics in practice are often highly malleable, *justifying* political decisions rather than *informing* them. Necessity is the mother of invention, in ethics as well as in other aspects of life. For example, in 1912, when the AMA thought salaried practice was a threat to the autonomy of the profession, its Code of Ethics pronounced it unethical for physicians to join group practices. Now, some 80 years later, we are again hearing that it is a matter of ethics for the medical profession to carry out what is essentially a political agenda. But ethics should be a little more stable than that. Ethics should be based on fundamental moral principles governing our behavior and obligations toward one another. If a doctor is ethically committed to care for the individual patient, that commitment should not be abridged lightly. And it should not be nullified by a budgetary crunch. Doctors should continue to care for each patient unstintingly, even while they join with other citizens to devise a more efficient and just health care system. To control costs effectively will in my view require a coherent national health care system, with a global cap and a single payer (Angell 1993). Only in this way can we have an affordable health care system that does not require doctors to be double agents.

ACKNOWLEDGMENT

This article is based on the annual Edmund D. Pellegrino Lecture at the Kennedy Institute of Ethics.

REFERENCES

Angell, Marcia. 1993. How Much Will Health Care Reform Cost? *New England Journal of Medicine* 328: 1778–79.

Blendon, Robert J. 1991. The Public View of Medicine. *Clinical Neurosurgery* 37: 2563–65.

Callahan, Daniel. 1990. *What Kind of Life? The Limits of Medical Progress.* New York: Simon & Schuster.

Daniels, Norman. 1986. Why Saying No to Patients in the United States Is So Hard: Cost Containment, Justice, and Provider Autonomy. *New England Journal of Medicine* 314: 1380–83.

Morreim, E. Haavi. 1991. *Balancing Act: The New Medical Ethics of Medicine's Economics.* Boston: Kluwer Academic Publishers.

Schieber, George J.; Poullier, Jean-Pierre; and Greenwald, Leslie M. 1992. U.S. Health Expenditure Performance: An International Comparison and Data Update. *Health Care Financing Review* 13 (4): 1–15.

Stoline, Anne M., and Weiner, Jonathan P. 1993. *The New Medical Marketplace: A Physician's Guide to the Health Care System in the 1990s.* Baltimore: Johns Hopkins University Press.

Woolhandler, Steffie, and Himmelstein, David. 1991. The Deteriorating Administrative Efficiency of the U.S. Health Care System. *New England Journal of Medicine* 324: 1253–58.

Patients' Obligations

Patients' Duties
Michael J. Meyer

Michael J. Meyer is associate professor of philosophy at Santa Clara University. His areas of specialization are ethics, philosophy of law, and political philosophy. He is the author of such articles as "The Idea of Selling in Surrogate Motherhood" and "Rights between Friends."

Meyer contends that the partnership between the autonomous patient and the health-care professional gives rise to certain patient duties. Observance of these duties, he argues, serves the patient's health interests while showing respect for the professional. Examples of patients' duties are a duty to be honest about the reasons for seeking care; a duty to learn about available treatments and their likely side effects; and, for patients with infectious disease, a duty to take measures to prevent further transmission.

I.

In the past twenty years discussion of patients' rights—an idea which would have seemed curious less than a century ago—has achieved unprecedented prominence in accounts of the moral and legal relationship between patients and health care professionals. If the sheer volume of literature is any indication, then there is presently a dominant concern with *patients'* rights and *professionals'* responsibilities.[1] Accounts of such rights and responsibilities range from the American Hospital Association's 'A patient's bill of rights', to the codes of ethics adopted by various health care associations, to the burgeoning legal and philosophical literature on the complex of ideas associated with patients' rights.[2]

Such emphasis also indicates that at least the winds of rhetoric are blowing steadily in favor of the patient; this is undoubtedly for good reason. In the past patients' rights have been ignored. Often in the spirit of paternal-

The Journal of Medicine and Philosophy, vol. 17 (October 1992), pp. 541–542, 549–553. © 1992 by Kluwer Academic Publishers. Reprinted by permission of Kluwer Academic Publishers.

ism, patients have been denied information about their own diagnosis, prognosis and treatment. Patients have even been used in medical experiments without their consent or often when consent has been obtained with at best a partial sense of the risks involved. Patients' rights are also deemed worthy of special attention because in the relationship with health care professionals, the patient is typically seen as in an inherently disadvantaged position. Though for such reasons the present focus on patients' rights is understandable—indeed laudable—some balance in this discussion is a necessity. In particular, what is needed is a corresponding account of patients' duties. . . .

[II.]

While patients' duties might be classified by some as either self-regarding duties or duties to others, especially to health care professionals, each of the duties described below fits *both* categories. Patients' duties do not admit of this simple traditional division because the source of those duties is the partnership between the autonomous patient and the health care professional. Compliance with patients' duties serves the legitimate interests of both the patient and the health care professional. While the observance of patients' duties is self-regarding—observing them is a way of honoring a commitment to one's own health—observing these same duties also shows the proper respect due to the conscientious health care professional. In addition, throughout this section one should recognize that such duties are *prima facie* duties. There are, no doubt, a variety of situations and reasonable arguments for not complying with one or another of these duties in particular cases. Finally, there is no suggestion here that a patient's failure to comply with his duties, for good reasons or not, entails that he thereby forfeits his rights.

First, the autonomous patient has a duty to communicate his own concerns openly. This includes: a duty to be honest about why the patient seeks the health care professional's assistance; a duty to give as good a medical history as possible; a duty, for ongoing patients, to tell the health care professional whether they are following previously agreed-upon procedures (and if not, offer some explanation, for instance a report on the side effects of a drug). This duty goes beyond the obligation to avoid lying. It includes a duty to avoid withholding information believed to be relevant, because this may ultimately affect the patient's participation in treatment.[3]

Such a duty is a self-regarding duty, and complying with it clearly benefits the patient. In fact, acting in accord with this duty is required by the autonomous patient's commitment to self-care. But this duty is also owed to the health care professional. Its observance directly benefits her as well. It is a duty to the health care professional because of what the good nurse or the good physician invests in the partnership with the autonomous patient. This includes a carefully directed expenditure of time and energy, a genuine concern for the patient's health, and an ongoing study and review of the course of a disease or a treatment. Such a commitment ought to be repaid by open communication. The autonomous patient should avoid presenting the health care professional with the dilemma of guessing what her client wants. Being a successful health care professional should not require—though in practice it seems that it often does—planning the patient's treatment without any direct input from the patient.

As the nature of his condition becomes clear the autonomous patient is also obliged to go beyond initial concerns with his symptoms and make responsible decisions about his own self-care. This entails: a duty to collect information on a range of available treatments, and

their likely side-effects; a duty to have an active interest in the effects of his condition on himself and others. These are constitutive features of the duty to make responsible decisions about self-care. There are, of course, special duties incumbent upon the patient who discovers he has a contagious condition or an infectious disease, be it rubella or AIDS. One of their most important responsibilities is to understand the means and the likelihood of transmission. This is *not* a duty to needlessly forsake the company of others, or to become social outcasts, but a duty to act upon that information which can best prevent further transmission.

The duty to engage in responsible self-care provides the patient with a direct payoff, but it is also a duty owed to others, including the health care professional. The health care professional has a legitimate interest in the patient's active participation in his own care. This is important because without the patient's inclination to self-care, the health care professional can not do his job well. Consider, by analogy, a music teacher and his student. Given that a good teacher carefully prepares his subject so as to instill in his apprentice a genuine love for music, a student's duty to practice in order to learn is owed not only to himself but also to his teacher. While it may be possible to train an animal without its cooperation—through the brute force of conditioned response—it is simply not possible to teach a complex discipline to any human being without his participation. Similarly, the health care professional can not provide assistance with self-care, if no self-care ever takes place. The autonomous patient's right to information implies an interest in self-care that overrides the inclination to paternalism. But paternalism can not be overcome without the patient's observance of the duties of self-care.

The autonomous patient also has a duty to cooperate on mutually agreed-upon goals (or to negotiate an adjustment of those goals). If the health care professional and the autonomous patient agree that his hypertension calls for a change in diet, then the patient has a duty to alter his diet in the appropriate fashion. Such a duty is a self-regarding duty; indeed it is the centerpiece of self-care. It is also a duty owed to the health care professional because she has a direct interest in the patient's health—that is, as a *professional* her interests transcend personal concerns like the advancement of her knowledge or her career. This duty does *not* override all the patient's liberties. It is clearly a *prima facie* duty based on the prior agreement to treatment (which is, of course, open to renegotiation). The patient always retains the liberty to seek a second opinion or even refuse professional treatment altogether.

The autonomous patient has no duty to follow a treatment regime he has good reason to avoid—for instance, one whose deleterious side effects outweigh its promised benefits. He simply has a duty to try a mutually agreed-upon treatment, or explain why he has not. This does entail that all excuses for failing to follow through with treatment are equally legitimate. The fact that a patient is too busy or too lazy to care for himself is an offense against the patient *and* the health care professional. This is an offense against the health care professional because in order to do his job well he needs patient cooperation, indeed some must have a great deal. The surgeon requires, at minimum, the signing of the appropriate consent forms, while the physical therapist or the psychologist rely upon frequent and considerable patient participation in self-care.

The autonomous patient has a duty to avoid regarding the health care professional as infallible. The patient ought to see nurses or doctors for what they are, skilled and concerned professionals with limited powers. This duty to recognize the limits of the health care professional is not a duty to overlook negligent behavior. It is simply a duty to avoid the assumption that this is the source of the patient's every problem. This duty goes to the heart of the autonomous patient's role in collaborative decision making. A fair and accurate view of the abilities of the health care professional is necessary to clarify the patient's own role in his health care. In this same vein the autonomous patient also has a duty to not ask the *autonomous* health care professional for clearly unprofessional treatment. As has been noted in this regard before: a "patient may knowingly decline treatment, but he may not demand mistreatment".[4]

In a sense the *autonomous* patient has a duty to avoid being a patient. The root meaning of 'patient' is "a person or thing that undergoes some action".[5] Literally a *patient* is the conceptual opposite of an *agent*, the person who bears responsibility for his actions. While it seems paradoxical to claim that the patient ought to avoid being a patient, this simply points up the paradox inherent in our conception of the patient—one which blurs the distinction between the unconscious patient in the operating room and the fully rational patient in the waiting room. The idea that the patient is not a responsible actor but an object to be acted upon has been the principal source of the modern collective vision of patienthood. It has also offered a clear rationale for the health care professional to practice paternalism.[6] At minimum the autonomous patient has a duty to avoid adopting a sick role solely as a way to shirk the difficult responsibilities of his life. And since the patient may at times be the only one who can see this, it's crucial that he be the first to recognize patients' duties.

Suggesting that the judicious patient ought to ask questions or ought to take an active role in his own care has become common. However, for the autonomous patient—armed as he should be with patients' rights—this is not only a prudential dictum but a moral requirement. It is not just the *perfect* patient, or the *virtuous* patient, who should ask questions or engage in self-care. All autonomous patients have a moral obligation to do so. Patients' duties are not suggestions on how to become the ideal patient, but minimum, general moral requirements. Patients' duties are moral obligations because their practice goes beyond the exercise of mere prudence. While these duties are protective of some of the patient's most basic interests, they are also duties to health care professionals. While the autonomous patient has no duty to spare the health care professional the frustration of having his advice questioned, the health care professional cannot be expected to provide for patient autonomy alone. Modern health care systems still struggle with paternalism and are plagued by the ever-escalating cost of health care, as well as a rash of malpractice litigation. While attention to patient duties and the recognition of health care as help with self-care will not solve these problems, they can never be fully resolved unless we formulate an adequate conception of the patient's responsibilities.[7]

NOTES

1 Examples of this one-sided emphasis are abundant. A few include: Thomas A. Mappes and Jane S. Zembaty (eds.), *Biomedical Ethics* 3rd ed., (New York: McGraw-Hill, 1990). Chapter 2 is titled 'Physician's obligations and patient's rights'. Tom L. Beauchamp and LeRoy Walters (eds.), *Contemporary Issues in Bioethics* 3rd ed., (Belmont, California: Wadsworth, 1989). Chapter 7 is titled 'Patient's rights and professional responsibilties'. Carol Levine (ed.), *Case Studies in Bioethics: Selections from the Hastings Center Report* (New York: St. Martins, 1988). Chapter 1 is entitled 'Health care professionals' responsibilities and patients' rights'. These divisions and the articles included in each case strongly suggest that *patients' duties* are not of pressing importance.

2 For the American Hospital Association's 'A patient's bill of rights' see Warren T. Reich *et al.*, (eds.), *Encyclopedia of Bioethics* Vol. 4 (New York: Free Press, 1978), pp. 1782–83; see also the U.S. Department of

Health, Education and Welfare's list of patients' rights, pp. 1783–87. For a history of patients' rights see George Annas 'Patients' rights movement' *Encyclopedia of Bioethics* Vol. 3, pp. 1201–1205, which includes a bibliography.

3 Here is a clear case where the duties at issue are *prima facie* duties. Clearly, there are cases where the revelation of information may conflict with the patient's rights—for example, a right to privacy. One must realize, however, that the right to privacy, however construed, is not absolute. And, in addition, that the *exercise* of any such right to privacy should be tempered by considerations of the partnership in question.

4 *United States V. George,* 239 F. Supp. 752, 754 (D. Conn. 1965).

5 *The Oxford English Dictionary* (Oxford: 1961), Vol. 7, p. 556.

6 For example, Terrance Ackerman claims "the institutional role of patient requires the physician to assume the responsibilities of making decisions" in 'Why doctors should intervene', *Hastings Center Report* 12, (August, 1982). p. 15.

7 I do thank Martin Gunderson, Carol White, Lori Zink, this journal's reviewers, and students in my medical ethics classes at the University of North Carolina at Chapel Hill and Santa Clara University for helpful discussions of issues raised in this paper.

REFERENCES

Ackerman, T.: 1982, 'Why doctors should intervene', *Hastings Center Report* 12, 14–17.

Beauchamp, T. & Walters, L. (eds.): 1989, *Contemporary Issues in Bioethics,* Wadsworth, Belmont, CA.

Levine, Carol (ed.): 1988, *Case Studies in Bioethics: Selections from the Hastings Center Report,* St. Martins, New York.

Mappes, T. A. & Zembaty, J. S. (eds.): 1990, *Biomedical Ethics,* McGraw-Hill, New York.

Reich, W. T., *et al.* (eds.): *Encyclopedia of Bioethics,* Free Press, New York.

ANNOTATED BIBLIOGRAPHY: CHAPTER 2

Beauchamp, Tom L.: "The Promise of the Beneficence Model for Medical Ethics," *Journal of Contemporary Health Law and Policy* 6 (spring 1990), pp. 145–155. Beauchamp presents a historical and conceptual overview of the beneficence and autonomy models of the physician-patient relationship, before critically evaluating the effort of Edmund D. Pellegrino to reconcile the two in a reconstructed beneficence model.

Bok, Sissela: *Lying: Moral Choice in Public and Private Life* (New York: Random House, 1978). In this classic book, Bok provides a highly detailed examination of ethical issues connected with lying.

Brody, Howard: "The Physician-Patient Relationship: Models and Criticisms," *Theoretical Medicine* 8 (June 1987), pp. 205–220. This article includes a very useful overview of some of the theoretical models for the physician-patient relationship. Brody suggests that an amalgamation of the contractarian model with elements from a virtue-based approach, combined with appropriate empirical investigation, may yield richer models.

Council on Ethical and Judicial Affairs, American Medical Association: "Conflicts of Interests: Physician Ownership of Medical Facilities," *JAMA* 267 (May 6, 1992), pp. 2366–2369. This AMA position paper argues that physicians generally should not refer patients to medical facilities at which they do not directly provide care if they have a financial interest in the facility. An exception is made, however, for cases in which the community has a demonstrated need for the facility and there is no alternative way to finance the facility.

Edelstein, Ludwig: *Ancient Medicine* (Baltimore: Johns Hopkins, 1967). In this book, Edelstein discusses the Hippocratic Oath and shows that it contains two distinct sets of obligations—those to the patient and those to the physician's teacher and the teacher's progeny.

Faden, Ruth R., and Tom L. Beauchamp: *A History and Theory of Informed Consent* (New York: Oxford University Press, 1986). This ambitious work spans the history, theory, and practice of informed consent in medicine, human behavioral research, philosophy, and law.

Fox, Daniel M.: "The Politics of Physicians' Responsibility in Epidemics: A Note on History," *Hastings Center Report* 18 (April/May 1988), pp. 5–10 of supplement. Fox addresses the following historical questions: How did the medical profession, collectively, behave toward patients with contagious diseases, and how did public policy affect that behavior?

Humber, James M., and Robert F. Almeder, eds.: *Biomedical Ethics Reviews, 1988: AIDS and Ethics* (Clifton, NJ: Humana Press, 1989). Among the articles in this issue, which is devoted to some of the most challenging questions raised by AIDS, is David T. Ozar's "AIDS, Risk, and the Obligations of Health Professionals." Ozar maintains that healthcare professionals have an obligation to run more than ordinary risks to their lives in the interest of those who need their care. However, he considers various scenarios to bring out the limits of this obligation.

Jennings, Bruce, Daniel Callahan, and Arthur L. Caplan: "Ethical Challenges of Chronic Illness," *Hastings Center Report* 18 (February/March 1988), pp. 3–10 of supplement. The authors explore the possibility that the special nature of chronic care and the experience of chronic illness may require a change in some of the assumptions made in bioethics about the goals of medicine as well as a revision of central concepts such as patient autonomy and best interests.

Lidz, Charles W., Paul S. Appelbaum, and Alan Meisel: "Two Models of Implementing Informed Consent," *Archives of Internal Medicine* 148 (June 1988), pp. 1385–1389. The authors provide detailed, contrasting descriptions of two ways of implementing the doctrine of informed consent: the event model and the process model. They argue in favor of the process model before noting some of its limitations.

President's Commission for the Study of Ethical Problems in Medicine and Biomedical and Behavioral Research: *Making Health Care Decisions: The Ethical and Legal Implications of Informed Consent in the Patient-Practitioner Relationship*, Vol. 1: *Report* (Washington, DC: U.S. Government Printing Office, 1982). This report presents the Commission's conclusions and recommendations regarding both the role of informed consent in the patient-practitioner relationship and the means to promote a fuller understanding by patients and professionals of their common enterprise.

————: *Making Health Care Decisions*, Vol. 2: *Appendices: Empirical Studies of Informed Consent*. This volume contains the empirical studies used by the President's Commission in formulating its conclusions.

————: *Making Health Care Decisions*, Vol. 3: *Studies in the Foundations of Informed Consent*. Viewpoints represented in this volume are those of a psychologist, a historian, an anthropologist, a sociologist, a pediatrician-oncologist, a philosopher, and a medical student.

Relman, Arnold S.: "Dealing with Conflicts of Interest," *The New England Journal of Medicine* 313 (September 19, 1985), pp. 749–751. Relman condemns what he sees as a new entrepreneurialism on the part of physicians that generates conflicts of interests between physicians' commercial interests and their loyalty to patients.

Rosoff, Arnold J.: *Informed Consent: A Guide for Health Care Providers* (Rockville, MD: Aspen, 1981). This is a reference book that contains a great deal of practical information. It (1) sets forth the law in the informed consent area, (2) provides a philosophical framework for understanding legal developments, and (3) lays a foundation for researching questions of patient-consent law in particular states.

Wicclair, Mark R.: "Patient Decision-Making Capacity and Risk," *Bioethics* 5 (April 1991), pp. 91–104. In this article, Wicclair criticizes "risk-related standards" of decision-making capacity (competence). His main target is the standard defended by Allen E. Buchanan and Dan W. Brock, which requires balancing the values of (1) respecting a patient's self-determination and (2) protecting his or her well-being.

CHAPTER 3

PROFESSIONALS' OBLIGATIONS, INSTITUTIONS, AND PATIENTS' RIGHTS

INTRODUCTION

Many who receive medical care today do so in hospitals, nursing homes, clinics, and other large institutions. Providers of health care include nurses, interns, staff physicians, operating room technicians, and other health-care professionals and paraprofessionals. Many medical-care providers are not private practitioners but employees of the kinds of institutions mentioned above. Under these circumstances, a discussion of patients' rights and health professionals' responsibilities must encompass much more than the moral considerations raised in Chapter 2, which center on the physician-patient relationship. This chapter explores the rights of hospital patients and the correlative responsibilities of professionals. In particular, it examines in depth the role and responsibilities of nurses, issues concerning the protection of patient confidentiality, and questions about the role of institutional ethics committees (IECs).

Professional Statements Regarding Patients' Rights and Professionals' Obligations

What rights do hospital patients have? Recent statements of patients' rights, such as the American Hospital Association's "A Patient's Bill of Rights," included in this chapter, attempt to answer this question. These documents, however, usually say nothing about the nature of the rights in question. They do not specify whether the statements of "rights" function as (1) analogues of professional codes of ethics providing guidelines for professional conduct, (2) formulations of moral rights, or (3) statements of legal rights granted by a particular legal system. Despite this ambiguity, statements of patients' rights serve as reminders to hospital patients and health professionals that patients are to be treated as persons; they are neither mere objects to be manipulated by professionals nor subservient individuals who have waived their right of self-determination and other rights simply by becoming hospital patients.

Statements of hospital patients' rights have been explicitly formulated only recently. Most of us would take the asserted rights for granted. They include, for example, patients' rights to confidentiality and to adequate information regarding their condition. The apparent need to make these rights explicit, however, may be due to an increased awareness of their importance and of their frequent institutional abuses. It is not uncommon today for hospital patients to suspect that hospital routines are often organized around staff convenience rather than patient comfort and that patients are often treated more as "cases" than as persons. One critic of hospital practices, Willard Gaylin, describes the situation as follows:

> A stay in a hospital exposes an individual to a condition of passivity and impotence unparalleled in adult life, this side of prison. You are dressed in an uncomfortable garment, leaving you exposed and ludicrous; told when you must sleep and when you must rise; informed of what you may eat and when you have to eat it; notified as to when you can have visitors, who they shall be, and how long they can stay. You are discussed in the third person in your presence as though you were some idiot child or inanimate object. If you are unfortunate enough to have an interesting case, you will be presented to a group of strangers who may take the invasion of your privacy as their privilege. Your chart, at the foot of the bed, will contain all the vital information that you would seem to be entitled to have; yet, should you attempt to examine it, you will be treated like a pre-pubescent caught with a copy of *Portnoy's Complaint.*
>
> Some of this may be necessary for health and some for convenience, but most of it is simply the inevitable result of an authoritative person dealing with people who unquestionably accept his authority.[1]

Gaylin is not impressed by the American Hospital Association's statement of rights. He considers it a weak document that simply reminds patients of their rights but does not take hospitals to task for their failure to respect patients' rights. George Annas, in contrast, maintains that although the document can be criticized on grounds of incompleteness, generality, and unenforceability, it does have tremendous symbolic value, especially since the rights it espouses are sometimes challenged.[2]

Whether in the hospital setting or elsewhere, patients' rights entail obligations on the part of health-care professionals. For example, the idea that patients have a right to confidentiality implies that professionals are obliged to respect their patients' confidentiality. However, professionals sometimes see themselves as having obligations not only to patients but also to other persons or groups as well. For example, the American Nurses' Association Code for Nurses, reprinted in this chapter, states obligations that nurses have to the nursing profession and to the public, as well as to patients—who are referred to as "clients." Interestingly, while other codes of nursing ethics have generally asserted an obligation to "carry out physicians' orders," this code does not. The omission seems to reflect convictions about the importance of *professional autonomy* and *patient (client) advocacy* that are implied in the document, as in this statement: "The nurse acts to safeguard the client and the public when health care and safety are affected by the incompetent, unethical, or illegal practice of any person."

The Role and Responsibilities of Nurses

Nurses face both a set of moral problems similar to those faced by physicians and a special set of problems related to their professional role. As with physicians, nurses are sometimes forced to choose between doing what they believe will promote patients' well-being and respecting patients' self-determination. Various models of the nurse-patient relationship are possible, including a paternalistic model and a very different contracted-clinician model, which respects both a patient's right of self-determination and a nurse's right of conscientious refusal.[3]

But nurses also face dilemmas not faced by physicians. These dilemmas result from the nurse's position within the system or unit in which nurses work—which may be regarded as a *hierarchy* or as a *team,* depending on which features are emphasized. Nurses in hospitals care for patients and supervise others giving that care. Usually, they are directly responsible both for patient care and for implementing therapy. At the same time, nurses often have very little influence in decision making regarding patients. Furthermore, they are generally regarded as subordinate to doctors, who make diagnoses and issue orders that nurses are expected to carry out. Under these circumstances, nurses are sometimes confronted with situations in which their obligations to patients seem to conflict with their obligations to physicians. The following questions exemplify the kinds of problems nurses face. (1) Should nurses follow physicians' orders when (*a*) they have good reason to believe that the orders are mistaken, (*b*) the physicians refuse to admit that they might be mistaken, and (*c*) following orders seems likely to jeopardize a patient's safety or well-being? (2) What should nurses do if they have good reason to believe that physicians are violating their patients' right of self-determination? For example, what should a nurse do when a physician lies or withholds information from a patient?

Developing themes emphasized in feminist ethics (as discussed in Chapter 1), Joy Kroeger-Mappes focuses on these sorts of questions in this chapter. She stresses the difficulties faced by nurses in our society when protecting patients' interests requires them to buck the system. Kroeger-Mappes underscores the hierarchical nature of this system and attributes a large part of the difficulty to classist and sexist forces in society. She implicitly defends the increasingly prominent ideal of the nurse as an autonomous professional who is prepared, under some circumstances, to challenge physicians' authority in advocating for patients' interests.

In response to this emerging ideal, Lisa H. Newton, in an article reprinted in this chapter, defends the traditional ideal of the nurse, whose role requires submission to the authority of physicians. In defending the role of the traditional nurse, Newton argues that hospitals can function properly only if professionals' roles are clearly recognized; since only physicians have the training required to deal with many medical situations, their authority must be respected. Moreover, hospital patients have emotional needs that are best met by nurses in their traditional role. (Newton's arguments suggest viewing the doctor much as a quarterback; in this view, a player who questions and interferes with the quarterback's play calling, is unlikely to help the team.)

James L. Muyskens in this chapter directly challenges the claim that the nature of nursing demands submission and subservience. He articulates various arguments against this assertion. Some stress objectionable ways in which the traditional conception invites us to perceive nurses; others develop the position (contrary to that of Newton) that efficient healthcare delivery requires replacing the traditional role with that of the client advocate. That nurses should advocate for patients is assumed by Amy M. Haddad, who, in this chapter, focuses on the details of nurse-physician interactions in ethical decision making. Haddad suggests that some common differences in the ethical perspectives of men and women may sometimes contribute to ethical conflicts that arise between physicians and nurses. Another factor she highlights is their differing degrees of power and authority. Haddad uses a case to illustrate strategies for protecting patients' interests without unnecessarily damaging professional relationships or compromising nurses' self-respect.

Confidentiality and Conflicting Obligations

Whatever the full complement of patients' rights may be, the right of privacy and the related principle of confidentiality deserve special discussion. The importance of the principle of confidentiality in medicine has long been recognized. It is affirmed in the Hippocratic Oath as well as in more recent professional codes and statements such as those of the American Medical Association and the American Nurses' Association. It is also recognized by the ethical codes of medical record librarians and social workers. The law also recognizes the importance of the patient's right to control information held by health professionals. It does so in two ways: (1) Physicians and psychotherapists are subject to legal sanctions if they reveal confidential information about patients; (2) Physicians and psychotherapists are exempt from giving testimony about their patients before a court of law. Most discussions of the moral significance of the principle of confidentiality in health care stress either the importance of protecting the trust essential to the professional-patient relationship or respect for the patient's autonomy and privacy. In this chapter, Morton E. Winston discusses the justifications advanced for the rule of confidentiality in the medical context.

Most commentators, including Winston, believe that, despite the importance of medical confidentiality, the duty to respect confidentiality is a prima facie one, that is, one that may sometimes be justifiably overridden when it conflicts with other moral duties. Winston's article and the opinions in *Tarasoff v. Regents of the University of California* focus on the moral dilemmas posed for health-care professionals when such conflicts arise. Winston's article deals with the moral problems posed for health-care professionals by patients who either have AIDS or are carriers of HIV, the virus that causes AIDS. Under what conditions, if any, may physicians and nurses, for example, disclose confidential information about HIV carriers and other patients to prevent harm to others? In the *Tarasoff* case, the conflict at issue was between a psychologist's duty to respect the confidence of a patient, Prosenjit Poddar, and his possible duty to warn a young woman, Tatiana Tarasoff, that Poddar might try to kill her. He did not warn the woman or her family, and Poddar did kill her. Did the psychologist have a duty to protect the life of a woman who was not his patient? If he did, should this duty have taken precedence over his duty to respect Poddar's confidences? The contrast between the majority and the dissenting opinions in the case serves to heighten awareness of the moral dilemmas raised for the professional who must choose between violating confidentiality and failing to perform an act that might save the life of another human being or otherwise prevent serious harm.

Additional problems are raised for the traditional right to confidentiality by current developments in medical care. Hospital medicine, the need to share information among health-care team members, the existence of third-party insurance programs, and the expanding limits of medicine all result in a wide dissemination of "confidential" information about patients. Mark Siegler, in this chapter, discusses some of these problems.

Hospital (Institutional) Ethics Committees

As the provision of medical care has become more complex and as awareness of ethical issues in medicine has evolved, more and more health-care institutions, including hospitals, have established institutional ethics committees (IECs) to help them address the ethical issues that arise. IECs are usually composed of both medical and nonmedical members. A typical IEC might consist of physicians, nurses, and one or more hospital administrators, attorneys, laypersons, as well as members of the clergy or ethicists. The major functions of IECs might include the following: (1) *education*—educating the hospital staff about ethical aspects of medical care; (2) *policy and guideline formulation*—developing mandatory or suggested institutional guidelines and policies regarding ethical issues; and (3) *consultation*—reviewing cases, either prospectively or retrospectively, and making recommendations to those directly involved and to hospital administrators and others if necessary; prospective reviews usually examine the options available in a single case, and retrospective reviews usually look at a group of cases as a class.

Despite the proliferation of IECs, their strengths and weaknesses—and proper role—remain a matter of dispute. While there appears to be consensus on the appropriateness of an educational role and near consensus on the role of policy and guideline formulation, the consultative role is more contentious. Those who see IECs as capable of serving usefully in this role note several benefits. In the case of retrospective reviews, the IEC can identify inappropriate decisions so that similar cases in the future can be better handled. In the case of prospective reviews, the IEC can facilitate communication by identifying ethical issues and spelling out the conflicting values and interests that may be at the heart of disagreements. An IEC can provide a forum in which disagreements among staff, patients, and patients' families can be discussed and resolved; an IEC can also provide support when hard decisions have to be made. In addition, the committee may help to prevent unnecessary litigation by aiding in the resolution of disagreements that might otherwise require judicial handling. The most controversial consultative function is that of (prospectively) making recommendations about, or even deciding, what professionals should do in particular cases. While relatively supportive of a consultative role for IECs, Bernard Lo raises important questions in this chapter about IECs' efficiency and ethicality. He expresses concern about the actual process of committee decision making and sees a need to ensure that patients' interests are adequately represented when IEC decisions are made.

Concerns about the adequacy of IECs to function in a consultative role have motivated the question of whether some other form of ethical case review in health-care institutions might be more helpful. An alternative to the use of committees that enjoys the favor of some physicians is the use of individual ethics consultants. In this chapter's final reading, Michael D. Swenson and Ronald B. Miller examine the advantages and disadvantages of both the committee and consultant models. While, in their view, each model is preferable in certain kinds of situations, some situations may call for a third model—that of a consulting team of three or four individuals from different disciplines.

D.D.

NOTES

1 Willard Gaylin, "The Patient's Bill of Rights," *Saturday Review of the Sciences* 1 (February 24, 1973), p. 22.
2 George J. Annas, "The Emerging Stowaway, Patients' Rights in the 1980s," in Bart Gruzalski and Carl Nelson, eds., *Value Conflicts in Health Care Delivery* (Cambridge, MA: Ballinger, 1982).
3 See Sheri Smith, "Three Models of the Nurse-Patient Relationship," in Stuart F. Spicker and Sally Gadow, eds., *Nursing: Images and Ideals* (New York: Springer Publishing Company, 1980), pp. 176–188.

Professional Statements

A Patient's Bill of Rights
American Hospital Association

This statement, issued by the American Hospital Association (AHA), was affirmed by the AHA House of Delegates on February 6, 1973. It makes explicit some moral rights that many would take for granted (such as the right to considerate and respectful care) and some legal rights that hospitals, as well as other institutions, must respect.

The American Hospital Association presents a Patient's Bill of Rights with the expectation that observance of these rights will contribute to more effective patient care and greater satisfaction for the patient, his physician, and the hospital organization. Further, the Association presents these rights in the expectation that they will be supported by the hospital on behalf of its patients, as an integral part of the healing process. It is recognized that a personal relationship between the physician and the patient is essential for the provision of proper medical care. The traditional physician-patient relationship takes on a new dimension when care is rendered within an organizational structure. Legal precedent has established that the institution itself also has a responsibility to the patient. It is in recognition of these factors that these rights are affirmed.

(1) The patient has the right to considerate and respectful care.

(2) The patient has the right to obtain from his physician complete current information concerning his diagnosis, treatment, and prognosis in terms the patient can be reasonably expected to understand. When it is not medically advisable to give such information to the patient, the information should be made available to an appropriate person in his behalf. He has the right to know, by name, the physician responsible for coordinating his care.

(3) The patient has the right to receive from his physician information necessary to give informed consent prior to the start of any procedure and/or treatment. Except in emergencies, such information for informed consent should include but not necessarily be limited to the specific procedure and/or treatment, the medically significant risks involved, and the probable duration of incapacitation. Where medically significant alternatives for care or treatment exist, or when the patient requests information concerning medical alternatives, the patient has the right to such information. The patient also has the right to know the name of the person responsible for the procedures and/or treatment.

(4) The patient has the right to refuse treatment to the extent permitted by law and to be informed of the medical consequences of his action.

(5) The patient has the right to every consideration of his privacy concerning his own medical care program. Case discussion, consultation, examination, and treatment are confidential and should be conducted discreetly. Those not directly involved in his care must have the permission of the patient to be present.

(6) The patient has the right to expect that all communications and records pertaining to his care should be treated as confidential.

(7) The patient has the right to expect that within its capacity a hospital must make reasonable response to the request of a patient for services. The hospital must provide evaluation, service, and/or referral as indicated by the urgency of the case. When medically permissible, a patient may be transferred to another facility only after he has received complete information and explanation concerning the needs for and alternatives to such a transfer. The institution to which the patient is to be transferred must first have accepted the patient for transfer.

(8) The patient has the right to obtain information as to any relationship of his hospital to other health care and educational institutions insofar as his care is concerned. The patient has the right to obtain information as to the existence of any professional relationships among individuals, by name, who are treating him.

(9) The patient has the right to be advised if the hospital proposes to engage in or perform human experimentation affecting his care or treatment. The patient has the right to refuse to participate in such research projects.

(10) The patient has the right to expect reasonable continuity of care. He has the right to know in advance what appointment times and physicians are available and where. The patient has the right to expect that the hospital will provide a mechanism whereby he is informed by his physician or a delegate of the physician of the patient's continuing health care requirements following discharge.

(11) The patient has the right to examine and receive an explanation of his bill regardless of source of payment.

(12) The patient has the right to know what hospital rules and regulations apply to his conduct as a patient.

No catalog of rights can guarantee for the patient the kind of treatment he has a right to expect. A hospital has many functions to perform, including the prevention and treatment of disease, the education of both health professionals and patients, and the conduct of clinical research. All these activities must be conducted with an overriding concern for the patient, and, above all, the recognition of his dignity as a human being. Success in achieving this recognition assures success in the defense of the rights of the patient.

American Nurses' Association Code for Nurses

This code of ethics, adopted by the American Nurses' Association, states some of the obligations nurses have to (1) their patients, (2) the nursing profession, and (3) the public. The word *patient,* however, is never used. Throughout the document, the recipient of nurses' professional services is referred to as the "client." Unlike other codes of nursing ethics, this code does not explicitly assert any obligation "to carry out physicians' orders." Rather, it emphasizes nurses' obligations to clients and views both nurses and clients as the bearers of both basic rights and responsibilities.

PREAMBLE

A code of ethics makes explicit the primary goals and values of the profession. When individuals become nurses, they make a moral commitment to uphold the values and special moral obligations expressed in their code. The Code for Nurses is based on a belief about the nature of individuals, nursing, health, and society. Nursing encompasses the protection, promotion, and restoration of health; the prevention of illness; and the alleviation of suffering in the care of clients, including individuals, families, groups, and communities. In the context of these functions, nursing is defined as the diagnosis and treatment of human responses to actual or potential health problems.

Since clients themselves are the primary decision makers in matters concerning their own health, treatment, and well-being, the goal of nursing actions is to support and enhance the client's responsibility and self-determination to the greatest extent possible. In this context, health is not necessarily an end in itself, but rather a means to a life that is meaningful from the client's perspective.

When making clinical judgments, nurses base their decisions on consideration of consequences and of universal moral principles, both of which prescribe and justify nursing actions. The most fundamental of these principles is respect for persons. Other principles stemming from this basic principle are autonomy (self-determination), beneficence (doing good), nonmaleficence (avoiding harm), veracity (truth-telling), confidentiality (respecting privileged information), fidelity (keeping promises), and justice (treating people fairly).

In brief, then, the statements of the code and their interpretation provide guidance for conduct and relationships in carrying out nursing responsibilities consistent with the ethical obligations of the profession and with high quality in nursing care.

Reprinted with permission from *Code for Nurses with Interpretive Statements* © 1985, American Nurses' Association, Kansas City, Mo., pp. i,1.

CODE FOR NURSES

1. The nurse provides services with respect for human dignity and the uniqueness of the client, unrestricted by considerations of social or economic status, personal attributes, or the nature of health problems.

2. The nurse safeguards the client's right to privacy by judiciously protecting information of a confidential nature.

3. The nurse acts to safeguard the client and the public when health care and safety are affected

by the incompetent, unethical, or illegal practice of any person.

4. The nurse assumes responsibility and accountability for individual nursing judgments and actions.

5. The nurse maintains competence in nursing.

6. The nurse exercises informed judgment and uses individual competence and qualifications as criteria in seeking consultation, accepting responsibilities, and delegating nursing activities to others.

7. The nurse participates in activities that contribute to the ongoing development of the profession's body of knowledge.

8. The nurse participates in the profession's efforts to implement and improve standards of nursing.

9. The nurse participates in the profession's efforts to establish and maintain conditions of employment conducive to high quality nursing care.

10. The nurse participates in the profession's effort to protect the public from misinformation and misrepresentation and to maintain the integrity of nursing.

11. The nurse collaborates with members of the health professions and other citizens in promoting community and national efforts to meet the health needs of the public.

The Role and Responsibilities of Nurses

Ethical Dilemmas for Nurses: Physicians' Orders versus Patients' Rights
Joy Kroeger-Mappes

Joy Kroeger-Mappes is associate professor of philosophy at Frostburg State University (Maryland). Working especially in feminist philosophy, she is the author of "The Ethic of Care vis-a-vis the Ethic of Rights: A Problem for Contemporary Moral Theory." In the past, she has worked as a registered nurse.

Kroeger-Mappes identifies two kinds of ethical dilemmas that arise for the hospital nurse. One kind of ethical dilemma arises in cases in which following a physician's orders (explicit or implicit) would violate the patient's right to adequate medical treatment. Although Kroeger-Mappes makes clear that the nurse can be faced with some difficult matters of judgment, she argues that the nurse is morally obligated to act on behalf of the patient in those cases in which there is good reason to think that the physician's orders are not in the best medical interest of the patient. A second kind of ethical dilemma arises in cases in which following a physician's orders would violate the patient's right of self-determination. In Kroeger-Mappes's view, this second class of cases is less problematic than the first, since the nurse is not faced with problematic judgments about the patient's best medical interest. She contends that the nurse is morally obliged to act to protect the patient's right of self-determination. However, emphasizing the classist and sexist forces that typically make it difficult for the nurse to act on behalf of the patient, she goes on to suggest that "changes must be made in the workplace."

The American Hospital Association in a widely promulgated statement entitled "A Patient's Bill of Rights," makes explicit a number of the generally recognized rights of hospitalized patients.[1] Among the rights expressly articulated in the AHA statement is a cluster of rights closely associated with a more general right, the right of self-determination. The "self-determination cluster" includes: (1) the right to information concerning diagnosis, treatment, and prognosis; (2) the right to information necessary to give informed consent; and (3) the right to refuse treatment. The AHA statement duly recognizes several other important patient rights but, importantly, fails to explicitly recognize the patient's right to adequate medical care.[2] Surely, if the purpose of a statement of patients' rights is to catalogue patients' rights, we ought not to overlook this one. After all, the patient has agreed to enter the hospital setting precisely for the purpose of obtaining medical treatment. To the extent that adequate medical care is not forthcoming, the patient has been done an injustice. That is, the patient's right to adequate medical care has been violated.

This paper explores two types of ethical dilemmas related to patients' rights that arise for the hospital nurse.[3] (1) The first set of dilemmas is related to the patient's basic right to adequate medical care. (2) The second set of dilemmas is related to the cluster of rights closely associated with the patient's right of self-determination. Dilemmas arise for a nurse if adequate medical care for a patient would be jeopardized by following the expressed or understood orders of a physician. Dilemmas also arise for a nurse if the patient's right to self-determination would be violated by following the expressed or understood orders of a physician. In each case, the logic of the dilemma is similar. The dilemma arises because the nurse's apparent obligation to follow the physician's order conflicts with his or her obligation to act in the interest of the patient. To carry out the physician's order would be to act against the interest of the patient. To act in the interest of the patient would be to disobey the physician's order.[4] I will argue that when this conflict arises the nurse's obligation to the patient is overriding and that nurses must act and be allowed and encouraged to act to protect the rights of the patient.

I   NURSING DILEMMAS AND THE PATIENT'S RIGHT TO ADEQUATE MEDICAL CARE

In a hospital the primary responsibility for a patient's care rests with a physician. Physicians determine the medical diagnosis, treatment, and prognosis of patients' illnesses and write orders to arrive at and effect these determinations. In general, physicians' orders govern what a patient is to do and what is to be done for a patient, i.e., the degree of activity, diet, medication, diagnostic and treatment procedures to be performed. Nurses carry out physicians' orders themselves, delegate tasks to others, or make the orders known to those responsible for carrying them out. They are not generally allowed by law to diagnose or prescribe.[5] Although this is a greatly oversimplified picture of what goes on, as anyone familiar at all with the functioning of a hospital will realize, at least some of the complexities involved in the interaction among physicians, nurses, and patients in a hospital setting will emerge as we proceed.

The complexity of the ethical dilemmas arising for nurses regarding the patient's right to adequate medical care can best be understood by examining various examples. The following are suggested as being not atypical of situations arising in hospitals:

(1) A patient who has had emphysema for a number of years is admitted to a cardiac unit for observation with a tentative diagnosis of myocardial infarction. Oxygen is ordered in a concentration commonly given for patients with this diagnosis. The nurse, knowing that oxygen is contraindicated for patients with emphysema, must decide whether to carry out or question the order through appropriate channels.

(2) A patient admitted to the hospital for a diagnostic work-up has been on a special and fairly extensive drug therapy regimen. This regimen is common to patients of a particular private physician, seemingly regardless of their diagnosis. The private physician orders the drug therapy program continued after admission. However, accepted medical practice would ordinarily call for ceasing as many drugs as is safely possible, thus avoiding unnecessary variables in arriving at an accurate diagnosis. In general the private physician is viewed by other physicians as incompetent. The nurse is aware that the orders do not reflect good medical practice, but also realizes that she[6] will be dealing with this physician as long as she works at that hospital. The nurse must decide whether to follow the orders or refuse to carry out the orders, attempting through channels to have the orders changed.

(3) A frail patient recovering from recent surgery has been receiving intra-muscular antibiotic injections four times a day. The injection sites are very tender, and though the patient now is able to eat without problems, the intern refuses to change the order to an oral route of administration of the antibiotic because the absorption of the medication would be slightly diminished.

The nurse must decide whether to follow the order as it stands or continue through channels to try to have the order changed.

(4) A nurse on the midnight shift of a large medical center is closely monitoring a patient's vital signs (blood pressure, pulse rate, respiratory rate). The physicians have been unable to diagnose the patient's illness. In reviewing the patient's record, the nurse thinks of a possible diagnosis. The patient's condition begins to worsen and the nurse phones the intern-on-call to notify him of the patient's condition. The nurse mentions that the record indicates that diagnosis X is possible. The intern dismisses the nurse's suggested diagnosis and instructs the nurse to follow existing orders. Concerned that the patient's condition will continue to deteriorate, the nurse contacts her supervisor who concurs with the intern. The patient's blood pressure gradually but steadily falls and the pulse increases. The nurse has contacted the intern twice since the initial call but the orders remain unchanged. The nurse must decide whether to pursue the matter further, e.g., calling the resident-on-call and/or the patient's private physician.[7]

What are the obligations of nurses in such cases? Under what circumstances are nurses obligated to rely on their judgment and to question the physician's order? To what extent must nurses pursue the questioning when, in their view, the patient's right to adequate medical care is being violated? It is often taken for granted that when the medical assessments of physician and nurse differ, "the physician knows best." In order to see both why this is thought, perhaps correctly so, to be generally true and yet why it is surely not always true, it is necessary to consider some of the factors that account for the difference in physician and nurse assessments.

A nurse's assessment of what constitutes adequate medical treatment may differ from a physician's assessment for at least three reasons. (a) There is a difference in the amount and the content of their formal training. Physicians generally have a number of years more formal training than nurses, though that difference is not as great as it once was. More nurses now continue formal training in various ways, i.e., by pursuing graduate work and/or by becoming nurse practitioners, nurse clinicians, or nurse anesthetists. In addition, proportionately more nurses than ever before are college graduates. However, a physician's formal training is more extensive and detailed. Moreover, and perhaps most importantly, physicians are explicitly trained in the diagnosis and treatment of illness, with the emphasis of the training placed on the hard sciences. Nurses are trained to be knowledgeable about illness in general, the symptoms and treatment of illness, and the complications and side effects of various forms of therapy. While this formal training includes both the hard sciences and the social (primarily behavioral) sciences, there is an emphasis on the behavioral sciences. Nurses are trained to concentrate on the overall well-being of the patient. (b) There may be a difference in the length or concentration of their experience. For example, nurses who have worked in special care units (in medical and surgical cardiac units, burn units, renal units, intensive care units) for a number of years acquire a great deal of knowledge which may not be possessed by interns, and perhaps even residents and nonspecialty private physicians. Nurses who have worked for years in small community hospitals may well be more knowledgeable in some areas than some physicians. (c) There may be a difference in their knowledge of the patient. Nurses often have more detailed knowledge about patients than do physicians, who often see a patient only once a day. Nurses who are "at the bedside" are thus in a position to recognize small changes as they happen. Because of the possibility of more detailed knowledge, nurse assessments may be more accurate than physician assessments. Where physician and nurse assessments differ then, it is not necessarily the case that the physician's assessment is the correct one simply because of the amount and content of the physician's formal training. Physicians do make mistakes and, when they do, nurses must be in a position to protect the patient.[8]

Ethical dilemmas of the kind typified in the above four examples arise when to follow physician's orders would be to act against the medical interest of the patient. Given the fact that the *basic* obligation of both the physician and the nurse is to act in the medical interest of the patient, it is rather striking that anyone should suppose that the nurse's obligation to follow the physician's orders should ever take precedence. What, after all, is the foundation of the nurse's obligation to follow the physician's orders? Presumably, the nurse's obligation to follow the physician's orders is grounded on the nurse's obligation to act in the medical interest of the patient. The point is that the nurse has an obligation to follow physicians' orders because, ordinarily, patient welfare (interest) thereby is ensured. Thus when a nurse's obligation to follow a physician's order comes into *direct* conflict with the nurse's obligation to act in the medical interest of the patient, it would seem to follow that the patient's interests should always take precedence.

For instance, Example 1 provides a clear case of a medically unsound order. In fact, it is such a clear case that a nurse not questioning the order would be judged incompetent. The medically unsound order may be the result of a medical mistake or of medical incompetence. If the order is the result of an oversight, the physician is likely to be grateful when (if) a nurse questions the order. If the order is a result of incompetence, the physician is not likely to be grateful. Whatever the reason for the medically unsound order, the nurse is obligated to question an order if it is clearly medically unsound. The nurse must refuse to carry out the order if it is not changed, and to press the matter through channels in order to protect the medical interest of the patient. Example 2 is similar to Example 1 in that it involves a medical practice that is clearly unsound. If the orders are questioned, the physician here again is not likely to be grateful. Indeed, since the physician's practice may ultimately be at stake, the pressures brought to bear on a nurse may be overwhelming, particularly if the physician's colleagues choose to defend him or her. It is undeniable, however, that medical incompetence is not in the best medical interest of patients, and thus that the nurse's obligation is to question the order. It is of course true that a nurse acting on behalf of the patient in this situation may pay a heavy price, perhaps his or her job, for protecting the medical interests of patients. However, the nurse's moral obligation is no less real on this account.

With Example 3 the murkiness begins, since it does not provide a clear case of unsound medical practice, though perhaps it presents us with a case in which the physician is operating with a too-narrow view of good medical practice. As I mentioned earlier, nurses often are more concerned with the overall well-being of the patient. Physicians often are concerned only with identifying the illness, treating it, and determining how responsive the illness is to the treatment. To the extent that Example 3 resembles Example 1, i.e., the lumps are very bad and the difference in the absorption of the medication in the two routes of administration is small, the nurse has an obligation to question the order. Example 4 is like Example 3 in that it does not provide a clear case of a medically unsound order. However, in Example 4, much more is at stake. Since life itself is involved, any decision must be considered very carefully. The problem here is not a problem of weighing or balancing but a problem of being either right or wrong. Both Examples 3 and 4 force a nurse to assess this question: "How strong are my grounds for thinking that the orders are not in tune with the patient's best medical interest?" The murkiness comes in knowing exactly when the physician's order is in direct conflict with the patient's medical interest. As the last two examples illustrate, it can be very difficult to know exactly what is in the best medical interest of the patient. To the extent that the nurse has carefully considered the situation and is sure that his or her view is in accord with good medical care, the order should be questioned. The less sure one is, the less clear it becomes whether the order should be questioned and the matter pressed through channels.

In arguing the above, I am not advocating uncritical questioning. Clearly, questioning at some point must cease. Otherwise, hospitals could not function efficiently and as a result the medical interest of all patients would suffer. But if there is little or no opportunity for nurses and other health professionals to contribute their knowledge to the care of the patient, or if they are directly or indirectly discouraged from contributing, it would seem that they will find it difficult, if not impossible, to fulfill their obligations with respect to the patient's right to adequate medical care.

II   NURSING DILEMMAS AND THE PATIENT'S RIGHT OF SELF-DETERMINATION

The complexity of the ethical dilemmas arising for nurses regarding the patient's right of self-determination can best be understood by examining various cases. Again, the following are suggested as being not atypical of situations arising in hospitals:

(1) A patient is scheduled for prostate surgery (prostatectomy) early in the morning. Because he is generally unaware of what is happening to him due to senility, he is judged incompetent to give informed consent for surgery. The patient's sister visits him in the evenings, but the physicians have not been available during those times for her to give consent. The physicians have asked the nurses to obtain consent from the patient's sister. When she arrives the evening before surgery is scheduled, the nurses explain to her that her brother is to have surgery and what it would entail. The sister had not been told that surgery was being considered and questions its necessity for her brother who has not experienced any real problems due to an enlarged prostate. She does not feel she can sign the consent form without talking with one of his physicians. Should the nurses encourage her to sign the consent form, as the physicians have requested, or call one of the physicians to speak with the patient's sister?

(2) A patient in the cardiac unit who was admitted with a massive myocardial infarction begins to show

signs of increased cardiac failure. The patient and the family have clearly expressed their desire to the medical and nursing staff to refrain from "heroics" should complications arise. The patient stops breathing and the intern begins to intubate the patient, requests the nurse's assistance, and orders a respirator. Should the nurse follow orders or attempt to convince the intern to reconsider, calling the resident-on-call should the intern refuse?

(3) A patient is hospitalized for a series of diagnostic tests. The tests, history, and physical pretty clearly indicate a certain diagnosis. The physicians only tell the patient that they are not yet sure of the diagnosis, reassuring the patient that he is in good hands. Each day after the physicians leave, the patient asks the nurse, coming in to give medications, what the tests have shown and what his diagnosis is. When the nurse encourages the patient to ask the physicians these questions, he says he feels intimidated by them and that when he does ask questions they simply say that everything will be fine. Should the nurse reinforce what the physicians have said or attempt to convince the physicians that the patient has a right to information about his illness, pressing the matter through channels if they do not agree?

(4) A patient suffering from cancer is scheduled for surgery in the morning. While instructing the patient not to eat or drink after a certain hour, the nurse realizes that the patient is unaware of the risks involved in having the surgery and of those involved in not having the surgery. In talking further, the nurse sees clearly that the option of not having surgery was never presented and that the patient has only a vague idea of what the surgery will entail. She also appears to be unaware of her diagnosis. The patient has signed the consent form for surgery. Should the nurse proceed in preparing the patient for surgery, or, proceeding through channels, attempt to provide for a genuinely informed consent for the surgery?

What are the obligations of nurses in examples such as these? To what extent must nurses pursue questioning when, in their view, the patient's right of self-determination is being violated? Unless we are willing to say that a patient upon entering a hospital surrenders the right of self-determination, it seems clear that physicians' orders, explicit and implied, should be questioned in all of the above examples. After all, in each of the above examples, one of the rights expressly outlined by the American Hospital Association is in danger of being abridged. The rights involved are (or should be) known by all to be possessed by all. Here a difference in the for-

mal training and knowledge based on experience is not relevant in any difference between a physician's and a nurse's assessment. No formal training in medicine is necessary to arrive at the conclusion that the patient's right of self-determination is endangered.

The tension that exists for nurses in situations typified in the above four examples is not really that of a moral dilemma, but rather, a tension between doing what is morally right and what is least difficult practically, a tension common in everyday life. The problem is not that the nurse's obligation is unclear, but that in actual situations fulfilling this moral obligation is extremely difficult. What we must consider now in some detail are the social forces that make it so difficult for a nurse to act on behalf of the patient.

III NURSING DILEMMAS AND THE IMPORTANCE OF A CLASSIST AND SEXIST CONTEXT

I have argued that when following a physician's order would violate the patient's right to adequate medical care or the patient's right of self-determination, the nurse's moral obligation is to question the order. If necessary, the matter should be pressed through channels. It is well and good to say what nurses should do. It is quite another thing, given the forces at work in the everyday world in which nurses must work, to expect nurses to do what they ought to do.

To begin with, we must recognize that there is an important class difference between physicians and nurses, the difference between the upper middle class or upper class of physicians and the lower middle class of nurses.[9] A large proportion of physicians both start out and end their lives in the upper class. Though the economic status of a physician is not as high as that of a high-level corporation executive, the social status of a physician is very high because of the prestige of the profession of medicine in the United States today.[10] Physicians have a high social status in American society and they understand and identify with people who have a similarly high status.[11] "Physicians talked with physicians; nurses talked with nurses," is an observation of one sociological study.[12] Generally physicians do not understand or identify with nurses (or with most patients), in part because of a difference in social status. Correspondingly there is an educational difference between physicians and nurses. As mentioned earlier, the formal educational training necessary for a physician is generally much longer than that necessary for a nurse, and their training differs in content.

The differences in the composition of each profession on the basis of sex is clear. Most physicians are male (93.1 percent) and most nurses are female (97.3 percent).[13] In accordance with traditional sex roles, physicians are encouraged to be decisive and to act with authority. Studies indicate that physicians view themselves as omnipotent.[14] Nurses are encouraged to be tactful, sensitive, and diplomatic. Tact and diplomacy are necessary to make a physician feel in control. Put another way, nurses' recommendations for patient treatment must take a particular form. These recommendations must appear to be initiated by the physician. Nurses are expected to take the initiative and are responsible for making recommendations, but at the same time must appear passive.[15] Nurses who see their roles, partially at least, as one of consultant must follow certain rules of the "game."[16] If they refuse to follow the rules, they will be made to suffer consequences such as snide remarks, ostracism, harassment, or job termination.

Again, in accordance with traditional sex roles, nurses in hospitals are viewed much the same as are wives and mothers in the family. This is the view of nursing held both by society and by physicians. Nurses as women are expected to be subservient to physicians as men, to provide "tender loving care" to whoever may be in need, and to be responsible and competent in the absence of physicians but to relinquish that responsibility upon request, i.e., when physicians are present.[17]

As in society, women in hospitals (here women nurses) are typically viewed as sex objects, a situation which encourages physicians to discount the input of nurses with regard to patient care. The observation that women are viewed by male physicians as sexual objects was prevalent in a project which studied the discriminatory practices and attitudes against women in forty-one United States medical schools as seen from questionnaires completed by 146 women medical students. As the author notes, "The open expression of the notion that any woman—even if she is a patient—is fair game for lecherous interests of all men (including physicians) is in some ways the most distressing fact of these student observations."[18] Responses showing the prevalent attitude of physicians toward women in general or toward women as patients included: "[I] often hear demeaning remarks, usually toward nurses offered by clinicians. . . ." "[There is] superficial discussion of topics related to women. . . . Basic assumption: women are not worth serious consideration." "[The] most frequent remarks concern female patients—women's illnesses are assumed psychosomatic until proven otherwise."[19] Perhaps the most frequent response of women medical students depicting the attitudes of male medical students, professors, and clinicians centered around the use of slides in class of parts of women's anatomy and slides of nude women from magazine centerfolds. Those slides were introduced by medical-student colleagues or instructors often to bait women medical students or belittle them. One student relates, "My own experience with [a professor who had included a "nudie" slide in his lecture] was an interesting and emotional comment ending on, 'Men need to look down on women, and that's why I show the slide.' "[20] The response of the male members of the class to the slides was generally one of unmitigated laughter and approval. With such a negative and restricted view of women as persons, nurses, not to mention all women, are at a disadvantage in dealing with most male physicians.

Another aspect of the sexism that permeates the physician-nurse relationship is reflected in divergent standards of mental health for men and women. A study of thirty-three female and forty-six male psychiatrists, psychologists, and social workers showed that they held a different standard of mental health for women and men. The standard agreed upon for mentally healthy men was basically the same as the standard for mentally healthy adults. The standard for mentally healthy women included being more easily influenced, less objective, etc., in general characteristics which are less socially desirable.[21] Women then who are mentally healthy women are mentally unhealthy adults and women who are mentally healthy adults are mentally unhealthy women. This is clearly a "no win" situation for all women. Women nurses are no exception.

It is the just described classist and sexist economic and social context of the physician-nurse relationship that often inhibits the nurse from effectively functioning on behalf of the patient. Nurses have a moral responsibility to act on behalf of the patient, but in order to expect them to carry out that responsibility, changes must be made in the workplace. Nurses must be in a position to act to protect the rights of patients. They must be allowed and encouraged to do so. Therefore, those operating and managing hospitals and those responsible for hospital policies must establish policies which make it possible for nurses to protect patients' rights without risking their present and future employment. Those operating and managing hospitals cannot eradicate classism and sexism, but they must be aware of the impact it has on patient care, for again the ultimate goal of everyone connected with hospitals is adequate medical care within the framework of patients' rights. As potential patients it is important to all of us.[22]

NOTES

1 The statement can be found, for example, in *Hospitals,* vol. 4 (Feb. 16, 1973).

2 I am aware of the difficulties in determining what constitutes adequate medical care. For example, is adequate medical care determined solely by reference to past and present medical practices, by the established wisdom of knowledgeable health professionals, or by knowledgeable recipients of medical care? And how is the standard for knowledgeability determined? I am presuming that problems such as these, though difficult, are not insoluble. I am also aware of the related difficulty in distinguishing medical care from health care. And what distinguishes medical care and health care from nursing care? In this paper, "medical care" will refer to the diagnosis and treatment of illness. Health professionals then, who aid physicians in the process of diagnosing and treating illness, aid in providing medical care.

3 A large majority of all working nurses work in hospitals.

4 The International Code of Nursing Ethics is ambiguous in addressing such a dilemma. The relevant section (#7) of the code merely states: "The nurse is under an obligation to carry out the physician's orders intelligently and loyally and to refuse to participate in unethical procedures." What exactly is the nurse supposed to do when to carry out the physician's orders is in effect to participate in unethical procedures? The most recent (1976) version of the *Code for Nurses* (available from the American Nurses' Association) adopted by the American Nurses' Association directly addresses this problem. Section 3 states, "The nurse acts to safeguard the client and the public when health care and safety are affected by the incompetent, unethical, or illegal practice of any person." The interpretive statement of section 3 begins, "The nurse's primary commitment is to the client's care and safety. Hence, in the role of client advocate, the nurse must be alert to and take appropriate action regarding any instances of incompetent, unethical, or illegal practice(s) by any member of the health-care team or the health-care system itself, or any action

on the part of others that is prejudicial to the client's best interests."

5 The area of practice which is solely that of the nurse and the area of practice which is solely that of the physician is presently in a state of flux. The submissive role that nursing has held in relation to the physician's practice of medicine is being rejected by the nursing profession. Nurse practice acts, which regulate the practice of nursing, in many states reflect the change toward an expanded and more independent role for nurses. For example, a definition of a nursing diagnosis, as distinct from a medical diagnosis, is a part of some nurse practice acts. Daniel A. Rothman and Nancy Lloyd Rothman, *The Professional Nurse and the Law* (Boston: Little, Brown, 1977), pp. 65–81.

6 The overwhelming majority of nurses are women and the overwhelming majority of physicians are men. Because the examples are intended to reflect the hospital situation as it exists, I will use the feminine pronoun to refer to nurses and the masculine pronoun to refer to physicians.

7 In an actual case of this description, the intern dismissed the nurse's diagnosis by asking if her woman's intuition told her that diagnosis X was the correct one. The nurse's decision was to not pursue the matter, and early in the morning the patient sustained a cardiac arrest and was unresponsive to resuscitation efforts by the resuscitation team.

8 Obviously, nurses also make mistakes, but physicians are clearly in a position to protect the patient when they become aware of nurses' mistakes.

9 Vicente Navarro, "Women in Health Care," *New England Journal of Medicine,* vol. 292 (Feb. 20, 1975), p. 400.

10 Barbara Ehrenreich and John Ehrenreich, "Health Care and Social Control," *Social Policy,* vol. 5 (May/June 1974), p. 33.

11 Raymond S. Duff and August Hollingshead, *Sickness and Society* (New York: Harper & Row, 1968), p. 371.

12 *Ibid.,* p. 376.

13 Navarro, p. 400.

14 Robert L. Kane and Rosalie A. Kane, "Physicians' Attitudes of Omnipotence in a University Hospital," *Journal of Medical Education,* vol. 44 (August 1969), pp. 684–690; and Trucia Kushner, "Nursing Profession: Condition Critical," *Ms,* vol. 2 (August 1973), p. 99.

15 Kushner, p. 99.

16 Leonard I. Stein, "The Doctor-Nurse Game," in

Edith R. Lewis, ed., *Changing Patterns of Nursing Practice: New Needs, New Roles* (New York: American Journal of Nursing Company, 1971), p. 227.

17 JoAnn Ashley, *Hospitals, Paternalism, and the Role of the Nurse* (New York: Teachers College, 1976), p. 17.

18 Margaret A. Campbell, *Why Would a Girl Go into Medicine?* (Old Westbury, N.Y.: Feminist Press, 1973), p. 73.

19 *Ibid.*, p. 74.

20 *Ibid.*, p. 26.

21 Inge K. Broverman, Donald M. Broverman, Frank E. Clarkson, Paul S. Rosenkrantz, and Susan R. Vogel, "Sex-Role Stereotypes and Clinical Judgments of Mental Health," *Journal of Consulting and Clinical Psychology*, vol. 34 (February 1970), pp. 1–7.

22 I wish to thank Jorn Bramann, Marilyn Edmunds, Jane Zembaty, and especially Tom Mappes for their helpful comments on earlier versions of this paper.

In Defense of the Traditional Nurse
Lisa H. Newton

Lisa H. Newton is professor of philosophy and director of the Program in Applied Ethics at Fairfield University. She is coauthor of *Watersheds: Classic Cases in Environmental Ethics* (1994), coeditor of *Taking Sides—Clashing Views on Controversial Issues in Business Ethics and Society* (2d ed., 1992), and the author of such articles as "Virtue and Role: Reflections on the Social Nature of Morality."

Newton counters the emerging ideal of the nurse as an autonomous professional who is prepared to challenge doctors' authority and advocate for patients' interests (an ideal that Kroeger-Mappes defends). In its place she urges "the traditional ideal of the skilled and gentle caregiver, whose role in health care requires submission to authority as an essential component." In defending the traditional nurse, Newton argues the following: (1) To run properly, hospital bureaucracies require clear roles and lines of authority; (2) only physicians are properly trained to handle serious medical situations that arise without warning; and (3) the vulnerable, compromised situation of hospital patients gives rise to emotional needs that can be met only by nurses, who serve (in some respects) as surrogate mothers. After exploring limits of the nurse-mother analogy, Newton responds to objections motivated by a feminist perspective. In this discussion she emphasizes that being an autonomous person is compatible with choosing a nonautonomous professional role, such as that of the nurse, and that support for men's participation in nursing would be liberating for them.

When a truth is accepted by everyone as so obvious that it blots out all its alternatives and leaves no respectable perspectives from which to examine it, it becomes the natural prey of philosophers, whose essential activity is to question accepted opinion. A case in point may be the ideal of the "autonomous professional" for nursing. The consensus that this ideal and image are appropri-

ate for the profession is becoming monolithic and may profit from the presence of a full-blooded alternative ideal to replace the cardboard stereotypes it routinely condemns. That alternative, I suggest, is the traditional ideal of the skilled and gentle caregiver, whose role in health care requires submission to authority as an essential component. We can see the faults of this traditional ideal very clearly now, but we may perhaps also be able to see virtues that went unnoticed in the battle to displace it. It is my contention that the image and ideal of

Reprinted from *Nursing Outlook*, vol. 29 (June 1981), pp. 348–354, with permission from Mosby-Year Book, Inc.

the traditional nurse contain virtues that can be found nowhere else in the health care professions, that perhaps make an irreplaceable contribution to the care of patients, and that should not be lost in the transition to a new definition of the profession of nursing. . . .

ROLE COMPONENTS

The first task of any philosophical inquiry is to determine its terminology and establish the meanings of the key terms for its own purposes. To take the first term, a *role* is a norm-governed pattern of action undertaken in accordance with social expectations. The term is originally derived from the drama, where it signifies a part played by an actor in a play. In current usage, any ordinary job or profession (physician, housewife, teacher, postal worker) will do as an example of a social role; the term's dramatic origin is nonetheless worth remembering, as a key to the limits of the concept.

Image and ideal are simply the descriptive and prescriptive aspects of a social role. The *image* of a social role is that role as it is understood to be in fact, both by the occupants of the role and by those with whom the occupant interacts. It describes the character the occupant plays, the acts, attitudes, and expectations normally associated with the role. The *ideal* of a role is a conception of what that role could or should be—that is, a conception of the norms that should govern its work. It is necessary to distinguish between the private and public aspects of image and ideal.

Since role occupants and general public need not agree either on the description of the present operations of the role or on the prescription for its future development, the private image, or self-image of the role occupant, is therefore distinct from the public image or general impression of the role maintained in the popular media and mind. The private ideal, or aspiration of the role occupant, is distinct from the public ideal or normative direction set for the role by the larger society. Thus, four role-components emerge, from the public and private, descriptive and prescriptive, aspects of a social role. They may be difficult to disentangle in some cases, but they are surely distinct in theory, and potentially in conflict in fact.

TRANSITIONAL ROLES

In these terms alone we have the materials for the problematic tensions within transitional social roles. Stable social roles should exhibit no significant disparities among images and ideals: what the public generally gets is about what it thinks it should get; what the job turns out to require is generally in accord with the role-occupant's aspirations; and public and role-occupant, beyond a certain base level of "they-don't-know-how-hard-we-work" grumbling, are in general agreement on what the role is all about. On the other hand, transitional roles tend to exhibit strong discrepancies among the four elements of the role during the transition; at least the components will make the transition at different times, and there may also be profound disagreement on the direction that the transition should take. . . .

BARRIERS TO AUTONOMY

The first contention of my argument is that the issue of autonomy in the nursing profession lends itself to misformulation. A common formulation of the issue, for example, locates it in a discrepancy between public image and private image. On this account, the public is asserted to believe that nurses are ill-educated, unintelligent, incapable of assuming responsibility, and hence properly excluded from professional status and responsibility. In fact they are now prepared to be truly autonomous professionals through an excellent education, including a thorough theoretical grounding in all aspects of their profession. Granted, the public image of the nurse has many favorable aspects—the nurse is credited with great manual skill, often saintly dedication to service to others, and, at least below the supervisory level, a warm heart and gentle manners. But the educational and intellectual deficiencies that the public mistakenly perceives outweigh the "positive" qualities when it comes to deciding how the nurse shall be treated, and are called upon to justify not only her traditionally inferior status and low wages, but also the refusal to allow nursing to fill genuine needs in the health care system by assuming tasks that nurses are uniquely qualified to handle. For the sake of the quality of health care as well as for the sake of the interests of the nurse, the public must be educated through a massive educational campaign to the full capabilities of the contemporary nurse; the image must be brought into line with the facts. On this account, then, the issue of nurse autonomy is diagnosed as a public relations problem: the private ideal of nursing is asserted to be that of the autonomous professional and the private image is asserted to have undergone a transition from an older subservient role to a new professional one but the public image of the nurse ideal is significantly not mentioned in this analysis.

An alternative account of the issue of professional autonomy in nursing locates it in a discrepancy between private ideal and private image. Again, the private ideal is that of the autonomous professional. But the actual performance of the role is entirely slavish, because of the way the system works—with its tight budgets, insane schedules, workloads bordering on reckless endangerment for the seriously ill, bureaucratic red tape, confusion, and arrogance. Under these conditions, the nurse is permanently barred from fulfilling her professional ideal, from bringing the reality of the nurse's condition into line with the self-concept she brought to the job. On this account, then, the nurse really is not an autonomous professional, and total reform of the power structure of the health care industry will be necessary in order to allow her to become one.

A third formulation locates the issue of autonomy in a struggle between the private ideal and an altogether undesirable public ideal: on this account, the public does not want the nurse to be an autonomous professional, because her present subservient status serves the power needs of the physicians; because her unprofessional remuneration serves the monetary needs of the entrepreneurs and callous municipalities that run the hospitals; and because the low value accorded her opinions on patient care protects both physicians and bureaucrats from being forced to account to the patient for the treatment he receives. On this account, the nurse needs primarily to gather allies to defeat the powerful interest groups that impose the traditional ideal for their own unworthy purposes, and to replace that degrading and dangerous prescription with one more appropriate to the contemporary nurse.

These three accounts, logically independent, have crucial elements of content in common. Above all, they agree on the objectives to be pursued: full professional independence, responsibility, recognition, and remuneration for the professional nurse. And as corollary to these objectives, they agree on the necessity of banishing forever from the hospitals and from the public mind that inaccurate and demeaning stereotype of the nurse as the Lady with the Bedpan: an image of submissive service, comforting to have around and skillful enough at her little tasks, but too scatterbrained and emotional for responsibility.

In none of the interpretations above is any real weight given to a public ideal of nursing, to the nursing role as the public thinks it ought to be played. Where public prescription shows up at all, it is seen as a vicious and false demand imposed by power alone, thoroughly illegitimate and to be destroyed as quickly as possible. The possibility that there may be real value in the traditional role of the nurse, and that the public may have good reasons to want to retain it, simply does not receive any serious consideration on any account. It is precisely that possibility that I take up in the next section.

DEFENDING THE "TRADITIONAL NURSE"

As Aristotle taught us, the way to discover the peculiar virtues of any thing is to look to the work that it accomplishes in the larger context of its environment. The first task, then, is to isolate those factors of need or demand in the nursing environment that require the nurse's work if they are to be met. I shall concentrate, as above, on the hospital environment, since most nurses are employed in hospitals.

The work context of the hospital nurse actually spans two societal practices or institutions: the hospital as a bureaucracy and medicine as a field of scientific endeavor and service. Although there is enormous room for variation in both hospital bureaucracies and medicine, and they may therefore interact with an infinite number of possible results, the most general facts about both institutions allow us to sketch the major demands they make on those whose function lies within them.

To take the hospital bureaucracy first: its very nature demands that workers perform the tasks assigned to them, report properly to the proper superior, avoid initiative, and adhere to set procedures. These requirements are common to all bureaucracies, but dramatically increase in urgency when the tasks are supposed to be protective of life itself and where the subject matter is inherently unpredictable and emergency prone. Since there is often no time to re-examine the usefulness of a procedure in a particular case, and since the stakes are too high to permit a gamble, the institution's effectiveness, not to mention its legal position, may depend on unquestioning adherence to procedure.

Assuming that the sort of hospital under discussion is one in which the practice of medicine by qualified physicians is the focal activity, rather than, say, a convalescent hospital, further contextual requirements emerge. Among the prominent features of the practice of medicine are the following: it depends on esoteric knowledge, which takes time to acquire and which is rapidly advancing; and, because each patient's illness is unique, it is uncertain. Thus, when a serious medical situation arises without warning, only physicians will know how to deal with it (if their licensure has any point), and they will not always be able to explain or justify their actions to nonphysicians, even those who are required to assist them in patient care.

If the two contexts of medicine and the hospital are superimposed, three common points can be seen. Both are devoted to the saving of life and health; the atmosphere in which that purpose is carried out is inevitably tense and urgent; and, if the purpose is to be accomplished in that atmosphere, all participating activities and agents must be completely subordinated to the medical judgments of the physicians. In short, those other than physicians, involved in medical procedures in a hospital context, have no right to insert their own needs, judgments, or personalities into the situation. The last thing we need at that point is another autonomous professional on the job, whether a nurse or anyone else.

PATIENT NEEDS: THE PRIME CONCERN

From the general characteristics of hospitals and medicine, that negative conclusion for nursing follows. But the institutions are not, after all, the focus of the endeavor. If there is any conflict between the needs of the patient and the needs of the institutions established to serve him, his needs take precedence and constitute the most important requirements of the nursing environment. What are these needs?

First, because the patient is sick and disabled, he needs specialized care that only qualified personnel can administer, beyond the time that the physician is with him. Second, and perhaps most obviously to the patient, he is likely to be unable to perform simple tasks such as walking unaided, dressing himself, and attending to his bodily functions. He will need assistance in these tasks, and is likely to find this need humiliating; his entire self-concept as an independent human being may be threatened. Thus, the patient has serious emotional needs brought on by the hospital situation itself, regardless of his disability. He is scared, depressed, disappointed, and possibly, in reaction to all of these, very angry. He needs reassurance, comfort, someone to talk to. The person he really needs, who would be capable of taking care of all these problems, is obviously his mother, and the first job of the nurse is to be a mother surrogate.

That conclusion, it should be noted, is inherent in the word "nurse" itself: it is derived ultimately from the Latin *nutrire,* "to nourish or suckle"; the first meaning of "nurse" as a noun is still, according to *Webster's New Twentieth Century Unabridged Dictionary* "one who suckles a child not her own." From the outset, then, the function of the nurse is identical with that of the mother, to be exercised when the mother is unavailable. And the meanings proceed in logical order from there: the second definitions given for both noun and verb involve caring for children, especially young children, and the third, caring for those who are childlike in their dependence—the sick, the injured, the very old, and the handicapped. For all those groups—infants, children, and helpless adults—it is appropriate to bring children's caretakers, surrogate mothers, nurses, into the situation to minister to them. It is especially appropriate to do so, for the sake of the psychological economies realized by the patient: the sense of self, at least for the Western adult, hangs on the self-perception of independence. Since disability requires the relinquishing of this self-perception, the patient must either discover conditions excusing his dependence somewhere in his self-concept, or invent new ones, and the latter task is extremely difficult. Hence the usefulness of the maternal image association: it was, within the patient's understanding of himself "all right" to be tended by mother; if the nurse is (at some level) mother, it is "all right" to reassume that familiar role and to be tended by her.

LIMITS ON THE "MOTHER" ROLE

The nurse's assumption of the role of mother is therefore justified etymologically and historically but most importantly by reference to the psychological demands of and on the patient. Yet the maternal role cannot be imported into the hospital care situation without significant modification—specifically, with respect to the power and authority inherent in the role of mother. Such maternal authority, includes the right and duty to assume control over children's lives and make all decisions for them; but the hospital patient most definitely does not lose adult status even if he is sick enough to want to. The ethical legitimacy as well as the therapeutic success of his treatment depend on his voluntary and active cooperation in it and on his deferring to some forms of power and authority—the hospital rules and the physician's sapiential authority, for example. But these very partial, conditional, restraints are nowhere near the threat to patient autonomy that the real presence of mother would be; maternal authority, total, diffuse, and unlimited, would be incompatible with the retention of moral freedom. And it is just this sort of total authority that the patient is most tempted to attribute to the nurse, who already embodies the nurturant component of the maternal role. To prevent serious threats to patient autonomy, then, the role of nurse must be from the outset, as essentially as it is nurturant, unavailable for such attribution of authority. Not only must the role of nurse not include authority; it must be incompatible with authority: essentially, a subservient role.

The nurse role, as required by the patient's situation, is the nurturant component of the maternal role and excludes elements of power and authority. A further advantage of this combination of maternal nurturance and subordinate status is that, just as it permits the patient to be cared for like a baby without threatening his autonomy, it also permits him to unburden himself to a sympathetic listener of his doubts and resentments, about physicians and hospitals in general, and his in particular, without threatening the course of his treatment. His resentments are natural, but they lead to a situation of conflict, between the desire to rebel against treatment and bring it to a halt (to reassert control over his life), and the desire that the treatment should continue (to obtain its benefits). The nurse's function speaks well to this condition: like her maternal model, the nurse is available for the patient to talk to (the physician is too busy to talk), sympathetic, understanding, and supportive; but in her subordinate position, the nurse can do absolutely nothing to change his course of treatment. Since she has no more control over the environment than he has, he can let off steam in perfect safety, knowing that he cannot do himself any damage.

The norms for the nurse's role so far derived from the patient's perspective also tally, it might be noted, with the restrictions on the role that arise from the needs of hospitals and medicine. The patient does not need another autonomous professional at his bedside, any more than the physician can use one or the hospital bureaucracy contain one. The conclusion so far, then is that in the hospital environment, the traditional (nurturant and subordinate) role of the nurse seems more adapted to the nurse function than the new autonomous role.

PROVIDER OF HUMANISTIC CARE

So far, we have defined the hospital nurse's function in terms of the specific needs of the hospital, the physician, and the patient. Yet there is another level of function

that needs to be addressed. If we consider the multifaceted demands that the patient's family, friends, and community make on the hospital once the patient is admitted, it becomes clear that this concerned group cannot be served exclusively by attending to the medical aspect of care, necessary though that is. Nor is it sufficient for the hospital-as-institution to keep accurate and careful records, maintain absolute cleanliness, and establish procedures that protect the patient's safety, even though this is important. Neither bureaucracy nor medical professional can handle the human needs of the human beings involved in the process.

The general public entering the hospital as patient or visitor encounters and reacts to that health care system as an indivisible whole, as if under a single heading of "what the hospital is like." It is at this level that we can make sense of the traditional claim that the nurse represents the "human" as opposed to "mechanical" or "coldly professional" aspect of health care, for there is clearly something terribly missing in the combined medical and bureaucratic approach to the "case": they fail to address the patient's fear for himself and the family's fear for him, their grief over the separation, even if temporary, their concern for the financial burden, and a host of other emotional components of hospitalization.

The same failing appears throughout the hospital experience, most poignantly obvious, perhaps, when the medical procedures are unavailing and the patient dies. When this occurs, the physician must determine the cause and time of death and the advisability of an autopsy, while the bureaucracy must record the death and remove the body; but surely this is not enough. The death of a human being is a rending of the fabric of human community, a sad and fearful time; it is appropriately a time of bitter regret, anger, and weeping. The patient's family, caught up in the institutional context of the hospital, cannot assume alone the burden of discovering and expressing the emotions appropriate to the occasion; such expression, essential for their own regeneration after their loss must originate somehow within the hospital context itself. The hospital system must, somehow, be able to share pain and grief as well as it makes medical judgments and keeps records.

The traditional nurse's role addresses itself directly to these human needs. Its derivation from the maternal role classifies it as feminine and permits ready assumption of all attributes culturally typed as "feminine": tenderness, warmth, sympathy, and a tendency to engage much more readily in the expression of feeling than in the rendering of judgment. Through the nurse, the hospital can be concerned, welcoming, caring, and grief-stricken; it can break through the cold barriers of efficiency essential to its other functions and share human feeling.

The nurse therefore provides the in-hospital health care system with human capabilities that would otherwise be unavailable to it and hence unavailable to the community in dealing with it. Such a conclusion is unattractive to the supporters of the autonomous role for the nurse, because the tasks of making objective judgments and of expressing emotion are inherently incompatible; and since the nurse shows grief and sympathy on behalf of the system, she is excluded from decision-making and defined as subordinate.

However unappealing such a conclusion may be, it is clear that without the nurse role in this function, the hospital becomes a moral monstrosity, coolly and mechanically dispensing and disposing of human life and death, with no acknowledgment at all of the individual life, value, projects, and relationships of the persons with whom it deals. Only the nurse makes the system morally tolerable. People in pain deserve sympathy, as the dead deserve to be grieved; it is unthinkable that the very societal institution to which we generally consign the suffering and the dying should be incapable of sustaining sympathy and grief. Yet its capability hangs on the presence of nurses willing to assume the affective functions of the traditional nursing role, and the current attempt to banish that role, to introduce instead an autonomous professional role for the nurse, threatens to send the last hope for a human presence in the hospital off at the same time.

THE FEMINIST PERSPECTIVE

From this conclusion it would seem to follow automatically that the role of the traditional nurse should be retained. It might be argued, however, that the value of autonomy is such that any nonautonomous role ought to be abolished, no matter what its value to the current institutional structure.

Those who aimed to abolish black slavery in the United States have provided a precedent for this argument. They never denied the slave's economic usefulness; they simply denied that it could be right to enslave any person and insisted that the nation find some other way to get the work done, no matter what the cost. On a totally different level, the feminists of our own generation have proposed that the traditional housewife and mother role for the woman, which confined women to domestic life and made them subordinate to men, has been very useful for everyone except the women trapped in it. All the feminists have claimed is that the profit of

others is not a sufficient reason to retain a role that demeans its occupant. As they see it, the "traditional nurse" role is analogous to the roles of slave and housewife—it is derived directly, in fact, as we have seen, from the "mother" part of the latter role—exploitative of its occupants and hence immoral by its very nature and worthy of abolition.

But the analogy does not hold. A distinction must be made between an autonomous person—one who, over the course of adult life, is self-determining in all major choices and a significant number of minor ones, and hence can be said to have chosen, and to be responsible for, his own life—and an autonomous *role*—a role so structured that its occupant is self-determining in all major and most minor role-related choices. An autonomous person can certainly take on a subordinate role without losing his personal autonomy. For example, we can find examples of slaves (in the ancient world at least) and housewives who have claimed to have, and shown every sign of having, complete personal integrity and autonomy with their freely chosen roles.

Furthermore, slave and housewife are a very special type of role, known as "life-roles." They are to be played 24 hours a day, for an indefinite period of time; there is no customary or foreseeable respite from them. Depending on circumstances, there may be de facto escapes from these roles, permitting their occupants to set up separate personal identities (some of the literature from the history of American slavery suggests this possibility), but the role-definitions do not contemplate part-time occupancy. Such life-roles are few in number; most roles are the part-time "occupational roles," the jobs that we do eight hours a day and have little to do with the structuring the rest of the twenty-four. An autonomous person can, it would seem, easily take up a subordinate role of this type and play it well without threat to personal autonomy. And if there is excellent reason to choose such a role—if, for example, an enterprise of tremendous importance derives an essential component of its moral worth from that role—it would seem to be altogether rational and praiseworthy to do so. The role of "traditional nurse" would certainly fall within this category.

But even if the traditional nurse role is not inherently demeaning, it might be argued further, it should be abolished as harmful to the society because it preserves the sex stereotypes that we are trying to overcome. "Nurse" is a purely feminine role, historically derived from "mother," embodying feminine attributes of emotionality, tenderness, and nurturance, and it is subordinate—thus reinforcing the link between femininity and subordinate status. The nurse role should be available to men, too, to help break down this unfavorable stereotype.

This objective to the traditional role embodies the very fallacy it aims to combat. The falsehood we know as sexism is not the belief that some roles are autonomous, calling for objectivity in judgment, suppression of emotion, and independent initiative in action, but discouraging independent judgment and action and requiring obedience to superiors; the falsehood is the assumption that only men are eligible for the first class and only women are eligible for the second class.

One of the most damaging mistakes of our cultural heritage is the assumption that warmth, gentleness, and loving care, such as are expected of the nurse, are simply impossible for the male of the species, and that men who show emotion, let alone those who are ever known to weep, are weaklings, "sissies," and a disgrace to the human race. I suspect that this assumption has done more harm to the culture than its more publicized partner, the assumption that women are (or should be) incapable of objective judgment or executive function. Women will survive without leadership roles, but it is not clear that a society can retain its humanity if all those eligible for leadership are forbidden, by virtue of that eligibility, to take account of the human side of human beings: their altruism, heroism, compassion, and grief, their fear and weakness, and their ability to love and care for others.

In the words of the current feminist movement, men must be liberated as surely as women. And one of the best avenues to such liberation would be the encouragement of male participation in the health care system, or other systems of the society, in roles like the traditional nursing role, which permit, even require, the expressive side of the personality to develop, giving it a function in the enterprise and restoring it to recognition and respectability.

CONCLUSIONS

In conclusion, then, the traditional nurse role is crucial to health care in the hospital context; its subordinate status, required for its remaining features, is neither in itself demeaning nor a barrier to its assumption by men or women. It is probably not a role that everyone would enjoy. But there are certainly many who are suited to it, and should be willing to undertake the job.

One of the puzzling features of the recent controversy is the apparent unwillingness of some of the current crop of nursing school graduates to take on the assignment for which they have ostensibly been prepared, at least until such time as it shall be redefined to accord more closely with their notion of professional. These frustrated nurses who do not want the traditional nursing role, yet wish to employ their skills in the health care system in some way, will clearly have to do something else. The health care industry is presently in the process of very rapid expansion and diversification, and has created significant markets for those with a nurse's training and the capacity, and desire, for autonomous roles. Moreover, the nurse in a position which does not have the "nurse" label, does not need to combat the "traditional nurse" image and is ordinarily accorded greater freedom of action. For this reason alone it would appear that those nurses intent on occupying autonomous roles and tired of fighting stereotypes that they find degrading and unworthy of their abilities, should seek out occupational niches that do not bear the label, and the stigma, of "nurse."

I conclude, therefore: that much of the difficulty in obtaining public acceptance of the new "autonomous professional" image of the nurse may be due, not to public ignorance, but to the opposition of a vague but persistent public ideal of nursing; that the ideal is a worthy one, well-founded in the hospital context in which it evolved; and that the role of traditional nurse, for which that ideal sets the standard, should therefore be maintained and held open for any who would have the desire and the personal and professional qualifications, to assume it. Perhaps the current crop of nursing school graduates do not desire it, but there is ample room in the health care system for the sort of "autonomous professional" they wish to be, apart from the hospital nursing role. Wherever we must go to fill this role, it is worth going there, for the traditional nurse is the major force remaining for humanity in a system that will turn into a mechanical monster without her.

The Role of the Nurse
James L. Muyskens

James L. Muyskens is professor of philosophy and dean of the college of liberal arts and sciences, University of Kansas. He is the author of *Moral Problems in Nursing: A Philosophical Investigation* (1982), from which this selection is taken. His published articles include "Nursing and Access to Health Care" and "No Easy Choice: Resolving Everyday Ethical Dilemmas."

Muyskens confronts the question of whether nursing, by its very nature, demands that its members play a subservient role (as argued by Newton). Many find traditional models of the nurse objectionable, he argues, for reasons that include the following: (1) The associated sex-role stereotyping has been challenged by feminists; (2) our understanding of proper family roles has changed; (3) technological advances in health care have, for practical reasons, resulted in delegating some duties to nurses that were formerly assumed only by physicians; and (4) the increasing proportion of elderly in the population has increased demand for services best provided by nursing. Thus, not only have traditional nursing *care* functions gained in importance, but also nurses participate increasingly in *cure* and other functions that were traditionally the sole province of physicians (e.g., initiating treatment in cardiac arrest and performing diagnostic procedures). In part because care remains the distinguishing feature of nursing, nurses are best regarded neither as surrogate mothers nor as extensions of physicians but rather as "client advocates."

. . . [O]ne of the sources of our moral directives is our role, whether it be professional, familial, or societal. In this chapter we shall examine the changing and expanding role of the nurse and see how these changes influence moral problems in nursing. The changes that have occurred and are occurring make it especially difficult to be clear about the nurse's role-related duties. At times such as these we get very little guidance from tradition and custom—for they, too, are being questioned. Nevertheless, a look at the traditional model of the nurse can help us understand how it is that we have come to be in the present state of flux.

Until recently nurses have been viewed (by the public and nurses themselves) as dependent functionaries, acting under the direction and supervision of physicians. In a recent study of hospitalized patients, those queried mentioned the following as nursing functions: taking doctors' orders, giving medications, serving meals, giving shots, and providing bedpans (Beletz, 1974). The nurse's role has frequently been viewed as

Reprinted with permission of the author from James L. Muyskens, *Moral Problems in Nursing: A Philosophical Investigation* (Rowman and Littlefield, 1982), pp. 30–39.

being analogous to that of the traditional wife and mother in a household.

> When the first American schools of nursing were established the family was the institutional model for the operation of hospitals. All policies and procedures formulated to guide management of the "household" were designed to look out for the overall interests of the institution. . . . The role of [nurses] was very early conceived as that of caring for the "hospital family" . . . Like mothers in a household, nurses were responsible for meeting the needs of all members of the hospital family—from patients to physicians [Ashley, 1977, p. 17].

The concept of the nurse as "surrogate mother" with the physician as (traditional) husband and father (i.e., as head of the household) and client as child has not only been widely held in the past, it continues to be held by many today.

A related model of the nurse—one that stresses even more than the surrogate mother model the nurse's dependency relationship to the physician—is that of "handmaiden of the physician" (female servant or attendant). The nurse is seen as the physician's personal assistant, who can provide technical and humane services which nurture the client. The nurse is not a decision-maker nor one to initiate treatment. She (or he) lacks the knowledge for that. She is able only to implement the physician's decisions.

With these two as the dominant models of nursing in early and mid-twentieth century, it is not surprising that 97 percent of nurses are women [Navarro, 1975, p. 400]. This, despite the fact that in earlier times men were much more prominent in the nursing profession. . . . [Aroskar, 1980, p. 21].

These days it is frequently argued . . . that nursing has come to be regarded as a feminine (passive, submissive) role because most nurses are women, and in a male-dominated, sexist society such as ours, women are seen as (and see themselves as) dependent and subservient. As Robert Baker has pointed out, however, another possible way to account for the disproportionate number of females in nursing is that they "have been channeled into nursing because the profession, *by its very nature,* requires its members to play a dependent and subservient role (i.e., the traditional female role in a sexist society)" [Baker, 1980, pp. 42–43].

Our task is not that of constructing the most adequate historical account of the fact that nursing in the mid-twentieth century is regarded as a feminine role. What is important for our purposes is to determine whether nursing, by its very nature, requires its members to play a dependent and subservient role. The moral duties one has as a "dependent professional" (the title of an editorial by Rozella Schlotfeldt, 1976) are quite different from those one has as an autonomous professional. The ANA *Code for Nurses* is premised on the notion of the nurse as an autonomous professional and on the concept of the nurse as client advocate [ANA, 1976]. One of the sharpest contrasts between it and the (earlier) *International Code of Nursing Ethics* is that of the view of the nurse presupposed by the codes. The International Code has not moved far from the traditional notion of dependency upon the physician. Whereas the ANA code entails that the nurse's primary duty is to the client, the International Code entails that her or his fundamental allegiance is to the physician. . . .

There are several reasons why many nurses and others who are interested in the well-being of the nursing profession favor a model of nursing such as that of client advocate, and who find the traditional surrogate mother and handmaiden of the physician models inadequate and objectionable. Most of these reasons . . . are nonmoral reasons (i.e., they are concerned with factors such as efficiency of care, political power, and so on). Yet they are relevant to our task because . . . the role-related duties a nurse has are contingent upon the role which has been adopted. Let us consider the variety of reasons the traditional models have lost favor with many.

A. The sex-role stereotyping with which these models are linked has been challenged by the women's liberation (feminist) movement. We have all seen that if we take away the blind, unthinking adherence to gender or sex-role stereotypes and eliminate the coercive practices that make it difficult for members of either sex to step beyond the cultural definitions of male and female work, many women are no longer content to play the submissive, passive role. We see that many more women than in the past are going into fields previously considered as male domains. But even those going into the traditional female occupations have changed. Students in baccalaureate nursing programs today appear to be less inclined to fall into a submissive role than did students ten or more years ago [Davis, 1969; DeLora and Moses, 1969].

B. Our concept of the proper roles of family members has changed. Many factors have produced this change in outlook: the breakdown of sex-role stereotypes (just discussed), changing economic circumstances (high percentages of two-income family units), changing birth rates (fewer children per couple), experimentation with alternative family structures (for example, a family unit headed by two females rather than a husband and a wife), and the breakdown of an increasingly large number of marriages, resulting in single-parent family units. With all these changes in the basic family model, it no longer seems obvious that other institutions need be patterned after the traditional model. Other models with rather different implications for the role of the nurse can now be considered. Experience has demonstrated that the mother's and the wife's role can be quite different from the traditional conception. So, too, can roles (e.g., nursing) that have been based on the models of mother and wife.

C. Technological advances in the care of the sick have also affected both the practice and the conception of the role of the nurse. Especially in hospital care, changing technology has resulted in extending the responsibility of nurses. Often for very practical reasons, nurses have been delegated authority to carry out duties initially assigned only to physicians. An example from one area of nursing is representative of a rather common phenomenon.

Careful research into the nurse's role in the coronary care unit indicates that it came about primarily as a result of default, dictate, *and* exigency, and not from careful analysis of the role by the nursing profession. Doctors staffed one of the original coronary care units that later served as the prototype of many other units, until they rebelled against the boredom and constant vigilance; then nurses, who are believed somehow different in temperament so that they really understand boring vigils, were assigned to replace the doctors. When it became obvious that the nurse's vigilance was not enough in the coronary care unit, it was conveniently reasoned that the same nurses, who throughout history were thought to be capable only of observing and reporting, could now not only detect a potentially fatal arrhythmia, but were capable also of terminating it with a complex electronic device—capable, that is, only in the event the physician did not arrive in the critical first two minutes [Berwind, 1975, p. 89].

D. The changing age distribution of the population has resulted in a greater need for the kinds of services nursing best provides. The number of people in the postretirement age group is rapidly increasing. People of advanced age are more likely than others to need the nurture, the care, the emotional support, the long-term monitoring, and the teaching necessary to cope with diminished capacities that nurses are well-suited to provide. The aged suffering from chronic illness need *care* and sustenance rather than *cure*. Often in these cases, the highly technical and interventionist skills of the physician are, in fact, ancillary to the caring functions of the nurse.

Of course, in reality the power has usually remained in the hands of the physician, whose position is securely buttressed by the law and tradition. But the physician's position as perpetual "captain of the team" appears to square with neither the way services are actually provided today nor efficiency in their delivery. The exalted position of physicians appears to have no basis other than their desire to hold on to a position of power and prestige. Those concerned with efficiency of health care delivery, cost-cutting, as well as the prestige and professional standing of nurses argue for an increasingly active and autonomous role for nurses in cases in which care rather than cure is the primary need. . . .

A case for the primacy of nursing care can be made not only for an increasing number of aged who are chronically ill but also for those (of any age) recognized as incurable. Such people are beyond the help of physicians but clearly are not beyond the help of nurses. . . . An example of nursing care as primary, with physician's care as ancillary, is the hospice movement, one of which is St. Christopher's.

St. Christopher's is a nursing facility for the incurably ill directed by Cicely Saunders—a nurse who, in order to have her theories of nursing the incurably ill listened to, had to qualify as a physician. At St. Christopher's, care of the sick is primary; disease *per se* is untreated, and physicians are indeed ancillary to nurses [Baker, 1980, p. 45].

These (A–D) and undoubtedly other factors have contributed to the dissatisfaction with the traditional conceptions of the nurse's role and the search for a more appropriate one. All seem to agree on at least one feature of an appropriate model, namely, that the nurse must be viewed as more than a dependent functionary. She or he may quite appropriately work at times under a physician. But that is not the defining characteristic of the profession.

A small number of nurses (nurse practitioners—about 13,000 of the 1.4 million licensed nurses) have extended the role of the nurse by adding to their functions many that traditionally have been done by physicians. They take clients' health histories, make referrals to physicians, perform diagnostic procedures, make initial house calls to assess a client's condition, initiate treatment in cardiac arrest, prescribe medications for certain conditions, and so on. All this is done under the supervision of a physician, but the nurse practitioner has considerable latitude. The greater responsibility and decision-making authority is what distinguishes the practitioner from the traditional nurse as "handmaiden of the physician." Yet she or he remains "an extension of the physician's hands."

There are two rather different, yet *not* necessarily incompatible, ways the search for a more adequate role has taken. On the one hand, as we saw earlier, the nurse's role can be *distinguished from* that of the physician. Whereas the physician's function is (roughly speaking) to cure, the nurse's is to care (the hospice movement is an example). On the other hand, as we have just seen with the nurse practitioner (which is modeled after, and very similar to, the physician's assistant program), the nurse's role can be seen as *identical with* a segment of the physician's traditional responsibilities.

The role of the nurse is expanding in both of these ways: traditional nursing *care* functions have increased in importance (for reasons already discussed), while the traditional function of assisting a physician has greatly gained in scope. An adequate understanding of the nurse's role must encompass both of these developments. Frequently, however, one of these dimensions of the expanding role is stressed at the expense of the other.

When similarities between nursing and medicine are emphasized, the role of the nurse can be expanded into those (a) areas and (b) functions which suffer as a result of the uneven distribution of, and lack of, general practitioners. Examples of (a) are the nurse practitioners with organizations such as the National Health Service who frequently are the only full-time health professional in a county which has no physician. Examples of (b) are nurse practitioners who perform the basic diagnostic functions of the general practitioner in order to admit clients into the health care network. That is, the nurse performs the "gate-keeping" function, determining who needs the services of the various professionals within the health care facility. It seems likely that nursing will continue to expand in these ways and that the nurse practitioner—many of whom may go into private practice—will play an ever-increasing role in the delivery of health care. One of many recent developments in which we can see this occurring is in the design of health maintenance organizations (HMOs). . . .

These are important developments and ones that promise greater efficiency and better use of personnel resources than will be the case if we continue to insist that these services remain in the sphere of the physician. The developments are also attractive to many nurses, who yearn for greater responsibility and opportunity. It would be a mistake to consider the nurse practitioner as the paradigm for the nurse of the future, however. Nursing is much broader than this. The most serious loss with such a concept of nursing would be the failure to capture the quality that sets nursing apart from the other health professions, namely, a special kind of client *care*.

We have compared the curative function of the physician with the care or nurturing function of the nurse. It is in this contrast with physicians that we touch the core of nursing, the feature that cannot be absent if nursing is present. The distinction between physician cure and nursing care developed earlier is most vividly captured by the image of the physician stopping momentarily by the bedside to see how the treatment plan is progressing, while the nurse is at the bedside 24 hours a day providing care, comfort, and compassion. The most vital human dimension of health care—a dimension which increases in importance as our society becomes increasingly dominated by technology—is what the nurse *qua* nurse has to offer. "In a society of machines, in institutions of healing run by machines, the nurse has a vital part to play in preserving the human aspects of patient care" [Wilson, 1974, p. 414].

Examination of the nurse's role reveals that its unique contribution to client care is maintaining the human element in what would otherwise become cold, uncaring, and depersonalized treatment. The nurse's role is, at its fundamental level, a moral one, one of ensuring the dignity and autonomy of the client in need. The fundamental question concerning the nurse's role is what conception of the nurse will likely result in the most effective and efficient exercising of this primary nursing responsibility to ensure humane, dignified care.

Rather than seeing oneself as a mother surrogate or as an extension of the physician, clearly a far better model for achieving the primary nursing care objective is that of the client's advocate. On this view, the nurse assumes the responsibility of assisting the client in meeting his or her health care needs. The nurse, in concert with other health care professionals, helps the client to understand what his or her needs really are, to know what possibilities are available for meeting these needs, to stand up to anyone who is threatening the client's autonomy or well-being, and to help the client help himself or herself. Thus the nurse makes it possible for a client to avail himself or herself of health care without having to lose the dignity and humanity concomitant with the exercise of autonomy. The client need not assume the role of the child. His or her status as a rational being is not threatened. Given the client's present condition (physical weakness, pain, anxiety, possibly confusion, and so on), the nurse is there to safeguard his or her status as an autonomous agent.

Nursing care, more than anything else, can contribute to diminishing the factors that (in many cases) inhibit the possibility of free, unfettered decision-making: the pain, the anxiety, the lack of knowledge of one's prognosis, one's alternatives, one's rights. If a client advocate instead of a parent surrogate, the nurse does not decide for the client. Rather, whenever possible, the nurse helps the client to decide. When that is not possible, the nurse takes those steps (a) which are likely to maximize the possibilities for the client's autonomous choice in the future or (b) which best express the client's wishes or aspirations (previously expressed by the client or inferred from past actions or information obtained from the client's family).

As mentioned, being a client advocate at times may entail standing up to other health professionals who are acting in ways that do not conform to the client's wishes or maximum autonomy. The nurse may also have to help the client so that she or he can insist on an alternative form of treatment or discontinuation of treatment or whatever. Indeed, it is also likely that the presence of nurses as effective client advocates would soon modify the behavior of any other health professionals who are inclined to act out of disregard for their client's autonomy. Quite likely they too would want to avoid unpleasant controversy and would take that into account in making their initial judgment. So the large number of unpleasant confrontations that are often imagined if nurses were generally to act as effective client advocates are just not at all probable. The claim that the delivery of health care would be hampered by nurses acting as client advocates just cannot be substantiated.

The nurse is ideally situated to perform the function of client advocate. The nurse's caring functions—attending to basic and intimate physical needs—put him or her in constant, close contact with the client. Frequently no other health care professional has anywhere near the same opportunities to observe and interact with the client. The nurse's professional training and position make it more possible for her or him than for family members to strike a balance between sensitive involvement with the client and a dispassionate, detached relationship. The nurse's training and experience also provide her or him with indispensable knowledge about prospects for cure, alternative modes of treatment, anticipated side-effects of treatments, and so on.

The conception of the nurse developed above is the one assumed by the framers of the ANA *Code of Ethics*. The nurse's first or primary obligation is to the client. . . .

One of the most controversial and divisive issues within the nursing profession in recent years has been that of educational requirements for the nurse [Fields, 1980a,b]. If the view of client advocate outlined here is to become the dominant model for nursing care, it is obvious that the nurse must be well educated. Nursing education must include teaching of basic nursing skills and technique but also nursing specialties, use of sophisticated equipment, and a broad understanding of the humanities, ethics, communication skills, and psychology. Precisely how the required education can best be accomplished is one of the main items on the agenda of nursing educators. What complicates the debate is the vested interests of the various types of degree programs, as well as the understandable concern of many graduates of diploma and associate degree programs when proposals are made to require nurses to have the baccalaureate degree to qualify as a "professional" nurse. If one considers oneself a professional and has for many years, to be placed in the bottom tier of a two-tier system and to be called a technical nurse is tantamount to a demotion. Also, such a person may be far better trained—through on-the-job experience and self-education—than those with baccalaureate degrees who are beginning their nursing careers. Accommodation, sensitivity, and creativity in dealing with these cases and in setting interim standards are not only necessary from the point of view of prudence (achieving the necessary good-will and votes to obtain the goal) but also from the point of view of morality (treating diploma and associate degree nurses fairly and with respect). Yet this does not in any way reduce the need for a rigorous and broad educational requirement.

Beside the fact that a liberal arts education combined with rigorous nursing courses and experience is likely to be the most efficient and effective way to gain the knowledge required to function effectively as a client advocate, another reason for establishing these (as is being done) as requirements for future entrants into the profession is that it is probably the only way nursing can achieve a standing of equality with other professions. That one can enter the profession of nursing without having completed a quality liberal arts education is a factor that sets nursing apart from most other professional groups. This is a dubious mark of distinction—and one that acts as a millstone around the neck of the profession.

If nurses are to be client advocates, their training also must instill a clear and affirmative self-concept. That is, they must understand and acknowledge their *own* moral rights. On the mother surrogate model and especially the handmaiden of the physician model, it is quite possible (even if not desirable) for the nurse to accept a subservient, even servile, role, to view herself or himself as standing lower than others, and to take a deferential attitude toward others due to ignorance or lack of understanding of one's own moral rights. But if one combines such an attitude with the client advocate model, it becomes a fatal flaw. . . .

Acknowledging fully one's own rights as a person and developing a concept of oneself as a moral agent may be the first steps to recognizing and honoring the rights of others. The training of a nurse should include moral education to encourage and promote such personal growth. One of the positive features of feminism has been that it has acted as a catalyst for many women and nurses, helping them to see the moral defects of servility [Hill, 1973]. A person with a developed moral sense satisfies one of the essential criteria for being an effective advocate for a sick person. Combine this with knowledge of the various basic technical skills, nurse specialties, related disciplines, and so on, and we have a nurse who meets all the conditions for effective client advocacy. . . .

BIBLIOGRAPHY AND REFERENCES

American Nurses' Association (ANA). 1976. *Code for Nurses with Interpretive Statements.* American Nurses' Association, Kansas City, Mo.

Aroskar, M. A. 1980. "The Fractured Image: The Public Stereotype of Nursing and the Nurse." In *Nursing: Images and Ideals,* edited by S. Gadow and S. Spicker, pages 18–34. New York: Springer Publishing Co.

Ashley, J. 1977. *Hospitals, Paternalism, and the Role of the Nurse.* New York: Teachers College Press.

Baker, R. 1980. "Care of the Sick and Cure of Disease: Comment on 'The Fractured Image'. In *Nursing: Images and Ideals,* edited by S. Gadow and S. Spicker, pages 41–48. New York: Springer Publishing Co.

Beletz, E. E. 1974. "Is Nursing's Public Image Up to Date?" *Nursing Outlook* 22, no. 7, (July): 432–35.

Berwind, A. 1975. "The Nurse in the Coronary Care Unit." In *The Law and the Expanding Nursing Role,* edited by B. Bullough, pages 82–94. New York: Appleton-Century-Crofts.

Davis, A. J. 1969. "Self-Concept, Occupational Role Expectation, and Occupational Choice in Nursing and Social Work." *Nursing Research* 18, no. 57 (January–February).

Delora, J. R., and Moses, D. V. 1969. "Specialty Preferences and Characteristics of Nursing Students in Baccalaureate Programs." *Nursing Research* 18, no. 2 (March–April): 137–44.

Fields, C. M. 1980a. "What Kind of Education for Nurses?" *The Chronicle of Higher Education,* February 11.

———. 1980b. "Drive to Require Bachelor's Degrees for Nurses Seen Heading to Some Questionable Programs." *The Chronicle of Higher Education,* April 21.

Hill, T. E., Jr. 1973. "Servility and Self-Respect." *The Monist* 57, no. 1 (January): 87–104.

Navarro, V. 1975. "Women in Health Care." *New England Journal of Medicine* 292 (February 20): 398–402.

Schlotfeldt, R. M. 1976. Editorial, "The Dependent Professional." *The American Nurse,* May 15, 1976.

Wilson, H. 1974. "A Case for Humanities in Professional Nursing Education." *Nursing Forum* 13, no. 4.

The Nurse/Physician Relationship and Ethical Decision Making
Amy M. Haddad

Amy M. Haddad is associate professor at the school of pharmacy and allied health professions and associate of the Creighton Center for Health Policy and Ethics at Creighton University. She is the coauthor of *Ethical and Legal Issues in Home Health Care* (1991). Her published articles include "Problematic Ethical Experiences: Stories from Nursing Practice" and "Ethical Problems in Home Healthcare."

Haddad explores the nurse-physician relationship in the context of ethical decision making. After describing differences in power and authority between physicians and nurses, Haddad argues that the divergent ways in which these professionals approach ethical problems may reflect differences in the characteristic ethical problem-solving styles of men and women (as stressed in the ethics of care). Haddad then explores a case involving a man of uncertain competence. She uses this case to illustrate the importance of (1) direct, nondeferential communication by nurses to physicians and (2) a vivid awareness of the effects of particular decisions on relationships within the health-care team and on the patient's quality of life.

Reprinted with permission of the publisher from *AORN Journal,* vol. 53 (January 1991), pp. 151–156.

. . .

FACTORS AFFECTING THE NURSE/PHYSICIAN RELATIONSHIP

In 1967, Leonard I. Stein, MD, identified a basic communication pattern that physicians and nurses used. He called it the "Doctor-Nurse Game."[1] The game is still played daily in many surgery departments. The object of the game is for the nurse to be bold, have initiative, and be responsible for making significant recommendations while appearing to be doing none of this. It should appear that it was the physician who made the recommendations.

Both the nurse and physician need to be acutely aware of subtle nonverbal cues and verbal nuances in the conversation. The major rule of the game is that open disagreement must be avoided at all costs. Nurses learn to make suggestions and ask for recommendations in a way that sounds like they are not doing so. It is interesting that Dr Stein and his colleagues revisited the Doctor-Nurse Game in 1990.[2] Twenty-three years later, they found only minor changes in the way the game is played.

Consequences of this indirect method of communication are that it is inefficient and stifles open communication that is essential in ethical decision making. The doctor-nurse game is similar to the superior-subordinate game that occurs in almost all organizational hierarchies. Subordinates often use the passive voice to make suggestions to superiors within the organization.

Stereotypes are oversimplified, unvarying conceptions about a person or a group. Traditional gender stereotypes in nursing, both positive (eg, ministering, self-sacrificing angels, nurturing mothers) and negative (eg, sexpots, battle axes), add a new dimension to the superior-subordinate game. Positive (eg, noble, decisive leaders; captain of the ship) and negative (eg, egotistical, arrogant dictators) stereotypes in medicine have the same effect. Unfortunately, negative stereotypes in nursing and medicine tend to mirror those of women and men in society at large.

Another influencing factor in the nurse/physician relationship arises from the inherent inequity in power and authority that each discipline exercises. Physicians exercise a great deal of direct power in the health care system. Even though some reimbursement systems have begun to erode the physician's role as gatekeeper, physicians still tend to determine who is admitted and what type of treatments and procedures are to be performed.

These decisions translate directly into revenue for the hospital.

Nurses are not a direct source of revenue for the hospital, but the hospital would not be able to function without them. Nurses' work is largely unseen but essential. Therefore, nurses, like others in traditionally female jobs, exercise little direct authority regarding decisions that affect their work or welfare. They generally receive little pay for the amount of responsibility associated with their work, and they receive little recognition and respect for their contribution to the enterprise as a whole.

Physicians, especially surgeons, earn more and generally are self-employed. The difference in income and employment status result in class barriers between physicians and nurses. The two groups rarely socialize with each other, which limits opportunities for informal discussions outside of the work setting. Informal discussions over coffee, at lunch, or during social activities, help individuals understand each other's values and motivations, which inevitably affect how the people work together.

Physicians and nurses also differ in educational preparation. Nurses generally have fewer years of formal education, which puts them at a disadvantage. Efforts to increase entry-level education in nursing have been strongly resisted by organized medicine. Physicians argue that increased education pulls nurses away from patient care. The more education a nurse has, however, the more she or he threatens the status quo and the authority of the physician. All of these factors influence the ability to collaborate and resolve ethical problems. The process becomes even more difficult because nurses and physicians usually do not perceive ethical problems in the same way.

APPROACHES TO ETHICAL DECISION MAKING

Carol Gilligan, PhD, noted some significant differences in how males and females reason morally.[3] One view predominant in females acknowledges that people's lives are embedded in relationships and that the relationships are central to moral decision making. People with this interdependent view are concerned about being responsible and responsive to others. They consider the specifics of a situation when making a decision. This view is most clearly reflected in the concept of mercy and commonly is used by nurses in making ethical decisions.

A counter view of moral reasoning consists of a rights and rules perspective and is directed toward justice and fair play. Males tend to use this type of moral reasoning. They seek a general rule that can be applied to specific situations. Physicians often take this approach when making ethical decisions.

These different attitudes affect ethical decision making. Nurses may appear unsure. They may seem overly concerned with details and the specifics of a situation and, therefore, slow to come to decisions. Nurses will identify interrelationships and include these as important factors when coming to a decision. They will ask how people are related and who will be affected by the decision and how. Often, nurses will consider quality of life and ability to function in ethical decision making.

Physicians, on the other hand, may have difficulty seeing the need for details and ambiguity. This is particularly true of surgeons who are rewarded, both financially and professionally, for their decisiveness and ability to act quickly under pressure. Because physicians are still trained in a reductionistic framework, they are likely to use a "rule out" approach to analyze ethical problems. Therefore, they have a tendency to break down the problem to its essential elements and dispense with all the extraneous details that nurses seem to believe are important. It is common for physicians to confuse professional expertise for moral authority. They often take it upon themselves to make ethical decisions with little or no collaboration or input.

CASE STUDY

The following case illustrates these different perspectives in action and how they affect ethical decision making. Dorothy Donahoe, RN, is assigned to complete the preoperative assessment on Wilford Cook, a 77-year-old patient in the intensive care unit. He is scheduled for spinal fusion. Dorothy reads through Wilford's clinical record and is overwhelmed at Wilford's course of treatment since he was admitted.

Wilford had no living relatives and had lived in a state institution for the mentally handicapped most of his life. With deinstitutionalization, he was placed in a group living setting in the community. To everyone's surprise, he surpassed all expectations regarding his functional abilities. Wilford learned to read and write, and he was able to work independently in the community.

Wilford had been admitted one month earlier for evaluation of chronic respiratory insufficiency and recurrent bronchitis and pneumonia. Dorothy notes that Wilford had carefully signed each permit for the various tests and procedures performed since his admission. Wilford had not, however, signed the surgical permit for removal of a mediastinal mass. On the line where his signature should have been are the words, "No, No, No." Below these words is the signature of the surgeon who had operated on Wilford and removed not only a malignant mediastinal mass but several vertebrae.

Since the surgery two weeks ago, Wilford has remained on a ventilator and in a semiconscious state. The head of the bed can be elevated only slightly because of the possibility of compressing the spinal cord. Dorothy decides to speak to the nurse in the critical care unit. He tells Dorothy the following:

Wilford didn't want the initial surgery. I believe he understood the risks and alternatives to surgery. I guess the surgeon thought Wilford wasn't capable of giving consent. Because Wilford doesn't have any family, I guess the surgeon thought he was acting in Wilford's best interest. Wilford hasn't done well since surgery.

Now the surgeon wants to put in Harrington rods to help support the spine so we can get Wilford up. If you ask me, I think that's too aggressive. However, when I suggested to Dr Anton that a tracheostomy would be easier to manage and more comfortable for Wilford, he told me that a tracheostomy was too aggressive!

Dorothy goes in to see Wilford. He has an endotracheal tube attached to the ventilator. Wilford responds to Dorothy's touch. Dorothy introduces herself and asks Wilford if he understands that the surgeon wants to take him back to the operating room and place support rods in his spine in place of the bones that were removed. Wilford nods. Dorothy asks, "Wilford, do you want to have this surgery?" Wilford shakes his head "no" slowly but purposefully.

Dorothy returns to the surgery department to speak to Dr Anton. She knows it is against hospital policy for a surgeon to sign a consent form unless it is an emergency procedure. She also thinks that Wilford needs someone to speak for him, but she is not certain how to go about finding someone. Dorothy finds Dr Anton and speaks to him. "Dr Anton, I have just been up to see Mr Cook in the critical care unit. Have you spoken to him about surgery?"

Dr Anton responds,

I see no point in talking to him. He has a long history of mental retardation. Without the support of Harrington rods, he'll never be able to sit up, let alone walk. He definitely needs the operation.

Dorothy has assisted with this type of procedure before. She knows it is an extremely complicated and lengthy operation that is hard on healthy adolescents, much less a terminally ill man who obviously does not want to go through the procedure. Dorothy hesitantly continues,

When I went in to see Mr Cook, he seemed to understand me and responded negatively when I brought up the surgery. I also noticed that the oncologist on the case doesn't think any treatment would be helpful at this point. The prognosis is very poor.

Dr Anton responds, "Just what are you saying? Are you suggesting that this operation is not indicated?"

What is Dorothy saying? She is using indirect communication patterns of the doctor-nurse game. Dr Anton has picked up on the underlying theme of her concerns and is directly challenging her.

Dorothy and the critical care nurse have demonstrated many characteristics of the interdependent view of ethical decision making. They are concerned about honoring the patient's wishes and about his quality of life. Hence, the critical care nurse saw the need for a tracheostomy to improve Wilford's quality of life. Dorothy expressed concern about a procedure that offered little benefit but would surely increase Wilford's pain and suffering in whatever time he has left.

The surgeon is concerned about Wilford's life and may believe that quality of life applies only if there is life. The surgeon has not only made a medical decision but an ethical one. He has decided what kind of life Wilford will have during his last days. It is obvious that the surgeon will do what he thinks is necessary to help this questionably competent patient, and he is willing to override any concerns expressed by the patient.

Neither Dorothy nor Dr Anton are completely right or wrong. To come to a decision that draws on the strengths of both perspectives, some fundamental changes must occur in the way they work together. The following changes in the nurse's attitude may help improve the nurse-physician relationship.

AREAS FOR CHANGE

Nurses must learn to be credible, articulate, knowledgeable, and strong. This means anticipating arguments and heated exchanges. One place to begin is with language. Nurses must practice assertiveness and avoid over-qualifying and hesitancy. This requires direct communication and an abandonment of the doctor-nurse game.

For example, in the exchange between Dr Anton and Dorothy, Dr Anton responded, "Just what are you saying? Are you suggesting that this operation is not indicated?"

Dorothy wants to avoid a confrontation about the efficacy of the surgery so she could respond with, "No, I'm not suggesting that. I am saying that Mr Cook has clearly communicated that he does not want to undergo surgery." This response is assertive and direct. Dorothy has focused her response on Mr Cook's expressed wishes, not the appropriateness of the operation. Now the discussion revolves around Mr Cook's competency. Since there is a disagreement regarding Mr Cook's competency, Dorothy could then pursue guardianship to protect Mr Cook's interests.

Other types of language that discredit the speaker, such as, "I think this is probably wrong, but . . ." or "I know you're terribly busy and I hate to bother you, but . . ." also should be eliminated. These phrases interpret for the listener and give the listener permission to discount what follows. Nurses' observations about the specific details of a patient's life are important and should be shared with clarity and conviction. Nursing contributions to the decision-making process must not be lost in deferential language. One way to change language is to listen to peers and correct usage that undermines the speaker's intent.

In addition to direct communication, nurses should use every available opportunity to teach physicians about their roles and responsibilities within the health care system. It is ironic, but frequently true, that health care professionals who work in close proximity are not remotely aware of what the other members of the team do.

Education can occur in interdisciplinary committees, during workshops and in-service programs, and especially during one-to-one interactions. On a more formal basis, a surgery department could set up an interdisciplinary ethics committee to review particularly troublesome cases and to establish guidelines for common ethical problems in surgery. The shared authority of the group process allows for better decisions to emerge. There also is greater commitment to the decision by those involved. The establishment of such a group can be an excellent source of support for nurses and physicians.

Finally, nurses must realize that the patterns of

interaction highlighted throughout this discussion are large trends and not just personal, isolated experiences. It is important for nurses to recognize the personal and structural aspects of people and situations at work. By doing this, they will learn to cut their losses and focus energy on relationships that are amenable to change. Because of their roles and expertise, nurses have access to information regarding patients' responses to health problems and the meaning patients give to the phrase *quality of life*. Both are major factors in all ethical decisions.

Because of their roles, physicians have expertise in diagnosis, prognosis, and treatment of disease and disability. Both aspects of these two essential health care professionals are necessary for humane and competent ethical decision making.

NOTES

1 L I Stein, "The doctor-nurse game," *Archives of General Psychiatry* 16 (June 1967) 699–703.
2 L I Stein, D T Watts, T Howell, "The doctor-nurse game revisited," *The New England Journal of Medicine* 322 (Feb 22, 1990) 546–549.
3 C Gilligan, *In a Different Voice: Psychological Theory and Women's Development* (Cambridge, Mass.: Harvard University Press, 1982).

Confidentiality

Majority Opinion in *Tarasoff v. Regents of the University of California*
Justice Mathew O. Tobriner

Mathew O. Tobriner was an associate justice of the Supreme Court of California from 1962 until 1981. Prior to his appointment to the Supreme Court of California, Justice Tobriner served as a judge in the District Court of Appeals, 1st District of California (1959–1962) and as a professor at the Hastings Law School (1958–1959). Justice Tobriner contributed to legal journals before his death in 1982.

Tatiana Tarasoff was murdered by Prosenjit Poddar, who was a patient of psychotherapists employed by the University of California Hospital. Her parents brought an action against the university regents, doctors, and campus police. The Tarasoffs complained that the doctors and police had failed to warn them that their daughter was in danger from Poddar. In finding for the Tarasoffs, Justice Tobriner argues that a doctor or psychotherapist treating a mentally ill patient has a duty to warn third parties of threatened dangers arising out of the patient's violent intentions. Responding to the defendants' appeal to the important role played by the principle of confidentiality in the psychotherapeutic situation, Tobriner argues that the public interest in safety from violent assault must be weighed against the patient's right to privacy.

On October 27, 1969, Prosenjit Poddar killed Tatiana Tarasoff. Plaintiffs, Tatiana's parents, allege that two months earlier Poddar confided his intention to kill Tatiana to Dr. Lawrence Moore, a psychologist employed by the Cowell Memorial Hospital at the University of California at Berkeley. They allege that on Moore's request, the campus police briefly detained Poddar, but released him when he appeared rational. They further claim that Dr. Harvey Powelson, Moore's superior, then directed that no further action be taken to detain Poddar. No one warned plaintiffs of Tatiana's peril. . . .

We shall explain that defendant therapists cannot

California Supreme Court; July 1, 1976. 131 California Reporter 14. Reprinted with permission of West Publishing Co.

escape liability merely because Tatiana herself was not their patient. When a therapist determines, or pursuant to the standards of his profession should determine, that his patient presents a serious danger of violence to another, he incurs an obligation to use reasonable care to protect the intended victim against such danger. The discharge of this duty may require the therapist to take one or more of various steps, depending upon the nature of the case. Thus it may call for him to warn the intended victim or others likely to apprise the victim of the danger, to notify the police, or to take whatever other steps are reasonably necessary under the circumstances. . . .

PLAINTIFFS' COMPLAINTS

. . . Plaintiffs' first cause of action, entitled "Failure to Detain a Dangerous Patient," alleges that on August 20, 1969, Poddar was a voluntary outpatient receiving therapy at Cowell Memorial Hospital. Poddar informed Moore, his therapist, that he was going to kill an unnamed girl, readily identifiable as Tatiana, when she returned home from spending the summer in Brazil. Moore, with the concurrence of Dr. Gold, who had initially examined Poddar, and Dr. Yandell, assistant to the director of the department of psychiatry, decided that Poddar should be committed for observation in a mental hospital. Moore orally notified Officers Atkinson and Teel of the campus police that he would request commitment. He then sent a letter to Police Chief William Beall requesting the assistance of the police department in securing Poddar's confinement.

Officers Atkinson, Brownrigg, and Halleran took Poddar into custody, but, satisfied that Poddar was rational, released him on his promise to stay away from Tatiana. Powelson, director of the department of psychiatry at Cowell Memorial Hospital, then asked the police to return Moore's letter, directed that all copies of the letter and notes that Moore had taken as therapist be destroyed, and "ordered no action to place Prosenjit Poddar in 72-hour treatment and evaluation facility."

Plaintiffs' second cause of action, entitled "Failure to Warn on a Dangerous Patient," incorporates the allegations of the first cause of action, but adds the assertion that defendants negligently permitted Poddar to be released from police custody without "notifying the parents of Tatiana Tarasoff that their daughter was in grave danger from Prosenjit Poddar." Poddar persuaded Tatiana's brother to share an apartment with him near Tatiana's residence; shortly after her return from Brazil, Poddar went to her residence and killed her.

Plaintiffs' third cause of action, entitled "Abandonment of a Dangerous Patient," seeks $10,000 punitive damages against defendant Powelson. Incorporating the crucial allegations of the first cause of action, plaintiffs charge that Powelson "did the things herein alleged with intent to abandon a dangerous patient, and said acts were done maliciously and oppressively."

Plaintiffs' fourth cause of action, for "Breach of Primary Duty to Patient and the Public," states essentially the same allegations as the first cause of action, but seeks to characterize defendants' conduct as a breach of duty to safeguard their patient and the public. Since such conclusory labels add nothing to the factual allegations of the complaint, the first and fourth causes of action are legally indistinguishable. . . .

. . . We direct our attention . . . to the issue of whether plaintiffs' second cause of action can be amended to state a basis for recovery.

PLAINTIFFS CAN STATE A CAUSE OF ACTION AGAINST DEFENDANT THERAPISTS FOR NEGLIGENT FAILURE TO PROTECT TATIANA

The second cause of action can be amended to allege that Tatiana's death proximately resulted from defendants' negligent failure to warn Tatiana or others likely to apprise her of her danger. Plaintiffs contend that as amended, such allegations of negligence and proximate causation, with resulting damages, establish a cause of action. Defendants, however, contend that in the circumstances of the present case they owed no duty of care to Tatiana or her parents and that, in the absence of such duty, they were free to act in careless disregard of Tatiana's life and safety.

In analyzing this issue, we bear in mind that legal duties are not discoverable facts of nature, but merely conclusory expressions that, in cases of a particular type, liability should be imposed for damage done. "The assertion that liability must . . . be denied because defendant bears no 'duty' to plaintiff 'begs the essential question—whether the plaintiff's interests are entitled to legal protection against the defendant's conduct. . . . [Duty] is not sacrosanct in itself, but only an expression of the sum total of those considerations of policy which lead the law to say that the particular plaintiff is entitled to protection.' "

In the landmark case of *Rowland v. Christian* (1968), Justice Peters recognized that liability should be imposed "for an injury occasioned to another by his want of ordinary care or skill" as expressed in section 1714 of the Civil Code. Thus, Justice Peters, quoting from *Heaven v. Pender* (1883) stated: " 'Whenever one person is by circumstances placed in such a position with regard to another . . . that if he did not use ordinary care and skill in his own conduct . . . he would cause danger of injury to the person or property of the other, a duty arises to use ordinary care and skill to avoid such danger.' "

We depart from "this fundamental principle" only upon the "balancing of a number of considerations"; major ones "are the foreseeability of harm to the plaintiff, the degree of certainty that the plaintiff suffered injury, the closeness of the connection between the defendant's conduct and the injury suffered, the moral blame attached to the defendant's conduct, the policy of preventing future harm, the extent of the burden to the defendant and consequences to the community of imposing a duty to exercise care with resulting liability for breach, and the availability, cost and prevalence of insurance for the risk involved."

The most important of these considerations in establishing duty is foreseeability. As a general principle, a "defendant owes a duty of care to all persons who are foreseeably endangered by his conduct, with respect to all risks which make the conduct unreasonably dangerous." As we shall explain, however, when the avoidance of foreseeable harm requires a defendant to control the conduct of another person, or to warn of such conduct, the common law has traditionally imposed liability only if the defendant bears some special relationship to the dangerous person or to the potential victim. Since the relationship between a therapist and his patient satisfies this requirement, we need not here decide whether foreseeability alone is sufficient to create a duty to exercise reasonable care to protect a potential victim of another's conduct.

Although, as we have stated above, under the common law, as a general rule, one person owed no duty to control the conduct of another nor to warn those endangered by such conduct, the courts have carved out an exception to this rule in cases in which the defendant stands in some special relationship to either the person whose conduct needs to be controlled or in a relationship to the foreseeable victim of that conduct. Applying this exception to the present case, we note that a relationship of defendant therapists to either Tatiana or Poddar will suffice to establish a duty of care; as

explained in section 315 of the Restatement Second of Torts, a duty of care may arise from either "(a) a special relation . . . between the actor and the third person which imposes a duty upon the actor to control the third person's conduct, or (b) a special relation . . . between the actor and the other which gives to the other a right of protection."

Although plaintiffs' pleadings assert no special relation between Tatiana and defendant therapists, they establish as between Poddar and defendant therapists the special relation that arises between a patient and his doctor or psychotherapist. Such a relationship may support affirmative duties for the benefit of third persons. Thus, for example, a hospital must exercise reasonable care to control the behavior of a patient which may endanger other persons. A doctor must also warn a patient if the patient's condition or medication renders certain conduct, such as driving a car, dangerous to others.

Although the California decisions that recognize this duty have involved cases in which the defendant stood in a special relationship *both* to the victim and to the person whose conduct created the danger, we do not think that the duty should logically be constricted to such situations. Decisions of other jurisdictions hold that the single relationship of a doctor to his patient is sufficient to support the duty to exercise reasonable care to protect others against dangers emanating from the patient's illness. The courts hold that a doctor is liable to persons infected by his patient if he negligently fails to diagnose a contagious disease, or having diagnosed the illness, fails to warn members of the patient's family.

Since it involved a dangerous mental patient, the decision in *Merchants Nat. Bank & Trust Co. of Fargo v. United States* (1967) comes closer to the issue. The Veterans Administration arranged for the patient to work on a local farm, but did not inform the farmer of the man's background. The farmer consequently permitted the patient to come and go freely during nonworking hours; the patient borrowed a car, drove to his wife's residence and killed her. Notwithstanding the lack of any "special relationship" between the Veterans Administration and the wife, the court found the Veterans Administration liable for the wrongful death of the wife.

In their summary of the relevant rulings Fleming and Maximov conclude that the "case law should dispel any notion that to impose on the therapists a duty to take precautions for the safety of persons threatened by a patient, where due care so requires, is in any way opposed to contemporary ground rules on the duty relationship. On the contrary, there now seems to be suffi-cient authority to support the conclusion that by enter-ing into a doctor-patient relationship the therapist becomes sufficiently involved to assume some responsi-bility for the safety, not only of the patient himself, but also of any third person whom the doctor knows to be threatened by the patient." [Fleming & Maximov, *The Patient or His Victim: The Therapist's Dilemma* (1974) 62 Cal. L. Rev. 1025, 1030.]

Defendants contend, however, that imposition of a duty to exercise reasonable care to protect third persons is unworkable because therapists cannot accurately pre-dict whether or not a patient will resort to violence. In support of this argument amicus representing the Amer-ican Psychiatric Association and other professional soci-eties cites numerous articles which indicate that thera-pists, in the present state of the art, are unable reliably to predict violent acts; their forecasts, amicus claims, tend consistently to overpredict violence, and indeed are more often wrong than right. Since predictions of vio-lence are often erroneous, amicus concludes, the courts should not render rulings that predicate the liability of therapists upon the validity of such predictions.

The role of the psychiatrist, who is indeed a practi-tioner of medicine, and that of the psychologist who performs an allied function, are like that of the physi-cian who must conform to the standards of the profes-sion and who must often make diagnoses and predic-tions based upon such evaluations. Thus the judgment of the therapist in diagnosing emotional disorders and in predicting whether a patient presents a serious danger of violence is comparable to the judgment which doc-tors and professionals must regularly render under accepted rules of responsibility.

We recognize the difficulty that a therapist encoun-ters in attempting to forecast whether a patient presents a serious danger of violence. Obviously we do not require that the therapist, in making the determination, render a perfect performance; the therapist need only exercise "that reasonable degree of skill, knowledge, and care ordinarily possessed and exercised by members of [that professional specialty] under similar circum-stances." Within the broad range of reasonable practice and treatment in which professional opinion and judg-ment may differ, the therapist is free to exercise his or her own best judgment without liability; proof, aided by hindsight, that he or she judged wrongly is insufficient to establish negligence.

In the instant case, however, the pleadings do not raise any question as to failure of defendant therapists to predict that Poddar presented a serious danger of vio-lence. On the contrary, the present complaints allege that defendant therapists did in fact predict that Poddar would kill, but were negligent in failing to warn.

Amicus contends, however, that even when a ther-apist does in fact predict that a patient poses a serious danger of violence to others, the therapist should be absolved of any responsibility for failing to act to pro-tect the potential victim. In our view, however, once a therapist does in fact determine, or under applicable professional standards reasonably should have deter-mined, that a patient poses a serious danger of violence to others, he bears a duty to exercise reasonable care to protect the foreseeable victim of that danger. While the discharge of this duty of due care will necessarily vary with the facts of each case, in each instance the ade-quacy of the therapist's conduct must be measured against the traditional negligence standard of the rendi-tion of reasonable care under the circumstances. As explained in Fleming and Maximov, *The Patient or His Victim: The Therapist's Dilemma* (1974), ". . . the ulti-mate question of resolving the tension between the con-flicting interests of patient and potential victim is one of social policy, not professional expertise. . . . In sum, the therapist owes a legal duty not only to his patient, but also to his patient's would-be victim and is subject in both respects to scrutiny by judge and jury." . . .

The risk that unnecessary warnings may be given is a reasonable price to pay for the lives of possible victims that may be saved. We would hesitate to hold that the therapist who is aware that his patient expects to attempt to assassinate the President of the United States would not be obligated to warn the authorities because the therapist cannot predict with accuracy that his patient will commit the crime.

Defendants further argue that free and open com-munication is essential to psychotherapy; that "unless a patient . . . is assured that . . . information [revealed by him] can and will be held in utmost confidence, he will be reluctant to make the full disclosure upon which diagnosis and treatment . . . depends." The giving of a warning, defendants contend, constitutes a breach of trust which entails the revelation of confidential com-munications.

We recognize the public interest in supporting effective treatment of mental illness and in protecting the rights of patients to privacy and the consequent pub-lic importance of safeguarding the confidential character of psychotherapeutic communication. Against this inter-est, however, we must weigh the public interest in safety from violent assault. The Legislature has undertaken the difficult task of balancing the countervailing concerns.

In Evidence Code section 1014, it established a broad rule of privilege to protect confidential communications between patient and psychotherapist. In Evidence Code section 1024, the Legislature created a specific and limited exception to the psychotherapist-patient privilege: "There is no privilege . . . if the psychotherapist has reasonable cause to believe that the patient is in such mental or emotional condition as to be dangerous to himself or to the person or property of another and that disclosure of the communication is necessary to prevent the threatened danger."

We realize that the open and confidential character of psychotherapeutic dialogue encourages patients to express threats of violence, few of which are ever executed. Certainly a therapist should not be encouraged routinely to reveal such threats; such disclosures could seriously disrupt the patient's relationship with his therapist and with the persons threatened. To the contrary, the therapist's obligations to his patient require that he not disclose a confidence unless such disclosure is necessary to avert danger to others, and even then that he do so discreetly, and in a fashion that would preserve the privacy of his patient to the fullest extent compatible with the prevention of the threatened danger.

The revelation of a communication under the above circumstances is not a breach of trust or a violation of professional ethics; as stated in the Principles of Medical Ethics of the American Medical Association (1957), section 9: "A physician may not reveal the confidence entrusted to him in the course of medical attendance . . . *unless he is required to do so by law or unless it becomes necessary in order to protect the welfare of the individual or of the community.*" (Emphasis added.) We conclude that the public policy favoring protection of the confidential character of patient-psychotherapist communications must yield to the extent to which disclosure is essential to avert danger to others. The protective privilege ends where the public peril begins.

Our current crowded and computerized society compels the interdependence of its members. In this risk-infested society we can hardly tolerate the further exposure to danger that would result from a concealed knowledge of the therapist that his patient was lethal. If the exercise of reasonable care to protect the threatened victim requires the therapist to warn the endangered party or those who can reasonably be expected to notify him, we see no sufficient societal interest that would protect and justify concealment. The containment of such risks lies in the public interest. For the foregoing reasons, we find that plaintiffs' complaints can be amended to state a cause of action against defendants Moore, Powelson, Gold, and Yandell and against the Regents as their employer, for breach of a duty to exercise reasonable care to protect Tatiana. . . .

Dissenting Opinion in *Tarasoff v. Regents of the University of California*
Justice William P. Clark

William P. Clark, who began practicing law in 1958, served as associate justice of the Supreme Court of California from 1973 to 1981. Subsequently, he was assistant to the president of the United States for national security affairs (1982–1983) and secretary of the interior (1983–1985).

Justice Clark, dissenting from Justice Tobriner's majority opinion, argues that confidentiality in the psychiatrist-patient relationship must be assured for three reasons. (1) Without the promise of such confidentiality, people needing treatment will be deterred from seeking it. (2) Effective therapy requires the patient's full disclosure of his or her innermost thoughts. Without the assurance that the thoughts disclosed will not be revealed by the therapist, the patient could not overcome the psychological barriers standing in the way of such revelations. (3) Successful treatment itself requires a relationship of trust between psychiatrist and patient.

California Supreme Court; July 1, 1976. 131 California Reporter 14. Reprinted with permission of West Publishing Co.

In light of these three reasons, Clark argues that if a duty to warn is imposed on psychiatrists, the result will be an increase in violent acts by persons who either don't seek help or whose therapy is unsuccessful. Furthermore, Clark holds, imposing such a duty on psychiatrists will result in an increase in the involuntary civil commitment of patients.

Until today's majority opinion, both legal and medical authorities have agreed that confidentiality is essential to effectively treat the mentally ill, and that imposing a duty on doctors to disclose patient threats to potential victims would greatly impair treatment. Further, recognizing that effective treatment and society's safety are necessarily intertwined, the Legislature has already decided effective and confidential treatment is preferred over imposition of a duty to warn.

The issue whether effective treatment for the mentally ill should be sacrificed to a system of warnings is, in my opinion, properly one for the Legislature, and we are bound by its judgment. Moreover, even in the absence of clear legislative direction, we must reach the same conclusion because imposing the majority's new duty is certain to result in a net increase in violence. . . .

COMMON LAW ANALYSIS

Entirely apart from the statutory provisions, the same result must be reached upon considering both general tort principles and the public policies favoring effective treatment, reduction of violence, and justified commitment.

Generally, a person owes no duty to control the conduct of another. Exceptions are recognized only in limited situations where (1) a special relationship exists between the defendant and injured party, or (2) a special relationship exists between defendant and the active wrongdoer, imposing a duty on defendant to control the wrongdoer's conduct. The majority does not contend the first exception is appropriate to this case.

Policy generally determines duty. Principal policy considerations include foreseeability of harm, certainty of the plaintiff's injury, proximity of the defendant's conduct to the plaintiff's injury, moral blame attributable to defendant's conduct, prevention of future harm, burden on the defendant, and consequences to the community.

Overwhelming policy considerations weigh against imposing a duty on psychotherapists to warn a potential victim against harm. While offering virtually no benefit to society, such a duty will frustrate psychiatric treatment, invade fundamental patient rights and increase violence.

The importance of psychiatric treatment and its need for confidentiallity have been recognized by this court. "It is clearly recognized that the very practice of psychiatry vitally depends upon the reputation in the community that the psychiatrist will not tell." [Slovenko, *Psychiatry and a Second Look at the Medical Privilege* (1960) 6 Wayne L. Rev. 175, 188.]

Assurance of confidentiality is important for three reasons.

Deterrence from Treatment

First, without substantial assurance of confidentiality, those requiring treatment will be deterred from seeking assistance. It remains an unfortunate fact in our society that people seeking psychiatric guidance tend to become stigmatized. Apprehension of such stigma—apparently increased by the propensity of people considering treatment to see themselves in the worst possible light—creates a well-recognized reluctance to seek aid. This reluctance is alleviated by the psychiatrist's assurance of confidentiality.

Full Disclosure

Second, the guarantee of confidentiality is essential in eliciting the full disclosure necessary for effective treatment. The psychiatric patient approaches treatment with conscious and unconscious inhibitions against revealing his innermost thoughts. "Every person, however well-motivated, has to overcome resistances to therapeutic exploration. These resistances seek support from every possible source and the possibility of disclosure would easily be employed in the service of resistance." (Goldstein & Katz, *Psychiatrist-Patient Privilege: The GAP Proposal and the Connecticut Statute*, 36 Conn. Bar J., 175, 179; see also, 118 Am. J. Psych. 734, 735.) Until a patient can trust his psychiatrist not to violate their confidential relationship, "the unconscious psychological control mechanism of repression will prevent the recall of past experiences." [Butler, *Psychotherapy and Griswold: Is Confidentiality a Privilege or a Right?* (1971) 3 Conn. L. Rev. 599, 604.]

Successful Treatment

Third, even if the patient fully discloses his thoughts, assurance that the confidential relationship will not be breached is necessary to maintain his trust in his psychiatrist—the very means by which treatment is effected. "[T]he essence of much psychotherapy is the contribution of trust in the external world and ultimately in the self, modelled upon the trusting relationship established during therapy" (Dawidoff, *The Malpractice of Psychiatrists,* 1966 Duke L. J. 696, 704). Patients will be helped only if they can form a trusting relationship with the psychiatrist. All authorities appear to agree that if the trust relationship cannot be developed because of collusive communication between the psychiatrist and others, treatment will be frustrated.

Given the importance of confidentiality to the practice of psychiatry, it becomes clear the duty to warn imposed by the majority will cripple the use and effectiveness of psychiatry. Many people, potentially violent—yet susceptible to treatment—will be deterred from seeking it; those seeking it will be inhibited from making revelations necessary to effective treatment; and, forcing the psychiatrist to violate the patient's trust will destroy the interpersonal relationship by which treatment is effected.

VIOLENCE AND CIVIL COMMITMENT

By imposing a duty to warn, the majority contributes to the danger to society of violence by the mentally ill and greatly increases the risk of civil commitment—the total deprivation of liberty—of those who should not be confined. The impairment of treatment and risk of improper commitment resulting from the new duty to warn will not be limited to a few patients but will extend to a large number of the mentally ill. Although under existing psychiatric procedures only a relatively few receiving treatment will ever present a risk of violence, the number making threats is huge, and it is the latter group—not just the former—whose treatment will be impaired and whose risk of commitment will be increased.

Both the legal and psychiatric communities recognize that the process of determining potential violence in a patient is far from exact, being fraught with complexity and uncertainty.[1]

In fact precision has not even been attained in predicting who of those having already committed violent acts will again become violent, a task recognized to be of much simpler proportions.

This predictive uncertainty means that the number of disclosures will necessarily be large. As noted above, psychiatric patients are encouraged to discuss all thoughts of violence, and they often express such thoughts. However, unlike this court, the psychiatrist does not enjoy the benefit of overwhelming hindsight in seeing which few, if any, of his patients will ultimately become violent. Now, confronted by the majority's new duty, the psychiatrist must instantaneously calculate potential violence from each patient on each visit. The difficulties researchers have encountered in accurately predicting violence will be heightened for the practicing psychiatrist dealing for brief periods in his office with heretofore nonviolent patients. And, given the decision not to warn or commit must always be made at the psychiatrist's civil peril, one can expect most doubts will be resolved in favor of the psychiatrist protecting himself.

Neither alternative open to the psychiatrist seeking to protect himself is in the public interest. The warning itself is an impairment of the psychiatrist's ability to treat, depriving many patients of adequate treatment. It is to be expected that after disclosing their threats, a significant number of patients, who would not become violent if treated according to existing practices, will engage in violent conduct as a result of unsuccessful treatment. In short, the majority's duty to warn will not only impair treatment of many who would never become violent but worse, will result in a net increase in violence.[2]

The second alternative open to the psychiatrist is to commit his patient rather than to warn. Even in the absence of threat of civil liability, the doubts of psychiatrists as to the seriousness of patient threats have led psychiatrists to overcommit to mental institutions. This overcommitment has been authoritatively documented in both legal and psychiatric studies. This practice is so prevalent that it has been estimated that "as many as twenty harmless persons are incarcerated for every one who will commit a violent act." [Steadman & Cocozza, *Stimulus/Response: We Can't Predict Who Is Dangerous* (Jan. 1975) 8 Psych. Today 32, 35.]

Given the incentive to commit created by the majority's duty, this already serious situation will be worsened. . . .

NOTES

1 A shocking illustration of psychotherapists' inability to predict dangerousness . . . is cited and discussed in Ennis, *Prisoners of Psychiatry: Mental Patients, Psychiatrists, and the Law* (1972): "In a well-known study, psychiatrists predicted that 989 persons were so dangerous that they could not be kept even in civil mental hospitals, but would have to be kept in maximum security hospitals run by the Department of Corrections. Then, because of a United States Supreme Court decision, those persons were transferred to civil hospitals. After a year, the Department of Mental Hygiene reported that one-fifth of them had been discharged to the community, and over half had agreed to remain as voluntary patients. During the year, only 7 of the 989 committed or threatened any act that was sufficiently dangerous to require retransfer to the maximum security hospital. Seven correct predictions out of almost a thousand is not a very impressive record.

"Other studies, and there are many, have reached the same conclusion: psychiatrists simply cannot predict dangerous behavior." (*Id.* at p. 227.)

2 The majority concedes that psychotherapeutic dialogue often results in the patient expressing threats of violence that are rarely executed. The practical problem, of course, lies in ascertaining which threats from which patients will be carried out. As to this problem, the majority is silent. They do, however, caution that the therapist certainly "should not be encouraged routinely to reveal such threats; such disclosures could seriously disrupt the patient's relationships, with his therapist and with the persons threatened."

Thus, in effect, the majority informs the therapists that they must accurately predict dangerousness—a task recognized as extremely difficult—or face crushing civil liability. The majority's reliance on the traditional standard of care for professionals that "therapist need only exercise 'that reasonable degree of skill, knowledge, and care ordinarily possessed and exercised by members of [that professional specialty] under similar circumstances' " is seriously misplaced. This standard of care assumes that, to a large extent, the subject matter of the specialty is ascertainable. One clearly ascertainable element in the psychiatric field is that the therapist cannot accurately predict dangerousness, which, in turn, means that the standard is inappropriate for lack of a relevant criterion by which to judge the therapist's decision. The inappropriateness of the standard the majority would have us use is made patent when consideration is given to studies, by several eminent authorities, indicating that "[t]he chances of a second psychiatrist agreeing with the diagnosis of a first psychiatrist 'are barely better than 50–50; or stated differently, there is about as much chance that a different expert would come to some different conclusion as there is that the other would agree.' " (Ennis & Litwack, *Psychiatry and the Presumption of Expertise: Flipping Coins in the Courtroom*, 62 Cal. L. Rev. 693, 701, quoting Ziskin, Coping with Psychiatric and Psychological Testimony, 126.) The majority's attempt to apply a normative scheme to a profession which must be concerned with problems that balk at standardization is clearly erroneous.

In any event, an ascertainable standard would not serve to limit psychiatrist disclosure of threats with the resulting impairment of treatment. However compassionate, the psychiatrist hearing the threat remains faced with potential crushing civil liability for a mistaken evaluation of his patient and will be forced to resolve even the slightest doubt in favor of disclosure or commitment.

AIDS, Confidentiality, and the Right to Know
Morton E. Winston

Morton E. Winston is associate professor of philosophy and religion at Trenton State College. He specializes in ethics, philosophy of science, and philosophy of mind. He is the coauthor of

Reprinted with permission from *Public Affairs Quarterly*, vol. 2 (April 1988), pp. 91–104.

a related article, "AIDS and the Duty to Protect," and the coeditor of *The Philosophy of Human Rights* (1988).

Winston addresses questions regarding the limits of medical confidentiality when third parties are at risk. He begins by discussing four arguments for the rule of medical confidentiality. Maintaining that these arguments establish at least a prima facie obligation to maintain confidentiality, Winston proceeds to argue that two principles can be used to delimit those cases where the strict observance of confidentiality cannot be ethically justified. The first principle, which he calls the "harm principle," "requires moral agents to refrain from acts and omissions which would foreseeably result in preventable wrongful harm to innocent others." The second, which he calls the "vulnerability principle," is used to give a more precise analysis of those circumstances in which there is a strict duty to protect others. The vulnerability principle states that "the duty to protect against harm tends to arise most strongly in contexts in which someone is specially dependent on others or in some way specially vulnerable to their choices and actions." Using these principles, Winston distinguishes cases in which breaches of confidentiality in regard to AIDS carriers are justified from other cases in which they are not.

In June of 1987, a young woman who was nine months pregnant was shot with an arrow fired from a hunting bow on a Baltimore street by a man who was engaged in an argument with another person. Emergency workers from the city fire fighting unit were called to the scene, administered resuscitation to the profusely bleeding woman and took her to a local hospital where she died shortly afterwards. Her child, delivered by emergency Caesarean section, died the next day.

This tragedy would have been quickly forgotten as yet another incident of random urban violence if it had not been later learned that the woman was infected with the AIDS virus. A nurse at the hospital decided on her own initiative that the rescue workers who had brought the woman to the emergency room should be informed that they had been exposed to HIV-infected blood and contacted them directly. Several days after this story hit the newspapers two state legislators introduced a bill adding AIDS to the list of diseases that hospitals would be required to inform workers about. A hospital spokeswoman was quoted in the newspaper as opposing the proposed legislation on the grounds that it would violate patient confidentiality, and that, "People taking care of patients should assume that everyone is a potential AIDS patient and take precautions. The burden is on you to take care of yourself."[1]

This case, and others like it, raises difficult and weighty ethical and public policy issues. What are the limits of medical confidentiality? Who, if anyone, has a right to know that they may have been exposed to AIDS or other dangerous infectious diseases? Whose responsibility is it to inform the sexual contacts of AIDS patients or others who may have been exposed to the infection? Can public health policies be framed which will effectively prevent the spread of the epidemic while also protecting the civil and human rights of its victims?

I THE LIMITS OF CONFIDENTIALITY

The rule of medical confidentiality enjoins physicians, nurses, and health care workers from revealing to third parties information about a patient obtained in the course of medical treatment. The rule protecting a patient's secrets is firmly entrenched in medical practice, in medical education, and receives explicit mention in all major medical oaths and codes of medical ethics. Sissela Bok has argued that the ethical justification for confidentiality rests on four arguments.[2]

The first and most powerful justification for the rule of confidentiality derives from the individual's right, flowing from autonomy, to control personal information and to protect privacy. The right of individuals to control access to sensitive information about themselves is particularly important in cases where revelation of such information would subject the individual to invidious discrimination, deprivation of rights, or physical or emotional harm. Since persons who are HIV-infected or who have AIDS or ARC (AIDS-Related Complex), are often subjected to discrimination, loss of employment, refusal of housing and insurance, many physicians believe that the confidentiality of HIV antibody test results and diagnoses of AIDS should be safeguarded under all circumstances. Since many infected persons and AIDS patients are members of groups which have traditionally been subject to discrimination or social disapproval—homosexuals, drug users, or prostitutes—the protection of confidentiality of patients who belong to these groups is especially indicated.

The second and third arguments for confidentiality concern the special moral relationship which exists between physicians and their patients. Medical practice requires that patients reveal intimate personal secrets to their physicians, and that physicians live up to the trust that is required on the part of patients to reveal such information; to fail to do so would violate the physician's duty of fidelity. Additionally, since medical practice is normally conducted under a tacit promise of confidentiality, physicians would violate this expectation by revealing their patients' secrets.

The fourth argument for confidentiality is based on utilitarian or broadly pragmatic considerations. Without a guarantee of confidentiality, potential patients in need of medical care would be deterred from seeking medical assistance from fear that sensitive personal information will be revealed to third parties thereby exposing the individual to the risk of unjust discrimination or other harm. Many physicians who work with AIDS patients find such pragmatic arguments particularly compelling, believing, perhaps correctly, that breaches of medical confidentiality concerning antibody status or a diagnosis of AIDS, would have a "chilling effect" preventing people in high-risk groups from seeking voluntary antibody testing and counselling. Since programs of education designed to encourage voluntary testing and voluntary behavior change are widely believed to be the only effective and ethically acceptable means to curtail the spread of the AIDS epidemic, measures which mandate testing for members of certain groups, and which permit disclosure of test results to third parties, are viewed as inimical to the medical communities' effort to control and treat this disease.[3]

Together, these four arguments present a compelling rationale for treating confidentiality as sacrosanct, particularly in the context of AIDS, and according to Bok, help to "explain the ritualistic tone in which the duty of preserving secrets is repeatedly set forth in professional oaths and codes of ethics."[4] But, she continues,

Not only does this rationale point to links with the most fundamental grounds of autonomy and relationship and trust and help; it also serves as a rationalization that helps deflect ethical inquiry. The very self-evidence that it claims can then expand beyond its legitimate applications. Confidentiality, like all secrecy, can then cover up for and in turn lead to a great deal of error, injury, pathology, and abuse.[5]

Bok believes that confidentiality is at best a prima facie obligation, one that while generally justified, can be overridden in certain situations by more compelling moral obligations. Among the situations which license breaches of confidentiality Bok cites are: cases involving a minor child or incompetent patient who would be harmed if sensitive information were not disclosed to a parent or guardian, cases involving threats of violence against identifiable third parties, cases involving contagious sexually transmitted diseases, and other cases where identifiable third parties would be harmed or placed at risk unknowingly by failure to disclose information known to a physician obtained through therapeutic communication.

In general, personal autonomy, and the derivative right of individuals to control personal information, is limited by the "Harm Principle" [HP], which requires moral agents to refrain from acts and omissions which would foreseeably result in preventable wrongful harm to innocent others. Bok argues that when HP (or a related ethical principle which I will discuss shortly) comes into play, "the prima facie premises supporting confidentiality are overridden," . . .[6] If this argument is correct, then the strict observance of confidentiality cannot be ethically justified in all cases, and physicians and nurses who invoke the rule of confidentiality in order to justify their not disclosing information concerning threats or risks to innocent third parties may be guilty of negligence.

Before accepting this conclusion, however, it is necessary that we clarify the force of HP in the context of the ethics of AIDS, and refine the analysis of the conditions under which breaches of confidentiality pertaining to a patient's antibody status or a diagnosis of AIDS may be ethically justifiable.

II VULNERABILITY, DISEASE CONTROL, AND DISCRIMINATION

Defenders of HP typically hold that all moral agents have a general moral obligation with respect to all moral patients to (a) avoid harm, (b) prevent or protect against harm, and (c) remove harm. One problem with HP is that not all acts and omissions which result in harm to others appear to be wrong. For instance, if I buy the last pint of Häagen-Dazs coffee ice cream in the store, then I have, in some sense, harmed the next customer who wants to buy this good. Similarly, if one baseball team defeats another, then they have harmed the other team. But neither of these cases represent *wrongful* harms. Why then are some harms wrongful and others not?

Robert Goodin has recently developed a theory which provides at least a partial answer to this question. According to Goodin, the duty to protect against harm tends to arise most strongly in contexts in which someone is specially dependent on others or in some way specially vulnerable to their choices and actions.[7] He dubs this the Vulnerability Principle [VP]. Vulnerability, implying risk or susceptibility to harm, should be understood in a relational sense: being vulnerable to another is a condition which involves both a relative inability of the vulnerable party to protect themselves from harm or risk, and a correlative ability of another individual to act (or refrain from actions) which would foreseeably place the vulnerable party in a position of harm or risk or remove them from such a position.

No one is completely invulnerable, and we are all to some extent dependent on the choices and actions of others. However, where there exists a rough parity of power among the parties to protect their own interests, VP does not apply. It only applies in cases where one party is *specially* vulnerable, the parties are unequal in their powers or abilities to protect their own interests, or where an inequality in knowledge or power gives one party an unfair advantage over the other.

The Vulnerability Principle is related to the Harm Principle in giving a more precise analysis of the circumstances in which a strict duty to protect others arises. For example, under HP it might be thought that individuals, qua moral agents, have a duty to ensure that persons be inoculated against contagious, preventable diseases, such as polio. However, while we have no strong obligations under HP to ensure that other adults have been inoculated, we *do* have a strong general obligation under VP to see to it that all young children are inoculated, and I have a special duty as a parent to see that my own children are inoculated. Children, as a class, are especially vulnerable and lack the ability to protect themselves. Being a parent *intensifies* the duty to prevent harm to children, by focusing the duty to protect the vulnerable on individuals who are specially responsible for the care of children. For other adults, on the other hand, I have no strong duty to protect, since I may generally assume that mature moral agents have both the ability and the responsibility to protect themselves.[8]

Viewed in this light, the remarks quoted earlier by the hospital spokeswoman take on new meaning and relevance. She argued that it is the responsibility of health care workers to protect themselves by taking appropriate infection control measures in situations in which they may be exposed to blood infected with HIV. This argument might be a good one if people who occupy these professional roles are trained in such measures and are equipped to use them when appropriate. If they were so equipped, then in the Baltimore case, the nurse who later informed the rescue workers of the patient's antibody status was *not* specially responsible to prevent harm; the paramedics were responsible for their own safety.

The main problem with this argument is that it is not always possible to assume that emergency workers and others who provide direct care to AIDS patients or HIV-infected individuals are properly trained and equipped in infection control, nor, even if they are, that it is always feasible for them to employ these procedures in emergency situations. The scene of an emergency is not a controlled environment, and while emergency and public safety workers may take precautions such as wearing gloves and masks, these measures can be rendered ineffective, say, if a glove is torn and the worker cut while wrestling someone from a mass of twisted metal that was a car. While *post hoc* notification of the antibody status of people whom public safety workers have handled may not prevent them from contracting infection, it can alert them to the need to be tested, and thus can prevent them from spreading the infection (if they are in fact infected) to others, e.g., their spouses.

Health care workers, public safety workers, paramedics, and others who come into direct contact with blood which may be infected with the AIDS virus represent a class of persons for whom the Vulnerability Principle suggests a special "duty to protect" is appropriate. It is appropriate in these cases because such workers are routinely exposed to blood in the course of their professional activities, and exposure to infected blood is one way in which people can become infected with the AIDS virus. Such workers could protect themselves by simply refusing to handle anyone whom they suspected of harboring the infection. Doing this, however, would mean violating their professional responsibility to provide care. Hence, morally, they can only protect themselves by reducing their risk of exposure, in this case, by employing infection control measures and being careful. In this respect, health care workers, whether they work inside or outside of the hospital, are in a relevantly different moral situation than ordinary people who are not routinely exposed to blood and who have no special duty to provide care, and this makes them specially vulnerable. It thus appears that the nurse who informed the emergency workers of their risk of exposure did the right thing in informing them, since in doing so she was discharging a duty to protect the vulnerable.[9]

But do similar conclusions follow with respect to "ordinary" persons who need not expose themselves to infection in the course of their professional activities? Consider the case in which a patient who is known to have a positive antibody status informs his physician that he does not intend to break off having sexual relations and that he will not tell his fiancée that he is infected with the AIDS virus.[10]

In this case, we have a known, unsuspecting party, the fiancée, who will be placed at risk by failure to discharge a duty to protect. The fiancée is vulnerable in this case to the infected patient, since it is primarily *his* actions or omissions which place her at risk. According to HP + VP, the patient has a strong special responsibility to protect those with whom he has or will have sexual relations against infection. There are a number of ways in which he can discharge this duty. For instance, he can break off the relationship, abstain from sexual intercourse, practice "safe sex," or he can inform his fiancée of his antibody status. This last option protects the fiancée by alerting her to the need to protect herself. But does the physician in this case also have a special responsibility to protect the fiancée?

She does, in this case, if she has good reason to believe that her patient will not discharge his responsibility to protect his fiancée or inform her of his positive antibody status. Since the physician possesses the information which would alert her patient's fiancée to a special need to protect herself, and the only other person who has this information will not reveal it, the fiancée is specially dependent upon the physician's choices and actions. Were she to fail to attempt to persuade her patient to reveal the information, or if he still refused to do so, to see to it that the patient's fiancée was informed, she would be acting in complicity with a patient who was violating his duty to prevent harm, and so would also be acting unethically under the Vulnerability Principle.

It thus appears that the rule of confidentiality protecting a patient's HIV antibody status cannot be regarded as absolute. There are several sorts of cases where HP + VP override the rule of confidentiality. However, finding there are justified exceptions to a generally justified rule of practice does not allow for unrestricted disclosure of antibody status to all and sundry. The basic question which must be answered in considering revealing confidential information concerning a patient's HIV antibody status is: *Is the individual to be notified someone who is specially vulnerable? That is, are they someone who faces a significant risk of exposure to the infection, and, will revealing confidential information to them assist them in reducing this risk to themselves or others?*

Answering this question is not always going to be easy, and applying HP + VP, and balancing its claims against those of confidentiality will require an extraordinary degree of moral sensitivity and discretion. Because the rule of confidentiality describes a valid prima facie moral responsibility of physicians, the burden of proof must always fall on those who would violate it in order to accommodate the claims of an opposing ethical principle. Perhaps this is why physicians tend to assume that if the rule of confidentiality is not absolute, it might as well be treated as such. Physicians, nurses, and others who are privy to information about patients' antibody status, by and large, are likely to lack the relevant degree of ethical sensitivity to discriminate the cases in which confidentiality can be justifiably violated from those where it cannot. So if we must err, the argument goes, it is better to err on the side of confidentiality.

Aside from underestimating the moral sensitivity of members of these professional groups, this argument fails to take into account that there are two ways of erring—one can err by wrongfully disclosing confidential information to those who have no right to know it, and one can err by failing to disclose confidential information to those who do have a right to know it. The harm that can result from errors of the first kind are often significant, and sometimes irreparable. But so are the harms that result from errors of the second kind. While the burden of proof should be placed on those who would breach the prima facie rule of confidentiality, it should sometimes be possible for persons to satisfy this burden and act in accordance with HP + VP without moral fault.

The strength of conviction with which many physicians in the forefront of AIDS research and treatment argue for the protection of confidentiality can be explained partly by recognizing that they view themselves as having a special responsibility to prevent harm to AIDS patients. The harm which they seek to prevent, however, is not only harm to their patients' health. It is also social harm caused by discrimination that these physicians are trying to prevent. This is yet a different application of HP + VP in the context of AIDS which merits close attention.

As was noted earlier, the particular strength of the pragmatic argument for confidentiality in the context of AIDS, derives from the fact that, because of the public hysteria about AIDS, HIV-infected persons or those with AIDS or ARC are likely to be subjected to invidious discrimination in housing, employment, access to insurance and other services, should the information that they are AIDS patients or are HIV-infected become widely known. These are clearly wrongful harms, but whose responsibility is it to prevent such harms? Generally speaking, preventing the harms which arise from injustice and disregard of civil and human rights is the proper responsibility of public officials. However, at present, only a few municipalities, San Francisco, New York City, and Washington, D.C. have enacted AIDS anti-discrimination legislation, and recently, the Reagan Administration has taken the position that it is not a Federal responsibility to do so.[11]

Because the efforts of public officials to pass and enforce effective AIDS anti-discrimination measures have been lackadaisical, many physicians feel that they have inherited the responsibility to protect their patients against the social harms caused by discrimination, and have acted on that conviction in the only way readily available to them, by insisting that the rule of confidentiality be strictly observed with respect to persons infected with HIV. Confidentiality of HIV antibody test results and diagnoses of AIDS is currently seen as the only effective barrier against unjust discrimination.

By relying exclusively on a guarantee of absolute confidentiality to protect people with AIDS from discrimination, we acknowledge the problem of harm caused by discrimination but do not effectively address it. The passage of anti-discrimination standards applying to HIV-infected persons, people with AIDS, ARC, and members of groups who are perceived as being infected, should be the first priority of all those who are concerned to prevent the spread of this disease. Such measures are justified not only on the grounds of human dignity, and human rights, but because in the context of the AIDS epidemic, they will also tend to function as effective public health measures by removing (or diminishing) one reason which deters persons at risk from seeking testing and counseling. Medical personnel and public health authorities who take the position that confidentiality is absolute in order to shield their patients from discrimination, will increasingly find themselves in the uncomfortable position of being accomplices to the irresponsible behavior of known noncompliant positives.

What is needed, then, is a finely drawn public policy that includes strong and effective anti-discrimination standards, a public education program which encourages individual and professional responsibility, and a set of clear effective guidelines for public health authorities concerning when and to whom confidential information necessary for disease control and the protection of those at risk may be revealed.

III   WHO HAS A RIGHT TO KNOW?

The Vulnerability Principle suggests that breaches of confidentiality may be justified in cases where the following conditions obtain: (1) there is an identifiable person or an identifiable group of people who are "at risk" of contracting AIDS from a known carrier, (2) the carrier has not or will not disclose his/her antibody status to those persons whom he/she has placed or will place at risk, and (3) the identity of the carrier and his/her antibody status is known to a physician, nurse, health care worker, public health authority, or another person privileged to this information. It is justifiable, under these circumstances, to reveal information which might enable others to identify an AIDS patient or HIV-infected person. Revelation of confidential information is justified under this rule by the fact that others are vulnerable to infection, or may be unknowingly infecting others, and the information to be revealed may serve as an effective means of protecting those at risk.

The phrase "at risk" is most significant since not everyone who comes into contact with AIDS patients and HIV-infected persons will be placed at risk. Those persons who are most at risk are sexual partners of persons who are infected, persons who are exposed to an infected person's blood, and the fetuses of infected women.[12] Because these are the only documented means of transmitting the disease, it is relatively easy in the case of AIDS to identify those individuals who are specially vulnerable, and to distinguish them from others who are not. In particular, persons who will at most have "casual contact" with the patient are not specially vulnerable.[13] Discrimination in housing or employment is, therefore, not justifiable since AIDS cannot be transmitted by merely working in the same office or living in the same house as an HIV-infected person. On the other hand, it is known that AIDS can be transmitted by sexual contact or by blood or blood products. Fears of contagion via these routes are not irrational, and public policies should address ways of preventing the further spread of the disease.

A policy option which has been suggested is mandatory HIV antibody testing for everyone, or for everyone in certain risk groups, or for people applying for marriage licenses, or as a preemployment screen. However, mandatory testing programs are fraught with ethical problems and, in general, are neither cost-effective nor just.[14] HIV testing should remain voluntary, but, if it is voluntary, and the onus of informing the sexual contacts of those who test positive is also voluntary, then some HIV-infected individuals will not be tested, and of those who are tested and are found to be positive, some will not inform their sexual partners.

A more justifiable policy would be to keep testing voluntary, but to urge those who test positive to disclose their antibody status to their known sexual contacts, or if they do not wish to or will not do this themselves, to ask them to supply the names of their partners so that notification of those at risk can proceed by other means. A number of states have instituted such programs of voluntary partner notification.[15] The ethical rationale supporting such measures derives a "right to know" another person's HIV antibody status from HP + VP, the fact that sexual transmission of HIV has been documented, and the assumption that notification will enable those who may have been exposed to the infection to protect themselves, and, if they are already infected, to protect others.

The main problem with reliance on voluntary personal disclosure is that there is no way to check to see whether or not the infected person has indeed complied and informed all of their contacts. Another way to carry out partner notification is to have the carrier voluntarily reveal the names of their sexual and drug contacts to physicians or nurses who will then personally notify partners. This method of contacting those at risk is preferable on two grounds: it may be emotionally easier for some people to have partner notification handled by third parties, and secondly, there is a way of checking to see that all identified sexual contacts have been notified.

The main problem with this proposal is that it places primary care providers in an uncomfortable "dual role." Instead of leaving this matter to the discretion of direct health care providers, procedures should be devised whereby physicians, nurses and other primary care personnel can avoid "dual roles" as caregivers and public health officers. One way to do this is to establish a special office in the state public health administration and to have public health authorities notify persons known to be at risk. Physicians and nurses can confidentially report cases of HIV infection to this office, and

public health officials can make the determination as to whether notification of partners is warranted in accordance with the Vulnerability Principle. Patients should always be informed that this is being done, and should sign a form releasing the information needed to notify contacts. Notification taking this form would not have to indicate the source of the information, a private physician or clinic, and this might help allay fears about a "chilling effect" on a particular physician's AIDS practice. The notification of contacts should also attempt to protect the identity of the carrier. In making a partner notification, personnel in the public health office can simply state that they have reason to believe that a person may have been exposed to HIV and to urge that they report for testing and counseling.

This method will work with respect to known positives who voluntarily comply, but can anything be done about those who refuse to reveal the names of their contacts, or reveal only some of them?

Noncompliance in supplying names of sexual or IV drug partners should not be associated with sanctions such as fines or short prison terms; we cannot extort or coerce this kind of information, and such measures will tend to discourage some persons from seeking testing and counseling. The appropriate response to this kind of noncompliance should be a warning that more active means of contact tracing which involve greater risk of disclosure or invasion of privacy, such as surveillance and investigation, may be employed. In extreme cases, e.g., where known carriers continue to engage in practices likely to infect others, e.g., prostitution, stronger remedies and sanctions, e.g., civil commitment, quarantine, or arrest, may be justified.

Some may argue that such programs of partner notification and limited contact tracing are unwise on the grounds that they will tend to deter individuals from being tested in the first place. The reply is that such programs will not deter individuals who are socially responsible and are willing to take steps to protect themselves and others from HIV infection, and it will tend to increase compliance with voluntary disease control measures among identified HIV-infected members of risk groups who are reluctant to accept their social responsibilities. However, such programs have little chance of success unless they are coupled with strong federal antidiscrimination policies which are strictly enforced.[16] Such measures would function analogously to infection control measures in reducing or removing the risk of harm caused by discrimination, thereby enabling people to act more responsibly.

Even so, programs of voluntary partner notification

and limited contact tracing for sexual and IV drug partners of known noncompliant positives will not prevent the infection from being transmitted. It is estimated that there are 1.5 million people in the United States currently infected with the virus and therefore capable of transmitting it. The overwhelming majority of those infected do not know that they are infected. Thus, the onus of responsibility for protecting people who are "at risk" rests primarily with those persons who engage in high risk behaviors, and only secondarily with other persons who have knowledge of infection or infectiousness such as health care providers and public health authorities. In some other cases, for instance, cases of pediatric AIDS, parents and classroom teachers will also have a "right to know" because they will be the ones responsible for the care and protection of minors. However, except in these cases, i.e., in cases where other individuals should have knowledge of HIV infection in order to protect themselves or specially vulnerable others from risk of infection, there is no generalized "right to know." Confidentiality should be protected in all other cases.[17]

NOTES

1 *The Baltimore Sun,* June 11, 1987, p. D1.
2 Sissela Bok, *Secrets: On the Ethics of Concealment and Revelation* (New York: Vintage Books, 1983); Chapter IX.
3 Sheldon Landesman presents this argument compellingly: "Any legally or socially sanctioned act that breaches confidentiality or imposes additional burdens (such as job loss or cancellation of insurance) acts as a disincentive to voluntary testing. Thus if all physicians were legally required to report HIV-positive persons to a health department or to inform sexual partners at risk from the HIV-positive person, no one would come forward for testing. This is especially true if the physician is known to treat many patients with AIDS and HIV infection. The public knowledge that such a physician has violated confidentiality would result (indeed, has resulted in several cases) in a sharp decline of potentially infected persons seeking counselling and testing. Consequently, a growing number of persons would remain ignorant of their infectiousness as would their sexual partners," *The Hastings Center Report,* Vol. 17 (1987), p. 25.
4 Bok, *Op. Cit.,* p. 123.
5 *Ibid.*

6 *Ibid.,* pp. 129–130. In a note at the end of this passage Bok concedes that the fourth premise involves important "line-drawing" problems which may vary among cases, a point that I will address shortly in the context of AIDS prevention and treatment.
7 Robert E. Goodin, *Protecting the Vulnerable: A Reanalysis of Our Social Responsibilities* (Chicago: The University of Chicago Press, 1985).
8 It follows on this view that I also have a responsibility to protect myself, or my future selves, from such preventable harms. Cf. M. E. Winston, "Responsibility to Oneself," unpublished paper presented at the American Philosophical Association, Pacific Division Meetings, March 27, 1987.
9 In fact, the fire fighters who provided emergency care to the wounded Baltimore woman were not wearing gloves. In this particular case a further reason for condoning the nurse's action might be found in the fact that the patient died. Is it possible to violate confidentiality when the person whose secret is revealed is dead? The pragmatic justifications for the rule of confidentiality would still apply in such cases, but it is a moot question as to whether the deceased individuals themselves can be harmed or wronged by revealing confidential information. See Joan Callahan, "Harming the Dead," *Ethics,* Vol. 97 (1987), pp. 341–352.
10 Cf. "AIDS and a Duty to Protect," *The Hastings Center Report,* Vol. 17 (1987), pp. 22–23.
11 *The New York Times,* September 21, 1987, p. A1.
12 The Center for Disease Control lists persons belonging to certain groups or who engage in certain types of behavior as having "high risk" of contracting HIV, and these include: homosexual/bisexual males, IV drug users, persons born in countries where heterosexual transmission is prevalent (e.g., Haiti and Central African countries), hemophiliacs, male and female prostitutes, sexual partners of members of high-risk groups, infants born to women in high-risk groups, and persons receiving blood transfusions before 1985 when screening for HIV began. [CDC. Additional Recommendations to Reduce Sexual and Drug Abuse-Related Transmission of Human T-[Lymphotropic Virus Type III/Lymphadenopathy-Associated Virus.] MMWR 1986, March 14; 152–155.] It is important to note that not everyone belonging to these groups is "at risk." Certain behaviors in certain contexts place individuals at risk, and other behaviors can reduce or remove these risks.
13 In an epidemiological study by Friedland, et al. of

the family members of 39 AIDS patients it was found that there were no instances of horizontal transmission of HIV to family members living in the same household. [Friedland, G. H., Saltzman, B. R., Rogers, M. S., Kahl, P. A., Lesser, M. L., Mayers, M. M., and Klein, R. S., "Lack of transmission of HTLV-III/LAV infection to household contacts of patients with AIDS or AIDS-related complex with oral candidiasis," *New England Journal of Medicine.* Vol. 314 (1986), pp. 344–349.] Additionally, there is no known risk of transmission of HIV in settings such as offices, schools, factories, or by personal services workers, such as beauticians and barbers or food service workers. [CDC. Recommendations for preventing transmission of infection with T-Lymphotropic Virus Type III/Lymphadenopathy-associated virus in the workplace. MMWR 1985, Vol. 34, no. 45, pp. 682–695.]

14 See Kenneth R. Howe, "Why Mandatory Screening for AIDS Is a Very Bad Idea." In Christine Pierce and Donald VanDeVeer (Eds.), *AIDS: Ethics and Public Policy* (Belmont: Wadsworth Publishing Co., 1988), pp. 140–149.

15 In Maryland, the Governor's Task Force on AIDS has recently recommended that, "Health care providers should strongly encourage HIV-infected patients to speak directly to and refer their own sexual and needle-sharing contacts for counselling and medical evaluation. There are instances, however, when these professionals may be *obligated* to notify persons *known* to have had significant exposures to HIV infection. In such cases, the duty to notify is a matter of good medical practice and supersedes the need to maintain confidentiality." *AIDS and Maryland: Policy Guidelines and Recommendations*, Report of the Governor's Task Force on Acquired Immune Deficiency Syndrome. December 1986.

16 Cf. Larry Gostin, "Time for Federal Laws on AIDS Discrimination," Letter to the Editor, *The New York Times,* October 1, 1987.

17 I am indebted to David Newell and to an anonymous reviewer for helpful comments on this paper.

Confidentiality in Medicine—A Decrepit Concept
Mark Siegler

A biographical sketch of Mark Siegler is found on page 64.

Siegler argues that hospital medicine, the rise of health-care teams, the existence of third-party insurance programs, and the expanding limits of medicine will necessarily modify our traditional understanding of medical confidentiality. He identifies two functions of confidentiality in medicine: (1) respect for the patient's sense of individuality and privacy and (2) the improvement of the patient's health care, which requires a bond of trust between the health professional and the patient. Siegler then proposes possible solutions to the problems raised by the developments in medical care cited above. He concludes by criticizing those violations of a patient's right of privacy that are due to careless indiscretion on the part of professionals.

Medical confidentiality, as it has traditionally been understood by patients and doctors, no longer exists. This ancient medical principle, which has been included

Reprinted by permission of the *New England Journal of Medicine,* vol. 307, pp. 1518–1521; 1982.

in every physician's oath and code of ethics since Hippocratic times, has become old, worn-out, and useless; it is a decrepit concept. Efforts to preserve it appear doomed to failure and often give rise to more problems than solutions. Psychiatrists have tacitly acknowledged the impossibility of ensuring the confidentiality of medical records by choosing to establish a separate, more secret record. The following case illustrates how the confidentiality principle is compromised systematically in the course of routine medical care.

A patient of mine with mild chronic obstructive pulmonary disease was transferred from the surgical intensive-care unit to a surgical nursing floor two days after an elective cholecystectomy. On the day of transfer, the patient saw a respiratory therapist writing in his medical chart (the therapist was recording the results of an arterial blood gas analysis) and became concerned about the confidentiality of his hospital records. The patient threatened to leave the hospital prematurely unless I could guarantee that the confidentiality of his hospital record would be respected.

This patient's complaint prompted me to enumerate the number of persons who had both access to his hospital record and a reason to examine it. I was amazed to learn that at least 25 and possibly as many as 100 health professionals and administrative personnel at our university hospital had access to the patient's record and that all of them had a legitimate need, indeed a professional responsibility, to open and use that chart. These persons included 6 attending physicians (the primary physician, the surgeon, the pulmonary consultant, and others); 12 house officers (medical, surgical, intensive-care unit, and "covering" house staff); 20 nursing personnel (on three shifts); 6 respiratory therapists; 3 nutritionists; 2 clinical pharmacists; 15 students (from medicine, nursing, respiratory therapy, and clinical pharmacy); 4 unit secretaries; 4 hospital financial officers; and 4 chart reviewers (utilization review, quality assurance review, tissue review, and insurance auditor). It is of interest that this patient's problem was straightforward, and he therefore did not require many other technical and support services that the modern hospital provides. For example, he did not need multiple consultants and fellows, such specialized procedures as dialysis, or social workers, chaplains, physical therapists, occupational therapists, and the like.

Upon completing my survey I reported to the patient that I estimated that at least 75 health professionals and hospital personnel had access to his medical record. I suggested to the patient that these people were all involved in providing or supporting his health-care services. They were, I assured him, working for him. Despite my reassurances the patient was obviously distressed and retorted, "I always believed that medical confidentiality was a part of a doctor's code of ethics. Perhaps you should tell me just what you people mean by 'confidentiality'!"

TWO ASPECTS OF MEDICAL CONFIDENTIALITY

Confidentiality and Third-Party Interests

Previous discussions of medical confidentiality usually have focused on the tension between a physician's responsibility to keep information divulged by patients secret and a physician's legal and moral duty, on occasion, to reveal such confidences to third parties, such as families, employers, public-health authorities, or police authorities. In all these instances, the central question relates to the stringency of the physician's obligation to maintain patient confidentiality when the health, well-being, and safety of identifiable others or of society in general would be threatened by a failure to reveal information about the patient. The tension in such cases is between the good of the patient and the good of others.

Confidentiality and the Patient's Interest

As the example above illustrates, further challenges to confidentiality arise because the patient's personal interest in maintaining confidentiality comes into conflict with his personal interest in receiving the best possible health care. Modern high-technology health care is available principally in hospitals (often, teaching hospitals), requires many trained and specialized workers (a "health-care team"), and is very costly. The existence of such teams means that information that previously had been held in confidence by an individual physician will now necessarily be disseminated to many members of the team. Furthermore, since health-care teams are expensive and few patients can afford to pay such costs directly, it becomes essential to grant access to the patient's medical record to persons who are responsible for obtaining third-party payment. These persons include chart reviewers, financial officers, insurance auditors, and quality-of-care assessors. Finally, as medicine expands from a narrow, disease-based model to a model that encompasses psychological, social, and economic problems, not only will the size of the health-care team and medical costs increase, but more sensitive information (such as one's personal habits and financial condition) will now be included in the medical record and will no longer be confidential.

The point I wish to establish is that hospital medicine, the rise of health-care teams, the existence of third-party insurance programs, and the expanding limits of medicine all appear to be responses to the wishes of people for better and more comprehensive medical care. But each of these developments necessarily modifies our traditional understanding of medical confidentiality.

THE ROLE OF CONFIDENTIALITY IN MEDICINE

Confidentiality serves a dual purpose in medicine. In the first place, it acknowledges respect for the patient's sense of individuality and privacy. The patient's most personal physical and psychological secrets are kept confidential in order to decrease a sense of shame and vulnerability. Secondly, confidentiality is important in improving the patient's health care—a basic goal of medicine. The promise of confidentiality permits people to trust (i.e., have confidence) that information revealed to a physician in the course of a medical encounter will not be disseminated further. In this way patients are encouraged to communicate honestly and forthrightly with their doctors. This bond of trust between patient and doctor is vitally important both in the diagnostic process (which relies on an accurate history) and subsequently in the treatment phase, which often depends as much on the patient's trust in the physician as it does on medications and surgery. These two important functions of confidentiality are as important now as they were in the past. They will not be supplanted entirely either by improvements in medical technology or by recent changes in relations between some patients and doctors toward a rights-based, consumerist model.

POSSIBLE SOLUTIONS TO THE CONFIDENTIALITY PROBLEM

First of all, in all nonbureaucratic, noninstitutional medical encounters—that is, in the millions of doctor-patient encounters that take place in physicians' offices, where more privacy can be preserved—meticulous care should be taken to guarantee that patients' medical and personal information will be kept confidential.

Secondly, in such settings as hospitals or large-scale group practices, where many persons have opportunities to examine the medical record, we should aim to provide access only to those who have "a need to know." This could be accomplished through such administrative changes as dividing the entire record into several sections—for example, a medical and financial section—and permitting only health professionals access to the medical information.

The approach favored by many psychiatrists—that of keeping a psychiatric record separate from the general medical record—is an understandable strategy but one that is not entirely satisfactory and that should not be generalized. The keeping of separate psychiatric records implies that psychiatry and medicine are different undertakings and thus drives deeper the wedge between them and between physical and psychological illness. Furthermore, it is often vitally important for internists or surgeons to know that a patient is being seen by a psychiatrist or is taking a particular medication. When separate records are kept, this information may not be available. Finally, if generalized, the practice of keeping a separate psychiatric record could lead to the unacceptable consequence of having a separate record for each type of medical problem.

Patients should be informed about what is meant by "medical confidentiality." We should establish the distinction between information about the patient that generally will be kept confidential regardless of the interest of third parties and information that will be exchanged among members of the health-care team in order to provide care for the patient. Patients should be made aware of the large number of persons in the modern hospital who require access to the medical record in order to serve the patient's medical and financial interests.

Finally, at some point most patients should have an opportunity to review their medical record and to make informed choices about whether their entire record is to be available to everyone or whether certain portions of the record are privileged and should be accessible only to their principal physician or to others designated explicitly by the patient. This approach would rely on traditional informed-consent procedural standards and might permit the patient to balance the personal value of medical confidentiality against the personal value of high-technology, team health care. There is no reason that the same procedure should not be used with psychiatric records instead of the arbitrary system now employed, in which everything related to psychiatry is kept secret.

AFTERTHOUGHT: CONFIDENTIALITY AND INDISCRETION

There is one additional aspect of confidentiality that is rarely included in discussions of the subject. I am referring here to the wanton, often inadvertent, but avoidable exchanges of confidential information that occur frequently in hospital rooms, elevators, cafeterias, doctors' offices, and at cocktail parties. Of course, as more people have access to medical information about the patient the potential for this irresponsible abuse of confidentiality increases geometrically.

Such mundane breaches of confidentiality are probably of greater concern to most patients than the broader issue of whether their medical records may be entered into a computerized data bank or whether a respiratory therapist is reviewing the results of an arterial blood gas determination. Somehow, privacy is violated and a sense of shame is heightened when intimate secrets are revealed to people one knows or is close to—friends, neighbors, acquaintances, or hospital roommates—rather than when they are disclosed to an anonymous bureaucrat sitting at a computer terminal in a distant city or to a health professional who is acting in an official capacity.

I suspect that the principles of medical confidentiality, particularly those reflected in most medical codes of ethics, were designed principally to prevent just this sort of embarrassing personal indiscretion rather than to maintain (for social, political, or economic reasons) the absolute secrecy of doctor-patient communications. In this regard, it is worth noting that Percival's Code of Medical Ethics (1803) includes the following admonition: "Patients should be interrogated concerning their complaint in a tone of voice which cannot be overheard."[1] We in the medical profession frequently neglect these simple courtesies.

CONCLUSION

The principle of medical confidentiality described in medical codes of ethics and still believed in by patients no longer exists. In this respect, it is a decrepit concept. Rather than perpetuate the myth of confidentiality and invest energy vainly to preserve it, the public and the profession would be better served if they devoted their attention to determining which aspects of the original principle of confidentiality are worth retaining. Efforts could then be directed to salvaging those.[2]

NOTES

1 Leake, C. D., ed., *Percival's medical ethics*. Baltimore, Williams & Wilkins, 1927.
2 Supported by a grant (OSS-8018097) from the National Science Foundation and by the National Endowment for the Humanities. The views expressed are those of the author and do not necessarily reflect those of the National Science Foundation or the National Endowment for the Humanities.

Hospital Ethics Committees

Behind Closed Doors: Promises and Pitfalls of Ethics Committees
Bernard Lo

Bernard Lo is professor of medicine and director of the program in medical ethics at the University of California Medical Center, San Francisco. His articles include "The Clinical Use of Advanced Directives" and "Assessing Decision-Making Capacity." He is also the author of *Resolving Ethical Dilemmas: A Guide for Clinicians* (1995).

Lo supports the continued existence of hospital ethics committees. However, he raises important questions about their ethicality, their effectiveness, and even the desirability of agreement by committee. Lo stresses the need for committees to define their goals more clearly and to establish procedures—especially regarding who will have access to committee proceedings—that will adequately protect the interests of patients. In discussing the ques-

Reprinted with permission from the *New England Journal of Medicine*, vol. 317 (1987), pp. 46–50. Copyright © Massachusetts Medical Society.

tionable nature of agreement by committee, Lo stresses the dangers of "groupthink," especially the fact that it may result in an inadequate consideration of patients' preferences. Lo concludes by recommending that ethics committees, like all other medical innovations, be subject to evaluation before consulting ethics committees is accepted as a standard decision-making procedure. He also suggests several criteria that could be used to evaluate both the process by which committees review cases and the results of their deliberations.

Hospital ethics committees have been hailed as providing a promising way to resolve ethical dilemmas in patient care. Although ethics committees may have various tasks, such as confirming prognoses, educating care givers, or developing hospital policies, their most innovative role is making recommendations in individual cases.[1-5] This role has been supported by the President's Commission for the Study of Ethical Problems in Medicine and Biomedical and Behavioral Research, the American Medical Association, and the American Hospital Association. Strictly speaking, such recommendations are not binding, but they undoubtedly carry great weight, especially if they are cogently justified.[6] It is predicted that most ethics committees will make recommendations in particular cases[3] and that the courts will respect them.[3]

Ethics committees may offer an attractive alternative to the courts.[3-5] The judicial system may be too slow for clinical decisions.[7,8] Moreover, the adversarial judicial process may polarize physicians, patients, and families,[9] whereas ethics committees may reconcile divergent views. The 1986 New York State Task Force on Life and the Law encouraged resolving patient care dilemmas at the hospital level, rather than turning to the courts, and suggested that ethics committees might mediate such disagreements.[10]

Although I support ethics committees, several questions trouble me. First, are these committees ethical? The goals and procedures of some committees may conflict with established ethical principles. Second, is agreement by committees always desirable? Group dynamics may lead to flawed information, reasoning, or recommendations. Third, are these committees effective? Like other medical innovations, they need to be rigorously evaluated.

GOALS AND PROCEDURES OF ETHICS COMMITTEES

The very name suggests that ethics committees base their recommendations on ethical principles and rational deliberation, rather than on mere custom, political power, or self-interest. A consensus on medical decision making has emerged in the medical literature, court decisions, and reports of the President's Commission.[1,7,8,11,12] According to this consensus, competent patients should give informed consent or refusal to the recommendations of physicians. Care givers need not accede to patient requests for treatments, however, if there are no medical indications. In cases in which patients are incompetent, decisions should be based on their previously expressed preferences or, if such preferences are unclear or unknown, on their best interests. The goals of some ethics committees, however, may conflict with these ethical guidelines. Goals vary substantially among committees.[1-3,13-15] Some do not have explicit goals. One committee has said, "We have never formally stated in writing the exact purpose or purposes of our committee but have decided to proceed in an informal manner. . . . We felt that to formalize our objectives might be counterproductive to the work of our committee."[14] But as ethics committees mature, and especially as they wish to serve as alternatives to the courts, they need to define their goals more clearly. Some so-called ethics committees have as goals confirming prognoses, providing emotional support for care givers, or reducing legal liability for physicians or hospitals.[1-3,13-15] One hospital administrator has even suggested that the ethics committee be used as a public relations "tool" for justifying unpopular decisions to discontinue unprofitable services.[16] Although committees on quality assurance, staff support, risk management, or public relations are important, there is little reason for patients, their surrogates, or the public to accept their recommendations about patient care.

After clarifying goals, committees can establish procedures. Ethics committees must decide who can refer cases or attend meetings. Many committees limit participation by patients and families. According to a 1982 survey, only 25 percent of ethics committees that reviewed cases allowed patients to bring cases to the committee. Only 19 percent of committees allowed patients to attend meetings, whereas 44 percent allowed family members to do so.[17] Limiting access to committee proceedings may seem desirable. It may be sound political strategy to overcome initial resistance to the ethics committee within the hospital. For example, attending physicians may fear that their authority will be undermined if patients, families, or nurses can ask the committee to review cases. Restricting access may also facilitate frank discussions by care givers and committee members about sensitive topics. In addition, discussions with other health professionals may help physicians to clarify their thinking before they talk to patients or families.

Restricted discussions, however, may not be accepted by patients, families, and society. Patients or surrogates who disagree with physicians are unlikely to regard the committee as impartial if they may not convene the committee or present their views directly, whereas physicians may do so. Disagreements that reach ethics committees usually involve important personal issues—even questions of life and death. In such vital decisions, patients and their proxies are not likely to accept recommendations by a committee whose members they have not met or that seems to meet behind closed doors.

The composition of ethics committees may not reassure patients that their wishes and interests are represented. Typically, most members of ethics committees are physicians, who may assess the importance of medical problems or the risks and benefits of treatment differently from patients.[18,19] Patients or surrogates who disagree with the committee's recommendations may say that the composition of the committee was biased against them.

Some committees meet with patients or family members who take the initiative and request meetings. But people who need the most help in expressing their preferences or interests may be the least likely to request a meeting. They may be cognitively impaired or unable to navigate the medical system, or there may be cultural, language, or educational barriers. Hence, it is desirable for the committee to take steps to inform patients, as well as care givers, of its work. Such information is particularly important if the committee can review a case without the consent of the parties. Mandatory review has been recommended, for example, when withholding life-sustaining treatment from neonates or from incompetent adults without surrogates is being considered.[20] A pamphlet about the committee might be distributed when patients are admitted. Patients or surrogates who are concerned that committee discussions or recommendations may invade

their privacy can then express those concerns in advance. Before the committee discusses a case, it should inform patients or surrogates and invite them to participate in the deliberations.

Most ethics committees also restrict the access of nurses. The 1982 survey found that only 31 percent of committees allowed nurses to present cases, and only 50 percent allowed nurses to attend meetings.[17] But it may be advisable to increase the access of nurses. Nurses have close contact with patients and families and may take the role of patient advocates.[21] They may raise previously overlooked issues, contribute new information, or express the questions and viewpoints of patients and families. Disagreements by nurses with physicians' orders often indicate a need to reconsider decisions.[22]

Because ethics committees are touted as an alternative to the courts, it may be useful to compare their safeguards with those in legal procedures.[23] The legal system notifies parties of the proceedings, allows them to give evidence, and ensures representation for patients. If the patient is incompetent, the court may appoint a guardian ad litem to represent the interests of the patient or to argue for continuing treatment. Moreover, parties are notified of the decision and the reasons for it, so that the decision can be reviewed or appealed. Ethics committees that make recommendations may not need safeguards that are as elaborate as those in a legal system that makes binding decisions. But for ethics committees to be accepted as a quicker and less acrimonious alternative to the courts, they must be perceived to be as fair as the courts.

In order for ethics committees to assist in decision making, their recommendations and the reasons for them must be known by all parties. In addition to communicating with the patient or surrogate and the attending physician, a representative of the committee might write a note in the medical record, so that nurses, consultants, and physicians understand the committee's recommendation and reasoning. Ethics committees, however, may seem reluctant to allow their recommendations to be reviewed. Some committees do not note their recommendations and reasoning in the medical record. In addition, articles about ethics committees discuss how to reduce the liability of individual committee members by keeping records from being "discoverable"—that is, from being subpoenaed in civil suits.[20,24] Such apparent secrecy may evoke the suspicion that the committee is more concerned with protecting physicians, the hospital, or itself than with helping patients.

PITFALLS OF COMMITTEE DISCUSSIONS

Pressures on ethics committees to reach agreement may lead to recommendations that are ethically questionable. Agreement or even consensus does not confer infallibility. For example, in the 1960s, hospital committees selected patients with chronic renal failure for treatment with life-prolonging dialysis machines, which were limited in number. When it was disclosed that criteria of social worth were implicitly applied, these committee decisions were criticized as being unfair and discriminatory.[25]

In some circumstances, committees may impair rather than improve decision making. Political scientists and psychologists have shown that committees may inadvertently pressure members to reach consensus, avoid controversial issues, underestimate risks and objections, or fail to consider alternatives or to search for additional information.[26,27] In other words, committees may not serve their intended function of considering diverse viewpoints and arguments. Such undesirable qualities of committee discussions, which have been called "groupthink," may lead to grave errors in judgment.

Ethics committees may fall victim to groupthink. First, these committees may reach consensus too easily, by not adequately considering patients' preferences. Despite the ideal of informed consent, patients are often not involved in decisions about their care.[28-30] Second, committees may accept secondhand information uncritically. Physicians appreciate that medical consultants should take new histories, examine patients, and review x-ray films and scans.[31,32] Similarly, an ethics committee should scrutinize information about the medical situation and the patient's preferences. Conclusions and inferences, rather than primary data, may be presented. For instance, patients may be described as "terminal" or "hopelessly ill," or it may be reported that an incompetent patient would not want "heroic care." Since such phrases are ambiguous and potentially misleading, committees should require and, if necessary, seek out more specific information. Third, ethics committees may overlook imaginative means of resolving disagreements. Disputes over patient care are not always caused by conflicts of ethical principles or obligations. They may also result from misunderstandings, stress, or lack of attention to the details of care.[22] Despite stalemates over conflicting ethical principles or duties, agreements on particular recommendations for patient care may be possible.[33]

Ethics committees should appreciate that they work under conditions that predispose them to groupthink. A rapid recommendation may be needed despite uncertain information and conflicting values and interests. Such clinical urgency may press the committee to reach agreement. The committee may feel attacked by various groups: attending physicians who fear that their power is being usurped, nurses who think that they are given unreasonable orders, administrators who wish to control costs, or risk managers who want to avoid legal difficulties. If committee chairpeople are forceful leaders who control discussions, they may unintentionally discourage frank debate and disagreement. Tendencies toward groupthink may be reinforced if access to the committee is limited.

Ethics committees that recognize the dangers of groupthink can take steps to avoid them. First, committees can guard against premature agreement. The chairperson may explicitly ask that doubts and objections be expressed or may appoint members to make the case against the majority. Second, committees can scrutinize any secondhand information they receive. To understand the patient's preferences, the committee might talk with the patient or proxy directly, invite the patient or surrogate to participate in some discussions, or assign a committee member to act as a patient advocate. Third, the committee can look for innovative ways to settle disputes. Improved communication may resolve disagreements. Families, nurses, or house staff may accept the attending physician's decision after they hear the reasons for it and have an opportunity to ask questions. Alternatively, a compromise may be negotiated.[34] For example, a patient who threatens to sign out of a cardiac care unit may agree to further treatment if he or she is given more control over the timing of the administration of medications and nursing care and if one physician and one nurse take responsibility for answering his or her questions.

EVALUATING ETHICS COMMITTEES

Ultimately, the question of whether ethics committees are useful is an empirical one. Before consulting ethics committees can be considered to be a standard decision-making procedure rather than a promising innovation, they need to be evaluated. Because enthusiastic anecdotes about innovations may not be confirmed in controlled trials, pleas have been made to evaluate new technological procedures, such as angioplasty, before they are accepted and put into wide use.[35] Institutional innovations should also be evaluated, even if they seem to be obviously beneficial. For instance, hospices were expected to provide more humane and less expensive care for patients with terminal illnesses. Controlled studies, however, suggest that hospice care may not differ substantially from current conventional care and may be more expensive.[36–38]

As in any evaluation, deciding on clinically meaningful outcomes and designing unbiased studies require thought and planning. I suggest several criteria for evaluating both the process by which ethics committees review cases and the results of their deliberations. First, patients and their surrogates should have access to the ethics committees. Specifically, they should be able to ask the committees to review their cases and to meet with the committees if they desire. Second, recommendations by the committee and the reasons for them should be available to the parties in each case. Generally, a note in the medical record would be required. Third, recommendations by ethics committees and actual decisions by attending physicians should be consistent with ethical and legal guidelines. The gold standard should be the widespread ethical consensus that has emerged on many issues.[39] Evaluations might focus on whether ethics committees reduce discrepancies between this consensus and actual decisions by physicians. For instance, studies indicate that care givers often fail to discuss management options with patients or the surrogates of incompetent patients.[28–30] Ethics committees should recommend such discussions when appropriate. If their recommendations have an effect on care givers, fewer decisions will be made without such discussions with patients or their surrogates. Committees should also increase informed refusals of care by patients. Moreover, committees should decrease decisions based on ambiguous or uncorroborated second-hand information about the indications for treatment or about patient preferences. Fourth, parties in disagreements should be satisfied with the process of review and with the recommendations of the ethics committee. Although the degree of satisfaction of care givers with ethics consultations has been studied,[40] it is also important to determine the reactions of patients or their surrogates. Finally, ethics committees that make recommendations should have their own internal systems of review, to ensure that the suggested criteria are met.

In summary, the promise that ethics committees will resolve dilemmas about patient care and avoid legal disputes needs to be examined critically. If recommendations by ethics committees are to be accepted by patients, families, society, and the courts, the wishes and interests of patients must be represented and ethical guidelines must be followed. Committees can take active steps to reduce the risk of groupthink. Empirical studies may indicate what kinds of committees improve decisions relating to patient care and in which clinical circumstances.

ACKNOWLEDGMENT

Supported in part by a grant (1 P50 MH42459-01) from the National Institute of Mental Health and a grant from the Commonwealth Foundation.

I am indebted to L. Dornbrand, J. Ungaretti, S. Cummings, S. Schroeder, and W. Strull for helpful suggestions.

REFERENCES

1 President's Commission for the Study of Ethical Problems in Medicine and Biomedical and Behavioral Research. Deciding to forego life-sustaining treatment: a report on the ethical, medical, and legal issues in treatment decisions. Washington, D.C.: Government Printing Office, 1983.

2 Cranford RE, Doudera AE, eds. Institutional ethics committees and health care decision making. Ann Arbor, Mich.: Health Administration Press, 1984.

3 Bayley SC, Cranford RE. Ethics committees: what we have learned. In: Friedman E, ed. Making choices: ethics issues for health care professionals. Chicago: American Hospital Publishing, 1986:193–9.

4 Lynn J. Roles and functions of institutional ethics committees: the President's Commission's view. In: Cranford RE, Doudera AE, eds. Institutional ethics committees and health care decision making. Ann Arbor, Mich.: Health Administration Press, 1984:22–30.

5 Committee on Ethics and Medical-Legal Affairs. Institutional ethics committee's [sic] roles, responsibilities, and benefits for physicians. Minn Med 1985; 68:607–12.

6 Siegler M. Ethics committees: decisions by bureaucracy. Hastings Cent Rep 1986; 16(3):22–4.

7 Lo B, Dornbrand L. The case of Claire Conroy: Will administrative review safeguard incompetent patients? Ann Intern Med 1986; 104:869–73.

8 Lo B. The Bartling case: protecting patients from harm while respecting their wishes. J Am Geriatr Soc 1986; 34:44–8.

9 Burt RA. Taking care of strangers: the rule of law in doctor-patient relations. New York: Free Press, 1979.

10 New York State Task Force on Life and the Law. Do not resuscitate orders: the proposed legislation and report of the New York State Task Force on Life and the Law, April 1986.

11 Wanzer SH, Adelstein SJ, Cranford RE, et al. The physician's responsibility towards hopelessly ill patients. N Engl J Med 1984; 310:955–9.

12 Lo B, Jonsen AR. Clinical decisions to limit treatment. Ann Intern Med 1980; 93:764–8.

13 Levine C. Questions and (some very tentative) answers about hospital ethics committees. Hastings Cent Rep 1984; 14(3):9–12.

14 Kushner T, Gibson JM. Institutional ethics committees speak for themselves. In: Cranford RE, Doudera AE, eds. Institutional ethics committees and health care decision making. Ann Arbor, Mich.: Health Administration Press, 1984:96–105.

15 Fost N, Cranford RE. Hospital ethics committees: administrative aspects. JAMA 1985; 253:2687–92.

16 Summers JW. Closing unprofitable services: ethical issues and management responses. Hosp Health Serv Adm 1985; 30:8–28.

17 Youngner SJ, Jackson DL, Coulton C, Juknialis BW, Smith E. A national survey of hospital ethics committees. Crit Care Med 1983; 11:902–5.

18 Friedin RB, Goldman L, Cecil RR. Patient-physician concordance in problem identification in the primary care setting. Ann Intern Med 1980; 93:490–3.

19 McNeil BJ, Weichselbaum R, Pauker SG. Fallacy of the five-year survival in lung cancer. N Engl J Med 1978; 299:1397–401.

20 Winslow GR. From loyalty to advocacy: a new metaphor for nursing. Hastings Cent Rep 1984; 14(3):32–40.

21 Robertson JA. Ethics committees in hospitals: alternative structures and responsibilities. Conn Med 1984; 48:441–4.

22 Lo B. The death of Clarence Herbert: withdrawing care is not murder. Ann Intern Med 1984; 101:248–51.

23 Baron C. The case for the courts. J Am Geriatr Soc 1984; 32:734–8.

24 Cranford RE, Hester FA, Ashley BZ. Institutional ethics committees: issues of confidentiality and immunity. Law Med Health Care 1985; 13:52–60.

25 Fox RC, Swazey JP, eds. The courage to fail: a social view of organ transplants and dialysis. Chicago: University of Chicago Press, 1974:240–79.

26 Janis IL, Mann L. Decision-making: a psychological analysis of conflict, choice, and commitment. New York: Free Press, 1977.

27 George A. Towards a more soundly based foreign policy. In: Commission on the Organization of the Government for the Conduct of Foreign Policy, appendix B. Washington, D.C.: Government Printing Office, 1975.

28 Lidz CW, Meisel A, Osterweis M, Holden JL, Marx JH, Munetz MR. Barriers to informed consent. Ann Intern Med 1983; 99:539–43.

29 Bedell SE, Pelle D, Maher PL, Cleary P. Do-not-resuscitate orders for critically ill patients in the hospital: How are they used and what is their impact? JAMA 1986; 256:233–7.

30 Goldman L, Lee T, Rudd P. Ten commandments for effective clinicians. Arch Intern Med 1983; 143:1753–5.

31 Lo B, Saika G, Strull W, Thomas E, Showstack J. 'Do not resuscitate' decisions: a prospective study at three teaching hospitals. Arch Intern Med 1985; 145:1115–7.

32 Tumulty PA. The effective clinician: his methods and approach to diagnosis and care. Philadelphia: W.B. Saunders, 1973:45–8.

33 Beauchamp TL, Childress J. Principles of biomedical ethics. 2nd ed. New York: Oxford University Press, 1983.

34 Steinbrook R, Lo B. The case of Elizabeth Bouvia: Starvation, suicide, or problem patient? Arch Intern Med 1986; 146:161–4.

35 Mock MB, Reeder GS, Schaff HV, et al. Percutaneous transluminal coronary angioplasty versus coronary artery bypass: Isn't it time for a randomized trial? N Engl J Med 1985; 312:916–9.

36 Kane RL, Wales J, Bernstein L, Leibowitz A, Kaplan S. A randomised controlled trial of hospice care. Lancet 1984; 1:890–4.

37 Kane RL, Bernstein L, Wales J, Rothenberg R. Hospice effectiveness in controlling pain. JAMA 1985; 253:2683–6.

38 Birnbaum HG, Kidder D. What does hospice cost? Am J Public Health 1984; 74:689–97.

39 Jonsen AR. A concord in medical ethics. Ann Intern Med 1983; 99:261–4.

40 Perkins HS, Saathoff BS. How do ethics consultations benefit clinicians? Clin Res 1986; 34:831A, abstract.

Ethics Case Review in Health Care Institutions: Committees, Consultants, or Teams?

Michael D. Swenson and Ronald B. Miller

Michael D. Swenson practices internal medicine for the Norton Sound Health Corporation in Nome, Alaska. He is the author of "Justice in Medicine" and "Scarcity in the Intensive Care Unit: Principles of Justice for Rationing ICU Beds." Ronald B. Miller is director of the Program in Medical Ethics and clinical professor of medicine at the University of California, Irvine. His coauthored articles include "A Paradigm Shift for Ethics Committees and Case Consultation" and "Improving Hospital Ethics Committees."

Swenson and Miller take up the question of whether ethics case review in health-care institutions is best conducted by hospital ethics committees or, as some have recently suggested, by individual ethics consultants. Starting with the assumption that the goal of ethics case review should be to facilitate ethical reflection and decision making, the authors explore the potential strengths and weaknesses of both the committee and consultant models. They argue that each is more appropriate than the other in certain types of situations. Additionally, they recommend a third model—that of a consulting team of three or four individuals from different disciplines—for situations in which it is possible to combine the advantages of both committees and consultants while avoiding the pitfalls of either.

Traditionally, review of difficult ethical problems that emerge in the care of patients has been performed by hospital ethics committees. It has been proposed that this case review would be more effectively conducted by individual clinicians who are skilled in ethical analysis, much as medical consultations are provided by specialists.[1,2] In this article, we will discuss the potential advantages and disadvantages of both the committee and consultant models for ethics case review in health care institutions. We suggest that neither model should be used exclusively, as each is more appropriate than the other under certain circumstances. Furthermore, we recommend that consideration be given to a third model, wherein cases are reviewed by a consulting team of three or four individuals of varied disciplines and expertise. The use of this alternative can retain the virtues of both committees and consultants without succumbing to the limitations of either.

There appears to be consensus in the literature that the goal of ethics case review, whether by committee or consultant, should be to facilitate ethical reflection and decision making by the persons involved in the case, rather than to impose a decision by discovering the

"truth" of the situation or the "right" moral solution.[3–7] The achievement of this goal involves many tasks: clarifying concepts and principles, describing precedents or applicable policies and laws, eliciting overlooked facts and perspectives, encouraging communication between involved parties, providing emotional support and reassurance, and resolving misunderstandings and disputes. The question then becomes: Are committees or consultants better equipped to achieve this goal and perform these tasks? Are there circumstances in which one model is more effective than the other?

WHEN CONSULTANTS ARE PREFERABLE TO COMMITTEES

What advantages might an ethics consultant have over an ethics committee? While members of a committee can (in principle) meet with the patient or his or her proxies, a consultant is more likely to have direct contact with the patient. This direct contact is desirable for a number of reasons. Dialogue can be held with the patient and/or proxies in an environment less threatening than that of a committee. The consulting clinician can gather data firsthand rather than relying on the interpretation of data from others, permitting verification of the diagnosis and prognosis, as well as eliciting pertinent values and attitudes. The patient's progress can be observed much more easily, and subsequent recommendations can be made if there is a change in the patient's condition or in the goals of therapy. The consultant has the opportunity to know the patient as a person, promoting integrity, compassion, and respect, and forming the basis for a therapeutic patient-consultant relationship.[8] Finally, bedside role modeling and teaching of clinical ethics to health care students and workers is facilitated when direct patient contact is possible.[8] Since a consultant is more likely to have direct contact with the patient or family than is a committee, the former model better realizes these desirable features.

Because fewer people are involved, consultants have a logistic advantage over committees. Even though consultants may face time constraints, it is often difficult to assemble a committee on short notice, and it generally takes longer for a committee to reach a consensus than for a consultant to make a recommendation. This would be important in a case where review is needed urgently—if, for example, a physician were unsure whether to initiate mechanical ventilation for a patient who was hopelessly ill. Individual consultants also would be able to monitor the patient's progress and update their recommendations on the basis of changes in the patient's clinical condition or in the patient's (and family's) preferences for treatment.

Furthermore, reasonable limits on the duration of a meeting may pressure the committee into a consensus that it would not make if it had more time for reflection and deliberation, and into a recommendation not easily changed, since to do so would require another meeting of the committee. Such a false consensus is an example of what Lo[9] termed *groupthink,* and it may be the result of time constraints, alternative agendas on the part of some committee members, or the varying political power that different members have. Other adverse effects of group dynamics include misinterpreting patient preferences, accepting secondhand information uncritically, and overlooking imaginative alternatives to resolving problems.[9]

Another potential liability of committees relates to the number of people involved and the understandable reluctance of some health care workers to bring cases before a committee. Speaking in front of a large group is intimidating, and most people are reluctant to have their decisions scrutinized by others. A recent study reported that 71% of physicians polled would prefer a single consultant over a committee when they needed help resolving an ethical dilemma.[10] Furthermore, the committee may wield more political power than it wishes or

intends, and it may be more likely than a consultant unintentionally to pressure the physician into an action with which he or she disagrees. Thus, there are a number of reasons for preferring the consultant model for case review.

WHEN COMMITTEES ARE PREFERABLE TO CONSULTANTS

On the other hand, there are circumstances in which committees are preferable to consultants. Ethical dilemmas that arise in the care of particular patients often lead to the revision or creation of hospital policy. Some of the earliest "do not resuscitate" policies, for example, were prompted by particular cases.[11] Hospitals understandably have an interest in the kind of health care that is practiced within their walls. If the care provided a particular patient has potentially negative consequences for the care that is provided to other patients, it is appropriate for some instrument of the hospital to review that case and formulate guidelines when necessary. Even those authors who advocate a strong role for ethics consultants concede that an ethics committee (at least in addition to a consultant) should be involved in reviewing cases with potential policy implications.[1,2]

A second virtue of committees is their multidisciplinary membership, with diverse expertise and points of view. From a practical perspective, this has several advantages. Nonphysicians may be more likely to seek the help of a committee than of a consultant: for example, a nurse faced with an ethical dilemma might be more likely to bring his or her concerns to another nurse who is a member of an ethics committee than to a physician consultant. Furthermore, a broad spectrum of expertise enables the committee to respond to various difficulties with more flexibility. Some problems require input from medical specialists, while others are better handled by chaplains or social workers. Representation of multiple disciplines ensures that more options will be conceived and considered, since an important goal in case review is creative conceptualization of as many possible actions as are ethically permissible.

From a theoretical perspective, there is good reason to believe that the multidisciplinary perspectives on a committee represent a more defensible forum for engaging in ethical reflection. Moreno[12,13] suggested that the pluralistic nature of our society makes breadth of membership crucial for a hospital ethics committee. He argued that a satisfactory representation of moral discourse in a pluralistic society would incorporate

Dewey's method of "social intelligence," and that a diverse array of professional expertise is necessary for this cooperative deliberation to succeed in health care settings. While a careful investigation into the nature of moral discourse would be necessary before Moreno's proposal could be confirmed, there is good reason to think that objectivity in ethics, if it exists at all, must be grounded in some sort of social consensus.[14] Assuming that this is the case, the diverse perspectives on an ethics committee might be expected to reflect moral "reality" more accurately than the deliberations of an individual consultant.

A similar concern was raised by Ross.[15] The selection of one model over the other conveys an important message to the hospital community. A preference for ethics consultants over committees conveys the message that ethics is to be done by experts, and that moral deliberation is a skill best left to those who possess a specialized body of knowledge. Such a concept is dangerous because it encourages health care practitioners and patients to defer to the "experts" in their moral judgments and responsibilities, thereby divorcing the practice of medicine from its inherently moral foundations. By having an ethics committee, a hospital sends a very different message: moral discourse is a community enterprise, an exercise in social intelligence that must not be divorced from everyday life and practice. The existence of a committee carries the message that

ethical reflection ought to find focus in a group of people representing the hospital community and not be relegated to the realm of experts.

To recapitulate, there are theoretical advantages and disadvantages to both models for "doing ethics" in health care contexts (Table 1). Consultants are more likely to have direct contact with patients, which provides a personal and humane disposition to individual case review and allows an impartial assessment of the medical facts on which diagnosis and prognosis are dependent; unfortunately, reliance on consultants runs the risk of separating ethical deliberation from the practice of medicine by allowing practitioners to refer their moral problems and to defer their moral responsibilities. Committees are better equipped to deal with ethical problems that have policy implications, but their inefficiency hampers their effectiveness when help in resolving an ethical dilemma is needed urgently. Case review may be less frequently sought by physicians if they are intimidated by the thought of presenting a case to a hospital committee; on the other hand, the diversity of such a committee may empower nonphysicians to seek its aid and make it more flexible in responding to those needs. The deliberations of committees may succumb to the dangers of *groupthink,* but if such pitfalls can be avoided, the process of moral deliberation that goes on in committees may be a more defensible method of ethical deliberation.

TABLE 1   Advantages and Disadvantages of Committees and Consultants

Advantages	Disadvantages
Consultants	
Direct contact with patients and families is possible	The consultant model conveys the message that ethical problems should be referred to an expert
Consultants are more flexible and efficient than committees	Seeking solutions from consultants may allow physicians to defer their moral responsibilities
Consultants may be preferred by physicians[13]	
Committees	
Issues with policy implications are more appropriately handled by committees	Committees are susceptible to the adverse effects of group dynamics
Multidisciplinary participation provides diverse viewpoints and conceptualization of alternatives	The size of the committee may be intimidating to those seeking case review
Committees provide a more appropriate forum for ethical reflection	Committees may have more political power than is appropriate

A POSSIBLE COMPROMISE

In the end, neither model is superior to the other in all instances, and further empiric studies are necessary before their respective impact on actual patient care can be fully assessed. We would like to suggest that an alternative model be considered, wherein case review would be done by a small team of committee members with clinical expertise who can comfortably visit the patient at the bedside. The exact composition of this team would depend on the talents available at the hospital and the needs of the case; in general, we envision such a team to be composed of a physician, a nurse, a chaplain, a social worker, and an ethicist (or some combination of these), all of whom have special interest and experience in the facilitation of moral discourse in clinical settings. For special problems, ad hoc members, such as a neurologist or lawyer, might also be considered. When a case review is requested, such a team could establish direct contact with the patient and family, either as a team or as individuals. This team would function closely with, but maintain a separate identity from, the hospital ethics committee. Discussion with our colleagues suggests that this model already is being used in many US hospitals, and similar models have been described in the literature.[16,17]

This alternative model preserves the virtues of both the committee and the consultant without succumbing to the limitations of either. Direct contact with the patient would take place, encouraging dialogue between consultants and patient, ensuring verification of medical facts, enabling observation of the patient's progress, enhancing bedside teaching of clinical ethics, and engendering respect for the patient as a person. The team could act quickly if necessary; one (or more) member could assess the situation nearly as efficiently as could an ethics consultant, and that member could rapidly transmit the relevant information to the other members. The diversity of the group would give it greater creativity in considering a variety of options for clinical ethical problems, as well as ensuring accessibility to all members of the health care team. This diversity of perspectives and expertise would make its deliberations more like the ideal

TABLE 2 Issues Appropriate for Ethics Committee, Consulting Team, or Consultant

Committee	Team or committee	Team or consultant	Consultant
When the issue has ethical or legal implications for hospital policy, allocation, or credibility	For complex issues and where there is lack of societal consensus	If direct contact with patient or staff is needed	When the patient, family, or physician prefers a consultant
If the issue threatens the hospital or significant relationships within it (whether interdepartmental or interpersonal)	If multiple perspectives or expertise are needed	If ongoing or repeated contact is needed	When the physician requests that a consultant help manage the case
When patient, family, or physician prefers a committee	For empowerment of a patient or nonphysician requesting the review	If the problem is urgent and the committee is not readily available	If the hospital ethics committee is ineffective
If the consultant is ineffective	When a personality conflict exists between the principals and consultant, or if a conflict of interests exists for the consultant	When the positions in a dispute are not yet entrenched or public	
	For retrospective review	For questions of fact regarding law, policy, or societal consensus	
	For surrogate decision making when there is no proxy	For evaluation of the decision-making capacity of the patient	

of ethical discourse as a community enterprise, and its form would send the message that ethical deliberation does benefit from a multiplicity of perspectives. Its relationship with the hospital ethics committee would permit it to call on the full committee for those problems that are especially difficult and complex, when consensus cannot be achieved by the members of the smaller team, when the case would have substantial policy or legal implications for the hospital, and for periodic review of the team's consultations. While interpersonal dynamics of the team might still make it subject to the dangers of *groupthink,* review by the full committee and familiarity among the members of the team should allow early recognition and correction of this problem.

We are not recommending that this interdisciplinary team replace either the consultant or the full ethics committees. Rather, we suggest that two models, or perhaps all three, might coexist productively within the same institution. Each model has its respective strengths and weaknesses, and the use of each would be more or less appropriate, depending on the particular situation (Table 2). Occasionally, more than one model might be useful for case review in a single patient. Problems requiring case review seem to exist along a continuum, with few situations at either extreme that can be handled solely by a consultant or a committee. A consulting team would be useful for dealing with the many cases between these extremes.

We do not imagine that Table 2 is exhaustive of all possible situations in which case review would be appropriate. Some problems may be handled best by calling a conference of the patient's primary caretakers, eg., when the primary issue is inadequate communication among those caretakers, or when a dispute arises among them that is not yet polarized. This patient care conference would include at least the physicians and nurses attending the patient, but it might also include the patient and family members, social worker, chaplain, or ethicist. Still other "ethical" problems might arise that would not be appropriate for any of the models described in this article (such as unethical behavior on the part of a physician that required disciplinary action), problems that might be better handled by the hospital administrator, chief of staff, department chairperson, institutional review board, or the legal office.

CONCLUSION

The need for careful ethical deliberation in case review will continue to increase as more and more treatment options become technically feasible. It will be important for physicians, patients, families, and other members of the health care team to have a resource to which they can turn when they are unclear about what is the "right thing to do." As we have seen, there are three models that can undertake case review; each has its respective strengths and limitations, and further empiric investigation is needed to determine the degree to which their respective characteristics impact on patient care. The committee model best represents our conviction that moral discourse is a community enterprise that ought not be relegated to "experts"; consequently, we urge that committees be central to any hospital's efforts at ethics case review. By adding a consulting team or a consultant (or both), the effectiveness of a hospital ethics committee can be enhanced in a wide range of ethical problems through improvements in efficiency, fact finding, and the quality of dialogue with patient, family, physician, and hospital staff.

ACKNOWLEDGMENT

We are grateful for the help we received on earlier drafts of this article from the following individuals: Carl Elliot, MD, PhD, Larry Feinberg, MD, John La Puma, MD, Alvin Moss, MD, Judith Wilson Ross, MA, Robert Schrier, MD, and Mark Siegler, MD.

REFERENCES

1 La Puma J, Toulmin SE. Ethics consultants and ethics committees. *Arch Intern Med.* 1989; 149:1109–1112.
2 La Puma J, Schiedermayer DL. Ethics consultation: skills, roles, and training. *Ann Intern Med.* 1991; 114:155–160.
3 Fleetwood JE, Arnold RM, Baron RJ. Giving answers or raising questions? The problematic role of institutional ethics committees. *J Med Ethics.* 1989; 15:137–142.
4 Ackerman TF. Conceptualizing the role of the ethics consultant: some theoretical issues. In: Fletcher JC, Quist N, Jonsen AR, eds. *Ethics Consultation in Health Care.* Ann Arbor, Mich: Health Administration Press; 1989:37–52.
5 Judicial Council of the AMA. Guidelines for ethics committees in health care institutions. *JAMA.* 1985; 253:2698–2699.
6 President's Commission for the Study of Ethical

Problems in Medicine and Biomedical and Behavioral Research. *Deciding to Forego Life-Sustaining Treatment.* US Government Printing Office; March 1983.

7 Siegler M, Singer PA. Clinical ethics consultation: godsend or 'God squad?' *Am J Med.* 1988;85:759–760.

8 La Puma J, Schiedermayer DL. Must the ethics consultant see the patient? *J Clin Ethics.* 1990;1:38–43.

9 Lo B. Behind closed doors: promises and pitfalls of ethics committees. *N Engl J Med.* 1987;317:46–50.

10 Perkins HS, Saathof BS. Impact of medical ethics consultations on physicians: an exploratory study. *Am J Med.* 1988;85:761–765.

11 Cassem NH. Confronting the decision to let death come. *Crit Care Med.* 1974;2:113–117.

12 Moreno JD. Ethics by committee: the moral authority of consensus. *J Med Phil.* 1988;13:411–432.

13 Moreno JD. What means this consensus? Ethics committees and philosophic tradition. *J Clin Ethics.* 1990;1:38–43.

14 Lovibond S. *Realism and Imagination in Ethics.* Minneapolis, Minn: University of Minnesota Press; 1983.

15 Ross JW. Case consultation: the committee or the clinical consultant? *HEC Forum.* 1990;2:289.

16 Fletcher JC, White ML, Foubert PJ. Biomedical ethics and an ethics consultation service at the University of Virginia. *HEC Forum.* 1990;2:89–99.

17 Wear S, Katz P, Andrzejewski B, Haryadi T. The development of an ethics consultation service. *HEC Forum.* 1990;2:75–87.

ANNOTATED BIBLIOGRAPHY: CHAPTER 3

Agich, George J., and Stuart Youngner: "For Experts Only?: Access to Hospital Ethics Committees," *Hastings Center Report* 21 (September-October 1991), pp. 17–25. The authors explore the issue of how much access patients should have to ethics committees. Should patients, for example, be able to initiate consultations and be informed about committee deliberations? Agich and Youngner argue that a responsibilities-based model is more useful than a patients-rights model in addressing these questions.

Annas, George J.: "The Emerging Stowaway: Patients' Rights in the 1980s." In Bart Gruzalski and Carl Nelson, eds., *Value Conflict in Health Care Delivery* (Cambridge, MA: Ballinger, 1982), pp. 89–100. Annas characterizes and criticizes the values and factual assumptions underlying the paternalistic attitudes that lead physicians to downplay patients' rights. He asserts five rights intended to humanize the hospital environment.

———: *The Rights of Patients,* 2d ed. (Totowa, NJ: Humana, 1992). This American Civil Liberties Union handbook on the rights of hospital patients is a guide for those directly affected by the problems discussed. Using a question-and-answer approach, the book provides a statement of patients' rights under the law.

Ashley, JoAnn: *Hospitals, Paternalism and the Role of the Nurse* (New York: Teachers College, 1976). This book is a study of the development of nursing in the United States. Ashley gives extensive historical documentation in showing that hospitals were established by male physicians and male hospital administrators to offer nursing care provided by women. Ashley documents overt and covert efforts to deny nurses any significant voice in establishing or changing hospital policies and practices.

Benjamin, Martin, and Joy Curtis: *Ethics in Nursing,* 3d ed. (New York: Oxford University Press, 1992). The intent of this book is to give nursing students and nurses an introduction to the identification and analysis of ethical issues in nursing. The book includes a large number of actual cases, many of which are explored in detail.

———: "Virtue and the Practice of Nursing." In Earl E. Shelp, ed., *Virtue in Medicine* (Boston: Kluwer, 1985), pp. 257–274. The authors use virtue ethics as a framework for understanding the role of the nurse in contemporary health care. The article includes fascinating historical data on the history of the nursing profession.

Cohen, Elliot D.: "Confidentiality, Counseling, and Clients Who Have AIDS," *Journal of Counseling & Development* 68 (January/February 1990), pp. 282–286. Cohen employs ethical theory in exploring the limits of confidentiality that mental-health professionals should observe in dealing with sexually active clients who have AIDS. He proposes a model rule to guide such decisions.

Corcoran, Sheila: "Toward Operationalizing an Advocacy Role," *Journal of Professional Nursing* 4 (July/August 1988), pp. 242–248. Corcoran begins by contrasting two models of nursing advocacy—the legal rights model and the existential advocacy model. Accepting the second model, Corcoran describes an approach that nurses might take when they attempt to perform the advocacy function of helping patients make decisions.

Cranford, Ronald E., and A. Edward Doudera, eds.: *Institutional Ethics Committees and Health Care Decision Making* (Ann Arbor, MI: Health Administration Press, 1984). Published in cooperation with the American Society of Law and Medicine, this collection of articles includes material on the development, roles, and functions of ethics committees as well as on their legal aspects, problems, and implementation. Descriptive summaries of existing institutional ethics committees and sample guidelines and policies are also included.

Daley, Dennis W.: "*Tarasoff v. Regents of the University of California* (Cal. 528 P2nd 553) and the Psychotherapist's Duty to Warn," *San Diego Law Review* 12 (July 1975), pp. 932–951. Daley analyzes the practical problems and potential consequences for psychiatry stemming from the *Tarasoff* decision. He discusses in more detail the same types of issues set forth in Justice Clark's dissenting opinion in the case, such as the difficulty of predicting violence and the importance of confidentiality in the patient-therapist relationship.

Macklin, Ruth: "HIV-Infected Psychiatric Patients: Beyond Confidentiality," *Ethics & Behavior* 1 (1991), pp. 3–20. Macklin examines ethical issues concerning HIV-infected psychiatric patients. Devoting most of her analysis to professionals' conflicting obligations of (1) confidentiality and (2) protecting persons at risk, she defends some limits to the first obligation before turning to other kinds of ethical dilemmas.

Salsberry, Pamela J.: "Caring, Virtue Theory, and a Foundation for Nursing Ethics," *Scholarly Inquiry for Nursing Practice* 6 (Summer 1992), pp. 155–167. Salsberry critically examines virtue ethics as a foundation for a nursing ethics based on the ideal of caring. She argues that, while virtue ethics can meet some of the conditions of an adequate foundation, it ultimately fails to provide a viable alternative to a duty-based approach as a foundation for nursing ethics.

Smith, Martin L., and Kevin P. Martin: "Confidentiality in the Age of AIDS: A Case Study in Clinical Ethics," *Journal of Clinical Ethics* 4 (Fall 1993), pp. 236–241. The authors explore a detailed case in examining the ethical dimensions of situations involving a conflict between the duty to protect the confidences of an AIDS patient and the duty to protect third parties. Their analysis is distinguished by its attention to salient details and nuances of such situations.

Swenson, Sara, et al., compilers: "Bibliography of Ethics Committees." (Briarcliff Manor, NY: The Hastings Center, Fall 1988.) This is an excellent annotated bibliography.

Winslow, Betty J., and Gerald R. Winslow: "Integrity and Compromise in Nursing Ethics," *Journal of Medicine and Philosophy* 16 (June 1991), pp. 307–323. The authors grapple with ethical issues that arise for nurses when they consider compromise as a means of resolving conflicts in which they are entangled. They argue that compromise is compatible with moral integrity if certain conditions are met.

Winslow, Gerald R.: "From Loyalty to Advocacy: A New Metaphor for Nursing," *Hastings Center Report* 14 (June 1984), pp. 32–39. Winslow argues that in the nursing literature two dominant metaphors have served as basic models of ideal nursing practice—a military metaphor, with its language of loyalty and obedience; and a legal metaphor, with its language of advocacy and rights.

CHAPTER 4

HUMAN AND ANIMAL EXPERIMENTATION

INTRODUCTION

The primary focus of this chapter is on ethical issues raised by biomedical experimentation (or research) using human subjects. Analyses of these issues employ some of the same ethical concepts and principles discussed in the previous two chapters. Here, too, appeal is made to the value of individual autonomy and to the requirements of informed consent and, for patients lacking competence, proxy consent. At the same time, a concern unique to experimentation is its potential benefits to society as a whole. In addition to dealing with issues related to the requirements of informed and proxy consent, this chapter features an extensive discussion of randomized clinical trials. It also takes up ethical issues raised by animal experimentation.

Conceptual Issues

Before examining some of the ethical issues raised by human experimentation, we should clarify the meaning of *human experimentation* (or *research using human subjects*) and the distinction often made between therapeutic and nontherapeutic experimentation (or research). In the biomedical context, *therapy* ordinarily refers to a set of activities whose primary purpose is to relieve suffering, restore or maintain health, or prolong life. Therapy takes many forms. Medical treatment, diagnosis, and even some preventive measures (e.g., vaccine injections) are all considered forms of therapy. It is important to notice that the primary aim of therapy is to benefit the recipient. In contrast, *research* or *experimentation* refers to a set of scientific activities whose primary purpose is to develop or contribute to generalizable knowledge about the chemical, physiological, or psychological processes involved in human (or sometimes animal) functioning. In *human experimentation*, human beings are used as subjects.

A distinction is commonly drawn between therapeutic and nontherapeutic research. *Therapeutic research,* like all research, is said to be concerned with the acquisition of generalizable knowledge. However, in therapeutic research the patient-subjects are themselves expected to benefit medically from the new drug, vaccine, treatment, or diagnostic procedure being tried. For example, the first patients on kidney dialysis machines and the first recipients of coronary bypass surgery were participants in medical experiments. The techniques involved had never been tried on human subjects, so the use of these techniques on these patient-subjects was experimental. Furthermore, the information gained by the medical professionals furthered their research and thus contributed to generalizable knowledge. At the same time, however, the new techniques provided a form of therapy designed to alleviate the patient-subjects' own medical problems. Thus the procedures were used on the patients for their benefit, because the procedures promised to be more effective than any other therapy available. By contrast, *nontherapeutic research* is said to be research whose *sole* aim is to provide information required by the researchers. Nontherapeutic research is not concerned with providing therapy for the research subjects.

In an article reprinted in this chapter, Donald F. Phillips describes several ethically troubling experiments, one of which will serve to illustrate the difference between therapeutic and nontherapeutic research. In the 1940s researchers at several American universities injected 18 patients with plutonium to observe where it would go in their bodies. The research was designed to determine the risk to workers exposed to plutonium. (Many of the patients and their families were never informed about the purpose of the studies.) This project provides a clear example of nontherapeutic research because there was no expectation that the subjects themselves might benefit from their participation.

In practice, it is difficult to draw a clear line between therapeutic and nontherapeutic research. Therapeutic research is not conducted *solely* to benefit the patient-subjects since the purpose of all research is to contribute to generalizable knowledge. In addition, the therapeutic project may require patient-subjects to undergo additional procedures unrelated to their own therapy. They may have to give blood samples or be catheterized, for example. Such additional procedures are nontherapeutic for the patients and may even carry some risks unrelated to their own therapy. Nontherapeutic research, in turn, may *indirectly* provide medical benefits (such as better medical care) for subjects. Despite these complications, which obscure somewhat the distinction between therapeutic and nontherapeutic research, many commentators find the distinction helpful in exploring ethical issues pertaining to research. For example, it is commonly believed that the degree of risk to patient-subjects in therapeutic research may ethically be somewhat higher than the degree of risk that is acceptable in research where subjects are not expected to benefit directly—that is, in nontherapeutic research. The acceptance of this distinction is reflected in codes of research ethics that continue to use it. One example of such a code is "The Declaration of Helsinki," reprinted in this chapter.

The Justifiability of Experimentation Using Human Subjects

Many biomedical research projects involve some risk to subjects. Drugs being tested may turn out to be toxic, for example. In some experiments, subjects may have to be deliberately exposed to a disease such as malaria before they can be used to test the efficacy of a new treatment. What moral justification can be offered for experimentation that puts human subjects at risk?

The most common justification offered for human experimentation is a utilitarian one, which features two main claims. First, human experimentation enhances the discovery of new diagnostic and therapeutic techniques. Past research, for example, has made possible cardiovascular surgery, renal transplantation, and the control of poliomyelitis. Second, controlled experiments are necessary for sound medical practice. Iatrogenic illnesses will be prevented only if clinical research provides necessary knowledge about human reactions to specific therapies. In the past, physicians employed many techniques that were of no benefit and sometimes even harmed patients. For example, neither the bloodletting common in the eighteenth century nor the practice of freezing the stomachs of patients with ulcers in the twentieth century proved to have any therapeutic value. Yet both practices were believed to be therapeutic. Well-designed, controlled research projects, it is argued, will help to minimize the use of worthless or harmful procedures. The utilitarian conclusion is that human experimentation is not just morally permissible but morally required because its harmful consequences for some will be far outweighed by its future benefits and prevention of harm to others.

Sometimes a different sort of argument, based on considerations of justice, is advanced to justify human experimentation and to defend the view that individuals have a duty to participate as research subjects. The argument is simple. We are the beneficiaries of advances made by past biomedical research. Without the use of human subjects, these advances would have been impossible. Since we have benefitted from the sacrifices made by past research subjects, we have a fairness-based obligation to reciprocate by serving as subjects ourselves. In reply to this argument, it has been claimed that medical progress is an optional goal, not an imperative, so that no obligation to participate in research can be derived from this goal.[1]

The Informed-Consent Requirement

Most of the literature on the ethics of human experimentation is concerned with specifying the *conditions* under which human experimentation is ethically acceptable. Since World War II, more than 30 different guidelines and codes of ethics identifying these conditions have been formalized. Foremost among these are the two codes included in this chapter—"The Nuremburg Code" and "The Declaration of Helsinki." Common to all these codes is the principle that experimentation may not be conducted on human subjects without their informed consent (or, as some codes allow, the consent—where appropriate—of a proxy). Discussions of this requirement are commonplace in the literature on human research, and some of the major topics connected with informed consent are treated in this chapter.

One major topic is the *justification* of the informed-consent requirement. The justifications offered for requiring that human beings not be used as research subjects without their informed consent are similar to those advanced to justify the requirement in the ordinary (nonresearch) biomedical context. The primary argument, advanced from a deontological perspective, rests on the principle of respect for autonomy, which is sometimes called the principle of respect for *persons*. Respect for human beings as persons requires that their autonomy be protected and promoted. Research that uses human subjects without their consent violates that autonomy and is, therefore, morally unacceptable. Paul Ramsey, a main proponent of this position, holds that informed consent is the "chief canon of loyalty" between the biomedical researcher and the patient-subject. It serves as a deontological check on any attempt to justify the use of human subjects solely on utilitarian grounds, insofar as it affirms that human beings are not objects to be used, without their consent, for others' benefit. In Ramsey's view, only individuals who are (1) capable of knowingly involving themselves in a common cause with the researcher and (2) willing to participate as research subjects may serve in that capacity.

Some of the literature on informed consent in research focuses on special causes for concern, including (1) egregious failures on the part of researchers to comply with the requirement (historical causes for concern) and (2) cultural complexities in implementing it (cultural causes for concern). Perhaps the most famous example of egregious noncompliance is that of the Nazi researchers, who performed many gruesome experiments on nonconsenting adults without any regard for their interests; "The Nuremburg Code" was written in the wake of these atrocities. In an article reprinted in this chapter, Donald F. Phillips describes several experiments (one of which provided an example of nontherapeutic research above) that were part of a group that has come to be known as "the radiation experiments." During the Cold War with the U.S.S.R., federal agencies funded and in some cases conducted research projects in which hundreds of Americans were exposed to high doses of radiation; often the subjects selected were from vulnerable groups, and frequently no consent was obtained. Another historical cause for concern is described briefly by Patricia A. King in this chapter: a federally funded, longitudinal study in Tuskegee, Alabama, of the consequences of untreated syphilis in which all of the subjects were black men. Among the shocking facts about this research is that, after penicillin was discovered, subjects were not informed of its availability, although it was known to be an effective treatment for syphilis. Because the violation of the subjects' right to self-determination appeared to be related to racism, this episode also suggests cultural reasons for concern about the implementation of the informed-consent requirement. In fact, King's article uses the Tuskegee experience as a backdrop to a broader cultural concern regarding the use of minority research subjects: an uncomfortable tension between avoiding the perpetuation of negative stereotyping while being prepared to note racially correlated differences that may be medically significant.

Proxy Consent for Research Subjects Incapable of Informed Consent

Since children, especially young children, cannot give informed consent because they lack the competence to assess information about research procedures, any research using them as subjects may seem to violate the informed-consent requirement. When the research project is primarily therapeutic and is reasonably expected to benefit the child, it is less troublesome. Here, as in the case of validated therapies, it is usually agreed that proxies, such as parents and guardians, can legitimately consent on the child's behalf. However, when the procedure is not intended to benefit the child directly but to acquire knowledge that will benefit future patients, the child's participation is more problematic. Is it ever morally correct for parents and guardians to consent on their children's behalf to the latter's participation in nontherapeutic research?

Proponents of research using children cite its benefits to children as a group. Children are not just "little adults" in sickness or in health. Results of studies on adults cannot be simply extrapolated to children. To cite just one example, it would be disasterous to administer intravenous fluids to infants and children on the basis of adult requirements. Children would be given too much or too little. The requirements for specific age groups can only be identified by studying the normal constituents of body fluids and metabolism in infants and children. There are also a number of diseases, such as infantile autism, that are unique to children. For these, as well as many other reasons, the use of children as research subjects is required for medical progress that will eventually benefit children as a group. In view of these potential gains, some proponents of research using children argue for the validity of proxy consent.

One such proponent, Richard A. McCormick, argues that parents can give a valid proxy consent to nontherapeutic pediatric research when (1) the risks of such research are minimal and (2) the potential benefits to *children as a group* are very great. McCormick's claim is based on his "natural law" ethics. By their very nature, human beings are social, interdependent beings. As such, they owe it to each other to perform certain minimum moral duties, including the duty to participate in minimally risky nontherapeutic research whose benefit to society may be very great. As members of society, even children have these obligations, so it is morally acceptable for their parents to consent to their participation in minimally risky experiments.[2]

Perhaps no one is more opposed to using children as subjects in nontherapeutic research than Ramsey, whose argument is included in a reading in this chapter. In Ramsey's view, it is always wrong to subject children to procedures that are neither intended nor reasonably expected to benefit them directly. An experimental procedure holds the promise of directly benefiting a child if the procedure is (1) seen as the best means of effecting the child's recovery or (2) intended to protect the child against some greater risk. Using young children in experimental trials of polio vaccines, for example, at a time when children were at risk of contracting the crippling disease summer after summer, was morally acceptable in Ramsey's view, because the risks of the experimental procedure had to be weighed against the dangers posed for the experimental subjects themselves by polio epidemics. However, Ramsey rejects the claim that using children as subjects in a nontherapeutic research project is morally acceptable when the intended beneficiaries are children as a group. His position is grounded in the claim (discussed earlier in this introduction) that all human experimentation must be a joint venture, freely undertaken by two autonomous persons. In keeping with this position, he refuses to recognize the validity of proxy consent to any nontherapeutic procedures.

Barry F. Brown's argumentation in this chapter stands in sharp contrast to Ramsey's. Brown focuses on incompetent adults, especially Alzheimer's patients, and defends their use in at least some nontherapeutic research projects. He develops a McCormick-type argument, maintaining that proxy consent to participation in nontherapeutic research may be morally legitimate in the case of those who are in the advanced stages of Alzheimer's, so long as the intended beneficiaries of the research are potential Alzheimer's patients. In his view, what directly benefits the latter *indirectly* benefits the research subjects insofar as they are all members of a community or group with a *common good*—the prevention of harm resulting from the disease.

Experimental Design and Randomized Clinical Trials

Questions about informed consent are also raised in discussions of randomized clinical trials (RCTs). Considered the "gold standard" of clinical research, the RCT is a comparison of two or more treatment arms—scientifically controlled with random assignment of subjects—to study the efficacy of new therapies. In one of this chapter's readings, Samuel Hellman and Deborah S. Hellman argue that RCTs present an ethical dilemma admitting of no comfortable solution. Typically, at the beginning of a study or at some point during the study, they maintain, researchers have an opinion about which treatment arm is preferable in terms of the patient-subjects' best interests. But while sharing that opinion seems required out of fidelity to the patient, doing so would ruin the study, according to the authors.

Although today it is widely appreciated that RCTs can place researchers in conflicting roles, not all commentators consider the problem as intractable as Hellman and Hellman do. Benjamin Freedman, for example, presents a contrasting analysis in an article reprinted in this chapter. He believes the ethical tension that can arise in RCTs has been blown out of proportion due to a misunderstanding of the concept of *equipoise,* which all commentators agree to be ethically required in RCTs, but most have taken to involve the individual investigator's beliefs. Freedman argues that a plausible understanding of equipoise largely removes the sense of conflict. Clinical equipoise exists when, within the expert medical community, there is genuine uncertainty about the relative merits of the treatments being compared, a situation that often occurs even though an individual investigator has an opinion one way or the other.

In another of this chapter's readings, Robert M. Veatch proposes a quite different approach. Veatch contends that when subjects who are among the least well-off in society strongly prefer one treatment arm in an RCT, justice requires turning the study into what he describes as a "semi-randomized clinical trial." Veatch argues that this innovation proves to be scientifically, as well as ethically, sound.

Animal Experimentation

The use of animals in biomedical experimentation intended to benefit humans raises its own set of troubling questions. Some questions concern the *importance of the research,* while others concern the *moral status of animals*. Regarding the importance of the research, is there a genuine need to use animals in experiments intended to benefit humans? More specifically, how valuable is the knowledge sought, and how necessary is the use of animals to obtain that knowledge? Regarding animals themselves, do they have moral status? If so, is their moral status the same as that of humans, such that whatever is morally impermissible in the case of humans is also impermissible in the case of animals? If not, in what respects do humans and animals have unequal moral status? In general, what characteristics must a being possess in order to be entitled to moral consideration?

Peter Singer in this chapter argues that the interests of animals must be given equal consideration to human interests. Failure to meet this standard, he contends, is *speciesism*, which is morally analogous to racism and sexism. Applying the principle of equal consideration, Singer condemns the vast bulk of animal experimentation for causing great harm to animals while rarely achieving important goals. He argues that the use of animals in research is justified only when using a human of comparable mental capacities would also be justified. In another of this chapter's readings, Christina Hoff Sommers supports the idea that animals' interests must be given serious consideration. However, emphasizing the claim that human lives have greater value than animal lives (even if humans and animals have a similar interest in avoiding suffering), she defends the use of research animals in some circumstances for important medical purposes. In this chapter's final reading, James Lindemann Nelson addresses ethical issues connected with an experimental technology that cuts across the research-therapy distinction—the transplantation of animal organs, such as livers or hearts, to humans whose own defective organs place them in desperate need.

D.D.

NOTES

1 Hans Jonas, "Philosophical Reflections on Experimenting with Human Subjects," in Paul Freund, ed., *Experimentation with Human Subjects* (New York: Braziller, 1970), pp. 1–31.
2 Richard A. McCormick, "Proxy Consent in the Experimentation Situation," *Perspectives in Biology and Medicine* 18 (Autumn 1974), pp. 2–20.

Ethical Codes

The Nuremberg Code

"The Nuremberg Code of Ethics in Medical Research" was developed by the Allies after the Second World War. During the war crimes trials in Germany, this code provided the standards against which the practices of Nazis involved in human experimentation were judged. The Nuremberg Code emphasizes the centrality of voluntary consent. Its first and longest article discusses consent in great detail. The code also sets forth other criteria that must be met before any experiment using human beings as subjects can be judged morally acceptable.

Reprinted from *Trials of War Criminals before the Nuremberg Military Tribunals* (Washington, DC: U.S. Government Printing Office, 1948).

1) The voluntary consent of the human subject is absolutely essential. This means that the person involved should have legal capacity to give consent; should be so situated as to be able to exercise free power of choice, without the intervention of any element of force, fraud, deceit, duress, overreaching, or other ulterior form of constraint or coercion; and should have sufficient knowledge and comprehension of the elements of the subject matter involved as to enable him to make an understanding and enlightened decision. This latter element requires that before the acceptance of an affirmative decision by the experimental subject there should be made known to him the nature, duration, and purpose of the experiment; the method and means by which it is to be conducted; all inconveniences and hazards reasonably to be expected; and the effects upon his health or person which may possibly come from his participation in the experiments.

The duty and responsibility for ascertaining the quality of the consent rests upon each individual who initiates, directs or engages in the experiment. It is a personal duty and responsibility which may not be delegated to another with impunity.

(2) The experiment should be such as to yield fruitful results for the good of society, unprocurable by other methods or means of study, and not random and unnecessary in nature.

(3) The experiment should be so designed and based on the results of animal experimentation and a knowledge of the natural history of the disease or other problem under study that the anticipated results [will] justify the performance of the experiment.

(4) The experiment should be so conducted as to avoid all unnecessary physical and mental suffering and injury.

(5) No experiment should be conducted where there is an a priori reason to believe that death or disabling injury will occur; except, perhaps, in those experiments where the experimental physicians also serve as subjects.

(6) The degree of risk to be taken should never exceed that determined by the humanitarian importance of the problem to be solved by the experiment.

(7) Proper preparations should be made and adequate facilities provided to protect the experimental subject against even remote possibilities of injury, disability, or death.

(8) The experiment should be conducted only by scientifically qualified persons. The highest degree of skill and care should be required through all stages of the experiment of those who conduct or engage in the experiment.

(9) During the course of the experiment the human subject should be at liberty to bring the experiment to an end if he has reached the physical or mental state where continuation of the experiment seems to him to be impossible.

(10) During the course of the experiment the scientist in charge must be prepared to terminate the experiment at any stage, if he has probable cause to believe, in the exercise of good faith, superior skill and careful judgment required of him that a continuation of the experiment is likely to result in injury, disability, or death to the experimental subject.

Declaration of Helsinki
World Medical Association

In 1964 the Eighteenth World Medical Assembly, meeting in Helsinki, Finland, adopted an ethical code to be used as a guide by medical doctors involved in biomedical research involving human subjects. This code has been revised several times, most recently in Hong Kong in 1989. The code reprinted here is the most recent version. It has much in common with the Nuremberg Code (e.g., the informed-consent requirement and the requirement that animal experimentation must precede human experimentation). The Helsinki Code, however, goes beyond the Nuremberg Code in certain important respects. Two differences are especially noteworthy. (1) The Helsinki Code distinguishes between clinical (therapeutic) and nonclinical (nontherapeutic) biomedical research and sets forth specific criteria of ethical acceptability for each, as well as other basic principles common to both. (2) The Nuremberg Code is silent regarding the informed-consent requirement in the case of the legally incompetent. The Helsinki Code addresses itself to such cases, asserting the ethical acceptability of what is sometimes called "proxy consent."

INTRODUCTION

It is the mission of the physician to safeguard the health of the people. His or her knowledge and conscience are dedicated to the fulfillment of this mission.

The Declaration of Geneva of the World Medical Assembly binds the physician with the words, "The health of my patient will be my first consideration," and the International Code of Medical Ethics declares that, "A physician shall act only in the patient's interest when providing medical care which might have the effect of weakening the physical and mental condition of the patient."

The purpose of biomedical research involving human subjects must be to improve diagnostic, therapeutic and prophylactic procedures and the understanding of the aetiology and pathogenesis of disease.

In current medical practice most diagnostic, therapeutic or prophylactic procedures involve hazards. This applies especially to biomedical research.

Medical progress is based on research which ultimately must rest in part on experimentation involving human subjects.

In the field of biomedical research a fundamental distinction must be recognized between medical research in which the aim is essentially diagnostic or therapeutic for a patient, and medical research, the essential object of which is purely scientific and without implying direct diagnostic or therapeutic value to the person subjected to the research.

Special caution must be exercised in the conduct of research which may affect the environment, and the welfare of animals used for research must be respected.

Because it is essential that the results of laboratory experiments be applied to human beings to further scientific knowledge and to help suffering humanity, the World Medical Association has prepared the following recommendations as a guide to every physician in biomedical research involving human subjects. They should be kept under review in the future. It must be stressed that the standards as drafted are only a guide to physicians all over the world. Physicians are not relieved from criminal, civil and ethical responsibilities under the laws of their own countries.

I. BASIC PRINCIPLES

1.   Biomedical research involving human subjects must conform to generally accepted scientific principles and should be based on adequately performed laboratory and animal experimentation and on a thorough knowledge of the scientific literature.

2.   The design and performance of each experimental procedure involving human subjects should be clearly formulated in an experimental protocol which should be transmitted for consideration, comment and guidance to a specially appointed committee independent of the investigator and the sponsor provided that this independent committee is in conformity with the laws and regulations of the country in which the research experiment is performed.

3.   Biomedical research involving human subjects should be conducted only by scientifically qualified persons and under the supervision of a clinically competent medical person. The responsibility for the human subject must always rest with a medically qualified person and never rest on the subject of the research, even though the subject has given his or her consent.

4.   Biomedical research involving human subjects cannot legitimately be carried out unless the importance of the objective is in proportion to the inherent risk to the subject.

5.   Every biomedical research project involving human subjects should be preceded by careful assessment of predictable risks in comparison with foreseeable benefits to the subject or to others. Concern for the interests of the subject must always prevail over the interests of science and society.

6.   The right of the research subject to safeguard his or her integrity must always be respected. Every precaution should be taken to respect the privacy of the subject and to minimize the impact of the study on the subject's physical and mental integrity and on the personality of the subject.

7.   Physicians should abstain from engaging in research projects involving human subjects unless they are satisfied that the hazards involved are believed to be predictable. Physicians should cease any investigation if the hazards are found to outweigh the potential benefits.

8. In publication of the results of his or her research, the physician is obliged to preserve the accuracy of the results. Reports of experimentation not in accordance with the principles laid down in this Declaration should not be accepted for publication.

9. In any research on human beings, each potential subject must be adequately informed of the aims, methods, anticipated benefits and potential hazards of the study and the discomfort it may entail. He or she should be informed that he or she is at liberty to abstain from participation in the study and that he or she is free to withdraw his or her consent to participation at any time. The physician should then obtain the subject's freely-given informed consent, preferably in writing.

10. When obtaining informed consent for the research project the physician should be particularly cautious if the subject is in a dependent relationship to him or her or may consent under duress. In that case the informed consent should be obtained by a physician who is not engaged in the investigation and who is completely independent of this official relationship.

11. In case of legal incompetence, informed consent should be obtained from the legal guardian in accordance with national legislation. Where physical or mental incapacity makes it impossible to obtain informed consent, or when the subject is a minor, permission from the responsible relative replaces that of the subject in accordance with national legislation.

Whenever the minor child is in fact able to give a consent, the minor's consent must be obtained in addition to the consent of the minor's legal guardian.

12. The research protocol should always contain a statement of the ethical considerations involved and should indicate that the principles enunciated in the present Declaration are complied with.

II. MEDICAL RESEARCH COMBINED WITH CLINICAL CARE (CLINICAL RESEARCH)

1. In the treatment of the sick person, the physician must be free to use a new diagnostic and therapeutic measure, if in his or her judgement it offers hope of saving life, reestablishing health or alleviating suffering.

2. The potential benefits, hazards and discomfort of a new method should be weighed against the advantages of the best current diagnostic and therapeutic methods.

3. In any medical study, every patient—including those of a control group, if any—should be assured of the best proven diagnostic and therapeutic method.

4. The refusal of the patient to participate in a study must never interfere with the physician-patient relationship.

5. If the physician considers it essential not to obtain informed consent, the specific reasons for this proposal should be stated in the experimental protocol for transmission to the independent committee (I, 2).

6. The Physician can combine medical research with professional care, the objective being the acquisition of new medical knowledge, only to the extent that medical research is justified by its potential diagnostic or therapeutic value for the patient.

III. NON-THERAPEUTIC BIOMEDICAL RESEARCH INVOLVING HUMAN SUBJECTS (NON-CLINICAL BIOMEDICAL RESEARCH)

1. In the purely scientific application of medical research carried out on a human being, it is the duty of the physician to remain the protector of the life and health of that person on whom biomedical research is being carried out.

2. The subjects should be volunteers—either healthy persons or patients for whom the experimental design is not related to the patient's illness.

3. The investigator or the investigating team should discontinue the research if in his/her or their judgement it may, if continued, be harmful to the individual.

4. In research on man, the interest of science and society should never take precedence over considerations related to the wellbeing of the subject.

Historical and Cultural Causes for Concern

Past Radiation Experiments May Lead to New Efforts for Informed Consent
Donald F. Phillips

Donald F. Phillips is managing editor of *Hospital Ethics*. His area of specialization is the evaluation of ethics committees. Phillips is the author of "Hospital Ethics Committees: Are They Evaluating Their Performance?", "Through the Looking Glass: New Voices Ask to Be Heard in Bioethics," and "Pastoral Care: Finding a Niche in Ethical Decision-Making."

Phillips examines a disturbing chapter in American research history that was recently revealed to the wider public and has relevance for informed consent today. For several decades during the Cold War, hundreds of Americans were exposed to harmful levels of radiation, often without their consent, in experiments funded and run by federal agencies. The subjects of the experiments were frequently vulnerable individuals who knew little or nothing about radiation. They included newborns, terminally ill patients, prisoners, mentally retarded persons, minorities, and the poor. After describing several of these studies, as well as the politics surrounding their revelation, Phillips explores the practical ramifications of the revelation. They include, in his view, the possibilities of (1) increased scrutiny of informed-consent procedures in other current and past experiments, (2) damaged trust in the American research enterprise, and (3) critical examination of the current system for reviewing research protocols.

Public disclosure by newspapers toward the end of 1993 that hundreds of Americans were exposed to harmful levels of radiation, sometimes without their permission, in experiments conducted and/or supported by federal agencies and universities left many Americans feeling that the public trust had been betrayed.

In December, President Clinton called for full disclosure of all federally funded radiation experiments conducted during the Cold War on at least 800 Americans. Soon after, Energy Secretary Hazel O'Leary called for the federal government to compensate those Americans who were unwittingly exposed to radiation during this period.

Scientists in federal agencies and universities have launched an intensive reexamination of experiments conducted over 30 years ago and there is some hope that attention to these studies may force greater scrutiny on today's procedures for obtaining informed consent.

What seems to be most disturbing about the past experiments is that the subjects chosen were people who

had little understanding of radiation and were highly vulnerable, namely, prisoners, the mentally retarded, newborn babies, the terminally ill, members of minority groups, and the indigent.

At the time of the experiments, the dangers of radiation were well known within the medical community. Furthermore, although many of the experiments claimed to be providing medical benefits to their subjects, they were often supported by the Department of Defense or the Atomic Energy Commission, not by health agencies. Such studies, critics say, should be looked at skeptically.

"For some reason, rich white people were deprived of all this wonderful research," says David S. Egilman, M.D., clinical assistant professor, Brown University, in his testimony before a congressional hearing in January on the past experiments.

Despite the known effects of radiation, experiments were deliberately intended to measure how radiation would affect tissue, bones, and organs. And even though some studies used radiation as experimental therapy, at least a few researchers knew that what they were doing would not benefit the subjects and might harm them.

Federal documents and newspaper reports describe researchers who went to ghoulish lengths to track radiation damage. In the 1970s, federal researchers who were following up on studies done in the 1940s that involved direct injections of plutonium asked permission from families of participants in the earlier studies to exhume their bodies so they could find out how much radioactive material was left.

STUDIES DESCRIBED

The current wave of interest in the issue of past experiments stems from investigative reporting by the *Albuquerque Tribune* and the *Boston Globe,* among other newspapers, which carried personal stories on those who allegedly suffered from the research. They include the following examples:

- From 1945 to 1947, researchers at the Universities of Rochester, California at San Francisco, and Chicago injected 18 men and women, said at the time to be terminally ill, with plutonium to determine where it would go in the body. The research was supported by the Manhattan Project and was aimed at assessing risk to workers exposed to plutonium. Recent investigations found that many of the patients and their families had not been told about the purpose of the studies, even during follow-up research in the early 1970s. Although the patients were originally categorized as terminally ill, many of them lived for years after the injections.

- In research supported by the Atomic Energy Commission (AEC), doses of radioactive radium and thorium were injected into or fed to 20 subjects aged 63 to 83 at the Massachusetts Institute of Technology (MIT) from 1961 to 1965. A congressional report states that the doses used were up to six times the maximum amount of internally deposited radioactive material that was determined later to be a safe dose.

- In another study sponsored by the AEC from 1963 to 1970, researchers from the University of Washington irradiated the testicles of 64 inmates at Washington State Prison to determine the smallest dose of radiation that would render someone sterile. The experiments were stopped after a university review board objected to them in 1969. All of the men were supposed to have had vasectomies after the radiation, but a few of them did not. Investigators from the Pacific Northwest Research Foundation conducted a similar study on 67 prisoners in Oregon State Prison.

- From 1946 to 1956, research teams from MIT and Harvard University fed radioactive iron and calcium to as many as 125 residents at a Massachusetts state school for the retarded to determine whether a diet rich in cereal would block the digestion of these two elements. The research was sponsored by the AEC and the Quaker Oats Company. Subsequent review of the work showed that although the doses were low, even by today's standards, at least some of the students and their parents were not told that exposure to radiation was part of the study.

- In the late 1960s, a study, sponsored by the Department of Defense and conducted by researchers at the Universities of Cincinnati and California at Irvine, exposed at least 16 cancer patients, 13 of whom were black with little education, to radiation to measure changes in the intellectual abilities of the patients. Finding any effects would have been very difficult in light of the fact that, according to the study's report, all of the patients had begun the study with relatively low intelligence quotients and strong evidence of "cerebral organic deficits."

POLITICAL VIEWS

Current efforts by federal officials and university administrators to right past wrongs committed by researchers is a distinct departure from previous political strategy. Energy Department documents obtained by the Associated Press showed that the Reagan Administration sought to play down the experiments, arguing against compensation or follow-up exams for the human subjects.

One other congressional investigation, held in 1986, which received little attention at the time, noted: "American citizens became nuclear calibration devices." That investigation, led by Rep. Edward J. Markey (D-MA), was blocked by the lack of cooperation from federal agencies, in particular the Department of Energy, the successor to the AEC. Today, Markey calls the experiments a "gruesome testament to the nuclear naivete and paranoia" of the Cold War's early years. He also noted that revelations that shock today's sensibilities were, just eight years ago, "a one-day story."

"There was a massive public relations partnership that existed between the [Reagan] administration, the defense contractors, and experimenters in America throughout the 1980s," Markey said. "It was an era that sanctified the nuclear arms race."

With the disclosure of the radiation experiments, a number of experts in human research are arguing that the studies need to be put into a historical context in which formal informed consent did not exist. Jay Katz, Ph.D., professor of law, medicine, and psychiatry, Yale University, and an authority on the ethics of experimentation with human subjects, says the requirements for informed consent were "very nebulous" in the 1940s and 50s. "There were a lot of studies going on with little regard for informed consent."

On the other hand, he points out that the Nuremberg Code was developed in 1947 in reaction to the gruesome experiments in Nazi concentration camps and was intended to end experimentation on humans without their full understanding and permission. The code was adopted by the AMA in the same year. "These old problems still haunt us," Katz said.

As to why there are headlines today, some think that it has a lot to do with radiation phobia—that is, in the minds of many people, all radiation is lumped together as bad or dangerous.

Another change in perspective over time is that the groups of people considered fair game for experimentation 40 years ago—the elderly, handicapped, disabled or mentally retarded (developmentally challenged), native Americans, women, children, prisoners—are now accorded special sensitivity.

In making her appeal for compensation during an interview with the *New York Times,* Energy Secretary O'Leary said she was persuaded to reverse the government's long-standing resistance to compensating thousands of people in the Southwest, known as "downwinders," who have asserted that they were harmed by radioactive fallout from open-air testing of atomic bombs in the 1950s and early '60s.

"I looked at the history of the Energy Department with the downwinders where the department for some years really did battle with these people to hold off their ability to make claims," O'Leary said, a posture that she does not want to take.

As to the radiation experiments, the secretary added, "It seems to me that my position ought to be: What does it take to make these people whole? If they can prove there was no consent for the experimentation and harm resulted from the experiments, they or members of their families are going to want more than a formal apology."

O'Leary's appeal for compensation puts her department in direct conflict with the Justice Department. In every case where Congress has considered legislation to compensate people exposed to harmful levels of radiation, including the Southwest's downwinders, the tort branch of the Justice Department's civil division has aggressively opposed this effort.

The department has also vigorously defended the government in lawsuits, dating from the early 1950s, in which ranchers, soldiers, uranium miners, and the industry's own workers asserted harm by radiation from the nuclear weapons industry.

Justice Department lawyers are currently defending the government in a Nevada case in which the families of more than 200 weapons industry workers, most of whom have died, contend that their relatives were injured or killed by radiation from atomic bomb testing at the Nevada Test Site northwest of Las Vegas.

In this case, which began December 13 in Las Vegas, several of the government's chief medical witnesses are physicians who conducted some of the previous radiation experiments now under O'Leary's scrutiny.

FUTURE FALLOUT

Some teaching hospitals and universities are starting searches of their records to help state and federal investigators and to notify those who were subjects of the research. Such searches will be difficult, not only because of the time that has passed, but also because individual scientists usually maintain their own research data, and many of them are now deceased.

Hospitals are required to keep medical data but could not make the names of those who have participated in past research public, since to do so would violate privacy laws. They might be able to make the records available to federal investigators.

As of the end of January, the Energy Department is still conducting more than 200 experiments involving humans, including many involving radiation, but O'Leary promises that strict ethical procedures and proper consent are being followed, generally under guidelines in effect since 1991.

At the January 21 hearing of the Senate Governmental Affairs Committee, chairman Sen. John Glenn (D-OH) asked O'Leary what assurances there were that "rogue operators" were not conducting experiments without proper patient consent.

She replied that, while conceding that she may have opened Pandora's box by pressing for a governmentwide records search on past radiation testing in humans, she expects President Clinton to direct all federal agencies to immediately halt any experiments where consent might be in question.

She later told reporters that the directive was being issued, in part, to respond to a request by Glenn and not because of any evidence that proper consent might not have been obtained. Within her department, she said, "we're pretty certain that everyone is following the spirit and intent" of rules on ethical conduct.

Federal and local investigations may expand beyond the radiation experiments and into the broader realm of research that has been conducted without informed consent. In Massachusetts, for example, area newspapers have begun to examine a broad variety of medical experiments that have been done without the permission of subjects at state prisons and a school for the retarded.

In the meantime, expect a slew of suits to be filed. For example, last month in Nashville, three women who said they were fed a solution containing radioactive iron as part of a nutrition study filed a lawsuit on behalf of more than 800 women who seek damages from Vanderbilt University, its medical center, and others for deaths, illnesses, and emotional suffering by women involved in a 1945–49 study of iron absorption in pregnant women to help establish nutritional guidelines for them. At the congressional hearing on January 25, one of the women said that the experiments caused the 1959 death of her daughter, who died from cancer at age 11.

The revelations about the radiation experiments may also shake the public's trust in the safety of current research. At the congressional hearing, Gerald Mousso, the nephew of a man injected with plutonium at the University of Rochester's teaching hospital in 1946, asked an oft-repeated question, "Can this happen today?" He said, "I think it's not likely, but I'm not sure."

Whether it does or not may depend on how well research proposals are critiqued at the institutional level. Since the late 1960s, universities and other institutions that receive federal funds have been required to have institutional review boards (IRBs) or research committees to ensure that the principle of informed consent is accounted for in research projects.

The manner by which informed consent is acquired is generally a quiet one—usually ironed out in private discussions between the IRBs, scientists, and subjects. Although some states require that IRB meetings be open to the public at state-supported hospitals and universities, few laymen ever attend.

Scientists' research plans are usually closely guarded in the university review process to prevent competitors from learning about the ideas involved. But notions of privacy may give way to more public review, following the adage that "sunlight is the best disinfectant."

"One of the most important lessons for me from these earlier studies," says LeRoy Walters, Ph.D., professor of Christian ethics, Georgetown University, "is how important it is that these things not be kept secret when they don't need to be kept secret."

Nonetheless, strong tensions exist between members of IRBs. Joan Rachlin, executive director of Public Responsibility in Medicine and Research (PRIM&R), Boston, says that committee members "walk a fine line between representing subjects and working for the institutions." IRBs are generally conscientious about their responsibilities. But, she adds, they are under enormous, but subtle, pressure not to slow down or stop research at a time when hospitals and universities are eager for every research dollar they can get.

Other critics of the IRB system note that university committees, in particular, are too heavily stacked with scientists who might eventually have their own research proposals reviewed, and are therefore more lenient toward others' proposals. It becomes, as one person at the congressional hearing observed, a case of "one hand washing the other."

Paula Knudson, executive coordinator for a 30-member committee for the protection of human subjects at the University of Texas Health Sciences Center, Houston, says that hospitals can run the risk of putting paper forms ahead of patients' interests. Her committee reviews more than 1,000 studies a year.

The world's best-designed informed consent form still means little, she says, "if a person in authority with a white coat and stethoscope walks into a room and tells a patient, 'I have a great study that is just right for you.'" The way in which a patient is told about a study, not the form itself, is the most important part of informed consent, Knudson says.

However, she doesn't believe that informed consent keeps the public safe from unnecessarily dangerous research. Rather, she says that a lot of responsibility rests on the shoulders of physicians and nurses, since review committees can't be in the room when potential subjects are told about research. "We can't be policemen," she notes. "We have to trust our investigators."

At the Harris County Psychiatric Center, a hospital affiliated with the University of Texas, Knudson is trying a new way to make sure patients get all their questions answered about research. An independent "research intermediary" talks to patients a day or so after they have signed informed consent forms to make sure they comprehend the research and their role in it. The intermediary also checks with patients during later stages of the research process to make sure they are still comfortable participating. Knudson says she hopes the concept of intermediaries will catch on elsewhere.

As complex treatments—from gene therapy to exotic methods of treating infertility—become more common, the pressure to ensure informed consent agreements will increase, Knudson says.

Many ethicists and physicians are using the controversy over the radiation experiments to revive a call for national guidance on the ethical predicaments that face local committees charged with protecting human subjects.

The Dangers of Difference
Patricia A. King

Patricia A. King is professor of law at Georgetown University Law Center. Her articles include "The Authority of Families to Make Medical Decisions for Incompetent Patients After the Cruzan Decision," "Helping Women Helping Children: Drug Policy and Future Generations," and "Searching for Consensus."

King cites the historically important case of the Tuskegee syphilis study—a federally funded study of the effects of untreated syphilis on black men, in which subjects were not informed of the availability of penicillin—in exploring an ethical dilemma concerning racial differences in scientific studies. In King's view, the dilemma arises as follows. If racial differences are ignored and all groups are treated equally, harm may result from a failure to recognize racially correlated factors. On the other hand, if differences are recognized and efforts are made to respond to past injustices or unique burdens, harmful stereotypes may be reinforced. As a strategy for managing this dilemma, King recommends beginning with the defeasible presumption that whites and blacks are biologically the same with respect to disease and treatment and looking for nonbiological factors before considering the possibility of biologically differentiated responses. As an example, she suggests that, "rather than trying to determine whether blacks and whites respond differently to AZT, attention should first be directed to learning whether the response to AZT is influenced by social, cultural, or environmental conditions."

It has been sixty years since the beginning of the Tuskegee syphilis experiment and twenty years since its existence was disclosed to the American public. The social and ethical issues that the experiment poses for medicine, particularly for medicine's relationship with African Americans, are still not broadly understood, appreciated, or even remembered.[1] Yet a significant aspect of the Tuskegee experiment's legacy is that in a racist society that incorporates beliefs about the inherent

Reprinted with permission of the author and the publisher from *Hastings Center Report*, vol. 22 (November–December 1992), pp. 35–38. © The Hastings Center.

inferiority of African Americans in contrast with the superior status of whites, any attention to the question of differences that may exist is likely to be pursued in a manner that burdens rather than benefits African Americans.

The Tuskegee experiment, which involved approximately 400 males with late-stage, untreated syphilis and approximately 200 controls free of the disease, is by any measure one of the dark pages in the history of American medicine. In this study of the natural course of untreated syphilis, the participants did not give informed consent. Stunningly, when penicillin was subsequently developed as a treatment for syphilis, measures were taken to keep the diseased participants from receiving it.

Obviously, the experiment provides a basis for the exploration of many ethical and social issues in medicine, including professional ethics,[2] the limitations of informed consent as a means of protecting research subjects, and the motives and methods used to justify the exploitation of persons who live in conditions of severe economic and social disadvantage. At bottom, however, the Tuskegee experiment is different from other incidents of abuse in clinical research because all the participants were black males. The racism that played a central role in this tragedy continues to infect even our current well-intentioned efforts to reverse the decline in health status of African Americans.[3]

Others have written on the scientific attitudes about race and heredity that flourished at the time that the Tuskegee experiment was conceived.[4] There has always been widespread interest in racial differences between blacks and whites, especially differences that related to sexual matters. These perceived differences have often reinforced and justified differential treatment of blacks and whites, and have done so to the detriment of blacks. Not surprisingly, such assumptions about racial differences provided critical justification for the Tuskegee experiment itself.

Before the experiment began a Norwegian investigator had already undertaken a study of untreated syphilis in whites between 1890 and 1910. Although there had also been a follow-up study of these untreated patients from 1925 to 1927, the original study was abandoned when arsenic therapy became available. In light of the availability of therapy a substantial justification for replicating a study of untreated syphilis was required. The argument that provided critical support for the experiment was that the natural course of untreated syphilis in blacks and whites was not the same.[5] Moreover, it was thought that the differences between blacks and whites were not merely biological but that they extended to psychological and social responses to the disease as well. Syphilis, a sexually transmitted disease, was perceived to be rampant among blacks in part because blacks—unlike whites—were not inclined to seek or continue treatment for syphilis.

THE DILEMMA OF DIFFERENCE

In the context of widespread belief in the racial inferiority of blacks that surrounded the Tuskegee experiment, it should not come as a surprise that the experiment exploited its subjects. Recognizing and taking account of racial differences that have historically been utilized to burden and exploit African Americans poses a dilemma.[6] Even in circumstances where the goal of a scientific study is to benefit a stigmatized group or person, such well-intentioned efforts may nevertheless cause harm. If the racial difference is ignored and all groups or persons are treated similarly, unintended harm may result from the failure to recognize racially correlated factors. Conversely, if differences among groups or persons are recognized and attempts are made to respond to past injustices or special burdens, the effort is likely to reinforce existing negative stereotypes that contributed to the emphasis on racial differences in the first place.

This dilemma about difference is particularly worrisome in medicine. Because medicine is pragmatic, it will recognize racial differences if doing so will promote health goals. As a consequence, potential harms that might result from attention to racial differences tend to be overlooked, minimized, or viewed as problems beyond the purview of medicine.

The question of whether (and how) to take account of racial differences has recently been raised in the context of the current AIDS epidemic. The participation of African Americans in clinical AIDS trials has been disproportionately small in comparison to the numbers of African Americans who have been infected with the Human Immunodeficiency Virus. Because of the possibility that African Americans may respond differently to drugs being developed and tested to combat AIDS,[7] those concerned about the care and treatment of AIDS in the African American community have called for greater participation by African Americans in these trials. Ironically, efforts to address the problem of underrepresentation must cope with the enduring legacy of the Tuskegee experiment—the legacy of suspicion and skepticism toward medicine and its practitioners among African Americans.[8]

In view of the suspicion Tuskegee so justifiably engenders, calls for increased participation by African Americans in clinical trials are worrisome. The question of whether to tolerate racially differentiated AIDS research testing of new or innovative therapies, as well as the question of what norms should govern participation by African Americans in clinical research, needs careful and thoughtful attention. A generic examination of the treatment of racial differences in medicine is beyond the scope of this article. However, I will describe briefly what has occurred since disclosure of the Tuskegee experiment to point out the dangers I find lurking in our current policies.

INCLUSION AND EXCLUSION

In part because of public outrage concerning the Tuskegee experiment,[9] comprehensive regulations governing federal research using human subjects were revised and subsequently adopted by most federal agencies.[10] An institutional review board (IRB) must approve clinical research involving human subjects, and IRB approval is made contingent on review of protocols for adequate protection of human subjects in accordance with federal criteria. These criteria require among other things that an IRB ensure that subject selection is "equitable." The regulations further provide that:

> [i]n making this assessment the IRB should take into account the purposes of the research and the setting in which the research will be conducted and should be particularly cognizant of the special problems of research involving vulnerable populations, such as women, mentally disabled persons, or economically or educationally disadvantaged persons.[11]

The language of the regulation makes clear that the concern prompting its adoption was the protection of vulnerable groups from exploitation. The obverse problem—that too much protection might promote the exclusion or underrepresentation of vulnerable groups, including African Americans—was not at issue. However, underinclusion can raise as much of a problem of equity as exploitation.[12]

A 1990 General Accounting Office study first documented the extent to which minorities and women were underrepresented in federally funded research. In response, in December 1990 the National Institutes of Health, together with the Alcohol, Drug Abuse and Mental Health Administration, directed that minorities and women be included in study populations,

> so that research findings can be of benefit to all persons at risk of the disease, disorder or condition under study; special emphasis should be placed on the need for inclusion of minorities and women in studies of diseases, disorders and conditions that disproportionately affect them.[13]

If minorities are not included, a clear and compelling rationale must be submitted.

The new policy clearly attempts to avoid the perils of overprotection, but it raises new concerns. The policy must be clarified and refined if it is to meet the intended goal of ensuring that research findings are of benefit to all. There are at least three reasons for favoring increased representation of African Americans in clinical trials. The first is that there may be biological differences between blacks and whites that might affect the applicability of experimental findings to blacks, but these differences will not be noticed if blacks are not included in sufficient numbers to allow the detection of statistically significant racial differences. The second reason is that race is a reliable index for social conditions such as poor health and nutrition, lack of adequate access to health care, and economic and social disadvantage that might adversely affect potential benefits of new interventions and procedures. If there is indeed a correlation between minority status and these factors, then African Americans and all others with these characteristics will benefit from new information generated by the research. The third reason is that the burdens and benefits of research should be spread across the population regardless of racial or ethnic status.[14] Each of these reasons for urging that representation of minorities be increased has merit. Each of these justifications also raises concern, however, about whether potential benefits will indeed be achieved.

The third justification carries with it the obvious danger that the special needs or problems generated as a result of economic or social conditions associated with minority status may be overlooked and that, as a result, African Americans and other minorities will be further disadvantaged. The other two justifications are problematic and deserve closer examination. They each assume that there are either biological, social, economic, or cultural differences between blacks and whites.

THE WAY OUT OF THE DILEMMA

Understanding how, or indeed whether, race correlates with disease is a very complicated problem. Race itself is a confusing concept with both biological and social connotations. Some doubt whether race has biological significance at all.[15] Even if race is a biological fiction, however, its social significance remains.[16] As Bob Blauner points out, "Race is an essentially political construct, one that translates our tendency to see people in terms of their color or other physical attributes into structures that make it likely that people will act for or against them on such a basis."[17]

In the wake of Tuskegee and, in more recent times, the stigma and discrimination that resulted from screening for sickle cell trait (a genetic condition that occurs with greater frequency among African Americans), researchers have been reluctant to explore associations between race and disease. There is increasing recognition, however, of evidence of heightened resistance or vulnerability to disease along racial lines.[18] Indeed, sickle cell anemia itself substantiates the view that biological differences may exist. Nonetheless, separating myth from reality in determining the cause of disease and poor health status is not easy. Great caution should be exercised in attempting to validate biological differences in susceptibility to disease in light of this society's past experience with biological differences. Moreover, using race as an index for other conditions that might influence health and well-being is also dangerous. Such practices could emphasize social and economic differences that might also lead to stigma and discrimination.

If all the reasons for increasing minority participation in clinical research are flawed, how then can we promote improvement in the health status of African Americans and other minorities through participation in clinical research while simultaneously minimizing the harms that might flow from such participation? Is it possible to work our way out of this dilemma?

An appropriate strategy should have as its starting point the defeasible presumption that blacks and whites are biologically the same with respect to disease and treatment. Presumptions can be overturned of course, and the strategy should recognize the possibility that biological differences in some contexts are possible. But the presumption of equality acknowledges that historically the greatest harm has come from the willingness to impute biological differences rather than the willingness to overlook them. For some, allowing the presumption to be in any way defeasible is troubling. Yet I do not believe that fear should lead us to ignore the possibility of biologically differentiated responses to disease and treatment, especially when the goal is to achieve medical benefit.

It is well to note at this point the caution sounded by Hans Jonas. He wrote, "Of the new experimentation with man, medical is surely the most legitimate; psychological, the most dubious; biological (still to come), the most dangerous."[19] Clearly, priority should be given to exploring the possible social, cultural, and environmental determinants of disease before targeting the study of hypotheses that involve biological differences between blacks and whites. For example, rather than trying to determine whether blacks and whites respond differently to AZT, attention should first be directed to learning whether response to AZT is influenced by social, cultural, or environmental conditions. Only at the point where possible biological differences emerge should hypotheses that explore racial differences be considered.

A finding that blacks and whites are different in some critical aspect need not inevitably lead to increased discrimination or stigma for blacks. If there indeed had been a difference in the effects of untreated syphilis between blacks and whites such information might have been used to promote the health status of blacks. But the Tuskegee experiment stands as a reminder that such favorable outcomes rarely if ever occur. More often, either racist assumptions and stereotypes creep into the study's design, or findings broken down by race become convenient tools to support policies and behavior that further disadvantage those already vulnerable.

REFERENCES

1 For earlier examples of the use of African Americans as experimental subjects see Todd L. Savitt, "The Use of Blacks for Medical Experimentation and Demonstration in the Old South," *Journal of Southern History* 48, no. 3 (1982): 331–48.

2 David J. Rothman, "Were Tuskegee & Willowbrook 'Studies in Nature'?" *Hastings Center Report* 12, no. 2 (1982): 5–7.

3 For an in-depth examination of the health status of African Americans see Woodrow Jones, Jr., and Mitchell F. Rice, eds. *Health Care Issues in Black America: Policies, Problems, and Prospects* (New York: Greenwood Press, 1987).

4 See for example Allan M. Brandt, "Racism and Research: The Case of the Tuskegee Syphilis Study," *Hastings Center Report* 8, no. 6 (1978): 21–29; and James H. Jones, *Bad Blood: The Tuskegee Syphilis Experiment* (New York: Free Press, 1981).

5 Jones, *Bad Blood*, p. 106.

6 Martha Minow, *Making All the Difference: Inclusion, Exclusion, and American Law* (Ithaca, N.Y.: Cornell University Press, 1990).

7 Wafaa El-Sadr and Linnea Capps, "The Challenge of Minority Recruitment in Clinical Trials for AIDS," *JAMA* 267, no. 7 (1992): 954–57.

8 See for example Stephen B. Thomas and Sandra Crouse Quinn, "Public Health Then and Now," *American Journal of Public Health* 81, no. 11 (1991): 1498–1505; Henry C. Chinn, Jr., "Remember Tuskegee," *New York Times*, 29 May 1992.

9 Tuskegee Syphilis Study Ad Hoc Advisory Panel, *Final Report of the Tuskegee Syphilis Study Ad Hoc Advisory Panel* (Washington, D.C.: U.S. Depart-

ment of Health, Education and Welfare, Public Health Service, 1973).

10 Federal Policy for the Protection of Human Subjects; Notices and Rules, *Federal Register* 56, no. 117 (1991): 28002.

11 45 *Code of Federal Regulations* §46.111(a)(3).

12 This problem is discussed in the context of research in prisons in Stephen E. Toulmin, "The National Commission on Human Experimentation: Procedures and Outcomes," in *Scientific Controversies: Case Studies in the Resolution and Closure of Disputes in Science and Technology,* ed. H. Tristram Engelhardt, Jr. and Arthur L. Caplan (New York: Cambridge University Press, 1987), pp. 602–6.

13 National Institutes of Health and Alcohol, Drug Abuse and Mental Health Administration, "Special Instructions to Applicants Using Form PHS 398 Regarding Implementation of the NIH/ADAMHA Policy concerning Inclusion of Women and Minorities in Clinical Research Study Populations," December 1990.

14 Arthur L. Caplan, "Is There a Duty to Serve as a Subject in Biomedical Research?" *IRB: A Review of Human Subjects Research* 6, no. 5 (1984): 1–5.

15 See J. W. Green, *Cultural Awareness in the Human Services* (Englewood Cliffs, N.J.: Prentice-Hall, 1982), p. 59; Bob Blauner, "Talking Past Each Other: Black and White Languages of Race," *American Prospect* 61, no. 10 (1992): 55–64.

16 Patricia A. King, "The Past as Prologue: Race, Class, and Gene Discrimination," in *Using Ethics and Law as Guides,* ed. George J. Annas and Sherman Elias (New York: Oxford University Press, 1992), pp. 94–111.

17 Blauner, "Talking Past Each Other," p. 16.

18 See for example James E. Bowman and Robert F. Murray, Jr., *Genetic Variation and Disorders in People of African Origin* (Baltimore, Md.: Johns Hopkins University Press, 1981); Warren W. Leary, "Uneasy Doctors Add Race-Consciousness to Diagnostic Tools," *New York Times,* 15 September 1990.

19 Hans Jonas, "Philosophical Reflections on Experimenting with Human Subjects," in *Experimentation with Human Subjects,* ed. Paul A. Freund (New York: George Braziller, 1970), p. 1. Recent controversy in genetic research makes Jonas's warning particularly timely. See Daniel Goleman, "New Storm Brews on Whether Crime Has Roots in Genes," *New York Times,* 15 September 1992.

Proxy Consent for Children and the Incompetent Elderly

Consent as a Canon of Loyalty with Special Reference to Children in Medical Investigations
Paul Ramsey

Paul Ramsey (1924–1988) was Harrington Spear Paine Professor of Religion at Princeton University. His books include *The Patient as Person: Explorations in Medical Ethics* (1970), *Fabricated Man: The Ethics of Genetic Control* (1970), *Ethics at the Edges of Life* (1978), and *Deeds and Rules in Christian Ethics* (1980). He was also the editor of *Jonathan Edwards: Ethical Writings* (1989).

According to Ramsey, the principle of informed consent is the "cardinal canon of loyalty," which joins people together in medical practice and investigation. In his view, experimentation on a human subject that is not for that subject's benefit can never be justified if it is performed without the subject's free and informed consent. Since young children are incapable of giving such consent, research involving children should never be allowed unless participation in such research benefits the child. The use of an experimental procedure on chil-

Reprinted with permission of the publisher from Paul Ramsey, *The Patient as a Person* (New Haven, Conn.: Yale University Press, 1970).

dren is morally justified only if the procedure is either (1) seen as the best means to effect the child's own recovery from an illness or disease or (2) intended to protect the child against some greater risk.

From consent as a canon of loyalty in medical practice it follows that children, who cannot give a mature and informed consent, or adult incompetents, should not be made the subjects of medical experimentation unless, other remedies having failed to relieve their grave illness, it is reasonable to believe that the administration of a drug as yet untested or insufficiently tested on human beings, or the performance of an untried operation, may further *the patient's own recovery.*

Now that is not a very elaborate moral rule governing medical practice in the matter of experiments involving children or incompetents as human subjects. It is a good example of the general claims of childhood specified for application in medical care and research. It is also a qualification immediately entailed by the meaning of consent in medical investigations as a joint undertaking between men. Again, one has to be prudent (which does not mean overcautious or scrupulous) in order to know how to care for child-patients in this way. One must know the possible relation of a proposed procedure to the child's own recovery, and also its likely effectiveness compared with other methods that have been or could be tried. These considerations may provide the doctor with necessary and sufficient reason for investigations upon children, perhaps even very hazardous ones. One has to proportion the peril to the diagnostic or therapeutic needs of the child.

Practical medical judgment has undeniable and ominous room for its determinations, since a "benefit" is whatever is *believed* to be of help to the child. Still the limits this rule imposes on practice are essentially clear; where there is no possible relation to the child's recovery, a child is not to be made a mere object in medical experimentation for the sake of good to come. The likelihood of benefits that could flow from the experiment for many other children is an equally insufficient warrant for child experimentation. The individual child is to be tended in illness or in dying, since he himself is not able to donate his illness or his dying to be studied and worked upon solely for the advancement of medicine. Again, future experience may tell us more about the meaning of this particular rule expressive of loyalty to a human child, and we may learn a great deal more about how to apply it in new situations with greater sensitivity and refinement—or we may learn more and

more how to practice violations of it. But we are committed to refraining from morally significant exceptions to this rule defining impermissible medical experimentation upon children.

To experiment on children in ways that are not related to them as patients is already a sanitized form of barbarism; it already removes them from view and pays no attention to the faithfulness-claims which a child, simply by being a normal or a sick or dying child, places upon us and upon medical care. We should expect no morally significant exceptions to this canon of faithfulness to the child. To expect future justifiable exceptions is, in some sense, already to have forgotten the child. . . .

To attempt to consent for a child to be made an experimental subject is to treat a child as not a child. It is to treat him as if he were an adult person who has consented to become a joint adventurer in the common cause of medical research. If the grounds for this are alleged to be the presumptive or implied consent of the child, that must simply be characterized as a violent and a false presumption. Nontherapeutic, nondiagnostic experimentation involving human subjects must be based on true consent if it is to proceed as a human enterprise. No child or adult incompetent can choose to become a participating member of medical undertakings, and no one else on earth should decide to subject these people to investigations having no relation to their own treatment. That is a canon of loyalty to them. This they claim of us simply by being a human child or incompetent. When he is grown, the child may put away childish things and become a true volunteer. This is the meaning of being a volunteer: that a man enter and establish a consensual relation in some joint venture for medical progress—where before he could not, nor could anyone else, "volunteer" him for submission to unknown possible hazards for the sake of good to come.

If the requirement of parents, investigators, and state authorities in regard to their wards is "Never subject children to the unknown possible hazards of medical investigations having no relation to their own treatment," we must understand that the maladies for which the individual needs treatment and protection need not already be resident within the compass of the child's own skin. He can properly be regarded as one of a population, and we can add to the foregoing words: "except in epidemic conditions." Dr. Salk tried his polio vaccine on himself and his own children first. Then it was tested on selected children within a normal population. This involved some risk for the children vaccinated, and for other children as well, that the disease *might* be contracted from the vaccine itself, or that there might be unexpected injurious results. But the normal population of children was already subjected to waves of crippling epidemic summer after summer. A parent consenting for his child to be used in this trial was balancing the risks from the trial against the hazards from polio itself for that same child.

Physician-investigators are often in a quandary in which they are torn between the warrants for giving an experimental drug, and the warrants for withholding it from anyone in order to test it. Neither act seems justified, or both acts are equally warranted, when there is no available remedy and the indications are that a new drug may succeed. This situation also justifies a parent or guardian in consenting for a child, since we are supposing the hazard of the proposed treatment to be less or no greater than the hazard of the disease itself when treated by the established procedures. That would be a medical trial having clear relation to the treatment or protection of the child himself. He is not made, without his consent, the subject of medical investigations of possible benefit only to other children, other patients, or for the future advancement of medical science.

These may have been the circumstances surrounding the field trial of the vaccine for rubella (German measles) made in Taiwan, if this was in epidemic conditions, or in expectation of epidemic conditions, early in 1968 by a medical team from the University of Washington, headed by Dr. Thomas Grayston.[1] The vaccine was given to 3,269 young grade-school boys in the cities of Taipei and Taichung, while roughly an equal number were left unvaccinated for comparison purposes. The latter group were given Salk polio vaccine so that they would derive some benefit from the experience to which they were subjected. This generous "payment" does not alter the moral dilemma of withholding the rubella vaccine from a selected group. Yet there may have been an equipoise between the hazards of contracting rubella or other damage from the vaccine and the hazards of contracting it if not vaccinated. There could have been a likelihood favoring the vaccinated of the two comparison groups.

These considerations, we may suppose, produced the quandary in the conscience of the investigators that was partially relieved by giving the unrelated Salk vaccine to the control group. Such equipoise alone would

warrant—and it would sufficiently warrant—a parent or guardian in consenting that his child or ward be used for these research purposes. In the face of actual or predictable epidemic conditions, this would be medical investigation having some measurable or immeasurable relation to a child's own treatment or protection, as surely as the catheterization of the heart of a child with congenital heart trouble may be needed in his own diagnosis and treatment; and to this type of treatment a parent may venture to consent in his child's behalf. If no gulf is to be fixed between maladies beneath the skin and diseases afflicting children as members of a population, then the consent-requirement means: "Never submit children to medical investigation not related to their own treatment, except in face of epidemic conditions, endangering also each individual child." This is simply the meaning of the consent-requirement in application, not a "quantity-of-benefit-to-come" exception clause or a violation of this canon of loyalty to child-patients.

Indeed, a stricter construction of the necessary connection between proxy consent and the foreseeable needs of the child would permit the use of only girl children in field trials of rubella vaccine. Rubella is not the most contagious type of measles. The benefit to the subjects used in these trials (which plus the consent of parents legitimated subjecting them to experiment) was mainly to prevent their giving birth to children with congenital malformations should they later contract rubella during pregnancy. Therefore, there was stronger argument for considering only girl children as part of a population in establishing the necessary connection between experiment and "treatment."

More questionable were the earlier trials of the rubella vaccine performed upon the inmates of a retarded children's home in Conway, Arkansas. These subjects were not specially endangered by an epidemic of rubella. Few of the girls among them will ever be able to become part of the population of child-bearing women, or be in danger of pregnancy while in institutions. Using them simply had the advantage that they were segregated from the rest of the population, and any degree of risk to them would not spread to other people, including women of child-bearing age.

If children are incapable of truly consenting to experiments having unknown hazards for the sake of good to come, and if no one else should consent for them in cases unrelated to their own treatment, then medical research and society in general must choose a perhaps more difficult course of action to gain the benefits we seek from medical investigations. Surely it was possible to secure normal adult volunteers to consent to segregate themselves from the rest of the population for the duration of a rubella trial.[2] That method was simply more costly and inconvenient. At the same time, this illustrates the general fact that if we as a society are to proceed to the conquest of diseases, indeed, if we are to teach medical skills with fairness and justice to the poor and the ward patients, and with no violation of the basic claims of childhood, then there must be far greater encouragement generally in our society of a willingness to engage as joint adventurers for medical progress than has been achieved, or believed morally required by the principle of consent, in the past. . . .

NOTES

1 *New York Times,* October 17, 1968.
2 *New York Times,* April 5, 1969, reported that a hundred monks and nuns, from both Anglican and Roman Catholic orders, living in enclosed communities, were the voluntary subjects in testing American, British, and Belgian vaccines against German measles. This project was organized and directed by Dr. J. A. Dudgeon of London's Great Ormond Street Hospital for Sick Children.

Proxy Consent for Research on the Incompetent Elderly
Barry F. Brown

Barry F. Brown is associate professor of philosophy at St. Michael's College, University of Toronto. His areas of specialization are metaphysics and ethics, including biomedical ethics. Brown is the author of *Accidental Being: A Study in the Metaphysics of St. Thomas Aquinas* (1985) and of "Canadian, U.S. Systems Face Off."

Brown argues (1) that some research using borderline or definitely incompetent elderly patients is justified and (2) that relatives can legitimately give proxy consent for patients' use as research subjects even though the patients cannot directly benefit from their participation. The moral legitimacy of proxy consent to participation in research that benefits the participant is taken for granted in Brown's argument. However, he widens the scope of relevant benefits so that it includes certain indirect benefits. Brown's argument is based on a conception of the relationship between the individual good and the societal or common good. He argues that research ethics require a conception of the *common good* that (1) is narrower than that of society as a whole yet transcends immediate benefit to an individual and (2) includes the individual's good rather than being in opposition to it. In Brown's analysis, if the "community" with which the research subject is identified consists of those who have a stake in the amelioration or prevention of the disease from which the individual suffers, then the subject who participates in research intended to benefit members of that community is indirectly benefited as a member of that group, since the good of the class is "his" good. Brown ends on a cautionary note, indicating the need for stringent protective procedures.

In the past decade, the ethical issues of research with the elderly have become of increasing interest in gerontology, medicine, law, and biomedical ethics. In particular, the issue has been raised whether the elderly deserve special protection as a dependent group (Ratzan 1980). One of the most profound difficulties in this area of reflection is that of the justification of proxy consent for research on borderline or definitely incompetent patients.

Some diseases of the elderly, such as Alzheimer's disease, cause senile dementia: devastating for the

From *Ethics and Aging: The Right to Live and the Right to Die,* edited by James E. Thornton and Earl R. Winkler, pp. 183–193. Copyright © 1988 by The University of British Columbia Press. Reprinted by permission of the publisher.

patient and family and, in future, a considerable burden for society. This condition, in turn, renders a patient incapable of giving informed, voluntary consent to research procedures designed to learn about the natural history of the disease, to control it, and to find a cure. The research must be done on human subjects, since there is not as yet a suitable animal model; indeed some feel that there never can be such a model. A protection of the patient, rooted in concern for his best interests, from procedures to which he cannot give consent gives rise to a paradox: "If we can only perform senile dementia research using demented patients, but should not allow them to participate because they are incompetent, then we are left in a quandary. We cannot ethically conduct senile dementia research using demented patients because they are incompetent; but we cannot technically perform it using competent subjects because they are not demented" (Ratzan 1980: 36). Such a position seems to protect demented patients at the expense of their exposure, as a class, to prolonged misery or death.

If the patient cannot give consent, is the proxy consent of relatives ethically valid? That is, do the relatives have the moral right or capacity to give consent for procedures that may not offer much hope for the patient in that they may not offer a direct benefit to him?

Such procedures have by recent convention been called non-therapeutic. They might offer a possible benefit for other sufferers in the future, but little hope of benefit for *this* patient, here and now.

At present, an impasse has developed regarding such research. It appears that such procedures might be illegal under criminal laws on assault. If the research is strictly non-therapeutic, then no benefit is to be found for the patient-subject. If the requirement of therapeutic experimentation is that a direct, or fairly immediate, improvement in the patient's condition is the sole benefit that could count, then it is difficult to see how this could be discovered. For unlike the case of a curable disease or research on preventive measures for childhood diseases, such as polio, the Alzheimer's patients suffer from a presently terminal illness. Studies of the causation of this condition may hold little or no hope of alleviating the condition in them. There appears to be no present or future benefit directly accruing to them. Others may benefit, but they likely will not. Thus, it seems, there is no benefit in view.

If, in fact, such procedures, even relatively innocuous ones, are illegal, then such research cannot go ahead. If so, such persons will remain "therapeutic orphans" just as surely as infants and children unless proxy consent is valid. If proxy consent is also legally

invalid, then the legal challenge to this impasse may be either legislative or judicial. In either case, ethical arguments must be offered as justification for the case that proxy consent is or ought to be legally valid. The following explorations are a contribution to that debate.

Can some kind of benefit for the demented be found in research that offers no immediate hope of improvement? I believe that it can, but the nature of that benefit will be unfamiliar or unacceptable to those who are sure that there are only two mutually exclusive alternatives: a utilitarian conception of the social good pitted against a deontological notion of the individual's rights.

Contemporary biomedical ethics routinely employs three principles in its effort to resolve such dilemmas (Reich 1978; Beauchamp & Childress 1983). These are the principle of beneficence, which demands that we do good and prevent harm; the principle of respect for persons (or the principle of autonomy), from which flows the requirement of informed consent; and the principle of justice, which demands the equitable distribution of the benefits and burdens of research. But the first two obviously conflict with each other in human experimentation: the principle of beneficence, which mandates research to save life and restore health, especially if this is seen as directed to the good of society, is in tension with the principle of respect for persons, which requires us to protect the autonomy of subjects. Moreover, the principle of beneficence requires us not only to benefit persons as patients through research, but also to avoid harming them as research subjects in the process. So there is an internal tension between moral demands created by the same principle. Finally, demented patients are no longer fully or sufficiently autonomous. Standard objections to paternalism do not apply. Consequently paternalism of the parental sort is not inappropriate, but rather necessary in order to protect the interest of the patient.

Simple application of these principles, therefore, will not provide a solution. Underlying the manner in which they are applied are radically different conceptions of the relationship of the individual good to the societal or common good.

In the present framework of philosophical opinion, there appear to be two major positions. On the one hand, some consequentialist arguments for non-therapeutic research justify non-consensual research procedures on the grounds that individual needs are subordinate to the general good conceived as an aggregate of individual goods. This good, that of the society as a whole, can easily be seen to take precedence over that of individuals. This is especially so if the disease being researched is conceptualized as an "enemy" of society. On the other hand, a deontological position argues that the rights of the individual take precedence over any such abstract general good as the advancement of science, the progress of medicine, or the societal good. In this view, to submit an individual incapable of giving or withholding consent to research procedures not for his own direct benefit is to treat him solely as a means, not as an end in himself. In this debate, one side characterizes the general good proposed by the other as much too broad and inimical to human liberty; the other sees the emphasis on individual rights as excessively individualistic or atomistic.

There are strengths and weaknesses in both approaches. The consequentialist rightly insists on a communal good, but justifies too much; the deontologist rightly protects individual interests, but justifies too little. I contend that if we are to resolve the dilemma concerning the incompetent "therapeutic orphan," it is necessary to go between these poles. In order to do so, I wish to draw upon and develop some recent explorations concerning non-therapeutic research with young children. In at least one important respect, that of incompetence, children and the demented are similar. We ought to treat similar cases similarly. I wish also to argue that research ethics requires: (1) a conception of the *common good* that is at once narrower than that of society as a whole and yet transcends immediate benefit to a single individual; and (2) a conception of the common good that sees it not in opposition to the individual good but including it, so that the good is seen as distributed to individuals.

THE LESSON OF RESEARCH WITH CHILDREN

As to the first, we may learn much from the discussions concerning research with children, particularly as they bear upon the distinction between therapeutic and non-therapeutic experimentation. In the 1970s a spirited debate took place between the noted ethicists Paul Ramsey and Richard McCormick on the morality of experimentation with children (Ramsey 1970, 1976, 1977; McCormick 1974, 1976). Ramsey presented a powerful deontological argument against non-therapeutic experimentation with children. Since infants and young children cannot give consent, an essential requirement of the canon of loyalty between researcher and subject, they cannot be subjected ethically to pro-

cedures not intended for their own benefit. To do so, he contended, is to treat children solely as means to an end (medical progress), not as ends in themselves (Ramsey 1970).

McCormick, arguing from a natural law position similar to that developed in the next section, argued that since life and health are fundamental natural goods, even children have an obligation to seek to preserve them. Medical research is a necessary condition of ensuring health, and this is a desirable social goal. Consequently children, as members of society, have a duty in social justice to wish to accept their share of the burdens of participating in research that promises benefit to society and is of minimal or no risk. Thus the parents' proxy consent is a reasonable presumption of the child's wishes if he were able to consent (McCormick 1974).

There are two major puzzles generated by this debate over non-therapeutic research in children. First, Ramsey stressed that the condition to which a child may be at risk need not reside within his skin, but could be an epidemic dread disease. Thus, testing of preventive measures such as polio vaccine on children is justified; indeed it counts for Ramsey as therapeutic. This is interesting for several reasons. First, the therapeutic benefit may be indirect or remote, not necessarily immediate. Second, it embodies the concept of a group or population at risk smaller than society as a whole. Third, it apparently allows for considerable risk. There was a risk of contracting polio from the vaccine. Although the risk might have been slight statistically, the potential damage was grave. By Ramsey's own account, a slight risk of grave damage is a grave risk. Thus, he was prepared to go beyond the limit of minimal or no risk on the grounds that the polio vaccine was *therapeutic,* while McCormick attempted to justify *non-therapeutic* research on children, but confined the risk to minimal or none. It is odd that in the subsequent protracted debate, this difference was not contested.

The second major puzzle arises from McCormick's view that fetuses, infants, and children ought to participate in low- or no-risk non-therapeutic research in order to share in the burden of social and medical progress in order that all may prosper. Note that only *burdens* are to be shared, not benefits. This is because the topic by definition was non-therapeutic experimentation. By putting it this way he seemed to many to be subordinating the interests of such subjects to a very broadly construed societal good. But let us remember that the argument for such research in the first place was that without it, infants and children would be "therapeutic orphans."

That is, without pediatric research, there could be fewer and slower advances in pediatric therapy.

Although not of direct benefit, such research is intended for the long-term benefit of children, and is thus indirectly or remotely therapeutic. It is not conducted for "the benefit of society" or for "the advancement of medical science"; it is for children in the future. Otherwise, it could be carried out on adults. Thus, such research should be construed as done not in view of broad social benefit but for the benefit of children as a group or a sub-set of society. Of course, if advances are made in medicine for the sake of children, society benefits as well, but this is incidental and unnecessary. The sole justification is provided by the benefits now and to come for *children*. At the same time, such benefits set one of the limits for such research: it should be confined to children's conditions, and should not be directed at conditions for which the research may be done on competent persons.

THE COMMON GOOD OF A DISEASE COMMUNITY

Some of the hints arising from the foregoing debate can now be developed. It is indeed wrong to experiment on an incompetent person for "the benefit of society" if the research is unrelated to that person's disease and he is made a subject simply because he is accessible and unresistant. But is it necessarily unethical to conduct experiments on an incompetent person which attempt to discover the cause of the condition which causes the incompetence, and which may cure it or prevent it in others, even if he will not himself be cured?

In a "third way" of conceptualizing the relation between the individual and the group, the good in view is neither that of society as a whole nor that of a single individual. It involves the group of persons with a condition, such as Alzheimer's disease. Here I turn to a conception of the common good articulated by John Finnis of Oxford. Finnis defines the common good not as the "greatest good for the greatest number" but as "a set of conditions which enables the members of a community to attain for themselves reasonable objectives, or to realize reasonably for themselves the value(s) for the sake of which they have reason to collaborate with each other (positively and/or negatively) in a community" (Finnis 1980: 155).

The community may be either the complete community or the political one, or it may be specialized, such as the medical community, the research community, or the community of children with leukemia, and so on. The common good is thus not the sum total of individual interests, but an ensemble of conditions which enable individuals to pursue their objectives or purposes, which enable them to flourish. The purposes are fundamental human goods: life, health, play, esthetic experience, knowledge, and others. Relevant to this discussion are life, health, especially mental integrity, and the consequent capacity for knowledge, all of which are threatened by diseases which cause dementia.

For my purposes, the community should be considered to be, at a minimum, those suffering from Alzheimer's disease. They have, even if they have never explicitly associated with each other, common values and disvalues: their lost health and the remaining health and vitality they possess. It could be said with McCormick that if they could do so, they would reasonably wish the good of preventing the condition in their relatives and friends.

But the community may be rightly construed more broadly than this. It naturally includes families with whom the patients most closely interact and which interact in voluntary agencies devoted to the condition, the physicians who treat them, the nurses, social workers, and occupational therapists who care for them, and the clinical and basic researchers who are working to understand, arrest, cure, and prevent the disease.

The participation of the patient, especially the demented patient, may be somewhat passive. He is a member of the specialized community by accident, not by choice, unless he has indicated his wish to become a research subject while still competent. Efforts to determine what a demented or retarded person would have wished for himself had he been competent have been made in American court decisions involving an incompetent patient's medical care. These "substituted judgment" approaches may have some worth, especially if the patient had expressed and recorded his wishes while still competent.

An individual might execute a document analogous to a human tissue gift—a sort of pre-dementia gift, in which he would officially and legally offer his person to medical research if and when he became demented. This might alleviate the problem of access to some extent, but it has its own difficulties. A pre-dementia volunteer cannot know in advance what types of research procedures will be developed in future, and so cannot give a truly informed consent except to either very specific procedures now known or to virtually anything. Such a pre-commitment may give some support to the decision to allow him to be a subject. But that decision, I contend, is justified by the claim, if valid, that it is for the common good of the dementia-care-research community, of which he is a member and to which, it is presumed, he would commit himself if he were capable of doing so at the time.

It is true, of course, that one might not ever have wished to participate in research procedures. In this case, the individual should be advised to register his or her objection in advance, along the lines that have been suggested for objection to organ donation in those countries that have a system of presumed consent for such donation. This can be achieved by carrying a card on which such an opt-out is recorded, or by placing one's name on a registry which might be maintained by support organizations. I suggest that unless one opt out in this manner, in the early stages of the disease, he or she be considered to have opted-in. That is, there should be a policy of presumed consent. In any event, as experience with organ retrieval has shown, in the final analysis it is the permission of relatives that is decisive in both those cases in which an individual has consented and those in which he or she has not made his or her wishes known.

The other members of the community may not all know each other. They do, however, have common values and, to a considerable degree, common objectives. There can be a high level of deliberate and active interaction, especially if there is close communication between the researchers, family, and volunteers in the voluntary health agencies.

What, then, is the ensemble of conditions which constitute the common good of the Alzheimer's community? Insofar as the purposes of collaboration include the effort to cure or to alleviate the disease, the common good would embrace, in addition to caring health professionals, a policy of promoting research, its ethical review, a sufficient number of committed clinical and scientific researchers, the requisite physical facilities and funding (some or all of which may be within other communities such as hospitals and medical schools), availability of volunteers for research, an atmosphere of mutual trust between researcher and subject, and finally ongoing research itself. This list is not exhaustive.

If access to the already demented is not allowed, and if this is essential for research on the disease to continue, it may well be impossible to find the answers to key questions about the disease. The common good of the Alzheimer's community would be damaged or insufficiently promoted. Since the goods of life and mental health are fundamental goods, this insufficiency would be profound.

One essential aspect of this common good is distributive justice. Each patient-subject shares not only in the burdens of research in order that all may prosper, but also the benefits. The benefits are not necessarily improved care or cure for the subject, but generally improved conditions for all such patient-subjects: a more aggressive approach to research, improved knowledge of the disease, increased probabilities for a cure, and others. Since the individual participates wholly in that good, he will be deprived of it in its entirety if it is not pursued. The common good is not so much a quantity of benefits as a quality of existence. It can therefore be distributed in its fullness to each member of the community. So, too, each can suffer its diminution.

Richard McCormick (1974) left his description of the common good unnecessarily broad and sweeping. According to some natural law theorists (Maritain 1947) the common good is always a distributed good, not simply the sum of parts. It is construed as flowing back upon the individual members of the community, who are not simply parts of a whole but persons, to whom the common good is distributed in its entirety. Thus, not only can the common good of which McCormick speaks be narrowed to that of children as a group (equivalent to Ramsey's population at risk) but the benefits of such research can be seen as redistributed to the individuals of the group. The benefits are not to be taken in the sense of an immediately available therapy, but in the sense of improved general conditions under which a cure, amelioration, or prevention for all is more likely.

CONCLUSION

Some of these observations can now be applied to the case of the elderly demented. First, the debate showed the inadequacy of the simple distinction between therapeutic and non-therapeutic experimentation, which has been challenged on several grounds in past years. For example, May (1976: 83) includes diagnostic and preventive types of research under therapeutic experimentation, whereas Reich (1978: 327) observes that the terms "therapeutic" and "non-therapeutic" are inadequate because they do not seem to include research on diagnostic and preventive techniques. In the area of the development of experimental preventive measures such as vaccines for epidemic diseases, and in the area of diseases in which research is carried out on terminal patients with little or no expectation of immediate benefit for these patients, the distinction is somewhat blurred. In each case, there is a defined population at risk: one without the disease but at great risk of contracting it, the other with a disease but with little hope of benefiting from the research.

Such types of research seem to constitute an intermediate category: the "indirectly therapeutic," involving the hope of either prevention or alleviation or cure. This category as applied to dementia shows some characteristics of therapeutic experimentation in the accepted sense, since it is carried out on persons who are ill and it is directed to their own illness. But it also shares some properties of non-therapeutic research, since it is not for their immediate treatment and, therefore, benefit. The good to be achieved is more remote, both in time and in application, since it is less sharply located in the individual than is therapy as such.

It must be admitted that there is a difference between the testing of a vaccine for prevention of disease in young, healthy children and research on elderly, seriously ill patients. In the former, the child-subjects will benefit if the vaccine is successful, or at least be protected from harm. In the latter, the subjects will not benefit by way of prevention or cure of their disease, but rather simply by being part of a community in which those goals are being actively pursued. The identification of the demented patient's good with that common good is doubtless less concrete than the identification of the child's good with that of his peers. But it seems to me that underlying both these cases is a notion of the common good required to justify all cases of research that do not promise a hope of direct benefit to a person who is, here and now, ill.

Years ago, Hans Jonas (1969) noted that a physician-researcher might put the following question to a dying patient: "There is nothing more I can do for you. But there is something you can do for me. Speaking no longer as your physician but on behalf of medical science, we could learn a great deal about future cases of this kind if you would permit me to perform certain experiments on you. It is understood that you yourself would not benefit from any knowledge we might gain; but future patients would." Although greatly vulnerable and deserving of maximum protection, such a patient might be ethically approached to be a research subject, because the benefits to future patients are in a way a value to him: "At least that residue of identification is left him that it is his own affliction by which he can contribute to the conquest of that affliction, his own kind of suffering which he helps alleviate in others; and so *in a sense it is his own cause*" (Jonas 1969: 532, emphasis mine).

In this case, the individual apprehends a good greater than his personal good, less than that of society: that of his disease class, which is *his* good. Of course, the identification of which Jonas speaks is psychological; he would likely not agree with the approach herein outlined and might require that such participation be through a conscious, free choice of the patient. Nevertheless, it is a real, objective good which justifies his choice and prevents us from asking him to participate in research unrelated to his disease. Can a relative, a son or daughter perhaps, ethically make that decision for an incompetent, demented Alzheimer's patient? If so, it is because, in a sense, it is the patient's cause, the patient's good as a member of a community which justifies that choice. It is not a matter of enforcing a social duty or minimal social obligation here, but seeking a good that lies in the relationship one has to others with the same disease. That same good, as noted above, limits the participation of the subject to research related precisely to his disease, not to anything else.

What is the implication of this for risk and the limits of risk? As has been seen, some wish to allow for exposure of subjects to greater than minimal risk provided only that it is classified as "therapeutic" (though the subjects are not ill). Others, in spite of the fact that the research is intended for the benefit of a group at risk, classify it as non-therapeutic and limit the acceptable risk to minimal levels. Are these the only alternatives? One advisory group has allowed, in the case of the mentally incompetent, for a "minor increase over minimal risk" in such circumstances (National Commission for the Protection of Human Subjects 1978: 16). This is presumably permitted because the research is "of vital importance for the understanding or amelioration of the type of disorder or condition of the subjects" or "may reasonably be expected to benefit the subjects in future" (17). But what counts as minor increase in risk? Proposed research into Alzheimer's might involve invasive procedures such as brain biopsies, implantation of electrodes, spinal taps, and injections of experimental drugs. Are these of greater risk than that specified by the National Commission simply because they are invasive of the human brain? Or is there clear statistical risk of serious added damage to the brain? These are matters for empirical study. The invasiveness per se should not rule out a procedure. The major limitations should be whether the procedure is painful, causes anxiety, or adds to the already serious damage to the brain. If research involving procedures of greater risk than "minor increase over minimal" is ever to be justified, it must be so by the intent to avert the proportional evils of death or mental incapacity. If these are insufficient, then I fail to see what grounds might be available upon which to base a case for legislative change.

It is clear, then, that should such research be acceptable, it also demands that stringent protective procedures be established in order to ensure that the demented are not drafted into research unrelated to their disease class. This is because the standard, being broader than that of "direct or fairly immediate benefit," is open to an accordionlike expansion, and therefore to abuse. Such safeguards could include: rigorous assurance that the proxy's consent (in reality, simply a permission) is informed and voluntary, the provision of a consent auditor, and various layers of administrative review and monitoring, from a local institutional review board up to a judicial review with a guardian appointed to represent the patient-subject's rights. These procedures may prove to be onerous. But we are on dangerous ground, and as we try to avoid overprotection, which may come at the expense of improved therapy for all, we must also avoid opening up a huge door to exploitation.

REFERENCES

Beauchamp, T.L., & Childress, J.F. (1983). *Principles of biomedical ethics.* 2nd ed. New York: Oxford University Press

Finnis, J. (1980). *Natural law and natural rights.* Oxford: Clarendon Press

Jonas, H. (1969). Philosophical reflections on experimenting with human subjects. In T. Beauchamp and L. Walters (Eds.), *Contemporary issues in bioethics.* 2nd ed. Belmont, CA: Wadsworth

Maritain, J. (1947). *The person and the common good.* New York: Charles Scribner's Sons

May, W. (1976). Proxy consent to human experimentation. *Linacre Quarterly, 43,* 73–84

McCormick, R. (1974). Proxy consent in the experimentation situation. *Perspectives in Biology and Medicine, 18,* 2–20

McCormick, R. (1976). Experimentation in children: sharing in sociality. *Hastings Center Report, 6,* 41–46

National Commission for the Protection of Human Subjects (1978). *Report and recommendations: Research involving those institutionalized as mentally infirm.* Washington, DC

Ramsey, P. (1970). *The patient as person.* New Haven: Yale University Press

Ramsey, P. (1976). The enforcement of morals: Nontherapeutic research on children. *Hastings Center Report, 4,* 21–30

Ramsey, P. (1977). Children as research subjects: a reply. *Hastings Center Report, 2,* 40–41

Ratzan, R. (1980). "Being old makes you different": The ethics of research with elderly subjects. *Hastings Center Report, 5,* 32–42

Reich, W. (1978). Ethical issues related to research involving elderly subjects. *Gerontologist, 18,* 326–37

Experimental Design and Randomized Clinical Trials

Of Mice But Not Men: Problems of the Randomized Clinical Trial
Samuel Hellman and Deborah S. Hellman

Samuel Hellman is A. N. Pritzker Distinguished Service Professor, Department of Radiation and Cellular Oncology, University of Chicago. He is the author of such articles as "The End of Inevitability, or Dr. Frankenstein and the Biological Revolution" and *"Fin de Siècle* Medicine. Avoiding the Unintended Consequences of Health Care Reform." Deborah S. Hellman is assistant professor of law at the University of Maryland. Her areas of specialization are ethics and jurisprudence.

Hellman and Hellman argue that an ethical dilemma confronts the use of randomized clinical trials, that is, controlled comparisons of two or more treatment arms (one of which

Reprinted by permission of the publisher from *The New England Journal of Medicine,* vol. 324 (May 30, 1991), pp. 1585–1589. © 1991 Massachusetts Medical Society.

may involve a placebo) in which subjects are randomly assigned to the different groups. According to the authors, such studies require researchers to enter into two largely incompatible roles. (1) As *physicians,* they are ethically required to act in their patients' best interests. (2) As *scientists,* they are expected to address rigorously the question of whether a particular therapy is effective, or how effective it is compared with others, in the hope of offering a genuine benefit to future patients. At some point in a study, the authors contend, researchers usually have an opinion about which treatment arm is more advantageous—but disclosing that judgment would ruin the study, while nondisclosure would mean failing to act in their patients' best interests. Hellman and Hellman conclude by suggesting that several research techniques might be sufficiently rigorous to offer viable alternatives to randomized clinical trials.

As medicine has become increasingly scientific and less accepting of unsupported opinion or proof by anecdote, the randomized controlled clinical trial has become the standard technique for changing diagnostic or therapeutic methods. The use of this technique creates an ethical dilemma.[1,2] Researchers participating in such studies are required to modify their ethical commitments to individual patients and do serious damage to the concept of the physician as a practicing, empathetic professional who is primarily concerned with each patient as an individual. Researchers using a randomized clinical trial can be described as physician-scientists, a term that expresses the tension between the two roles. The physician, by entering into a relationship with an individual patient, assumes certain obligations, including the commitment always to act in the patient's best interests. As Leon Kass has rightly maintained, "the physician must produce unswervingly the virtues of loyalty and fidelity to his patient."[3] Though the ethical requirements of this relationship have been modified by legal obligations to report wounds of a suspicious nature and certain infectious diseases, these obligations in no way conflict with the central ethical obligation to act in the best interests of the patient medically. Instead, certain nonmedical interests of the patient are preempted by other social concerns.

The role of the scientist is quite different. The clinical scientist is concerned with answering questions—i.e., determining the validity of formally constructed hypotheses. Such scientific information, it is presumed, will benefit humanity in general. The clinical scientist's role has been well described by Dr. Anthony Fauci, director of the National Institute of Allergy and Infectious Diseases, who states the goals of the randomized clinical trial in these words: "It's not to deliver therapy. It's to answer a scientific question so that the drug can

be available for everybody once you've established safety and efficacy."[4] The demands of such a study can conflict in a number of ways with the physician's duty to minister to patients. The study may create a false dichotomy in the physician's opinions: according to the premise of the randomized clinical trial, the physician may only know or not know whether a proposed course of treatment represents an improvement; no middle position is permitted. What the physician thinks, suspects, believes, or has a hunch about is assigned to the "not knowing" category, because knowing is defined on the basis of an arbitrary but accepted statistical test performed in a randomized clinical trial. Thus, little credence is given to information gained beforehand in other ways or to information accrued during the trial but without the required statistical degree of assurance that a difference is not due to chance. The randomized clinical trial also prevents the treatment technique from being modified on the basis of the growing knowledge of the physicians during their participation in the trial. Moreover, it limits access to the data as they are collected until specific milestones are achieved. This prevents physicians from profiting not only from their individual experience, but also from the collective experience of the other participants.

The randomized clinical trial requires doctors to act simultaneously as physicians and as scientists. This puts them in a difficult and sometimes untenable ethical position. The conflicting moral demands arising from the use of the randomized clinical trial reflect the classic conflict between rights-based moral theories and utilitarian ones. The first of these, which depend on the moral theory of Immanuel Kant (and seen more recently in neo-Kantian philosophers, such as John Rawls[5]), asserts that human beings, by virtue of their unique capacity for rational thought, are bearers of dignity. As such, they ought not to be treated merely as means to an end; rather, they must always be treated as ends in themselves. Utilitarianism, by contrast, defines what is right as the greatest good for the greatest number—that is, as social utility. This view, articulated by Jeremy Bentham and John Stuart Mill, requires that pleasures (understood broadly, to include such pleasures as health and well-being) and pains be added together. The morally correct act is the act that produces the most pleasure and the least pain overall.

A classic objection to the utilitarian position is that according to that theory, the distribution of pleasures and pains is of no moral consequence. This element of the theory severely restricts physicians from being utilitarians, or at least from following the theory's dictates. Physicians must care very deeply about the distribution of pain and pleasure, for they have entered into a relationship with one or a number of individual patients. They cannot be indifferent to whether it is these patients or others that suffer for the general benefit of society. Even though society might gain from the suffering of a few, and even though the doctor might believe that such a benefit is worth a given patient's suffering (i.e., that utilitarianism is right in the particular case), the ethical obligation created by the covenant between doctor and patient requires the doctor to see the interests of the individual patient as primary and compelling. In essence, the doctor-patient relationship requires doctors to see their patients as bearers of rights who cannot be merely used for the greater good of humanity.

As Fauci has suggested,[4] the randomized clinical trial routinely asks physicians to sacrifice the interests of their particular patients for the sake of the study and that of the information that it will make available for the benefit of society. This practice is ethically problematic. Consider first the initial formulation of a trial. In particular, consider the case of a disease for which there is no satisfactory therapy—for example, advanced cancer or the acquired immunodeficiency syndrome (AIDS). A new agent that promises more effectiveness is the subject of the study. The control group must be given either an unsatisfactory treatment or a placebo. Even though the therapeutic value of the new agent is unproved, if physicians think that it has promise, are they acting in the best interests of their patients in allowing them to be randomly assigned to the control group? Is persisting in such an assignment consistent with the specific commitments taken on in the doctor–patient relationship? As a result of interactions with patients with AIDS and their advocates, Merigan[6] recently suggested modifications in the design of clinical trials that attempt to deal

with the unsatisfactory treatment given to the control group. The view of such activists has been expressed by Rebecca Pringle Smith of Community Research Initiative in New York: "Even if you have a supply of compliant martyrs, trials must have some ethical validity."[4]

If the physician has no opinion about whether the new treatment is acceptable, then random assignment is ethically acceptable, but such lack of enthusiasm for the new treatment does not augur well for either the patient or the study. Alternatively, the treatment may show promise of beneficial results but also present a risk of undesirable complications. When the physician believes that the severity and likelihood of harm and good are evenly balanced, randomization may be ethically acceptable. If the physician has no preference for either treatment (is in a state of equipoise[7,8]), then randomization is acceptable. If, however, he or she believes that the new treatment may be either more or less successful or more or less toxic, the use of randomization is not consistent with fidelity to the patient.

The argument usually used to justify randomization is that it provides, in essence, a critique of the usefulness of the physician's beliefs and opinions, those that have not yet been validated by a randomized clinical trial. As the argument goes, these not-yet-validated beliefs are as likely to be wrong as right. Although physicians are ethically required to provide their patients with the best available treatment, there simply is no best treatment yet known.

The reply to this argument takes two forms. First, and most important, even if this view of the reliability of a physician's opinions is accurate, the ethical constraints of an individual doctor's relationship with a particular patient require the doctor to provide individual care. Although physicians must take pains to make clear the speculative nature of their views, they cannot withhold these views from the patient. The patient asks from the doctor both knowledge and judgment. The relationship established between them rightfully allows patients to ask for the judgment of their particular physicians, not merely that of the medical profession in general. Second, it may not be true, in fact, that the not-yet-validated beliefs of physicians are as likely to be wrong as right. The greater certainty obtained with a randomized clinical trial is beneficial, but that does not mean that a lesser degree of certainty is without value. Physicians can acquire knowledge through methods other than the randomized clinical trial. Such knowledge, acquired over time and less formally than is required in a randomized clinical trial, may be of great value to a patient.

Even if it is ethically acceptable to begin a study,

one often forms an opinion during its course—especially in studies that are impossible to conduct in a truly double-blinded fashion—that makes it ethically problematic to continue. The inability to remain blinded usually occurs in studies of cancer or AIDS, for example, because the therapy is associated by nature with serious side effects. Trials attempt to restrict the physician's access to the data in order to prevent such unblinding. Such restrictions should make physicians eschew the trial, since their ability to act in the patient's best interests will be limited. Even supporters of randomized clinical trials, such as Merigan, agree that interim findings should be presented to patients to ensure that no one receives what seems an inferior treatment.[6] Once physicians have formed a view about the new treatment, can they continue randomization? If random assignment is stopped, the study may be lost and the participation of the previous patients wasted. However, if physicians continue the randomization when they have a definite opinion about the efficacy of the experimental drug, they are not acting in accordance with the requirements of the doctor–patient relationship. Furthermore, as their opinion becomes more firm, stopping the randomization may not be enough. Physicians may be ethically required to treat the patients formerly placed in the control group with the therapy that now seems probably effective. To do so would be faithful to the obligations created by the doctor–patient relationship, but it would destroy the study.

To resolve this dilemma, one might suggest that the patient has abrogated the rights implicit in a doctor–patient relationship by signing an informed-consent form. We argue that such rights cannot be waived or abrogated. They are inalienable. The right to be treated as an individual deserving the physician's best judgment and care, rather than to be used as a means to determine the best treatment for others, is inherent in every person. This right, based on the concept of dignity, cannot be waived. What of altruism, then? Is it not the patient's right to make a sacrifice for the general good? This question must be considered from both positions— that of the patient and that of the physician. Although patients may decide to waive this right, it is not consistent with the role of a physician to ask that they do so. In asking, the doctor acts as a scientist instead. The physician's role here is to propose what he or she believes is best medically for the specific patient, not to suggest participation in a study from which the patient cannot gain. Because the opportunity to help future patients is of potential value to a patient, some would say physicians should not deny it. Although this point

has merit, it offers so many opportunities for abuse that we are extremely uncomfortable about accepting it. The responsibilities of physicians are much clearer; they are to minister to the current patient.

Moreover, even if patients could waive this right, it is questionable whether those with terminal illness would be truly able to give voluntary informed consent. Such patients are extremely dependent on both their physicians and the health care system. Aware of this dependence, physicians must not ask for consent, for in such cases the very asking breaches the doctor–patient relationship. Anxious to please their physicians, patients may have difficulty refusing to participate in the trial the physicians describe. The patients may perceive their refusal as damaging to the relationship, whether or not it is so. Such perceptions of coercion affect the decision. Informed-consent forms are difficult to understand, especially for patients under the stress of serious illness for which there is no satisfactory treatment. The forms are usually lengthy, somewhat legalistic, complicated, and confusing, and they hardly bespeak the compassion expected of the medical profession. It is important to remember that those who have studied the doctor–patient relationship have emphasized its empathetic nature.

> [The] relationship between doctor and patient partakes of a peculiar intimacy. It presupposes on the part of the physician not only knowledge of his fellow men but sympathy. . . . This aspect of the practice of medicine has been designated as the art; yet I wonder whether it should not, most properly, be called the essence.[9]

How is such a view of the relationship consonant with random assignment and informed consent? The Physician's Oath of the World Medical Association affirms the primacy of the deontologic view of patients' rights: "Concern for the interests of the subject must always prevail over the interests of science and society."[10]

Furthermore, a single study is often not considered sufficient. Before a new form of therapy is generally accepted, confirmatory trials must be conducted. How can one conduct such trials ethically unless one is convinced that the first trial was in error? The ethical problems we have discussed are only exacerbated when a completed randomized clinical trial indicates that a given treatment is preferable. Even if the physician believes the initial trial was in error, the physician must indicate to the patient the full results of that trial.

The most common reply to the ethical arguments has been that the alternative is to return to the physician's intuition, to anecdotes, or to both as the basis of medical opinion. We all accept the dangers of such a practice. The argument states that we must therefore accept randomized, controlled clinical trials regardless of their ethical problems because of the great social benefit they make possible, and we salve our conscience with the knowledge that informed consent has been given. This returns us to the conflict between patients' rights and social utility. Some would argue that this tension can be resolved by placing a relative value on each. If the patient's right that is being compromised is not a fundamental right and the social gain is very great, then the study might be justified. When the right is fundamental, however, no amount of social gain, or almost none, will justify its sacrifice. Consider, for example, the experiments on humans done by physicians under the Nazi regime. All would agree that these are unacceptable regardless of the value of the scientific information gained. Some people go so far as to say that no use should be made of the results of those experiments because of the clearly unethical manner in which the data were collected. This extreme example may not seem relevant, but we believe that in its hyperbole it clarifies the fallacy of a utilitarian approach to the physician's relationship with the patient. To consider the utilitarian gain is consistent neither with the physician's role nor with the patient's rights.

It is fallacious to suggest that only the randomized clinical trial can provide valid information or that all information acquired by this technique is valid. Such experimental methods are intended to reduce error and bias and therefore reduce the uncertainty of the result. Uncertainty cannot be eliminated, however. The scientific method is based on increasing probabilities and increasingly refined approximations of truth.[11] Although the randomized clinical trial contributes to these ends, it is neither unique nor perfect. Other techniques may also be useful.[12]

Randomized trials often place physicians in the ethically intolerable position of choosing between the good of the patient and that of society. We urge that such situations be avoided and that other techniques of acquiring clinical information be adopted. For example, concerning trials of treatments for AIDS, Byar et al.[13] have said that "some traditional approaches to the clinical-trials process may be unnecessarily rigid and unsuitable for this disease." In this case, AIDS is not what is so different; rather, the difference is in the presence of AIDS activists, articulate spokespersons for the ethical problems created by the application of the randomized clinical trial to terminal illnesses. Such arguments are equally applicable to advanced cancer and other serious illnesses. Byar et al. agree that there are even circumstances in which uncontrolled clinical trials may be justified: when there is no effective treatment to use as a control, when the prognosis is uniformly poor, and when there is a reasonable expectation of benefit without excessive toxicity. These conditions are usually found in clinical trials of advanced cancer.

The purpose of the randomized clinical trial is to avoid the problems of observer bias and patient selection. It seems to us that techniques might be developed to deal with these issues in other ways. Randomized clinical trials deal with them in a cumbersome and heavy-handed manner, by requiring large numbers of patients in the hope that random assignment will balance the heterogeneous distribution of patients into the different groups. By observing known characteristics of patients, such as age and sex, and distributing them equally between groups, it is thought that unknown factors important in determining outcomes will also be distributed equally. Surely, other techniques can be developed to deal with both observer bias and patient selection. Prospective studies without randomization, but with the evaluation of patients by uninvolved third parties, should remove observer bias. Similar methods have been suggested by Royall.[12] Prospective matched-pair analysis, in which patients are treated in a manner consistent with their physician's views, ought to help ensure equivalence between the groups and thus mitigate the effect of patient selection, at least with regard to known covariates. With regard to unknown covariates, the security would rest, as in randomized trials, in the enrollment of large numbers of patients and in confirmatory studies. This method would not pose ethical difficulties, since patients would receive the treatment recommended by their physician. They would be included in the study by independent observers matching patients with respect to known characteristics, a process that would not affect patient care and that could be performed independently any number of times.

This brief discussion of alternatives to randomized clinical trials is sketchy and incomplete. We wish only to point out that there may be satisfactory alternatives, not to describe and evaluate them completely. Even if randomized clinical trials were much better than any alternative, however, the ethical dilemmas they present may put their use at variance with the primary obligations of the physician. In this regard, Angell cautions, "If this commitment to the patient is attenuated, even for so good a cause as benefits to future patients, the implicit assumptions of the doctor–patient relationship are violated."[14] The risk of such attenuation by the randomized trial is great. The AIDS activists have brought this dramatically to the attention of the academic medical community. Techniques appropriate to the laboratory may not be applicable to humans. We must develop and use alternative methods for acquiring clinical knowledge.

REFERENCES

1 Hellman S. Randomized clinical trials and the doctor–patient relationship: an ethical dilemma. Cancer Clin Trials 1979; 2:189–93.

2 *Idem.* A doctor's dilemma: the doctor-patient relationship in clinical investigation. In: Proceedings of the Fourth National Conference on Human Values and Cancer, New York, March 15–17, 1984. New York: American Cancer Society, 1984:144–6.

3 Kass LR. Toward a more natural science: biology and human affairs. New York: Free Press, 1985:196.

4 Palca J. AIDS drug trials enter new age. Science 1989; 246:19–21.

5 Rawls J. A theory of justice. Cambridge, Mass.: Belknap Press of Harvard University Press, 1971:183–92, 446–52.

6 Merigan TC. You *can* teach an old dog new tricks—how AIDS trials are pioneering new strategies. N Engl J Med 1990; 323:1341–3.

7 Freedman B. Equipoise and the ethics of clinical research. N Engl J Med 1987; 317:141–5.

8 Singer PA, Lantos JD, Whitington PF, Broelsch CE, Siegler M. Equipoise and the ethics of segmental liver transplantation. Clin Res 1988; 36:539–45.

9 Longcope WT. Methods and medicine. Bull Johns Hopkins Hosp 1932; 50:4–20.

10 Report on medical ethics. World Med Assoc Bull 1949; 1:109, 111.

11 Popper K. The problem of induction. In: Miller D, ed. Popper selections. Princeton, N.J.: Princeton University Press, 1985:101–17.

12 Royall RM. Ethics and statistics in randomized clinical trials. Stat Sci 1991; 6(1):52–62.

13 Byar DP, Schoenfeld DA, Green SB, et al. Design considerations for AIDS trials. N Engl J Med 1990; 323:1343–8.

14 Angell M. Patients' preferences in randomized clinical trials. N Engl J Med 1984; 310:1385–7.

Equipoise and the Ethics of Clinical Research
Benjamin Freedman

Benjamin Freedman is professor at the McGill Center for Medicine, Ethics, and Law and clinical ethicist at Sir Mortimer B. Davis Jewish General Hospital, Montreal, Canada. He is the author of such articles as "AIDS and the Ethics of Clinical Trials," "Violating Confidentiality to Warn of a Risk of HIV Infection," and "Is There a Duty to Provide Medical Care to HIV-Infected Patients?"

Freedman disputes the thesis that randomized clinical trials entail an ethically unmanageable conflict for investigators (as Hellman and Hellman argue). The ethics of clinical research, he notes, requires *equipoise,* "a state of genuine uncertainty on the part of the clinical investigator regarding the comparative therapeutic merits of each arm in a trial"; the discovery that one treatment is superior requires the investigator to offer it. Freedman argues that, while equipoise is usually understood to be disrupted if the investigator forms a treatment preference, a plausible interpretation of equipoise blocks this implication: *Clinical equipoise* exists when there is genuine uncertainty in the medical community about which treatment is preferable, even if the individual investigator has a preference.

Reprinted by permission of the publisher from *The New England Journal of Medicine,* vol. 317 (July 16, 1987), pp. 141–145. © 1987 Massachusetts Medical Society.

There is widespread agreement that ethics requires that each clinical trial begin with an honest null hypothesis.[1,2] In the simplest model, testing a new treatment B on a defined patient population P for which the current accepted treatment is A, it is necessary that the clinical investigator be in a state of genuine uncertainty regarding the comparative merits of treatments A and B for population P. If a physician knows that these treatments are not equivalent, ethics requires that the superior treatment be recommended. Following Fried, I call this state of uncertainty about the relative merits of A and B "equipoise."[3]

Equipoise is an ethically necessary condition in all cases of clinical research. In trials with several arms, equipoise must exist between all arms of the trial; otherwise the trial design should be modified to exclude the inferior treatment. If equipoise is disturbed during the course of a trial, the trial may need to be terminated and all subjects previously enrolled (as well as other patients within the relevant population) may have to be offered the superior treatment. It has been rigorously argued that a trial with a placebo is ethical only in investigating conditions for which there is no known treatment[2]; this argument reflects a special application of the requirement for equipoise. Although equipoise has commonly been discussed in the special context of the ethics of randomized clinical trials,[4,5] it is important to recognize it as an ethical condition of all controlled clinical trials, whether or not they are randomized, placebo-controlled, or blinded.

The recent increase in attention to the ethics of research with human subjects has highlighted problems associated with equipoise. Yet, as I shall attempt to show, contemporary literature, if anything, minimizes those difficulties. Moreover, there is evidence that concern on the part of investigators about failure to satisfy the requirements for equipoise can doom a trial as a result of the consequent failure to enroll a sufficient number of subjects.

The solutions that have been offered to date fail to resolve these problems in a way that would permit clinical trials to proceed. This paper argues that these problems are predicated on a faulty concept of equipoise itself. An alternative understanding of equipoise as an ethical requirement of clinical trials is proposed, and its implications are explored.

Many of the problems raised by the requirement for equipoise are familiar. Shaw and Chalmers have written that a clinician who "knows, or has good reason to believe," that one arm of the trial is superior may not ethically participate.[6] But the reasoning or preliminary results that prompt the trial (and that may themselves be ethically mandatory)[7] may jolt the investigator (if not his or her colleagues) out of equipoise before the trial begins. Even if the investigator is undecided between A and B in terms of gross measures such as mortality and morbidity, equipoise may be disturbed because evident differences in the quality of life (as in the case of two surgical approaches) tip the balance.[3–5,8] In either case, in saying "we do not know" whether A or B is better, the investigator may create a false impression in prospective subjects, who hear him or her as saying "no evidence leans either way," when the investigator means "no controlled study has yet had results that reach statistical significance."

Late in the study—when P values are between 0.05 and 0.06—the moral issue of equipoise is most readily apparent,[9,10] but the same problem arises when the earliest comparative results are analyzed.[11] Within the closed statistical universe of the clinical trial, each result that demonstrates a difference between the arms of the trial contributes exactly as much to the statistical conclusion that a difference exists as does any other. The contribution of the last pair of cases in the trial is no greater than that of the first. If, therefore, equipoise is a condition that reflects equivalent evidence for alternative hypotheses, it is jeopardized by the first pair of cases as much as by the last. The investigator who is concerned about the ethics of recruitment after the penultimate pair must logically be concerned after the first pair as well.

Finally, these issues are more than a philosopher's nightmare. Considerable interest has been generated by a paper in which Taylor et al.[12] describe the termination of a trial of alternative treatments for breast cancer. The trial foundered on the problem of patient recruitment, and the investigators trace much of the difficulty in enrolling patients to the fact that the investigators were not in a state of equipoise regarding the arms of the trial. With the increase in concern about the ethics of research and with the increasing presence of this topic in the curricula of medical and graduate schools, instances of the type that Taylor and her colleagues describe are likely to become more common. The requirement for equipoise thus poses a practical threat to clinical research.

RESPONSES TO THE PROBLEMS OF EQUIPOISE

The problems described above apply to a broad class of clinical trials, at all stages of their development. Their resolution will need to be similarly comprehensive. However, the solutions that have so far been proposed address a portion of the difficulties, at best, and cannot be considered fully satisfactory.

Chalmers' approach to problems at the onset of a trial is to recommend that randomization begin with the very first subject.[11] If there are no preliminary, uncontrolled data in support of the experimental treatment B, equipoise regarding treatments A and B for the patient population P is not disturbed. There are several difficulties with this approach. Practically speaking, it is often necessary to establish details of administration, dosage, and so on, before a controlled trial begins, by means of uncontrolled trials in human subjects. In addition, as I have argued above, equipoise from the investigator's point of view is likely to be disturbed when the hypothesis is being formulated and a protocol is being prepared. It is then, before any subjects have been enrolled, that the information that the investigator has assembled makes the experimental treatment appear to be a reasonable gamble. Apart from these problems, initial randomization will not, as Chalmers recognizes, address disturbances of equipoise that occur in the course of a trial.

Data-monitoring committees have been proposed as a solution to problems arising in the course of the trial.[13] Such committees, operating independently of the investigators, are the only bodies with information concerning the trial's ongoing results. Since this knowledge is not available to the investigators, their equipoise is not disturbed. Although committees are useful in keeping the conduct of a trial free of bias, they cannot resolve the investigators' ethical difficulties. A clinician is not merely obliged to treat a patient on the basis of the information that he or she currently has, but is also required to discover information that would be relevant to treatment decisions. If interim results would disturb equipoise, the investigators are obliged to gather and use that information. Their agreement to remain in ignorance of preliminary results would, by definition, be an unethical agreement, just as a failure to call up the laboratory to find out a patient's test results is unethical. Moreover, the use of a monitoring committee does not solve problems of equipoise that arise before and at the beginning of a trial.

Recognizing the broad problems with equipoise, three authors have proposed radical solutions. All three think that there is an irresolvable conflict between the requirement that a patient be offered the best treatment known (the principle underlying the requirement for equipoise) and the conduct of clinical trials; they there-fore suggest that the "best treatment" requirement be weakened.

Schafer has argued that the concept of equipoise, and the associated notion of the best medical treatment, depends on the judgment of patients rather than of clinical investigators.[14] Although the equipoise of an investigator may be disturbed if he or she favors B over A, the ultimate choice of treatment is the patient's. Because the patient's values may restore equipoise, Schafer argues, it is ethical for the investigator to proceed with a trial when the patient consents. Schafer's strategy is directed toward trials that test treatments with known and divergent side effects and will probably not be useful in trials conducted to test efficacy or unknown side effects. This approach, moreover, confuses the ethics of competent medical practice with those of consent. If we assume that the investigator is a competent clinician, by saying that the investigator is out of equipoise, we have by Schafer's account said that in the investigator's professional judgment one treatment is therapeutically inferior—for that patient, in that condition, given the quality of life that can be achieved. Even if a patient would consent to an inferior treatment, it seems to me a violation of competent medical practice, and hence of ethics, to make the offer. Of course, complex issues may arise when a patient refuses what the physician considers the best treatment and demands instead an inferior treatment. Without settling that problem, however, we can reject Schafer's position. For Schafer claims that in order to continue to conduct clinical trials, it is ethical for the physician to offer (not merely accede to) inferior treatment.

Meier suggests that "most of us would be quite willing to forego a modest expected gain in the general interest of learning something of value."[15] He argues that we accept risks in everyday life to achieve a variety of benefits, including convenience and economy. In the same way, Meier states, it is acceptable to enroll subjects in clinical trials even though they may not receive the best treatment throughout the course of the trial. Schafer suggests an essentially similar approach.[5,14] According to this view, continued progress in medical knowledge through clinical trials requires an explicit abandonment of the doctor's fully patient-centered ethic.

These proposals seem to be frank counsels of desperation. They resolve the ethical problems of equipoise by abandoning the need for equipoise. In any event, would their approach allow clinical trials to be conducted? I think this may fairly be doubted. Although many people are presumably altruistic enough to forgo the best medical treatment in the interest of the progress of science, many are not. The numbers and proportions required to sustain the statistical validity of trial results suggest that in the absence of overwhelming altruism, the enrollment of satisfactory numbers of patients will not be possible. In particular, very ill patients, toward whom many of the most important clinical trials are directed, may be disinclined to be altruistic. Finally, as the study by Taylor et al.[12] reminds us, the problems of equipoise trouble investigators as well as patients. Even if patients are prepared to dispense with the best treatment, their physicians, for reasons of ethics and professionalism, may well not be willing to do so.

Marquis has suggested a third approach. "Perhaps what is needed is an ethics that will justify the conscription of subjects for medical research," he has written. "Nothing less seems to justify present practice."[4] Yet, although conscription might enable us to continue present practice, it would scarcely justify it. Moreover, the conscription of physician investigators, as well as subjects, would be necessary, because, as has been repeatedly argued, the problems of equipoise are as disturbing to clinicians as they are to subjects. Is any less radical and more plausible approach possible?

THEORETICAL EQUIPOISE VERSUS CLINICAL EQUIPOISE

The problems of equipoise examined above arise from a particular understanding of that concept, which I will term "theoretical equipoise." It is an understanding that is both conceptually odd and ethically irrelevant. Theoretical equipoise exists when, overall, the evidence on behalf of two alternative treatment regimens is exactly balanced. This evidence may be derived from a variety of sources, including data from the literature, uncontrolled experience, considerations of basic science and fundamental physiologic processes, and perhaps a "gut feeling" or "instinct" resulting from (or superimposed on) other considerations. The problems examined above arise from the principle that if theoretical equipoise is disturbed, the physician has, in Schafer's words, a "treatment preference"—let us say, favoring experimental treatment B. A trial testing A against B requires that some patients be enrolled in violation of this treatment preference.

Theoretical equipoise is overwhelmingly fragile; that is, it is disturbed by a slight accretion of evidence favoring one arm of the trial. In Chalmers' view, equipoise is disturbed when the odds that A will be

more successful than B are anything other than 50 percent. It is therefore necessary to randomize treatment assignments beginning with the very first patient, lest equipoise be disturbed. We may say that theoretical equipoise is balanced on a knife's edge.

Theoretical equipoise is most appropriate to one-dimensional hypotheses and causes us to think in those terms. The null hypothesis must be sufficiently simple and "clean" to be finely balanced: Will A or B be superior in reducing mortality or shrinking tumors or lowering fevers in population P? Clinical choice is commonly more complex. The choice of A or B depends on some combination of effectiveness, consistency, minimal or relievable side effects, and other factors. On close examination, for example, it sometimes appears that even trials that purport to test a single hypothesis in fact involve a more complicated, portmanteau measure—e.g., the "therapeutic index" of A versus B. The formulation of the conditions of theoretical equipoise for such complex, multidimensional clinical hypotheses is tantamount to the formulation of a rigorous calculus of apples and oranges.

Theoretical equipoise is also highly sensitive to the vagaries of the investigator's attention and perception. Because of its fragility, theoretical equipoise is disturbed as soon as the investigator perceives a difference between the alternatives—whether or not any genuine difference exists. Prescott writes, for example, "It will be common at some stage in most trials for the survival curves to show visually different survivals," short of significance but "sufficient to raise ethical difficulties for the participants."[16] A visual difference, however, is purely an artifact of the research methods employed: when and by what means data are assembled and analyzed and what scale is adopted for the graphic presentation of data. Similarly, it is common for researchers to employ interval scales for phenomena that are recognized to be continuous by nature—e.g., five-point scales of pain or stages of tumor progression. These interval scales, which represent an arbitrary distortion of the available evidence to simplify research, may magnify the differences actually found, with a resulting disturbance of theoretical equipoise.

Finally, as described by several authors, theoretical equipoise is personal and idiosyncratic. It is disturbed when the clinician has, in Schafer's words, what "might even be labeled a bias or a hunch," a preference of a "merely intuitive nature."[14] The investigator who ignores such a hunch, by failing to advise the patient that because of it the investigator prefers B to A or by recommending A (or a chance of random assignment to A) to the patient, has violated the requirement for equipoise and its companion requirement to recommend the best medical treatment.

The problems with this concept of equipoise should be evident. To understand the alternative, preferable interpretation of equipoise, we need to recall the basic reason for conducting clinical trials: there is a current or imminent conflict in the clinical community over what treatment is preferred for patients in a defined population P. The standard treatment is A, but some evidence suggests that B will be superior (because of its effectiveness or its reduction of undesirable side effects, or for some other reason). (In the rare case when the first evidence of a novel therapy's superiority would be entirely convincing to the clinical community, equipoise is already disturbed.) Or there is a split in the clinical community, with some clinicians favoring A and others favoring B. Each side recognizes that the opposing side has evidence to support its position, yet each still thinks that overall its own view is correct. There exists (or, in the case of a novel therapy, there may soon exist) an honest, professional disagreement among expert clinicians about the preferred treatment. A clinical trial is instituted with the aim of resolving this dispute.

At this point, a state of "clinical equipoise" exists. There is no consensus within the expert clinical community about the comparative merits of the alternatives to be tested. We may state the formal conditions under which such a trial would be ethical as follows: at the start of the trial, there must be a state of clinical equipoise regarding the merits of the regiments to be tested, and the trial must be designed in such a way as to make it reasonable to expect that, if it is successfully concluded, clinical equipoise will be disturbed. In other words, the results of a successful clinical trial should be convincing enough to resolve the dispute among clinicians.

A state of clinical equipoise is consistent with a decided treatment preference on the part of the investigators. They must simply recognize that their less-favored treatment is preferred by colleagues whom they consider to be responsible and competent. Even if the interim results favor the preference of the investigators, treatment B, clinical equipoise persists as long as those results are too weak to influence the judgment of the community of clinicians, because of limited sample size, unresolved possibilities of side effects, or other factors. (This judgment can necessarily be made only by those who know the interim results—whether a data-monitoring committee or the investigators.)

At the point when the accumulated evidence in favor of B is so strong that the committee or investiga-

tors believe no open-minded clinician informed of the results would still favor A, clinical equipoise has been disturbed. This may occur well short of the original schedule for the termination of the trial, for unexpected reasons. (Therapeutic effects or side effects may be much stronger than anticipated, for example, or a definable subgroup within population P may be recognized for which the results demonstrably disturb clinical equipoise.) Because of the arbitrary character of human judgment and persuasion, some ethical problems regarding the termination of a trial will remain. Clinical equipoise will confine these problems to unusual or extreme cases, however, and will allow us to cast persistent problems in the proper terms. For example, in the face of a strong established trend, must we continue the trial because of others' blind fealty to an arbitrary statistical bench mark?

Clearly, clinical equipoise is a far weaker—and more common—condition than theoretical equipoise. Is it ethical to conduct a trial on the basis of clinical equipoise, when theoretical equipoise is disturbed? Or, as Schafer and others have argued, is doing so a violation of the physician's obligation to provide patients with the best medical treatment?[4,5,14] Let us assume that the investigators have a decided preference for B but wish to conduct a trial on the grounds that clinical (not theoretical) equipoise exists. The ethics committee asks the investigators whether, if they or members of their families were within population P, they would not want to be treated with their preference, B? An affirmative answer is often thought to be fatal to the prospects for such a trial, yet the investigators answer in the affirmative. Would a trial satisfying this weaker form of equipoise be ethical?

I believe that it clearly is ethical. As Fried has emphasized,[3] competent (hence, ethical) medicine is social rather than individual in nature. Progress in medicine relies on progressive consensus within the medical and research communities. The ethics of medical practice grants no ethical or normative meaning to a treatment preference, however powerful, that is based on a hunch or on anything less than evidence publicly presented and convincing to the clinical community. Persons are licensed as physicians after they demonstrate the acquisition of this professionally validated knowledge, not after they reveal a superior capacity for guessing. Normative judgments of their behavior—e.g., malpractice actions—rely on a comparison with what is done by the community of medical practitioners. Failure to follow a "treatment preference" not shared by this community and not based on information that would convince it could not be the basis for an allegation of legal or ethical malpractice. As Fried states: "[T]he conception of what is good medicine is the product of a professional consensus." By definition, in a state of clinical equipoise, "good medicine" finds the choice between A and B indifferent.

In contrast to theoretical equipoise, clinical equipoise is robust. The ethical difficulties at the beginning and end of a trial are therefore largely alleviated. There remain difficulties about consent, but these too may be diminished. Instead of emphasizing the lack of evidence favoring one arm over another that is required by theoretical equipoise, clinical equipoise places the emphasis in informing the patient on the honest disagreement among expert clinicians. The fact that the investigator has a "treatment preference," if he or she does, could be disclosed; indeed, if the preference is a decided one, and based on something more than a hunch, it could be ethically mandatory to disclose it. At the same time, it would be emphasized that this preference is not shared by others. It is likely to be a matter of chance that the patient is being seen by a clinician with a preference for B over A, rather than by an equally competent clinician with the opposite preference.

Clinical equipoise does not depend on concealing relevant information from researchers and subjects, as does the use of independent data-monitoring committees. Rather, it allows investigators, in informing subjects, to distinguish appropriately among validated knowledge accepted by the clinical community, data on treatments that are promising but are not (or, for novel therapies, would not be) generally convincing, and mere hunches. Should informed patients decline to participate because they have chosen a specific clinician and trust his or her judgment—over and above the consensus in the professional community—that is no more than the patients' right. We do not conscript patients to serve as subjects in clinical trials.

THE IMPLICATIONS OF CLINICAL EQUIPOISE

The theory of clinical equipoise has been formulated as an alternative to some current views on the ethics of human research. At the same time, it corresponds closely to a preanalytic concept held by many in the research and regulatory communities. Clinical equipoise serves, then, as a rational formulation of the approach of many toward research ethics; it does not so much change things as explain why they are the way they are.

Nevertheless, the precision afforded by the theory of clinical equipoise does help to clarify or reformulate some aspects of research ethics; I will mention only two.

First, there is a recurrent debate about the ethical propriety of conducting clinical trials of discredited treatments, such as Laetrile.[17] Often, substantial political pressure to conduct such tests is brought to bear by adherents of quack therapies. The theory of clinical equipoise suggests that when there is no support for a treatment regimen within the expert clinical community, the first ethical requirement of a trial—clinical equipoise—is lacking; it would therefore be unethical to conduct such a trial.

Second, Feinstein has criticized the tendency of clinical investigators to narrow excessively the conditions and hypotheses of a trial in order to ensure the validity of its results.[18] This "fastidious" approach purchases scientific manageability at the expense of an inability to apply the results to the "messy" conditions of clinical practice. The theory of clinical equipoise adds some strength to this criticism. Overly "fastidious" trials, designed to resolve some theoretical question, fail to satisfy the second ethical requirement of clinical research, since the special conditions of the trial will render it useless for influencing clinical decisions, even if it is successfully completed.

The most important result of the concept of clinical equipoise, however, might be to relieve the current crisis of confidence in the ethics of clinical trials. Equipoise, properly understood, remains an ethical condition for clinical trials. It is consistent with much current practice. Clinicians and philosophers alike have been premature in calling for desperate measures to resolve problems of equipoise.

ACKNOWLEDGMENTS

Supported in part by a research grant from the Social Sciences and Humanities Research Council of Canada.

I am indebted to Robert J. Levine, M.D., and to Harold Merskey, D.M., for their valuable suggestions.

REFERENCES

1 Levine RJ. Ethics and regulation of clinical research. 2nd ed. Baltimore: Urban & Schwarzenberg, 1986.
2 *Idem.* The use of placebos in randomized clinical trials. IRB: Rev Hum Subj Res 1985; 7(2):1–4.
3 Fried C. Medical experimentation: personal integrity

and social policy. Amsterdam: North-Holland Publishing, 1974.

4 Marquis D. Leaving therapy to chance. Hastings Cent Rep 1983: 13(4):40–7.

5 Schafer A. The ethics of the randomized clinical trial. N Engl J Med 1982; 307:719–24.

6 Shaw LW, Chalmers TC. Ethics in cooperative clinical trials. Ann NY Acad Sci 1970; 169:487–95.

7 Hollenberg NK, Dzau VJ, Williams GH. Are uncontrolled clinical studies ever justified? N Engl J Med 1980; 303:1067.

8 Levine RJ, Lebacqz K. Some ethical considerations in clinical trials. Clin Pharmacol Ther 1979; 25:728–41.

9 Klimt CR, Canner PL. Terminating a long-term clinical trial. Clin Pharmacol Ther 1979; 25:641–6.

10 Veatch RM. Longitudinal studies, sequential designs and grant renewals: what to do with preliminary data. IRB: Rev Hum Subj Res 1979; 1(4):1–3.

11 Chalmers T. The ethics of randomization as a decision-making technique and the problem of informed consent. In: Beauchamp TL, Walters L, eds. Contemporary issues in bioethics. Encino, Calif.: Dickenson, 1978:426–9.

12 Taylor KM, Margolese RG, Soskolne CL. Physicians' reasons for not entering eligible patients in a randomized clinical trial of surgery for breast cancer. N Engl J Med 1984; 310:1363–7.

13 Chalmers TC. Invited remarks. Clin Pharmacol Ther 1979; 25:649–50.

14 Schafer A. The randomized clinical trial: for whose benefit? IRB: Rev Hum Subj Res 1985; 7(2):4–6.

15 Meier P. Terminating a trial—the ethical problem. Clin Pharmacol Ther 1979; 25:633–40.

16 Prescott RJ. Feedback of data to participants during clinical trials. In: Tagnon HJ, Staquet MJ, eds. Controversies in cancer: design of trials and treatment. New York: Masson Publishing, 1979:55–61.

17 Cowan DH. The ethics of clinical trials of ineffective therapy. IRB: Rev Hum Subj Res 1981; 3(5):10–1.

18 Feinstein AR. An additional basic science for clinical medicine. II. The limitations of randomized trials. Ann Intern Med 1983; 99:544–50.

Justice and the Semi-Randomized Clinical Trial
Robert M. Veatch

Robert M. Veatch is director and professor of medical ethics, Kennedy Institute of Ethics, Georgetown University. Very widely published in biomedical ethics, he is the author of *Death, Dying, and the Biomedical Revolution* (1976), *A Theory of Medical Ethics* (1981), *The Patient as Partner: A Theory of Human Experimentation Ethics* (1987), and *The Patient-Physician Relation* (1991).

Veatch contends that, when subjects have a strong preference for one treatment arm in a randomized clinical trial and are among the least well-off in the population, justice requires that researchers switch to a "semi-randomized clinical trial." As defined by Veatch, such a trial differs from a randomized clinical trial in two ways. (1) Those persons who initially refuse to be randomized are offered the standard treatment and asked for permission to be followed as part of the study. (2) Before randomization, subjects are given the option to drop out of the group to be randomized, receive the experimental therapy, and be followed. The important ethical result, Veatch argues, is that someone (e.g., a cancer patient) who is among the least well-off and believes it is in his or her interests to have the experimental therapy (perhaps for reasons relating to the patient's nonmedical values) will be able to select it; giving patients this option not only respects their autonomy but also promotes justice by benefiting the least

Reprinted with permission of Indiana University Press from Robert M. Veatch, *The Patient as Partner: A Theory of Human-Experimentation Ethics* (1987), pp. 130–135.

well-off. Veatch also makes the case that the semi-randomized trial proves to be better science.

If the [principles of autonomy, beneficence, and justice] are to be the core of an ethic for research involving human subjects in which the subject is a partner in the research, a number of important implications follow for the design of research and the recruitment of subjects. . . . [S]ome of these implications will be explored. One complicated example of a problem arises when subjects have a strong preference for one treatment arm in a randomized clinical trial. The problem is even more complex if the subjects are so poorly off that, for purposes of consideration of the principle of justice, they can be considered among the least well-off of the population. In such circumstances researchers working with subjects may have to shift to what I shall call a "semi-randomized clinical trial."

Consider a typical study on a chronically ill patient with a terminal illness such as cancer. To what extent does justice require that subjects in the typical oncology protocol have access to whichever treatment arm they prefer? Should an IRB insist, contrary to common practice and FDA regulation, that oncology patients be allowed to receive the experimental compound in a clinical trial if the subjects are convinced they would be better off receiving it? The argument favoring this policy would be that the oncology patient who is a member of a least well-off group (compared with others who might be touched by the protocol) should have his or her judgment on available treatment respected since this would predictably improve the lot of a least well-off person. Justice, therefore, would require this policy.

I assume that most persons find this implication absurd. Most will probably find the subject's action irrational. The modification is at least contrary to standard research practice and thought to be potentially damaging to good research. The argument is that such choice is irrational on the part of the subject since research cannot morally be conducted unless there is a legitimate scientific doubt about which of two (or more) treatment options is in the patient's interest. Patients thus have no basis for preferring the experimental treatment. Should they prefer it, they then have been misled by the hope for success.

I am convinced this argument is erroneous. For a protocol to be justified there must be legitimate scientific doubt about which option is medically preferable. It does not follow, though, that individual patients may not have legitimate idiosyncratic, perhaps psychological, reasons for preferring one arm of the study over the other. Some individuals are conservative in their biases and would prefer not to participate in research until the intervention in question is tested further. We recognize the right of such patients to refuse to participate in the study, in effect acting on their conservative world view. Other patients may have uniquely interventionistic world views. They take the view that when in doubt, they should gamble with the high-risk high-gain option. There is nothing irrational about patients, based on their unique psychological world views, preferring one treatment arm over another in spite of the fact that there is no objective *medical* difference known to exist between them. Right now the conservative least well-off patient has the right to withdraw from the study and get the standard treatment, but the interventionistic patient does not have the right to withdraw and get the experimental treatment. If such a patient may rationally prefer that course, justice requires that he be given that opportunity.

I propose that we consider a "semi-randomized clinical trial." Before I discuss its merits, it will be useful to review the ways it differs from the traditional trial. This latter trial begins with a sample whose members are asked to consent to be randomized, let us say, between control or standard treatment and experimental treatment. Some in the sample drop out. They receive some version of the standard treatment, but are not followed. They constitute group 1 in Figure 1. Those who consent are then randomized into the two treatment arms (groups 2a and 2b in Figure 1), and results are compared.

I propose two modifications, which will result in what I call a "semi-randomized clinical trial," in order to fulfill the requirements of justice. First, those who presently refuse randomization (group 1) should be given the option of a standardized form of the usual treatment and should be asked to consent to have their case followed as part of the study. Those who consent remain in the study as group 1b; those refusing (group 1a) are, of course, lost to the follow-up. Second, before randomization, subjects should also be given the option to drop out of the randomization, receive the experi-

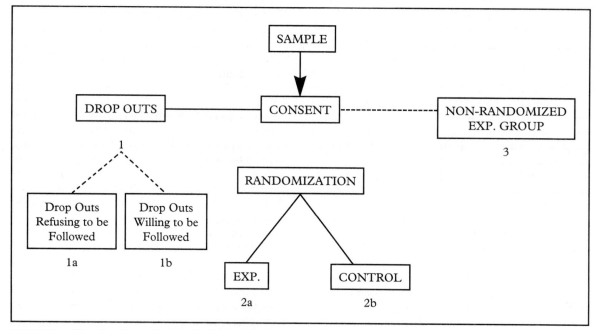

FIGURE 1   The Semi-randomized Clinical Trial. Reprinted from Clinical Research. Vol. 31, No. 1, February, 1983. Published by Charles B. Slack, Inc., Medical Publisher. © AFCR.

mental treatment, and be followed like the non-ran-domized standard treatment group. They would form a new non-randomized experimental group (group 3). The result will be two non-randomized groups (groups 1b and 3) and two randomized ones (groups 2a and 2b), each pair containing a standard treatment group and an experimental treatment group. The result will be that one group of least well-off patients (group 3), which is now deprived of a treatment it desires for good reason, will have an opportunity to have their interests served, thus meeting the demands of the principle of equity.

The main argument against this semi-randomized trial is a scientific one—that the sample is contaminated by the opportunity to opt for the experimental treatment without randomization. To this may be added the argument from efficiency that it will take longer to get an adequate randomized sample. It should be recognized that these are both arguments from beneficence, that is, they are arguments that less benefit will come or greater costs will be incurred if these patients are given this opportunity. As an argument from beneficence, how-ever, it does not cut against the concern for equity or justice upon which the proposal of a semi-randomized trial is based. Just as the right of patients to consent

(based on autonomy) cannot be overridden by consid-eration of good research design (beneficence), so the right of a least well-off group to be benefited (based on justice) cannot be overridden on beneficence grounds.

The researcher and the IRB remain faced with the unhappy conflict between the claims of good science (beneficence) and the claims of justice. This dilemma persists unless it can be shown that the semi-random-ized design turns out to be better science as well as bet-ter ethics. I think this position can be defended.

The scientific argument for use of semi-randomized design is longer and more complicated than the ethical argument, and, in the end, the claim of justice is inde-pendent of the argument about scientific validity. Here we might have just another example of what morality requires being scientifically unacceptable and what sci-ence requires being morally unacceptable.

We need to review the scientific argument for the semi-randomized trial. It is well recognized by persons sophisticated in research design that in order to general-ize findings of such a randomized clinical trial to gen-eral clinical use, some critical assumptions must be made.[1] Among these is the assumption that the results obtained from a randomized experimental group (group 2a) are comparable to the ones that would be obtained from medically identical patients who had not been randomized—patients such as those who might eventually receive the treatment in routine clinical practice. Likewise, it must be assumed that the randomized control (or standard treatment) group (group 2b) produced results that are identical to those that would be found in a non-randomized group receiving the standard treatment. While these assumptions are plausible, they are not necessarily true. In fact subtle differences among populations is the reason for adopting the randomization strategy in the first place.

It would be nice—scientifically more elegant—if we had some partial test to assess the truth of these assumptions. I therefore propose following the dropouts, creating a second control group (the non-randomized group 1b). With these two control groups (1b and 2b) one could test the hypothesis that the medical and social characteristics of those willing to be randomized (2b) and those not so willing (1b) are identical. One could also compare the results of the two groups. Additional techniques designed to test the impact of both physician and patient preferences have been suggested by Freireich.[2]

A study by the Boston Inter-Hospital Liver Group on "Therapeutic Portacaval Anastomosis" published in 1974 in *Gastroenterology* produced a startling conclusion. Patients were randomized between surgical and medical treatment options. Some patients who were randomized into the surgery group nevertheless refused the surgery. To everyone's surprise, it was found that "those patients who were selected for surgery, but who refused it, inexplicably had the best survival of any group in the study."[3]

Those who were randomized to surgery but insisted on medical treatment did better than those randomized to medical treatment. The results were replicated at two separate institutions.[4] Were no data collected on the experimental surgery group dropouts, a remarkable conclusion would have been missed. If dropouts (before and after randomization) are followed, we have the opportunity to test whether a randomized group is identical in relevant diagnostic and outcome variables to a group of non-randomized patients who choose the treatment option because they are convinced it is better for them. If the result is a difference between the randomized and non-randomized groups (for example, between 2b and 1b or between 2a and 3), we may legitimately ask if the data from the randomized group can justifiably be applied to the general population. We, of course, should not conclude that the non-randomized group is identical to the general population of potential users. If a difference in the two control groups (1b and

2b) appears, we are left with the puzzle of which is the more appropriate group for comparing to the general population.

If the randomized and non-randomized groups appear identical in composition and results, we have some tentative supportive evidence to back what otherwise is a blind assumption: that the randomized group is similar to the rest of the population. Since the non-randomized controls (1b) are there for the asking, it is hard to see why they are not followed. Good science and good ethics as well would seem to demand making the comparison.

Likewise, once the problem is realized it seems clear that good science would also require comparing a randomized experimental group (2a) to a non-randomized one (3) made up of patients who, for one reason or another, believe the experimental treatment is good for them. The results of the comparison would help support or call into question what until now is a blind, unwarranted assumption: that patients willing to be randomized who are getting the experimental treatment (2a) are in all relevant respects like the eventual patient in the general population who may receive the treatment on a non-randomized basis. The comparison at least permits us to test whether the willingness to be randomized is itself a critical variable.

The size of the non-randomized experimental group (3) may present some unexpected problems. If a large number of subjects choose the non-randomized experimental treatment, the IRB should be concerned that the initial judgments justifying randomization (that experimental and control options are similar in benefit-harm ratios) may not be warranted. If the research is legitimately undertaken only when there is real doubt on the part of the researchers which treatment is better, we can expect that most potential subjects will likewise be indifferent and therefore will not object to being randomized. In fact, they may have no basis for expressing a preference. If that is the case, our non-randomized experimental group (3) may be shockingly small. If that is the result, I am contending it may lead to worse science. The non-randomized experimental group (3) may not be large enough to test the hypothesis that it is identical to the randomized experimental group (2a). To that I would reply that ethics nevertheless requires that if no one wants to enter the non-randomized experimental group (3), then no one should have to enter it.

At the present time, a random sample is already contaminated by the requirement that patients should be permitted to drop out and receive the standard treatment. We often fail to take advantage of the valuable data the dropout could contribute. I am now arguing that giving patients the opportunity to drop out in favor of the experimental treatment would only contaminate the sample somewhat more. In the exchange we would gain two things: First we would have modified the research design so as to benefit a least well-off group. That is the important change. But second, we would gain the opportunity to test hypotheses about the contamination. We could compare randomized and non-randomized groups in a way never possible before, and we would increase our warrant for the assumption that the results of the protocol can be transferred to the general population.

FINAL TEST

Let us test the semi-randomized design against the three basic principles of ethics of the Belmont Report. First,[5] . . . there can be no doubt that the semi-randomized trial enhances autonomy of subjects, compared to the forced-choice standard randomized design, where in order to get a chance at the experimental treatment patients have to agree to the coercive offer in which they will be randomized and run a risk of being placed in the control group.

The test of beneficence is ambiguous. The semi-randomized trial will require a somewhat larger sample because there is an extra experimental group. It will also require following the group presently refusing randomization and dropping out of the study. It will be seen as contaminating the sample by permitting additional dropouts. But the sample is already contaminated by the dropouts who refuse to consent to be randomized. Furthermore, as never before, the researcher has a chance to study the contamination. He or she has both experimental and control groups (3 and 1b) that are non-randomized so a direct comparison can be made. Moreover, he or she gains some preliminary evidence for what until now has been only a blind assumption about the relationship between the randomized group and the general population. On balance it is debatable whether the semi-randomized design is more beneficial than the full randomization. I am inclined to think semi-randomization is better science, but others might balance the benefits of the alternatives differently.

When the criterion of justice is added to the calculation, the result becomes lopsided in favor of semi-randomization. Now one group of least well-off patients gets to choose its preferred course by dropping out of the study and getting the standard treatment. The other group of least well-off, however, is forced into randomization with all the trauma that may involve for some who desperately want the experimental treatment. Justice—in terms of serving the interests of the least well-off—seems to come down strongly on the side of permitting this small subgroup to choose the experimental arm.

. . . [T]he Belmont Report force[s] researchers and IRBs to move beyond autonomy (or respect for persons) and beneficence to a consideration of justice—justice in the selection of subjects and justice in designing research protocols. Justice is therefore a new item on the agenda. The implications are enormous. It will certainly mean different evaluations of protocols. It may even turn out—if I am correct—that promoting justice in this case also produces better science.

ACKNOWLEDGMENT

The author is grateful to Robert J. Levine and Emil Freireich for helpful comments on an earlier draft of this paper.

NOTES

1 E. J. Freireich and E. A. Gehan, "The Limitations of the Randomized Clinical Trial," *Methods in Cancer Research* 17:277–309.

2 E. J. Freireich, "Informed Consent versus Pre-randomization," in *Adjuvant Therapy of Cancer III,* ed. S. E. Salmon and S. E. Jones (New York: Grune & Stratton, Inc., 1981), pp. 53–62.

3 H. O. Conn, "Therapeutic Portacaval Anastomosis: To Shunt or Not to Shunt," *Gastroenterology* (1974):1067.

4 *Ibid.,* p. 1070.

5 U.S. National Commission for the Protection of Human Subjects, *The Belmont Report: Ethical Principles and Guidelines for the Protection of Human Subjects of Research* (Washington, DC: U.S. Government Printing Office, 1978).

Animal Experimentation

All Animals Are Equal
Peter Singer

Peter Singer is professor of philosophy and director of the Centre for Human Bioethics at Monash University, Victoria, Australia. He is the author of such books as *Animal Liberation* (2d ed., 1990) and *Practical Ethics* (2d ed., 1993). He is coauthor of *Should the Baby Live?* (1985) and coeditor of the journal *Bioethics*.

Singer argues that *speciesism*—a prejudice in favor of the interests of members of one's own species and against those of members of other species—is morally analogous to racism and sexism. Just as we have a moral obligation to give equal consideration to the interests of all human beings, regardless of skin color or sex, we also have an obligation to give equal consideration to the interests of animals. Insofar as animals share with humans the capacity to suffer, they have an interest in not suffering. To discount that interest is speciesist and therefore unethical. In conjunction with his critique of speciesism, Singer attacks our current practice of using animals in experiments that frequently inflict tremendous suffering, often for trivial reasons. As a guideline for determining when an experiment using animals is morally justifiable, he suggests that an experiment is justifiable only if it is so important that it would be justified to use a human being of mental capacities comparable to those of the animals in question.

"Animal Liberation" may sound more like a parody of other liberation movements than a serious objective. The idea of "The Rights of Animals" actually was once used to parody the case for women's rights. When Mary Wollstonecraft, a forerunner of today's feminists, published her *Vindication of the Rights of Woman* in 1792, her views were widely regarded as absurd, and before long an anonymous publication appeared entitled *A Vindication of the Rights of Brutes*. The author of this satirical work (now known to have been Thomas Taylor, a distinguished Cambridge philosopher) tried to refute Mary Wollstonecraft's arguments by showing that they could be carried one stage further. If the argument for equality was sound when applied to women, why should it not be applied to dogs, cats, and horses? The reasoning seemed to hold for these "brutes" too; yet to hold that brutes had rights was manifestly absurd. Therefore the reasoning by which this conclusion had been reached must be unsound, and if unsound when applied to brutes, it must also be unsound when applied to women, since the very same arguments had been used in each case.

Reprinted with permission of the author from *Animal Liberation*, New York Review, second edition (1990), pp. 1–9, 36–37, 40, 81–83, 85–86.

In order to explain the basis of the case for the equality of animals, it will be helpful to start with an examination of the case for the equality of women. Let us assume that we wish to defend the case for women's rights against the attack by Thomas Taylor. How should we reply?

One way in which we might reply is by saying that the case for equality between men and women cannot validly be extended to nonhuman animals. Women have a right to vote, for instance, because they are just as capable of making rational decisions about the future as men are; dogs, on the other hand, are incapable of understanding the significance of voting, so they cannot have the right to vote. There are many other obvious ways in which men and women resemble each other closely, while humans and animals differ greatly. So, it might be said, men and women are similar beings and should have similar rights, while humans and nonhumans are different and should not have equal rights.

The reasoning behind this reply to Taylor's analogy is correct up to a point, but it does not go far enough. There are obviously important differences between humans and other animals, and these differences must give rise to some differences in the rights that each have. Recognizing this evident fact, however, is no barrier to the case for extending the basic principle of equality to nonhuman animals. The differences that exist between men and women are equally undeniable, and the supporters of Women's Liberation are aware that these differences may give rise to different rights. Many feminists hold that women have the right to an abortion on request. It does not follow that since these same feminists are campaigning for equality between men and women they must support the right of men to have abortions too. Since a man cannot have an abortion, it is meaningless to talk of his right to have one. Since dogs can't vote, it is meaningless to talk of their right to vote. There is no reason why either Women's Liberation or Animal Liberation should get involved in such nonsense. The extension of the basic principle of equality from one group to another does not imply that we must treat both groups in exactly the same way, or grant exactly the same rights to both groups. Whether we should do so will depend on the nature of the members of the two groups. The basic principle of equality does not require equal or identical *treatment;* it requires equal consideration. Equal consideration for different beings may lead to different treatment and different rights.

So there is a different way of replying to Taylor's attempt to parody the case for women's rights, a way that does not deny the obvious differences between human beings and nonhumans but goes more deeply into the question of equality and concludes by finding nothing absurd in the idea that the basic principle of equality applies to so-called brutes. At this point such a conclusion may appear odd; but if we examine more deeply the basis on which our opposition to discrimination on grounds of race or sex ultimately rests, we will see that we would be on shaky ground if we were to demand equality for blacks, women, and other groups of oppressed humans while denying equal consideration to nonhumans. To make this clear we need to see, first, exactly why racism and sexism are wrong. When we say that all human beings, whatever their race, creed, or sex, are equal, what is it that we are asserting? Those who wish to defend hierarchical, inegalitarian societies have often pointed out that by whatever test we choose it simply is not true that all humans are equal. Like it or not we must face the fact that humans come in different shapes and sizes; they come with different moral capacities, different intellectual abilities, different amounts of benevolent feeling and sensitivity to the needs of others, different abilities to communicate effectively, and different capacities to experience pleasure and pain. In short, if the demand for equality were based on the actual equality of all human beings, we would have to stop demanding equality.

Still, one might cling to the view that the demand for equality among human beings is based on the actual equality of the different races and sexes. Although, it may be said, humans differ as individuals, there are no differences between the races and sexes as such. From the mere fact that a person is black or a woman we cannot infer anything about that person's intellectual or moral capacities. This, it may be said, is why racism and sexism are wrong. The white racist claims that whites are superior to blacks, but this is false; although there are differences among individuals, some blacks are superior to some whites in all of the capacities and abilities that could conceivably be relevant. The opponent of sexism would say the same: a person's sex is no guide to his or her abilities, and this is why it is unjustifiable to discriminate on the basis of sex.

The existence of individual variations that cut across the lines of race or sex, however, provides us with no defense at all against a more sophisticated opponent of equality, one who proposes that, say, the interests of all those with IQ scores below 100 be given less consideration than the interests of those with ratings over 100. Perhaps those scoring below the mark would, in this society, be made the slaves of those scoring higher. Would a hierarchical society of this sort really be so much better than one based on race or sex? I think not. But if we tie the moral principle of equality to the factual equality of the different races or sexes, taken as a whole, our opposition to racism and sexism does not provide us with any basis for objecting to this kind of inegalitarianism.

There is a second important reason why we ought not to base our opposition to racism and sexism on any kind of factual equality, even the limited kind that asserts that variations in capacities and abilities are spread evenly among the different races and between the sexes: we can have no absolute guarantee that these capacities and abilities really are distributed evenly, without regard to race or sex, among human beings. So far as actual abilities are concerned there do seem to be certain measurable differences both among races and between sexes. These differences do not, of course, appear in every case, but only when averages are taken. More important still, we do not yet know how many of these differences are really due to the different genetic endowments of the different races and sexes, and how many are due to poor schools, poor housing, and other factors that are the result of past and continuing discrimination. Perhaps all of the important differences will eventually prove to be environmental rather than genetic. Anyone opposed to racism and sexism will certainly hope that this will be so, for it will make the task of ending discrimination a lot easier; nevertheless, it would be dangerous to rest the case against racism and sexism on the belief that all significant differences are environmental in origin. The opponent of, say, racism who takes this line will be unable to avoid conceding that if differences in ability did after all prove to have some genetic connection with race, racism would in some way be defensible.

Fortunately there is no need to pin the case for equality to one particular outcome of a scientific investigation. The appropriate response to those who claim to have found evidence of genetically based differences in ability among the races or between the sexes is not to stick to the belief that the genetic explanation must be wrong, whatever evidence to the contrary may turn up; instead we should make it quite clear that the claim to equality does not depend on intelligence, moral capacity, physical strength, or similar matters of fact. Equality is a moral idea, not an assertion of fact. There is no logically compelling reason for assuming that a factual difference in ability between two people justifies any difference in the amount of consideration we give to their needs and interests. *The principle of the equality of human beings is not a description of an alleged actual equality among humans: it is a prescription of how we should treat human beings.*

Jeremy Bentham, the founder of the reforming utilitarian school of moral philosophy, incorporated the essential basis of moral equality into his system of ethics by means of the formula: "Each to count for one and none for more than one." In other words, the interests of every being affected by an action are to be taken into account and given the same weight as the like interests of any other being. A later utilitarian, Henry Sidgwick, put the point in this way: "The good of any one individual is of no more importance, from the point of view (if I may say so) of the Universe, than the good of any other." More recently the leading figures in contemporary moral philosophy have shown a great deal of agreement in specifying as a fundamental presupposition of their moral theories some similar requirement that works to give everyone's interests equal consideration— although these writers generally cannot agree on how this requirement is best formulated.[1]

It is an implication of this principle of equality that our concern for others and our readiness to consider their interests ought not to depend on what they are like or on what abilities they may possess. Precisely what our concern or consideration requires us to do may vary according to the characteristics of those affected by what we do: concern for the well-being of children growing up in America would require that we teach them to read; concern for the well-being of pigs may require no more than that we leave them with other pigs in a place where there is adequate food and room to run freely. But the basic element—the taking into account of the interests of the being, whatever those interests may be— must, according to the principle of equality, be extended to all beings, black or white, masculine or feminine, human or nonhuman.

Thomas Jefferson, who was responsible for writing the principle of the equality of men into the American Declaration of Independence, saw this point. It led him to oppose slavery even though he was unable to free himself fully from his slaveholding background. He wrote in a letter to the author of a book that emphasized the notable intellectual achievements of Negroes in order to refute the then common view that they had limited intellectual capacities:

> Be assured that no person living wishes more sincerely than I do, to see a complete refutation of the doubts I myself have entertained and expressed on the grade of understanding allotted to them by nature, and to find that they are on a par with ourselves . . . but whatever be their degree of talent it is no measure of their rights. Because Sir Isaac Newton was superior to others in understanding, he was not therefore lord of the property or persons of others.[2]

Similarly, when in the 1850s the call for women's rights was raised in the United States, a remarkable black feminist named Sojourner Truth made the same point in more robust terms at a feminist convention:

> They talk about this thing in the head; what do they call it? ["Intellect," whispered someone nearby.] That's it. What's that got to do with women's rights or Negroes' rights? If my cup won't hold but a pint and yours holds a quart, wouldn't you be mean not to let me have my little half-measure full?[3]

It is on this basis that the case against racism and the case against sexism must both ultimately rest; and it is in accordance with this principle that the attitude that we may call "speciesism," by analogy with racism, must also be condemned. Speciesism—the word is not an attractive one, but I can think of no better term—is a prejudice or attitude of bias in favor of the interests of members of one's own species and against those of members of other species. It should be obvious that the fundamental objections to racism and sexism made by Thomas Jefferson and Sojourner Truth apply equally to speciesism. If possessing a higher degree of intelligence does not entitle one human to use another for his or her own ends, how can it entitle humans to exploit nonhumans for the same purpose?[4]

Many philosophers and other writers have proposed the principle of equal consideration of interests, in some form or other, as a basic moral principle; but not many of them have recognized that this principle applies to members of other species as well as to our own. Jeremy Bentham was one of the few who did realize this. In a forward-looking passage written at a time when black slaves had been freed by the French but in the British dominions were still being treated in the way we now treat animals, Bentham wrote:

> The day *may* come when the rest of the animal creation may acquire those rights which never could have been withholden from them but by the hand of tyranny. The French have already discovered that the blackness of the skin is no reason why a human being should be abandoned without redress to the caprice of a tormentor. It may one day come to be recognized that the number of the legs, the villosity of the skin, or the termination of the *os sacrum* are reasons equally insufficient for abandoning a sensitive being to the same fate. What else is it that should trace the insuperable line? Is it the faculty of reason, or perhaps the faculty of discourse? But a full-grown horse or dog is beyond comparison a more rational, as well as a more conversable animal, than an infant of a day or a week or even a month, old. But suppose they were otherwise, what would it avail? The question is not, Can they *reason?* nor Can they *talk?* but, Can they *suffer?*[5]

In this passage Bentham points to the capacity for suffering as the vital characteristic that gives a being the right to equal consideration. The capacity for suffering—or more strictly, for suffering and/or enjoyment or happiness—is not just another characteristic like the capacity for language or higher mathematics. Bentham is not saying that those who try to mark "the insuperable line" that determines whether the interests of a being should be considered happen to have chosen the wrong characteristic. By saying that we must consider the interests of all beings with the capacity for suffering or enjoyment Bentham does not arbitrarily exclude from consideration any interests at all—as those who draw the line with reference to the possession of reason or

language do. The capacity for suffering and enjoyment is *a prerequisite for having interests at all*, a condition that must be satisfied before we can speak of interests in a meaningful way. It would be nonsense to say that it was not in the interests of a stone to be kicked along the road by a schoolboy. A stone does not have interests because it cannot suffer. Nothing that we can do to it could possibly make any difference to its welfare. The capacity for suffering and enjoyment is, however, not only necessary, but also sufficient for us to say that a being has interests—at an absolute minimum, an interest in not suffering. A mouse, for example, does have an interest in not being kicked along the road, because it will suffer if it is.

Although Bentham speaks of "rights" in the passage I have quoted, the argument is really about equality rather than about rights. Indeed, in a different passage, Bentham famously described "natural rights" as "nonsense" and "natural and imprescriptable rights" as "nonsense upon stilts." He talked of moral rights as a shorthand way of referring to protections that people and animals morally ought to have; but the real weight of the moral argument does not rest on the assertion of the existence of the right, for this in turn has to be justified on the basis of the possibilities for suffering and happiness. In this way we can argue for equality for animals without getting embroiled in philosophical controversies about the ultimate nature of rights.

In misguided attempts to refute the arguments of this book, some philosophers have gone to much trouble developing arguments to show that animals do not have rights.[6] They have claimed that to have rights a being must be autonomous, or must be a member of a community, or must have the ability to respect the rights of others, or must possess a sense of justice. These claims are irrelevant to the case for Animal Liberation. The language of rights is a convenient political shorthand. It is even more valuable in the era of thirty-second TV news clips than it was in Bentham's day; but in the argument for a radical change in our attitude to animals, it is in no way necessary.

If a being suffers there can be no moral justification for refusing to take that suffering into consideration. No matter what the nature of the being, the principle of equality requires that its suffering be counted equally with the like suffering—insofar as rough comparisons can be made—of any other being. If a being is not capable of suffering, or of experiencing enjoyment or happiness, there is nothing to be taken into account. So the limit of sentience (using the term as a convenient if not strictly accurate shorthand for the capacity to suffer and/or experience enjoyment) is the only defensible boundary of concern for the interests of others. To mark this boundary by some other characteristic like intelligence or rationality would be to mark it in an arbitrary manner. Why not choose some other characteristic, like skin color?

Racists violate the principle of equality by giving greater weight to the interests of members of their own race when there is a clash between their interests and the interests of those of another race. Sexists violate the principle of equality by favoring the interests of their own sex. Similarly, speciesists allow the interests of their own species to override the greater interests of members of other species. The pattern is identical in each case.

ANIMALS AND RESEARCH

Most human beings are speciesists. . . . Ordinary human beings—not a few exceptionally cruel or heartless humans, but the overwhelming majority of humans—take an active part in, acquiesce in, and allow their taxes to pay for practices that require the sacrifice of the most important interests of members of other species in order to promote the most trivial interests of our own species. . . .

The practice of experimenting on nonhuman animals as it exists today throughout the world reveals the consequences of speciesism. Many experiments inflict severe pain without the remotest prospect of significant benefits for human beings or any other animals. Such experiments are not isolated instances, but part of a major industry. In Britain, where experimenters are required to report the number of "scientific procedures" performed on animals, official government figures show that 3.5 million scientific procedures were performed on animals in 1988.[7] In the United States there are no figures of comparable accuracy. Under the Animal Welfare Act, the U.S. secretary of agriculture publishes a report listing the number of animals used by facilities registered with it, but this is incomplete in many ways. It does not include rats, mice, birds, reptiles, frogs, or domestic farm animals used for experimental purposes; it does not include animals used in secondary schools; and it does not include experiments performed by facilities that do not transport animals interstate or receive grants or contracts from the federal government.

In 1986 the U.S. Congress Office of Technology Assessment (OTA) published a report entitled "Alternatives to Animal Use in Research, Testing and Education." The OTA researchers attempted to determine the number of animals used in experimentation in the U.S. and reported that "estimates of the animals used in the United States each year range from 10 million to upwards of 100 million." They concluded that the estimates were unreliable but their best guess was "at least 17 million to 22 million."[8]

This is an extremely conservative estimate. In testimony before Congress in 1966, the Laboratory Animal Breeders Association estimated that the number of mice, rats, guinea pigs, hamsters, and rabbits used for experimental purposes in 1965 was around 60 million.[9] In 1984 Dr. Andrew Rowan of Tufts University School of Veterinary Medicine estimated that approximately 71 million animals are used each year. In 1985 Rowan revised his estimates to distinguish between the number of animals produced, acquired, and actually used. This yielded an estimate of between 25 and 35 million animals used in experiments each year.[10] (This figure omits animals who die in shipping or are killed before the experiment begins.) A stock market analysis of just one major supplier of animals to laboratories, the Charles River Breeding Laboratory, stated that this company alone produced 22 million laboratory animals annually.[11]

The 1988 report issued by the Department of Agriculture listed 140,471 dogs, 42,271 cats, 51,641 primates, 431,457 guinea pigs, 331,945 hamsters, 459,254 rabbits, and 178,249 "wild animals": a total of 1,635,288 used in experimentation. Remember that this report does not bother to count rats and mice, and covers at most an estimated 10 percent of the total number of animals used. Of the nearly 1.6 million animals reported by the Department of Agriculture to have been used for experimental purposes, over 90,000 are reported to have experienced "unrelieved pain or distress." Again, this is probably at most 10 percent of the total number of animals suffering unrelieved pain and distress—and if experimenters are less concerned about causing unrelieved pain to rats and mice than they are to dogs, cats, and primates, it could be an even smaller proportion.

Other developed nations all use large numbers of animals. In Japan, for example, a very incomplete survey published in 1988 produced a total in excess of eight million.[12] . . .

Among the tens of millions of experiments performed, only a few can possibly be regarded as contributing to important medical research. Huge numbers of animals are used in university departments such as forestry and psychology; many more are used for commercial purposes, to test new cosmetics, shampoos, food coloring agents, and other inessential items. All this can happen only because of our prejudice against taking seriously the suffering of a being who is not a member of our own species. Typically, defenders of experiments on animals do not deny that animals suffer. They cannot deny the animals' suffering, because they need to stress the similarities between humans and other animals in order to claim that their experiments may have some relevance for human purposes. The experimenter who forces rats to choose between starvation and electric shock to see if they develop ulcers (which they do) does so because the rat has a nervous system very similar to a human being's, and presumably feels an electric shock in a similar way.

There has been opposition to experimenting on animals for a long time. This opposition has made little headway because experimenters, backed by commercial firms that profit by supplying laboratory animals and equipment, have been able to convince legislators and the public that opposition comes from uninformed fanatics who consider the interests of animals more important than the interests of human beings. But to be opposed to what is going on now it is not necessary to insist that all animal experiments stop immediately. All we need to say is that experiments serving no direct and urgent purpose should stop immediately, and in the remaining fields of research, we should whenever possible, seek to replace experiments that involve animals with alternative methods that do not. . . .

When are experiments on animals justifiable? Upon learning of the nature of many of the experiments carried out, some people react by saying that all experiments on animals should be prohibited immediately. But if we make our demands as absolute as this, the experimenters have a ready reply: Would we be prepared to let thousand of humans die if they could be saved by a single experiment on a single animal?

This question is, of course, purely hypothetical. There has never been and never could be a single experiment that saved thousands of lives. The way to reply to this hypothetical question is to pose another: Would the experimenters be prepared to carry out their experiment on a human orphan under six months old if that were the only way to save thousands of lives?

If the experimenters would not be prepared to use a human infant then their readiness to use nonhuman animals reveals an unjustifiable form of discrimination on the basis of species, since adult apes, monkeys, dogs, cats, rats, and other animals are more aware of what is happening to them, more self-directing, and, so far as

we can tell, at least as sensitive to pain as a human infant. (I have specified that the human infant be an orphan, to avoid the complications of the feelings of parents. Specifying the case in this way is, if anything, overgenerous to those defending the use of nonhuman animals in experiments, since mammals intended for experimental use are usually separated from their mothers at an early age, when the separation causes distress for both mother and young.)

So far as we know, human infants possess no morally relevant characteristic to a higher degree than adult nonhuman animals, unless we are to count the infants' potential as a characteristic that makes it wrong to experiment on them. Whether this characteristic should count is controversial—if we count it, we shall have to condemn abortion along with experiments on infants, since the potential of the infant and the fetus is the same. To avoid the complexities of this issue, however, we can alter our original question a little and assume that the infant is one with irreversible brain damage so severe as to rule out any mental development beyond the level of a six-month-old infant. There are, unfortunately, many such human beings, locked away in special wards throughout the country, some of them long since abandoned by their parents and other relatives, and, sadly, sometimes unloved by anyone else. Despite their mental deficiencies, the anatomy and physiology of these infants are in nearly all respects identical with those of normal humans. If, therefore, we were to force-feed them with large quantities of floor polish or drip concentrated solutions of cosmetics into their eyes [as has been done in experiments using animals], we would have a much more reliable indication of the safety of these products for humans than we now get by attempting to extrapolate the results of tests on a variety of other species. . . .

So whenever experimenters claim that their experiments are important enough to justify the use of animals, we should ask them whether they would be prepared to use a brain-damaged human being at a similar mental level to the animals they are planning to use. I cannot imagine that anyone would seriously propose carrying out the experiments described in this chapter on brain-damaged human beings. Occasionally it has become known that medical experiments have been performed on human beings without their consent; one case did concern institutionalized intellectually disabled children, who were given hepatitis. When such harmful experiments on human beings become known, they usually lead to an outcry against the experimenters, and rightly so. They are, very often, a further example of the arrogance of the research worker who justifies everything on the grounds of increasing knowledge. But if the experimenter claims that the experiment is important enough to justify inflicting suffering on animals, why is it not important enough to justify inflicting suffering on humans at the same mental level? What difference is there between the two? Only that one is a member of our species and the other is not? But to appeal to that difference is to reveal a bias no more defensible than racism or any other form of arbitrary discrimination. . . .

We have still not answered the question of when an experiment might be justifiable. It will not do to say "Never!" Putting morality in such black-and-white terms is appealing, because it eliminates the need to think about particular cases; but in extreme circumstances, such absolutist answers always break down. Torturing a human being is almost always wrong, but it is not absolutely wrong. If torture were the only way in which we could discover the location of a nuclear bomb hidden in a New York City basement and timed to go off within the hour, then torture would be justifiable. Similarly, if a single experiment could cure a disease like leukemia, that experiment would be justifiable. But in actual life the benefits are always more remote, and more often than not they are nonexistent. So how do we decide when an experiment is justifiable?

We have seen that experimenters reveal a bias in favor of their own species whenever they carry out experiments on nonhumans for purposes that they would not think justified them in using human beings, even brain-damaged ones. This principle gives us a guide toward an answer to our question. Since a speciesist bias, like a racist bias, is unjustifiable, an experiment cannot be justifiable unless the experiment is so important that the use of a brain-damaged human would also be justifiable.

This is not an absolutist principle. I do not believe that it could never be justifiable to experiment on a brain-damaged human. If it really were possible to save several lives by an experiment that would take just one life, and there were no other way those lives could be saved, it would be right to do the experiment. But this would be an extremely rare case. Admittedly, as with any dividing line, there would be a gray area where it was difficult to decide if an experiment could be justified. But we need not get distracted by such considerations now. . . . We are in the midst of an emergency in which appalling suffering is being inflicted on millions of animals for purposes that on any impartial view are obviously inadequate to justify the suffering. When we have ceased to carry out all those experiments, then there will be time enough to discuss what to do about the remaining ones which are claimed to be essential to save lives or prevent greater suffering. . . .

NOTES

1 For Bentham's moral philosophy, see his *Introduction to the Principles of Morals and Legislation,* and for Sidgwick's see *The Methods of Ethics,* 1907 (the passage is quoted from the seventh edition; reprint, London: Macmillan, 1963), p. 382. As examples of leading contemporary moral philosophers who incorporate a requirement of equal consideration of interests, see R. M. Hare, *Freedom and Reason* (New York: Oxford University Press, 1963), and John Rawls, *A Theory of Justice* (Cambridge: Harvard University Press, Belknap Press, 1972). For a brief account of the essential agreement on this issue between these and other positions, see R. M. Hare, "Rules of War and Moral Reasoning," *Philosophy and Public Affairs* 1 (2) (1972).

2 Letter to Henry Gregoire, February 25, 1809.

3 Reminiscences by Francis D. Gage, from Susan B. Anthony, *The History of Woman Suffrage,* vol. 1; the passage is to be found in the extract in Leslie Tanner, ed., *Voices From Women's Liberation* (New York: Signet, 1970).

4 I owe the term "speciesism" to Richard Ryder. It has become accepted in general use since the first edition of this book, and now appears in *The Oxford English Dictionary,* second edition (Oxford: Clarendon Press, 1989).

5 *Introduction to the Principles of Morals and Legislation,* chapter 17.

6 See M. Levin, "Animal Rights Evaluated," *Humanist* 37:14–15 (July/August 1977); M. A. Fox, "Animal Liberation: A Critique," *Ethics* 88: 134–138 (1978); C. Perry and G. E. Jones, "On Animal Rights," *International Journal of Applied Philosophy* 1: 39–57 (1982).

7 *Statistics of Scientific Procedures on Living Animals, Great Britain, 1988,* Command Paper 743 (London: Her Majesty's Stationery Office, 1989).

8 U.S. Congress Office of Technology Assessment, *Alternatives to Animal Use in Research, Testing and Education* (Washington, D.C.: Government Printing Office, 1986), p. 64.

9 Hearings before the Subcommittee on Livestock and Feed Grains of the Committee on Agriculture, U.S. House of Representatives, 1966, p. 63.

10 See A. Rowan, *Of Mice, Models and Men* (Albany: State University of New York Press, 1984), p. 71; his later revision is in a personal communication to the Office of Technology Assessment; see *Alternatives to Animal Use in Research, Testing and Education,* p. 56.

11 OTA, *Alternatives to Animal Use in Research, Testing and Education,* p. 56.

12 *Experimental Animals* 37: 105 (1988).

Immoral and Moral Uses of Animals
Christina Hoff Sommers

Christina Hoff Sommers is associate professor of philosophy, Clark University. Her areas of specialization are ethics, feminism, and the philosophy of education. She is author of *Who Stole Feminism?: How Women Have Betrayed Women* (1994), coeditor of *Vice and Virtue in Everyday Life* (3d ed., 1993), and the author of such articles as "Teaching the Virtues."

Sommers explores the issue of what uses of animals in research, if any, are morally justified. After rebutting some common arguments for the view that the use of animals raises no significant ethical issues, she contends that the capacity to suffer—a capacity that at least mammals and birds have—confers some degree of moral status. However, in Sommer's view, recognizing that animals are entitled to moral consideration, and in particular that their interest in avoiding the trauma of pain is similar to ours, is consistent with recognizing differences in the comparative value of human and animal lives; for, unlike the case of killing an animal, when we kill a human, "[h]is projects, his friendships, and his sense of himself as a human being are also terminated." Sommers draws out the implications of her analysis, arguing that in certain circumstances harming animals for very serious medical purposes is morally defensible. In response to the objection that her view implicitly justifies the harming of certain mentally impaired humans for research purposes (an implication Singer would emphasize), Sommers argues that the likely abuses of any policy allowing the harmful use of humans justify prohibiting such use.

One can do something wrong to a tree, but it makes no sense to speak of wronging it. Can one wrong an animal? Many philosophers think not, and many research scientists adopt the attitude that the use of laboratory animals raises no serious moral questions. It is understandable that they should do so. Moral neutrality toward the objects of one's research is conducive to scientific practice. Scientists naturally wish to concentrate on their research and thus tend not to confront the problems that may arise in the choice of techniques. In

Reprinted by permission of the publisher from *The New England Journal of Medicine,* vol. 302 (January 10, 1980), pp. 115–118. © 1980 Massachusetts Medical Society.

support of this attitude of indifference, they could cite philosophers who point to features peculiar to human life, by virtue of which painful experimentation on unwilling human beings is rightly to be judged morally reprehensible and that on animals not. What are these features?

Rationality and the ability to communicate meaningfully with others are the most commonly mentioned differentiating characteristics. Philosophers as diverse as Aristotle, Aquinas, Descartes, and Kant point to man's deliberative capacities as the source of his moral preeminence. Animals, because they are irrational, have been denied standing. The trouble is that not all human beings are rational. Mentally retarded or severely brain-damaged human beings are sometimes much less intelligent than lower primates that have been successfully taught to employ primitive languages and make simple, logical inferences beyond the capacity of the normal three-year-old child. The view that rationality is the qualifying condition for moral status has the awkward consequence of leaving unexplained our perceived obligations to nonrational humanity.

Some philosophers have therefore argued that man's privileged moral status is owed to his capacity for suffering. To be plausible, this way of explaining man's position as the only being who can be wronged must discount the apparent suffering of mammals and other highly organized creatures. It is sometimes assumed that the subjective experience of pain is quite different for animals and human beings. Descartes, for example, maintains that animals are machines: he speaks of tropisms of avoidance and desire rather than pleasure and pain.[1] Although it is true that human beings can suffer in ways that animals cannot, the idea that animals and human beings experience physical pain differently is physiologically incoherent. We know that animals feel pain because of their behavioral reactions (including writhing, screaming, facial contortions, and desperate efforts to escape the source of pain), the evidence of their nervous systems, and the evolutionary value of pain. (By "animals" I mean mammals, birds, and other organisms of comparable evolutionary complexity.)

There are other sources of human suffering besides pain, but they too are not peculiarly human. One has only to consult the reports of naturalists or go to the zoo or own a pet to learn that the higher animals, at least, can suffer from loneliness, jealousy, boredom, frustration, rage, and terror. If, indeed, the capacity to suffer is the morally relevant characteristic, then the facts determine that animals, along with all human beings, are the proper subjects of moral consideration.

There is, however, another common way of defending human privilege. It is sometimes asserted that "just being human" is a sufficient basis for a protected moral status, that sheer membership in the species confers exclusive moral rights. Each human life, no matter how impoverished, has a depth and meaning that transcends that of even the most gifted dolphin or chimpanzee. One may speak of this as the humanistic principle. Cicero was one of its earliest exponents: "Honor every human being because he is a human being."[2] Kant called it the Principle of Personality and placed it at the foundation of his moral theory.[3] The principle appears evident to us because it is embodied in the attitudes and institutions of most civilized communities. Although this accounts for its intuitive appeal, it is hardly an adequate reason to accept it. Without further argument the humanistic principle is arbitrary. What must be adduced is an acceptable criterion for awarding special rights. But when we proffer a criterion based, say, on the capacity to reason or to suffer, it is clearly inadequate either because it is satisfied by some but not all members of the species *Homo sapiens,* or because it is satisfied by them all—and many other animals as well.

Another type of argument for denying equal consideration to animals goes back at least to Aristotle. I refer to the view that man's tyranny over animals is natural because his superiority as an animal determines for him the dominant position in the natural scale of things. To suggest that man give up his dominance over animals is to suggest that he deny his nature. The argument assumes that "denial of nature" is ethically incoherent. But conformity with nature is not an adequate condition for ethical standards. Being moral does not appear to be a question of abiding by the so-called laws of nature; just as often it seems to require us to disregard what is "natural" in favor of what is compassionate. We avoid slavery and child labor, not because we have discovered that they are unnatural, but because we have discovered that slaves and children have their own desires and interests and they engage our sympathy. Social Darwinism was an ethical theory that sought to deduce moral rules from the "facts" of nature. Wealthy 19th-century industrialists welcomed a theory that seemed to justify inhumane labor practices by reference to the "natural order of things." It has become clear that these so-called "laws" of nature cannot provide an adequate basis for a moral theory, if only because they may be cited to support almost any conceivable theory.

It is fair to say that no one has yet given good reasons to accept a moral perspective that grants a privileged moral status to all and only human beings. A crucial moral judgment is made when one decides that a given course of action with respect to a certain class of beings does not fall within the range of moral consideration. Historically, mistakes at this level have proved dangerous: they leave the agent free to perpetrate heinous acts that are not regarded as either moral or immoral and are therefore unchecked by normal inhibition. The exclusion of animals from the moral domain may well be a similar and equally benighted error. It is, in any case, arbitrary and unfounded in good moral argument.

Whatever belongs to the moral domain can be wronged. But if one rejects the doctrine that membership in the moral domain necessarily coincides with membership in the human species, then one must state a satisfactory condition for moral recognition. Bentham offers an intuitively acceptable starting point. "The question is not, Can they *reason*?, nor, Can they *talk*? but Can they *suffer*?"[4] The capacity to suffer confers a minimal prima facie moral status on any creature, for it seems reasonable that one who is wantonly cruel to a sentient creature wrongs that creature. Animals too can be wronged; the practical consequences of such a moral position are, however, not as clear as they may seem. We must consider what we may and may not do to them.

I begin with a word about the comparative worthiness of human and animal life. Although animals are entitled to moral consideration, it does not follow that animals and human beings are always equal before the moral law. Distinctions must still be made. One may acknowledge that animals have rights without committing oneself to a radical egalitarianism that awards to animals complete parity with human beings. If hunting animals for sport is wrong, hunting human beings for the same purpose is worse, and such a distinction is not inconsistent with recognizing that animals have moral status. Although some proponents of animal rights would deny it, there are morally critical differences between animals and human beings. Animals share with human beings a common interest in avoiding pain, but the complexities of normal human life clearly provide a relevant basis for assigning to human beings a far more serious right to life itself. When we kill a human being, we take away his physical existence (eating, sleeping, and feeling pleasure and pain), but we deprive him of other things as well. His projects, his friendships, and his sense of himself as a human being are also terminated. To kill a human being is not only to take away his life, but to impugn the special meaning of his life. In contrast, an animal's needs and desires are restricted to his place in time and space. He lives "the life of the moment." Human lives develop and unfold; they have a direction. Animal lives do not. Accordingly, I suggest the following differential principle of life worthiness: Human lives are generally worthier than animal lives, and the right to life of a human being generally supersedes the right to life of an animal.

This differential principle rejects the Cartesian thesis, which totally dismisses animals from moral consideration, and it is consistent with two other principles that I have been tacitly defending: animals are moral subjects with claims to considerations that should not be ignored; and an animal's experience of pain is similar to a human being's experience of pain.

In the light of these principles I shall try to determine what general policies we ought to adopt in regulating the use of animals in experimental science. I am limiting myself to the moral questions arising in the specific area of painful or fatal animal experimentation, but some of the discussion will apply to other areas of human interaction with animals. Space does not allow discussion of killing animals for educational purposes.

Scientists who perform experiments on animals rarely see the need to justify them, but when they do they almost always stress the seriousness of the research. Although it may be regrettable that animals are harmed, their suffering is seen as an unavoidable casualty of scientific progress. The moral philosopher must still ask: is the price in animal misery worth it?

That the ends do not always justify the means is a truism, and when the means involve the painful treatment of unwilling innocents, serious questions arise. Although it is notoriously difficult to formulate the conditions that justify the consequences, it is plausible that desired ends are not likely to justify onerous means in the following situations: when those who suffer the means are not identical with those who are expected to enjoy the ends; when there is grave doubt that the justifying ends will be brought about by the onerous means; and when the ends can be achieved by less onerous means.

When a competent surgeon causes pain he does not run afoul of these conditions. On the other hand, social policies that entail mass misery on the basis of tenuous sociopolitical assumptions of great future benefits do run afoul of the last two conditions and often of the first as well. The use of laboratory animals often fails to satisfy these conditions of consequential justification; the first is ignored most frequently (I shall argue that this can often be justified), but scientists often violate the others as well when they carry out painful or fatal experiments with animals that are poorly designed or could have been just as well executed without intact living animals.

We can be somewhat more specific in formulating guidelines for animal experimentation if we consider the equality of animals and human beings with respect to pain. Because there are no sound biologic reasons for the idea that human pain is intrinsically more intense than animal pain, animals and men may be said to be equals with respect to pain. Equality in this case is a measure of their shared interest in avoiding harm and discomfort. The evil of pain, unlike the value of life, is unaffected by the identity of the individual sufferer.

Animals and human beings, however, do differ in

their experience of the aftereffects of pain. When an injury leaves the subject cosmetically disfigured, for example, a human being may suffer from a continuing sense of shame and bitterness, but for the animal the trauma is confined to the momentary pain. Even the permanent impairment of faculties has more serious and lasting aftereffects on human beings than on animals. It can be argued that a person who is stricken by blindness suffers his loss more keenly than an animal similarly stricken.

More important than the subjective experience of privation is the objective diminishment of a valuable being whose scope of activity and future experience have been severely curtailed. In terms of physical privation animals and human beings do not differ, but the measure of loss must be counted far greater in human beings. To sum up: human beings and animals have a parity with respect to the trauma of a painful episode but not with respect to the consequences of the trauma. Yet when an experiment involves permanent impairment or death for the subject and thus considerations of differential life worthiness make it wrong to use most human beings, the pain imposed on the animals should still be counted as intrinsically bad, as if human beings had been made to suffer it, regardless of the aftereffects.

Although I believe that the general inferiority of animal lives to human life is relevant to the formation of public policy, I cannot accept the view that their relative inferiority licenses harming animals except for very serious purposes in rather special circumstances. However, the special circumstances are not necessarily extraordinary. Many experiments, although not as many as is generally supposed, are medically important and needed. The researcher who is working to control cancer and other fatal and crippling diseases may be able to satisfy the conditions that justify the use of laboratory animals. Because I believe that normal human lives are of far greater worth than animal lives, I accept a policy in which those who suffer the means are not those who may enjoy the ends, which violates the first of the conditions of consequential justification mentioned above, by permitting the infliction of pain on animals to save human lives or to contribute substantially to their welfare. However, when researchers intend to harm an animal, they need more than a quick appeal to the worthiness of human life. They ought to be able to show that the resulting benefits are outstandingly compensatory; if the scientist cannot make a good case for the experiment, it should be proscribed. (On the other hand, if suffering is the main consideration in judging the admis-

sibility of experiments with animals, then nonpainful experiments, even fatal ones, may be under fewer constraints than painful, nonfatal experiments. Although this idea may seem paradoxical, it is in accord with the common moral intuition that condones those who put a kitten "to sleep" while condemning those who torment one.) The implementation of this policy raises questions that cannot be dealt with here. Yet one might expect that research proposals involving painful animal experimentation should be reviewed by a panel of experts, perhaps composed of two scientists in the field of the experiment and a scientifically knowledgeable philosopher versed in medical ethics.

In closing, I wish to indicate how I would deal with a possible objection. It may appear that my criteria of life worthiness place human idiots on a par with animals. On what grounds could I prohibit the painful or fatal experimental use of human subjects whose capacity does not differ from that of many animals? I would be prepared to rethink or even abandon a position that could not distinguish between animal and human experimentation. Fortunately, this distinction can be made.

I oppose painful or fatal experimentation on defective, nonconsenting human beings not because I believe that any person, just because he is human, has a privileged moral status, but because I do not believe that we can safely permit anyone to decide which human beings fall short of worthiness. Judgments of this kind and the creation of institutions for making them are fraught with danger and open to grave abuse. It is never necessary to show that an animal's life is not as valuable as that of a normal human being, but just such an initial judgment of exclusion would have to be made for idiots. Because there is no way to circumvent this problem, experiments on human beings are precluded and practically wrong. There are other arguments against experimenting on mentally feeble human beings, but this one seems to me to be the strongest and to be sufficient to support the view that whereas animal experimentation is justifiable, no dangerous or harmful experiments involving unwilling human subjects could be.

Accordingly, I have reached the following conclusions concerning the painful exploitation of animals for human rewards. Animals should not be used in painful experiments when substantial benefits are not expected to result. Even when the objective is important, there is a presumption against the use of animals in painful and dangerous experiments that are expected to yield tenuous results of doubtful value. Animals but not human beings may be used in painful and dangerous experiments that are to yield vital benefits for human beings (or other animals).

Vast numbers of animals are currently being used in all kinds of scientific experiments, many of which entail animal misery. Some of these studies, unfortunately, do not contribute to medical science, and some do not even require the use of intact animals. Even the most conservative corrective measures in the implementation of a reasonable and morally responsible policy would have dramatic practical consequences.

REFERENCES

1 Descartes R. Letter to the Marquess of Newcastle. In: Kenny A, ed. Philosophical letters. Oxford: Oxford University Press, 1970.
2 Cicero. de Finibus.
3 Kant I. In: Paton HJ, ed. Groundwork for a metaphysic of morals.
4 Bentham J. The principles of morals and legislation. New York: Hafner Publishing, 1948:311n.

Transplantation through a Glass Darkly

James Lindemann Nelson

James Lindemann Nelson is associate for ethical studies at The Hastings Center. He is the author of such articles as "Publicity and Pricelessness: Grassroots Decisionmaking and Justice in Rationing," "Moral Sensibilities and Moral Standing: Caplan on Xenograft 'Donors'," and "Making Peace in Gestational Conflicts."

Nelson examines the question of whether baboon organs should be used for transplantation into humans when spare human organs are unavailable. Noting that this question provokes the broader issue of the moral status of animals, he argues that animals, like fetuses, are "moral outliers" in the sense that we are not even close to having a consensus on their moral status. Nelson criticizes numerous arguments supporting xenografts (animal-to-human transplants) without taking a definite position on the moral status of animals. He concludes that, in the absence of clarity on that issue, we should drop xenograft research and therapy—not the least because we have done so little to engage human altruism in obtaining the organs most suitable for transplant, those of human cadavers.

Bioethical problems take many different forms, and fascinate many different kinds of people. Physicians and philosophers, lawyers and theologians, policy analysts and talk show hosts are all drawn by the blend of practical urgency and moral complexity that characterize these issues.

But there seem to be only two kinds of bioethical problems that typically pull into their orbits not only theorists and practitioners, but pickets and protesters as well. When it comes to the treatment of fetuses and animals, people take to the streets. On the same day that

Reprinted with permission of the author and the publisher from *Hastings Center Report*, vol. 22 (September–October 1992), pp. 6–8. © The Hastings Center.

demonstrators on both sides of the abortion issue lamented the Supreme Court's decision in *Casey*, representatives of PETA (People for the Ethical Treatment of Animals) gathered at the University of Pittsburgh to protest the implantation of a baboon's liver in a thirty-five-year-old man—the father of two children—whose own liver had been destroyed by hepatitis B virus.

There is, of course, a big difference in the way the disputes are perceived: abortion's bona fides as a central ethical issue are well established, but despite an upsurge of interest among ethicists over the past decade and a half, concern about animals still seems a bit quirky, too exclusively the domain of zealots who maintain the moral equality of all species, and thereby mark themselves as fundamentally out of sympathy with our basic ethical traditions. Here I try to pull moral consideration of nonhumans closer to the ethical center, arguing that thinking about the fate of nonhumans at our hands shares with abortion—indeed, with many of our culture's most difficult moral issues—a fundamental problem: we don't really know what we are talking about. More concretely, we're at a loss to say what it is about baboons that makes their livers fair game, when we wouldn't dare take vital organs from those of our own species whose abilities to live rich, full lives are no greater than those of the nonhumans we seem so willing to prey upon. Unless we're able to isolate and defend the relevant moral distinction, we should reject the seductive image of solving the problem of organ shortage by maintaining colonies of animals at the ready for transplantation on demand.

MORAL OUTLIERS

Public protest about abortion is not galvanized by concern about the quality of informed consent, or its impact on the doctor-patient relationship. What *does* lie at the center of the dispute is an absolutely crucial kind of ignorance. As a society, we don't know what fetuses are, and, in an important sense, we don't know what pregnant women are either. Are fetuses babies or tissue? Are pregnant women mothers bound by special duties to their unborn children, or independent adults exercising their right to make important self-regarding decisions under the protection of a mantle of privacy? Because we don't know these things, and they matter so much, we have a hard time imagining what responsible compromise might really be like.

And what gets people out into the streets in response to a daring attempt to rescue from certain death a young father of two? What, for that matter, causes medical research advocacy organizations to spend large amounts of money, not on research, but on full-page ads in the *New York Times* defending what scientists do? Is it concerns about justice in the allocation of medical resources? Doubts about the "courage to fail" ethos? Misgivings centered around the independence of IRB review? Surely not. The ground of protest and counterprotest is a similar kind of ignorance about the fundamental terms of the relevant moral discourse: we don't know what animals are, either. We treat them as if they were morally protean; we mold them into anything from much-loved companions and symbols of virtue to mere machines for making food and instruments for scientific research.

Our ignorance as a society about these dark corners of our moral commitments, our lack of consensus about where outliers really fit, is extremely divisive when coupled with individual assurance that there is in fact available knowledge about these matters, that the answers are of surpassing importance, and that there is something suspicious, if not downright evil, about the people who don't get it. While such conclusions cripple civility, and should of course be resisted, our history should be making us nervous. We have so often gotten matters of who counts morally just flatly wrong, and have exacted horrible prices from those shuffled unjustly to the margins of our moral concern.

What fetuses are has at least received a thorough airing in the bioethics literature. Gravid women we still find quite puzzling apparently, as witness current concerns about "forced cesareans" and "maternal-fetal conflict," but at least there is an awareness that getting clear about the moral character of pregnancy is a key to understanding the morality of pregnancy terminations. But despite their ubiquity in medical research and practice, determining what animals are is not thought of as a paradigmatic bioethics issue. Yet seeing animals clearly is likely to be at least as difficult as the analogous tasks for fetuses and pregnant women. After all, we have a strong stake in the presumption that nonhumans are things whose moral status is at our discretion: the looser we can keep the moral constraints, the freer we are to do as we like with these extremely useful creatures. Further, there is a sense in which animals really are protean. Human beings are animals; so are protozoa. Drawing some moral distinctions is inescapable when facing such a range, and if there's to be a bright line between entities that really matter and those that don't, the human species may very well seem a reasonable place to draw it.

Choosing this line may appear suspiciously self-serving. Yet, at least at first glance, it looks as though there really could be something ethically serious to be said for us. We don't have to rely on the brute fact that we've got all the power; this is a comfort, as "might makes right" has a dubious history as a basis for moral distinctions. Nor do we have to resort to the bare fact of our common species membership—again, all to the good, as such purely biological bases for moral categorization also have a simply horrifying pedigree. Further, we can avoid invoking the soul as a sort of special moral talisman whose possession elevates us above all others: purely metaphysical entities aren't much use when we're trying to do ethics with an eye to public policy in a pluralistic society. Besides, imagine what we would do if someone were to argue that the subjugation of women was justified on the grounds that all and only men possess "schmouls," an empirically undetectable entity that inexplicably gives them extra moral worth.

The distinction we wish to draw between humans and the rest of creation seems much more respectable than distinctions based on might, on species, or on sectarian metaphysics. One could say that the appeal to such things as the range and power of the human intellect, the complexity and depth of our interpersonal relationships, our passions, both personal and aesthetic, our sense of morality, and of tragedy makes good sense. If these abilities and vulnerabilities don't matter morally, it's hard to imagine what would.

But if these are the characteristics that matter morally, it is not only baboons who lack them; not all of us humans have them either. Many humans have lost, or will never have, powerful intellects, deep relationships, rich passions, or the intimations of mortality. Think of the profoundly mentally ill, the comatose, and those who have sustained severe brain injuries. While such humans are themselves instances of tragedy, they have no sense of what tragedy is.

Despite this sad fact, our convictions about the importance of simply being human are so strong that we hesitate to use organs from newborns with anencephaly, a condition incompatible with either sensation or life. Given this hesitation, one can imagine the response if a leading transplant surgeon were to call for the maintenance of colonies of mentally handicapped orphans, to be well cared for until needed, but whose organs would then be "humanely" harvested for use in dying but otherwise "normal" people—infants with hypoplastic left heart syndrome, young fathers with HVB. Yet this scenario—with baboons and other primates substituting for handicapped orphans—is precisely what some transplant surgeons have been advocating since at least the 1960s, and is quite explicitly part of the agenda underlying the recent effort in Pittsburgh. If we are morally repulsed by a call to use handicapped orphans, but are eager to see whether colonies of baboons mightn't become a solution to our endemic lack of transplantable organs, it surely behooves us to have a good answer to the question, "What's so different about the two kinds of creature?"

Perhaps there is a good answer to that question—a difference, or set of overlapping differences, that will end up ethically supporting our practice. Perhaps we could, without arbitrary prejudice, keep all mentally handicapped humans, no matter how damaged or how alone in the world they might be, in the ethical family,

so to speak. Perhaps it's appropriate to see all nonhumans, no matter how intelligent or complex their lives might be, as largely discretionary items, to be cast into the outer darkness if anything approaching a serious purpose seems to demand it. Or perhaps the real moral of the story here is that it is not baboons we should respect more, but humans who are their emotional and intellectual peers we should respect less; consider the research and therapeutic bonanza *that* would yield! But defending either of these conclusions would take a powerful argument, and there's very little evidence that any of the people most enthusiastically thumping the tub for more and better xenotransplantation have come up with reasons of the kind that are needed. Typically, their strategy is simply to point to the human cost of not pushing the xenograft agenda—the "three people who die every day waiting for a necessary organ" argument—without any serious attempt to balance that cost against the debit incurred to the victims of those grafts. Nor do we see much effort to set the xenograft strategy against the costs and benefits incurred by trying to enforce the required request laws that are already on the books, or to enact "presumed consent" or "routine retrieval" policies for organ procurement.

DISCERNMENT IN THE DARK

This, of course, returns us to our original problem: we don't even know how to begin that balancing act, and it seems that we aren't very keen on learning. A simple reliance on our moral intuitions isn't enough. As the history of medical research in the nineteenth and even twentieth century reveals, we have been more than willing to subject those who were "clearly less valuable" to the rigors of research—only then, the ones who were obviously less valuable were Jewish, or people of color. Our gut instincts simply aren't good enough as reliable moral guides when we're dealing with those whom we've pushed to the margin of moral discourse. The question is not whether we're generally able to move deftly within our ordinary understanding of morality, but whether, when it comes to the moral outliers, that ordinary understanding itself is adequate.

Cross-species transplantation crystallizes a certain kind of moral conflict between humans and other animals—perhaps too sharply. Pitting the life of the father of two against that of a baboon is sure to strike most of us as no contest. The glare of the contrast distracts us from such realities as the fact that, at the point of decisionmaking, the animal's death buys only a chance, not a guarantee, or that the outcome of acting is not always better than the outcome of refraining, even when death is inevitable if we stay our hand. If we reflect about our moral duties and liberties more broadly, it may strike us that we are apparently quite comfortable allowing many tragic deaths to occur daily, when what it would take to stop them is not the life of an intelligent animal, but merely the cost of drinks after work.

On the other hand, if we do refuse to take the baboon's life in an effort to save the human's out of a sense that the moral parity between baboons and mentally handicapped humans leaves us no other option, then we need to ask what else that sense of parity implies. The animal who provided the liver in the Pittsburgh case was at least killed in an effort to save the life of an identifiable person. But most of what we do with the lives of animals is—at best—only distantly related to the lives and health of people in general. If it is wrong to kill a baboon to try to save a man's life, is it wrong to kill a pig because sausages taste so good? To kill a kid to make elegant gloves? Critics of xenograft whose main concern is with the "sacrificed" animal may find it relatively easy to adopt vegan diets and eschew wearing leather. But do they really advocate that ill people begin a wholesale boycott of a medical system in which the training and research leading up to its quite standard offerings are, as it were, drenched in the blood of nonhumans?

The implications of all this for the development of xenograft and the creation of "donor" colonies are comparatively clear. There are numerous ways in which we might strive to save and enhance lives, including many that are more efficient than killing animals who resemble us in no small degree—ways that do not burden us by reinforcing our commitment to moral positions we do not fully understand, and may not be able to maintain. If we feel morally constrained to continue organ transplantation as an important way of saving and enhancing human lives, we ought not to try to respond to that moral challenge with the technological fix of a better antirejection drug that will allow us to use nonhumans as organ sources, but rather by figuring out better ways to engage the altruism of the human community, until at last it strikes us all as mighty peculiar that anyone would want to hang on to her organs after death, when she has no conceivable use for them.

We ought to drop xenograft research and therapy, investing the resources of human effort, ingenuity, and money it consumes elsewhere. We don't now know what the judgment of history regarding our relationship with nonhumans will be, but there's no reason to be sanguine about it. What this uncertainty says for our overall relationship with animals may still be a matter for debate, but there's no compelling need to make matters any worse.

ANNOTATED BIBLIOGRAPHY: CHAPTER 4

Appelbaum, Paul S., et al.: "False Hopes and Best Data: Consent to Research and the Therapeutic Misconception," *Hastings Center Report* 17 (April 1987), pp. 20–24. The authors focus on the potential conflict, in randomized clinical trials, between seeking generalizable knowledge and serving patients' best interests. After arguing that patient-subjects commonly labor under the "therapeutic misconception"—the denial of the possibility that one's participation in RCTs can be seriously disadvantageous to oneself—the authors maintain that proper educational efforts can dispel this misconception for many subjects.

Bateson, Patrick: "When to Experiment on Animals," *New Scientist* 20 (February 1986), pp. 30–32. Bateson proposes a framework for managing the conflict between the potential benefits of animal research and ethical concerns about using animals. His analysis of when animal research is justified is summarized in a decision cube that represents the dimensions of (1) quality of research, (2) certainty of medical benefit, and (3) animal suffering.

DeGrazia, David: "The Moral Status of Animals and Their Use in Research: A Philosophical Review," *Kennedy Institute of Ethics Journal* 1 (March 1991), pp. 48–70. DeGrazia summarizes five leading theories about the moral status of animals and traces their implications for the use of research animals. After arguing that these theories converge in some of their implications, he identifies several leading issues for future investigation.

Erwin, Edward, Sidney Gendin, and Lowell Kleiman, eds.: *Ethical Issues in Scientific Research: An Anthology* (New York: Garland, 1994). This anthology includes articles on a wide range of ethical issues in research, including such topics as fraud and deception in research, research on humans, animal research, genetic research, and controversial topics such as the debate over the inheritability of intelligence.

Greenwald, Robert A., Mary Kay Fyan, and James E. Mulvihill: *Human Subjects Research: A Handbook for Institutional Review Boards* (New York: Plenum, 1982). This is a useful, practical handbook for members of institutional review boards (IRBs) as well as for those engaged in research using human subjects.

Holmes, Helen Bequaert: "Can Clinical Research Be Both Ethical and Scientific?", *Hypatia* 4 (Summer 1989), pp. 154–165. Holmes argues that conflicts between physicians' therapeutic and research obligations in clinical research may result, in part, from excessive faith in the objectivity of science and in statistics. She contends that feminist approaches to clinical research hold promise for more satisfactorily dealing with the ethical and scientific issues involved.

IRB: A Review of Human Subjects Research (Briarcliff Manor, NY: The Hastings Center). This periodical, published ten times a year, is devoted to articles dealing with the ethical aspects of research involving human subjects.

Jonas, Hans: "Philosophical Reflections on Experimenting with Human Subjects," in Paul Freund, ed., *Experimentation with Human Subjects* (New York: Braziller, 1970), pp. 1–31. In this classic essay, Jonas challenges common arguments for the view that the use of human subjects in medical experimentation is morally justified. While Jonas does not argue that all such research is unjustified, he maintains that researchers and other scientists should be the first volunteers in justifiable research.

Journal of Medicine and Philosophy 11 (November 1986). This issue, entitled "Ethical Issues in the Use of Clinical Controls," is edited by Kenneth F. Schaffner. Schaffner himself provides a historical and methodological context for the essays in this volume, and the essays deal with some of the problems posed by clinical trials in general as well as by RCTs and prerandomized clinical trials in particular.

Journal of Medicine and Philosophy 13 (May 1988). This issue, "Animals in Research," is edited by Tom L. Beauchamp and Tom Regan. The essays explore such issues as whether any use of animals in research is justified, what standards should guide the use of animals, and what sort of ethical review of animal research is appropriate.

Katz, Jay, with Alexander M. Capron and Eleanor Swift Glass, eds.: *Experimentation with Human Beings: The Authority of the Investigator, Subject, Professions, and State in the Human Experimentation Process* (New York: Russell Sage, 1972). This excellent, well-organized collection of edited materials includes discussions of the function and limitations of informed consent, of research on specific subject groups, and of many other research-related topics.

Kodish, Eric, John D. Lantos, and Mark Siegler: "The Ethics of Randomization," *CA— A Cancer Journal for Clinicians* 41 (May/June 1991), pp. 180–187. The authors explore ethical issues arising from the randomization of subjects in randomized clinical trials. Drawing from two important cases—the AZT study and a major study of breast-cancer patients— they argue for restrictive conditions on the use of RCTs.

Marquis, Don: "Leaving Therapy to Chance," *Hastings Center Report* 13 (August 1983), pp. 40–47. Marquis argues that RCTs as presently conducted are unethical despite providing important benefits.

National Commission for the Protection of Human Subjects of Biomedical and Behavioral Research: *The Belmont Report: Ethical Principles and Guidelines for the Protection of Human Subjects of Research.* DHEW (OS) 78-0012. *The Belmont Report. Appendix,* Vols. 1,2.

DHEW (OS) 78-0013, 78-0014. (Bethesda, MD, 1978). This report was put out by a commission established under the National Research Act (P.L. 93-348). The commission's purpose was to develop ethical guidelines for the conduct of research involving human subjects and to make recommendations for the application of these guidelines to research conducted or supported by the Department of Health, Education, and Welfare. *The Belmont Report* is the commission's final and most general report. The appendices to this report contain useful papers and other materials that were reviewed by the commission prior to formulating its recommendations.

Smith, Jane A., and Kenneth M. Boyd: *Lives in the Balance: The Ethics of Using Animals in Biomedical Research* (Oxford: Oxford University Press, 1991). This book is a report of a working party of the Institute of Medical Ethics (Great Britain) that met 18 times to examine ethical issues related to animal research. Notable for both thoroughness and moderation, the book is especially helpful in addressing scientific aspects of the study of animals' mental states.

Taylor, Kathryn M., Richard G. Margolese, and Colin L. Soskolne: "Physicians' Reasons for Not Entering Eligible Patients in a Randomized Clinical Trial of Surgery for Breast Cancer," *New England Journal of Medicine* 310 (May 24, 1984), pp. 1363–1367. This report illustrates some of the ethical problems raised by RCTs. The reasons identified for physicians' reluctance include (1) concern about the effect that the RCT would have on the doctor-patient relationship, (2) difficulties with informed consent, and (3) perceived conflicts between the roles of clinician and scientist.

Warren, John W., et al.: "Informed Consent by Proxy: An Issue in Research with Elderly Patients," *New England Journal of Medicine* 315 (October 30, 1986), pp. 1124–1128. The authors studied the proxy decisions made on behalf of 168 nursing home patients whose participation was requested in a study involving minimal risk. They discuss the reasons that led almost half of the proxies to refuse consent.

CHAPTER 5

MENTAL ILLNESS, DEMENTIA, AND MENTAL RETARDATION

INTRODUCTION

What social policies are appropriate in regard to persons whose autonomy is diminished due to internal factors such as mental illness, dementia, and mental retardation? Policies have a great impact on the roles played by professionals in the lives of such individuals. However, policies by no means entirely determine these roles or answer all related ethical questions. This chapter focuses on several ethical issues involving policies and less formal strategies for dealing with different types of mentally impaired persons.

Mental Illness and Involuntary Civil Commitment

Mental illness poses both personal and social problems. On the personal level, mental illness can severely incapacitate individuals, disrupt family relationships, and make everyday living a hazardous, torturous affair. Mentally ill individuals who are seriously disoriented or deluded may be unable to care for their routine needs and may thus pose a significant risk to their own well-being. Those who are profoundly depressed may run the risk of committing suicide. Extremely agitated or confused individuals may pose a threat of substantial harm not just to themselves but to their families as well. On a wider social level, the mentally ill may be nuisances, may disrupt social activities, and may engage in antisocial behavior. In light of all this, questions arise concerning the state's legitimate role regarding those classified as mentally ill. Does morality permit—or perhaps even require—laws that give representatives of the state, such as judges and psychiatrists, the power to control the lives of the mentally ill? This power is exercised when patients are committed to psychiatric hospitals (or psychiatric units on hospitals) against their will; it is also exercised when patients are treated without their informed and voluntary consent.

The Concept of Mental Illness   The ethics of state interference in the lives of the mentally ill is complicated by the difficulty of defining *mental illness*. In modern physiological medicine, a patient might be diagnosed as suffering from leukemia. The patient is said to have a certain pathological condition, a physical disease. He or she is physically ill. In modern psychiatry, a patient might be diagnosed as suffering from a type of schizophrenia. The patient is said to have a certain psychopathological condition, a mental disease. He or she is mentally ill.

In our culture, when labels such as *insane* or *sick* are applied so casually to human behavior or mental functioning, it is easy to feel puzzled in the face of the concepts of mental health and mental illness. Our difficulty, however, is not limited to the confusion that is produced by the offhand misuse of such labels. If we had access to a firmly entrenched, widely accepted theory of mental health, we would probably feel ourselves to be on firmer ground. But that is just the problem. Mental health professionals subscribe to widely varying theories of mental health. Moreover, psychiatrists in the same school of thought often disagree about whether or not a particular diagnosis is applicable in an individual case.

It is sometimes alleged, most prominently in the work of psychiatrist Thomas S. Szasz, that mental illness is a myth. According to Szasz, as reflected in his selection in this chapter, the concept of mental illness has no scientific or descriptive content whatsoever and thus ought to be abandoned. Although it masquerades as a scientific concept, it functions in an exclusively normative way. When someone is labeled "mentally ill," Szasz holds, it is solely because that individual has deviated from certain ethical, political, or social norms. A more common view, however—one assumed by Paul Chodoff in a reading reprinted here—is that mental illness is a medical reality, however difficult it may be to define.

Involuntary Civil Commitment   Views on the justifiability of involuntary civil commitment often reflect underlying conceptions of mental illness. For example, Szasz argues that involuntary civil commitment is a crime against humanity and should be abolished.[1] Szasz's stance is clearly related to his "social deviance model" of mental illness. However, those who believe that mental illness is a definable reality rather than a myth are typically inclined to consider involuntary civil commitment justifiable in some circumstances. Chodoff discusses both the abolitionist position on involuntary civil commitment and the contrasting views of those who, like him, adopt a medical model of mental illness.

Clearly, those involved in disputes about the ethics of involuntary civil commitment often disagree about the concept of mental illness. They also often disagree on empirical issues, such as the "dangerousness" of mentally ill persons or the extent of their competence. The bearing of these empirical disagreements on moral positions regarding involuntary civil commitment emerges in the following discussion concerning the kinds of moral justifications advanced for the practice.

Explorations of the ethics of involuntary civil commitment usually involve implicit or explicit discussion of the liberty-limiting principles presented in Chapter 1. Should those classified as mentally ill be committed on any of the following grounds: (1) to keep them from substantially harming others (the harm principle), (2) to prevent them from offending others (the offense principle), (3) to keep them from harming themselves (the principle of paternalism), or (4) to benefit them (the principle of extreme paternalism)?

In assessing attempted justifications of involuntary civil commitment, we must keep two other questions in mind. (1) Which of the preceding principles are morally acceptable liberty-limiting principles? (2) Which principle is actually being used (explicitly or implicitly) to justify commitment? In regard to the first question, for example, if the principles of paternalism are *not* acceptable liberty-limiting principles, involuntary civil commitment cannot be justified on paternalistic grounds. Regarding the second, critics of involuntary civil commitment often argue that although it is not uncommon to commit individuals to psychiatric hospitals simply because their behavior is offensive, the attempt to justify their commitment is made on inapplicable grounds, such as their supposed dangerousness. Much of the behavior that earns the mentally ill the label *dangerous* is at most offensive to others. Shouting harangues on street corners and other bizarre behaviors, although offensive to some, pose no threat of serious harm. If offensive behavior is the real basis for committing someone, then the justifying ground would have to be provided by the offense principle and not the harm principle. However, few of us would hold that offensive behavior alone justifies significant deprivations of liberty. Therefore, exposing the actual reasons for commitment in certain cases may lead to the conclusion that interference in these cases is not justified.

Dangerousness and the Harm Principle   Since the harm principle is a widely accepted liberty-limiting principle, that principle would provide a strong ground for the involuntary civil commitment of mentally ill persons *if* they pose a serious threat of harm to others. It is not surprising, then, that the harm principle is often invoked, implicitly or explicitly, to justify involuntary civil commitment procedures. But are the mentally ill so dangerous that their commitment is necessary to protect others from harm? To answer this question, it is necessary to distinguish between different kinds of cases.

In some cases there is very little doubt that those labeled "mentally ill" are dangerous and pose a *serious threat of physical harm to others*. One example is a schizophrenic who attempts to carry out the commands of a disembodied voice ordering the execution of parents or siblings. Another example is a paranoid individual with a history of violent and apparently irrational acts who gives every indication of being ready to repeat such acts. Thus, in cases involving either great likelihood of substantial physical violence or its actual occurrence, involuntary civil commitment seems to be justified by the harm principle. Still, not everyone would agree with this conclusion. Abolitionists such as Szasz, for example, want no special treatment for those considered mentally ill. If they perform acts forbidden by law, they should be subject to the same legal sanctions as anyone else. However, if they break no laws, the state has no moral right to interfere with their freedom.

Even if this point of view is wrong, however, and the harm principle is correctly invoked in justifying *some* involuntary civil commitments, it does not follow that it justifies the commitment of everyone who is labeled "mentally ill"—or even everyone labeled both "mentally ill" and "dangerous." Studies have been conducted that suggest either that psychiatric patients as a group are no more dangerous than others[2] or that, if they are, the differences are so small that they allow very little success in prediction.[3] Moreover, while responsible mental health professionals today attribute dangerousness only to certain mentally ill individuals (rather than assuming that the mentally ill are generally dangerous), there has been considerable controversy regarding the accuracy or inaccuracy of such attributions.[4] If attributions of dangerousness are highly inaccurate yet are accepted as sufficient justification for involuntary commitment, then many nondangerous individuals will be committed on grounds that, in fact, do not apply.

Paternalism and Autonomy   As we saw in Chapter 1, taking decisions out of people's hands for their own good is paternalistic. When individuals are incapable of making decisions about their own well-being, there is no usurpation of autonomy, since the conditions for acting autonomously are absent. In these cases it would be incorrect to hold that the individual's autonomy has been infringed, interfered with, or limited. Problematic cases arise, however, when an individual's abilities to deliberate effectively and make decisions are diminished by delusions, compulsions, or other internal factors associated with mental illness—yet the person is an adult capable of understanding enough about his or her situation to refuse commitment. How much weight should be given to a refusal in such cases? Proponents of paternalistic interventions sometimes argue as follows. Suppose individuals reject commitment or psychiatric help because their present condition renders them incapable of realizing that such measures are in their own long-term interest. If they were thinking more clearly, if they were not confused or severely depressed, would they not want the benefits involved? Would they not want others to keep them from running the risks entailed by their rejection of commitment? Would they not want the treatment that would restore their competence for rational decision making—a competence that is presently limited by internal factors? Those who argue in this way believe that the autonomy of those diagnosed as mentally ill is sometimes sufficiently diminished to justify their involuntary commitment not only to keep them from harming themselves but also to help them in regaining lost autonomy.

Managing Mental Illness and Dementia

The compromised cognitive functioning of many mentally ill persons is chronic in nature. The cognitive deficits of persons suffering from dementia (a general mental deterioration, typically due to organic factors and characterized by memory loss) are also usually chronic. Many schizophrenics cannot be cured but can, under optimal conditions, be more or less stabilized; the same is true for many persons with bipolar (manic-depressive) disorder. Dementia in elderly persons might not be reversible but some of them might be able to cope relatively well with their deficits. Thus, for many chronically mentally ill or demented persons, a realistic goal is *managing*, rather than *curing*, their conditions.

The idea of managing mental illness and dementia has another important aspect. Whereas policies regarding individuals with cognitive deficits set certain *clear boundaries* for acceptable professional behavior—such as prohibiting involuntary civil commitment unless certain conditions are met—policies do not provide answers for many of the difficult ethical and practical issues concerning these individuals. For this reason, it is sometimes necessary for involved persons to work *creatively and resourcefully*, within limits set by relevant policies, in an effort to cope with the challenges that arise; in this sense, too, they must manage mental illness or dementia. Some of the ethical issues that arise in the effort to manage mental illness and dementia are taken up in this chapter.

In the 1960s and 1970s, in the movement toward deinstitutionalization, many of those who had been committed to psychiatric hospitals were released and returned to the community. In contrast to involuntary civil commitment, the ideal of deinstitutionalization, which incorporates an emphasis on community health-care centers, held out a promise that the chronically mentally ill would receive care without infringement of their civil rights. Deinstitutionalization was officially defined by E. Fuller Torrey, director of the National Institute of Mental Health, as follows:

> (1) The prevention of inappropriate mental hospital admissions through the provision of community alternatives for treatment, (2) the release to the community of all institutionalized patients who have been given adequate preparation for such a change, and (3) the establishment and maintenance of community support systems for noninstitutionalized people receiving mental health services in the community.[5]

Whatever the original ideal, deinstitutionalization has in fact resulted in a massive dumping of the chronically ill into communities with few facilities and little aftercare. Between 1955 and 1984, 433,407 psychiatric hospital beds were taken out of use.[6] In addition, many state psychiatric hospitals were closed, in effect leaving many of the long-term mentally ill with nowhere to go.

In his book *Nowhere to Go,* Torrey maintains that the effects of the policy of deinstitutionalization include the following:

(1) There are at least twice as many seriously mentally ill individuals living on streets and in shelters as there are in public mental hospitals. (2) There are increasing numbers of seriously mentally ill individuals in the nation's jails and prisons. (3) Seriously mentally ill individuals are regularly released from hospitals with little or no provision for aftercare or followup treatment. . . . (4) Laws designed to protect the rights of the seriously mentally ill primarily protect their right to remain mentally ill. . . . (5) The majority of mentally ill individuals discharged from hospitals have been officially lost. Nobody knows where they are.[7]

In one of this chapter's readings, H. Richard Lamb discusses deinstitutionalization. Although he believes that many things have gone right with deinstitutionalization, he points out some of its unfortunate results and discusses changes that need to be made. His article is addressed primarily to mental-health professionals whose task he sees as maximizing the benefits of deinstitutionalization for those who suffer from long-term mental illness and yet are capable of living as part of the community. Like Chodoff, however, Lamb holds that there are some long-term mentally ill individuals who, for either long or short periods of time, need highly structured care. Such care, Lamb notes, can only be provided in a hospital or in some alternative setting such as California's locked, skilled-nursing facilities, which have special programs for psychiatric patients.

Deinstitutionalization raises ethical questions regarding those chronically mentally ill individuals who are affected by this movement—in particular, those who must manage their conditions on the "outside" with less than ideal sources of support. Other ethical questions arise in conjunction with the management of specific conditions related to mental illness, such as suicidality. In an article reprinted in this chapter, Samuel L. Pauker and Arnold M. Cooper explore the implications of psychiatry's limited ability to care for suicidal patients, whose behavior can defy predictions and whose conditions are not always treatable. It is tempting for mental-health professionals, the authors note, to be extremely protective of patients at high risk for suicide (e.g., putting them under constant observation). However, they argue, often such protectiveness causes further psychological deterioration, diminished functioning, and loss of autonomy. Pauker and Cooper contend that keeping the patient alive is not the only goal of psychiatric treatment; since psychological health and independent functioning are also important goals, the most appropriate management of suicidal patients may entail taking some risks with their lives.

In addition to mental illness and specific conditions such as suicidality, dementia poses ethical and practical challenges to afflicted persons and those trying to assist them. In one of this chapter's readings, David T. Watts, Christine K. Cassel, and Timothy Howell discuss issues that arise in connection with demented elderly persons whose diminished competence appears to put them at risk of harm yet who resist liberty-limiting safety measures. As with the suicidal patients just discussed, promoting or respecting the autonomy of these individuals may require accepting some risk of serious harm or death. In the authors' view, resolving the dilemmas posed by such demented persons requires nuanced and creative responses to the specifics of each case.

The Mentally Retarded—Sterilization and Rights

The mentally ill are not the only group whose members have at times been almost routinely institutionalized in the past or whose freedoms have been limited because of their presumed incompetence in decision making. Many mentally retarded individuals have spent their lives in institutions. Many have been denied educational and other opportunities. Some have been sterilized without their consent. In many states today, even the mildly retarded, if considered legally incompetent, cannot marry, have children, live alone, or enter into any contractual relations without a guardian's consent. As in the case of the mentally ill, the usual reason given for denying even those who are mildly retarded the freedom of decision possessed by other adults is the purported danger they pose to themselves and others. Competence, however, is not all or nothing. Individuals may lack the cognitive skills to solve a geometric problem yet have sufficient cognitive ability to make everyday decisions about housing, meals, and other practical affairs. More than three-quarters of those considered retarded in our society are classified as "mildly retarded." Those who fit this classification have an IQ range of 52–68 as measured on the Stanford-Binet scale, and their ability to function on a day-to-day level differs widely, depending on their education, training, and experience.

The routine paternalistic treatment of the mentally retarded, especially of the mildly retarded, has been increasingly challenged. One practice around which challenges have been centered is involuntary sterilization. Robert Neville, however, offers arguments in this chapter for sterilizing the mentally retarded without their consent. Neville sees involuntary sterilization as morally justified when it is in the best interests of mildly retarded persons who lack the capacity to give or withhold informed consent because they do not understand the issues involved. He grants, however, that many empirical questions about the competence of mentally retarded individuals remain to be answered.

Recent developments in implantable drug-delivery systems may offer an alternative to surgical sterilization as a means of preventing pregnancies in mentally retarded individuals. At face value, the implantable contraceptive device seems much less ethically problematic than surgical sterilization, since such a device neither requires a major medical intervention nor results in permanent sterilization. However, as Eric T. Juengst and Ronald A. Siegel contend in a reading in this chapter, despite its advantages, the implantation of the device without the consent of the mentally retarded individual raises some of the same ethical problems as involuntary surgical sterilization.

If they are to develop and exercise their autonomy to the fullest extent possible, the retarded have problems that require special attention. Yet advocates for the retarded sometimes argue that those who are intellectually disadvantaged should be treated just like everyone else, with the same basic rights as all other citizens. This point of view is expressed in a code of rights proclaimed at a 1981 conference on mental retardation. The code demands "the closing of all institutions for intellectually disadvantaged persons."[8] While this statement was not the first articulated demand for a shift from custodialism to community care for the mentally retarded, it was the first code incorporating such demands written by "intellectually disadvantaged" representatives. In asserting their right to make their own choices about employment, housing, and so forth, the delegates argued, "We are humans first and disadvantaged second."[9] Another code, proclaimed by the International League of Societies for the Mentally Handicapped and reprinted in this chapter, asserts (1) the same basic rights for the mentally retarded as those held by other citizens of the same country and age, and (2) a set of special rights.

T.A.M. and D.D.

NOTES

1 See, e.g., Thomas S. Szasz, *Ideology and Insanity* (New York: Doubleday, 1970), especially pp. 113–139.

2 Jonas R. Rappeport, ed., *The Clinical Evaluation of the Dangerousness of the Mentally Ill* (Springfield, IL: Charles C. Thomas, 1967), pp. 72–80.

3 Alan A. Stone, *Mental Health and Law: A System in Transition* (Rockville, MD: Center for Studies of Crime and Delinquency, National Institute of Mental Health, DHEW Publication No. [ADM] 75–176, 1975).

4 For a discussion that is highly critical of psychiatrists' attributions of dangerousness, see Henry J. Steadman, "The Right Not to Be a False Positive: Problems in the Application of the Dangerousness Standard," *Psychiatric Quarterly* 52 (Summer 1980), pp. 84–99. For a discussion that presents such attributions in a more favorable light, see Charles W. Lidz, Edward P. Mulvey, Paul S. Appelbaum, and Sarah Cleveland, "Commitment: The Consistency of Clinicians and the Use of Legal Standards," *American Journal of Psychiatry* 146 (February 1989), pp. 176–181.

5 E. Fuller Torrey, *Nowhere to Go: The Tragic Odyssey of the Homeless Mentally Ill* (New York: Harper and Row, 1988), p. 4.

6 *Ibid.*, p. 139.

7 *Ibid.*, pp. 5–6.

8 The Australian Voice of Intellectually Disadvantaged Citizens, "Code of Rights," (Resolutions of the Second South Pacific Conference on Mental Retardation, Melbourne, Australia, presented by members of the Fifth Strand to Senator Fred Chaney, Federal Social Security Minister, August 28, 1981).

9 Stanley S. Herr, *Rights and Advocacy for Retarded People* (Lexington, MA: Lexington Books, 1983), p. 37.

Mental Illness and Involuntary Civil Commitment

The Myth of Mental Illness
Thomas S. Szasz

Thomas S. Szasz is professor emeritus of psychiatry at the State University of New York Health Sciences Center in Syracuse. A cofounder of the American Association for the Abolition of Involuntary Mental Hospitalization, he has long been an outspoken critic of contemporary psychiatric practice. Among his numerous published works are *The Ethics of Psychoanalysis* (1965), *The Manufacture of Madness* (1970), *Heresies* (1976), and *Insanity: The Idea and Its Consequences* (1987).

Szasz contends that there is no such thing as mental illness. In his view, the concept of mental illness has no cognitive (descriptive) content, functioning instead as a myth. Although he maintains that the term *mental illness* is unnecessary and misleading when used to refer to brain diseases, he especially objects to the term's being used to refer to alleged deformities of personality. Szasz maintains that, whereas physical illness may be ascribed on the basis of deviation from the norm of structural and functional integrity of the body, mental illness is ascribed solely on the basis of deviation (of personal behavior) from certain ethical, political, or social norms. According to Szasz, psychiatrists are mistaken in thinking that they are engaged in diagnosing and treating medical illness. Their patients do not have mental diseases but rather are experiencing "problems in living."

I

At the core of virtually all contemporary psychiatric theories and practices lies the concept of mental illness. A critical examination of this concept is therefore indispensable for understanding the ideas, institutions, and interventions of psychiatrists.

My aim in this essay is to ask if there is such a thing as mental illness and to argue that there is not. Of course, mental illness is not a thing or physical object; hence it can exist only in the same sort of way as do other theoretical concepts. Yet, to those who believe in them, familiar theories are likely to appear, sooner or later, as "objective truths" or "facts." During certain historical periods, explanatory concepts such as deities, witches, and instincts appeared not only as theories but as *self-evident causes* of a vast number of events. Today mental illness is widely regarded in a similar fashion, that is, as the cause of innumerable diverse happenings.

As an antidote to the complacent use of the notion of mental illness—as a self-evident phenomenon, theory, or cause—let us ask: What is meant when it is asserted that someone is mentally ill? In this essay I shall describe the main uses of the concept of mental illness, and I shall argue that this notion has outlived whatever cognitive usefulness it might have had and that it now functions as a myth.

II

The notion of mental illness derives its main support from such phenomena as syphilis of the brain or delirious conditions—intoxications, for instance—in which persons may manifest certain disorders of thinking and behavior. Correctly speaking, however, these are diseases of the brain, not of the mind. According to one school of thought, *all* so-called mental illness is of this type. The assumption is made that some neurological defect, perhaps a very subtle one, will ultimately be found to explain all the disorders of thinking and behavior. Many contemporary physicians, psychiatrists, and other scientists hold this view, which implies that people's troubles cannot be caused by conflicting personal needs, opinions, social aspirations, values, and so forth. These difficulties—which I think we may simply call *problems in living*—are thus attributed to physico-chemical processes that in due time will be discovered (and no doubt corrected) by medical research.

Mental illnesses are thus regarded as basically similar to other diseases. The only difference, in this view, between mental and bodily disease is that the former, affecting the brain, manifests itself by means of mental symptoms; whereas the latter, affecting other organ systems—for example, the skin, liver, and so on—manifests itself by means of symptoms referable to those parts of the body.

In my opinion, this view is based on two fundamental errors. In the first place, a disease of the brain, analogous to a disease of the skin or bone, is a neurological defect, not a problem in living. For example, a *defect* in a person's visual field may be explained by correlating it with certain lesions in the nervous system. On the other hand, a person's *belief*—whether it be in Christianity, in Communism, or in the idea that his internal organs are rotting and that his body is already dead—cannot be explained by a defect or disease of the nervous system. Explanations of this sort of occurrence—assuming that one is interested in the belief itself and does not regard it simply as a symptom or expression of something else that is more interesting—must be sought along different lines.

The second error is epistemological. It consists of interpreting communications about ourselves and the world around us as symptoms of neurological functioning. This is an error not in observation or reasoning, but rather in the organization and expression of knowledge. In the present case, the error lies in making a dualism between mental and physical symptoms, a dualism that is a habit of speech and not the result of known observations. Let us see if this is so.

In medical practice, when we speak of physical disturbances we mean either signs (for example, fever) or symptoms (for example, pain). We speak of mental symptoms, on the other hand, when we refer to a patient's communications about himself, others, and the world about him. The patient might assert that he is Napoleon or that he is being persecuted by the Communists. These would be considered mental symptoms only if the observer believed that the patient was *not* Napoleon or that he was *not* being persecuted by the Communists. This makes it apparent that the statement "X is a mental symptom" involves rendering a judgment that entails a covert comparison between the patient's ideas, concepts, or beliefs and those of the observer and the society in which they live. The notion of mental symptom is therefore inextricably tied to the social, and particularly the ethical, context in which it is made, just as the notion of bodily symptom is tied to an anatomical and genetic context.[1]

To sum up: For those who regard mental symptoms as signs of brain disease, the concept of mental illness is unnecessary and misleading. If they mean that people so labeled suffer from diseases of the brain, it would seem better, for the sake of clarity, to say that and not something else.

III

The term "mental illness" is also widely used to describe something quite different from a disease of the brain. Many people today take it for granted that living is an arduous affair. Its hardship for modern man derives, moreover, not so much from a struggle for biological survival as from the stresses and strains inherent in the social intercourse of complex human personalities. In this context, the notion of mental illness is used to identify or describe some features of an individual's so-called personality. Mental illness—as a deformity of the personality, so to speak—is then regarded as the cause of human disharmony. It is implicit in this view that social intercourse between people is regarded as something inherently harmonious, its disturbance being due solely to the presence of "mental illness" in many people. Clearly, this is faulty reasoning, for it makes the abstraction "mental illness" into a cause of, even though this abstraction was originally created to serve only as a shorthand expression for, certain types of human behavior. It now becomes necessary to ask: What kinds of behavior are regarded as indicative of mental illness, and by whom?

The concept of illness, whether bodily or mental, implies deviation from some clearly defined norm. In the case of physical illness, the norm is the structural and functional integrity of the human body. Thus, although the desirability of physical health, as such, is an ethical value, what health is can be stated in anatomical and physiological terms. What is the norm, deviation from which is regarded as mental illness? This question cannot be easily answered. But whatever this norm may be, we can be certain of only one thing: namely, that it must be stated in terms of psychosocial, ethical, and legal concepts. For example, notions such as "excessive repression" and "acting out an unconscious impulse" illustrate the use of psychological concepts for judging so-called mental health and illness. The idea that chronic hostility, vengefulness, or divorce are indicative of mental illness is an illustration of the use of ethical norms (that is, the desirability of love, kindness, and a stable marriage relationship). Finally,

the widespread psychiatric opinion that only a mentally ill person would commit homicide illustrates the use of a legal concept as a norm of mental health. In short, when one speaks of mental illness, the norm from which deviation is measured is a *psychosocial and ethical* standard. Yet, the remedy is sought in terms of *medical* measures that—it is hoped and assumed—are free from wide differences of ethical value. The definition of the disorder and the terms in which its remedy are sought are therefore at serious odds with one another. The practical significance of this covert conflict between the alleged nature of the defect and the actual remedy can hardly be exaggerated.

Having identified the norms used for measuring deviations in cases of mental illness, we shall now turn to the question, Who defines the norms and hence the deviation? Two basic answers may be offered: First, it may be the person himself—that is, the patient—who decides that he deviates from a norm; for example, an artist may believe that he suffers from a work inhibition; and he may implement this conclusion by seeking help *for himself* from a psychotherapist. Second, it may be someone other than the "patient" who decides that the latter is deviant—for example, relatives, physicians, legal authorities, society generally; a psychiatrist may then be hired by persons other than the "patient" to do something *to him* in order to correct the deviation.

These considerations underscore the importance of asking the question, Whose agent is the psychiatrist? and of giving a candid answer to it. The psychiatrist (or non-medical mental health worker) may be the agent of the patient, the relatives, the school, the military services, a business organization, a court of law, and so forth. In speaking of the psychiatrist as the agent of these persons or organizations, it is not implied that his moral values, or his ideas and aims concerning the proper nature of remedial action, must coincide exactly with those of his employer. For example, a patient in individual psychotherapy may believe that his salvation lies in a new marriage; his psychotherapist need not share this hypothesis. As the patient's agent, however, he must not resort to social or legal force to prevent the patient from putting his beliefs into action. If his *contract* is with the patient, the psychiatrist (psychotherapist) may disagree with him or stop his treatment, but he cannot engage others to obstruct the patient's aspirations.[2] Similarly, if a psychiatrist is retained by a court to determine the sanity of an offender, he need not fully share the legal authorities' values and intentions in regard to the criminal, nor the means deemed appropriate for dealing with him; such a psychiatrist cannot testify, however, that the accused is not insane, but that the legislators are—for passing the law that decrees the offender's actions illegal.[3] This sort of opinion could be voiced, of course—but not in a courtroom, and not by a psychiatrist who is there to assist the court in performing its daily work.

To recapitulate: In contemporary social usage, the finding of mental illness is made by establishing a deviance in behavior from certain psychosocial, ethical, or legal norms. The judgment may be made, as in medicine, by the patient, the physician (psychiatrist), or others. Remedial action, finally, tends to be sought in a therapeutic—or covertly medical—framework. This creates a situation in which it is claimed that psychosocial, ethical, and legal deviations can be corrected by medical action. Since medical interventions are designed to remedy only medical problems, it is logically absurd to expect that they will help solve problems whose very existence have been defined and established on non-medical grounds.

IV

Anything that people *do*—in contrast to things that *happen* to them[4]—takes place in a context of value. Hence, no human activity is devoid of moral implications. When the values underlying certain activities are widely shared, those who participate in their pursuit often lose sight of them altogether. The discipline of medicine—both as a pure science (for example, research) and as an applied science or technology (for example, therapy)—contains many ethical considerations and judgments. Unfortunately, these are often denied, minimized, or obscured, for the ideal of the medical profession as well as of the people whom it serves is to have an ostensibly value-free system of medical care. This sentimental notion is expressed by such things as the doctor's willingness to treat patients regardless of their religious or political beliefs. But such claims only serve to obscure the fact that ethical considerations encompass a vast range of human affairs. Making medical practice neutral with respect to some specific issues of moral value (such as race or sex) need not mean, and indeed does not mean, that it can be kept free from others (such as control over pregnancy or regulation of sex relations). Thus, birth control, abortion, homosexuality, suicide, and euthanasia continue to pose major problems in medical ethics.

Psychiatry is much more intimately related to problems of ethics than is medicine in general. I use the word "psychiatry" here to refer to the contemporary discipline concerned with problems in living, and not with diseases of the brain, which belong to neurology. Difficulties in human relations can be analyzed, interpreted, and given meaning only within specific social and ethical contexts. Accordingly, the psychiatrist's socioethical orientations will influence his ideas on what is wrong with the patient, on what deserves comment or interpretation, in what directions change might be desirable, and so forth. Even in medicine proper, these factors play a role, as illustrated by the divergent orientations that physicians, depending on their religious affiliations, have toward such things as birth control and therapeutic abortion. Can anyone really believe that a psychotherapist's ideas on religion, politics, and related issues play no role in his practical work? If, on the other hand, they do matter, what are we to infer from it? Does it not seem reasonable that perhaps we ought to have different psychiatric therapies—each recognized for the ethical positions that it embodies—for, say, Catholics and Jews, religious persons and atheists, democrats and Communists, white supremacists and Negroes, and so on? Indeed, if we look at the way psychiatry is actually practiced today, especially in the United States, we find that the psychiatric interventions people seek and receive depend more on their socioeconomic status and moral beliefs than on the "mental illnesses" from which they ostensibly suffer.[5] This fact should occasion no greater surprise than that practicing Catholics rarely frequent birth-control clinics, or that Christian Scientists rarely consult psychoanalysts.

V

The position outlined above, according to which contemporary psychotherapists deal with problems in living, not with mental illnesses and their cures, stands in sharp opposition to the currently prevalent position, according to which psychiatrists treat mental diseases, which are just as "real" and "objective" as bodily diseases. I submit that the holders of the latter view have no evidence whatever to justify their claim, which is actually a kind of psychiatric propaganda: their aim is to create in the popular mind a confident belief that mental illness is some sort of disease entity, like an infection or a malignancy. If this were true, one could *catch* or *get* a mental illness, one might *have* or *harbor* it, one might *transmit* it to others, and finally one could *get rid* of it. Not only is there not a shred of evidence to support this idea, but, on the contrary, all the evidence is the other way and supports the view that what people now call mental illnesses are, for the most part, *communications* expressing unacceptable ideas, often framed in an unusual idiom.

This is not the place to consider in detail the similarities and differences between bodily and mental illnesses. It should suffice to emphasize that whereas the term "bodily illness" refers to physicochemical occurrences that are not affected by being made public, the term "mental illness" refers to sociopsychological events that are crucially affected by being made public. The psychiatrist thus cannot, and does not, stand apart from the person he observes, as the pathologist can and often does. The psychiatrist is committed to some picture of what he considers reality, and to what he thinks society considers reality, and he observes and judges the patient's behavior in the light of these beliefs. The very notion of "mental symptom" or "mental illness" thus implies a covert comparison, and often conflict, between observer and observed, psychiatrist and patient. Though obvious, this fact needs to be re-emphasized, if one wishes, as I do here, to counter the prevailing tendency to deny the moral aspects of psychiatry and to substitute for them allegedly value-free medical concepts and interventions.

Psychotherapy is thus widely practiced as though it entailed nothing other than restoring the patient from a state of mental sickness to one of mental health. While it is generally accepted that mental illness has something to do with man's social or interpersonal relations, it is paradoxically maintained that problems of values—that is, of ethics—do not arise in this process. Freud himself went so far as to assert: "I consider ethics to be taken for granted. Actually I have never done a mean thing."[6] This is an astounding thing to say, especially for someone who had studied man as a social being as deeply as Freud had. I mention it here to show how the notion of "illness"—in the case of psychoanalysis, "psychopathology," or "mental illness"—was used by Freud, and by most of his followers, as a means of classifying certain types of human behavior as falling within the scope of medicine, and hence, by fiat, outside that of ethics. Nevertheless, the stubborn fact remains that, in a sense, much of psychotherapy revolves around nothing other than the elucidation and weighing of goals and values— many of which may be mutually contradictory—and the means whereby they might best be harmonized, realized, or relinquished.

Because the range of human values and of the methods by which they may be attained is so vast, and

because many such ends and means are persistently unacknowledged, conflicts among values are the main source of conflicts in human relations. Indeed, to say that human relations at all levels—from mother to child, through husband and wife, to nation and nation—are fraught with stress, strain, and disharmony is, once again, to make the obvious explicit. Yet, what may be obvious may be also poorly understood. This, I think, is the case here. For it seems to me that in our scientific theories of behavior we have failed to accept the simple fact that human relations are inherently fraught with difficulties, and to make them even relatively harmonious requires much patience and hard work. I submit that the idea of mental illness is now being put to work to obscure certain difficulties that at present may be inherent—not that they need to be unmodifiable—in the social intercourse of persons. If this is true, the concept functions as a disguise: Instead of calling attention to conflicting human needs, aspirations, and values, the concept of mental illness provides an amoral and impersonal "thing"—an "illness"—as an explanation for problems in living. We may recall in this connection that not so long ago it was devils and witches that were held responsible for man's problems of living. The belief in mental illness, as something other than man's trouble in getting along with his fellow man, is the proper heir to the belief in demonology and witchcraft. Mental illness thus exists or is "real" in exactly the same sense in which witches existed or were "real."

VI

While I maintain that mental illnesses do not exist, I obviously do not imply or mean that the social and psychological occurrences to which this label is attached also do not exist. Like the personal and social troubles that people had in the Middle Ages, contemporary human problems are real enough. It is the labels we give them that concern me, and, having labeled them, what we do about them. The demonologic concept of problems in living gave rise to therapy along theological lines. Today, a belief in mental illness implies—nay, requires— therapy along medical or psychotherapeutic lines.

I do not here propose to offer a new conception of "psychiatric illness" or a new form of "therapy." My aim is more modest and yet also more ambitious. It is to suggest that the phenomena now called mental illnesses be looked at afresh and more simply, that they be removed from the category of illnesses, and that they be regarded as the expressions of man's struggle with *the problem of how he should live.* This problem is obviously a vast one, its enormity reflecting not only man's inability to cope with his environment, but even more his increasing self-reflectiveness.

By problems in living, then, I refer to that explosive chain reaction that began with man's fall from divine grace by partaking of the fruit of the tree of knowledge. Man's awareness of himself and of the world about him seems to be a steadily expanding one, bringing in its wake an even larger *burden of understanding.*[7] This burden is to be expected and must not be misinterpreted. Our only rational means for easing it is more understanding, and appropriate action based on such understanding. The main alternative lies in acting as though the burden were not what in fact we perceive it to be, and taking refuge in an outmoded theological view of man. In such a view, man does not fashion his life and much of his world about him, but merely lives out his fate in a world created by superior beings. This may logically lead to pleading non-responsibility in the face of seemingly unfathomable problems and insurmountable difficulties. Yet, if man fails to take increasing responsibility for his actions, individually as well as collectively, it seems unlikely that some higher power or being would assume this task and carry this burden for him. Moreover, this seems hardly a propitious time in human history for obscuring the issue of man's responsibility for his actions by hiding it behind the skirt of an all-explaining conception of mental illness.

VII

I have tried to show that the notion of mental illness has outlived whatever usefulness it may have had and that it now functions as a myth. As such, it is a true heir to religious myths in general, and to the belief in witchcraft in particular. It was the function of these belief-systems to act as social tranquilizers, fostering hope that mastery of certain problems may be achieved by means of substitutive, symbolic-magical, operations. The concept of mental illness thus serves mainly to obscure the everyday fact that life for most people is a continuous struggle, not for biological survival, but for a "place in the sun," "peace of mind," or some other meaning or value. Once the needs of preserving the body, and perhaps of the race, are satisfied, man faces the problem of personal significance: What should he do with himself? For what should he live? Sustained adherence to the myth

of mental illness allows people to avoid facing this problem, believing that mental health, conceived as the absence of mental illness, automatically insures the making of right and safe choices in the conduct of life. But the facts are all the other way. It is the making of wise choices in life that people regard, retrospectively, as evidence of good mental health!

When I assert that mental illness is a myth, I am not saying that personal unhappiness and socially deviant behavior do not exist; what I am saying is that we categorize them as diseases at our own peril.

The expression "mental illness" is a metaphor that we have come to mistake for a fact. We call people physically ill when their body-functioning violates certain anatomical and physiological norms; similarly, we call people mentally ill when their personal conduct violates certain ethical, political, and social norms. This explains why many historical figures, from Jesus to Castro, and from Job to Hitler, have been diagnosed as suffering from this or that psychiatric malady.

Finally, the myth of mental illness encourages us to believe in its logical corollary: that social intercourse would be harmonious, satisfying, and the secure basis of a good life were it not for the disrupting influences of mental illness, or psychopathology. However, universal human happiness, in this form at least, is but another example of a wishful fantasy. I believe that human happiness, or well-being, is possible—not just for a select few, but on a scale hitherto unimaginable. But this can be achieved only if many men, not just a few, are willing and able to confront frankly, and tackle courageously, their ethical, personal, and social conflicts. This means having the courage and integrity to forego waging battles on false fronts, finding solutions for substitute problems—for instance, fighting the battle of stomach acid and chronic fatigue instead of facing up to a marital conflict.

Our adversaries are not demons, witches, fate, or mental illness. We have no enemy that we can fight, exorcise, or dispel by "cure." What we do have are problems in living—whether these be biologic, economic, political, or socio-psychological. In this essay I was concerned only with problems belonging in the last-mentioned category, and within this group mainly with those pertaining to moral values. The field to which modern psychiatry addresses itself is vast, and I made no effort to encompass it all. My argument was limited to the proposition that mental illness is a myth, whose function it is to disguise and thus render more palatable the bitter pill of moral conflicts in human relations.

NOTES

1 See Szasz, T. S.: *Pain and Pleasure: A Study of Bodily Feelings* (New York: Basic Books, 1957), especially pp. 70–81; "The problem of psychiatric nosology." *Amer. J. Psychiatry*, 114:405–13 (Nov.), 1957.
2 See Szasz, T. S.: *The Ethics of Psychoanalysis: The Theory and Method of Autonomous Psychotherapy* (New York: Basic Books, 1965).
3 See Szasz, T. S.: *Law, Liberty, and Psychiatry: An Inquiry into the Social Uses of Mental Health Practices* (New York: Macmillan, 1963).
4 Peters, R. S.: *The Concept of Motivation* (London: Routledge & Kegan Paul, 1958), especially pp. 12–15.
5 Hollingshead, A. B., and Redlich, F. C.: *Social Class and Mental Illness* (New York: Wiley, 1958).
6 Quoted in Jones, E.: *The Life and Work of Sigmund Freud* (New York: Basic Books, 1957), Vol. III, p. 247.
7 In this connection, see Langer, S. K.: *Philosophy in a New Key* [1942] (New York: Mentor Books, 1953), especially Chaps. 5 and 10.

Majority Opinion in *O'Connor v. Donaldson*
Justice Potter Stewart

Potter Stewart (1915–1985) served as associate justice of the United States Supreme Court from 1958 until 1981. Prior to that appointment, he spent some years in private practice and served as judge on the United States Circuit Court of Appeals for the 6th District (1954–1958).

In 1943 Kenneth Donaldson's parents asked a judge to commit their 34-year-old son to a mental institution for treatment. They did this after Donaldson's fellow workers apparently knocked him unconscious after he made a political comment. Once Donaldson was institutionalized and his reactions to what he perceived as injustices were diagnosed as pathological, he was given electroconvulsive therapy (ECT). After 11 weeks of ECT, he was released. In 1956 Donaldson visited his parents in Florida. During his visit, he made some complaints, which led his father to request a sanity hearing for his son. The senior Donaldson argued that his son was suffering from a "persecution complex." As a result of this complaint, Donaldson was arrested, jailed, and diagnosed as "paranoid schizophrenic" by a sheriff and two physicians. The physicians, each of whom spoke to Donaldson for less than two minutes, were not psychiatrists. Later a judge visited him and informed him that he would be sent to Florida State Hospital. This decision was based on the physicians' conclusions. Donaldson's requests for a judicial hearing and a lawyer were granted, but the hearing was held in jail, the physicians did not attend, and Donaldson's lawyer left while Donaldson was still testifying. Donaldson was sent to the hospital for a "few weeks' rest." He remained there for 15 years, never seeing a judge and seeing a psychiatrist only a few times a year. During those 15 years, Donaldson petitioned various courts 18 times, asking for a hearing. All but one of these requests were dismissed on the basis of physicians' reports and his previous institutionalization. When his case was finally going to be heard in 1971, Donaldson was released and certified as "no longer incompetent." However, he continued his suit, asking $100,000 in damages for the 15 years he had been committed without treatment. He won his case against J. B. O'Connor,

United States Supreme Court; June 26, 1975, 422 U.S. 563. 95 S.Ct. 2486.

the superintendent of the institution, and a codefendant physician, although only $38,500 was granted in damages.

The case was ultimately appealed to the United States Supreme Court. In handing down its 1975 landmark decision, the court ruled that a finding of mental illness alone is insufficient grounds for confining a nondangerous individual who has the capacity to survive safely in freedom, either by himself or with the help of responsible and willing relatives or friends.

I

Donaldson's commitment was initiated by his father, who thought that his son was suffering from "delusions." After hearings before a county judge of Pinellas County, Fla., Donaldson was found to be suffering from "paranoid schizophrenia" and was committed for "care, maintenance, and treatment" pursuant to Florida statutory provisions that have since been repealed. The state law was less than clear in specifying the grounds necessary for commitment, and the record is scanty as to Donaldson's condition at the time of the judicial hearing. These matters are, however, irrelevant, for this case involves no challenge to the initial commitment, but is focused, instead, upon the nearly 15 years of confinement that followed.

The evidence at the trial showed that the hospital staff had the power to release a patient, not dangerous to himself or others, even if he remained mentally ill and had been lawfully committed. Despite many requests, O'Connor refused to allow that power to be exercised in Donaldson's case. At the trial, O'Connor indicated that he had believed that Donaldson would have been unable to make a "successful adjustment outside the institution," but could not recall the basis for that conclusion. O'Connor retired as superintendent shortly before the suit was filed. A few months thereafter, and before the trial, Donaldson secured his release and a judicial restoration of competency, with the support of the hospital staff.

The testimony at the trial demonstrated, without contradiction, that Donaldson had posed no danger to others during his long confinement, or indeed at any point in his life. O'Connor himself conceded that he had no personal or secondhand knowledge that Donaldson had ever committed a dangerous act. There was no evidence that Donaldson had ever been suicidal or been thought likely to inflict injury upon himself. One of O'Connor's codefendants acknowledged that Donaldson could have earned his own living outside the hospital. He had done so for some 14 years before his com-

mitment, and immediately upon his release he secured a responsible job in hotel administration.

Furthermore, Donaldson's frequent requests for release had been supported by responsible persons willing to provide him any care he might need on release. In 1963, for example, a representative of Helping Hands, Inc., a halfway house for mental patients, wrote O'Connor asking him to release Donaldson to its care. The request was accompanied by a supporting letter from the Minneapolis Clinic of Psychiatry and Neurology, which a codefendant conceded was a "good clinic." O'Connor rejected the offer, replying that Donaldson could be released only to his parents. That rule was apparently of O'Connor's own making. At the time, Donaldson was 55 years old, and, as O'Connor knew, Donaldson's parents were too elderly and infirm to take responsibility for him. Moreover, in his continuing correspondence with Donaldson's parents, O'Connor never informed them of the Helping Hands offer. In addition, on four separate occasions between 1964 and 1968, John Lembcke, a college classmate of Donaldson's and a longtime family friend, asked O'Connor to release Donaldson to his care. On each occasion O'Connor refused. The record shows that Lembcke was a serious and responsible person, who was willing and able to assume responsibility for Donaldson's welfare.

The evidence showed that Donaldson's confinement was a simple regime of enforced custodial care, not a program designed to alleviate or cure his supposed illness. Numerous witnesses, including one of O'Connor's codefendants, testified that Donaldson had received nothing but custodial care while at the hospital. O'Connor described Donaldson's treatment as "milieu therapy." But witnesses from the hospital staff conceded that, in the context of this case, "milieu therapy" was a euphemism for confinement in the "milieu" of a mental hospital. For substantial periods, Donaldson was simply kept in a large room that housed 60 patients, many of whom were under criminal commitment. Donaldson's requests for ground privileges, occupational training, and an opportunity to discuss his case with O'Connor or other staff members were repeatedly denied.

At the trial, O'Connor's principal defense was that he had acted in good faith and was therefore immune from any liability for monetary damages. His position, in short, was that state law, which he had believed valid, had authorized indefinite custodial confinement of the "sick," even if they were not given treatment and their release could harm no one.

The trial judge instructed the members of the jury that they should find that O'Connor had violated Donaldson's constitutional right to liberty if they found that he had

> confined [Donaldson] against his will, knowing that he was not mentally ill or dangerous or knowing that if mentally ill he was not receiving treatment for his alleged mental illness. . . .
>
> Now, the purpose of involuntary hospitalization is treatment and not mere custodial care or punishment if a patient is not a danger to himself or others. Without such treatment there is no justification from a constitutional stand-point for continued confinement unless you should also find that [Donaldson] was dangerous to either himself or others.

The trial judge further instructed the jury that O'Connor was immune from damages if he

> reasonably believed in good faith that detention of [Donaldson] was proper for the length of time he was so confined. . . .
>
> However, mere good intentions which do not give rise to a reasonable belief that detention is lawfully required cannot justify [Donaldson's] confinement in the Florida State Hospital.

The jury returned a verdict for Donaldson against O'Connor and a codefendant, and awarded damages of $38,500, including $10,000 in punitive damages.

The Court of Appeals affirmed the judgment of the District Court in a broad opinion dealing with "the far-reaching question whether the Fourteenth Amendment guarantees a right to treatment to persons involuntarily civilly committed to state mental hospitals." The appellate court held that when, as in Donaldson's case, the rationale for confinement is that the patient is in need of treatment, the Constitution requires that minimally adequate treatment in fact be provided. The court further expressed the view that, regardless of the grounds for involuntary civil commitment, a person confined against his will at a state mental institution has "a constitutional right to receive such individual treatment as will give him a reasonable opportunity to be cured or to improve his mental condition." Conversely, the court's opinion implied that it is constitutionally permissible for a State to confine a mentally ill person against his will in order to treat his illness, regardless of whether his illness renders him dangerous to himself or others.

II

We have concluded that the difficult issues of constitutional law dealt with by the Court of Appeals are not presented by this case in its present posture. Specifically, there is no reason now to decide whether mentally ill persons dangerous to themselves or to others have a right to treatment upon compulsory confinement by the State, or whether the State may compulsorily confine a nondangerous, mentally ill individual for the purpose of treatment. As we view it, this case raises a single, relatively simple, but nonetheless important question concerning every man's constitutional right to liberty.

The jury found that Donaldson was neither dangerous to himself nor dangerous to others, and also found that, if mentally ill, Donaldson had not received treatment. That verdict, based on abundant evidence, makes the issue before the Court a narrow one. We need not decide whether, when, or by what procedures, a mentally ill person may be confined by the State on any of the grounds which, under contemporary statutes, are generally advanced to justify involuntary confinement of such a person—to prevent injury to the public, to ensure his own survival or safety,[1] or to alleviate or cure his illness. For the jury found that none of the above grounds for continued confinement was present in Donaldson's case.

Given the jury's findings, what was left as justification for keeping Donaldson in continued confinement? The fact that state law may have authorized confinement of the harmless mentally ill does not itself establish a constitutionally adequate purpose for the confinement. Nor is it enough that Donaldson's original confinement was founded upon a constitutionally adequate basis, if in fact it was, because even if his involuntary confinement was initially permissible, it could not constitutionally continue after that basis no longer existed.

A finding of "mental illness" alone cannot justify a State's locking a person up against his will and keeping him indefinitely in simple custodial confinement. Assuming that that term can be given a reasonably precise content and that the "mentally ill" can be identified with reasonable accuracy, there is still no constitutional basis for confining such persons involuntarily if they are dangerous to no one and can live safely in freedom.

May the State confine the mentally ill merely to ensure them a living standard superior to that which they enjoy in the private community? That the State has a proper interest in providing care and assistance to the unfortunate goes without saying. But the mere presence of mental illness does not disqualify a person from preferring his home to the comforts of an institution. Moreover, while the State may arguably confine a person to save him from harm, incarceration is rarely if ever a necessary condition for raising the living standards of those capable of surviving safely in freedom, on their own or with the help of family or friends.

May the State fence in the harmless mentally ill solely to save its citizens from exposure to those whose ways are different? One might as well ask if the State, to avoid public unease, could incarcerate all who are physically unattractive or socially eccentric. Mere public intolerance or animosity cannot constitutionally justify the deprivation of a person's physical liberty.

In short, a State cannot constitutionally confine without motive a nondangerous individual who is capable of surviving safely in freedom by himself or with the help of willing and responsible family members or friends. Since the jury found, upon ample evidence, that O'Connor, as an agent of the State, knowingly did so confine Donaldson, it properly concluded that O'Connor violated Donaldson's constitutional right to freedom.

III

O'Connor contends that in any event he should not be held personally liable for monetary damages because his decisions were made in "good faith." Specifically, O'Connor argues that he was acting pursuant to state law which, he believed, authorized confinement of the mentally ill even when their release would not compromise their safety or constitute a danger to others, and that he could not reasonably have been expected to know that the state law as he understood it was constitutionally invalid. A proposed instruction to this effect was rejected by the District Court.

The District Court did instruct the jury, without objection, that monetary damages could not be assessed against O'Connor if he had believed reasonably and in good faith that Donaldson's continued confinement was

"proper," and that punitive damages could be awarded only if O'Connor had acted "maliciously or wantonly or oppressively." The Court of Appeals approved those instructions. But that court did not consider whether it was error for the trial judge to refuse the additional instruction concerning O'Connor's claimed reliance on state law as authorization for Donaldson's continued confinement. Further, neither the District Court nor the Court of Appeals acted with the benefit of this Court's most recent decision on the scope of the qualified immunity possessed by state officials. . . . [*Wood v. Strickland* (1975)]

Under that decision, the relevant question for the jury is whether O'Connor "knew or reasonably should have known that the action he took within his sphere of official responsibility would violate the constitutional rights of [Donaldson], or if he took the action with the malicious intention to cause a deprivation of constitutional rights or other injury to [Donaldson]." For the purposes of this question, an official has, of course, no duty to anticipate unforeseeable constitutional developments.

Accordingly, we vacate the judgment of the Court of Appeals and remand the case to enable that court to consider, in light of *Wood v. Strickland,* whether the District Judge's failure to instruct with regard to the effect of O'Connor's claimed reliance on state law rendered inadequate the instructions as to O'Connor's liability for compensatory and punitive damages.[2]

It is so ordered.

Vacated and remanded.

NOTES

1 The judge's instructions used the phrase "dangerous to himself." Of course, even if there is no foreseeable risk of self-injury or suicide, a person is literally "dangerous to himself" if for physical or other reasons he is helpless to avoid the hazards of freedom either through his own efforts or with the aid of willing family members or friends. While it might be argued that the judge's instructions could have been more detailed on this point, O'Connor raised no objection to them, presumably because the evidence clearly showed that Donaldson was not "dangerous to himself" however broadly that phrase might be defined.

2 Upon remand, the Court of Appeals is to consider only the question whether O'Connor is to be held liable for monetary damages for violating Donald-

son's constitutional right to liberty. The jury found, on substantial evidence and under adequate instructions, that O'Connor deprived Donaldson, who was dangerous neither to himself nor to others and was provided no treatment, of the constitutional right to liberty. That finding needs no further consideration. If the Court of Appeals holds that a remand to the District Court is necessary, the only issue to be determined in that court will be whether O'Connor is immune from liability for monetary damages.

Of necessity our decision vacating the judgment of the Court of Appeals deprives that court's opinion of precedential effect, leaving this Court's opinion and judgment as the sole law of the case.

The Case for Involuntary Hospitalization of the Mentally Ill
Paul Chodoff

Paul Chodoff is clinical professor of psychiatry and behavioral sciences at George Washington University School of Medicine. Chodoff, who also maintains a private practice, is coeditor of *Psychiatric Ethics* (2d ed., 1991) and the author of such articles as "A Critique of Freud's Theory of Infantile Sexuality," "Psychiatric Aspects of Nazi Persecution," and "Treatment of the Histrionic Personality Disorder."

Chodoff is concerned with the question of the justifiability of involuntary civil commitment. He presents a number of cases as examples of behavior that most of us would agree differs significantly from the norm. He uses these cases as a background for his analysis and evaluation of three stances that are often taken toward involuntary civil commitment. The three stances are those of (1) abolitionists, (2) medical-model psychiatrists, and (3) civil liberties lawyers.

I will begin this paper with a series of vignettes designed to illustrate graphically the question that is my focus: under what conditions, if any, does society have the right to apply coercion to an individual to hospitalize him against his will, by reason of mental illness?

Case 1   A woman in her mid 50s, with no previous overt behavioral difficulties, comes to believe that she is worthless and insignificant. She is completely preoccupied with her guilt and is increasingly unavailable for the ordinary demands of life. She eats very little because of her conviction that the food should go to others whose need is greater than hers, and her physical condition progressively deteriorates. Although she will talk to others about herself, she insists that she is not

The American Journal of Psychiatry, vol. 133, no. 5 (May 1976), pp. 496–501. Copyright © 1976, The American Psychiatric Association. Reprinted by permission.

sick, only bad. She refuses medication, and when hospitalization is suggested she also refuses that on the grounds that she would be taking up space that otherwise could be occupied by those who merit treatment more than she.

Case 2   For the past 6 years the behavior of a 42-year-old woman has been disturbed for periods of 3 months or longer. After recovery from her most recent episode she has been at home, functioning at a borderline level. A month ago she again started to withdraw from her environment. She pays increasingly less attention to her bodily needs, talks very little, and does not respond to questions or attention from those about her. She lapses into a mute state and lies in her bed in a totally passive fashion. She does not respond to other people, does not eat, and does not void. When her arm is raised from the bed it remains for several minutes in the position in which it is left. Her medical history and a physical examination reveal no evidence of primary physical illness.

Case 3 A man with a history of alcoholism has been on a binge for several weeks. He remains at home doing little else than drinking. He eats very little. He becomes tremulous and misinterprets spots on the wall as animals about to attack him, and he complains of "creeping" sensations in his body, which he attributes to infestation by insects. He does not seek help voluntarily, insists there is nothing wrong with him, and despite his wife's entreaties he continues to drink.

Case 4 Passersby and station personnel observe that a young woman has been spending several days at Union Station in Washington, D.C. Her behavior appears strange to others. She is finally befriended by a newspaper reporter who becomes aware that her perception of her situation is profoundly unrealistic and that she is, in fact, delusional. He persuades her to accompany him to St. Elizabeth's Hospital, where she is examined by a psychiatrist who recommends admission. She refuses hospitalization and the psychiatrist allows her to leave. She returns to Union Station. A few days later she is found dead, murdered, on one of the surrounding streets.

Case 5 A government attorney in his late 30s begins to display pressured speech and hyperactivity. He is too busy to sleep and eats very little. He talks rapidly, becomes irritable when interrupted, and makes phone calls all over the country in furtherance of his political ambitions, which are to begin a campaign for the Presidency of the United States. He makes many purchases, some very expensive, thus running through a great deal of money. He is rude and tactless to his friends, who are offended by his behavior, and his job is in jeopardy. In spite of his wife's pleas he insists that he does not have the time to seek or accept treatment, and he refuses hospitalization. This is not the first such disturbance for this individual; in fact, very similar episodes have been occurring at roughly 2-year intervals since he was 18 years old.

Case 6 Passersby in a campus area observe two young women standing together, staring at each other, for over an hour. Their behavior attracts attention, and eventually the police take the pair to a nearby precinct station for questioning. They refuse to answer questions and sit mutely, staring into space. The police request some type of psychiatric examination but are informed by the city attorney's office that state law (Michigan) allows persons to be held for observation only if they appear obviously dangerous to themselves or others. In this case, since the women do not seem homicidal or suicidal, they do not qualify for observation and are released.

Less than 30 hours later the two women are found on the floor of their campus apartment, screaming and writhing in pain with their clothes ablaze from a self-made pyre. One woman recovers; the other dies. There is no conclusive evidence that drugs were involved (1).

Most, if not all, people would agree that the behavior described in these vignettes deviates significantly from even elastic definitions of normality. However, it is clear that there would not be a similar consensus on how to react to this kind of behavior and that there is a considerable and increasing ferment about what attitude the organized elements of our society should take toward such individuals. Everyone has a stake in this important issue, but the debate about it takes place principally among psychiatrists, lawyers, the courts, and law enforcement agencies.

Points of view about the question of involuntary hospitalization fall into the following three principal groups: the "abolitionists," medical model psychiatrists, and civil liberties lawyers.

THE ABOLITIONISTS

Those holding this position would assert that in none of the cases I have described should involuntary hospitalization be a viable option because, quite simply, it should never be resorted to under any circumstances. As Szasz (2) has put it, "we should value liberty more highly than mental health no matter how defined" and "no one should be deprived of his freedom for the sake of his mental health." Ennis (3) has said that the goal "is nothing less than the abolition of involuntary hospitalization."

Prominent among the abolitionists are the "antipsychiatrists," who, somewhat surprisingly, count in their ranks a number of well-known psychiatrists. For them mental illness simply does not exist in the field of psychiatry (4). They reject entirely the medical model of mental illness and insist that acceptance of it relies on a fiction accepted jointly by the state and by psychiatrists as a device for exerting social control over annoying or unconventional people. The antipsychiatrists hold that these people ought to be afforded the dignity of being held responsible for their behavior and required to accept its consequences. In addition, some members of this group believe that the phenomena of "mental illness" often represent essentially a tortured protest against the insanities of an irrational society (5). They maintain that society should not be encouraged in its oppressive course by affixing a pejorative label to its victims.

Among the abolitionists are some civil liberties lawyers who both assert their passionate support of the magisterial importance of individual liberty and react with repugnance and impatience to what they see as the abuses of psychiatric practice in this field—the commitment of some individuals for flimsy and possibly self-serving reasons and their inhuman warehousing in penal institutions wrongly called "hospitals."

The abolitionists do not oppose psychiatric treatment when it is conducted with the agreement of those being treated. I have no doubt that they would try to gain the consent of the individuals described earlier to undergo treatment, including hospitalization. The psychiatrists in this group would be very likely to confine their treatment methods to psychotherapeutic efforts to influence the aberrant behavior. They would be unlikely to use drugs and would certainly eschew such somatic therapies as ECT.* If efforts to enlist voluntary compliance with treatment failed, the abolitionists would not employ any means of coercion. Instead, they would step aside and allow social, legal, and community sanctions to take their course. If a human being should be jailed or a human life lost as a result of this attitude, they would accept it as a necessary evil to be tolerated in order to avoid the greater evil of unjustified loss of liberty for others (6).

THE MEDICAL MODEL PSYCHIATRISTS

I use this admittedly awkward and not entirely accurate label to designate the position of a substantial number of psychiatrists. They believe that mental illness is a meaningful concept and that under certain conditions its existence justifies the state's exercise, under the doctrine of parens patriae, of its right and obligation to arrange for the hospitalization of the sick individual even though

---

*Editors' note: Electroconvulsive therapy (ECT) involves direct intervention into the brain. In ECT, electric currents applied to the front of the patient's head induce convulsions and unconsciousness.

coercion is involved and he is deprived of his liberty. I believe that these psychiatrists would recommend involuntary hospitalization for all six of the patients described earlier.

The Medical Model

There was a time, before they were considered to be ill, when individuals who displayed the kind of behavior I described earlier were put in "ships of fools" to wander the seas or were left to the mercies, sometimes tender but often savage, of uncomprehending communities that regarded them as either possessed or bad. During the Enlightenment and the early nineteenth century, however, these individuals gradually came to be regarded as sick people to be included under the humane and caring umbrella of the Judeo-Christian attitude toward illness. This attitude, which may have reached its height during the era of moral treatment in the early nineteenth century, has had unexpected and ambiguous consequences. It became overextended and partially perverted, and these excesses led to the reaction that is so strong a current in today's attitude toward mental illness.

However, reaction itself can go too far, and I believe that this is already happening. Witness the disastrous consequences of the precipitate dehospitalization that is occurring all over the country. To remove the protective mantle of illness from these disturbed people is to expose them, their families, and their communities to consequences that are certainly maladaptive and possibly irreparable. Are we really acting in accordance with their best interests when we allow them to "die with their rights on" (1) or when we condemn them to a "preservation of liberty which is actually so destructive as to constitute another form of imprisonment" (7)? Will they not suffer "if [a] liberty they cannot enjoy is made superior to a health that must sometimes be forced on them" (8)?

Many of those who reject the medical model out of hand as inapplicable to so-called "mental illness" have tended to oversimplify its meaning and have, in fact, equated it almost entirely with organic disease. It is necessary to recognize that it is a complex concept and that there is a lack of agreement about its meaning. Sophisticated definitions of the medical model do not require only the demonstration of unequivocal organic pathology. A broader formulation, put forward by sociologists and deriving largely from Talcott Parsons' description of the sick role (9), extends the domain of illness to encompass certain forms of social deviance as well as biological disorders. According to this definition, the medical model is characterized not only by organicity but also by being negatively valued by society, by "non-voluntariness," thus exempting its exemplars from blame, and by the understanding that physicians are the technically competent experts to deal with its effects (10).

Except for the question of organic disease, the patients I described earlier conform well to this broader conception of the medical model. They are all suffering both emotionally and physically, they are incapable by an effort of will of stopping or changing their destructive behavior, and those around them consider them to be in an undesirable sick state and to require medical attention.

Categorizing the behavior of these patients as involuntary may be criticized as evidence of an intolerably paternalistic and antitherapeutic attitude that fosters the very failure to take responsibility for their lives and behavior that the therapist should uncover rather than encourage. However, it must also be acknowledged that these severely ill people are not capable at a conscious level of deciding what is best for themselves and that in order to help them examine their behavior and motivation, it is necessary that they be alive and available for treatment. Their verbal message that they will not accept treatment may at the same time be conveying other more covert messages—that they are desperate and want help even though they cannot ask for it (11).

Although organic pathology may not be the only determinant of the medical model, it is of course an important one and it should not be avoided in any discussion of mental illness. There would be no question that the previously described patient with delirium tremens is suffering from a toxic form of brain disease. There are a significant number of other patients who require involuntary hospitalization because of organic brain syndrome due to various causes. Among those who are not overtly organically ill, most of the candidates for involuntary hospitalization suffer from schizophrenia or one of the major affective disorders. A growing and increasingly impressive body of evidence points to the presence of an important genetic-biological factor in these conditions; thus, many of them qualify on these grounds as illnesses.

Despite the revisionist efforts of the antipsychiatrists, mental illness *does* exist. It does not by any means include all of the people being treated by psychiatrists (or by non-psychiatrist physicians), but it does encompass those few desperately sick people for whom involuntary commitment must be considered. In the words of a recent article, "The problem is that mental illness is not a myth. It is not some palpable falsehood propagated among the populace by power-mad psychiatrists, but a cruel and bitter reality that has been with the human race since antiquity" (12, p. 1483).

Criteria for Involuntary Hospitalization

Procedures for involuntary hospitalization should be instituted for individuals who require care and treatment because of diagnosable mental illness that produces symptoms, including marked impairment in judgment, that disrupt their intrapsychic and interpersonal functioning. All three of these criteria must be met before involuntary hospitalization can be instituted.

1. Mental Illness This concept has already been discussed, but it should be repeated that only a belief in the existence of illness justifies involuntary commitment. It is a fundamental assumption that makes aberrant behavior a medical matter and its care the concern of physicians.

2. Disruption of Functioning This involves combinations of serious and often obvious disturbances that are both intrapsychic (for example, the suffering of severe depression) and interpersonal (for example, withdrawal from others because of depression). It does not include minor peccadilloes or eccentricities. Furthermore, the behavior in question must represent symptoms of the mental illness from which the patient is suffering. Among these symptoms are actions that are imminently or potentially dangerous in a physical sense to self or others, as well as other manifestations of mental illness such as those in the cases I have described. This is not to ignore dangerousness as a criterion for commitment but rather to put it in its proper place as one of a number of symptoms of the illness. A further manifestation of the illness, and indeed, the one that makes involuntary rather than voluntary hospitalization necessary, is impairment of the patient's judgment to such a degree that he is unable to consider his condition and make decisions about it in his own interests.

3. Need for Care and Treatment The goal of physicians is to treat and cure their patients; however, sometimes they can only ameliorate the suffering of their patients and sometimes all they can offer is care. It is not possible to predict whether someone will respond to treatment; nevertheless, the need for treatment and the availability of facilities to carry it out constitute essential preconditions that must be met to justify requiring anyone to give up his freedom. If mental hospital patients have a right to treatment, then psychiatrists have a right to ask for treatability as a front-door as well as a back-door criterion for commitment (7). All of the six individuals I described earlier could have been treated with a reasonable expectation of returning to a more normal state of functioning.

I believe that the objections to this formulation can be summarized as follows.

1. The whole structure founders for those who maintain that mental illness is a fiction.

2. These criteria are also untenable to those who hold liberty to be such a supreme value that the presence of mental illness per se does not constitute justification for depriving an individual of his freedom; only when such illness is manifested by clearly dangerous behavior may commitment be considered. For reasons to be discussed later, I agree with those psychiatrists (13, 14) who do not believe that dangerousness should be elevated to primacy above other manifestations of mental illness as a sine qua non for involuntary hospitalization.

3. The medical model criteria are "soft" and subjective and depend on the fallible judgment of psychiatrists. This is a valid objection. There is no reliable blood test for schizophrenia and no method for injecting grey cells into psychiatrists. A relatively small number of cases will always fall within a grey area that will be difficult to judge. In those extreme cases in which the question of commitment arises, competent and ethical psychiatrists should be able to use these criteria without doing violence to individual liberties and with the expectation of good results. Furthermore, the possible "fuzziness" of some aspects of the medical model approach is certainly no greater than that of the supposedly "objective" criteria for dangerousness, and there is little reason to believe that lawyers and judges are any less fallible than psychiatrists.

4. Commitment procedures in the hands of psychiatrists are subject to intolerable abuses. Here, as Peszke said, "It is imperative that we differ-

entiate between the principle of the process of civil commitment and the practice itself" (13, p. 825). Abuses can contaminate both the medical and the dangerousness approaches, and I believe that the abuses stemming from the abolitionist view of no commitment at all are even greater. Measures to abate abuses of the medical approach include judicial review and the abandonment of indeterminate commitment. In the course of commitment proceedings and thereafter, patients should have access to competent and compassionate legal counsel. However, this latter safeguard may itself be subject to abuse if the legal counsel acts solely in the adversary tradition and undertakes to carry out the patient's wishes even when they may be destructive.

Comment

The criteria and procedures outlined will apply most appropriately to initial episodes and recurrent attacks of mental illness. To put it simply, it is necessary to find a way to satisfy legal and humanitarian considerations and yet allow psychiatrists access to initially or acutely ill patients in order to do the best they can for them. However, there are some involuntary patients who have received adequate and active treatment but have not responded satisfactorily. An irreducible minimum of such cases, principally among those with brain disorders and process schizophrenia, will not improve sufficiently to be able to adapt to even a tolerant society.

The decision of what to do at this point is not an easy one, and it should certainly not be in the hands of psychiatrists alone. With some justification they can state that they have been given the thankless job of caring, often with inadequate facilities, for badly damaged people and that they are now being subjected to criticism for keeping these patients locked up. No one really knows what to do with these patients. It may be that when treatment has failed they exchange their sick role for what has been called the impaired role (15), which implies a permanent negative evaluation of them coupled with a somewhat less benign societal attitude. At this point, perhaps a case can be made for giving greater importance to the criteria for dangerousness and releasing such patients if they do not pose a threat to others. However, I do not believe that the release into the community of these severely malfunctioning individuals will serve their interests even though it may satisfy formal notions of right and wrong.

It should be emphasized that the number of individuals for whom involuntary commitment must be considered is small (although, under the influence of current pressures, it may be smaller than it should be). Even severe mental illness can often be handled by securing the cooperation of the patient, and certainly one of the favorable efforts. However, the distinction between voluntary and involuntary hospitalization is sometimes more formal than meaningful. How "voluntary" are the actions of an individual who is being buffeted by the threats, entreaties, and tears of his family?

I believe, however, that we are at a point (at least in some jurisdictions) where, having rebounded from an era in which involuntary commitment was too easy and employed too often, we are now entering one in which it is becoming very difficult to commit anyone, even in urgent cases. Faced with the moral obloquy that has come to pervade the atmosphere in which the decision to involuntarily hospitalize is considered, some psychiatrists, especially younger ones, have become, as Stone (16) put it, "soft as grapes" when faced with the prospect of committing anyone under any circumstances.

THE CIVIL LIBERTIES LAWYERS

I use this admittedly inexact label to designate those members of the legal profession who do not in principle reject the necessity for involuntary hospitalization but who do reject or wish to diminish the importance of medical model criteria in the hands of psychiatrists. Accordingly, the civil liberties lawyers, in dealing with the problem of involuntary hospitalization, have enlisted themselves under the standard of dangerousness, which they hold to be more objective and capable of being dealt with in a sounder evidentiary manner than the medical model criteria. For them the question is not whether mental illness, even of disabling degree, is present, but only whether it has resulted in the probability of behavior dangerous to others or to self. Thus they would scrutinize the cases previously described for evidence of such dangerousness and would make the decision about involuntary hospitalization accordingly. They would probably feel that commitment is not indicated in most of these cases, since they were selected as illustrative of severe mental illness in which outstanding evidence of physical dangerousness was not present.

The dangerousness standard is being used increasingly not only to supplement criteria for mental illness but, in fact, to replace them entirely. The recent Supreme Court decision in *O'Connor v. Donaldson* (17)

is certainly a long step in this direction. In addition, "dangerousness" is increasingly being understood to refer to the probability that the individual will inflict harm on himself or others in a specific physical manner rather than in other ways. This tendency has perhaps been carried to its ultimate in the *Lessard v. Schmidt* case (18) in Wisconsin, which restricted suitability for commitment to the "extreme likelihood that if the person is not confined, he will do immediate harm to himself or others." (This decision was set aside by the U.S. Supreme Court in 1974.) In a recent Washington, D.C., Superior Court case (19) the instructions to the jury stated that the government must prove that the defendant was likely to cause "substantial physical harm to himself or others in the reasonably foreseeable future."

For the following reasons, the dangerousness standard is an inappropriate and dangerous indicator to use in judging the conditions under which someone should be involuntarily hospitalized. Dangerousness is being taken out of its proper context as one among other symptoms of the presence of severe mental illness that should be the determining factor.

1. To concentrate on dangerousness (especially to others) as the sole criterion for involuntary hospitalization deprives many mentally ill persons of the protection and treatment that they urgently require. A psychiatrist under the constraints of the dangerousness rule, faced with an out-of-control manic individual whose frantic behavior the psychiatrist truly believes to be a disguised call for help, would have to say, "Sorry, I would like to help you but I can't because you haven't threatened anybody and you are not suicidal." Since psychiatrists are admittedly not very good at accurately predicting dangerousness to others, the evidentiary standards for commitment will be very stringent. This will result in mental hospitals becoming prisons for a small population of volatile, highly assaultive, and untreatable patients (14).

2. The attempt to differentiate rigidly (especially in regard to danger to self) between physical and other kinds of self-destructive behavior is artificial, unrealistic, and unworkable. It will tend to confront psychiatrists who want to help their patients with the same kind of dilemma they were faced with when justification for therapeutic abortion on psychiatric grounds depended on evidence of suicidal intent. The advocates of the

dangerousness standard seem to be more comfortable with and pay more attention to the factor of dangerousness to others even though it is a much less frequent and much less significant consequence of mental illness than is danger to self.

3. The emphasis on dangerousness (again, especially to others) is a real obstacle to the right-to-treatment movement since it prevents the hospitalization and therefore the treatment of the population most amenable to various kinds of therapy.

4. Emphasis on the criterion of dangerousness to others moves involuntary commitment from a civil to a criminal procedure, thus, as Stone (14) put it, imposing the procedures of one terrible system on another. Involuntary commitment on these grounds becomes a form of preventive detention and makes the psychiatrist a kind of glorified policeman.

5. Emphasis on dangerousness rather than mental disability and helplessness will hasten the process of deinstitutionalization. Recent reports (20, 21) have shown that these patients are not being rehabilitated and reintegrated into the community, but rather, that the burden of custodialism has been shifted from the hospital to the community.

6. As previously mentioned, emphasis on the dangerousness criterion may be a tactic of some of the abolitionists among the civil liberties lawyers (22) to end involuntary hospitalization by reducing it to an unworkable absurdity.

DISCUSSION

It is obvious that it is good to be at liberty and that it is good to be free from the consequences of disabling and dehumanizing illness. Sometimes these two values are incompatible, and in the heat of the passions that are often aroused by opposing views of right and wrong, the partisans of each view may tend to minimize the importance of the other. Both sides can present their horror stories—the psychiatrists, their dead victims of the failure of the involuntary hospitalization process, and the lawyers, their Donaldsons. There is a real danger that instead of acknowledging the difficulty of the problem, the two camps will become polarized, with a consequent rush toward extreme and untenable solutions rather than working toward reasonable ones.

The path taken by those whom I have labeled the abolitionists is an example of the barren results that ensue when an absolute solution is imposed on a complex problem. There are human beings who will suffer greatly if the abolitionists succeed in elevating an abstract principle into an unbreakable law with no exceptions. I find myself oppressed and repelled by their position, which seems to stem from an ideological rigidity which ignores that element of the contingent immanent in the structure of human existence. It is devoid of compassion.

The positions of those who espouse the medical model and the dangerousness approaches to commitment are, one hopes, not completely irreconcilable. To some extent these differences are a result of the vantage points from which lawyers and psychiatrists view mental illness and commitment. The lawyers see and are concerned with the failures and abuses of the process. Furthermore, as a result of their training, they tend to apply principles to classes of people rather than to take each instance as unique. The psychiatrists, on the other hand, are required to deal practically with the singular needs of individuals. They approach the problem from a clinical rather than a deductive stance. As physicians, they want to be in a position to take care of and to help suffering people whom they regard as sick patients. They sometimes become impatient with the rules that prevent them from doing this.

I believe we are now witnessing a pendular swing in which the rights of the mentally ill to be treated and protected are being set aside in the rush to give them their freedom at whatever cost. But is freedom defined only by the absence of external constraints? Internal physiological or psychological processes can contribute to a throttling of the spirit that is as painful as any applied from the outside. The "wild" manic individual without his lithium, the panicky hallucinator without his injection of fluphenazine hydrochloride and the understanding support of a concerned staff, the sodden alcoholic—are they free? Sometimes, as Woody Guthrie said, "Freedom means no place to go."

Today the civil liberties lawyers are in the ascendancy and the psychiatrists on the defensive to a degree that is harmful to individual needs and the public welfare. Redress and a more balanced position will not come from further extension of the dangerousness doctrine. I favor a return to the use of medical criteria by psychiatrists—psychiatrists, however, who have been chastened by the buffeting they have received and are quite willing to go along with even strict legal safeguards as long as they are constructive and not tyrannical.

REFERENCES

1 Treffert, D. A.: "The practical limits of patients' rights." *Psychiatric Annals* 5(4):91–96, 1971.

2 Szasz, T.: *Law, Liberty and Psychiatry,* New York, Macmillan Co., 1963.

3 Ennis, B.: *Prisoners of Psychiatry,* New York, Harcourt Brace Jovanovich, 1972.

4 Szasz, T.: *The Myth of Mental Illness,* New York, Harper & Row, 1961.

5 Laing, R.: *The Politics of Experience,* New York, Ballantine Books, 1967.

6 Ennis, B.: "Ennis on 'Donaldson'." *Psychiatric News,* Dec. 3, 1975, pp. 4, 19, 37.

7 Peele, R., Chodoff, P., Taub, N.: "Involuntary hospitalization and treatability. Observations from the DC experience." *Catholic University Law Review* 23:744–753, 1974.

8 Michels, R.: "The right to refuse psychotropic drugs." *Hastings Center Report,* Hastings-on-Hudson, NY, 1973.

9 Parsons, T.: *The Social System.* New York, Free Press, 1951.

10 Veatch, R. M.: "The medical model; its nature and problems." *Hastings Center Studies* 1(3):59–76, 1973.

11 Katz, J.: "The right to treatment—an enchanting legal fiction?" *University of Chicago Law Review* 36:755–783, 1969.

12 Moore, M. S.: "Some myths about mental illness." *Arch Gen Psychiatry* 32:1483–1497, 1975.

13 Peszke, M. A.: "Is dangerousness an issue for physicians in emergency commitment?" *Am J Psychiatry* 132:825–828, 1975.

14 Stone, A. A.: "Comment on Peszke, M. A.: Is dangerousness an issue for physicians in emergency commitment?" Ibid. 829–831.

15 Siegler, M., Osmond, H.: *Models of Madness, Models of Medicine.* New York, Macmillan Co., 1974.

16 Stone, A. A.: Lecture for course on The Law, Litigation, and Mental Health Services. Adelphi, Md., Mental Health Study Center, September 1974.

17 *O'Connor v Donaldson,* 43 USLW 4929 (1975).

18 *Lessard v Schmidt,* 349 F Supp 1078, 1092 (ED Wis 1972).

19 In re Johnnie Hargrove, Washington, DC, Superior Court Mental Health number 506–75, 1975.

20 Rachlin, S., Pam, A., Milton, J.: "Civil liberties versus involuntary hospitalization." *Am J Psychiatry* 132:189–191, 1975.

21 Kirk, S. A., Therrien, M. E.: "Community mental health myths and the fate of former hospitalized patients." *Psychiatry* 38:209–217, 1975.

22 Dershowitz, A. A.: "Dangerousness as a criterion for confinement." *Bulletin of the American Academy of Psychiatry and the Law* 2:172–179, 1974.

Managing Mental Illness and Dementia

Deinstitutionalization at the Crossroads
H. Richard Lamb

H. Richard Lamb is professor of psychiatry at the University of Southern California School of Medicine. He is the author of *Treating the Long-Term Mentally Ill* (1982) and the editor of *The Homeless Mentally Ill: A Task Force Report of the American Psychiatric Association* (1984). His published articles include "Some Reflections on Treating Schizophrenics" and "Structure: The Neglected Ingredient of Community Treatment."

Lamb, while acknowledging that many things have gone right with deinstitutionalization, points out some of its unfortunate results—the problem of the homeless mentally ill, for example. His special concern is with the long-term mentally ill, a nonhomogeneous group whose various members have very different needs. A minority of the long-term mentally ill need a highly structured, locked, 24-hour environment for the adequate intermediate- or long-term management of their illness. Deinstitutionalization for them may be a disservice. However, the majority of the long-term mentally ill are able to live in the community, although the needs of members of this group are also very diverse. Lamb argues that a comprehensive system of care for those able to live in the community must be established, but such a system must recognize their heterogeneity. He concludes with a number of recommendations for mental-health professionals. The recommendations are calculated to maximize the benefits of deinstitutionalization for individuals with very different needs.

Probably nothing more graphically illustrates the problems of deinstitutionalization than the shameful and incredible phenomenon of the homeless mentally ill. The conditions under which they live are symptomatic of the lack of a comprehensive system of care for the long-term mentally ill in general. Though the homeless mentally ill have become an everyday part of today's society, they are nameless; the great majority are not on the caseload of any mental health professional or mental health agency. Hardly anyone is out looking for them, for they are not officially missing. By and large the system does not know who they are or where they came from.

We can see first hand society's reluctance to do anything definitive for them: for instance, stopgap measures such as shelters may be provided, but the underlying problem of a lack of a comprehensive system of care is not addressed (1). We can see our own ambivalence about taking the difficult stands that need to be taken—as, for instance, advocating changes in the laws for involuntary treatment and the ways these laws are administered.

When we get to know homeless mentally ill persons as individuals, we often find that they are not able to meet the criteria for the programs that most appeal to us as professionals. For the citizenry generally, the homeless mentally ill represent everything that has gone wrong with deinstitutionalization, and their circumstances have persuaded many that deinstitutionalization was a mistake.

Many things have gone right with deinstitutionalization. For instance, the chronically mentally ill have much more liberty, in the majority of cases appropriately so, than when they were institutionalized; we have learned what is necessary to meet their needs in the

Hospital and Community Psychiatry, vol. 39 (September 1988), pp. 941–945. Copyright © 1988, The American Psychiatric Association. Reprinted by permission.

community; and we have begun to understand the plight of families and how to enlist their help in the treatment process. But the purpose of this paper is twofold: to examine the problems of deinstitutionalization—not just with regard to the homeless mentally ill but for the long-term mentally ill generally—and to draw upon our experience, especially our clinical experience, in working with them in order to make recommendations about what we should do.

HOSPITAL AND COMMUNITY

Has deinstitutionalization gone too far in attempting to treat long-term mentally ill persons in the community? We now have more than three decades of experience to guide us. Some long-term mentally ill persons require a highly structured, locked, 24-hour setting for adequate intermediate or long-term management (2). For those who need such care, do we not have a professional obligation to provide it (3), either in a hospital or in an alternative setting such as California's locked skilled nursing facilities with special programs for psychiatric patients (4)?

Where to treat should not be an ideological issue; it is a decision best based on the clinical needs of each person. Unfortunately deinstitutionalization efforts have, in practice, too often confused locus of care and quality of care (5). Where mentally ill persons are treated has been seen as more important than how they are treated. Care in the community has often been assumed almost by definition to be better than hospital care. In actuality, poor care can be found in both hospital and community settings. But the other issue that requires attention is appropriateness. The long-term mentally ill are not a homogeneous population; what is appropriate for some is not appropriate for others.

For instance, what of those persons who are characterized by such problems as assaultive behavior;

severe, overt major psychopathology; lack of internal controls; reluctance to take psychotropic medications; inability to adjust to open settings; problems with drugs and alcohol; and self-destructive behavior? When attempts have been made to treat some of these persons in open community settings, they have required an inordinate amount of time and effort from mental health professionals, various social agencies, and the criminal justice system. Many have been lost to the mental health system and are on the streets or in jail.

Moreover, both mentally ill persons and mental health professionals have often considered these results as evidence of failures by both groups. As a consequence, many long-term mentally ill persons have become alienated from a system that has not met their needs, and some mental health professionals have become disenchanted with their treatment. Unfortunately the heat of the debate over whether to provide intermediate and long-term hospitalization for such patients has tended to obscure the benefits of community treatment for the great majority of the long-term mentally ill who do not require such highly structured 24-hour care.

SOME BASIC QUESTIONS

What about the majority of long-term mentally ill persons who are able to live in the community? First and foremost, we need to ask ourselves if we have truly established this group as the highest-priority population in public mental health.

If so, does this priority include commitments of our resources and our funding, as well as our concern? We have learned a great deal about the needs of the long-term mentally ill in the community. Thus we know that this population needs a comprehensive and integrated system of care (6); such a system would include an adequate number and range of supervised, supportive housing settings; adequate, comprehensive, and accessible crisis intervention, both in the community and in hospitals; and ongoing treatment and rehabilitative services, all provided assertively through outreach when necessary.

We know the importance of a system of case management in which every long-term mentally ill person is on the caseload of a mental health agency that will take full responsibility for individualized treatment planning, linking patients to needed resources and monitoring them so that they not only receive the services they need but are not lost to the system. Have we done enough to put our knowledge into practice? For most parts of this nation, the answer is clearly no (7).

THERAPEUTIC BUT REALISTIC OPTIMISM

Nothing is more important than therapeutic optimism if we are to work successfully with the long-term mentally ill. But equally important is a need for a realistic appraisal of these persons' capacities. With such an appraisal we can mount vigorous treatment and rehabilitation efforts for those with the potential for high levels of functioning and strive for other goals, such as improving quality of life, when patients have less potential.

An important issue related to goal setting is that the kinds of criteria that theorists, researchers, policy-makers, and clinicians use to assess social integration have a distinct bias in favor of the values held by these professionals and by middle-class society generally (8). Thus holding a job, increasing one's socialization and relationships with other people, and living independently may be goals that are not shared by a large proportion of the long-term mentally ill.

Likewise, what makes the patient happy may be unrelated to these goals. Patients may want (or need) to avoid the stress of competitive employment, or even sheltered employment, and of living independently. They may experience more anxiety than gratification from the threat of intimacy that accompanies increased involvement with other people. Furthermore, many relatives may be primarily interested in the simple provision of decent custodial care (9).

Moreover, if we use expectations applicable to the higher-functioning patients as our only model, we will neglect the large population who are lower functioning and cannot respond to these expectations. And, in fact, in many jurisdictions this population has been neglected. We can only speculate about why.

One possible reason is the failure by some mental health professionals to recognize that there are many different kinds of long-term patients who vary greatly in their capacity for rehabilitation and for change (10). Long-term mentally ill persons differ in their ability to cope with stress without decompensating and developing psychotic symptoms. They differ too in the kinds of stress and pressure they can handle; for instance, some who are amenable to social rehabilitation cannot handle the stresses of vocational rehabilitation, and vice versa. What may appear, at first glance, to be a homogeneous group turns out to be a group that ranges from persons who can tolerate almost no stress at all to those who can, with some assistance, cope with most of life's demands.

Such a view is supported by the very marked variations of course and outcome in both the shorter-term follow-up studies of schizophrenia (11, 12) and the longer-term studies discussed later. For some long-term patients, competitive employment, independent living, and a high level of social functioning are realistic goals; for others, just maintaining their present level of functioning should be considered a success (13).

Dependency, and the reactions of professionals to it, may well be another important factor. To gratify dependency needs and to nurture are crucial activities in the helping professions. And we learn to do this in such a way that patients do not experience a loss of self-esteem from knowing that they need our help and support (14). Not only may this process be draining to professionals, but in addition when we nurture, we expect growth, and we are sorely disappointed when we do not get it, even though the potential for the growth we seek may not be there. As a result, lower-functioning patients may receive less of our attention, our resources, and our efforts.

Moreover, most of us, as products of our culture and our society, tend to morally disapprove of persons who have "given in" to their dependency needs, who have adopted a passive, inactive life-style, and who have accepted public support instead of working (10). Perhaps this moral disapproval helps to explain why programs whose goals are rehabilitating patients to high levels of functioning, or "mainstreaming" them, attract the most attention and the most funding. Such programs are very much needed. If, however, professionals attempt to raise patients' low-functioning adaptations to the pressures of life, without making a realistic appraisal of the capabilities of each individual, an acute exacerbation of psychosis may result. Probably no problems are more difficult to overcome in the treatment of the long-term mentally ill than those of professionals having to come to terms with the fact that some persons are unable, or unwilling, or both to give up a life of dependency.

The matter of independence presents similar problems. Society generally, including professionals, highly values independence. And yet nothing is more difficult for many long-term mentally ill persons to attain and sustain (15). The issue of supervised versus unsupervised housing provides an example. Professionals want to see their patients living in their own apartments, managing on their own, perhaps with some outpatient support. But the experience of deinstitutionalization has been that most long-term mentally ill persons living in unsupervised settings in the community find the ordinary stresses of managing on their own more than they can handle. After a while they tend to not take their medications, to neglect their nutrition, and to let their lives unravel and become disorganized. Eventually they find their way back to the hospital or the streets (1).

Mentally ill persons highly value independence, but they very often underestimate their dependency needs. Professionals need to be realistic about their patients' potential for independence, even if the patients are not.

Still another factor that may contribute to the focus on higher-functioning patients is some professionals' lack of appreciation of the rewards of treating patients who function less well and of forming a relationship over many years with both patient and family. Even when the potential for higher functioning is limited, we can derive an immense amount of satisfaction from helping to transform chaotic, dysphoric life-styles into stable ones, with at least some opportunity for pleasure and contentment for both the mentally ill person and the family.

LONG-TERM OUTCOME AND EXPECTATIONS

Some mental health professionals believe that long-term follow-up studies of schizophrenia indicate that we should raise our expectations of how schizophrenics will function in the community. Such a conclusion requires closer scrutiny. These studies, with mean lengths of follow-up ranging from 22.4 to 36.9 years, have demonstrated considerable degrees of improvement and even "recovery" over time (16–20).

These findings are not surprising, for they are consistent with everyday clinical experience that schizophrenia in the patient's middle and later years tends to be more benign and far less stormy than in the earlier years. In contrast, younger schizophrenics are faced with the same concerns and life-cycle stresses as others in their age group. They strive for independence, satisfying relationships, a sense of identity, and vocational success. Many, lacking the ability to withstand stress and intimacy, struggle and often repeatedly fail. The result is anxiety, depression, psychotic episodes, and hospitalization. Denial of illness and the rebelliousness of youth often compound the problems.

As the years go by, schizophrenics and those around them tend to come to terms with the illness.

Goals are lowered, and expectations are lessened. Under these circumstances many persons with limited abilities to cope and deal with stress gradually become able to function in both vocational and domestic roles, meeting lowered expectations of others and themselves. With time the fires of youth burn lower. Increasing maturity is still another factor. Thus older patients with schizophrenia may present a far different picture than when they were younger, less mature, and striving to meet higher aspirations.

There is a danger, however, in using the word recovery rather than remission when referring to improved or even normal functioning. Recovery implies eradication of the illness. The evidence is compelling that schizophrenia, with its predisposition to decompensation under stress, is a genetically determined illness (21). There is no evidence that patients' genetic predisposition to decompensate under stress disappears. Moreover, as important as these long-term findings are, they should not mislead clinicians working with schizophrenics in their twenties or thirties to expect short- or intermediate-term results that are beyond individual patients' capabilities within shorter time frames.

PROBLEMS OF THE CITIES

What are the practical limits of what our nation, and in particular our largest cities, can and will do to serve the long-term mentally ill? The greatest number of these persons are in our largest cities, but it is here that the politics are most complex, the bureaucracies largest and most cumbersome, the battles for power and turf fiercest (22, 23). Here too the administrative costs of providing care tend to be high, often more than 50 percent of the budget, leaving an insufficient amount for actual services to patients. It is in the largest cities, too, that resistance to change tends to be strongest and most stubborn. These factors, if not corrected, inevitably lead to inadequate care of the long-term mentally ill.

INVOLUNTARY TREATMENT

Involuntary treatment presents us with an extremely difficult dilemma. Our beliefs in civil liberties come into conflict with our concern for the welfare of our patients. This dilemma can be resolved if we believe that the mentally ill have a right to involuntary treatment (24, 25) when, because of severe mental illness, they present a serious threat to their own welfare or that of others

and at the same time are not mentally competent to make a rational decision about accepting treatment.

Reaching out to patients and working to encourage them to accept help on a voluntary basis is certainly an important first step. But if it fails and the patient is at serious risk, helping professionals need to see that ethically we cannot simply stop there. Is it not our obligation to advocate for changes in the laws that will facilitate involuntary treatment for such persons, or changes in the way the laws for involuntary treatment are administered? These changes would result in patients' prompt return to acute inpatient treatment when it is clinically indicated, and ongoing measures, such as conservatorship, court-mandated outpatient treatment, and appointment of a payee for the patient's Supplemental Security Income check, when they are indicated.

What is needed is a treatment philosophy recognizing that such external controls are a positive, even crucial, therapeutic approach for those in the long-term mentally ill population who lack the internal controls to deal with their impulses and to organize themselves to cope with life's demands. Such external controls may interrupt the self-destructive, chaotic life of a patient who is on the streets and in and out of jails and hospitals.

For instance, in some parts of California, conservatorship has become an important therapeutic modality for such persons. It is particularly useful when conservators are psychiatric social workers or persons with similar backgrounds and skills who use their court-granted authority to become a crucial source of stability and support for chronically mentally ill persons. Conservatorship thus can enable persons who might otherwise be long-term residents of hospitals to live in the community and achieve a considerable measure of autonomy and satisfaction in their lives.

If we do not take a firm stand on these issues, we risk being seen by society, not to mention by the long-term mentally ill themselves, as uncaring and even inhumane. The homeless mentally ill dramatically illustrate this issue.

THE TASKS AHEAD OF US

What do we need to do to get deinstitutionalization back on course? The following strategies should be considered.

- We should acknowledge that while deinstitutionalization was a positive step and the correct thing to do, it has gone too far.

- Of the long-term mentally ill now in the community, only some need intermediate or long-term highly structured 24-hour residential care. For those who need such care, however, we should provide it. When we do not, the resulting problems and debate obscure the benefits of community treatment for the great majority who do not require highly structured 24-hour care.
- We should truly make the long-term mentally ill our highest priority in public mental health in terms of both resources and funding. In making this commitment, we should join with our natural allies, the families.
- We should establish a comprehensive and coordinated system of care for the long-term mentally ill.
- We should not settle for stop-gap solutions, as, for instance, relying on a system of shelters for the homeless mentally ill instead of dealing with the underlying problem of the lack of a comprehensive system of care for the long-term mentally ill generally.
- We should have the needed therapeutic optimism to treat the long-term mentally ill, but temper this optimism with realistic, individualized goals.
- We should emphasize that the long-term mentally ill are a highly heterogeneous population.
- We should be aware that the values and goals of psychiatrically disabled persons may be different from those projected onto them by well-meaning professionals.
- We should continue to mount a vigorous rehabilitation effort aimed at achieving higher levels of functioning, both social and vocational, for those long-term mentally ill persons who can benefit from it.
- We should also give high priority to those among the long-term mentally ill who function at lower levels and not focus only on persons with higher functioning.
- We should realize the gratification we can derive from helping to change the chaotic and painful life of a patient who is on the streets and in and out of jails and hospitals into a stable life that offers the possibility of at least some contentment, even if we cannot rehabilitate that patient to a high level of functioning.
- We should not confuse the more favorable long-term outcome of schizophrenia over 20 or more years with the lesser improvements that can be accomplished over the short or intermediate term.
- We should come to grips with the bureaucracy, politics, and inefficiency of our largest cities, where so many long-term mentally ill persons live. It may be that these problems cannot be solved and that in some instances the responsibility for the long-term mentally ill should be taken away from the cities and another administrative solution found—as, for instance, turning this responsibility over to the states.
- We as mental health professionals should actively advocate involuntary treatment, both emergency and ongoing, for persons for whom it is clinically indicated.

We have now had more than three decades of experience with deinstitutionalization. Most of what we know about community treatment of the long-term mentally ill we have learned the hard way—through experience. We need to be guided by that hard-won knowledge, look at each long-term mentally ill person as an individual with unique strengths, weaknesses, and needs, and do what our experience and clinical judgment tell us needs to be done to maximize the benefits of deinstitutionalization for each individual.

REFERENCES

1 Lamb HR (ed): The Homeless Mentally Ill: A Task Force Report of the American Psychiatric Association. Washington, DC, American Psychiatric Association, 1984

2 Dorwart RA: A ten-year follow-up study of the effects of deinstitutionalization. Hospital and Community Psychiatry 39:287–291, 1988

3 Group for the Advancement of Psychiatry: The Positive Aspects of Long Term Hospitalization in the Public Sector for Chronic Psychiatric Patients. New York, Mental Health Materials Center, 1982

4 Lamb HR: Structure: the neglected ingredient of community treatment. Archives of General Psychiatry 37:1224–1228, 1980

5 Bachrach LL: A conceptual approach to deinstitutionalization. Hospital and Community Psychiatry 29:573–578, 1978

6 Bachrach LL: The challenge of service planning for chronic mental patients. Community Mental Health Journal 22:170–174, 1986

7 Talbott JA: The fate of the public psychiatric system. Hospital and Community Psychiatry 36:46–50, 1985

8 Shadish WR Jr, Bootzin RR: Nursing homes and

chronic mental patients. Schizophrenia Bulletin 7:488–498, 1981

9 Thomas S: A survey of the relative importance of community care facility characteristics to different consumer groups. Presented at the Midwestern Psychological Association, St Louis, 1980

10 Lamb HR: Treating the Long-Term Mentally Ill. San Francisco, Jossey-Bass, 1982

11 World Health Organization: Schizophrenia: An International Follow-Up Study. New York, Wiley, 1979

12 Hawk AB, Carpenter WT, Strauss JS: Diagnostic criteria and five-year outcome in schizophrenia: a report from the International Pilot Study of Schizophrenia. Archives of General Psychiatry 32:343–347, 1975

13 Solomon EB, Baird B, Everstine L, et al: Assessing the community care of chronic psychotic patients. Hospital and Community Psychiatry 31:113–116, 1980

14 Lamb HR: Some reflections on treating schizophrenics. Archives of General Psychiatry 43:1007–1011, 1986

15 Harris M, Bergman HC: Differential treatment planning for young adult chronic patients. Hospital and Community Psychiatry 38:638–643, 1987

16 Bleuler M: A 23-year longitudinal study of 208 schizophrenics and impressions in regard to the nature of schizophrenia, in The Transmission of Schizophrenia. Edited by Rosenthal D, Kety SS. Oxford, England, Pergamon, 1968

17 Huber G, Gross G, Schuttler R, et al: Longitudinal studies of schizophrenic patients. Schizophrenia Bulletin 6:592–605, 1980

18 Ciompi L: Catamnestic long-term study on the course of life and aging of schizophrenics. Schizophrenia Bulletin 6:606–618, 1980

19 Tsuang M, Woolson R., Fleming J: Long-term outcome of major psychoses, I: schizophrenia and affective disorders compared with psychiatrically symptom-free surgical conditions. Archives of General Psychiatry 36:1295–1301, 1979

20 Harding CM, Brooks GW, Ashikaga T, et al: The Vermont longitudinal study of persons with severe mental illness, II: long-term outcome of subjects who retrospectively met DSM-III criteria for schizophrenia. American Journal of Psychiatry 144:727–735, 1987

21 Kety SS, Rosenthal D, Wender PH, et al: Studies based on a total sample of adopted individuals and their relatives: why they were necessary, what they demonstrated and failed to demonstrate. Schizophrenia Bulletin 2:413–428, 1976

22 Keill SL: Politics and public psychiatric programs. Hospital and Community Psychiatry 36:1143, 1985

23 Elpers JR: Dividing the mental health dollar: the ethics of managing scarce resources. Hospital and Community Psychiatry 37:671–672, 1986

24 Rachlin S: One right too many. Bulletin of the American Academy of Psychiatry and the Law 3:99–102, 1975

25 Lamb HR, Mills MJ: Needed changes in law and procedure for the chronically mentally ill. Hospital and Community Psychiatry 37:475–480, 1986

Paradoxical Patient Reactions to Psychiatric Life Support: Clinical and Ethical Considerations

Samuel L. Pauker and Arnold M. Cooper

Samuel L. Pauker is assistant clinical professor of psychiatry at Cornell University Medical College and assistant attending psychiatrist at the Payne Whitney Clinic, New York Hospital. He is coauthor of *The First Year of Marriage* (1987) and coeditor of *The Columbia Psychoanalytic Newsletter*. Arnold M. Cooper is Stephen P. Topin and Dr. Arnold M. Cooper Professor Emeritus in Consultation-Liason Psychiatry, Cornell University Medical College. He is

The American Journal of Psychiatry, vol. 147 (April 1990), pp. 488–491. Copyright © 1990, The American Psychiatric Association. Reprinted by permission.

deputy editor of *The American Journal of Psychiatry* and his articles include "Will Neurobiology Influence Psychoanalysis?"

Pauker and Cooper explore the clinical and ethical implications of two commonly overlooked facts: (1) Psychiatry's capacity to keep suicidal patients alive is limited; (2) in the case of some suicidal patients, constant observation and other measures designed to protect them from self-harm can sometimes exacerbate psychological symptoms and lessen the chances for autonomous functioning. In the authors' view, these facts suggest that "sometimes our efforts to foster patient improvement entail taking potentially life-threatening risks." Pauker and Cooper examine the clinical details of two cases that support their contention.

The two clinical situations we present in this article are not new to clinicians; indeed, they are all too familiar. These two clinical challenges consume much inpatient staff time and energy in the form of deliberation and concern. In one case, this deliberation was prospective: How should we proceed with a suicidal patient who reacted negatively to our efforts to keep her alive? The other involved a retrospective evaluation of what was done for a suicidal patient who seemed to be improving but then precipitously committed suicide.

We present these cases because we feel there is an important clinical reality that tends to be overlooked and/or denied and may be integrated in the thinking of clinicians and of society at large. It is that there is a limit to the powers of our current clinical art and science to keep psychiatric patients alive and sometimes our efforts to foster patient improvement entail taking potentially life-threatening risks. Taking such risks is inherent in good care, given the limits of our current therapeutic capacity.

Few clinical situations are as difficult and frightening to psychiatrists as the care of the seriously suicidal patient who fails to respond to treatment. Some patients remain overtly suicidal despite great efforts to provide treatment and life support. In fact, at times our attempts to guarantee survival by the use of life support systems—such as constant observation—may exacerbate psychopathology or deprive the patient of an opportunity to achieve a reasonable level of autonomy.

By "psychiatric life support" we mean procedures that keep psychiatric patients alive but are not directed at ameliorating psychopathology. While medical life support usually entails complex modern technologies, psychiatric life support involves one-to-one monitoring of suicidal patients and the interventions required to restrain patients from harming themselves, such as physical restraint or sedation. Psychopharmacology,

psychotherapy, and other psychosocial interventions are also used in this effort and are usually aimed at modifying the course of a disorder, in contrast to life support, which is intended to keep a patient alive until the course of illness is modified. There are patients, however, whose underlying disorders are refractory to the treatment interventions currently known to us. We may observe these patients for long periods of time, get to know them as well as we can, and apply successive therapeutic regimens as intensively as possible, and the patient may still remain suicidal (1–4).

The cases of two patients follow. For the first, extended life support seemed to inhibit recovery. In the second, additional life support might have prevented a suicide.

CASE REPORTS

Case 1: The Treatment-Refractory Suicidal Patient

Ms. A, an unmarried 29-year-old woman, had been given diagnoses of dysthymic disorder and mixed personality disorder. This was her fifth psychiatric hospitalization for depression and suicidality, which had followed the breakup of her relationship with a boyfriend. Ms. A's hospital care included multiple drug treatments for her depression (including phenelzine, lithium, L-triiodothyronine, trazodone, lorazepam, alprazolam, and various combinations of these agents) and intensive psychotherapy, with little improvement. She required $3^{1}/_{2}$ months of almost continuous observation because of her increasingly life-threatening acting out. Multiple consultations were sought regarding both drug treatment and her milieu treatment with maximum observation. A senior consultant felt that the maximum observation had become countertherapeutic, causing Ms. A to regress in the hospital, and that the somatic and psychotherapeutic modalities were providing her little benefit, as she continued to be actively suicidal.

Since the life support was felt to be harming rather than helping, it was decided to gradually reduce the observation. Ms. A and her family were carefully apprised of the reasons for this course of action and the significant risks involved. As this treatment plan proceeded, Ms. A was observed to be "re-organizing" herself, functioning in a less dependent manner, and exhibiting less sadomasochistic acting out. During this period she superficially cut her wrists and hinted at a plan to hang herself, but the staff felt that these were more attention-seeking gestures than truly suicidal endeavors. Mobilization proceeded and Ms. A was eventually able to be discharged to an outpatient therapist with whom she had a close working alliance.

This case illustrates that our usual hospital treatment modalities may exacerbate rather than ameliorate a patient's condition, creating an environment that induces clinical regression and the potential for further life-threatening behavior. The multiple expert consultations requested reflect the extreme danger that the staff perceived for this patient. Ultimately the staff recognized that their best treatment efforts had been ineffective and that providing a risk-free environment was antitherapeutic. They then attempted to fashion a treatment that might help to promote the patient's well-being by enhancing her autonomy and responsibility, rather than providing total protection from risk. The treatment team also appreciated that the risks of this decision must be shared with the patient and her family.

As the staff's adoption of Ms. A's ego functions was cautiously reversed and monitoring was withdrawn, she made a series of suicidal gestures that, fortunately but not predictably, were of minimal seriousness. The treatment strategy was successful in this instance. Ms. A had a good therapeutic alliance with an outpatient psychiatric psychotherapist, which helped sustain her during this process, and she was eventually able to be discharged. We emphasize, however, that the patient might have killed herself, and that other patients in similar circumstances have done so and will do so in the future.

In the following case vignette, the patient appeared to be doing better than Ms. A but killed herself when life support was tapered.

Case 2: The Suicidal Patient Who Seems to Be Improving

Ms. B, a young unmarried woman, had been admitted for psychiatric hospitalization because of acute psychosis and suicidal ideation. Her adolescence had been marked by multiple symptoms, including sexual promiscuity, religiosity, rebellion against her parents, substance abuse (marijuana and some cocaine), and bulimia. She had also exhibited bizarre behaviors, such as stating that she could communicate with tiny creatures, having odd decorations in her room, and treating pet animals sadistically. Ms. B's one prior psychiatric hospitalization had been related to her eating disorder; she believed her "stomach was connected to the center of the earth." Before her current hospitalization she had been paranoid and said she was being manipulated by the television and radio. The bizarre nature and chronicity of her symptoms and a prior poor response to lithium led to the diagnosis of schizophrenia.

After her workup, Ms. B was treated with neuroleptics, psychotherapy, and various milieu therapeutic modalities. Given the protracted nature of her illness, after due consideration the staff believed that Ms. B's best chance for both survival and achievement of the maximum level of adaptation of which she was capable would be best served by long-term hospitalization.

Ms. B's initial hospital course was unremarkable. Although she was psychotic (i.e., had ideas of reference, thought others were speaking her thoughts, and exhibited paranoia) and suicidal, Ms. B was able to come to the staff when feeling suicidal, was reassured by their attention, and responded well to restriction to the unit's central lounge.

On hospital day 13, Ms. B came in contact with an elderly depressed male patient, which seemed to upset her greatly. Afterward she precipitously and surreptitiously eloped with a strong intent to obtain razor blades and to swallow them and kill herself. She was found and brought back to the hospital by her mother. After her return, she continued to be psychotic and suicidal. Her neuroleptic dose was increased. The elopement was felt by the staff to signal a significant change; Ms. B could no longer be counted on to come to the staff for help when feeling acutely suicidal. From day 13 on, therefore, she was placed on round-the-clock observation.

With the increased neuroleptic dose, Ms. B's paranoid ideation diminished. Her active suicidal ideation persisted, however, and the maximum observation was continued. ECT was considered but postponed in the belief that it might interfere with efforts to facilitate Ms. B's transfer for long-term care. Indeed, with the higher dose of neuroleptic her mood began to brighten. She rejoined activities and was much less suicidal.

After 22 days of round-the-clock observation her status was downgraded, and her monitoring was decreased to checks every 15 minutes during the day and constant observation at night. For 12 days, at this level of monitoring, Ms. B was able to participate in some activities and was more communicative with the staff, in whom she could now confide her periodic passive suicidal ideation.

On hospital day 47, after 34 days of total or partial observation, it was felt that maximum observation could be discontinued. Three days later Ms. B continued to appear to be doing well. After a pleasant telephone call with her mother and a conversation with a staff nurse, neither of whom detected any special difficulty, with no evident precipitant Ms. B went into a bathroom stall, put a plastic bag over her head, and asphyxiated herself. She was found a short time later and was given cardiopulmonary resuscitation but was eventually found to be brain dead.

A follow-up mortality and morbidity conference was held, as is the hospital's usual procedure after a death. It was uniformly thought that Ms. B's diagnosis and treatment had been appropriate. Her diagnosis (schizophrenia) and demoralization were seen as high-risk factors in the case. However, Ms. B had seemed to be doing better at the time of her suicide and during the days before it, after maximum observation had been withdrawn.

This case highlights a number of clinical and ethical points. Despite our best clinical efforts we cannot always predict underlying suicidality, especially in our schizophrenic patients (5, 6). When a patient is improving, as Ms. B was, and we are trying to switch the patient to less restrictive long-term treatment, we attempt to transfer self-care functions back to the patient.

Cases such as this one make us wonder if extending monitoring for suicidality beyond the point of apparent clinical improvement would prevent many suicides. Despite the potential merits of such an option, clinicians would generally find this an ill-advised and unacceptable clinical precaution. Unlike the monitoring of patients who have had myocardial infarctions, who may experience life-threatening arrhythmias, psychiatric life support may be an invasive procedure associated with morbidity itself and may delay the patient's reacquisi-

tion of self-care capabilities or, as in the first case, stimulate regressive self-destructive acts.

DISCUSSION

We have identified two kinds of suicidal patients who are difficult to manage. The first type seems to worsen with maximum observation and improve when it is terminated and the patient is given increased responsibility for his or her own care. The second type seems to be improving but is at risk for unexpected suicide when maximum observation is withdrawn. Currently there are no means of identifying either type of patient despite careful clinical attention. Careful study and research are needed to diminish the time required to identify the first type of patient and to devise some form of extended observation or monitoring for the second. Despite our best efforts, however, we are faced with and will continue to be faced with a central clinical ethical dilemma. Psychiatric recovery entails the patient's eventually regaining responsibility for his or her own care. Since this is an important part of the recovery process, some small percentage of patients will at some point present the kind of risk described in case 2.

The question of when life support may ethically be discontinued has preoccupied medicine since technology has been able to sustain physiological functioning in patients who are no longer sentient or whose hopelessness and suffering—and their wish for relief from the pain of life—would lead to a wished-for death in the absence of life support (7). The comparable response in psychiatry is not technologic; rather, it invokes a social procedure—maximum observation—to maintain life in a patient whose psychiatric disorder leads to the determination to die and who does not respond to available treatments. A psychiatric hospital has an obligation to 1) provide a safe haven for the patient, 2) carefully consider all diagnostic possibilities, 3) offer all appropriate treatments, 4) work assiduously at understanding the patient and family to help them overcome any resistance to compliance, 5) alert the patient and family to the risks and limitations, as well as benefits, of any treatment effort, 6) take steps to protect the patient with all available life support measures pending successful treatment, and 7) recognize when a treatment has failed or is contributing further to morbidity.

As psychiatrists, we may find it difficult to accept that a small percentage of our suicidal patients are refractory to the currently available interventions and that acceptance of this risk is a critical part of the care of psychiatric patients. Like their counterparts in oncology and other medical and surgical subspecialties that deal with the severely and terminally ill, some of these patients, despite our best efforts, will die. Our task is to maximize life support for those who will benefit from our treatments while, with the greatest caution, we attempt to identify that small group who cannot benefit from and may be harmed by prolonged psychiatric life support procedures. At some point in the care of the nonpsychotic, chronically suicidal patient, we must examine whether life support measures are contributing to the patient's morbidity and whether their usefulness justifies the drain on the resources available for the care of other patients.

Paradoxically, some patients appear to do worse with maximum observation and respond well to the judicious return of self-care functions (as in case 1), while some who seem to be improving surprise us with impulsive lethal acts (as in case 2). Clearly, both groups deserve additional study and research. Until we better understand the nature of the impulsive, "unpredictable" suicide and since we cannot and should not keep all improving patients under extended maximum observa-

tion, we must accept that facilitating patient improvement and autonomy will engender a small but significant unavoidable risk of mortality.

REFERENCES

1 Robins LN, Kulbok PA: Methodological strategies in suicide, in Psychobiology of Suicidal Behavior. Edited by Mann JJ, Stanley M. New York, Annals of the New York Academy of Sciences, 1986

2 Linehan MM: Suicidal people: one population or two? Ibid

3 Cohen J: Statistical approaches to suicidal risk factor analysis. Ibid

4 Pfeffer CR: Suicide prevention: current efficacy and future promise. Ibid

5 Johns CA, Stanley M, Stanley B: Suicide in schizophrenia. Ibid

6 Salama AA: Depression and suicide in schizophrenic patients. Suicide Life Threat Behav 1988; 18:379–384

7 Rachels J: Barney Clark's key. Hastings Cent Rep 1983; 13(2):17–19

Dangerous Behavior in a Demented Patient: Preserving Autonomy in a Patient with Diminished Competence

David T. Watts, Christine K. Cassel, and Timothy Howell

David T. Watts is associate professor of medicine at the University of Wisconsin, Madison. He is the author of such articles as "The Family's Will or the Living Will: Patient Self-Determination in Doubt." Christine K. Cassel is professor of medicine and public policy and chief of the section of general internal medicine at the University of Chicago. Her many articles include "Physician-Assisted Suicide: Are We Asking the Right Questions?" Timothy Howell is professor of psychiatry and family medicine at the University of Wisconsin, Madison. He practices psychiatry at the Mendota Mental Health Institute and his coauthored articles include (with Watts) "Assisted Suicide Is Not Voluntary Active Euthanasia."

Watts, Cassel, and Howell examine an ethical dilemma that frequently arises with demented elderly persons who exhibit dangerous behavior but resist placement in a safer environment: how to reconcile their desire for freedom and independence with professionals' belief that they have an obligation to help such persons. In the authors' view, the dilemma is especially acute when the demented person is neither clearly competent nor clearly incompetent. After exploring in depth a case involving an elderly man with mild to moderate demen-

Reprinted with permission of the publisher from *Journal of the American Geriatrics Society*, vol. 37 (July 1989), pp. 658–662.

tia, the authors conclude that such situations "call for interventions which are both medically and ethically creative, and the marshalling of resources to maintain the individual's autonomy for as long as possible."

Dementia has been termed the "silent epidemic."[1] With increasing numbers of very aged persons in our society, the health care system is challenged to deal more effectively with dementia, one of the major afflictions of the elderly. While the cognitive impairment of dementia may progress insidiously, its behavioral complications often manifest acutely and require physician intervention. Dangerous behaviors can include reckless driving, combativeness, wandering, careless smoking, unsafe use of cooking or heating devices, or neglect of personal health or well-being.[2]

Such behavior may result from the loss of memory itself, a decline in ability to recognize or appreciate consequences, or a lack of insight about physical or mental impairments. Concurrent medical conditions may also aggravate cognitive impairment and precipitate dangerous behavior.

Dangerous behavior often leads to medical intervention, as caregivers find it difficult to cope or to accept the risks involved. Restrictions on activities of daily living, or even placement in a nursing care facility, may be considered as possible solutions. Such considerations are complex, involving divergent views and conflicting values,[3] as efforts to reduce risks may compromise individual liberties and self-esteem. The following case highlights these issues.

J.E., a 94-year-old man, was brought to the hospital by a neighbor after causing a fire while attempting to dry his clothes in his gas oven. The neighbor reported other instances suggesting the patient's judgment was diminished. As J.E. was a widower living alone, it appeared to the hospital staff that nursing home placement might be necessary to provide adequate supervision. However, J.E. refused to consider this and insisted on returning to his own house.

IMPLICATIONS OF HOSPITALIZATION FOR THE VERY OLD

Hospital admission removed J.E. from his familiar surroundings and accentuated his dependency. Though he had clung precariously to his independent lifestyle, it now appeared that he would need placement in a nurs-

ing care facility. Such "decisions to leave home" require sensitivity to the broader issue of preserving the individual's quality of life.[4]

When he refused nursing home placement, J.E. was transferred to the Geriatric Evaluation Unit (GEU) for evaluation by a team consisting of geriatric physicians, nurses, psychiatrist, social worker, and rehabilitative therapists. The team delved into J.E.'s private life, his psyche, and critically examined the circumstances under which he lived. Though J.E. wanted to return home, his dangerous behavior presented the risk of serious personal harm, and raised difficult questions of ethical responsibility and legal liability for staff. The dilemma was how to preserve his autonomy while at the same time providing him with the health care and support he needed.

A major therapeutic goal in working with demented patients is to maintain their autonomy as long as possible. Preserving an individual's autonomy requires respecting his or her values and preferences. Hence it is important to ascertain what those values are. The ethical obligation to determine a patient's wishes does not depend on whether he asserts his right to self determination.[5] Hospitalized elders may have difficulty expressing their preferences due to illness (especially dementia), frailty, or psychosocial factors.[6] This makes it incumbent upon the staff to elicit, if possible, a patient's own values and preferences, even where these are not volunteered. A GEU provides an environment in which a cognitively-impaired patient's desire to return home can be thoroughly evaluated.

Had J.E. acquiesced to institutionalization, presumably the machinery would have moved smoothly forward. Hospital staff would have felt reassured that he was "safe," and that hospital resources had been conserved by a timely transfer. His intransigence forced the system to pause and consider the causes and implications of his dangerous behavior. The question became, Would it be possible to respect his wish to return home?

ETHICAL OBLIGATIONS IN EVALUATING DANGEROUS BEHAVIOR

Accurate descriptions of dangerous behavior are essential for evaluating the level of cognitive impairment, degree of risk, possible causes of the behavior, and course of action. Eyewitness accounts need to be obtained directly from caregivers, neighbors, or police.

The context of the behavior, including the patient's level of cognitive functioning, is important. Can the patient remember, describe, and explain the incident in question? Deficits in memory or judgment may be apparent from the patient's account. Alternatively, the patient may have a cogent explanation for seemingly bizarre behavior. Other signs of behavioral deterioration may occur in a patient with moderate dementia. A careful mental status examination, including assessment of orientation, memory, intellect, judgment, affect, and screening for the presence of agitation, delusions, hallucinations, mood disturbance, or anxiety, are necessary to elucidate possible causes of dangerous behavior. A rapid deterioration in cognition suggests an acute medical illness causing delirium. Physical and laboratory assessment should focus on reversible conditions that can adversely affect cognition.

J.E. stated that his dryer had broken, and he therefore had used the oven to dry his clothes. He minimized the seriousness of the incident, stating that there had not really been a fire, "just some smoke," and no serious danger. It was verified that no one else had been placed in jeopardy.

The geriatric psychiatrist found J.E. to be attentive, but not always well-oriented. His speech was difficult to understand, due to mandibular resorption from a long-standing absence of teeth. His hearing was poor. His memory was variable, and his insight and judgment were marginal. He scored 23 correct on the 30-item Folstein Mini-Mental status exam.

The assessment was that J.E. had mild to moderate dementia. The psychiatrist concluded that J.E. could not, by himself, adequately integrate all the information needed to assist in planning for medical care upon discharge. Medical evaluation found a urinary tract infection, for which antibiotics were prescribed. He also had weakness due to cervical myelopathy which limited his ambulation to crawling.

It was recommended that discharge to his home be contingent upon demonstration of self-care skills. But J.E. insisted on returning to his home, without further evaluation by the hospital staff.

J.E. had the right to refuse further treatment and leave the hospital. He was temporarily unable to exercise these rights, however, due to his physical and mental impairments. The health care team felt obligated to further evaluate J.E.'s dangerous behavior, yet discomfited by his daily demands to leave the hospital. He was a challenge for the health professionals to understand. He had lived alone and isolated within the community for decades. To the staff, he represented someone from an earlier time, a different culture, a sort of Rip Van Winkle. That J.E. was not allowed to leave the hospital seemed to reflect the "parentalistic" attitudes of relatively youthful health professionals toward very frail elderly persons.

THE OBLIGATION TO EVALUATE RISK

Several factors enter into consideration of the risks posed by patients' dangerous behaviors: the immediacy of danger, the seriousness of the consequences to themselves and others, their ability to evaluate the risks involved, and their values.

Immediacy of danger concerns the likelihood of hazardous incidents. Concurrent psychosis, delirium, alcohol abuse, or a recurrent pattern all raise the risks. Often, however, there are only isolated instances, scattered in time, which make it difficult to determine when or if the dangerous behavior will recur. Severe potential consequences may dictate a full evaluation of even rare instances of dangerous behavior. A particularly problematic area, as J.E.'s case exemplified, is an elderly person's misuse of heating or cooking devices. The potential consequences of fire include serious harm or death to the individual or others living in the same building. Yet, the use of cooking devices is necessary for independent living, and is a fundamental prerogative of competent adults. Therefore, the burden is on health professionals to demonstrate, to a reasonable degree of medical certainty, that there is an urgent threat of serious harm to self or others before restricting use of the stove. The risk can be decreased by modifying the stove with safety switches, automatic shutoff, warning alarms, or adding smoke detectors, but these measures depend on the impaired person's ability to respond appropriately to the different signals.

A cognitively-impaired patient's ability to evaluate risk is a crucial point. J.E.'s judgment was highly suspect, since he had been using an inappropriate appliance to dry his clothes. Was the fire an unpredictable outcome, or did he fail to take adequate care? Had J.E., for example, insisted on driving when it was clear he could no longer do so safely, restriction of his driving would be justified because of the great risk to himself and others.

The risks of dangerous behavior need to be considered in the context of the person's values. Staff appreciation for J.E.'s values developed during his evaluation on the GEU. Those who worked closely with J.E. described him as proud, independent, a "fighter." He had demonstrated resiliency and coping skills by remaining at home despite his disabilities. He had had virtually no contact with the health care system, and disdained the institutional environment. He had bought his house 30 years earlier, planning to live with his wife there all their lives; she had died there 20 years ago. In J.E.'s mind these factors weighed strongly in considering the relative risks and benefits of returning home.

J.E.'s desire to live at home was a dilemma for some team members, who believed he needed supervision to support him and prevent him from harming himself. Others felt that the health care system had no right to restrict him against his will. One solution would be to coerce him to accept protective services through the legal system, but this would undermine his autonomy. Another would be to let him go his own way, but this would amount to abandoning him. But such situations need not devolve into all or nothing decisions. To accommodate conflicting values, one can forge a compromise. Such a compromise depends not only on team members' expertise in rehabilitative, social work, psychiatric, nursing, and medical disciplines, but on their experience in resolving such ethical dilemmas. The team process in developing a compromise can provide a way in which conflicting values are balanced in an optimal manner.

Sympathy with J.E.'s independent spirit was a deciding factor in assisting his return home. A plan was devised to meet his essential needs, including assistance with meal preparation, housekeeping services to maintain safety and sanitation, and nursing visits to monitor health status. J.E. acquiesced to the home care plan. He wanted to leave the hospital, and cooperation with home services seemed a precondition.

REFUSAL OF HOME CARE: ETHICAL ISSUES

Soon after he returned home, problems arose in providing J.E.'s care. He was rude and gruff to homemaker personnel. When they encouraged him to eat, he became hostile and verbally aggressive towards them. The visiting nurse described conditions in the home as "intolerable." Meat was left sitting out to spoil; prepared food was left uneaten. He resisted help in bathing or transfers, and often seemed disoriented or unaware of his surroundings.

The hoped-for improvements in J.E.'s performance on returning home were not realized. The conditions in which he lived were probably no worse than they had been prior to hospitalization, but his privacy had been irretrievably lost. The risks in his situation could not be ignored by the health care team, and they considered several further options: institutional placement, disengagement, or modification of home care.

Institutional Placement   The health care system, through legal agency, *could* have removed J.E. to an institution for protective placement. He met the nominal criterion for incompetence under Wisconsin statutes, insofar as he was "substantially incapable of managing his property or caring for himself by reason of infirmities of aging. . . ."[7] This legal standard of competency hinges on whether a person can care for himself without substantial risk of harm. In many areas of health care decision-making, however, a different notion of competency is used. In those contexts, competency depends on the person's ability to understand and weigh information, and make choices with an awareness of the likely consequences. [For example, in Wisconsin, a patient is considered "not competent to refuse medication if because of mental illness . . . the individual is incapable of expressing an understanding of the advantages and disadvantages of accepting treatment, and the alternatives to accepting the particular treatment offered . . ." Wisconsin Statutes, Sec. 51.61(3)(g).]

The health care team's dilemma was that while J.E. could express a preference to live independently, he lacked the capacity to provide for his own daily needs. Court proceedings in such circumstances, whereby infirm elderly persons may become the object of protective efforts by well-meaning family members or social service professionals, are seen by some as a serious threat to the civil liberties of aged persons.[8] Legal interventions such as guardianship or protective placement may be arbitrarily applied, and may also depend on random medical events which bring the individual to the attention of the health care system.

Thus, depending upon how the statutory language was interpreted, J.E. could have been declared incompetent and protectively placed. However, this seemed too great an insult, considering his age, expressed preferences, and personality. Adversarial guardianship proceedings, physical removal from his home, placement in a strange setting—all these would likely have killed J.E., in spirit if not in fact. It seemed unlikely that someone as independent and obstinate as J.E. would adapt well to a nursing home.[9]

Disengagement   The right of a competent adult to refuse medical therapy is now generally recognized, even if such refusal would lead to death. The legal emergence of this right, however, has been relatively recent. An example is the 1984 case of a 70-year-old man with respiratory failure, whose right to discontinue ventilatory support was upheld. The court determined that the man wanted to live, but not if this meant continued dependence on a ventilator. He clearly understood that without a ventilator, he would die. He preferred death to "intolerable" life maintained by a ventilator, and this was respected.[10]

These issues are less clear for an elderly person risking death through a behavioral consequence of dementia, who may or may not appreciate the consequences of his behavior. To J.E., an existence dependent on institutional care was unacceptable. He even found health care in the home intrusive and burdensome. But did J.E. understand that he risked an earlier death without home care? A physician interviewed J.E. at home and found that he understood the risks and was willing to take them. The physician believed J.E. had sufficient understanding of his situation and the possible consequences of his actions to make an informed choice. J.E. further stated he would rather not return to the hospital even if seriously ill, and would prefer to die at home. Thus, J.E. was competent to refuse care, in that he displayed sufficient understanding and appreciation of the risks involved.

Preference for less than the usual amount of medical attention has been described in other elderly patients.[11] These individuals object to the intrusion of routine, ordinary medical care into their daily lives, and prefer to live and die in familiar surroundings. Family and friends typically favor more vigorous medical intervention. Nonetheless, health professionals are obliged to respect the considered preferences of competent individuals, whether reasonable or irrational, to limit medical or social interventions. Even incompetent patients' clearly stated preferences should be given substantial weight in treatment decisions.[12]

Modification of Home Care   Though J.E. had consistently expressed the wish to be left alone, it was the consensus of health care team members that he needed a minimal degree of supervision to reduce significant risks to his person. Thus, the team decided to modify their earlier compromise and stay involved with him to the extent he would permit.

J.E.'s home services were changed to ensure minimal intrusion into his personal activities. Caregivers were selected for their rapport with J.E., including a sympathetic neighbor who assisted with meals and safety supervision. The overall goals of providing care were redefined so that safety concerns were balanced against J.E.'s desire for independence. J.E. appeared to develop a tolerance, and sometimes even appreciation, of the system of care that was developed for him.

Home services for frail elderly persons are sanctioned by protective services legislation. Usually such services are received voluntarily, and indeed, welcomed.[13] But involuntary services or placement may be ordered for incompetent persons where there is "substantial risk of physical harm or deterioration."[14] A hostile reaction to attempts to provide needed care may be cited as justification for involuntary services.[15] Over 95% of petitions under Wisconsin's protective services legislation have led to a protective *placement,* either in the person's home with services or in an institution (residential facility or nursing home).[16] Thus the prospect of involuntary placement, expressed or implied, lies behind the provision of voluntary services to frail elderly persons. Careful, respectful negotiation of supportive interventions can sometimes obviate the need for legal resources.

SUMMARY AND CONCLUSION

J.E.'s wishes became more articulate during the course of his involvement with the health care system. Ultimately, he stated that he would rather die at home than return to the hospital. Despite his apparent desire to be unencumbered by outside assistance, the health professionals believed their ethical obligations prohibited absolute disengagement. Another way of framing the dilemma here is that there are different legal concepts of competence which can be applied to J.E.'s case. To the extent that he was able to appreciate the risks, benefits, and alternatives to treatment interventions, he was competent, in one sense of the law. But to the extent that he was substantially incapable of caring for himself, in another sense of the law, he was incompetent. J.E.'s situation was that he was only marginally competent with regard to his mental status, and marginally incompetent with regard to his physical condition. His physical limitations impaired his ability to exercise what competency he retained. Situations such as these call for interventions which are both medically and ethically creative, and the marshalling of resources to maintain the individual's autonomy for as long as possible.

Had J.E.'s dangerous behavior put anyone else in jeopardy, the ethical dilemma would have been somewhat different. If he had risked setting fire to an apartment building, for example, the health professionals should rightly consider the interests of the community in preserving its safety. While an individual may be willing to risk his own life, a person who puts others in danger needs to be held to a higher standard of safe behavior.

The solution for J.E. was neither simple nor neat, nor likely to be very long-lasting. As his needs changed, new compromises would have to be negotiated, calling for continuing availability and flexibility from the health professionals. Mutually acceptable compromises cannot be achieved in all such situations. The desire to remain independent may far overreach the capacity. The danger to self or others may be too great, or too poorly perceived. Needed supportive services may be unavailable or refused. Protective services or placement may be necessary and appropriate. For both patients and health care providers, there may be significant ambivalence concerning which values should have priority. Whatever the clinical situation, health professionals need to be especially sensitive to the evolving needs and desires of elderly patients with dementia, and compassionately work to preserve their autonomy.

REFERENCES

1 Beck JC (moderator): Dementia in the elderly: the silent epidemic. Ann Intern Med 97:231, 1982

2 Howell T, Watts DT: Behavioral complications of dementia. (Manuscript in preparation)

3 Meier DE, Cassel CK: Nursing home placement and the demented patient: a case presentation and ethical analysis. Ann Intern Med 104:98, 1986

4 Stollerman GH: Decisions to leave home. J Am Geriatr Soc 36:375, 1988

5 Cassel CK, Jameton AL: Dementia in the elderly: an analysis of medical responsibility. Ann Intern Med 94:802, 1981

6 Jackson DL, Youngner S: Patient autonomy and "death with dignity": some clinical caveats. N Engl J Med 301:404, 1979

7 Wisconsin State Statutes, Sec. 880.01(4)

8 Regan JJ: Protecting the elderly: the new paternalism. Hastings Law Journal 32:34, 1981

9 Rodin J: Aging and health: effects of the sense of control. Science 233:1271, 1986

10 *Bartling vs. Super. Ct.* (Glendale Adven. Med.) 209 Cal. Rptr. 220 (Cal. App. 2 Dist 1984)

11 Hershkowitz M: To die at home. J Am Geriatr Soc 32:457, 1984

12 (Anon) State Court: incompetent has say in her treatment. American College of Physicians, *Observer* April 1985, p. 14

13 Kapp MB: Adult protective services: convincing the patient to consent. Law, Medicine, and Health Care 11:163, 1983

14 Wisconsin State Statutes, Sec. 55.05(2)(d)

15 Center for Public Representation (Madison, Wisconsin): A Plain-Language Legal Guide to Helping the Elderly Client. 1985, pp. 78–79

16 Regan JJ: Adult protective services: an appraisal and prospectus, *in* Regan JJ: Improving Protective Services for Older Americans (monograph series), 1982, pp. 12–18

Sterilization and the Rights of the Mentally Retarded

Sterilizing the Mildly Mentally Retarded without Their Consent
Robert Neville

Robert Neville is dean of the school of theology and professor of religion, philosophy, and theology at Boston University. He is the editor of *New Essays in Metaphysics* (1987) and the

From *Mental Retardation and Sterilization,* edited by Ruth Macklin and Willard Gaylin (New York: Plenum Press, 1981), pp. 181–193. Copyright © 1981 The Hastings Center. Reprinted with permission of the author and The Hastings Center.

author of several books, including *Creativity and God* (1980), *The Tao and the Daimon* (1982), and *Eternity and Time's Flow* (1993).

Neville maintains that it is sometimes morally permissible to sterilize mildly retarded individuals without their consent. He advances, and argues for, two claims: (1) involuntary sterilization is in the best interests of some mildly mentally retarded persons because it will maximize their freedom to enjoy heterosexual activity; (2) involuntary sterilization enhances the dignity of the mildly mentally retarded's position in the moral community insofar as it fosters and encourages their capacity for moral behavior.

Under certain specific circumstances it is morally permissible to sterilize some mildly mentally retarded people without their consent. At the outset of my argument I want to acknowledge that there is a grave difficulty, conceptually and empirically, in identifying which individuals belong to the relevant class of the mentally retarded. If that class is either conceptually so vague or empirically so confused that individuals who do not belong in it are inadvertently placed there, then it would be ethically impermissible to subject the class to involuntary sterilization. But let me put that difficulty aside until the end, and proceed with the argument as if we knew with acceptable exactness who the mildly mentally retarded are and which of them meet the specified requirements for sterilization.

THE HUMBLE ARGUMENT

My argument is really two arguments, one nested in the other. The first can be called the "humble argument" for involuntary sterilization, and it attempts to make the case that involuntary sterilization is in the best interest of certain mildly mentally retarded people. The second can be called the "philosophical argument," and it interprets the "humble argument" as a problem of rights and responsibilities, and attempts to show that involuntary sterilization in the right cases fosters rather than denies the membership of the mildly mentally retarded in the moral community.

The humble argument begins with certain observations. First, at least some mildly mentally retarded people are capable of engaging in and taking pleasure in heterosexual intercourse. My following remarks concern only this group; presumably those incapable of such intercourse would not need sterilization; those who, because of inexperience, do not know their capacities for pleasure should be viewed as capable of engaging in and taking pleasure from sexual activity until proved otherwise.

Second, for some mildly retarded people sexual activity is capable of being integrated into emotional aspects of affection, which can in turn contribute to positive, rewarding fulfillments of personal and social life. Freed from pregnancy, childbearing, and child rearing, an active heterosexual life can enrich the existence of some mildly mentally retarded people in much the way it can that of so-called "normals." Other things being equal, mildly mentally retarded people can benefit from and have a right to sexual activity and the social forms sexual relationships can involve, such as marriage. Capacities for marriage and long-lasting affection do not have to be clearly present, however, for the retarded to have a claim on sexual activity for purposes of pleasure alone.

Third, what begins to make the situation for the retarded "not equal" to that for "normals"? For mildly mentally retarded women the physiological and emotional changes that take place during pregnancy, and the violence of childbirth, are often experienced as disorienting and terrifying traumata. To the extent that a retarded man participates in the process, he too can be disoriented and lose his personal equilibrium.

Fourth, child rearing is sometimes beyond the capacities of mildly mentally retarded people precisely because of the characteristics of their retardation. The fact that child rearing is in practice also beyond the emotional capacities of many normal people should not obscure the overwhelming difficulty that it often poses for the retarded. Now it seems a prima facie argument that children ought not be conceived if there is not some reasonable expectation that they will receive minimal care. (Note that this is not an argument that conceived children should be aborted, which is more difficult to sustain.)

Fifth, mildly mentally retarded people have very great difficulty in managing impermanent forms of contraception. I am assuming that sterilization is the only permanent contraceptive; at least it cannot be reversed without medical help. Therefore, if these mildly mentally retarded people are to engage in sexual intercourse, which is otherwise desirable, without fear of the woman becoming pregnant, sterilization seems the only responsible contraceptive choice.

The humble argument, then, puts together these observations and says that the mildly mentally retarded people to whom these conditions apply should be sterilized so that they may enjoy heterosexual activity if they are so inclined. If they were not sterilized they would have to be prevented from engaging in sexual activity, or conditioned to homosexual or autoerotic sexual activity exclusively, which would be hard to guarantee. If their sex lives were not so controlled, they would run the risk of pregnancy with likely trauma for themselves and improper care for their child. If the retarded people do not or cannot give consent, then someone should have the standing to insist that the retarded be sterilized involuntarily.

An added consideration may be raised at the level of the humble argument. Who is to be sterilized, men, women, or both? The answer to that question clearly depends on the circumstances—whether the candidates are living in an institution, whether that institution is highly regulated or more informal in its management of personal associations; or, if the candidates are living outside institutions, in what kinds of settings. But generally the point of sterilization is to maximize the freedom of the mildly mentally retarded in sexual matters, and it is relevant to administer the procedure to any candidate meeting the conditions who stands to suffer harm or loss of freedom without it.

THE PHILOSOPHICAL ARGUMENT

The humble argument is a fairly straightforward, prudential argument operating within the limits and categories generally taken for granted when dealing with the mildly mentally retarded. The philosophical argument differs by calling into question the limits and categories otherwise taken for granted.

My philosophical argument consists of two main parts. The first considers the objection that sterilization of the mildly mentally retarded is wrong if done involuntarily because it would thereby deny the subjects their proper place in the moral community, treating them as means only and not ends in themselves. I shall argue on the contrary that the procedure enhances the dignity of their position in the moral community. The second part raises the very large problem of who decides about ster-

ilization in the context of the mildly mentally retarded. Whereas some people might argue that no third party has sufficient standing in the matter to warrant doing violence to the candidate, I shall argue that it is the responsibility (a) of the moral community to establish policy creating such standing, and (b) of its properly delegated representatives to carry out the policy subject to a variety of checks.

Membership in the Moral Community

In that tradition of Western theory which takes most seriously the dignity of the human individual, the Kantian, one of the central concepts is that of the moral community. The dignity that should be accorded to each person as a human being consists in being regarded as a member of the moral community. Membership in that community means that a person is held to be morally responsible for his or her actions and life, and is to be held responsible by the rest of the community for assuming that responsibility.

With respect to human dignity, the grave danger is that a person will be treated as a thing rather than a responsible agent. This may happen when someone or some group treats a person merely as a means toward their own ends; this was Immanuel Kant's particular worry. It may also happen when the community simply fails to recognize the person as a moral agent, which happens most often when people's behavior is explained in such a way as to shift responsibility onto causes other than themselves. This objectification or alienation has been a primary worry of existentialists and many other social critics. In a strict philosophical sense (deriving from Aristotle), violence is done to people when they are prevented by external forces from fulfilling their basic or natural goals; one form of violence is to prevent someone from exercising membership in the moral community.

The mildly retarded suffer enough from their incapacities that special care should be taken to ensure them as full a membership in the moral community as possible. To sterilize them involuntarily, some people argue, is to do them unnecessary and dehumanizing violence. It is to regard them first of all as incapable of making a responsible decision about sterilization, thus ruling them out of membership in this respect; no defender of involuntary sterilization could deny this fact. It is, second, to regard their sex lives and childbearing and child rearing lives as so controlled by irresponsible impulses that the people may just as well be managed like objects in those areas of life. Third, it is quite possible and indeed likely, according to this position, that sterilization is sought for the mildly mentally retarded in order to make their custody easier, in which cases the people are treated in that respect as means only, not as ends in themselves.

In answer to these arguments let me point out three characteristics of the moral community. First, membership in the moral community is relative to the capacity for taking moral responsibility; there is no membership in the moral community under ordinary circumstances in the respects in which there is no capacity for taking responsibility. Second, most capacities for taking moral responsibility need to be developed; ordinary socialization develops most of them. The state of moral adulthood can be defined as being in possession of the capacity to take responsibility for developing the other capacities for responsible action that might be called upon. Third, a general moral imperative for any community is that its structures and practices foster the development of the capacities for responsible behavior wherever possible, and avoid hindering that development.

The idea of a moral community is an ideal that exists in pure form only in the imagination. When the ideal is applied to actual communities, it must be tailored to the fact that some people can have only partial memberships because of limited capacity for morally responsible behavior. Children, for example, only slowly take on the capacities for full membership in the moral community, and come to be treated as full members by degrees. Ordinarily we think of young children as full human beings because of their potential to develop into adults with full capacity for responsible action; when the coherence of their lives is extended over a reasonable life span, they can be expected to have moral capacities in due season.

Other people have other sorts of limited capacities for responsible behavior, such as those resulting from mental illness or senility, in which certain areas of life may involve severe incapacities for responsible behavior whereas others do not. In these cases, we usually regard people as fully human members of the moral community by according them the rights of responsibility where they do in fact have the capacity and by assigning to other people the responsibilities of proxy in areas of incapacity. The concept of a proxy, in the restrictive use of my distinction, is that of an agent who fits into the patient's overall moral responsibility as a substitute in a certain area or under certain circumstances; the concept of proxy is used to maintain and support the notion that a person is a member of the

moral community in circumstances where the direct capacity for that is lacking.

The case of the mildly mentally retarded is somewhat different from that of children and from the limited capacity of the mentally ill or senile. Like children, their capacities for development may be far greater than would have been imagined a few years ago. But unlike children, the pacing and sequencing of their development does not lead to emotional maturity at the same time they reach bodily maturity. For instance, the emotional and intellectual capacities to manage conventional birth control methods, to adjust to pregnancy, or to raise children do not develop by the time their physical development and their social peers among nonretarded people are ready for sexual activity.

Neither, sometimes, does the capacity to make informed decisions about sterilization. Indeed, if one were to say that heterosexual activity should be prevented among certain mildly mentally retarded people until such time as they develop the capacities for responsible behavior regarding pregnancy, or for consenting to surgical sterilization, the result is very likely to be the prevention of heterosexual activity altogether. As the humble argument says, this approach would amount to preventing the development of an important capacity for responsible behavior in areas that would be possible if an active sex life were possible, and would therefore be contrary to the imperative that the moral community foster such capacities.

Mildly mentally retarded people are like certain kinds of mentally ill people in that, from the adult perspective, there are certain areas of life in which they may lack capacities for responsible behavior and other areas where they may have them. But they are unlike mentally ill people in an important respect. A mentally ill person is conceived to be a member of the moral community because even though a proxy might exercise some of his or her responsibilities, he or she is believed to have the structure of a person who possesses the capacities for those responsibilities.

This belief is based on the fact, for instance, that the person once exercised those responsibilities before becoming ill. With the help of a proxy, almost as a prosthetic device, a mentally ill person can be presented to the moral community as a fully responsible moral agent. A mildly mentally retarded person, however, lacks the full personality structure that would come from having had the capacities for morally responsible behavior in the past. Although another person might make decisions in areas in which the retarded person is incapacitated, that would not strictly speaking be a case of proxy because the retarded person does not have a personality structured around the capacity for which a proxy might have to substitute.

Paternalism and proxy are models for enabling persons—children and the mentally ill, respectively—to enjoy membership in the moral community when they themselves have capacities for only partial membership. Another model is needed for the limited capacity of mildly mentally retarded people, one which I propose to call the model of "involuntary restrictive conditions." The model depicts mildly mentally retarded people as members of the moral community on the condition that they meet certain restrictions. Just as people with bad eyesight may be licensed to drive with the restriction that they wear glasses, so mildly mentally retarded people may be required to meet certain restrictions in order to be members of the moral community.

The analogy with driver's licenses is imperfect, however, because a person with bad eyesight can always choose not to drive and thereby not to need to wear glasses. But a person cannot choose to be in or out of the moral community; one is either in the position to be held responsible or one is not. Mildly mentally retarded people, and perhaps other groups, must meet the restrictions as conditions for being in the community. Therefore, from the standpoint of mildly mentally retarded people, the restrictive conditions are involuntary.

In a moment I shall urge that sterilization may be a proper involuntary restrictive condition for membership in the moral community for mildly mentally retarded people, subject to the limitations mentioned in connection with the humble argument. Before that, however, I want to address the question of who decides about involuntary restrictive conditions.

Who Should Decide?

Whether a certain restrictive condition does indeed foster the capacity for responsible moral behavior is an empirical question. The suggestion has been made that, with sterilization, mildly mentally retarded people will be able to engage in the kind of sex life that can develop their capacities for responsible behavior in various human relationships. Without sterilization they either would be prevented from having sex, and therefore would not develop those capacities for sexual affection and comradeship, or they would have sex and find themselves in such trouble that sexual affection and companionship would again be beyond them.

Furthermore, this empirical argument suggests that behavior having to do with sexual affection and companionship is more important than what mildly mentally retarded people might gain from opportunities for pregnancy, childbirth, and child rearing. The first "who decides" question is: Who decides whether that empirical argument is right? I suggest that this decision is a broad social one, which should be as informed as possible by experts in all the relevant fields, including both mental retardation and ethics. Clearly that argument will always be under redefinition and refinement.

But the next "who decides" question is: Who sets the policies regarding the treatment of the mildly mentally retarded? The answer is that the decision must come from the political process (again informed by relevant experts, and formulated by broad intellectual dialogue). The reason for locating the decision in the political process is that that is the only legitimate way by which individuals can be dealt with against their wills by due process. But there are two normative factors within the political process. One is that the process should conform to whatever political norm structures it—for instance, that of a representative democracy. According to this factor, what the political process decides about mildly mentally retarded people is legitimate if due political procedures have been followed. The other normative factor, however, is the demands of being a moral community, since the political process is the vehicle for actualizing those demands. A political decision is moral if it accords with what is required as a minimum for a moral community.

If the sterilization of mildly mentally retarded people, subject to appropriate limitations, does indeed foster important capacities for morally responsible behavior, and if a moral community ought to foster such capacities where possible, the warrant for politically deciding to sterilize certain mildly mentally retarded people is a moral one, not merely one of political legitimacy. There is a prima facie obligation to foster people's capacity for responsibility, since this capacity is the basis of their membership in the moral community. Paradoxically, to refrain from sterilization is to do them the violence of preventing them from participating in the moral community in one of the important respects of which they are capable.

Assuming that the political process results in a sterilization policy, by what procedures and what officers should decisions be made about particular candidates? That is a prudential political question that I shall not attempt to address. It is necessary at this point, however, to refer to what Hastings Center lore calls the "klutz factor," namely, that translating a theoretical moral argument into a public policy with significant effects is likely to lead to blunders and abuse. Because of the "klutz factor," prudence may very well dictate that policies should be far more conservative than morality otherwise would dictate.

For instance, as I stated in the "humble argument," the candidates for involuntary sterilization should include those who are capable of engaging in and taking pleasure in heterosexual activity, and yet who are incapable of taking responsibility for this activity in regards to pregnancy and the rest. This is a positive argument for sterilizing a class of people. In light of the "klutz factor," according to which the wrong people might be sent to the surgeon, perhaps it would be a prudent extra restriction to insist that candidates have demonstrated their need for sterilization by having already gotten into trouble by their sexual activity. I am not sure how to prevent such a restriction from being turned into a punitive measure against the retarded, however.

In general, with regard to all the "who decides" questions, it is important to make sure that the process of decision is self-critical and that opposition to any point of view is always funded as a corrective support.

UNIFYING THE ARGUMENTS

The philosophical side of the argument has intended to show that, contrary to the beliefs of some, involuntary sterilization does not involve treating the mildly mentally retarded as if they were not members of the moral community; rather, it acknowledges real incapacities and neutralizes their effects, thereby enabling other capacities to be realized. Furthermore, if sterilization does in some important ways lead to the development of greater capacities for responsibility, then it is part of the obligation a society owes to its potential members to provide it, subject to appropriate protections against abuse. If a mildly mentally retarded person lacks the capacity to give or withhold informed consent because he or she does not understand the subtle issues involved, then having the decision made by the society's agents is one of the involuntary restrictive conditions that might help place the person in the community. The society has the prima facie obligation to make that decision and should do so unless other considerations prevail.

The basic philosophical principle involved in this argument is that a moral community has the social responsibility to foster capacities for morally responsible behavior. It should do so paternalistically in the case of children; it should do so with appropriate proxies in the case of impaired capacities; and it should do so through the institution of involuntary restrictive conditions in the case of basic human capacities that are undevelopable only in a future that is too late for other valuable capacities to be developed that otherwise would have been possible.

This reasoning brings us back to the "humble argument." From a philosophical point of view, the humble argument might well be valid. At least it is not wrong by virtue of violating the canons of membership in the moral community; it does not deny human dignity. Indeed, the structure of the humble argument is to provide for the dignity of humane heterosexual relations by removing the unbearable complications of potential pregnancy. Whether its premises are valid is an empirical matter.

Let me close by dealing with the question of adequate diagnosis of the appropriate conditions for involuntary sterilization. Some structure must be worked out to determine appropriate subjects. We have seen that to do so requires two sorts of determinations. The first is whether informed and emotionally balanced decisions regarding sterilization are within the capacities of the candidates; if they are, then the candidates' word should be decisive, and if they prefer nonsterilization then society should respect that choice, whatever other compensatory restrictions it requires (such as no sexual activity). The second is whether the candidates are capable of heterosexual intercourse but not capable of coping adequately with pregnancy, childbirth, and child rearing. Not all mentally retarded people would fall into this category, and specific empirical criteria would have to be developed before a program of involuntary sterilization could be instituted.

If no mildly mentally retarded people can be found who fall into this category, then none of them should be involuntarily sterilized. The consequence of this requirement is that the validity of involuntary-sterilization programs depends upon the development of criteria and diagnostic skills sufficient to discriminate the proper category of people. There have been disagreements concerning whether the definitions of relevant characteristics, and diagnostic skills for discerning them, are sufficiently developed to provide a capacity for responsible programs. In the face of excessive modesty and caution it should be pointed out that people are now classified as mildly mentally retarded and subjected to programs intended to help them.

There is one final point. It is sometimes believed that there is a totalitarian impetus lurking in any social policy that might require people to be good—in this case, to submit to involuntary restrictive conditions in order to develop the amiable responsibilities of a decent sex life. I admit that there is a danger, but urge that it be guarded against by specific safeguards and internal critical mechanisms rather than by a blanket rejection. If people could be whole and fully responsible by themselves, society would have no positive responsibilities, only negative, peace-keeping ones. But because people become responsible through the grace of social life, and because some people need special help in exercising responsibility, society does have positive duties in developing the capacity for responsible moral behavior.

Subtracting Injury from Insult: Ethical Issues in the Use of Pharmaceutical Implants
Eric T. Juengst and Ronald A. Siegel

Eric T. Juengst, a bioethicist, is associate professor of biomedical ethics, Center for Biomedical Ethics, Case Western Reserve School of Medicine. He is the coeditor of *The Meaning of AIDS* (1989) and the author of articles such as "Germ-Line Gene Therapy: Back to Basics" and "Prenatal Diagnosis and the Ethics of Uncertainty." Ronald A. Siegel is associate professor of pharmacy and pharmaceutical chemistry at the University of California at San Francisco. His research interests lie in the physical chemistry of polymers, the applications of these polymers in drug delivery, and the general design of drug-delivery systems.

Juengst and Siegel discuss some ethical issues raised by implantable drug-delivery systems when those receiving the implants are the mentally ill and the mentally retarded. The first drug implant they consider works as a relatively long-term contraceptive and might be seen as an alternative to sterilization for mentally retarded adolescents. The second drug implant they consider delivers a behavior control drug and might be seen as an alternative to psychosurgery for severely mentally ill patients whose behavior is consistently violent and yet who refuse to comply with a regimen of antipsychotic drugs. Juengst and Siegel strike a cautionary note. They maintain that the noninvasiveness and reversibility of pharmaceutical implants, although genuine virtues, are insufficient to eliminate all the ethical problems raised by involuntary sterilization and involuntary psychosurgery.

Ten years ago, psychosurgery . . . and surgical sterilization received considerable attention in bioethics. These interventions provided riveting examples of the kinds of questions that the young field took as its domain: questions about the ethical boundaries of biomedicine's power to modify bodies and minds. The focus of the field has since shifted. Soon, however, the concerns of

Reprinted with permission of the authors and the publisher from *Hastings Center Report,* vol. 18 (December 1988), pp. 41–46.

the last decade may be raised again, from a quite different corner of biomedicine. Advances in biomedical engineering and pharmaceutical chemistry are converging to produce devices that can be implanted in the body to deliver controlled doses of drugs automatically for months at a time.[1] These implants could be used to produce the *effects* of psychosurgery [and] surgical sterilizations . . . without their irrevocable invasions of bodily integrity. For contemporary pharmaceutical engineers, and for clinicians of the 1990s, the question is how well the earlier exploration of biomedicine's moral boundaries provides guidance in this new pharmacologic terrain.

In one respect, the discussion of the ethical issues raised by the surgeries does provide important precedents for the ethics of drug implantation: its analyses do map the relevant moral ground. However, the language of those analyses, while nicely crafted for their contexts, could seriously mislead efforts to evaluate the use of drug implants. Its dominant metaphors—trespass, unjust punishment, and irretractable offense—can be misread to imply that the clinical virtues of implantation—noninvasiveness, efficiency, and reversibility—allow this practice to escape the moral pitfalls encountered by the surgeries. To follow the lead of the earlier discussion successfully requires a critical rereading of its metaphors that can distinguish between their clinical and moral meanings.

IMPLANTABLE DRUG DELIVERY SYSTEMS

In the next two decades we may expect a revolution in drug therapy. In addition to the new hormones, enzymes, and vaccines that the biotechnology industry is producing, new techniques for drug delivery are being introduced. One idea that has received considerable attention from academic and industrial researchers is the development of implantable devices designed to release a drug into the body in a controlled manner. A well known example is the mechanical insulin pump carried by some diabetics.[2] Subcutaneous reservoirs, which deliver drugs passively into the blood stream, have been under development since the late 1960s.[3] "NORPLANT" (R), the implantable contraceptive device developed by The Population Council, is a more recent example. This small plastic rod infused with a contraceptive steroid is inserted subcutaneously under local anesthetic. The device is physically unobtrusive and can automatically release preset contraceptive doses for five years after implantation.[4] Current research is also aimed at developing self-regulated implants capable of interacting with their environment to meet the body's fluctuating pharmacologic needs.[5]

The reversibility and longevity of an implant depends on its design. In principle, implants can be designed to release drugs over virtually any duration, although most current devices have life spans measured in months rather than years. Some systems, like NORPLANT, are designed to remain intact throughout the release process and must be removed surgically when

exhausted. Others are designed to degrade into nontoxic by-products as the drug is released. Because they often lose their mechanical integrity during erosion, degradable devices may not be removable once implanted. Thus, while they may be more convenient than nondegradable devices, they may preclude other treatment choices for considerable periods of time.

In part, implantation is attractive because the traditional routes for drug delivery—ingestion or injection—are not well suited to the administration of new, genetically engineered biologicals. Such drugs are usually proteins and would be digested if taken orally. They also usually require regular administration, burdening patients with the inconvenience and discomfort of living with a prolonged course of injections. Implantable devices, by providing for the measured, subcutaneous release of a drug, are designed to obviate these problems.

Implantation holds advantages for other classes of drugs as well. Because they can be implanted near their target organs, less drug is required to achieve the same effect as oral or intravenous administration. "Organ targeting" has also been shown to avoid many of the side effects of oral administration by reducing the drug's dispersal and absorption in other parts of the body.[6]

Finally, developing improved pharmaceutical implants is attractive for more prosaic reasons. The process of developing, screening, clinically testing, and obtaining regulatory approval for a new drug often requires decades. Yet patent protection is relatively short (seventeen years), and must often overlap with several stages of the process. Drug companies are finding it less lucrative to develop new drugs than to seek new delivery methods for existing ones.

All these considerations may drastically change our view of what it means to be "taking drugs" for a medical problem. The combination of implantation's efficiency (in terms of enhanced drug efficacy, reduced side effects, greater convenience, and better compliance), with its relative noninvasiveness and reversibility give the technology distinct clinical advantages. There is a danger, though, that these virtues could distract us from other problems that could arise in prescribing this technology.

THE DOUBLE-EDGED VIRTUES OF IMPLANTATION TECHNOLOGY

As a novel therapeutic tool, any new implantable drug delivery device will present the same ethical questions that attend other clinical innovations: Its introduction will be marked by uncertainty about safety and efficacy, and its use will entail predictable risks as well as benefits. Drug implantation, in other words, is a double-edged technology in the usual sense of having both virtues and vices as a clinical tool. But these are not the issues that we address here. Drug implantation may also face ethical questions precisely when its virtues recommend its use. To the extent that they cause us to neglect those questions, implantation's virtues themselves may be double-edged. Ironically, their distracting potential is probably greatest where these questions are most pressing, because of the way our moral metaphors exacerbate it. Under their influence, implantation's clinical virtues appear to condone its use in cases where any intervention would be morally problematic.

NONINVASIVENESS

One of the primary reasons contraceptive implants are attractive is that they provide the long-term prophylaxis of surgical sterilization without requiring a major medical intervention. But consider the following scenario:

> The parents of an eighteen-year-old girl with Down syndrome come to their physician for help. Their daughter is sexually mature, and has an IQ of sixty-five. She is able to get about on her own and attends a special school each day. Her parents had hoped to place her in an adult group home when she completed school, but fear that she may well become pregnant and that this will be a very upsetting experience for her. They have tried oral contraceptives, which the girl refuses to take without a daily struggle, and they do not wish to subject her to the risks of an IUD. They feel that sterilization through tubal ligation is the only answer. However, they are relieved to learn about the existence of a biologically implantable device like NORPLANT that will have the same effect, and request it from their physician.[7]

Ethical debate on surgical sterilization for retarded adolescents usually contrasts the psychological burden of pregnancy and the potential psychosocial benefits of sexual activity with the surgery's harm to the patient's reproductive capacity, the lack of her consent to the procedure, and the foreclosure of her future reproductive options.[8] The issue turns on which course seems better to promote the patient's autonomy: to exercise, on her behalf, her right to sterilization, or to defend, since she cannot, the privacy of her reproductive choices.[9]

All of these considerations would also be present in a decision to fit the patient with a long-term contraceptive implant. The patient would be rendered infertile without her consent, and in a way that she would be powerless to change for an extended period. The problem of determining her competency to make reproductive choices and raise children remains, as well as the prospect of infringing unjustifiably on a very important sphere of personal decisionmaking.

However, the implant will not sterilize the patient permanently, as tubal ligation would. Moreover, implantation entails neither the dramatic invasion of bodily integrity of surgery nor the recurrent struggle of administering oral contraceptives. It is a minor procedure, performed in the doctor's office and then forgotten. Do these clinical advantages help ameliorate the physician's ethical problem?

Those concerned about surgical sterilization of the retarded often cite the bodily injury of the procedure in the same breath with its insult to the patient's autonomy. For example, one cautious critic of sterilization argues that:

> A just cause is required because sterilization in the absence of consent constitutes a significant invasion of the body and a rather massive intrusion into the sphere of reproductive privacy.[10]

Here, the "trespass" metaphors of "invasion" and "intrusion" provide useful but complementary descriptions of both the physical harms and moral wrongs involved in involuntary sterilization.

Nevertheless, "trespass" metaphors do tend to focus on the consequences of surgery for (structural) bodily integrity rather than for (functional) reproductive capacity. The prospect of minimally invasive implantable contraceptive devices forces us to ask which of these harms is really of central concern. If the decisive ethical issue is how best to promote the subject's reproductive autonomy, how relevant is the fact that involuntary implantation can compromise reproductive function without a "significant invasion of the body"?

The "bodily invasion" of surgery provides a graphic symbol of trespass, but it is the intervention's *functional* effects that intrude furthest into the subject's reproductive privacy. Of course, invasive surgery is riskier than subcutaneous implantation: the noninvasiveness of the implant gives it a genuine clinical advantage, which counts ethically in its favor. However, to the extent that the noninvasiveness of the implantable contraceptive is viewed as the *decisive* ethical consideration in cases like this, the language of the surgical sterilization debate will have misled our moral reflection. In this debate, appeals to bodily integrity play a primarily rhetorical role; they are designed to invoke the metaphors of trespass that underscore the importance of the reproductive function at stake . . .

REVERSIBILITY

It is easy to see how invasiveness . . . play[s] [an] important symbolic [role] in ethical debates over involuntary sterilization. . . . But is the clinical irreversibility of [the] intervention merely a rhetorically useful side issue as well? The reversibility of implantation seems to speak most directly to the ethical issues in [this case] because it provides a way to proceed in the face of moral uncertainty. For example, consider the case for using implants as an alternative to psychosurgery. . . .

> A long-term inpatient at a mental institution with a history of paranoia and violent behavior consistently refuses to comply with a regimen of anti-psychotic drugs. Electroencephalographic examination of the patient shows brain activity compatible with temporal lobe epilepsy. Because of this finding, the institution's medical staff discusses psychosurgery as an alternative to the patient's forced medication. However, since the patient's medications, once administered, do seem effective in controlling his behavior, they are hesitant to proceed. As a third option, a consulting pharmacologist suggests that an implantable drug delivery system be used to supply the patient's regimen of anti-psychotic medication automatically for months at a time.

The ethics of psychosurgical intervention oscillates around two related issues: distinguishing the cure of behavioral pathology from unjustified behavior control, and determining a psychiatric patient's authority to refuse (or consent to) this kind of treatment.[11] Neither of these issues is peculiar to psychosurgery and a decision to use a pharmaceutical implant raises exactly the same questions about how best to promote and protect this patient's interests. However, commentators usually argue that psychosurgery is a paradigm for ethical conflicts in behavior control techniques because of its invasiveness, destructiveness, and irreversibility:

> Psychosurgery is perhaps the most dramatic of all medically based individual therapies for mental and behavioral deviance. It goes directly to the physical seat of experience, and makes irreversible destructive lesions. Because of its dramatic quality, psychosurgery focuses with great intensity the fundamental problem of all behavior control: by what values should behavior be controlled?[12]

What is special about psychosurgery, then, is the way it metaphorically underscores its own moral dangers: Not only does it offend the patient's integrity, but its insult is one that can never be retracted. Psychosurgery's irreversibility, like its invasiveness, neatly dramatizes the seriousness of the moral hazards it shares with . . . surgical sterilization: the misuse of medical expertise and the violation of the patient's personal autonomy. The question raised by the prospect of a pharmaceutical implant is whether the permanence of psychosurgery has any other moral significance, against which the implant's reversibility measures favorably.

Clearly, there are clinical situations in which the implant's reversibility would make it the intervention of choice. For example, lucid patients might be given the opportunity to commit themselves to a "Ulysses contract," with the option of renegotiating at the end of each cycle.[13] However, in our case, the staff must still face the central issues of whether the goal of the intervention is therapeutic or coercive, and how to respond when the patient refuses it. If the staff's intent is coercive or the patient's refusal valid, the fact that the implant's behavioral effects are reversible will not undo the wrong that forced implantation would represent. Could we justify denying individuals the right to vote by pointing out that they will get another chance in the next election?

Of course, the implant could be proposed simply to test the validity of the patient's refusal. If it were used to enhance our confidence in the patient's capacity for self-determination and to allow him to make an authoritative decision about further treatment, the moral importance of its reversibility would increase. In fact, if the goal of such a test is to return control to the patient, the preference should be for the most readily reversible intervention that would work: for example, a course of traditionally administered medication. Here, the convenience of the implant may recommend its use . . . , but its relative longevity and irreversibility actually militate against it.

More important, just why does the moral significance of reversibility increase when implantation is used to resolve our uncertainty about the patient's capacity? In this situation, the implant's reversibility opens the possibility of making amends for the moral insult of its imposition on the patient. But the significance of this is only that it allows us to apologize for imposing the test, not that it renders apologies unnecessary. The implant's reversibility does not allow us to avoid inflicting the insult in the first place, any more than it speaks to the question of whether behavior control is the appropriate prescription for this patient's problems. Once again, it would be a mistake to let the prominence of the "irreversibility" rhetoric in the psychosurgery debate suggest that the reversibility of pharmaceutical implants allows us to avoid all the serious ethical concerns of psychosurgery.

MORAL AND CLINICAL MEANINGS

The noninvasiveness, increased efficiency, and reversibility of pharmaceutical implants will make implantation technology the preferred approach to drug delivery in an increasing number of situations, and rightly so: they are genuine virtues. Implantable devices can accomplish the goals of surgical sterilization . . . and psychosurgery without the invasiveness . . . or irreversibility that serve as graphic reminders of the moral issues these latter interventions raise. But having subtracted the injuries of those interventions from their insults, drug implantation can still leave clinicians facing the most serious moral problems of the surgeries: the conflicts between visions of personal autonomy and difficulties in distinguishing the appropriate therapeutic uses of medical knowledge from its abuses on behalf of social prejudices and priorities.

To remain sensitive to these problems, it is important to be able to distinguish the moral and the clinical meanings of the metaphors that give implantation's virtues their appearance of moral force. It is natural that biomedicine should focus on the clinical interpretations of "trespass," "unjust punishment," and "irrevocable insult," and seek therapeutic strategies, like drug implantation, that can address them. But this search risks distracting us from the moral dangers the metaphors warn against. To the extent that drug implantation will be contemplated in cases like those examined above, these hazards still exist in the moral terrain this technology must cross. The charts of this terrain provided by its pioneers will be invaluable in that crossing, but only if we translate their signs and symbols correctly.

REFERENCES

1 See A.C. Tanquary and R.E. Lacey, eds., *Controlled Release of Biologically Active Agents* (New York: Plenum Press, 1974); Perry J. Blackshear, "Implantable Drug Delivery Systems," *Scientific American* 241:6 (December 1979), 66–73; Joseph Kost and Robert Langer, "Controlled Release of Bioactive Agents," *Trends in Biotechnology* 2 (1984), 47–51.

2 Michael Sefton, "Implantable Pumps," CRC *Critical Reviews in Biomedical Engineering* 14 (1987), 201–40.

3 Robert A. Ratcheson and Ayub K. Ommaya, "Experience with the Subcutaneous Cerebrospinal-Fluid Reservoir: Preliminary Report of 60 Cases," *New England Journal of Medicine* 279:19 (November 7, 1968), 1025–31.

4 Irving Civin, "Clinical Effects of NORPLANT Subdermal Implants for Contraception," *Advances in Human Fertility and Reproductive Endocrinology* 2 (1982), 89–116.

5 Seo Y. Jeong *et al.,* "Self-Regulating Insulin Delivery Systems," *Journal of Controlled Release* 2 (1985), 143–52.

6 B.B. Pharris *et al.,* "Progestasert: A Uterine Therapeutic System for Long Term Contraception," *Fertility and Sterility* 25:11 (November 1974), 915–21.

7 We are indebted to Adele Hoffman and James Morrissey for this case, which we have adapted for our purposes.

8 Ruth Macklin and Willard Gaylin, eds., *Mental Retardation and Sterilization: A Problem of Competency and Paternalism* (New York: Plenum Press, 1981).

9 Daniel Wikler, "Paternalism and the Mildly Retarded," *Philosophy and Public Affairs* 8 (1979), 915–21.

10 LeRoy Walters, "Sterilizing the Retarded Child," *Hastings Center Report* 6:2 (April 1976), 13–15.

11 Ruth Macklin, *Man, Mind and Morality: The Ethics of Behavior Control* (Englewood Cliffs, NJ: Prentice-Hall, 1982), 15–18.

12 Robert Neville, "Psychosurgery," in *The Encyclopedia of Bioethics,* ed. Warren Reich (New York: Macmillan, 1978), 1387.

13 See also Rebecca Dresser, "Bound to Treatment: The Ulysses Contract," *Hastings Center Report* 14:3 (June 1984), 13–17.

Declaration of General and Special Rights of the Mentally Retarded
International League of Societies for the Mentally Handicapped

The International League of Societies for the Mentally Handicapped, now known as the International League of Societies for Persons with Mental Handicap, was founded in 1960. Its founders included representatives of parent organizations and professional groups as well as individuals concerned with the interests of the mentally handicapped.

This declaration of rights was officially proclaimed in 1968 at a meeting of the league. In 1971 it was adopted almost word for word by the United Nations General Assembly. Among the positive rights it asserts are the rights to economic security, a decent standard of living, and the education, training, habilitation, and guidance requisite to develop abilities and potentials to the fullest possible extent.

Whereas the universal declaration of human rights, adopted by the United Nations, proclaims that all of the human family, without distinction of any kind, have equal and inalienable rights of human dignity and freedom;

Whereas the declaration of the rights of the child, adopted by the United Nations, proclaims the rights of the physically, mentally or socially handicapped child to special treatment, education and care required by his particular condition.

Now therefore, The International League of Societies for the Mentally Handicapped expresses the general and special rights of the mentally retarded as follows:

ARTICLE I.

The mentally retarded person has the same basic rights as other citizens of the same country and same age.

ARTICLE II.

The mentally retarded person has a right to proper medical care and physical restoration and to such education, training, habilitation and guidance as will enable him to develop his ability and potential to the fullest possible extent, no matter how severe his degree of disability. No mentally handicapped person should be deprived of such services by reason of the costs involved.

Reprinted with the permission of the International League of Societies for Persons with Mental Handicap.

ARTICLE III.

The mentally retarded person has a right to economic security and to a decent standard of living. He has a right to productive work or to other meaningful occupation.

ARTICLE IV.

The mentally retarded person has a right to live with his own family or with fosterparents; to participate in all aspects of community life, and to be provided with appropriate leisure time activities. If care in an institution becomes necessary it should be in surroundings and under circumstances as close to normal living as possible.

ARTICLE V.

The mentally retarded person has a right to a qualified guardian when this is required to protect his personal wellbeing and interest. No person rendering direct services to the mentally retarded should also serve as his guardian.

ARTICLE VI.

The mentally retarded person has a right to protection from exploitation, abuse and degrading treatment. If accused, he has a right to a fair trial with full recognition being given to his degree of responsibility.

ARTICLE VII.

Some mentally retarded persons may be unable, due to the severity of their handicap, to exercise for themselves all their rights in a meaningful way. For others, modification of some or all of these rights is appropriate. The procedure used for modification or denial of rights must contain proper legal safeguards against every form of abuse, must be based on an evaluation of the social capability of the mentally retarded person by qualified experts and must be subject to periodic reviews and to the right of appeal to higher authorities.

Above all—The mentally retarded person has the right to respect.

ANNOTATED BIBLIOGRAPHY: CHAPTER 5

Appelbaum, Paul S.: *Almost a Revolution: Mental Health Law and the Limits of Change* (New York: Oxford University Press, 1994). Appelbaum investigates four major areas of reform in mental-health law over the past two decades: (1) involuntary hospitalization, (2) professional liability for predictable violent acts by patients, (3) the right to refuse treatment, and (4) the insanity defense. He argues that less real change has occurred for the mentally ill than most experts predicted; when the law seems to oppose good sense, judges, lawyers, psychiatrists, family members, and others work together in an extra-legal way to achieve what they think is sensible for mentally ill persons.

Bloch, Sidney, and Paul Chodoff, eds.: *Psychiatric Ethics*, 2d ed. (New York: Oxford University Press, 1991). Each essay in this comprehensive anthology treats some aspect of the ethics of psychiatric treatment and research. Topics include the ethics of suicide, confidentiality in psychiatry, ethical issues in child psychiatry, and the psychiatrist's responsibility to society.

Brock, Dan W.: "A Proposal for the Use of Advanced Directives in the Treatment of Incompetent Mentally Ill Persons," *Bioethics* 7 (April 1993), pp. 247–256. Brock argues that mentally ill persons could use advanced directives, which they would formulate at a time when they were competent and their disease was in remission, to give prior consent to treatment in cases where they would become incompetent and noncompliant with the treatment regimen.

Callahan, Joan C.: "Liberty, Beneficence, and Involuntary Confinement," *Journal of Medicine and Philosophy* 9 (August 1984), pp. 261–293. Callahan specifies a set of conditions that must be satisfied to justify paternalistic treatment of mentally ill adults. She also provides a critique of contemporary commitment criteria.

Culver, Charles M., and Bernard Gert: *Philosophy in Medicine: Conceptual and Ethical Issues in Medicine and Psychiatry* (New York: Oxford University Press, 1982). This excellent, well-written book demonstrates the possibility of clarifying conceptual and moral issues by careful philosophical analysis. The authors provide especially useful chapters on mental maladies, volitional disabilities, and the ethics of involuntary hospitalization.

Edwards, Rem B., ed.: *Psychiatry and Ethics: Insanity, Autonomy, and Mental Health Care* (Buffalo, NY: Prometheus Books, 1982). This well-organized collection of articles includes chapters on the concept of mental illness, the therapist-patient relationship and rights, the informed-consent requirement, coercion in commitment and therapy, controversial behavior-control therapies, the insanity defense, and deinstitutionalization. The authors include psychologists, psychiatrists, sociologists, lawyers, surgeons, medical directors, and political scientists.

Goffman, Erving: *Asylums* (New York: Doubleday Anchor, 1961). Goffman provides a detailed examination of life in institutions in general and psychiatric institutions in particular.

Hasker, William: "The Critique of 'Mental Illness': Conceptual and/or Ethical Crisis?" *Journal of Psychology and Theology* 5 (Spring 1977), pp. 110–124. After analyzing Szasz's attack on the concept of mental illness, Hasker argues that Szasz's critique has not as yet received a satisfactory response. Hasker contends that the most promising strategy of response is to try to define "a limited concept of mental illness."

Herr, Stanley S.: *Rights and Advocacy for Retarded People* (Lexington, MA: Lexington Books, 1983). This is a comprehensive, coherent review of the legal and judicial processes that have shaped the field of mental retardation. Herr provides a historical background, identifies the assumptions that underlie our treatment of the mentally retarded, and suggests a future agenda for those who serve as advocates for the mentally retarded.

Macklin, Ruth, and Willard Gaylin, eds.: *Mental Retardation and Sterilization: A Problem of Competency and Paternalism* (New York: Plenum Press, 1981). The product of interdisciplinary meetings conducted by The Hastings Center in 1976 and 1977, this book contains the outcome of participants' deliberations, several articles written by participants, and excerpts from court cases involving the sterilization of mentally retarded persons.

Moore, Michael S.: "Some Myths about 'Mental Illness,'" *Inquiry* 18 (Autumn 1975), pp. 233–265. Maintaining that mental illness is a "cruel and bitter reality," Moore identifies and rejects various versions of the argument that mental illness is a myth.

Mulvey, Edward P., Jeffrey L. Geller, and Loren H. Roth: "The Promise and Peril of Involuntary Outpatient Commitment," *American Psychologist* 42 (June 1987), pp. 571–584. The authors examine arguments for and against involuntary outpatient commitment—in which patients meeting criteria for "dangerousness" or "need for treatment" could be legally compelled to participate in community treatment programs. The article's final section discusses legal and practical issues concerning the implementation of any such policy.

Rosenhan, D. L.: "On Being Sane in Insane Places," *Science* 179 (January 19, 1973), pp. 250–258. This much discussed article describes the results of an experiment in which sane people gained admittance to psychiatric hospitals. Once inside a hospital, they were perceived as insane, leading Rosenhan to conclude that in psychiatric hospitals we cannot distinguish sane from insane.

Schafer, Arthur: "Civil Liberties and the Elderly Patient," in James E. Thornton and Earl R. Winkler, eds., *Ethics and Aging: The Right to Live, the Right to Die* (Vancouver: University of British Columbia Press, 1988), pp. 208–214. Schafer examines and criticizes some of the justifications used for limiting the freedom of elderly patients. His analysis shows the similarities between these justifications and those used for depriving the mentally ill of civil liberties.

Scott, Elizabeth S.: "Sterilization of Mentally Retarded Persons: Reproductive Rights and Family Privacy," *Duke Law Journal* 806 (1986), pp. 806–865. In this lengthy article, Scott develops an alternative to the paternalistic approach in regard to the sterilization of retarded persons. Her approach is based on the primacy of individual and family autonomy.

Szasz, Thomas S.: "Involuntary Mental Hospitalization: A Crime Against Humanity," in Thomas S. Szasz, *Ideology and Insanity* (New York: Doubleday, 1970), pp. 113–139. Szasz argues that the practice of involuntary mental hospitalization should be abolished. In his view, there is a strong analogy between the practice of involuntary mental hospitalization and the institution of slavery.

Torrey, E. Fuller: *Nowhere to Go: The Tragic Odyssey of the Homeless Mentally Ill* (New York: Harper and Row, 1988). Concerned with the effects of deinstitutionalization, Torrey discusses nineteenth- and twentieth-century U.S. social policies regarding the mentally ill and the changes in society's thinking about mental illness in this century. He condemns both the warehousing of patients in psychiatric institutions when institutionalization was in vogue and the dumping of patients without adequate supporting mechanisms in the deinstitutionalization movement. Torrey closes by recommending changes to improve the services available to the mentally ill.

CHAPTER 6

DEATH AND DECISIONS REGARDING LIFE-SUSTAINING TREATMENT

INTRODUCTION

Decisions regarding life-sustaining treatment frequently emerge from a complex dynamic involving physicians, patients, and families. A wide range of ethical questions and concerns can be raised about such decisions. This chapter begins by engaging a closely associated conceptual issue—the definition of death. Attention is then focused on the refusal of life-sustaining treatment by competent adults. Another focal point of discussion in this chapter is the ethics of resuscitation decisions, involving in particular a consideration of the underlying basis of do-not-resuscitate (DNR) orders. Finally, in conjunction with a consideration of surrogate decision making for incompetent adults, substantial attention is given to the topic of advance directives.

The Definition of Death

Two groups of patients are at the center of controversy in recent discussions of the definition of death. In the first group are patients whose *entire* brain has irreversibly ceased functioning. They are irreversibly unconscious, but cardiopulmonary function (heartbeat and respiration) is successfully maintained by a respirator and allied technology. These patients are usually identified either as "brain-dead" or "whole brain-dead." They will be referred to here as "brain-dead." In a second group of patients, brainstem function is sufficient to sustain respiration and heartbeat, but irreversible damage to "the higher brain," the cerebral cortex, is so severe that these patients are suspended in what is called a "persistent vegetative state" (PVS). Consciousness, and thus cognition, has been *irreversibly* lost.[1] Are the patients in each of these groups alive or dead? In any case, what is the morally appropriate treatment for patients in each group?

The traditional standard for the determination of death is the permanent absence of respiration and pulsation. According to this standard, brain-dead patients are alive so long as technological support systems sustain cardiopulmonary functioning. In 1968 an ad hoc committee of the Harvard Medical School issued a very influential report. In this report, the ad hoc committee specified a set of tests for the identification of a permanently nonfunctioning (whole) brain—that is, the condition of brain death. In the view of the ad hoc committee, when this condition has been diagnosed, "death is to be declared and *then* the respirator turned off."[2] In essence, then, the ad hoc committee advanced a new standard for the determination of death. A brain-dead patient is a dead patient, even if cardiopulmonary function is being maintained by artificial means.

It is a matter of substantial importance whether brain-dead patients are alive or dead. For example, taking the vital organs of these patients for transplantation purposes is morally unproblematic if they are dead, presuming of course that appropriate consent procedures have been followed. If they are alive, however, taking their vital organs would (presumably) be the cause of their death. There are other important implications for the way we think and the way we talk. When a respirator is withdrawn from a brain-dead patient, how are we to conceptualize this action? If the patient is still alive, then it is appropriate to describe the removal of the respirator as the withdrawal of life-sustaining treatment, and it makes sense to say that we are allowing the patient to die. However, if the patient is already dead when we remove the respirator, it does not make sense to say that we are allowing the patient to die.

The substance of the Harvard proposal is reflected in the approach taken by the President's Commission for the Study of Ethical Problems in Medicine and Biomedical and Behavioral Research. In its 1981 report, *Defining Death,* the Commission recommends the adoption by all states of the Uniform Determination of Death Act:

> An individual who has sustained either (1) irreversible cessation of circulatory and respiratory functions, or (2) irreversible cessation of all functions of the entire brain, including the brain stem, is dead. A determination of death must be made in accordance with accepted medical standards.

The whole-brain conception (standard) of death that is built into the Uniform Determination of Death Act has achieved widespread public acceptance in the United States. In fact, it is frequently said that a virtual consensus now exists in support of a whole-brain definition of death. Yet a substantial number of critics, including Robert M. Veatch in this chapter, continue to insist that the whole-brain approach to the definition of death is fundamentally flawed.

Charles M. Culver and Bernard Gert, in one of this chapter's selections, provide an analysis that ultimately factors out as an expression of the whole-brain approach. In their view, a patient who has undergone a permanent loss of functioning of the entire brain is dead, but a patient in a persistent vegetative state is not dead, even though, as they say, the organism has ceased to be a person. Indeed, insisting that "we must not confuse the death of an organism which was a person with an organism's ceasing to be a person," Culver and Gert explicitly argue against the higher-brain approach to the definition of death that is favored by Veatch. In accordance with a higher-brain approach, the permanent loss of consciousness is sufficient for death; thus it follows that a patient in PVS is already dead. Of course, if patients in PVS are already dead, then nothing that subsequently happens could be the cause of their death. In particular, it would be wrong to conceptualize the act of inducing cardiac arrest as killing the patient. Similarly, since the patient is already dead, the removal of organs for transplantation could not coherently be understood as an action tantamount to killing the patient.

Culver and Gert, committed to the more common view that the PVS patient is still alive, also consider the issue of morally appropriate treatment. Although they are uncomfortable with the idea of killing a patient in PVS, they endorse allowing the patient to die by discontinuing all care, even "ordinary and routine care." Presumably, the discontinuance of ordinary and routine care would include the withholding of nutrition and hydration—that is, "food and water."

Competent Adults and the Refusal of Life-Sustaining Treatment

Regarding the refusal of life-sustaining treatment by competent adults, there seem to be noteworthy differences among the following: (1) cases in which a patient, by accepting life-sustaining treatment, would return to a state of health; (2) cases in which a patient, by accepting life-sustaining treatment, would simply continue a severely compromised existence; and (3) cases in which a terminally ill patient, by accepting life-sustaining treatment, would merely *prolong the dying process.*

Refusal of treatment in cases of the first type is relatively uncommon but typically dramatic. The most discussed example involves a Jehovah's Witness who refuses to accept a blood transfusion for religious reasons. In one of this chapter's readings, Ruth Macklin argues—principally on the basis of individual autonomy—that the right of a competent adult Jehovah's Witness to refuse a life-sustaining blood transfusion should be respected.

In conjunction with ongoing developments in the courts, refusal of treatment in cases of the second type is probably becoming increasingly common. By and large, the law now recognizes the right of a competent adult—and not just one who is terminally ill or in the process of dying—to refuse life-sustaining treatment. Consider in this regard the example of a patient whose life is severely compromised by the presence of painful and debilitating arthritis. This patient is being treated for pneumonia and is temporarily respirator-dependent until the antibiotics have a chance to take effect. The pneumonia is entirely curable and the patient, however much compromised from a quality-of-life standpoint, is not in the process of dying. If the patient now decides to forgo the respirator, we cannot simply say that the patient has chosen not to prolong the dying process. Accordingly, although considerations of individual autonomy provide a strong moral warrant for the right to refuse life-sustaining treatment in general, some commentators would take issue with the right to refuse treatment in this kind of case because they are concerned about the implications of accepting quality-of-life considerations.[3]

Refusal of treatment in the third type of case has a strong foundation in both morality and law and is certainly very common. In many cases of terminal illness, "aggressive" treatment is capable of warding off death—for a time. However, it is often questionable whether such treatment is in a patient's best interest, and a competent adult is generally considered to have both a moral and a legal right to refuse treatment that would merely prolong the dying process.

Depending on a patient's particular circumstances, life-sustaining treatment can take a variety of forms—for example, mechanical respiration, cardiopulmonary resuscitation, kidney dialysis, surgery, antibiotics, and artificial nutrition and hydration. It is sometimes claimed that the provision of food and water is so fundamentally different from other forms of life-sustaining treatment that it may never be omitted. Those who systematically oppose withholding nutrition and hydration often call attention to the symbolic significance of food and water— their intimate connection with notions of care and concern. However, most commentators insist that there is no reason to apply a different standard to artificial nutrition and hydration. In their view, artificial nutrition and hydration—just like other life-sustaining treatments—will sometimes fail to offer a patient a net benefit, and the decision of a competent patient to refuse them must be respected.

In one of the selections in this chapter, the AMA Council on Ethical and Judicial Affairs acknowledges and endorses the right of competent patients to forgo life-sustaining treatment. The Council explicitly argues against the view that it is never permissible to forgo artificial nutrition and hydration. One other issue discussed by the Council is worthy of note. Although it is clear that medical decision making is sometimes influenced by the fact that many physicians are more comfortable with *withholding* a life-sustaining treatment to begin with rather than *withdrawing* it once it has been initiated, the Council insists that there is no ethically significant distinction between withholding and withdrawing life-sustaining treatment.

Resuscitation Decisions, DNR Orders, and Judgments of Futility

When a terminally ill patient undergoes cardiac arrest, resuscitation techniques can sometimes restore heartbeat and thereby prolong life. Yet, in many cases, the patient does not desire and cannot benefit from resuscitation. Of course, in other cases, the patient does desire and can benefit from resuscitation. In still other cases, the appropriateness of resuscitation is more in doubt. Perhaps the patient has been ambivalent in expressing a preference about resuscitation. Perhaps the physician is uncertain whether or not resuscitation would be of genuine benefit to the patient. Perhaps the physician believes that resuscitation is in the patient's best interest, but the patient has expressed a preference not to be resuscitated. Alternatively, perhaps the physician believes that resuscitation is not in the patient's best interest, but the patient has expressed a preference to be resuscitated. In one of this chapter's readings, the President's Commission for the Study of Ethical Problems in Medicine and Biomedical and Behavioral Research provides an extensive analysis of ethical considerations relevant to resuscitation decisions. According to the Commission, patient self-determination is the single most important ethical consideration in resuscitation decisions, although the physician's assessment of benefit to the patient, which is sometimes in conflict with a patient's preference, is also relevant. In proposing an overall scheme to guide decision making, the Commission attempts to come to grips not only with the conflicts that may arise between a patient's preference and a physician's assessment of the benefit but also with the uncertainties that may arise from either perspective.

In another reading, Tom Tomlinson and Howard Brody identify three distinct rationales for do-not-resuscitate (DNR) orders. Two of the identified rationales involve quality-of-life judgments. Insisting that quality-of-life judgments must ultimately be made by the patient or the patient's family (if the patient is incompetent), Tomlinson and Brody argue that it is inappropriate in such cases for a physician to write a DNR order without the *permission* of the patient or family. With regard to a third rationale, however, they contend that there is no need for the physician to secure the permission of the patient or family before writing a DNR order. They rely at this point on the concept of futility. In their view, it is sometimes the case that "resuscitation would almost certainly not be successful," and the "decision that CPR is unjustified because it is futile is a judgment that falls entirely within the physician's technical expertise."

If patients desire treatments considered futile by physicians, are physicians obligated to provide them? Clearly, Tomlinson and Brody would respond in the negative. Yet the meaning of *futility* is presently the source of intense controversy in biomedical ethics, as is the ethical significance of the concept. In one of this chapter's selections, Mark R. Wicclair distinguishes various senses of *futility* and ultimately recommends that physicians avoid the language of futility in expressing their opposition to a given treatment.

Advance Directives and Treatment Decisions for Incompetent Adults

The rigors of incurable illness and the dying process frequently deprive previously competent patients of their decision-making capacity. How can a person best ensure that his or her personal wishes with regard to life-sustaining treatment (in various possible circumstances) will be honored even if decision-making capacity is lost? Although communication of one's attitudes and preferences to one's physician, family, and friends surely provides some measure of protection, it is frequently asserted that the most effective protection comes through the formation of *advance directives*.

There are two basic types of advance directives, and each has legal status in a large majority (if not all) of the states. In executing an *instructional* directive, a person specifies instructions about his or her care in the event that decision-making capacity is lost. Such a directive, especially when it deals specifically with a person's wishes regarding life-sustaining treatment in various possible circumstances, is commonly called "a living will." In executing a *proxy* directive, a person specifies a surrogate decision maker to make health-care decisions for him or her in the event that decision-making capacity is lost. The legal mechanism for executing a proxy directive is called a "durable power of attorney" for health care. Since purging ambiguities from even the most explicit written directives is difficult, as is foreseeing all the contingencies that might give rise to a need for treatment decisions, many commentators recommend the execution of a durable power of attorney for health care even if a person has already executed a living will.

If a patient lacks decision-making capacity, a surrogate decision maker must be identified, and this will ordinarily be a member of the family or a close personal friend. If the patient has provided an instructional directive, the surrogate is of course expected to follow the stated instructions. However, sometimes an instructional directive provides insufficient guidance for the treatment decision at hand, and frequently a surrogate decision maker must function in the absence of any explicit directive. In applying the *substituted-judgment* standard, the surrogate decision maker is expected to consider the patient's preferences and values and make the decision that the patient would have made if she or he were able to choose. If no reliable basis exists to infer what the patient would have chosen, then the surrogate decision maker is expected to retreat to the *best-interests* standard. In applying the best-interests standard, the surrogate decision maker is expected to choose what a rational person in the patient's circumstances would choose. In one of this chapter's readings, Dan W. Brock suggests an overall ethical framework for surrogate decision making with regard to incompetent adults.

The Patient Self-Determination Act, passed by Congress in October 1990, requires all health-care institutions (e.g., hospitals and nursing homes) receiving federal funds to inform patients of their right to formulate advance directives. Nevertheless, advance directives remain problematic in many ways. Especially worrisome are concerns that can be raised about the construction, implementation, and force of instructional directives. For one thing, many of the living will forms that have emerged in conjunction with state statutes can be activated only upon the diagnosis of a "terminal illness," a category that has usually been interpreted to exclude both a patient in a persistent vegetative state and one who is existing in a severely compromised state as a result of a progressively debilitating disease (e.g., Alzheimer's). Other phrases commonly found in suggested living will forms are also problematic. For example, suppose a patient signs a form that authorizes withholding or withdrawing life-sustaining treatment if there is "no reasonable expectation that I will regain a meaningful quality of life." Unless a person provides a further specification of what counts for him or her as "a meaningful quality of life," numerous problems of interpretation can arise.

Is the refusal to follow the provisions of a patient's instructional directive ever justified? In some cases, there may be good reason to believe that a patient would not really want a certain provision (e.g., a systematic rejection of mechanical ventilation) to be followed in the particular circumstances that have emerged. Another problematic kind of case involves what might be called the "past wishes versus present interests problem." Suppose someone has unambiguously stipulated that life-sustaining treatments should not be provided if she becomes mentally debilitated. Suppose further that she is now severely debilitated but that she is "pleasantly demented" and does not appear to be suffering. In such a case, life-sustaining treatments may well be in her present interests, although they are clearly incompatible with her past wishes.[4]

In "Why I Don't Have a Living Will," Joanne Lynn gives voice to a series of concerns about the employment of living wills. Norman L. Cantor, on the other hand, is convinced of the importance of instructional directives. Mindful of the various inadequacies associated with "short-form" living wills, he provides us with a sophisticated example of an advance directive document that is tailored to the author's precise concerns. Although Cantor refers to this document as his living will, it has been designed to include a proxy directive as well as an extensive instructional directive.

T.A.M.

NOTES

1 There is a crucial ambiguity in the phrase *persistent vegetative state* (PVS). When a patient's vegetative state is identified as "persistent," it is certainly implied that the vegetative state has endured for a significant period of time. Is it also implied that the vegetative state is irreversible, that is, permanent? Many writers in biomedical ethics speak of a patient's vegetative state as "persistent" only when it is believed that the condition is permanent. Throughout this introduction, *persistent vegetative state* is used in this sense. That is, a *persistent* vegetative state entails that the condition is permanent.

    It is important to recognize, however, that many writers use the phrase *persistent vegetative state* in a contrasting way. For them, *persistent* vegetative state does not entail that the condition is permanent. When PVS is understood in this way, there is no contradiction in saying that a patient has recovered from PVS. Of course, whenever a patient has been in a vegetative state for a significant period of time, a medical determination of irreversibility is of central practical importance.

2 The Ad Hoc Committee of the Harvard Medical School to Examine the Definition of Brain Death, "A Definition of Irreversible Coma," *JAMA* 205 (August 6, 1968), p. 338.

3 It might also be argued that the refusal of life-sustaining treatment in this kind of case is tantamount to suicide. (The morality of suicide is discussed in Chapter 7.)

4 A related issue involves the concept of personal identity. If mental deterioration is so severe that there is good reason to doubt that the present patient is the *same person* as the one who executed the instructional directive, then what is the moral authority of the one to determine what happens to the other? For an extensive discussion of this issue, see Allen E. Buchanan and Dan W. Brock, *Deciding for Others: The Ethics of Surrogate Decision Making* (New York: Cambridge University Press, 1989), Chapter 3, "Advance Directives, Personhood, and Personal Identity."

Why "Update" Death?

President's Commission for the Study of Ethical Problems in Medicine and Biomedical and Behavioral Research

A descriptive account of the President's Commission is found on page 89.

In this selection, taken from the first chapter of its report, *Defining Death,* the Commission provides a compact account of both (1) the interrelationships of brain, heart, and lung functions and (2) the loss of brain functions. Emphasis is placed on the difference between "whole brain death" and a "persistent vegetative state" in which brainstem function persists. Although reference is made to the Commission's view that "the cessation of the vital functions of the entire brain [is] the only proper neurologic basis for declaring death," the analysis and argumentation the Commission presents in support of this view is found only in subsequent chapters of the report.

For most of the past several centuries, the medical determination of death was very close to the popular one. If a person fell unconscious or was found so, someone (often but not always a physician) would feel for the pulse, listen for breathing, hold a mirror before the nose to test for condensation, and look to see if the pupils were fixed. Although these criteria have been used to determine death since antiquity, they have not always been universally accepted.

DEVELOPING CONFIDENCE IN THE HEART-LUNG CRITERIA

In the eighteenth century, macabre tales of "corpses" reviving during funerals and exhumed skeletons found to have clawed at coffin lids led to widespread fear of premature burial. Coffins were developed with elaborate escape mechanisms and speaking tubes to the world above, mortuaries employed guards to monitor the newly dead for signs of life, and legislatures passed laws requiring a delay before burial. . . .

. . . The invention of the stethoscope in the mid-nineteenth century enabled physicians to detect heartbeat with heightened sensitivity. The use of this instrument by a well-trained physician, together with other

Reprinted from President's Commission for the Study of Ethical Problems in Medicine and Biomedical and Behavioral Research, *Defining Death* (1981), pp. 13–20.

clinical measures, laid to rest public fears of premature burial. The twentieth century brought even more sophisticated technological means to determine death, particularly the electrocardiograph (EKG), which is more sensitive than the stethoscope in detecting cardiac functioning.

THE INTERRELATIONSHIPS OF BRAIN, HEART, AND LUNG FUNCTIONS

The brain has three general anatomic divisions: the cerebrum, with its outer shell called the cortex; the cerebellum; and the brainstem, composed of the midbrain, the pons, and the medulla oblongata. Traditionally, the cerebrum has been referred to as the "higher brain" because it has primary control of consciousness, thought, memory and feeling. The brainstem has been called the "lower brain," since it controls spontaneous, vegetative functions such as swallowing, yawning and sleep-wake cycles. It is important to note that these generalizations are not entirely accurate. Neuroscientists generally agree that such "higher brain" functions as cognition or consciousness probably are not mediated strictly by the cerebral cortex; rather, they probably result from complex interrelations between brainstem and cortex.

Respiration is controlled in the brainstem, particularly the medulla. Neural impulses originating in the respiratory centers of the medulla stimulate the diaphragm and intercostal muscles, which cause the lungs to fill with air. Ordinarily, these respiratory centers adjust the rate of breathing to maintain the correct levels of carbon dioxide and oxygen. In certain circumstances, such as heavy exercise, sighing, coughing or sneezing, other areas of the brain modulate the activities of the respiratory centers or even briefly take direct control of respiration.

Destruction of the brain's respiratory center stops respiration, which in turn deprives the heart of needed oxygen, causing it too to cease functioning. The traditional signs of life—respiration and heartbeat—disappear: the person is dead. The "vital signs" traditionally used in diagnosing death thus reflect the direct interdependence of respiration, circulation and the brain.

The artificial respirator and concomitant life-support systems have changed this simple picture. Normally, respiration ceases when the functions of the diaphragm and intercostal muscles are impaired. This results from direct injury to the muscles or (more commonly) because the neural impulses between the brain and these muscles are interrupted. However, an artificial respirator (also called a ventilator) can be used to compensate for the inability of the thoracic muscles to fill the lungs with air. Some of these machines use negative pressure to expand the chest wall (in which case they are called "iron lungs"); others use positive pressure to push air into the lungs. The respirators are equipped with devices to regulate the rate and depth of "breathing," which are normally controlled by the respiratory centers in the medulla. The machines cannot compensate entirely for the defective neural connections since they cannot regulate blood gas levels precisely. But, provided that the lungs themselves have not been extensively damaged, gas exchange can continue and appropriate levels of oxygen and carbon dioxide can be maintained in the circulating blood.

Unlike the respiratory system, which depends on the neural impulses from the brain, the heart can pump blood without external control. Impulses from brain centers modulate the inherent rate and force of the heartbeat but are not required for the heart to contract at a level of function that is ordinarily adequate. Thus, when artificial respiration provides adequate oxygenation and associated medical treatments regulate essential plasma components and blood pressure, an intact heart will continue to beat, despite loss of brain functions. At present, however, no machine can take over the functions of the heart except for a very limited time and in limited circumstances (e.g., a heart-lung machine

used during surgery). Therefore, when a severe injury to the heart or major blood vessels prevents the circulation of the crucial blood supply to the brain, the loss of brain functioning is inevitable because no oxygen reaches the brain.

LOSS OF VARIOUS BRAIN FUNCTIONS

The most frequent causes of irreversible loss of functions of the whole brain are: (1) direct trauma to the head, such as from a motor vehicle accident or a gunshot wound, (2) massive spontaneous hemorrhage into the brain as a result of ruptured aneurysm or complications of high blood pressure, and (3) anoxic damage from cardiac or respiratory arrest or severely reduced blood pressure.

Many of these severe injuries to the brain cause an accumulation of fluid and swelling in the brain tissue, a condition called cerebral edema. In severe cases of edema, the pressure within the closed cavity increases until it exceeds the systolic blood pressure, resulting in a total loss of blood flow to both the upper and lower portions of the brain. If deprived of blood flow for at least 10–15 minutes, the brain, including the brainstem, will completely cease functioning. Other pathophysiologic mechanisms also result in a progressive and, ultimately, complete cessation of intracranial circulation.

Once deprived of adequate supplies of oxygen and glucose, brain neurons will irreversibly lose all activity and ability to function. In adults, oxygen and/or glucose deprivation for more than a few minutes causes some neuron loss. Thus, even in the absence of direct trauma and edema, brain functions can be lost if circulation to the brain is impaired. If blood flow is cut off, brain tissues completely self-digest (autolyze) over the ensuing days.

When the brain lacks all functions, consciousness is, of course, lost. While some spinal reflexes often persist in such bodies (since circulation to the spine is separate from that of the brain), all reflexes controlled by the brainstem as well as cognitive, affective and integrating functions are absent. Respiration and circulation in these bodies may be generated by a ventilator together with intensive medical management. In adults who have experienced irreversible cessation of the functions of the entire brain, this mechanically generated functioning can continue only a limited time because the heart usually stops beating within two to ten days. (An infant or small child who has lost all brain functions will typically suffer cardiac arrest within several weeks, although respiration and heartbeat can sometimes be maintained even longer.)

Less severe injury to the brain can cause mild to profound damage to the cortex, lower cerebral structures, cerebellum, brainstem, or some combination thereof. The cerebrum, especially the cerebral cortex, is more easily injured by loss of blood flow or oxygen than is the brainstem. A 4–6 minute loss of blood flow—caused by, for example, cardiac arrest—typically damages the cerebral cortex permanently, while the relatively more resistant brainstem may continue to function.

When brainstem functions remain, but the major components of the cerebrum are irreversibly destroyed, the patient is in what is usually called a "persistent vegetative state" or "persistent noncognitive state." Such persons may exhibit spontaneous, involuntary movements such as yawns or facial grimaces, their eyes may be open and they may be capable of breathing without assistance. Without higher brain functions, however, any apparent wakefulness does not represent awareness of self or environment (thus, the condition is often described as "awake but unaware"). The case of Karen Ann Quinlan has made this condition familiar to the general public. With necessary medical and nursing care—including feeding through intravenous or nasogastric tubes, and antibiotics for recurrent pulmonary infections—such patients can survive months or years, often without a respirator. (The longest survival exceeded 37 years.)

CONCLUSION: THE NEED FOR RELIABLE POLICY

Medical interventions can often provide great benefit in avoiding *irreversible* harm to a patient's injured heart, lungs, or brain by carrying a patient through a period of acute need. These techniques have, however, thrown new light on the interrelationship of these crucial organ systems. This has created complex issues for public policy as well.

For medical and legal purposes, partial brain impairment must be distinguished from complete and irreversible loss of brain functions or "whole brain death." The President's Commission, as subsequent chapters explain more fully, regards the cessation of the vital functions of the entire brain—and not merely portions thereof, such as those responsible for cognitive functions—as the only proper neurologic basis for declaring death. This conclusion accords with the overwhelming consensus of medical and legal experts and the public.

Present attention to the "definition" of death is part of a process of development in social attitudes and legal rules stimulated by the unfolding of biomedical knowledge. In the nineteenth century increasing knowledge and practical skill made the public confident that death could be diagnosed reliably using cardiopulmonary criteria. The question now is whether, when medical intervention may be responsible for a patient's respiration and circulation, there are other equally reliable ways to diagnose death. . . .

The Definition and Criterion of Death
Charles M. Culver and Bernard Gert

Charles M. Culver, formerly professor of psychiatry at Dartmouth Medical School, teaches bioethics at the Minetti Foundation in LaPlata, Argentina. He is the editor of *Ethics at the Bedside* (1990). Bernard Gert is The Eunice and Julian Cohen Professor for the Study of Ethics and Human Values, Dartmouth College. He is the author of *The Moral Rules* (1970) and *Morality: A New Justification of the Moral Rules* (1988). Culver and Gert are the coauthors of *Philosophy in Medicine: Conceptual and Ethical Issues in Medicine and Psychiatry* (1982).

Culver and Gert consider it essential to distinguish among the *definition* of death, the *criterion* of death, and the *tests* of death. In discussing the definition of death, they begin by giving reasons why death must be considered an event rather than a process. They define death as the permanent cessation of functioning of the *organism as a whole,* and they argue against a competing definition according to which the permanent loss of consciousness and cognition is sufficient for death. In their view, patients who are in a chronic (permanent) vegetative state are alive but are no longer persons, and it is morally justifiable to allow them to die by discontinuing even "ordinary and routine care." With regard to the *criterion* of death, Culver and Gert maintain that the correct criterion is the permanent loss of functioning of the entire brain, *not* the permanent loss of cardiopulmonary function. They conclude with a brief discussion of the appropriate *tests* of death.

Much of the confusion arising from the current brain death controversy is due to the failure to distinguish three distinct elements: (1) the definition of death; (2) the medical criterion for determining that death has occurred; and (3) the tests to prove that the criterion has been satisfied. We shall first define death in a way which makes its ordinary meaning explicit, then provide a criterion of death which fulfills this definition, and finally, indicate which tests have demonstrated perfect validity in determining that the criterion of death is satisfied.[1]

The definitions of death which appear in legal dictionaries and the new statutory definitions of death do not say what the layman actually means by death but merely set out the criteria by which physicians legally determine when death has occurred. *Death,* however, is not a technical term but a common term in everyday use. We believe that a proper understanding of the ordinary meaning of this word or concept must be developed before a medical criterion is chosen. We must decide what is ordinarily meant by death before physicians can decide how to measure it.

Agreement on the definition and criterion of death is literally a life-and-death matter. Whether a spontaneously breathing patient in a chronic vegetative state is classified as dead or alive depends on our understanding of the definition of death. Even given the definition, the status of a patient with a totally and permanently nonfunctioning brain who is being maintained on a ventilator depends on the criterion of death employed. Defining death is primarily a philosophical task; providing the criterion of death is primarily medical; and choosing the tests to prove that the criterion is satisfied is solely a medical matter.

THE DEFINITION OF DEATH

Death as a Process or an Event

It has been claimed that death is a process rather than an event (Morison, 1971). This claim is supported by the fact that a standard series of degenerative and destructive changes occurs in the tissues of an organism, usually following but sometimes preceding the irreversible cessation of spontaneous ventilation and circulation. These changes include: necrosis of brain cells, necrosis of other vital organ cells, cooling, rigor mortis, dependent lividity, and putrefaction. This process actually persists for years, even centuries, until the skeletal remains have disintegrated, and could even be viewed as beginning with the failure of certain organ systems during life. Because these changes occur in a fairly regular and ineluctable fashion, it is claimed that the stipulation of any particular point in this process as the moment of death is arbitrary.

The following argument, however, shows the theoretical inadequacy of any definition which makes death a process. If we regard death as a process, then either (1) the process starts when the person is still living, which confuses the process of death with the process of dying, for we all regard someone who is dying as not yet dead, or (2) the process of death starts when the person is no longer alive, which confuses the process of death with the process of disintegration. Death should be viewed not as a process but as the event that separates the process of dying from the process of disintegration.

On a practical level, regarding death as a process

makes it impossible to declare the time of death with any precision. This is not a trivial issue. There are pressing medical, legal, social, and religious reasons to declare the time of death with some precision, including the interpretation of wills, burial times and procedures, mourning times, and decisions regarding the aggressiveness of medical support. There are no countervailing practical or theoretical reasons for regarding death as a process rather than an event in formulating a definition of death. We shall say that death occurs at some definite time, although this time may not always be specifiable with complete precision.

Choices for a Definition of Death

The definition of death must capture our ordinary use of the term, for *death,* as noted earlier, is a word used by everyone and is not primarily a medical or legal term. In this ordinary use, certain facts are assumed, and we shall assume them as well. Therefore we shall not apply our analysis to science fiction speculations, for example, about brains continuing to function independently of the rest of the organism (Gert, 1967, 1971). Thus we shall assume that all and only living organisms can die, that the living can be distinguished from the dead with very good reliability, and that the moment when an organism leaves the former state and enters the latter can be determined with a fairly high degree of precision. We shall regard death as permanent. We know that some people claim to have been dead for several minutes and then to have returned to life, but we regard this as only a dramatic way of saying that consciousness was temporarily lost (for example, because of a brief episode of cardiac arrest).

Although there are religious theories that death involves the soul leaving the body, we know that religious persons and secularists do not disagree in their ordinary application of the term *dead.* We acknowledge that the body can remain physically intact for some time after death and that some isolated parts of the organism may continue to function (for example, it is commonly believed that hair and nails continue to grow after death). We shall now present our definition of death and contrast it to a proposed alternative.

We define death as the permanent cessation of functioning of the organism as a whole. By the organism as a whole, we do not mean the whole organism, that is, the sum of its tissue and organ parts, but rather the highly complex interaction of its organ subsystems. The organism need not be whole or complete—it may

have lost a limb or an organ (such as the spleen)—but it still remains an organism.

By the functioning of the organism as a whole, we mean the spontaneous and innate activities of integration of all or most subsystems (for example, neuroendocrine control) and at least limited response to the environment (for example, temperature change). However, it is not necessary that all of the subsystems be integrated. Individual subsystems may be replaced (for example, by pacemakers, ventilators, or pressors) without changing the status of the organism as a whole.

It is possible for individual subsystems to function for a time after the organism as a whole has permanently ceased to function. Spontaneous ventilation ceases either immediately after or just before the permanent cessation of functioning of the organism as a whole, but spontaneous circulation, with artificial ventilation, may persist for up to two weeks after the organism as a whole has ceased to function.

An example of an activity of the organism as a whole is temperature regulation. The control of this complex process is located in the hypothalamus and is important for normal maintenance of all cellular processes. It is lost when the organism as a whole has ceased to function.

Consciousness and cognition are sufficient to show the functioning of the organism as a whole in higher animals, but they are not necessary. Lower organisms never have consciousness and even when a higher organism is comatose, evidence of the functioning of the organism as a whole may still be evident, for example, in temperature regulation.

We believe that the permanent cessation of the functioning of the organism as a whole is what has traditionally been meant by death. This definition retains death as a biological occurrence which is not unique to human beings; the same definition applies to other higher animals. We believe that death is a biological phenomenon and should apply equally to related species. When we talk of the death of a human being, we mean the same thing as we do when we talk of the death of a dog or a cat. This is supported by our ordinary use of the term *death*, and by law and tradition. It is also in accord with social and religious practices and is not likely to be affected by future changes in technology.

An alternative definition of death as the irreversible loss of that which is essentially significant to the nature of man has been proposed by Veatch (1976). Though this definition initially seems very attractive, it does not state what we ordinarily mean when we speak of death.

It is not regarded as self-contradictory to say that a person has lost that which is essentially significant to the nature of man, but is still alive. For example, we all acknowledge that permanently comatose patients in chronic vegetative states are sufficiently brain-damaged that they have irreversibly lost all that is essentially significant to the nature of man but we still consider them to be living (for example, Karen Ann Quinlan; see Beresford, 1977).

The patients described by Brierley and associates (1971) are also in this category. These patients had complete neocortical destruction with preservation of the brainstem and diencephalic (posterior brain) structures. They had isoelectric (flat) electroencephalograms (EEGs) (indicating neocortical death) and were permanently comatose, although they had normal spontaneous breathing and brainstem reflexes; they were essentially in a permanent, severe, chronic vegetative state (Jennett and Plum, 1972). They retained many of the vital functions of the organism as a whole, including neuroendocrine control (that is, homeostatic interrelationships between the brain and various hormonal glands) and spontaneous circulation and breathing.

This alternative definition actually states what it means to cease to be a person rather than what it means for that person to die. *Person* is not a biological concept but rather a concept defined in terms of certain kinds of abilities and qualities of awareness. It is inherently vague. Death is a biological concept. Thus in a literal sense, death can be applied directly only to biological organisms and not to persons. We do not object to the phrase "death of a person," but the phrase in common usage actually means the death of the organism which was the person. For example, one might overhear in the hospital wards, "The person in room 612 died last night." In this common usage, one is referring to the death of the organism which was a person. By our analysis, Veatch (1976) and others have used the phrase "death of a person" metaphorically, applying it to an organism which has ceased to be a person but has not died.

Without question, consciousness and cognition are essential human attributes. If they are lost, life has lost its meaning. A patient in a chronic vegetative state is usually regarded as living in only the most basic biological sense. But it is just this basic biological sense that we want to capture in our definition of death. We must not confuse the death of an organism which was a person with an organism's ceasing to be a person. We are immediately aware of the loss of personhood in these patients and are repulsed by the idea of continuing to treat them as if they were persons. But were we to consider these chronic vegetative patients as actually dead, serious problems would arise. First, a slippery slope condition would be introduced wherein the question could be asked: How much neocortical damage is necessary before we declare a patient dead? Surely patients in a chronic vegetative state, although usually not totally satisfying the tests for neocortical destruction, have permanently lost their consciousness and cognition. Then what about the somewhat less severely brain-damaged patient?

By considering permanent loss of consciousness and cognition as a criterion for ceasing to be a person and not for death of the organism as a whole, the slippery slope phenomenon is put where it belongs: not in the definition of death, but in the determination of possible grounds for nonvoluntary euthanasia, that is, providing possible grounds for killing the organism, or allowing it to die, in those instances in which the organism is no longer a person. The justification of nonvoluntary euthanasia must be kept strictly separate from the definition of death. Most of us would like our organism to die when we cease to be persons, but this should not be accomplished by blurring the distinctions between biological death and the loss of personhood.

When an organism ceases to be a person, that is, when it permanently loses all consciousness and cognition, then practical problems arise. How are we to treat this organism? (1) Should we treat it just as we treat a person, making every effort to keep it alive? (2) Should we cease caring for it, either in part or at all, and allow it to die? (3) Should we kill it?

In our view, an organism that is no longer a person has no claim to be treated as a person. But just as one treats a corpse with respect, even more so would one expect that such a living organism be treated with respect. This does not mean, however, that one should strive to keep the organism alive. No one benefits by doing this; on the contrary, given the care needed to keep such an organism alive, it seems an extravagant waste of both economic and human resources to attempt to do so. On the other hand, it seems unjustified to require anyone to actively kill it. Even though the organism is no longer a person, it still looks like a person, and unless there are overwhelming reasons for killing it, it seems best not to do anything that might weaken the prohibition against killing. This leaves the second alternative, discontinuing all care and allowing the patient to die. This can take either of two forms: discontinuing medical treatment or discontinuing all ordinary and routine care. The latter is the position we favor.

It is important to note that the patient will not suffer from lack of care, for since the patient is no longer a person this means that it has permanently lost all consciousness and cognition. Any patient who retains even the slightest capacity to suffer pain or discomfort of any kind remains a person and must be treated as such. We make this point to emphasize our position that only patients who have completely and permanently lost all consciousness and cognition should have all care discontinued. We believe that discontinuing all care and allowing the patient who is no longer a person to die is the preferred alternative, and the one that should be recommended to the legal guardian or next of kin as the course of action to be followed.

THE CRITERION OF DEATH

We have argued that the correct definition of death is permanent cessation of functioning of the organism as a whole. We will now inspect the two competing criteria of death: (1) the permanent loss of cardiopulmonary functioning and (2) the total and irreversible loss of functioning of the whole brain.

Characteristics of Optimum Criteria and Tests

Given that death is the permanent cessation of functioning of the organism as a whole, a criterion will yield a false-positive if it is satisfied, and yet it would still be possible for that organism to function as a whole. By far the most important requirement for a criterion of death is that it yield no false-positives.

A criterion of death, however, cannot have any exceptions; this is what enables it to serve as a legal definition of death. It is not sufficient that the criterion be correct 99.99 percent of the time. This means that not only can the criterion yield no false-positives, it can also yield no false-negatives. A criterion of death yields a false-negative if it is not satisfied and yet the organism as a whole has irreversibly ceased to function. Of course, one may sometimes determine death without using the criterion, but it can never be that the criterion is satisfied and yet the person is not dead, or that the criterion is not satisfied and the person is dead. This is why it is so easy to mistake a criterion for an ordinary definition; it is rather a kind of operational definition, and serves as part of the legal definition, but the real operational definition is provided by the tests which show whether or not the criterion is satisfied.

Permanent Loss of Cardiopulmonary Functioning

Permanent termination of heart and lung function has been used as a criterion of death throughout history. The ancients observed that all other bodily functions ceased shortly after cessation of these vital functions, and the irreversible process of bodily disintegration inevitably followed. Thus permanent loss of spontaneous cardiopulmonary function was found to predict permanent nonfunctioning of the organism as a whole. Further, if there were no permanent loss of spontaneous cardiopulmonary function, then the organism as a whole continued to function. Therefore permanent loss of cardiopulmonary function served as an adequate criterion of death.

Because of current ventilation/circulation technology, permanent loss of spontaneous cardiopulmonary functioning is no longer necessarily predictive of permanent nonfunctioning of the organism as a whole. Consider a conscious, talking patient who is unable to breathe because of suffering from poliomyelitis and who requires an iron lung (thus having permanent loss of spontaneous pulmonary function), who has also developed asystole (loss of spontaneous heartbeat) requiring a permanent pacemaker (thus having permanent loss of spontaneous cardiac function). It would be absurd to regard such a person as dead.

It might be proposed that it is not the permanent loss of *spontaneous* cardiopulmonary function that is the criterion of death, but rather the permanent loss of all cardiopulmonary function, whether spontaneous or artificially supported. But now that ventilation and circulation can be mechanically maintained, an organism with permanent loss of whole brain functioning can have permanently ceased to function as a whole days to weeks before the heart and lungs cease to function with artificial support. Thus this supposed criterion would not be satisfied, yet the person would be dead. The heart and lungs now seem to have no unique relationship to the functioning of the organism as a whole. Continued artificially supported cardiopulmonary function is no longer perfectly correlated with life, and permanent loss of spontaneous cardiopulmonary functioning is no longer perfectly correlated with death.

Total and Irreversible Loss of Whole Brain Functioning

The criterion for the cessation of functioning of the organism as a whole is the permanent loss of functioning of the entire brain. This criterion is perfectly correlated with the permanent cessation of functioning of the organism as a whole because it is the brain that is necessary for the functioning of the organism as a whole. It integrates, generates, interrelates, and controls complex bodily activities. A patient on a ventilator with a totally destroyed brain is merely a preparation of artificially maintained subsystems since the organism as a whole has ceased to function.

The brain generates the signal for breathing through brainstem ventilatory centers and aids in the control of circulation through brainstem blood pressure control centers. Destruction of the brain produces apnea (inability to breath) and generalized vasodilation (opening of the peripheral blood vessels); in all cases, despite the most aggressive support, the adult heart stops within a week and that of the child within two weeks (Ingvar et al., 1978). Thus when the organism as a whole has ceased to function, the artificially supported vital subsystems quickly fail. Many other functions of the organism as a whole, including neuroendocrine control, temperature control, food-searching behaviors, and sexual activity, reside in the more primitive regions (hypothalamus, brainstem) of the brain. Thus total and irreversible loss of functioning of the whole brain and not merely the neocortex is required as the criterion for the permanent loss of the functioning of the organism as a whole.

Using permanent loss of functioning of the whole brain as the criterion for death of the organism as a whole is also consistent with tradition. Throughout history, whenever a physician was called to ascertain the occurrence of death, his examination included the following important signs indicative of permanent loss of functioning of the whole brain: unresponsivity, lack of spontaneous movements including breathing; and absence of pupillary light response. Only one important sign, lack of heartbeat, was not directly indicative of whole brain destruction. But since the heartbeat stops within several minutes of apnea, permanent absence of the vital signs is an important sign of permanent loss of whole brain functioning. Thus, in an important sense, permanent loss of whole brain functioning has always been the underlying criterion of death.

THE TESTS OF DEATH

Given the definition of death as the permanent cessation of functioning of the organism as a whole, and the criterion of death as the total and irreversible cessation

of functioning of the whole brain, the next step is the examination of the available tests of death. The tests must be such that they will never yield a false-positive result. Of secondary importance, they should produce few and relatively brief false-negatives.

Cessation of Heartbeat and Ventilation

The physical findings of permanent absence of heartbeat and respiration are the traditional tests of death. In the vast majority of deaths not complicated by artificial ventilation, these classic tests are still applicable. They show that the criterion of death has been satisfied since they always quickly produce permanent loss of functioning of the whole brain. However, when mechanical ventilation is being used, these tests lose most of their utility due to the production of numerous false-negatives for as long a time as one to two weeks, that is, death of the organism as a whole with still intact circulatory-ventilatory subsystems. Thus though the circulation-ventilation tests will suffice in most instances of death, if there is artificial maintenance of circulation or ventilation the special tests for permanent cessation of whole brain functioning will be needed.

Irreversible Cessation of Whole Brain Functioning

Numerous formalized sets of tests have been established to determine that the criterion of permanent loss of whole brain functioning has been met. These include, among others, tests described by the Harvard Medical School Ad Hoc Committee (Beecher, 1968) and the National Institutes of Health Collaborative Study of Cerebral Survival (1977). They have all been recently reviewed (Black, 1978; Molinari, 1978). What we call tests have sometimes been called "criteria," but it is important to distinguish these second-level criteria from the first-level criteria. While the first-level criteria must be for the death of the organism and must be understandable by the layman, the second-level criteria (tests) determine the permanent loss of functioning of the whole brain and need not be understandable by anyone except qualified clinicians. To avoid confusion, we prefer to use the designation "tests" for the second-level criteria.

All the proposed tests require total and permanent absence of all functioning of the brainstem and both hemispheres. They vary slightly from one set to another, but all require unresponsivity (deep coma), absent pupillary light reflexes, apnea (inability to breathe), and absent brainstem reflexes. They also require the absence of drug intoxication and low body temperature, and the newer sets require the demonstration that a lesion of the brain exists. Isoelectric (flat) EEGs are generally required, and tests disclosing the absence of cerebral blood flow are of confirmatory value (NIH Collaborative Study, 1977). All tests require the given loss of function to be present for a particular time interval, which in the case of the absence of cerebral blood flow may be as short as thirty minutes.

Current tests of irreversible loss of whole brain function may produce many false-negatives of a sort during the thirty-minute to twenty-four-hour interval between the successive neurologic examinations which the tests require. Certain sets of tests, particularly those requiring electrocerebral silence by EEG, may produce false-negatives if an EEG artifact is present and cannot confidently be distinguished from brain wave activity. Generally, a few brief false-negatives are tolerable and even inevitable, since tests must be delineated conservatively in order to eliminate any possibility of false-positives.

There are many studies which show perfect correlation between the loss of whole brain function tests of the Ad Hoc Committee of the Harvard Medical School and total brain necrosis at postmortem examination. Veith et al. (1977a) conclude that "the validity of the criteria [tests] must be considered to be established with as much certainty as is possible in biology or medicine" (p. 1652). Thus, when a physician ascertains that a patient satisfies the validated loss of whole brain function tests, he can be confident that the loss of whole brain functioning is permanent. Physicians should apply only tests which have been completely validated. . . .

NOTE

1 This [article] is adapted in part from Bernat, Culver, and Gert (1981).

REFERENCES

American Bar Association. House of Delegates redefines death, urges redefinition of rape, and undoes the Houston amendments. *American Bar Association Journal*, 1975, *61*, 463–464.

Beecher, Henry K. A definition of irreversible coma: report of the Ad Hoc Committee of the Harvard Medical School to examine the definition of brain death. *Journal of the American Medical Association*, 1968, *205*, 337–340.

Beresford, H. Richard. The Quinlan decision: problems and legislative alternatives. *Annals of Neurology*, 1977, *2*, 74–81.

Bernat, James L., Culver, Charles M., and Gert, Bernard. On the definition and criterion of death. *Annals of Internal Medicine*, 1981, *94*, 389–394.

Black, Peter M. Brain death. *New England Journal of Medicine*, 1978, *299*, 338–344, 393–401.

Brierley, J.B., Adams, J.H., Graham, D.I., and Simpson, J.A. Neocortical death after cardiac arrest. *Lancet*, 1971, *2*, 560–565.

Capron, Alexander M., and Kass, Leon R. A statutory definition of the standards for determining human death: an appraisal and a proposal. *University of Pennsylvania Law Review*, 1972, *121*, 87–118.

Gert, Bernard. Can the brain have a pain? *Philosophy and Phenomenological Research*, 1967, *27*, 432–436.

Gert, Bernard. Personal identity and the body. *Dialogue*, 1971, *10*, 458–478.

Hastings Center Task Force on Death and Dying. Refinements in criteria for the determination of death: an appraisal. *Journal of the American Medical Association*, 1972, *221*, 48–53.

Ingvar, David H., Brun, Arne, Johansson, Lars, and Sammuelsson, Sven M. Survival after severe cerebral anoxia with destruction of the cerebral cortex: the apallic syndrome. *Annals of the New York Academy of Science*, 1978, *315*, 184–214.

Jennett, B., and Plum, F. Persistent vegetative state after brain damage. A syndrome in search of a name. *Lancet*, 1972, *1*, 734–737.

Jonas, Hans. *Philosophical Essays: From Ancient Creed to Technological Man*. Englewood Cliffs, N.J.: Prentice-Hall, 1974, pp. 134–140.

Law Reform Commission of Canada. *Criteria for the Determination of Death*. Ottawa: Law Reform Commission of Canada, 1979.

Molinari, Gaetano F. Review of clinical criteria of brain death. *Annals of the New York Academy of Science*, 1978, *315*, 62–69.

Morison, Robert S. Death: process or event? *Science*, 1971, *173*, 694–698.

NIH Collaborative Study of Cerebral Survival. An appraisal of the criteria of cerebral death: a summary statement. *Journal of the American Medical Association*, 1977, *237*, 982–986.

President's Commission for the Study of Ethical Problems in Medicine and Biomedical and Behavioral

Research. *"Defining Death," a Report on the Medical, Legal and Ethical Issues in the Determination of Death.* Washington, D.C., 1981.

Veatch, Robert M. *Death, Dying and the Biological Revolution: Our Last Quest for Responsibility.* New Haven, Conn.: Yale University Press, 1976.

Veith, Frank J., Fein, Jack M., Tendler, Moses D., Veatch, Robert M., Kleiman, Marc A., and Kalkines, George. Brain death I. A status report of medical and ethical considerations. *Journal of the American Medical Association,* 1977a, *238,* 1651–1655.

Veith, Frank J., Fein, Jack M., Tendler, Moses D., Veatch, Robert M., Kleiman, Marc A., and Kalkines, George. Brain death II. A status report of legal considerations. *Journal of the American Medical Association,* 1977b, *238,* 1744–1748.

The Impending Collapse of the Whole-Brain Definition of Death
Robert M. Veatch

A biographical sketch of Robert M. Veatch is found on page 230.

Veatch favors a "higher-brain" definition of death over a "whole-brain" definition. He presents objections to the whole-brain approach and responds to a set of arguments commonly made against the higher-brain approach. Veatch pays particular attention to the charge that the higher-brain approach can be undermined by a slippery-slope argument. In his view, it is not the higher-brain approach but the whole-brain approach that is vulnerable to slippery-slope considerations. Although Veatch personally favors a higher-brain definition, he believes that each individual in a pluralistic society should be allowed to choose for herself or himself a definition of death that is responsive to that individual's religious and philosophical convictions. Thus, in terms of social policy, Veatch favors the incorporation of a "conscience clause" in any statute that defines death. According to him, an ideal social policy would identify a higher-brain definition as the default position, but it would also allow individuals to stipulate for themselves either the whole-brain standard or the more traditional (cardiopulmonary) standard.

For many years there has been lingering doubt, at least among theorists, that the currently fashionable "whole-brain-oriented" definition of death has things exactly right. I myself have long resisted the term "brain death" and will use it only in quotation marks to indicate the still common, if ambiguous, usage. The term is ambiguous because it fails to distinguish between the biological claim that the brain is dead and the social/legal/moral claim that the individual as a whole is dead because the brain is dead. An even greater problem with the term arises from the lingering doubt that individuals with dead brains are really dead. Hence,

Reprinted with permission of the author and the publisher from *Hastings Center Report,* vol. 23 (July/August 1993), pp. 18–24. © The Hastings Center.

even physicians are sometimes heard to say that the patient "suffered brain death" one day and "died" the following day. It is better to say that he "died" on the first day, the day the brain was determined to be dead, and that the cadaver's other bodily functions ceased the following day. For these reasons I insist on speaking of persons with dead brains as individuals who are dead, not merely persons who are "brain dead."

The presently accepted standard definition, the Uniform Determination of Death Act, specifies that an individual is dead who has sustained "irreversible cessation of all functions of the entire brain, including the brain stem."[1] It also provides an alternative definition specifying that an individual is also dead who has sustained "irreversible cessation of circulatory and respiratory functions." The President's Commission for the

Study of Ethical Problems in Medicine and Biomedical and Behavioral Research made clear, however, that circulatory and respiratory function loss are important only as indirect indicators that the brain has been permanently destroyed (p. 74).

DOUBTS ABOUT THE WHOLE-BRAIN-ORIENTED DEFINITION

It is increasingly apparent, however, that this consensus is coming apart. As long ago as the early 1970s some of us doubted that literally the entire brain had to be dead for the individual as a whole to be dead.[2]

From the early years it was known, at least among neurologists and theorists who read the literature, that individual, isolated brain cells could be perfused and continue to live even though integrated supercellular brain function had been destroyed. When the uniform definition of death said *all functions of the entire brain* must be dead, there was a gentleman's agreement that cellular level functions did not count. The President's Commission recognized this, positing that "cellular activity alone is irrelevant" (p. 75). This willingness to write off cellular level functions is more controversial than it may appear. After all, the law does not grant a dispensation to ignore cellular level functions, no matter how plausible that may be. Keep in mind that critics of soon-to-be-developed higher brain definitions of death would need to emphasize that the model statute called for loss of *all* functions.

By 1977 an analogous problem arose regarding electrical activity. The report of a multicenter study funded by the National Institutes of Neurological Diseases and Stroke found that all of the functions it considered important could be lost irreversibly while very small (2 microvolt) electrical potentials could still be obtained on EEG. These were not artifact but real electrical activity from brain cells. Nevertheless, the committee concluded that there could be "electrocerebral silence" and therefore the brain could be considered "dead" even though these small electrical charges could be recorded.[3]

It is possible that the members of the committee believed that these were the result of nothing more than cellular level functions, so that the same reasoning that permitted the President's Commission to write off little functions as unimportant would apply. However, no evidence was presented that these electrical potentials were arising exclusively from cellular level functions. It

could well be that the reasoning in this report expanded the existing view that cellular functions did not count to the view that some minor supercellular functions could be ignored as long as they were small.

More recently the neurologist James Bernat, a defender of the whole-brain-oriented definition of death, has acknowledged that:

> the bedside clinical examination is not sufficiently sensitive to exclude the possibility that small nests of brain cells may have survived . . . and that their continued functioning, although not contributing significantly to the functioning of the organism as a whole, can be measured by laboratory techniques. Because these isolated nests of neurons no longer contribute to the functioning of the organism as a whole, their continued functioning is now irrelevant to the dead organism.[4]

The idea that functions of "isolated nests of neurons" can remain when an individual is declared dead based on whole-brain-oriented criteria certainly stretches the plain words of the law that requires, without qualification, that *all functions of the entire brain* must be gone. That exceptions can be granted by individual private citizens based on their personal judgments about which functions are "contributing significantly" certainly challenges the integrity of the idea that the whole brain must be dead for the individual as a whole to be dead.

There is still another problem for those who favor what can now be called the "whole-brain definition of death." It is not altogether clear that the "death of the brain" is to be equated with the "irreversible loss of function." At least one paper appears to hold out not only for loss of function but also for destruction of anatomical structure.[5] Thus we are left with a severely nuanced and qualified whole-brain-oriented definition of death. For it to hold as applied in the 1990s, one must assume that function rather than structure is irreversibly destroyed and that not only can certain cellular-level functions and microvolt-level electrical functions be ignored as "insignificant," but also certain "nests of cells" and associated supercellular-level functions can as well.

By the time the whole-brain-oriented definition of death is so qualified, it can hardly be referring to the death of the whole brain any longer. What is particularly troublesome is that private citizens—neurologists, philosophers, theologians, and public commentators—seem to be determining just which brain functions are insignificant.

THE HIGHER-BRAIN-ORIENTED ALTERNATIVE

The problem is exacerbated when one reviews the early "brain death" literature. Writers trying to make the case for a brain-based definition of death over a heart-based one invariably pointed out that certain functions were irreversibly lost when the brain was gone. Then, implicitly or explicitly, they made the moral/philosophical/religious claim that individuals who have irreversibly lost these key functions should be treated as dead.

While this function-based defense of a brain-oriented definition of death served the day well, some of us realized that the critical functions cited were not randomly distributed throughout the brain. For instance, Henry Beecher, the chair of the Harvard Ad Hoc Committee, identified the following functions as critical: "the individual's personality, his conscious life, his uniqueness, his capacity for remembering, judging, reasoning, acting, enjoying, worrying, and so on."[6]

Of course, all these functions are known to require the cerebrum. If these are the important functions, the obvious question is why any lower brain functions would signal the presence of a living individual. This gave rise to what is now best called the *higher-brain-oriented definition of death:* that one is dead when there is irreversible loss of all "higher" brain functions.[7] At first this was referred to as a cerebral or a cortical definition of death, but it seems clear that just as some brain stem functions may be deemed insignificant, likewise, some functions in the cerebrum may be as well. Moreover, it is not clear that the functions of the kind Beecher listed are always necessarily localized in the cerebrum or the cerebral cortex. At least in theory someday we may be able to build an artificial neurological organ that could replace some functions of the cerebrum. Someone who was thinking, feeling, reasoning, and carrying on a conversation through the use of an artificial brain would surely be recognized as alive even if the cerebrum that it had replaced was long since completely dead. I have preferred the purposely ambiguous term "higher brain function," as a way to make clear that the key philosophical issue is which of the many brain functions are really important.

Although that way of putting the question may offend the defenders of the more traditional whole-brain definition of death, once they have made the move of excluding the cellular, electrical, and supercellular functions they consider "insignificant," they are hardly in a position to complain about the project of sorting functions into important and unimportant ones.

CRITICISMS OF THE HIGHER BRAIN FORMULATIONS

Several defenders of the whole-brain-oriented concept have claimed that defining death in terms of loss of certain significant brain functions involves a change in the concept of death. This, however, rests on the implausible claim of Alex Capron, the executive director of the President's Commission, that the move from a heart-oriented to a whole-brain-oriented definition of death is not a change in concept at all, but merely the recognition of new diagnostic measures for the traditional concept of death (p. 41). It is very doubtful, however, that the move to a whole-brain-oriented concept of death is any less of a fundamental change in concept than movement to a higher-brain-oriented one. From the beginning of the debate many people with beating hearts and dead brains would have been alive under the traditional concept of death focusing on fluid flow, but are clearly dead based on a then-newer whole-brain-oriented concept. Most understood this as a significant change in concept. In any case, even if there is a greater change in moving to a definition of death that identifies certain functions of the brain as significant, the mere fact that it is a conceptual change should not count against it. Surely, the critical question is which concept is right, not which concept squares with traditional views.

A second major charge against the higher-brain-oriented formulations has been that we are unable to measure precisely the irreversible loss of these higher functions based on current neurophysiological techniques (p. 40). By contrast it has been assumed that the irreversible loss of all functions of the entire brain is measurable based on current techniques.

Although lay people generally do not realize it, the measurement of death based on any concept can never be 100 percent accurate. The greatest error rates have certainly been with the heart-oriented concepts of death. Many patients have been falsely determined to have irreversibly lost heart functions. In earlier days we simply did not have the capacity to measure precisely. Even today there may be no reason to determine precisely whether the heart could be restarted in the case of a terminally ill, elderly patient who is ready to die.

There is even newly found ambiguity in the notion of irreversibility.[8] We are moving rapidly toward the day when organs for transplant will be obtained from non-heart-beating cadavers who have been determined to be dead based on heart function loss. It will be important for death to be pronounced as quickly as possible after the heart function has been found irreversibly lost. It is not clear, however, whether death should be pronounced when the heart has permanently stopped (say, following a decision based on an advance directive to withdraw a ventilator), but could be started again. In the minutes when it could be started, but will not be because the patient has refused resuscitation, can we say that the individual is dead?

Likewise, it is increasingly clear that we must acknowledge some, admittedly very small, risk of error in measuring the irreversible loss of all functions of the entire brain. Alan Shewmon has argued that the determination of the death of the entire brain cannot be made with as great a certainty as some neurologists would claim.[9] Some neurologists have persisted in claiming that brains are dead (or have irreversibly lost all function) even though electrical function still remains.[10] Clearly, brains with electrical function must have some living tissues; claims these brains are dead must rest on the assumption that remaining functions are insignificant.

None of this should imply that the death of the brain cannot be measured with great accuracy. But it is wrong to assume that similar or greater levels of accuracy cannot be obtained in measuring the irreversible loss of key higher functions, including consciousness. The literature on the persistent vegetative state repeatedly claims that we can know with great accuracy that consciousness is irreversibly lost.[11] The AMA's Councils on Scientific Affairs and Ethical and Judicial Affairs have concluded that the diagnosis can be made with an error rate of less than one in a thousand.[12] In fact the President's Commission itself said that "the Commission was assured that physicians with experience in this area can reliably determine that some patients' loss of consciousness is permanent."[13]

Even if we could not presently measure accurately the loss of key higher functions such as consciousness, that would have a bearing only on the clinical implementation of the higher-brain-oriented definition, not the validity of the concept itself. Defenders of the higher brain formulation might continue to use the now old-fashioned measures of loss of all function, but only because of the assurance that if all functions are lost, the higher functions certainly are. Such a conservative policy would leave open the question of whether we could some day measure the loss of higher functions accurately enough to use the measures clinically.

Still another criticism is the claim that any higher brain formulation would rely on a concept of personhood or personal identity that is philosophically contro-

versial (pp. 38–39). Personhood theories are notoriously controversial. It is simply wrong, however, to claim that any higher-brain-oriented concept of death is based on either personhood or personal identity theories. I, for one, have acknowledged the possibility that there are living human beings who do not satisfy the various concepts of personhood. As long as the law is only discussing whether someone is a living individual, the debate over personhood is irrelevant.

Perhaps the most serious charge against the higher-brain-oriented formulations is that they are susceptible to the so-called slippery slope argument.[14] Once one yields on the insistence that all functions of the entire brain must be irreversibly gone before an individual is considered dead, there seems to be no stopping the slide of eliminating functions considered insignificant. The argument posits that once totally and permanently unconscious individuals who have some other brain functions (such as brain stem reflexes) remaining are considered dead, someone will propose that those with only marginal consciousness similarly lack significant function and soon all manner of functionally compromised humans will be defined as dead. Since being labelled dead is normally an indicator that certain moral and legal rights cease, such a slide toward considering increasing numbers of marginally functional humans as dead would be morally horrific.

But is the slippery slope argument plausible? In its most significant form, such an argument involves a claim that the same principle underlying one apparently tolerable judgment also entails other, clearly unacceptable judgments. For example, imagine we were trying to determine whether the elderly could be excluded from access to certain health care services based on the utilitarian principle of choosing the course that produced the maximum aggregate good for society. The slippery slope argument might be used to show that the same principle entails implications presumed clearly unacceptable, such as excluding health care from the socially unproductive. To the extent that one is certain that the empirical assumptions are correct (for example, that the utilitarian principle does entail excluding care from the unproductive) and one is confident that such an outcome would be morally unacceptable, then one might attempt to use slippery slope arguments to challenge the proposal to withhold health care from the elderly. The same principle used to support one policy also entails other policies that are clearly unacceptable.

The slippery slope argument is valid insofar as it shows that the principle used to support one policy under consideration entails clearly unacceptable implications when applied to different situations. In principle, there is no difference between the small, potentially tolerable move and the more dramatic, unacceptable move. However, as applied to the definition of death debate, the slippery slope argument can actually be used to show that the whole-brain-oriented definition of death is less defensible than the higher-brain-oriented one.

As we have seen, the whole-brain-oriented definition of death rests on the claim that irreversible loss of all functions of the entire brain is necessary and sufficient for an individual to be dead. That, in effect, means drawing a sharp line between the top of the spinal cord and the base of the brain (i.e., the bottom of the brain stem). But is there any principled reason why one would draw a line at that point?

In the early years of the definition of death debate, the claim was made that an individual was dead when the central nervous system no longer retained the capacity for integration. It was soon discovered, however, that this could be taken to imply that one was "alive" as long as some spinal cord function remained. That was counterintuitive (and also made it more difficult to obtain organs for transplant). Hence, very early on it was agreed that simple reflexes of the spinal cord did not count as an indicator of life. Presumably the principle was that reflex arcs that do not integrate significant bodily functions are to be ignored.

But why then do brain stem reflexes mediated through the base of the brain stem count? By the same principle, if spinal reflexes can be ignored, it would seem that some brain stem reflexes might be as well. An effort to show that brain stem reflexes are more integrative of bodily function is doomed to fail. At most there are gradual, imperceptible gradations in complexity between the reflexes of the first cervical vertebra and those of the base of the brain stem. Some spinal reflexes that trigger extension of the foot while the contralateral arm is withdrawn certainly cover larger distances.

Whatever principle could be used to exclude the spinal reflexes surely can exclude some brain stem reflexes as well. We have seen that the defenders of the whole-brain-oriented position admit as much when they start excluding cellular level functions and electrical functions. Certainly, those who exclude "nests of cells" in the brain as insignificant have abandoned the whole brain position and are already sliding along the slippery slope.

By contrast the defenders of the higher-brain-oriented definition of death can articulate a principle that avoids such slipperiness. Suppose, for example, they rely on classical Judeo-Christian notions that the human is essentially the integration of the mind and body and that the existence of one without the other is not sufficient to constitute a living human being. Such a principle provides a bright line that would clearly distinguish the total and irreversible loss of consciousness from serious but not total mental impairments.

Likewise, the integration of mind and body provides a firm basis for telling which functions of nests of brain cells count as significant. It avoids the hopeless task of trying to show why brain stem reflexes count more than spinal ones or trying to show exactly how many cells must be in a nest before it is significant. There is no subjective assessment of different bodily functions, no quibble about how much integration there must be for the organism to function as a whole. The principle is simple. It relies on qualitative considerations: when, and only when, there is the capacity for organic (bodily) and mental function present together in a single human entity is there a living human being. That, I would suggest, is the philosophical basis for the higher-brain-oriented definition of death. It avoids the slippery slope on which the defenders of the whole-brain-oriented position have found themselves; it, and only it, provides a principled reason for avoiding the slippery slope.

CONSCIENCE CLAUSES

There is one final development that signals the demise of the whole-brain-oriented definition of death as the single basis for declaring death. It should be clear by now that the definition of death debate is actually a debate over the moral status of human beings. It is a debate over when humans should be treated as full members of the human community. When humans are living, full moral and legal human rights accrue. Saying people are alive is simply shorthand for saying that they are bearers of such rights. That is why the definition of death debate is so important. It is also why, in principle, there is no scientific way in which the debate can be resolved. The determination of who is alive—who has full moral standing as a member of the human community—is fundamentally a moral, philosophical, or religious determination, not a scientific one.

In a pluralistic society, we are not likely to reach agreement on such moral questions, which is why no one definition of death has carried the day thus far. When one realizes that there are many variants on each of the three major definitions of death, each of which has some group of adherents, it seems unlikely that any one position is likely to gain even a majority any time soon. For example, defense of the higher-brain-oriented position stands or falls on the claim that the essence of the human being is the integration of a mind and a body, a position reflecting religious and philosophical assumptions that are not beyond dispute. (Other defenders of the higher brain position, for example, are more Manichaean, holding that only the mind is important; they apparently are committed to a view that a human memory transferred to a computer with a capacity to continue mental function would still have all the essential ingredients of humanness and that the same living human being continues to live on the computer hard drive.) These are disputes not likely to be resolved soon.

As a society we have a method for dealing with fundamental disputes in religion and philosophy. We tolerate diversity and affirm the right of conscience to hold minority beliefs as long as actions based on those beliefs do not cause insurmountable problems for the rest of society. That is precisely what in 1976 I proposed doing in the dispute over the definition of death.[15] I proposed a definition of death with a conscience clause that would permit individuals to choose their own definition of death based on their religious and philosophical convictions. I did not say at the time, but should have, that the choices would have to be restricted to those that avoid violating the rights of others and avoid creating insurmountable social problems for the rest of society. For example, I assume that people would not be able to pick a definition that required society to treat them as dead even though they retained cardiac, respiratory, mental, and neurological integrating functions. Likewise, I assume that people would not be permitted to pick a definition that would insist that they treated as alive when all these functions were absent. There are minimal public health considerations that would set limits on the choices available, but certainly the three major options would be tolerable: heart-, whole-brain-, and higher-brain-oriented definitions.

The state of New Jersey has gone part of the way recently by adopting a law with a conscience clause that would permit religious objectors to designate in advance that a heart-oriented definition should be used in pronouncing their deaths. Since it is now widely accepted that anyone can write an advance directive mandating withdrawal of life support once one is permanently unconscious, any persons who favor a higher-brain-oriented definition of death already have the legal right to make choices that end up with them dead in anyone's

sense of the term very shortly after they had lost higher brain functions. Permitting them to designate that they be called dead when they are permanently unconscious changes very little.

There is a litany of worries over conscience clauses that defenders of the whole-brain-oriented definitions cite. They worry about life insurance paying off at different times, depending on which definition is chosen, and about homicide charges being dependent on such choices, but these are already with us when people are permitted to use advance directives to control the timing of their deaths. They worry about health insurance costs, but for those who choose a higher-brain-oriented formulation the only implication is lower costs. For those who choose a heart-oriented definition potentially higher health insurance costs could result, but that position is held only by a small minority, and it is technically so difficult to maintain a beating heart in someone whose brain is dead that the costs will probably not be significant. If they were, the problem could be addressed by clarifying that standard health insurance would not cover the medical costs for maintaining someone who is "alive with a dead brain." None of these problems has arisen in New Jersey, and none is likely to arise. In short, there is no reason to suspect that the use of a conscience clause will result in social chaos—only in greater respect for minority religious and philosophical views that would otherwise be suppressed by the tyranny of the majority. For convenience it would probably be prudent to adopt a single "default definition" favored by a majority; it would make little difference which definition is used as long as the minority who had strong preference for an alternative had the right to designate in advance its choice of another definition. As with surrogate decisionmaking for terminal care and the procurement of cadaver organs, I think it would be reasonable for the next of kin to have the right of surrogate decisionmaking in the case of minors or mentally incompetent individuals who had not expressed a preference while competent.

CRAFTING NEW PUBLIC LAW

Changing current law to conform to these suggestions will be complex and should be done with deliberate speed, but it should be done. Two changes would be needed in the current definition of death: (1) incorporating the higher brain function notion and (2) incorporating some form of the conscience clause.

Present law makes persons dead when they have

lost all functions of the entire brain. It is uniformly agreed that the law should incorporate only this basic concept of death, not the precise criteria or tests needed to determine that the whole brain is dead. That is left up to the consensus of neurological experts.

All that would be needed to shift to a higher brain formulation is a change in the wording of the law to replace "all functions of the entire brain" with some relevant, more limited alternative. There are at least three options: references to higher brain functions, cerebral functions, or consciousness. While we could simply change the wording to read that an individual is dead when there is irreversible cessation of all higher brain functions, that poses a serious problem. We are now suffering from the problems created by the vagueness of the referring to "all functions of the entire brain." Even though referring to "all higher brain functions" would be conceptually correct, it would be even more ambiguous. It would lack needed specificity.

This specificity could be achieved by referring to irreversible loss of cerebral functions, but we have already suggested two problems with that wording. Just as we now know there are some isolated functions of the whole brain that should be discounted, so there are probably some isolated cerebral functions that most would not want to count either. For example, if, hypothetically, an isolated "nest" of cerebral motor neurons were perfused so that if stimulated the body could twitch, that would be a cerebral function, but not a significant one for determining life any more than a brain stem reflex is. Second, in theory some really significant functions such as consciousness might some day be maintainable even without a cerebrum—if, for example, a computer could function as an artificial center for consciousness. The term "cerebral function" adds specificity but is not satisfactory.

The language that seems best if integration of mind and body is what is critical is "irreversible cessation of the capacity for consciousness." That is, after all, what the defenders of the higher brain formulations really have in mind. (If someone were to claim that some other "higher" function is critical, that alternative could simply be plugged in.) As is the case now, the specifics of the criteria and tests for measuring irreversible loss of capacity for consciousness would be left up to the consensus of neurological expertise, even though measuring irreversible loss of capacity for a brain function such as consciousness involves fundamentally nonscientific value judgments. If the community of neurological expertise claims that irreversible loss of consciousness cannot be measured, so be it. We will at least have clarified the

concept and set the stage for the day when it can be measured with sufficient accuracy. We have noted, however, that neurologists presently claim they can in fact measure irreversible loss of consciousness accurately.

A second significant change in the definition of death would be required to incorporate the conscience clause. It would permit individuals, while competent, to execute documents choosing alternative definitions of death that are, within reason, not threatening to significant interests of others. While the New Jersey law permits only the alternative of a heart-oriented definition, my proposal, assuming irreversible loss of consciousness were the default definition, would permit choosing either heart-oriented or whole-brain-oriented definitions as alternatives.

The New Jersey law presently permits only competent adults to execute such conscience clauses. This, of course, excludes the possibility of parents choosing alternative definitions for their children. I had long ago proposed that, just as legal surrogates have the right to make medical treatment decisions for their wards provided the decisions are within reason, so they should be permitted to choose alternative definitions of death provided the individual had never expressed a preference. This would, for example, permit Orthodox Jewish parents to require that the state continue to treat their child as alive even though he or she had suffered irreversible loss of consciousness or of total brain function. (Whether the state also requires insurers to continue paying for support of these individuals deemed living is a separate policy issue.) While the New Jersey law tolerates only variation with an explicitly religious basis, I would favor variation based on any conscientiously formulated position.

As a short-cut the law could state that patients who had clearly irreversibly lost consciousness because heart and lung function had stopped could continue to be pronounced dead based on criteria measuring heart and lung function. That this was simply an alternative means for measuring permanent loss of consciousness would have to be set out more clearly than in the present Uniform Determination of Death Act. I see no reason to continue including the alternative measurement in the legal definition. I would simply allow it to fall under the criteria to be articulated by the consensus of experts. This leads to a proposal for a new definition of death, which would read as follows:

> An individual who has sustained irreversible loss of consciousness is dead. A determination of death must be made in accordance with accepted medical standards.

However, no individual shall be considered dead based on irreversible loss of consciousness if he or she, while competent, has explicitly asked to be pronounced dead based on irreversible cessation of all functions of the entire brain or based on irreversible cessation of circulatory and respiratory functions.

Unless an individual has, while competent, selected one of these definitions of death, the legal guardian or next of kin (in that order) may do so. The definition selected by the individual, legal guardian or next of kin shall serve as the definition of death for all legal purposes.

If one favored only the shift to consciousness as a definition of death without the conscience clause, only paragraph one would be necessary. One could also craft a similar definition using the whole-brain-oriented definition of death as the default definition. Some have proposed an additional paragraph prohibiting a physician with a conflict of interest (such as an interest in the organs of the deceased) from pronouncing death. I am not convinced that paragraph is needed, however.

A PRINCIPLED REASON FOR DRAWING THE LINE

It has been puzzling why what at first seemed like a rather minor debate over when a human was dead should have persisted as long as it has. Many thought the definition of death debate was a technical argument that would be resolved in favor of the more fashionable, scientific, and progressive brain-oriented definition as soon as the old romantics attached to the heart died off. It is now clear that something much more complex and more fundamental is at stake. We have been fighting over the question of who has moral standing as a full member of the human moral community, a matter that forces on us some of the most basic questions of human existence: the relation of mind and body, the rights of religious and philosophical minorities, and the meaning of life itself.

I am not certain whether some version of the higher-brain-oriented definition of death will be adopted in any legal jurisdiction anytime soon, but I am convinced that the now old-fashioned whole-brain-oriented definition of death is becoming less and less plausible as we realize that no one really believes that literally all functions of the entire brain must be irreversibly lost for an individual to be dead. Unless there is some public consensus expressed in state or federal law conveying agreement upon exactly which brain functions are insignificant, we will all be vulnerable to a slippery slope in which private practitioners choose for themselves exactly where from the top of the cerebrum to caudal end of the spinal cord to draw the line. There is no principled reason to draw it exactly between the base of the brain and the top of the spine. Better that we have a principled reason for drawing it. To me, the principle is that for human life to be present—that is, for the human to be treated as a member in full standing of the human moral community—there must be integrated functioning of mind and body. That means some version of a higher-brain-oriented formulation.

REFERENCES

1 President's Commission for the Study of Ethical Problems in Medicine and Biomedical and Behavioral Research, *Defining Death: Medical, Legal and Ethical Issues in the Definition of Death* (Washington, D.C.: U.S. Government Printing Office, 1981), p. 2. Page numbers for subsequent citations are in the text.

2 Robert M. Veatch, "The Whole-Brain-Oriented Concept of Death: An Outmoded Philosophical Formulation," *Journal of Thanatology* 3 (1975): 13–30.

3 Earl A. Walker et al., "An Appraisal of the Criteria of Cerebral Death: A Summary Statement," *JAMA* 237 (1977): 982–86, at 983.

4 James L. Bernat, "How Much of the Brain Must Die on Brain Death?" *The Journal of Clinical Ethics* 3, no. 1 (1992): 21–26, at 25.

5 Paul A. Byrne, Sean O'Reilly, and Paul M. Quay, "Brain Death: An Opposing Viewpoint," *JAMA* 242 (1979): 1985–90.

6 Cited in Robert M. Veatch, *Death, Dying, and the Biological Revolution* (New Haven: Yale University Press, 1976), p. 38.

7 Robert M. Veatch, "Whole-Brain, Neocortical, and Higher Brain Related Concepts," in *Death: Beyond Whole-Brain Criteria,* ed. Richard M. Zaner (Dordrecht, Holland: D. Reidel Publishing Company, 1988), pp. 171–86.

8 David J. Cole, "The Reversibility of Death," *Journal of Medical Ethics* 18 (1992): 26–30.

9 Alan D. Shewmon, "Caution in the Definition and Diagnosis of Infant Brain Death," in *Medical Ethics: A Guide for Health Professionals,* ed. John F. Monagle and David C. Thomasma (Rockville, Md.: Aspen Publishers, 1988), pp. 38–57.

10 Stephen Ashwal and Sanford Schneider, "Failure of Electroencephalography to Diagnose Brain Death in Comatose Patients," *Annals of Neurology* 6 (1979): 512–17.

11 Ronald B. Cranford and Harmon L. Smith, "Some Critical Distinctions between Brain Death and the Persistent Vegetative State," *Ethics in Science and Medicine* 6 (Winter 1979): 199–209; Phiroze L. Hansotia, "Persistent Vegetative State," *Archives of Neurology* 42 (1985): 1048–52.

12 Council on Scientific Affairs and Council on Ethical and Judicial Affairs, "Persistent Vegetative State

and the Decision to Withdraw or Withhold Life Support," *JAMA* 263 (1990): 426–30, at 428.

13 President's Commission for the Study of Ethical Problems in Medicine and Biomedical and Behavioral Research, *Deciding to Forego Life-Sustaining Treatment: Ethical, Medical, and Legal Issues in Treatment Decisions* (Washington, D.C.: U.S. Government Printing Office, 1983), p. 177.

14 Bernat, "How Much of the Brain Must Die on Brain Death?" pp. 21–26.

15 Veatch, *Death, Dying, and the Biological Revolution,* pp. 72–76.

Competent Adults and the Refusal of Life-Sustaining Treatment

Consent, Coercion, and Conflicts of Rights
Ruth Macklin

Ruth Macklin is professor of bioethics at Albert Einstein College of Medicine, New York. Widely published in biomedical ethics, she is the author of *Man, Mind and Morality: The Ethics of Behavior Control* (1982), *Mortal Choices: Bioethics in Today's World* (1987) and *Enemies of Patients* (1993).

Macklin focuses attention on the moral issues raised by the case of the Jehovah's Witness who desires to refuse a blood transfusion for religious reasons. In her analysis, the right to refuse blood transfusions may be defended not only by appeal to the right to exercise one's religious beliefs but also by appeal to the autonomy of the patient qua person, that is, to the individual's right to decide matters affecting his or her own life and death. In direct conflict with these rights, however, is the right of the doctor to do what correct medical practice dictates. Macklin argues that it is morally justifiable to administer blood transfusions to minor children against the religious objections of parents. It is also morally justifiable to administer blood transfusions to *incompetent* adult patients. However, she insists, the only justification for compelling a competent adult Jehovah's Witness to accept blood transfusions is a paternalistic one, and such a paternalistic intervention is morally unjustified. Still, the doctor's right to do what correct medical practice dictates must be respected. "A patient can knowingly refuse treatment, but he cannot demand mistreatment."

Cases of conflict of rights are not infrequent in law and morality. A range of cases that has gained increasing prominence recently centers around the autonomy of

Reprinted with permission of the author and the publisher from *Perspectives in Biology and Medicine,* vol. 20, no. 3 (Spring 1977), pp. 360–371. Copyright © 1977 by the University of Chicago.

persons and their right to make decisions in matters affecting their own life and death. This paper will focus on a particular case of conflict of rights: the case of Jehovah's Witnesses who refuse blood transfusions for religious reasons and the question of whether or not there exists a right to compel medical treatment. The Jehovah's Witnesses who refuse blood transfusions do not do so because they want to die: in most cases, however, they appear to believe that they will die if their blood is not transfused. Members of this sect are acting on what is generally believed to be a constitutionally guaranteed right: freedom of religion, which is said to include not only freedom of religious belief, but also the right to act on such beliefs.

This study will examine a cluster of moral issues surrounding the Jehovah's Witness case. Some pertain to minor children of Jehovah's Witness parents, while others concern adult Witnesses who refuse treatment for themselves. The focus will be on the case as a moral one rather than a legal one, although arguments employed in some of the legal cases will be invoked. This is an issue at the intersection of law and morality—one in which the courts themselves have rendered conflicting decisions and have looked to moral principles for guidance. As is usually the case in ethics, whatever the courts may have decided does not settle the moral dispute, but the arguments and issues invoked in legal disputes often mirror the ethical dimensions of the case. The conflict—in both law and morals—arises out of a religious prohibition against blood transfusions, a prohibition that rests on an interpretation of certain scriptural passages by the Jehovah's Witness sect.

THE RELIGIOUS BASIS FOR THE PROHIBITION OF BLOOD TRANSFUSIONS

The Witnesses' prohibition of blood transfusions derives from an interpretation of several Old Testament passages, chief among which is the following from Lev. 17:10–14:

> And whatsoever man there be of the house of Israel, or of the strangers that sojourn among you, that eateth any manner of blood: I will even set my face against that soul that eateth blood, and will cut him off from among his people. . . .

The question immediately arises, On what basis do the Jehovah's Witnesses construe intravenous blood transfusions as an instance of eating blood? Witnesses sometimes claim that the prohibition against transfusions arises out of a literal interpretation of the relevant biblical passages, but the interpretation in question seems anything but "literal." One explanation for this is as follows: "Since they have been prohibited by the Bible from eating blood, they steadfastly proclaim that intravenous transfusion has no bearing on the matter, as it basically makes no difference whether the blood enters by the vein or by the alimentary tract. In their widely quoted reference *Blood, Medicine, and the Law of God* they constantly refer to the medical printed matter which early in the 20th century declared that blood transfusions are nothing more than a source of nutrition by a shorter route than ordinary" [1, p. 539]. Whether based on a literal interpretation of the Bible or not, the Witnesses' prohibition against transfusions extends not only to whole blood, but also to any blood derivative, such as plasma and albumin (blood substitutes are, however, quite acceptable) [1, p. 539].

This brief account of the basis of the religious prohibition has not yet addressed the moral issues involved: but for the sake of completeness, let us note two additional features of the Jehovah's Witness view—features that bear directly on the moral conflict.

The first point concerns the Witnesses' belief about the consequences of violating the prohibition: Receiving blood transfusions is an unpardonable sin resulting in withdrawal of the opportunity to attain eternal life [2]. In particular, the transgression is punishable by being "cut off": "Since the Witnesses do not believe in eternal damnation, to be 'cut off' signifies losing one's opportunity to qualify for resurrection" [3, p. 75]. A second, related feature of the Witnesses' belief system is their view that man's life on earth is not important: "They fervently believe that they are only passing through and that the faithful who have not been corrupted nor polluted will attain eternal life in Heaven" [1, p. 539]. This belief is important in the structure of a moral argument that pits the value of preservation of life on earth against other values, for example, presumed eternal life in Heaven. Put another way, the Witnesses can argue that the duty to preserve or prolong human life is always overridden by their perceived duty to God, so in a case of conflict, duty to God dictates the right course of action.

THE ADULT JEHOVAH'S WITNESS PATIENT

Freedom to exercise one's religious beliefs is one important aspect of the moral and legal issues involved in these cases. But in addition to this specific constitutionally guaranteed right, there are other rights and moral values that would be relevant even if religious freedom were not at issue. Even in cases that do not involve religious freedom at all, the question of the right to compel medical treatment against a patient's wishes raises some knotty moral problems. The Jehovah's Witness case may prove instructive for the range of cases in which religious freedom is not at issue.

Just which rights or values are involved in the adult Jehovah's Witness case, and how do they conflict? We shall return later to the right to act on one's religious beliefs, but first let us look at other moral concepts that enter into Witnesses' moral defense. Chief among these is the notion of autonomy. Does the patient in a medical setting have the autonomy that we normally accord persons simply by virtue of their being human? Or does one's status as a *patient* deprive him of a measure of autonomy normally accorded him as a nonpatient *person?* Many medical practitioners tend to argue for decreased autonomy of patients, while some religious ethicists, a number of moral philosophers, and a small number of physicians defend autonomous decision making on the part of patients. So one clearly identifiable moral issue concerns the autonomy of a person who becomes a patient. Does he or she have the right to make decisions about the details of medical treatment and about whether some treatments are to be undertaken at all? One may defend the Witnesses' right to refuse blood transfusions by appealing to the autonomy of the patient *qua* person solely on moral grounds, without even invoking First Amendment freedoms (i.e., freedom of religion).

The right of autonomous decision making on the part of the patient is in direct conflict with a right claimed on behalf of the treating physician: the "professional" right (duty, perhaps) of a doctor to do what correct medical practice dictates. As one writer notes: "In our society, medical treatment is a right which is guaranteed to every citizen, regardless of his religious tenets. But it is also the physician's inherent, albeit uncodified, right not to have constraints applied to a therapeutic program, which he regards as necessary for the patient's welfare or survival" [3, p. 73]. Unlike other sorts of cases involving refusal of medical treatment on religious grounds (notably, Christian Scientists' refusal to accept any medical treatment), Jehovah's Witnesses are opposed only to one specific treatment regimen: transfusion of whole blood or blood fractions. As a result, Witnesses visit doctors, voluntarily enter hospitals, and submit themselves to the usual range of treatments, with the singular exception of accepting transfusions. The question arises, then, Does the physician have a duty to do everything for a patient that is dictated by accepted medical practice? In a court case in 1965 (*United States v. George,* 33 LW 2518), the court argued that "the patient voluntarily submitted himself to and insisted on medical treatment. At the same time, he sought to dictate a course of treatment to his physician which amounted to malpractice. The court held that under these circumstances, a physician cannot be required to ignore the mandates of his own conscience, even in the name of the exercise of religious freedom. A patient can knowingly refuse treatment, but he cannot demand mistreatment" [3, p. 78].

The right or duty of a physician, as described here, does seem to be in direct conflict with both (1) the religious freedom of the Jehovah's Witness patient and (2) the autonomy of the patient as a person, or his right to decide on matters affecting his own life and death. The worth of human life and the duty to preserve it are usually viewed as paramount moral values in our culture. Since those arguing in favor of the right to compel medical treatment will invoke this important value in their defense, the moral dilemma has no clear solution.

It is worth noting briefly several additional moral issues involved in the adult Jehovah's Witness case. One is the issue of informed consent. Because of the refusal of Jehovah's Witnesses to grant consent to transfuse themselves or their relatives (including minor children), physicians may not (morally or legally) act contrary to the patient's wishes. But a court order may be obtained authorizing the physician to transfuse the patient. What, then, is the status of the requirement for "informed consent" in medical matters if the patient's publicly expressed wishes can be overridden by a doctor who obtains a court order? A second relevant moral issue concerns the competency of the Jehovah's Witness patient to make the decision about transfusion at the time that decision needs to be made. Is a semicomatose person competent to make decisions? Is a person in excruciating pain competent? A person suffering from mild shock? Surely, an unconscious person is not. In this last case, and perhaps the preceding ones as well, someone other than the patient must make the decision to refuse transfusion for him. Perhaps the patient, with death as the consequence of refusing treatment, would abandon his religious tenet in favor of the desire to live. Ought a family member decide for the patient, when the patient is unable to decide for himself? There is, obviously, no easy solution to these moral dilemmas. Arguments that rest on sound moral principles can be constructed to support either view, and such arguments have been embodied in several legal cases in the past few years. We shall return to these considerations in the final section, but first we turn to the overlapping, yet somewhat different set of issues concerning minor children of Jehovah's Witnesses.

TRANSFUSING MINOR CHILDREN OF JEHOVAH'S WITNESSES

The moral principles involved in the case of minor children of Jehovah's Witnesses differ in some important respects from principles that enter into the case of adult Witnesses who refuse transfusions for themselves. It is worth noting that all legal cases in which the transfusion of minor children was at issue were decided in favor of transfusing the child, against the religious objections of the parents. In these cases, the arguments given by the courts are a mixture of citation of legal statutes and precedents and appeal to moral principles. In one case in Ohio the court argued as follows: ". . . While [parents] may, under certain circumstances, deprive [their child] of his liberty or his property, under no circumstances, with or without religious sanction, may they deprive him of his life!" [4, p. 131]. In this and other legal decisions, the religious right of the parents is seen as secondary to the right to life and health on the part of the child. . . .

It might be argued that Jehovah's Witness parents, in refusing permission for blood to be given to their child, are acting in accordance with their perceived duty to God, as dictated by their religion, and that this duty to God overrides whatever secular duties they may have to preserve the life and health of their child. Here it can only be replied that when an action done in accordance with perceived duties to God results in the likelihood of harm or death to another person (whether child or adult), then the duties to preserve life here on earth take precedence. The duties of a physician are to preserve and prolong life and to alleviate suffering. These duties are not in the least mitigated by considerations of God's will, the possibility of life after death, or a view that God at some later time rewards those who suffer here on earth. Freedom of religion does not include the right to act in a manner that will result in harm or death to others.

If the parents refuse to grant permission for blood to be given to their child when failure to give blood will result in death or severe harm to the child, their *prima facie* right to retain control over their child no longer exists. Whatever the parents' reasons for refusing to allow blood to be given, and whether the parents believe that the child will survive or not, the case sufficiently resembles that of child neglect (in respect to harm to the child): in the absence of fulfillment of their primary duties, it is morally justifiable to take control of the child away from parents and administer blood transfusions against the parents' wishes and contrary to their religious convictions.

RIGHTS AND THE CONFLICT OF RIGHTS

It is evident that the case of the adult Jehovah's Witness who refuses blood transfusions for himself is a good deal more complicated than that of minor children of Jehovah's Witness parents. The arguments—both moral and legal—in the case of children rest largely on the moral belief that no one has the right or authority to make life-threatening decisions for persons unable to make those decisions for themselves. If this analysis is sound, it supplies a principle for dealing with the case of the adult patient who is not in a position to state his wishes at the time the treatment is medically required. This principle is avowedly paternalistic but is intended to be applied in those cases where a measure of paternalism seems morally justifiable. To the extent that a person is unable or not fully competent to decide for himself at the time transfusion is needed, it seems appropriate for medical personnel to decide in favor of life-saving treatment. Whatever a person may have claimed prior to an emergency in which death is imminent, and regardless of what relatives may claim on his behalf, it is morally wrong for others to act in a manner that will probably result in his death.

The task of ascertaining a person's competence to make decisions for himself presents a myriad of problems, some of them moral, some epistemological, and some conceptual. These problems are no different, in principle, from the difficulty of ascertaining the competency of retarded persons, the mentally ill, aged senile persons, and others. This is not to suggest that no difficulty exists but, rather, that similar problems arise in many other sorts of cases where competency needs to be ascertained for moral or legal or practical reasons.

There are several recent court cases dealing with adult Jehovah's Witness patients. In some of these cases the court refused the request to transfuse the patient: in others, the court decided that transfusion was warranted, despite the religious objections. The case of *John F. Kennedy Memorial Hospital v. Heston* was one of those in which transfusion was ordered, contrary to the patient's religious convictions. But it is important to note that the patient was deemed incompetent to make the decision for herself at the time transfusion was needed. The judge who delivered the court's opinion stated:

> Delores Heston, age 22 and unmarried, was severely injured in an automobile accident. She was taken to the plaintiff hospital where it was determined that she would

expire unless operated upon for a ruptured spleen and that if operated upon she would expire unless whole blood was administered. . . . Miss Heston insists she expressed her refusal to accept blood, but the evidence indicated she was in shock on admittance to the hospital and in the judgment of the attending physicians and nurses was then or soon became disoriented and incoherent. Her mother remained adamant in her opposition to a transfusion, and signed a release of liability for the hospital and medical personnel. Miss Heston did not execute a release; presumably she could not. Her father could not be located. [5, p. 671]

This case, then, fits the principle suggested above: To the extent that a person is unable or not fully competent to decide for himself at the time transfusion is needed, it seems appropriate for medical personnel to decide in favor of life-saving treatment.

In another case, *In re Osborne,* the court decided against transfusion. But here it was ascertained that the patient was not impaired in his ability to make judgments, that he "understood the consequences of his decision, and had with full understanding executed a statement refusing the recommended transfusion and releasing the hospital from liability" [6, p. 373]. This decision might be defended, in a moral argument, by appealing to the notion of the autonomy of persons; the legal defense rests, however, on the constitutionally guaranteed freedom of religion. A footnote in the court's opinion in *Osborne* says: "No case has come to light where refusal of medical care was based on individual choice absent religious convictions." But whether based on the moral concept of autonomy, or on the legal and moral right to act on one's religious beliefs, the right of a person (whose competency has been ascertained) to refuse medical treatment must be viewed as a viable moral alternative. Such a right rests on the precept of individual liberty that protects persons of sound mind against paternalistic interference by others.

CONCLUSION

It seems apparent that the only justification that can be offered for the coercive act of administering a blood transfusion without a person's consent and against his will is a paternalistic one. I follow that characterization of paternalism put forth by Gerald Dworkin: "the interference with a person's liberty of action justified by reasons referring exclusively to the welfare, good, happiness, needs, interests or values of the person being

coerced" [7, p. 65]. Now a person's life is involved in his welfare or good in the extreme—so much so, it might be argued, that it is not on a par with other things that contribute to one's welfare. Indeed, the existence of life is a necessary condition for there being any welfare, happiness, needs, interests, or values at all. Still, interference with a person's (presumably rational) decision to end his life or allow it to end presupposes a belief on the part of the interferer that he knows what is best for the person. This would, in fact, be the case if a Jehovah's Witness patient believed that he would not die if he were not transfused in cases where informed medical opinion predicts the reverse. But the Witness who accepts the high probability of his own death and still refuses transfusion does not disagree concerning matters of empirical fact with those who wish to interfere on his behalf. Dworkin identifies this as a value conflict, a case in which "a value such as health—or indeed life— may be overridden by competing values. Thus the problem with the [Jehovah's Witness] and blood transfusions. It may be more important for him to reject 'impure substances' than to go on living" [7, p. 78]. But Dworkin is wrong if he construes this as solely a question of conflict in values, and he is also mistaken in identifying one of the competing values as rejection of "impure substances." It is, rather, eternal life over against mortal life that the Jehovah's Witness is weighing, and rather than risk being "cut off" he opts to allow his mortal life to terminate.

It would appear, then, that beliefs about metaphysical matters of fact—as well as competing values—are involved in the Jehovah's Witness's decision. That such beliefs may be mistaken or ill founded is not sufficient warrant for paternalistic interference, unless it can be shown that persons who entertain such beliefs are irrational. But it would fly in the face of longstanding traditions and practices—especially in America—to deem persons irrational solely on the basis of religious convictions that differ from our own. If, however, the Witnesses are not to be judged irrational by virtue of their religious belief system, then the one clearly acceptable ground for paternalistic intervention is pulled out from under. Medical practitioners are sometimes criticized for acting in a paternalistic manner toward patients, so it is not surprising to see physicians advocate a course of action that overrides a patient's expressed wishes. But if the patient is deemed competent or rational (by whatever practical criteria are employed or ought to be adopted), then there is no warrant for interfering with his decisions, even those that affect his continued existence. Unless all decisions to end one's life (or allow it to terminate) are viewed as *ex hypothesi* irrational, interference with a person's liberty to choose in favor of what he believes to take precedence over continued mortal existence is an act of unjustified paternalism. Paternalism may be considered justifiable in cases where the agent is incompetent to make informed or rational judgments about his own welfare. The Jehovah's Witness who refuses a blood transfusion may be *mistaken* about what is in his long-range welfare, but he is not incompetent to make judgments based on his belief system. It is only if we decide that his particular set of religious beliefs constitutes good evidence for his overall irrationality that we are justified in interfering paternalistically with his liberty. While I am personally inclined to view such religious belief systems as irrational (because they are not warranted on the evidence), I do not thereby deem their proponents irrational *in a general sense* for holding such beliefs. And this, it seems, is the correct way of looking at the case of adult Jehovah's Witnesses who are deemed mentally competent (according to the usual medical criteria) and yet who refuse blood transfusions. Only if we are prepared to accept paternalistic interference with the liberty of (otherwise) rational or competent adults in similar cases are we justified in transfusing these patients against their expressed wishes.

We cannot let the matter rest here, however, because of the problems this solution would pose for medical practice. It has been argued above that the physician has a "right not to have constraints applied to a therapeutic program, which he regards as necessary for the patient's welfare or survival"; and one court opinion stated that "a physician cannot be required to ignore the mandates of his own conscience, even in the name of the exercise of religious freedom. A patient can knowingly refuse treatment, but he cannot demand mistreatment." Jehovah's Witnesses who present themselves for treatment and who are judged rational or competent to give or withhold consent should be given the option of either (*a*) being treated in accordance with the dictates of accepted medical practice, including blood transfusion if necessary; or (*b*) refusing in advance any treatment in which transfusion is normally a necessary component or is likely to be required in the case at hand. Presenting these options to the patient preserves his decision-making autonomy while not requiring the physician to embark on a treatment that amounts to malpractice.

If it is objected that this proposed solution violates the precepts of accepted medical practice, I can only reply that those precepts embody a measure of paternalism that is unjustifiable when judged against a principle of individual liberty that mandates autonomy of decision making for rational adult persons. Moreover, the precepts of accepted medical practice have been known to change, varying with the introduction of new medical technology, transformations in social consciousness, and other alterations in the status quo. Not all patients who can be treated vigorously are so treated; one aspect of current debates focuses on the moral dilemmas surrounding patient autonomy—the sorts of problems addressed in this paper. Consistent with the decision-making autonomy accorded a patient who is deemed rational enough to offer informed consent is the right of a physician to refuse to be dictated to in matters of medical competence. Once treatment is undertaken, the judgment that a blood transfusion is necessary would seem to be a judgment requiring medical competence. The decision to undertake treatment at all in such cases is not a purely medical matter but might well be decided by a patient who has full knowledge of the consequences yet who insists nonetheless on what amounts to partial treatment or mistreatment by attending physicians.

I have argued that the autonomy of patients, as rational persons, ought to be respected. But this autonomy implies a responsibility for one's decision—a responsibility that entails acceptance of the consequences. And these consequences include the right of physicians to reject a treatment regimen proposed by the patient, which is contrary to sound medical practice. If, faced with this consequence, some Jehovah's Witnesses opt for treatment with transfusion rather than no treatment at all, so much the better for such cases of conflict of rights. Those Witnesses who remain steadfast in their refusal to accept transfusions are exercising their right of autonomous decision making in matters concerning their own welfare—in the words of Justice Louis Brandeis, "the right to be let alone." In a judicial opinion rendered in a case involving a Jehovah's Witness who refused transfusion, Justice Warren Burger recalled Brandeis's view as follows: "Nothing in [his] utterance suggests that Justice Brandeis thought an individual possessed these rights only as to *sensible* beliefs, *valid* thoughts, *reasonable* emotions, or *well-founded* sensations. I suggest he intended to include a great many foolish, unreasonable, and even absurd ideas which do not conform, such as refusing medical treatment even at great risk"[8]. The risks are indeed great in the cases we have been discussing. But the sorts of risks to health or life a person may take, in the interest of something he considers worth the risk, appear to know no bounds. If an adult agent is rational and competent to make decisions, the risks are his to take.

REFERENCES

1 I. G. Thomas, R. W. Edmark, and T. W. Jones. *Am. Surg.*, 34:538, 1968.
2 W. T. Fitts, Jr., and M. J. Orloff. *Surg. Gynecol. Obstet.*, 180:502, 1959.
3 D. C. Schechter. *Am. J. Surg.*, 116:73, 1968.

4 *In re* Clark, 185 N.E. 2d 128, 1962.
5 John F. Kennedy Memorial Hospital *v* Heston, 279 A. 2d 670, 1971.
6 *In re* Osborne, 294 A. 2d 372, 1972.
7 G. Dworkin. *Monist*, 56:64, 1972.
8 Application of President and Directors of Georgetown College, 331 F. 2n 1010 (D.C. Cir.), 1964.

Withholding and Withdrawing Life-Sustaining Treatment
Council on Ethical and Judicial Affairs, American Medical Association

In this brief excerpt from a much longer report, the AMA Council on Ethical and Judicial Affairs presents a series of clarifications related to the right of a competent patient to forgo life-sustaining treatment. In conjunction with a consideration of the traditional distinction between ordinary and extraordinary treatments, the Council rejects the idea that it is never permissible to forgo artificial nutrition and hydration. Also rejected is the view that there is an ethically significant distinction between *withholding* and *withdrawing* life-sustaining treatment.

The principle of patient autonomy requires that physicians respect a competent patient's decision to forgo any medical treatment. This principle is not altered when the likely result of withholding or withdrawing a treatment is the patient's death.[1] The right of competent patients to forgo life-sustaining treatment has been upheld in the courts (for example, *In re Brooks Estate*, 32 Ill2d 361, 205 NE2d 435 [1965]; *In re Osborne*, 294 A2d 372 [1972]) and is generally accepted by medical ethicists.[1]

Decisions that so profoundly affect a patient's well-being cannot be made independent of a patient's subjective preferences and values.[2] Many types of life-sustaining treatments are burdensome and invasive, so that the choice for the patient is not simply a choice between life and death.[3] When a patient is dying of cancer, for example, a decision may have to be made whether to use a regimen of chemotherapy that might prolong life for several additional months but also would likely be painful, nauseating, and debilitating. Similarly, when a patient is dying, there may be a choice between returning home to a natural death, or

Reprinted with permission of the AMA from "Decisions Near the End of Life," *JAMA*, vol. 267, no. 16 (April 22/29, 1992), pp. 2229–2233.

remaining in the hospital, attached to machinery, where the patient's life might be prolonged a few more days or weeks. In both cases, individuals might weigh differently the value of additional life vs the burden of additional treatment.

The withdrawing or withholding of life-sustaining treatment is not inherently contrary to the principles of beneficence and nonmaleficence. The physician is obligated only to offer sound medical treatment and to refrain from providing treatments that are detrimental, on balance, to the patient's well-being. When a physician withholds or withdraws a treatment on the request of a patient, he or she has fulfilled the obligation to offer sound treatment to the patient. The obligation to offer treatment does not include an obligation to impose treatment on an unwilling patient. In addition, the physician is not providing a harmful treatment. Withdrawing or withholding is not a treatment, but the forgoing of a treatment.

Some commentators argue that if a physician has a strong moral objection to withdrawing or withholding life-sustaining treatment, the physician may transfer the patient to another physician who is willing to comply with the patient's wishes.[1] It is true that a physician does not have to provide a treatment, such as an abortion, that is contrary to his or her moral values. However, if a physician objects to withholding or withdrawing the treatment and forces unwanted treatment on a patient, the patient's autonomy will be inappropriately violated even if it will take only a short time for the patient to be transferred to another physician.

Withdrawing or withholding some life-sustaining treatments may seem less acceptable than others. The distinction between "ordinary" vs "extraordinary" treatments has been used to differentiate ethically obligatory vs ethically optional treatments.[4] In other words, ordinary treatments must be provided, while extraordinary treatment may be withheld or withdrawn. Varying criteria have been proposed to distinguish ordinary from extraordinary treatment. Such criteria include customariness, naturalness, complexity, expense, invasiveness, and balance of likely benefits vs burdens of the particular treatment.[4,5] The ethical significance of all these criteria essentially are subsumed by the last criterion—the balance of likely benefits vs the burdens of the treatment.[4]

When a patient is competent, this balancing must ultimately be made by the patient. As stated earlier, the evaluation of whether life-sustaining treatment should be initiated, maintained, or forgone depends on the values and preferences of the patient. Therefore, treatments are not objectively ordinary or extraordinary. For example, artificial nutrition and hydration have frequently been cited as an objectively ordinary treatment which, therefore, must never be forgone. However, artificial nutrition and hydration can be very burdensome to patients. Artificial nutrition and hydration immobilize the patient to a large degree, can be extremely uncomfortable (restraints are sometimes used to prevent patients from removing nasogastric tubes), and can entail serious risks (for example, surgical risks from insertion of a gastrostomy tube and the risk of aspiration pneumonia with a nasogastric tube).

Aside from the ordinary vs extraordinary argument, the right to refuse artificial nutrition and hydration has also been contested by some because the provision of food and water has a symbolic significance as an expression of care and compassion.[6] These commentators argue that withdrawing or withholding food and water is a form of abandonment and will cause the patient to die of starvation and/or thirst. However, it is far from evident that providing nutrients through a nasogastric tube to a patient for whom it is unwanted is comparable to the typical human ways of feeding those who are hungry.[5] In addition, discomforting symptoms can be palliated so that a death that occurs after forgo-

ing artificial nutrition and/or hydration is not marked by substantial suffering.[7,8] Such care requires constant attention to the patient's needs. Therefore, when comfort care is maintained, respecting a patient's decision to forgo artificial nutrition and hydration will not constitute an abandonment of the patient, symbolic or otherwise.

There is also no ethical distinction between withdrawing and withholding life-sustaining treatment.[1,4,9] Withdrawing life support may be emotionally more difficult than withholding life support because the physician performs an action that hastens death. When life-sustaining treatment is withheld, on the other hand, death occurs because of an omission rather than an action. However, as most bioethicists now recognize, such a distinction lacks ethical significance.[1,4,9] First, the distinction is often meaningless. For example, if a physician fails to provide a tube feeding at the scheduled time, would it be a withholding or a withdrawing of treatment? Second, ethical relevance does not lie with the distinction between acts and omissions, but with other factors such as the motivation and professional obligations of the physician. For example, refusing to initiate ventilator support despite the patient's need and request because the physician has been promised a share of the patient's inheritance is clearly ethically more objectionable than stopping a ventilator for a patient who has competently decided to forgo it. Third, prohibiting the withdrawal of life support would inappropriately affect a patient's decision to initiate such treatment. If treatment cannot be stopped once it is initiated, patients and physicians may be more reluctant to begin treatment when there is a possibility that the patient may later want the treatment withdrawn.[1]

While the principle of autonomy requires that physicians respect competent patients' requests to forgo life-sustaining treatments, there are potential negative consequences of such a policy. First, deaths may occur as a result of uninformed decisions or from pain and suffering that could be relieved with measures that will not cause the patient's death. Further, subtle or overt pressures from family, physicians, or society to forgo life-sustaining treatment may render the patient's choice less than free. These pressures could revolve around beliefs that such patients' lives no longer possess social worth and are an unjustifiable drain of limited health resources.

The physician must ensure that the patient has the capacity to make medical decisions before carrying out the patient's decision to forgo (or receive) life-sustaining treatment. In particular, physicians must be aware that the patient's decision-making capacity can be diminished by a misunderstanding of the medical prognosis and options or by a treatable state of depression. It is also essential that all efforts be made to maximize the comfort and dignity of patients who are dependent on life-sustaining treatment and that patients be assured of these efforts. With such assurances, patients will be less likely to forgo life support because of suffering or anticipated suffering that could be palliated.

The potential pressures on patients to forgo life-sustaining treatments are an important concern. The Council believes that the medical profession must be vigilant against such tendencies, but that the greater policy risk is of undermining patient autonomy.

REFERENCES

1 *Deciding to Forego Life-Sustaining Treatment: A Report on the Ethical, Medical, and Legal Issues in Treatment Decisions.* Washington, DC: President's Commission for the Study of Ethical Problems in Medicine and Biomedical and Behavioral Research; 1987.

2 Brock DW. Death and dying. In: Veatch RM, ed. *Medical Ethics.* Boston, Mass: Jones & Bartlett Publishing Inc; 1989.

3 Office of Technology Assessment Task Force. *Life-Sustaining Technologies and the Elderly.* Philadelphia, Pa: Science Information Resource Center; 1988.

4 Beauchamp TL, Childress JF. *Principles of Biomedical Ethics.* 3rd ed. New York, NY: Oxford University Press; 1989.

5 Lynn J, Childress JF. Must patients always be given food and water? *Hastings Cent Rep.* October 1983:17–21.

6 Ramsey P. *The Patient as Person.* New Haven, Conn: Yale University Press; 1970:113–129.

7 Schmitz P, O'Brien M. Observations on nutrition and hydration in dying patients. In: Lynn J, ed. *By No Extraordinary Means: The Choice to Forego Life-Sustaining Food and Water.* Bloomington, Ind: Indiana University Press; 1986.

8 Billings JA. Comfort measures for the terminally ill: is dehydration painful? *J Am Geriatr Soc.* 1985;33:808–810.

9 *Guidelines on the Termination of Life-Sustaining Treatment and the Care of the Dying: A Report by the Hastings Center.* Briarcliff Manor, NY: Hastings Center; 1987.

Resuscitation Decisions, DNR Orders, and Judgments of Futility

Resuscitation Decisions for Hospitalized Patients

President's Commission for the Study of Ethical Problems in Medicine and Biomedical and Behavioral Research

A descriptive account of the President's Commission is found on page 89.

Emphasizing the importance of advance deliberation, the Commission provides an extensive analysis of ethical considerations relevant to resuscitation decisions. In the view of the Commission, patient self-determination is the most important ethical consideration. Accordingly, the decision of a competent patient should ordinarily be accepted. However, the Commission also recognizes another important ethical consideration—a patient's well-being. Will resuscitation, in the judgment of the physician, promote a patient's welfare? After rejecting the idea that it is also appropriate to consider the costs of resuscitation in arriving at resuscitation decisions, the Commission proposes an overall scheme to guide decision making, taking into account both the competent and the incompetent patient.

Reprinted from President's Commission for the Study of Ethical Problems in Medicine and Biomedical and Behavioral Research, *Deciding to Forego Life-Sustaining Treatment* (1983), chapter 7, pp. 234–236, 239–248.

Resuscitation after a cardiac arrest involves a series of steps directed toward sustaining adequate circulation of oxygenated blood to vital organs while heartbeat is restored.

Efforts typically involve the use of cardiac massage or chest compression and the delivery of oxygen under compression through an endo-tracheal tube into the lungs. An electrocardiogram is connected

> to guide the resuscitation team. . . . Various plastic tubes are usually inserted intravenously to supply medications or stimulants directly to the heart. Such medications can also be supplied by direct injection into the heart. . . . A defibrillator may be used, applying electric shock to the heart to induce contractions. A pacemaker . . . may be fed through a large blood vessel directly to the heart's surface. . . . These procedures, to be effective, must be initiated with a minimum of delay. . . . Many of the procedures are obviously highly intrusive, and some are violent in nature. The defibrillator, for example, causes violent (and painful) muscle contractions which . . . may cause fracture of vertebrae or other bones.[1]

Though initially developed for otherwise healthy persons whose heartbeat and breathing failed following surgery or near-drowning, resuscitation procedures are now used with virtually everyone who has a cardiac arrest in a hospital. The initial success rate for in-hospital resuscitation is about one in three for all victims and two in three for patients hospitalized with irregularities of heart rhythm. Among patients who are successfully resuscitated, about one in three recovers enough to be discharged from the hospital eventually. Especially when used on the general hospital population, long-term success is fairly rare. In the past decade, health care providers have begun to express concern that resuscitation is being used too frequently and sometimes on patients it harms rather than benefits.

Special Characteristics of CPR

Cardiopulmonary resuscitation of hospitalized patients has certain special features that must be taken into account in both individual and institutional decision-making:

- Cardiac arrest occurs at some point in the dying process of every person, whatever the underlying cause of death. Hence the decision whether or not to attempt resuscitation is potentially relevant for all patients.
- Without a heartbeat, a person will die within a very few minutes (that is, heartbeat and breathing will both irreversibly cease).
- Once a patient's heart has stopped, any delay in resuscitation greatly reduces the efficacy of the effort. Hence a decision about whether to resuscitate ought to be made in advance.
- Although resuscitation grants a small number of patients both survival and recovery, attempts at it usually fail; even when they reestablish heartbeat, they can cause substantial morbidity.
- Clinical signs during resuscitation efforts do not reliably predict functional recovery of a patient. Thus it is difficult to apply the sorts of adjustment and reconsideration that other interventions receive to a decision to resuscitate. Usually, the full range of efforts has to be applied until it is clear whether heartbeat can be restored.
- The conjectural nature of advance deliberations about whether or not to resuscitate may make the discussions difficult for the patient, family, and health care professionals.

Policies on Orders Not to Resuscitate

Pioneering policies on "No Code" orders ("code" being the shorthand term for the emergency summoning of a "resuscitation team" by the announcement of "Code Blue" over a hospital's public address system) or "DNR orders" (for "Do Not Resuscitate") were published by several hospitals in 1976.[2] The policies followed the recognition by professional organizations that nonresuscitation was appropriate when well-being would not be served by an attempt to reverse cardiac arrest. . . .

ETHICAL CONSIDERATIONS

The Presumption Favoring Resuscitation

Resuscitation must be instituted immediately after cardiac arrest to have the best chance of success. Because its omission or delayed application is a grievous error when it should have been used to attempt to save a life, most hospitals now provide for the rapid assembling of a team of skilled resuscitation professionals at the bedside of any patient whose heart stops.

When there has been no advance deliberation, this presumption in favor of resuscitation is justified. Although the concern a few years ago was about overtreatment, some health care professionals are now worried about unwarranted undertreatment—a weakening of the presumption in favor of resuscitation. Very different presuppositions are involved when a physician feels a need to justify resuscitating as opposed to not resuscitating someone. In either case, however, the risks of an inappropriate decision with grave consequences for a patient are great if the issues are not properly addressed according to well-developed criteria. In order to avoid using resuscitation in circumstances when it would be appropriate to omit it, advance deliberation on the subject is indicated in most cases. As in all decisions in medicine, the basic issue should be what medical interventions, if any, serve a particular patient's interests and preferences best. When a person's interests or preferences cannot be known under the circumstances, a presumption to sustain the patient's life is warranted.

The Values at Stake

In considering the relative merits of a decision to resuscitate a patient, concerns arise from each of three value considerations—self-determination, well-being, and equity.

Self-Determination Patient self-determination is especially important in decisions for or against resuscitation. Such decisions require that the value of extending life—usually for brief periods and commonly under conditions of substantial disability and suffering—be weighed against that of an earlier death. Different patients will have markedly different needs and concerns at the end of their lives; having a few more hours, days, or even weeks of life under constrained conditions can be much less important to some people than to others. In decisions concerning competent patients, therefore, first importance should be accorded to patient self-determination, and the patient's own decision should be accepted.

This great weight accorded to competent patients' self-determination means that attending physicians have a duty to ascertain patients' preferences,[3] which involves informing each patient of the possible need for CPR and of the likely consequences (both beneficial and harmful) of either employing or foregoing it if the need arises. When cardiac arrest is considered a significant possibility for a competent patient, a DNR order should be entered in the patient's hospital chart only after the patient has decided that is what he or she wants. When resuscitation is a remote prospect, however, the physician need not raise the issue unless CPR is known to be a subject of particular concern to the patient or to be against the patient's wishes. Some patients in the final stages of a terminal illness would experience needless harm in a detailed discussion of resuscitation procedures and consequences.[4] In such cases, the physician might discuss the situation in more general terms, seeking to elicit the individual's general preferences concerning "vigorous" or "extraordinary" efforts and inviting any further questions he or she may have.[5]

Well-Being A second important ethical consideration is whether resuscitation will promote a patient's welfare. A physician's assessment of "benefit" to a patient incorporates both objective facts, based on the physician's evaluation of the patient's physical status before and following resuscitation, and subjective values, in considering whether resuscitation or nonresuscitation best serves the patient's own values and goals. In virtually all cases the attending physician is in a better position to evaluate the former, while a competent patient is best able to determine the relative value of alternative outcomes.

Even though decisions about resuscitation should recognize the importance of patients' self-determination it may sometimes be necessary to question patients' choices on the grounds of protecting well-being. First, a patient may be mistaken about the course of treatment that will actually achieve the end he or she desires. Even a competent patient may initially misunderstand the nature of alternative outcomes or their relationship to his or her values because of the complexity of the alternatives, the psychological barriers to understanding information, and so forth. Dissonance between the physician's and the patient's assessments of benefit point to the need for such steps as further discussion, reexamination of the patient's decisionmaking capacity, and reassessment of the physician's understanding of patient's goals and values; indeed, in some cases patients may even wish to evaluate their values and goals.

Second, decisions may have to be based on "well-being" because "self-determination" is not possible under the circumstances. Many patients for whom a decision not to resuscitate is indicated have inadequate decisional capacity, often due to their underlying illnesses. In these cases, providers and surrogates must assess whether resuscitation—like any other medical intervention—is or is not likely to benefit the patient. Of course, physicians face many of the same difficulties in deciding that patients do, and their attempts to assess "benefit" will not always lead to clear conclusions.

Equity   The Commission has concluded previously that "society has an ethical obligation to ensure equitable access to . . . an adequate level of care without excessive burdens."[6] Should resuscitation always be considered part of the "adequate level"? Resuscitation decisions are currently made with little regard to the costs incurred or to the manner in which costs are distributed, except when competent patients decide to include such considerations as a reflection of their own concern for family well-being or for distributional justice. The Commission heard from a number of people, however, who wondered if providers and others should consider whether the costs of resuscitation are warranted for those patients for whom survival is very unlikely and who would, in any case, suffer overwhelming disabilities and diseases.

To determine whether cardiac resuscitation is a component of care that all hospitalized patients should have access to, the predicted value of this procedure would have to be compared with other medical procedures that generate comparable expenses and burdens. It is the Commission's sense that, at the moment, resuscitation efforts usually provide benefits that justify their cost, and thus resuscitation services generally should continue to be provided when desired by a patient or an appropriate surrogate. When, in a particular case, an attempt to resuscitate would clearly be against the patient's stated wishes or best interests, then the reason for not resuscitating does not arise from concerns for equitable use of societal resources, though it may incidentally help conserve them.

Of course, a more refined analysis of whether particular cases or categories of cases should be excluded under the definition of "adequate care" might be attempted. A controversial step would be to attempt to eliminate resuscitations that, while advancing a patient's interests or in accord with a patient's preferences, sustained a very marginal existence at a very high cost.[7]

However, the negative consequences of trying to discern such categories in a workable way provide strong arguments against adopting such policies. Explicitly precluding resuscitation for some categories of patients would almost certainly be insensitive to their values, denigrating to their self-esteem, and distressing to health care professionals. Also, the uncertainties over

prognosis with resuscitation for each individual patient would make it very difficult to write clear and workable categories. It is unlikely that the costs incurred by marginally beneficial resuscitation are so substantial that their reduction should be a higher priority than the reduction of other well-documented kinds of wasteful or expensive and marginally beneficial care.

GUIDANCE FOR DECISIONMAKING

Competent Patients

When a competent patient's preference about resuscitation and a physician's assessment of its probable benefits coincide, the decision should simply be in accord with that agreement (see Table 1). When a physician is unclear whether resuscitation would benefit a patient but a competent patient has a clear preference on the subject, the moral claim of autonomy supports acting in accord with the patient's preference. Self-determination also supports honoring a previously competent patient's instructions.

Some patients, although apparently competent, do not express a preference for one course over another. Such patients may not have reached a judgment in their own minds (saying, for example, merely, "whatever you think, Doc") or they may simply be unwilling to articulate a view one way or the other. Provided that the patient's unwillingness to declare a view at the moment does not reflect incompetence, the physician should not immediately ask family members to substitute their views for those of the patient, but should instead seek to involve family members in other useful ways (assuming that the patient does not object to their participation), comparable to the roles sometimes played by clergy, nurses, and other professionals. First, the family may be able to facilitate communication between the hospital staff and the patient, making sure that the issues to be addressed have been understood and helping to overcome any barriers to understanding. Second, they may be able to help the patient to make his or her preferences known to the care giving professionals. Ideally, these efforts will lead the patient to express a preference for or against resuscitation.

Of course, it is necessary to have some operative policy while a patient is being encouraged to make a choice, and patients should be informed about what that will be. Until the person expresses a clear preference, the policy in effect should be based on the physician's

TABLE 1   Resuscitation (CPR) of Competent Patients—Physician's Assessment in Relation to Patient's Preference

Physician's assessment	Patient favors CPR*	No preference	Patient opposes CPR*
CPR would benefit patient	Try CPR	Try CPR	Do not try CPR; review decision**
Benefit of CPR unclear	Try CPR	Try CPR	Do not try CPR
CPR would not benefit patient	Try CPR; review decision**	Do not try CPR	Do not try CPR

*Based on an adequate understanding of the relevant information.

**Such a conflict calls for careful reexamination by both patient and physician. If neither the physician's assessment nor the patient's preference changes, then the competent patient's decision should be honored.

assessment of benefit to the patient; when it is unclear whether an attempt at CPR would be beneficial, there should be a presumption in favor of trying resuscitation.

When physicians and patients disagree about resuscitation, further discussion is warranted. Each can explain the basis of his or her position and why the other person's judgment seems unwarranted or mistaken. In some cases, consultation with experts may be helpful to resolve doubts about the facts of the case. Together, such steps often produce agreement.

Although disagreement in no way implies that a patient is incompetent, it will often be appropriate for the physician, and perhaps consultants or an advisory committee, to reexamine this issue if discussion does not lead to agreement between patient and physician—and also for the physician to reexamine his or her own thinking and to talk with advisors about it. The serious consequences of the patient's choice—which may include severe disability if resuscitation is tried or death if it is foregone—demand that this process be carried out with care. Once the adequacy of the patient's decisionmaking capacity is confirmed, then the patient's preference should be honored on grounds of self-determination, especially since the choice touches such important subjective values.

If a physician finds the course of action preferred by a competent patient to be medically or morally unacceptable and is unwilling to participate in carrying out the choice, he or she should help the patient find another physician. Indeed, such a change should be explored even when the physician is prepared to carry out the patient's wishes despite an initial disagreement if the difference of opinion created barriers to a good relationship.

Incompetent Patients

Decisionmaking for incompetent patients parallels that for competent ones except that when a physician or surrogate decisionmaker believes that resuscitation is not likely to benefit the patient, there are some additional constraints (see Table 2). Whenever a surrogate and physician disagree, as when only one thinks that resuscitation is warranted, the case should receive careful review, initially through intrainstitutional consultation or ethics committees. Urgent situations, however, or disagreements that are not resolved in this way should go to court. During such proceedings, resuscitation should be attempted if cardiac arrest occurs.

The review entailed will vary. When a physician feels that there is no benefit, a surrogate may either concur after additional consultations or may find another physician, especially if a consulting physician disagrees with the doctor who initially attended the patient. When a surrogate opposes resuscitation that a physician feels is beneficial, discussing the reasons in an impartial setting may uncover erroneous presuppositions, misunderstandings, or self-interested motives and allow for a resolution that is in the patient's best interests. When a surrogate is ambivalent, confirmation of the expected value of resuscitation by a consultant may be persuasive; continued ambivalence may signal the need for a new surrogate. The hospital will have to be able to ensure that helpful and effective responses are provided for these various situations.

If a patient has no surrogate and orders against resuscitation are contemplated, at least a *de facto* surrogate should be designated. When the physician feels that the decision against resuscitation is quite uncontrover-

TABLE 2   Resuscitation (CPR) of Incompetent Patients—Physician's Assessment in Relation to Surrogate's Preference

Physician's assessment	Surrogate favors CPR*	No preference	Surrogate opposes CPR*
CPR would benefit patient	Try CPR	Try CPR	Try CPR until review of decision
Benefit of CPR unclear	Try CPR	Try CPR	Try CPR until review of decision
CPR would not benefit patient	Try CPR until review of decision	Try CPR until review of decision	Do not try CPR

*Based on an adequate understanding of the relevant information.

sial, a consultation with another physician, professional staff consensus, or agreement from an institutionally designated patient advocate can provide suitable confirmation of the initial judgment. Decisions like these are made commonly and should be within the scope of medical practice rather than requiring judicial proceedings. Decisions that are more complex or uncertain should occasion more formal intrainstitutional review and sometimes judicial appointment of a guardian.

Judicial Oversight

As made clear throughout this Report, the Commission believes that decisionmaking about life-sustaining care is rarely improved by resort to courts. Although physicians might want court adjudication when they believe that a patient's decision against resuscitation is clearly and substantially against his or her interests, courts are unlikely to require people to submit to such an intrusive and painful therapy unless they conclude that the patient is incompetent. Some form of review mechanism within a hospital is generally more appropriate and desirable for such disagreements. The courts are sometimes the appropriate forum for serious, intractable disagreements between a patient's surrogate and physician, however. When intrainstitutional procedures have not led to agreement in such cases, judges may well have to decide between two differing accounts of a patient's interests.

NOTES

1 *In re Dinnerstein*, 380 N.E.2d 134, 135–36 (Mass. App. 1978).
2 Mitchell T. Rabkin, Gerald Gillerman, and Nancy R. Rice, *Orders Not to Resuscitate*, 295 NEW ENG. J. MED.

364 (1976); Optimum Care for Hopelessly Ill Patients: A Report of the Critical Care Committee of the Massachusetts General Hospital, 295 NEW ENG. J. MED. 362 (1976). . . .
3 Although the attending physician bears the responsibility, often others among the care giving professionals, religious advisors, or family members are in a good or better position to discuss the issues and convey the information. This is to be encouraged, but the physician is still obliged to see that it is done well.
4 *See, e.g.,* "Such explanations to the patient, on the other hand, are thoughtless to the point of being cruel, unless the patient inquires, which he is extremely unlikely to do." Steven S. Spencer, *"Code" or "No Code": A Non Legal Opinion,* 300 NEW ENG. J. MED. 138, 139 (1979). *But see* "The physician and family often underestimate the patient's ability to handle this issue and participate in the decision." Steven H. Miles, Ronald E. Cranford, and Alvin L. Schultz, *The Do-Not-Resuscitate Order in a Teaching Hospital,* 96 ANNALS INT. MED. 660, 661 (1982).
5 "Sometimes it seems cruel and unnecessary. Other times it is just difficult, in the midst of what is usually a very emotional and difficult time, to get around to the question of whether you want us pumping on your chest when you die. . . . Having taken care of someone for some period of time has usually generated prior tacit, if not overt, understanding between the patient and me on these issues.

(Michael Van Scoy-Mosher, *An Oncologist's Case for No-Code Orders,* in A. Edward Doudera and J. Douglas Peters, eds., LEGAL AND ETHICAL ASPECTS OF TREATING CRITICALLY AND TERMINALLY ILL PATIENTS, AUPHA Press, Ann Arbor, Mich. (1982) at 16. . . .)

6 President's Commission for the Study of Ethical Problems in Medicine and Biomedical and Behavioral Research, SECURING ACCESS TO HEALTH CARE, U.S. Government Printing Office, Washington (1983) at 4.

7 Resuscitation efforts themselves commonly cost over $1000 and usually entail substantial derivative costs in caring for the surviving patients who suffer side effects.

Ethics and Communication in Do-Not-Resuscitate Orders
Tom Tomlinson and Howard Brody

A biographical sketch of Tom Tomlinson is found on page 105. A biographical sketch of Howard Brody is found on page 83.

Tomlinson and Brody emphasize the importance of distinguishing among three distinct rationales for DNR orders: (1) CPR would be futile and thus offer no medical benefit; (2) there would be an unacceptable quality of life *after* CPR; (3) there is presently—*before* CPR—an unacceptable quality of life. In their view, whereas the first rationale involves a purely medical judgment, the second and third involve judgments that are properly made by the patient or the patient's family. Also, whereas the first and second do not imply that other forms of life-prolonging treatment are inappropriate, the third does have such an implication. The authors analyze the proper purposes of physician communication with patients and families by reference to the underlying rationale of a DNR order. They also argue that failure to make clear the underlying rationale of a DNR order is a potent source of confusion among professional staff.

Despite the extensive literature devoted to do-not-resuscitate (DNR) orders, they continue to raise vexing problems for physicians, house staff, nurses, and policy makers. The difficulties include physicians' ambivalence about who should be consulted before a DNR order is written, the frustration of house officers and nurses who are asked to continue complicated or invasive treatments of a patient for whom a DNR order has been written, and hospital administrators' uncertainty and confusion over what their DNR policies should be.

Many of these problems arise from the failure to distinguish among three distinct rationales for DNR orders and to appreciate their differing implications. Although some commentators, notably Annas,[1] have insisted that different justifications for a DNR order should be explicitly distinguished, the majority view has lumped them all together uncritically:

A decision not to resuscitate is considered for a variety of reasons: a request by a patient or family; advanced age of the patient; poor prognosis; severe brain damage; extreme suffering or disability in a chronically or terminally ill patient; and in some instances, the enormous cost and personnel commitment as opposed to the low probability of patient recovery.[2]

Each of the reasons listed may be good in one circumstance or another. But this shopping-list approach hides important differences among three distinct rationales that need to be better articulated and understood.

THREE RATIONALES FOR DNR

No Medical Benefit

A commonly accepted ethical principle is that physicians have no obligation to provide, and patients and families have no right to demand, medical treatment

Reprinted with permission of the publisher from the *New England Journal of Medicine*, vol. 318, no. 1 (January 7, 1988), pp. 43–46.

that is of no demonstrable benefit.[3] Patients or families may wrongly imagine that a futile treatment would be beneficial, but this imagined benefit does not generate a right to receive treatment; otherwise, patients would be entitled to demand and receive laetrile and other quack therapies from their physicians.[4]

Although published data on survival after cardiopulmonary resuscitation (CPR) will not always be decisive in individual cases,[5,6] we believe there are circumstances when a DNR order is justified because resuscitation would almost certainly not be successful, and so would be of no benefit to the patient. This rationale for DNR orders has been discussed by Blackhall.[7]

Poor Quality of Life after CPR

A second reason for withholding CPR is that the quality of life that would result after the cardiac arrest and the subsequent CPR effort is unacceptable, even though survival might be prolonged. The life that would remain might be of little or no benefit to the patient (as with permanent loss of consciousness), or the benefits might be far outweighed by likely burdens. For example, a patient who is physically disabled after a previous arrest may still have a life whose quality is acceptable to him or his family; but it can be predicted that if he should have another arrest, he would almost certainly deteriorate further into a condition he would consider unacceptable. The crucial feature of this rationale is that the arrest, the resuscitation effort, or both threaten a change in the patient's quality of life, from one that is at least minimally acceptable to one that is unacceptable.

Poor Quality of Life before CPR

The third rationale also involves a judgment about the quality of life, but here the judgment concerns the patient's current quality of life—before any anticipated arrest and resuscitation. Although the patient may survive the resuscitation, his current quality of life is judged to be unacceptable, either to him or to his family if he is incompetent. This rationale might be applied to a patient who was severely incapacitated, mentally or physically, or who suffered intolerably from a terminal or chronic disease. The crucial difference between this and the second rationale is that the judgment here concerns the patient's current quality of life, not merely the quality of life after an arrest.

With these distinctions in hand, it becomes apparent how vague many previous recommendations have been concerning the proper use of resuscitation. An example is the maxim advocated by the National Council on Cardiopulmonary Resuscitation and Emergency Cardiac Care, and often quoted with approval: "The purpose of CPR is the prevention of sudden, unexpected death. CPR is not indicated in certain situations, such as in cases of terminal irreversible illness where death is not unexpected."[1,8] "Cases of terminal irreversible illness" do not unequivocally exemplify just one kind of rationale for DNR orders, as this principle would suggest. A terminally ill patient may reasonably be given a DNR order for any of the three reasons just described, depending on the facts of the case. There could even be cases of terminal irreversible illness in which a DNR order would *not* be justified, because the resuscitation would not be futile and the patient would judge the quality of life both before and after the arrest to be acceptable.

This last possibility suggests the ethical danger of applying a single rule for the use of CPR unambiguously to all terminally ill patients, and also the ethical importance of the distinctions we have made. In what follows, we will substantiate the claim that these are distinctions that make a difference—for the ethics of DNR decisions, for communication with patients and families, for communication among health professionals, and for hospital policies. In these discussions, we will refer to two important contrasts among the three rationales.

CONTRASTS AMONG THE THREE RATIONALES

Relevance of Patient's Values

The first important difference among the rationales concerns the relevance of the patient's or family's values to the justification for the DNR decision. When the decision is based on there being no medical benefit in resuscitation, then the value that the patient or the patient's family might place on the patient's life after an arrest is irrelevant: resuscitation would not provide any meaningful prolongation of the patient's life and so could not provide anything that the patient or his family could reasonably value. Consequently, when resuscitation offers no medical benefit, the physician can make a reasoned determination that a DNR order should be written without any knowledge of the patient's values in the matter.

The decision that CPR is unjustified because it is futile is a judgment that falls entirely within the physician's technical expertise.

By contrast, when the rationale depends on an assessment of the patient's quality of life, either before or after CPR, it requires the application of a set of values that determine whether the benefit of continued life outweighs any associated harm such as pain or disability. Since the physician's values may well differ from those of the patient or the patient's family acting as proxy, and since the patient has both a legal and a moral right to accept or refuse treatment in accordance with his or her values, the values used to make these quality-of-life determinations are properly the patient's. Therefore, the justification of a DNR order on the basis of either one of the quality-of-life rationales described above is not purely a matter for expert judgment: it requires that the decision be based on the values of the individual patient.

Generalizability to Other Treatments

The other important area of contrast among the three rationales concerns their specificity to the event of an arrest and subsequent resuscitation, and the generalizations they allow about the appropriateness of treatment options besides CPR.

Both "no medical benefit" and "poor quality of life after CPR" are rationales that limit the scope of their judgments to resuscitation. A decision that resuscitation will be futile concerns that treatment alone and does not imply futility for other life-prolonging treatments. So too, the judgment that an arrest and subsequent resuscitation would result in an unacceptable quality of life for the patient pertains to the undesirable consequences of those specific events; it implies nothing about the consequences of other life-threatening events and their related treatments.

On the other hand, a DNR order based on the unacceptable quality of a patient's current life, before an anticipated or possible arrest, does not involve a judgment tied exclusively to the arrest and to CPR. Instead, it is a judgment that death would be preferable to continued survival, because of the burdens imposed either by disease or by necessary life-prolonging treatment. Therefore, the same logic that supports the DNR order also supports the withholding or withdrawing of other life-prolonging measures, other things being equal.

These contrasts are summarized in Table 1.

TABLE 1   Contrasts among Rationales for DNR Orders

Rationale	Patient's values relevant?	Implications for other treatments?
No medical benefit	No	No
Poor quality of life after CPR	Yes	No
Poor quality of life before CPR	Yes	Yes

COMMUNICATION WITH PATIENTS AND FAMILIES

The differences we have described among the three rationales have implications for the proper purposes of communicating with patients and families about DNR decisions. They also provide a basis for evaluating some of the published research in this area.

When the absence of medical benefit is the rationale for a DNR order, communication with the patient or family should aim at securing an understanding of the decision the physician has already made. Eliciting the patient's values or involving the family in the decision is not required because the decision is based on medical expertise. Rather, the discussion should inform them of the medical realities and attempt to persuade them of the reasonableness of the DNR order. (This is not to say that the physician should callously override or ignore the wishes of a patient or family that insists on resuscitation.)

When one of the quality-of-life rationales is involved, discussions with the patient or family have a different objective. Contemplating a DNR order justified by a quality-of-life rationale, a physician needs the patient's or family's permission (as an exercise of their rights), not merely their understanding (out of concern for their welfare). In such cases, it is inappropriate for the physician to begin by trying to persuade the patient or family to agree to the DNR order. It is presumptuous for the physician to believe that a DNR order is justified before he or she has knowledge of the only set of values—the patient's—that is relevant to a quality-of-life decision.

If we are correct on these points, then the President's Commission is wrong in claiming, with regard to all resuscitation decisions, that "the great weight accorded to competent patients' self-determination means that attending physicians have a duty to ascertain patients' preferences."[8] The right of self-determination, as well as the patient's preferences, is irrelevant to the determination that resuscitation would be of no medical benefit. When this is the rationale for a DNR decision, the physician has no duty to ascertain the patient's preferences.

Charlson et al. err on the other side by suggesting that DNR decisions should be discussed only with "patients whose hospital course is characterized by a slow, progressive deterioration," because statistically such patients account for the lowest post-CPR success and survival rates.[6] But these facts support their recommendation only on the false assumption that the sole valid reason for giving a DNR order is that CPR would be of no medical benefit.

Several recent studies of doctor-patient communication in DNR decisions are unhelpful when they do not distinguish among rationales. What, for example, should be made of the study[9] that indicated that one third of the DNR orders documented no discussion with either patient or family? We don't know how many of these cases involved DNR decisions based on the lack of medical benefit. In such cases, there would be no need for discussion, since the justification for the order would not rest on information about the patient's values or preferences. Other data showing a higher rate of communication[10] cannot be applauded until we know whether the communication had the proper objectives, pursuing understanding or permission only when each was appropriate. Future empirical studies in this area need to account explicitly for the ethical differences among the three rationales.

COMMUNICATION AMONG PHYSICIANS AND STAFF

In our experience, DNR orders can be potent sources of misunderstanding, dissension, and anger among the professional staff. These problems arise at least partly from uncertainty about which of the three rationales is being applied in a particular case.

An example is the case, described by Stuart Youngner,[11] of an elderly woman who had had a series of strokes but remained mentally alert. Both she and her family requested that if she should have a cardiac arrest, no resuscitative efforts should be made. Accordingly, she was given a DNR order. When she had a cardiac arrhythmia, however, she was successfully defibrillated.

Both the patient and the family were very upset at what they considered a violation of their directive. Some physicians agreed; others did not consider the arrhythmia an arrest and so disagreed that the patient's wishes had been violated.

Youngner uses this case simply to illustrate that there can be disagreement over what constitutes a cardiac arrest. But this way of framing the problem makes the dispute seem semantic and legalistic, when it is more than that. The question of whether defibrillation fell under the scope of the DNR order is better answered by looking to the rationale behind the request of the patient and family and their physician's agreement. Was the order made because resuscitation was thought to be of no medical benefit? If so, defibrillation might not be covered under that rationale, if it were the physician's judgment that a fibrillation could be treated more successfully than another arrest mechanism, such as a complete heart block. Was the issue worry about the quality of life after an arrest? Again, it might be thought that damage after a successful resuscitation from fibrillation would be less severe than that after other forms of arrest. Only if the original order were grounded in concern for the patient's quality of life before CPR would its interpretation be unambiguous. In that case, no life-prolonging treatment for any form of cardiac arrest would be acceptable, because the life to be prolonged had been judged as unacceptable by the patient, independently of any further facts about the mechanism of the arrest or the characteristics of the resuscitation.

As this example illustrates, proper understanding or interpretation of a DNR order is impossible without knowing the rationale behind it. Unfortunately, one study reports that for almost half of DNR orders there is no written explanation or justification to serve as a guide.[9] Another study revealed that physicians writing DNR orders invariably intended the order to include other interventions besides CPR—antibiotics, blood transfusions, antiarrhythmic drugs. Nevertheless, 43 percent of the patients' charts failed to mention these other interventions.[12] Lipton found that in "60 percent of the cases physicians did not specify the intent or philosophy of the overall treatment plan subsequent to DNR designation" and that in only 35 percent of the cases was there any mention of other specific types of care to be either continued or withdrawn.[13]

In practice, clearly, the terms "DNR" or "no code" are left both ambiguous and vague. The ambiguity arises from the existence of two meanings—the explicit "no CPR" and the often inferred "no extraordinary measures." The vagueness arises under both meanings because the other treatments to be withheld, if any, can only be guessed at when the rationale for the order is missing. It is therefore not surprising that if three staff members hear that a patient has been assigned a "no code," they will each construct an idea of what the patient's true management plan is, and the three imagined plans may be radically different.

HOSPITAL POLICY

Some proposed DNR policies have tried to avoid both ambiguity and vagueness by insisting that a DNR order should have no implication for the continuation of other treatments besides CPR.[2,8] As the data show, this has simply not worked, for an obvious reason. One of the three rationales for DNR—indeed, the one that may be used most frequently—does have implications for other modes of treatment. If it does not, the DNR order is illogical or unfounded. Thus, hospital staff members who continue to believe that at least some DNR orders imply conclusions about other management options are correct, formal hospital policies notwithstanding. We therefore reject this principle as invalid for guiding hospital DNR policies.

DNR forms that simply include options for withholding other types of treatment besides CPR[12] are also inadequate. When they offer options independently of the overall rationale for the DNR order, the forms invite the automatic withholding of other treatments whenever a DNR decision is made, even when the rationale for that decision may not readily generalize to other life-prolonging treatments.

Finally, our analysis also suggests difficulties with DNR policies that combine categories of patient care with resuscitation status. A typical scheme divides patients into groups assigned to receive "full support, including CPR," "full support, excluding CPR," or "modified support, excluding CPR."[14] The trouble with such schemes is that they do not connect the use of the no-CPR categories to the rationale for the decision not to use CPR, which leads to incoherent treatment plans or unjustified generalization from the patient's no-CPR status. Thus, a patient whose no-CPR order was based on an unacceptable quality of life before CPR could be placed in the category requiring full support, excluding CPR. This would require nursing and medical staff to continue other treatments that were also unjustified, leading to the miscommunication and anger we have

mentioned. Also, a patient could be assigned to the "modified support, excluding CPR" category merely on the basis of his or her no-CPR status, when such a generalization was unjustified by the rationale for the resuscitation decision.

REFERENCES

1 Annas GJ. CPR: when the beat should stop. Hastings Cent Rep 1982; 12(5):30–1.
2 Miles SH, Cranford R, Schultz AL. The do-not-resuscitate order in a teaching hospital: considerations and a suggested policy. Ann Intern Med 1982; 96:660–4.
3 President's Commission for the Study of Ethical Problems in Medicine and Biomedical and Behavioral Research. Making health care decisions: a report on the ethical and legal implications of informed consent in the patient-practitioner relationship. Vol. 1. Washington, D.C.: Government Printing Office, 1982:43–4. (Publication no. 0-383-515/8673.)
4 Brett AS, McCullough LB. When patients request specific interventions: defining the limits of the physician's obligation. N Engl J Med 1986; 315:1347–51.
5 Bedell SE, Delbanco TL, Cook EF, Epstein FH. Survival after cardiopulmonary resuscitation in the hospital. N Engl J Med 1983; 309:569–76.
6 Charlson ME, Sax FL, MacKenzie CR, Fields SD, Braham RL, Douglas RG Jr. Resuscitation: How do we decide? A prospective study of physicians' preferences and the clinical course of hospitalized patients. JAMA 1986; 255:1316–22.
7 Blackhall LJ. Must we always use CPR? N Engl J Med 1987; 317:1281–5.
8 President's Commission for the Study of Ethical Problems in Medicine and Biomedical and Behavioral Research. Deciding to forego life-sustaining treatment. Washington, D.C.: Government Printing Office, 1983. (Publication no. 0-402-884.)
9 Youngner SJ, Lewandowski W, McClish DK, Juknialis BW, Coulton C, Bartlett ET. 'Do not resuscitate' orders: incidence and implications in a medical intensive care unit. JAMA 1985; 253:54–7.
10 Bedell SE, Pelle D, Maher PL, Cleary PD. Do-not-resuscitate orders for critically ill patients in the hospital: How are they used and what is their impact? JAMA 1986; 256:233–7.

11 Youngner SJ. Do-not-resuscitate orders: no longer secret, but still a problem. Hastings Cent Rep 1987; 17(1):24–33.

12 Uhlmann RE, Cassel CK, McDonald WJ. Some treatment-withholding implications of no-code orders in an academic hospital. Crit Care Med 1984; 12:879–81.

13 Lipton HL. Do-not-resuscitate decisions in a community hospital: incidence, implications, and outcomes. JAMA 1986; 256:1164–9.

14 Daila F, Boisaubin EV, Sears DA. Patient care categories: an approach to do-not-resuscitate decisions in a public teaching hospital. Crit Care Med 1986; 14:1066–7.

Medical Futility: A Conceptual and Ethical Analysis
Mark R. Wicclair

Mark R. Wicclair is professor of philosophy at West Virginia University. He is also adjunct professor of medicine and associate of the Center for Medical Ethics, University of Pittsburgh. Wicclair is the author of *Ethics and the Elderly* (1993). His published articles include "Patient Decision-Making Capacity and Risk" and "Preferential Treatment and Desert."

Wicclair explores some of the difficulties associated with the view that judgments of futility can provide a justification for the refusal of physicians to make certain treatments available to patients. His analysis is developed by reference to three senses of futility: (1) physiological futility; (2) futility in relation to the patient's goals; and (3) futility in relation to standards of professional integrity. In Wicclair's view, judgments of futility almost always involve a reference to evaluative standards. Thus, since he believes that the language of futility tends to communicate a false sense of scientific objectivity, he ultimately recommends that physicians not use such language in expressing their opposition to providing certain treatments.

There is a growing consensus that patients who possess decision-making capacity have an ethical and legal right to accept or refuse medical interventions, including life-sustaining treatment.[1] Advance directives enable persons to express their wishes before losing decision-making capacity, and when patients who lack decision-making capacity have not executed advance directives with unambiguous instructions, surrogates can accept or refuse medical interventions on their behalf. However, a right to accept or refuse treatments *if they are offered* by physicians does not entail a right to demand or receive treatments that physicians are unwilling to offer. In fact, there is increasing support for the position that physicians are not obligated to give patients or their surrogates an opportunity to accept or refuse *medically futile* treatments.[2]

Adapted from *Ethics and the Elderly* by Mark R. Wicclair. Copyright © 1993 by Oxford University Press, Inc. Reprinted by permission.

It might be thought that physicians are uniquely qualified to make determinations of medical futility because such judgments are based on knowledge and expertise that physicians possess and patients and surrogates lack. But is this belief correct? To answer this question, it is necessary to distinguish three senses of "futility": (1) Physiological futility: A medical intervention is futile if there is no reasonable chance that it will achieve its direct physiological (medical) objective.[3] For example, CPR is futile in this sense if there is no reasonable chance that it will succeed in restoring cardiopulmonary function; dialysis is futile if there is no reasonable chance that it will succeed in cleansing the patient's blood of toxins; and tube feeding is futile if there is no reasonable chance that it will succeed in providing the patient with life-sustaining nutrition. (2) Futility in relation to the patient's goals: A medical intervention is futile if there is no reasonable chance that it will achieve the patient's goals. For example, if the patient's goal is to survive to leave the hospital, CPR is futile in this sense if there is no reasonable chance that it will enable the patient to do so. (3) Futility in relation to standards of professional integrity: A medical intervention is futile if there is no reasonable chance that it will achieve any goals that are compatible with norms of professional integrity.[4]

1. PHYSIOLOGICAL FUTILITY

Judgments of futility in the first sense (i.e., physiological futility) appear to be based on expertise that physicians possess and patients and surrogates typically lack. Physicians have scientific and clinical expertise that enables them to ascertain the likely physiological effects of medical interventions, and most patients and surrogates lack this ability. Consequently, if anyone is capable of determining that a medical intervention (e.g., CPR, chemotherapy, or dialysis) is unlikely to have a specified physiological effect in a particular case, it is the physician and not the patient or the patient's surrogate. However, there are still two reasons for doubting that the scientific and clinical expertise of physicians uniquely qualifies them to make futility judgments in this sense.

First, although their scientific and clinical expertise enables physicians to determine whether, in relation to a particular standard of reasonableness, there is a reasonable chance that a specified physiological outcome will occur, setting the standard of reasonableness involves a value judgment that goes beyond such expertise. Suppose a 79-year-old severely demented man is hospitalized with pneumonia. He appears to be responding to intravenous antibiotics. His physician believes that it is important to decide whether CPR should be initiated in the event of a cardiopulmonary arrest. The physician's scientific and clinical expertise uniquely qualifies her to determine whether the chance of restoring cardiopulmonary function is greater than X percent. However, unless X equals zero, that expertise does not uniquely qualify her to determine whether the chance of restoring cardiopulmonary function is reasonable or worthwhile only if it is greater than X percent.

Second, although the scientific and clinical expertise of physicians enables them to determine whether a medical intervention is likely to achieve a specified outcome, determining whether a particular outcome is an appropriate objective for a medical intervention involves value judgments that go beyond that expertise. Suppose a physician concludes that it would be futile to amputate the leg of a terminally ill cancer patient because an amputation would neither prevent the spread of the cancer nor significantly reduce pain. But the patient wants an amputation because he is disgusted by the thought of having a cancerous leg. Insofar as an amputation would achieve the patient's objective of removing a source of disgust and extreme displeasure, it would not be futile to the patient. The scientific and clinical expertise of the physician uniquely qualifies her to determine whether an amputation is likely to prevent the spread of the cancer or significantly reduce pain. However, that expertise does not uniquely qualify her to evaluate the patient's goal and to determine that the amputation is futile (inappropriate) even if there is a reasonable chance of achieving the patient's goal.

If a patient or surrogate wants a medical intervention that the physician deems to be futile because she concludes that there is no reasonable chance that the intervention will achieve its direct physiological (medical) objective, the physician can attempt to justify not offering it by citing standards of professional integrity. For example, the physician can claim that it is incompatible with those norms either (1) to attempt resuscitation when there is less than an X percent chance that it will restore cardiopulmonary function or (2) to amputate a limb because it disgusts a patient. However, the physician's decision not to offer a treatment would then involve a judgment of futility in the third sense (which will be considered later).

2. FUTILITY IN RELATION TO THE PATIENT'S GOALS

A medical intervention is futile in the second sense if there is no reasonable chance that it will achieve the patient's goals. Patients and surrogates may require assistance in identifying and clarifying goals, and physicians can sometimes provide such assistance. However, ordinarily physicians are not uniquely qualified to identify a patient's goals.

Even when patients or their surrogates and physicians agree on goals, there are two possible sources of disagreement about whether a treatment is futile in relation to those goals. First, the patient or surrogate and the physician might disagree about the *probability* of achieving the patient's goals by means of the treatment. Suppose that the patient's primary goal is to survive to leave the hospital. The physician concludes that the chance of achieving this goal by means of CPR if the patient were to experience cardiac arrest is close to nil. The patient agrees that CPR would be futile if the physician were right, but the patient refuses to accept the physician's conclusion. Instead, he insists that there is a very good chance that he would survive to leave the hospital if he were to receive CPR after experiencing cardiac arrest. In such cases, the disputed judgments call for scientific and clinical expertise that physicians have and patients and surrogates typically lack. Consequently, in situations of this kind, the expertise of physicians appears to uniquely qualify them to make futility determinations.

Second, even if a patient or surrogate and the physician agree on the probability of achieving the patient's goals, they might disagree about whether the probability is high enough to warrant treatment. Whereas a physician might conclude that treatment is futile because of the low probability of achieving the patient's goals, the patient or surrogate might believe that despite the poor odds, it is still worth a try. As it is sometimes put, "there is always a chance for a miracle," and the patient or surrogate may not want to foreclose whatever slim chance there is. This disagreement between the physician and the patient or surrogate concerns the standard for determining whether the probability of achieving a specified outcome is "reasonable." To recall what was said in relation to the first sense of futility, although the scientific and clinical expertise of physicians enables them to determine whether, in relation to a particular standard of reasonableness, a chance of producing a specified outcome is reasonable, setting that standard involves a value judgment that goes beyond such expertise. Again, the physician can attempt to justify a particular standard of reasonableness by citing standards of professional integrity. However, the physician's decision to not offer treatment would then involve a judgment of futility in the third sense.

3.   FUTILITY IN RELATION TO STANDARDS OF PROFESSIONAL INTEGRITY

The reasoning underlying the claim that physicians are uniquely qualified to make determinations of futility in the third sense is as follows. Since the best treatment choice for patients is a function of their individual preferences and values, the scientific and clinical expertise of physicians ordinarily does not uniquely qualify them to make treatment decisions for patients. However, as practitioners of medicine, physicians have a special responsibility to uphold standards of professional integrity. These are standards for the medical profession, and not merely personal standards of individual

physicians. For example, performing abortions or withdrawing life support might be contrary to the personal standards of a particular physician, but she might not hold that it is improper for *any* physician to perform an abortion or withdraw life support. That is, she need not believe that it is wrong to perform such actions *as a physician.*

Among other things, standards of professional integrity identify the proper goals of medicine and the appropriate objectives and uses of medical interventions. These standards provide a basis for claiming, say, that whereas certain surgical procedures (e.g., surgically altering the size and shape of a person's nose) are properly used for cosmetic purposes, others (e.g., an amputation of a healthy leg or arm) are not.

Of more relevance to futility determinations, standards of professional integrity might provide a basis for a principle such as the following: A medical intervention is futile if the probability of achieving any appropriate treatment goal by means of that intervention is too low. Suppose a physician recommends a Do Not Resuscitate (DNR) order to a patient with widely metastasized liver cancer. The patient responds that she *wants* CPR if she suffers cardiopulmonary arrest. The physician carefully explains the burdens of CPR and states that it is futile because the patient is within a group that has less than a 1 percent chance of surviving to leave the hospital. The patient responds that any chance of extending her life, even if it will be spent in the hospital, is worthwhile to her, and clearly outweighs the burdens of CPR. The physician can still maintain that CPR is futile because resuscitative efforts would be incompatible with norms of professional integrity. In effect, the physician would be claiming that the use of CPR in this case would constitute a *misuse* of that medical procedure.

It is important to recognize that this account of futility decisions is not based on the presumed special scientific and clinical expertise of physicians. Rather, it is based on norms associated with standards of professional integrity and the alleged special responsibility of physicians to uphold those norms. The term "standards of professional integrity" is ambiguous. It can be used descriptively or prescriptively (in an evaluative sense). Descriptively, "standards of professional integrity" can refer to: (1) an individual physician's standards (i.e., the physician's conception of the proper goals of medicine, the appropriate objectives and uses of medical interventions, and so forth), or (2) customary or currently accepted standards relating to the proper goals of medicine, the appropriate objectives and uses of medical interventions, and so forth. On some questions (e.g., whether Laetrile is an appropriate treatment for cancer) there may be enough agreement among members of the medical profession to warrant referring to "customary or currently accepted standards." However, on other questions (e.g., whether tube feeding is appropriate for patients who have been in a persistent vegetative state for over a month), there may be insufficient agreement. Prescriptively, "standards of professional integrity" refers to *valid* or *legitimate* standards. Such standards are valid if and only if their content is *worthy* of being adopted and maintained by members of the medical profession.[5]

If determinations that medical interventions are futile in the third sense can justify decisions to deny patients or their surrogates an opportunity to accept or refuse treatments, it can only be when futility judgments are based on *valid* standards of professional integrity.[6] Suppose Ms. P is a 76-year-old patient with lung cancer who suffers renal failure. Her physician is Dr. Q, and dialyzing patients under these circumstances is contrary to Dr. Q's conception of the appropriate objectives and uses of dialysis. Suppose it is not contrary to valid standards of professional integrity to dialyze Ms. P. If Dr. Q offers to refer Ms. P or her surrogate to a nephrologist who would be willing to dialyze Ms. P, then Dr. Q might justifiably assert that *he* is not obligated to dialyze her. However, Dr. Q cannot justifiably claim that Ms. P or her surrogate should be denied an opportunity to accept or refuse dialysis because dialyzing Ms. P would violate *his* and/or *customary* standards of professional integrity.

CONCLUSION

It is beyond the scope of this essay to provide criteria for identifying valid standards of professional integrity. By way of a modest conclusion about determinations of medical futility, however, I will suggest the following. The statement that a medical intervention is futile communicates a sense of scientific objectivity and finality and tends to suggest that clinical data alone can decisively demonstrate that it is justified to deny patients or surrogates an opportunity to accept or refuse the treatment. However, standards of professional integrity almost always are an essential component of judgments of futility in every sense, and these standards are *evaluative*. Whereas a medical intervention may be futile in relation to one conception of the proper goals of medicine and the appropriate objectives and uses of that intervention, it may not be futile in relation to another

conception. For example, according to one conception of the proper objectives and uses of mechanical ventilation, it may be futile for patients with advanced Alzheimer's disease; and according to another conception, ventilatory support may not be futile for such patients. Similarly, according to one conception of the proper objectives and uses of CPR, resuscitative efforts can be futile if the probability of survival until discharge is less than 2 percent; and according to another conception, resuscitative efforts may not be futile in the same circumstances. A key issue, then, is whether or not the medical intervention is *appropriate* from the perspective of valid standards of professional integrity.

Since the term "futility" tends to communicate a false sense of scientific objectivity and finality and to obscure the evaluative nature of the corresponding judgments, it is recommended that physicians avoid using the term to justify not offering medical interventions. Instead of saying, "life-extending treatment is not an option because it is futile," it is recommended that physicians explain the specific grounds for concluding that life-support generally, or a particular life-sustaining measure, is inappropriate in the circumstances. Whereas the statement that life-sustaining treatment is futile tends to discourage discussion, explaining the grounds for concluding that (some or all) life-extending interventions are inappropriate in the circumstances tends to invite discussion and point it in the right direction.

NOTES

1 See Alan Meisel, "The Legal Consensus About Forgoing Life-Sustaining Treatment: Its Status and Prospects," *Kennedy Institute of Ethics Journal,* Vol. 2, No. 4 (December 1992), pp. 309–45.

2 See, for example, Tom Tomlinson and Howard Brody, "Futility and the Ethics of Resuscitation," *Journal of the American Medical Association,* Vol. 264, No. 10 (Sept. 12, 1990), pp. 1276–1280; Lawrence J. Schneiderman, Nancy S. Jecker, and Albert R. Jonsen, "Medical Futility: Its Meaning and Ethical Implications," *Annals of Internal Medicine,* Vol. 112, No. 12 (June 15, 1990), pp. 949–954; and Steven H. Miles, "Medical Futility," *Law, Medicine & Health Care,* Vol. 20, No. 4 (Winter 1992), pp. 310–15.

3 This sense of futility might be further identified as *"specific* physiological futility" to distinguish it from *"general* physiological futility." A medical intervention is futile in the latter sense if there is no reasonable

chance that it will have *any* physiological effect. However, it is rarely, if ever, the case that a medical intervention is unlikely to have *any* physiological effect. For example, although a blood transfusion or chemotherapy may not extend a patient's life, each is likely to produce some physiological changes (e.g., an alteration in blood count).

4 See Tomlinson and Brody, "Futility and the Ethics of Resuscitation."

5 Alternatively, validity can be understood as a *procedural* concept. For example, it might be said standards are valid if: (1) they were adopted through a fair democratic process open to physicians and the general public, or (2) they would be adopted if such a process were followed.

6 Even if physicians are not obligated to *offer* medically futile treatments to patients or their surrogates, it may still be appropriate to *discuss* treatment goals and plans with patients or their surrogates before implementing a decision to forgo such treatments. As Youngner puts it, "Don't offer, perhaps, but please discuss." Stuart J. Youngner, "Futility in Context," *Journal of the American Medical Association*, Vol. 264, No. 10 (Sept. 12, 1990), p. 1296.

Advance Directives and Treatment Decisions for Incompetent Adults

Surrogate Decision Making for Incompetent Adults: An Ethical Framework
Dan W. Brock

A biographical sketch of Dan W. Brock is found on page 100.

Brock briefly considers the problem of determining when an adult patient is incompetent to make a particular treatment decision. He also addresses the problem of selecting an appropriate surrogate for such a patient, paying particular attention to the sense behind the presumption that a close family member is ordinarily the most appropriate surrogate. In considering the standards that a surrogate is expected to follow in making a decision for an incompetent patient, Brock specifies a set of three principles, arranged in order of priority: (1) the advance directive principle, (2) the substituted judgment principle, and (3) the best interests principle.

My role in this discussion is to add a philosphical perspective to the consideration of surrogate decision making. In the medical ethics literature a substantial, though not universal, consensus has developed that health care decision making should be shared between the physician and the competent patient. Typically, in medical practice, the physician brings his or her knowledge, training, expertise, and experience to the diagnosis of the patient's condition and provides the prognoses associated with different treatment alternatives, including the alternative of no treatment. The patient brings his or her own aims and values to the decision-making process and ideally evaluates the alternatives, with their particular mixes of benefits and risks (1).

What values underlie a commitment to shared decision making, and what ends are we seeking to promote with it? The first, and most obvious, is the promotion and protection of the patient's well-being. Shared decision making rests in part on the presumption that competent patients who have been suitably informed by their physicians about the treatment choice they face are generally, though of course not always, the best judges of what treatment will most promote their overall well-being (2). The other value is respecting the patient's self-determination. I mean by self-determination the interest of ordinary persons in making significant deci-

Reprinted with permission of the author and the publisher from *The Mount Sinai Journal of Medicine*, vol. 58, no. 5 (1991), pp. 388–392.

sions about their own lives themselves and according to their own values. It is by exercising self-determination that we have significant control over our lives and take responsibility for our lives and the kind of person we become. These then are the values that guide shared decision making.

For incompetent patients we still want shared decision making, but then the patient lacks the capacity to participate and a surrogate must take the patient's place. My aim in this paper is, therefore, to sketch an ethical framework for surrogate decision making about medical treatment for incompetent adults and for thinking about the ethical issues that arise in that decision making (3). Surrogate decision making should seek to extend the ideals of health care decision making for competent adults, with suitable changes required by and reflecting the patient's incompetence. Before considering who should be a surrogate and how the surrogate should decide, we must consider which patients should have a surrogate to decide for them.

DETERMINING INCOMPETENCE

In health care, if the patient is competent, the patient is entitled to decide and to give or refuse informed consent to treatment. If the patient is incompetent, a surrogate must be selected to decide for the patient. The concept, standards, and determination of competence are complex; and there is space here to emphasize only a few important points about competence and incompetence (see especially 3, ch. 1). Adults are presumed to be competent unless and until found to be incompetent. In questionable or borderline cases, competence should be understood as decision-relative, that is, a patient may be competent to make one decision but not another. First, decisions can vary in the demands they make on a patient, for example, in the complexity of the information relevant to the choice. Second, from the effects of medications, disease, and other factors, patients can change over time in the capacities they bring to the decision-making process.

Three distinct capacities are needed for competence in treatment decision making: the capacity for understanding and communication; the capacity for reasoning and deliberation; the capacity to have and apply a set of values or conception of one's good. Though people possess these capacities in different degrees, it is important to recognize that the determination of competence is not a comparative judgment. Because the competence determination in health care (and in the law) is used to sort the patient into either the class of patients who are competent to decide for themselves or into the class of patients who must have a surrogate to decide for them, it must be recognized as a threshold determination. The crucial question about competence in borderline cases then is how defective or impaired a person's decision making must be to warrant a determination of incompetence.

Two central values are at stake when a patient is judged competent or incompetent, and so two kinds of dangers should be balanced in that determination. One value is protecting the patient from the harmful consequences of his or her choice when the patient's decision making is seriously impaired. The other value is respecting the patient's interest in deciding for him or herself. The dangers to be considered are failing adequately to protect the patient from the harmful consequences of a seriously impaired choice, which must be balanced against failing to permit the patient to decide for him or herself when sufficiently able to do so. There is no unique objectively correct balancing of these two values and dangers. Instead, the proper balancing is inherently an ethically controversial choice.

Process as the Standard The evaluation of a patient's competence should address and evaluate the *process* of the patient's decision making; the standard should not be an outcome standard that simply looks to the content of the patient's choice. Given the values at stake in the competence determination, it follows that the standard for competence should vary according to the consequences for the patient's well-being of accepting his or her choice. The standard should vary along a continuum from high (when the choice appears to be seriously in conflict with the patient's well-being) to moderate (when the patient's choice appears to be comparable to other alternatives in its effect on the patient's well-being) to low (when the choice will clearly best serve the patient's well-being).

One controversial consequence of this account of the competence determination is that a patient might be competent to consent to a particular treatment, but not to refuse it, and vice versa. This follows from two facts. First, the process of reasoning to be evaluated will inevitably be different if it leads to a different choice. Second, the effects on one of the values to be balanced (the patient's well-being—if the patient's choice is accepted) can be radically different depending on whether the patient has consented to or refused the recommended treatment. Treatment refusal may reasonably trigger an evaluation of the patient's competence, though it should also trigger a revaluation by the physician both of the treatment recommendation and of the communication of that recommendation to the patient; some studies have shown that the most common cause of treatment refusals is failure of communication between physician and patient, and most refusals are consequently withdrawn when the recommendation is better explained (4).

The critical question to answer is, Does the patient's choice sufficiently accord with the patient's own underlying and enduring aims and values for it to be accepted and honored, even if others, including the physician, may think it not the best choice?

SELECTING A SURROGATE

Assume now that a patient has been found incompetent to make a particular treatment choice, so that a surrogate must act for the patient. Who should serve as surrogate? What standards should guide the surrogate's decision? If we are to respect the incompetent patient's wishes, then the surrogate should be the person the patient would have wanted to act as surrogate. In a number of states, by executing a Durable Power of Attorney for Health Care (DPOA), it is possible for a person, while competent, to legally designate a surrogate who will make health care decisions in the event of later incompetence. This document also allows a person to give instructions to the surrogate about one's wishes concerning treatment. Ethically, an oral designation by a person of a surrogate should have nearly the same weight as a formal DPOA. Competent patients should be encouraged to designate who will decide for them in the case of later incompetence. In fact, physicians have a responsibility to seek this information early in treatment and while patients are still competent, especially if a period of later incompetence is likely.

Often an incompetent patient will not have explicitly designated a surrogate. It is then reasonable and common to act on a presumption that a patient's close family member is the appropriate surrogate. (In most jurisdictions, a close family member lacks explicit legal authority to act as the patient's surrogate until formally appointed by a court as the guardian. States should consider adopting legislation like the recently enacted Health Care Decisions Act in the District of Columbia which formally authorizes a family member to act as surrogate for an incompetent patient without recourse to guardianship proceedings.) Only the most important considerations that support this presumption for a fam-

ily member acting as surrogate can be discussed here. First, usually a family member will be the person the patient would have wanted to act as surrogate for him or her. Second, the family member will know the patient best and will be most concerned for the patient's welfare. It is important to underline that the claim is only that the *practice* of using a close family member as surrogate will result overall in better decisions for patients than any feasible alternative practice, such as appointing an attorney to act as the patient's guardian. Third, in our society the family is the central social and moral unit assigned responsibilities to care for its dependent members. Although dependent children are the most obvious example, dependent adults are another important instance of this responsibility. The family is also the main place in which most people pursue and realize the values of intimacy and privacy. Both to fulfill these responsibilities and to realize these values, the family must be accorded significant, though not unlimited, freedom from external oversight, intrusion, and control.

These grounds for presuming a close family member to be an incompetent patient's surrogate do not imply that such a surrogate must always make the optimal choice. On the other hand they also make it clear that family members' authority as surrogate decision makers is limited. When the grounds do not hold—for example, when there is no close relation between patient and family member, or when there is a clear conflict of interest between patient and family member—the presumption for family members as surrogates can be rebutted. In such cases, an incompetent patient's physician can have a positive responsibility not to allow the family member to act as surrogate.

Sometimes no family member is available to serve as surrogate. Most reasons that support a family member serving as surrogate will then also support using a close friend who is available and willing to serve. When no family member or friend is available, institutional flexibility is desirable because of the wide range of different decisions that must be made. Institutions only need a settled and public policy insuring that decision making in such cases does not become paralyzed from lack of a natural surrogate. For example, a hospital might have a policy for a specified range of decisions (such as decisions to forgo life-sustaining treatment or resuscitation) requiring that the attending physician's proposed decision be referred to the chief of service who could review the decision and take any further steps deemed appropriate (perhaps referral to an ethics committee or to the courts).

HOW SURROGATES SHOULD DECIDE

Advance Directives   What standards should a surrogate employ in deciding for an incompetent patient? Three ordered principles can guide decision making: advance directive; substituted judgment; best interest. These are ordered principles in the sense that the surrogate should employ the first if possible; if not it, then the second if possible; and if neither the first or second can be used, then the third.

The advance directive principle tells the surrogate that if there is a valid advance directive from the patient, there is a strong presumption that it should be followed. Formal advance directives take two principal forms, living wills and durable powers of attorney for health care. Living wills are given legal force in approximately 40 states; DPOAs at present have legal force in far fewer jurisdictions.

Several common features limit the usefulness of living wills. I shall mention two. First, they are usually formulated in vague terms for describing both the patient conditions ("terminally ill") and the treatments ("extraordinary measures," "aggressive treatment"). Because they are executed well in advance of the decision to be made, this is to some extent inevitable and means that others must interpret how they should now apply. Second, probably in response to worries about potential abuses, enabling statutes in many states place limitations on the circumstances in which living wills can either be executed (for example, the person must already have been diagnosed as terminally ill with death imminent) or applied (for example, the decision cannot cover nutrition and hydration). When persons follow these restrictions and limitations, in many circumstances their living wills will fail to apply. Since living wills are rarely brought into court for enforcement, but function primarily as a means of informing others about the patient's wishes, restrictive formulations may be inadvisable.

Except for those who have no surrogate, DPOAs are the more desirable form of advance directive for most persons. First, they allow a person to give more detailed instructions to the surrogate about wishes regarding treatment, though it is important to avoid letting greater detail narrow the application of the instructions. Second, they address the issue of later interpreting the patient's instructions by allowing the patient to designate the interpreter.

Although there is a strong presumption that a valid advance directive should be followed, there are reasons why advance directives should not have the same degree of binding force as the contemporaneous decision of a competent patient. The decision of a competent patient can be made attending to the full and detailed context, whereas advance directives must inevitably be formulated before the precise context of future decisions is known. This means that occasionally a treatment decision will arise in circumstances radically different from those imagined by the patient when executing the advance directive; in such cases, following the letter of the directive may be contrary to following its spirit. Moreover, concern over whether the patient would have changed his or her mind about treatment does not arise for a competent patient. Finally, a decision by a competent patient that appears significantly contrary to his or her interests usually will be challenged by the care givers, thereby testing understanding and resolve to an extent not possible with advance directives. Despite these limitations, there are good reasons to accord a strong presumption to any patient's advance directive.

Substituted Judgment   At present, and probably for the forseeable future, most patients do not have advance directives. Then the substituted judgment principle should be followed. This principle tells the surrogate to attempt to decide as the patient would have decided, if competent, in the circumstances that now obtain. In effect, the principle directs the surrogate to use his or her knowledge of the patient and the patient's aims and values to infer what the patient's choice would have been.

Physicians have an important responsibility in helping surrogates to understand their role in applying substituted judgment. Rather than asking, "What do you now want us to do for your mother?" the physician should say, "You, of course, knew your mother better than I did, so help us decide together what she would have wanted done for her now." Confirmation that asking the right question matters in the choices surrogates make can be found in Tomlinson (5). This substituted judgment approach is helpful for arriving at decisions which are more in accordance with the patient's wishes. The approach also has the practical advantage of making the psychological and emotional burdens easier for surrogates to carry and facilitating their effective participation in decision making.

"Do everything" is nearly always an inadequate and unhelpful answer. Surrogates should be assured that appropriate care will always be given, including all care needed to maintain the patient's comfort and dignity. But what care is appropriate will often change with changes in the patient's condition and prognosis, and surrogates must be helped to understand that all possible care is not automatically appropriate care.

Two features of substituted-judgment decision making should be explicitly noted. First, the substituted-judgment model will let surrogates take account of how the interests of others will be affected by the decision, to the extent there is evidence that the patient would have weighed those interests. Second, it will allow surrogates to assess the patient's quality of life, both at present and as it will be affected by treatment decisions, according to the patient's own values. For consideration of forgoing life-sustaining treatment only a limited judgment of quality of life is relevant: Is the best anticipated quality of life with life-sustaining treatment sufficiently poor that the patient would have judged it to be worse than no further life at all? No judgments about social worth or the social value of the patient are warranted under substituted judgment.

Best Interest When no information is available about what this particular patient would have wanted in the situation at hand, the "best interests" principle directs the surrogate to select the alternative that furthers the patient's best interests. This, in effect, amounts to asking how most reasonable persons would decide in these circumstances, an approach which is justified by the absence of any information about how this patient differs from others. Treatment choices based on best interests can be especially difficult when reasonable persons can and do disagree about the choice. It is, therefore, important, where possible, to avoid having to appeal to best interests by determining patients' wishes about future treatment options when patients are still competent.

Ordering These Three Principles Strict ordering of these guidance principles would be an oversimplification. Evidence bearing on the patient's wishes concerning the decision at hand, whether from an advance directive or from the surrogate's knowledge of the patient, is not either fully determinate and decisive on the one hand, or completely absent on the other. Instead, such evidence ranges along a broad continuum in how strongly it supports a particular choice. In all cases physicians and surrogates should seek confidence that the choice made is reasonably in accord with the patient's wishes or interests. The better the evidence about what this particular patient would have wanted, the more one can rely on it. The less the information and evidence about what this patient would have wanted, the more others must reason in terms of what most persons would want.

What constitutes adequate evidence about the patient's wishes has been an issue in several recent court cases, most notably the O'Connor case in New York and the Cruzan case in Missouri, recently upheld by the U.S. Supreme Court (6). In the New York case the court imposed an extremely high standard of evidence for forgoing life-sustaining treatment by surrogate order, requiring clear and convincing proof that the patient had made a settled commitment, while competent, to reject the particular form of treatment under circumstances such as those now obtaining. Where there is any significant doubt, the court reasoned, the decision must be on the side of preserving life. This decision set a very difficult standard in New York for patients and their surrogates to satisfy, and thereby establishes a strong presumption in favor of extending the lives of incompetent patients with life-sustaining treatment. In Cruzan, the U.S. Supreme Court upheld the right of the State of Missouri to impose this same strong presumption, though without endorsing the wisdom of doing so.

Such a presumption undervalues patients' interest in self-determination and fails to recognize adequately the extent to which patients' well-being is determined by their own aims and values. But is it not reasonable, the Court might ask, always to err on the side of preserving life when there is any doubt about the patient's wishes? Several decades ago, when medicine only rarely had the capacity to extend life in circumstances where doing so would have been unwanted and no benefit to patients, such a policy would have been reasonable. Medicine, however, has vastly enlarged its capacities to extend life. Patients' lives can now often be extended when they would not want this done, and, as a result, New York's and Missouri's strong presumption in favor of extending life, when there is any significant doubt about the patient's wishes, can no longer be justified. Though the U.S. Supreme Court found no constitutional bar to the clear and convincing evidence standard, good reasons remain for other states not to adopt it.

CONCLUSION

I want to conclude with a plea for "preventive ethics" aimed at reducing the necessity to resort to surrogate decision making. This can only be accomplished by persons, while still competent, talking with their physicians and families about their treatment wishes should they become seriously ill. Such preventive measures are especially appropriate for persons with chronic, progressive diseases in which both a possible period of incompetence and the nature of later treatment decisions likely to arise are relatively predictable. Physicians have an important role in encouraging their patients to reflect on their wishes and to make those wishes known to those who are likely to be involved in their treatment decisions. The need for surrogate decision making in health care will never be eliminated, nor can all difficult decisions be avoided. But it should be possible greatly to reduce the number of cases in which physicians and surrogates must decide about an incompetent patient's care in the absence of knowledge of the patient's wishes when that information could have been obtained earlier had it been sought.

REFERENCES

1 Some respects in which this division of labor is oversimplified are explored in Brock DW. Facts and values in the physician/patient relationship. In: Veatch R, Pellegrino E, eds. Ethics, trust, and the professions. Washington, DC: Georgetown University Press, 1991.

2 For a discussion of different kinds of cases in which competent patients make irrational choices, and the responsibilities of their physicians in such circumstances, see Brock DW, Wartman SA. When competent patients make irrational choices. N Engl J Med 1990; 322 (May 31):1595–1599.

3 I draw freely here on prior published work I have done on this topic, some of it collaborative work with Allen Buchanan. See especially Buchanan AE, Brock DW. Deciding for others: the ethics of surrogate decision-making. Cambridge, England: Cambridge University Press, 1989.

4 Applebaum PS, Roth LS. Treatment refusal in the medical hospital. In: President's Commission for the Study of Ethical Problems in Medicine and Biomedical and Behavioral Research. Making health care decisions: the ethical and legal implications of informed consent in the patient-practitioner relationship, vol. 2 Appendices. Washington DC: U.S. Government Printing Office, 1982.

5 Tom Tomlinson, et al. An empirical study of proxy consent for elderly persons. Gerontologist 1990; 30(1):54–60.

6 In re O'Connor, No. 312 (NY Court of Appeals, October 14, 1988); Cruzan v. Director, Missouri Department of Health, 110 Sct 2841 (1990).

Why I Don't Have a Living Will
Joanne Lynn

Joanne Lynn is presently professor of medicine and of community and family medicine, Center for Evaluative Clinical Sciences, Dartmouth Medical School. She has also served as assistant director on the staff of the President's Commission for the Study of Ethical Problems in Medicine and Biomedical and Behavioral Research, and she is the editor of *By No Extraordinary Means* (1986). Lynn's many articles in biomedical ethics include "Procedures for Making Medical Decisions for Incompetent Adults."

Lynn articulates a wide range of concerns and problems related to the employment of living wills. She is especially critical of "standard form" living wills, but some of her arguments are directed against more sophisticated living wills as well. Lynn points out that there are two groups of patients who are fundamentally unsympathetic to the construction of advance directives. In the first group are patients who are uneasy with the very idea that their choices could have an impact on the length of their lives. In the second group (which includes Lynn herself) are patients who simply prefer to entrust future decision making to family or community.

Reprinted with permission of the author and the American Society of Law, Medicine & Ethics from *Law, Medicine & Health Care*, vol. 19, nos. 1–2 (1991), pp. 101–104.

Lynn concludes by acknowledging that there are "four good uses for formal advance directives." (1) In some cases, a person is clearly well served by executing a durable power of attorney for health care. (2) Formal advance directives can effectively function to document unusual or very specific preferences. (3) They can sometimes function to alleviate patient and family anxieties. (4) The task of preparing a formal advance directive is sometimes a natural focal point for organizing a discussion of the patient's priorities and preferences.

For a dozen years, my clinical practice has been largely with dying patients, my academic pursuits have focused on medical ethics, and my public service has been mostly at the interface of medicine and law. One would think that I would have "done the right thing" long ago and signed a living will. I have not. This essay is meant to illuminate my reasons. Some of my reasons may apply to others, and I will also mention some concerns that affect others but not me. However, I do not oppose the growth and development of advance directives. Rather, I hope to open the public and professional discussion of how to make decisions for incompetent adults in order to include more varieties of formal and informal advance directives and to force policy-makers to consider how to make decisions for incompetent adults who have no advance directives.

As a physician, I do use advance directives, both formal and informal, with many patients in all of my clinical settings. I have supported the Patient Self-Determination Act[1] and the distribution of living wills by Concern for Dying, and I have pushed for health care durable power of attorney legislation in my local jurisdictions. My endorsement of and enthusiasm for advance directives might well lead some to think that I am merely extraordinarily inefficient and imprudent in regard to my own affairs when they discover that I do not have a living will. While I may have these flaws of character, this particular behavior is not evidence for them.

I do not have a living will because I fear that the effects of having one would be worse, in my situation, than not having one. How could this be? A living will of the standard format attends to priorities that are not my own, addresses procedures rather than outcomes, and requires substantial interpretation without guaranteeing a reliable interpreter. Of course, a highly individualized formal advance directive might be able to escape these concerns, as is addressed below. First, however, I will consider the merits of a "standard" living will, such as is available in stationery stores and through the mail.

On its face, a "living will" purports to instruct care-givers to provide no life-sustaining treatment if the person signing it ever were on the verge of dying, with or without treatment, and were unable to make decisions for himself or herself. On the one hand, this is hardly a surprising instruction. Some combination of short life, interminable personal suffering, and adverse effects upon others is enough that virtually all persons would prefer to have had the opportunity to avoid this outcome, even at the cost of an earlier death. I have seen enough suffering that I can readily list all manner of existences that would induce me to accept death rather than have medical treatment to extend life. Not just in my case but in most cases, the text of a living will in standard format rarely tells the physician anything that was not nearly as likely to be true without it. The fact that a person took the time and trouble to sign one and get it to the physician does imply something about that person's character and the seriousness with which he or she approaches these issues, but not much about the individual's preferences and priorities.

As a physician, I use the fact that a person presents a standard-format living will as an opportunity to explore what he or she really means to avoid, what is really feared and hoped for, and who would be trusted to make decisions. This use is exceedingly valuable, but requires no legal standing for the document and does not require that it be treated as the definitive statement of what should be done.

However, many persons believe that they accomplish some very different ends by signing a living will. They believe they keep themselves from ever ending up like Nancy Cruzan or Karen Quinlan, or like a family member who had a particularly gruesome end of life in an intensive care unit. That belief is wrong. The public use of the standard living will is largely premised on an implicit promise that the document cannot ensure. Standard form living wills *should* have virtually no impact upon the care of persistent vegetative state patients, persons receiving vigorous therapy for potentially reversible physiologic imbalance, or persons with no clearly progressive and irreversible course toward imminent death, for none of these people clearly meet the requirement of dying soon irrespective of treatment. When people feel, as they commonly seem to, that having signed a living will serves to ensure that they will avoid medical torment of all sorts, they are misconstruing the document.

Nevertheless, sometimes living wills do have an impact upon the care plan of all sorts of patients because physicians and other providers inattentively overgeneralize. All too commonly, someone who has a living will is assumed to have requested hospice-type care including a "Do not resuscitate" order, to prefer not to use intensive care, and to have refused curative treatments. This assumption can obviously shape the care plan without there being explicit confirmatory discussion with patient or surrogate. Thus, the living will can also lead to errors of undertreatment.

The standard form living will is thoroughly disappointing as a legal document. It does not reliably shape the care plan as intended and carries risks of affecting the care plan adversely. Unless it is used as a trigger for further communication, it has little justification. As a patient, I do not believe I will need to have that trigger.

The "standard-form" living will may be an unfair target for my critique, as there have been many efforts made to personalize and expand living wills,[2] especially by incorporating the designation of a proxy (which has conventionally been perceived as part of the durable power of attorney). While some of these are quite good, all entail some serious remaining difficulties that would preclude my using them and that should occasion some care in their use by others.

For example, a living will entails a construction of reality that identifies, at any one time, a group of persons who are "dying." The rest of us, in this conception, are not. Only if one is among the dying is the living will in effect. I cannot accept this construction of reality. Working with persons with advanced years, advanced cancer, and advanced AIDS has illuminated the hubris of this cultural view. Classifying some persons as "dying" does function to protect people, most of their lives, against recognizing that there is a death in store for each of us. The boundary between being merely mortal (like all humans) and being in the "dying" category is a boundary that people want desperately to find (and to find themselves in the "non-dying" group).

However, the schism simply does not exist. We all are dying. As the likely time of death comes closer, some issues tend to be more important, but there is no clear dividing line. Sometimes persons far from death are mainly concerned with comfort or spiritual concerns; sometimes persons facing death in the next few hours are still completing business deals. Pretending that there is a morally important demarcation between the merely mortal and the dying leads to harmful policies and practices generally. One stunning example is the societal support for hospice through Medicare which serves mostly relatively well-off cancer patients with homes, in contrast with the societal denial of adequate support for long term care for those who are severely disabled and alone.

Also, the way that living wills have generally come to be constructed has focused attention on the patient's status (dying soon no matter what is done) and the procedures to be forgone (those that are artificial and "only" serve to prolong dying, sometimes expressed as a list of medical procedures). These two attributes of the standard living will subtly distort good decision-making. Good decision-making rests primarily in pursuing the best possible future, from among those plans of care that can be effectuated, and with the "best possible" being defined from the patient's perspective to the extent possible. Nothing in this model needs to turn on the proximity to death or the nature of the procedure involved, except as these considerations shape the desirability of various future courses to the patient. Sometimes ventilators are morally required, but sometimes even changing the sheets is contraindicated. For someone to be asked to decide in advance whether he or she would want dialysis, ventilator, or feeding tubes, without knowing what using these procedures would yield, is incomprehensible.

In addition, the issues that have become conventional to deal with in extended-version living wills are but a frail reflection of the concerns that very sick patients actually express. In fact, some of their real concerns have almost completely lost a place in the discussion of any kind of formal advance directives. Many patients are concerned about the emotional, physical, and financial burdens that their prolonged existence might entail for family. So often one hears, with real sincerity, "I don't want to be a burden," and so often we fail to have the ability, within this culture, to acknowledge and explore that sentiment. Perhaps, if we all learned how to carry on the discussions, many persons would be found to be more concerned about the issues around imposing burdens on others than are concerned about the ignominy of persistent vegetative state or the torment of long-term ventilator use. Certainly, I would. However, this we do not talk about and we do not include in conventional advance directives.

Many people may also have a high preference for

being able to choose a course of care that will never look foolish. Many persons seem to be more concerned to do the conventional thing, to be supported by friends and family as having "done his best," and never to have to feel that one bears much of the responsibility for the outcomes that one must endure. For example, I accepted a widely-used protocol for the treatment of a family member's illness, even though I knew that there was no data to support using some of the particularly onerous components of the protocol. The reason was largely because refusing those components would leave me bearing the responsibility for any adverse outcome. Even a maximally creative living will is likely to have difficulty expressing this particular sentiment; the formal prose itself tends to make the author look silly.

A number of factors that are known to affect decision-making are not regularly given voice through living wills. How is a person to write a living will that would ask for his family to seek divine guidance in prayer, or to ensure that her death is as dramatic and public as the rest of her life has been? Certainly, doing so would be difficult with any form that I have seen. In fact, much of what people ordinarily take to be important in their other choices is shunned in the conventional living will and the process of writing it. There is little passion or pathos, only the clean, sterile, black and white of choices made and enforced. Perhaps that is not how some, or most, of us would choose to die, if all choices were available. I, for example, would hope that my family would be emotional about the choices to be made, not simply concerned with the application of my advance directives to my situation.

Although my personal concerns do not include the first of these, two special classes of patient refuse to be involved in living will negotiations because of a fundamental discord between their model of how life is to be lived and the decision-analysis model that informs advance directives discussions. A substantial number of patients simply find it incomprehensible or distasteful to imagine that their choices have an impact upon the length of life. Even if this counts as a denial of the facts of the situation, it still is cause for concern that there are a lot of people who refuse to "play the game" for what amounts to religious reasons. Such persons commonly state, "It's up to God." Surely they do not therefore gain the obligation to be tormented by modern medicine; but, at least under some legal conditions, that is their only option if they lose competence without giving advance directives limiting life-sustaining treatment.[3]

The other group who refuse to be involved in advance directives includes those who simply want to be able to live in the moment and to have a community and family that is trustworthy about making future choices. I personally have a great deal of sympathy with this claim. Why is it that the society wants individuals to get clear about their preferences and priorities and to express them in detail—only about life-sustaining medical treatment? Why can potential future patients not just trust that caregivers and family will make "about" the right choice? I prefer to believe that the "system" is caring and compassionate rather than that it is a cafeteria of services that can freely be chosen or forgone. One might well want to imagine that one's "circle of friends" would be affected by one's plight and motivated to ensure that the best possible choices were made. A survey of the competent residents of a nursing home that I served found that none of the residents' advance decisions (formal or informal) were known to all relevant caregivers and decision-makers, yet every resident was highly confident that the right choices would be made. Is this a less good state of affairs than if as many decisions as possible were made in advance and these choices were well-known and documented, but the system of care was feared by the clients? I think not. Of course, perhaps we can have trustworthy systems of care *and* formal advance directives; but, very likely, requiring formal advance directives before reasonable plans of care can be implemented for a variety of situations will prove an obstacle to a sense of trustworthiness.

I, and surely some other patients, prefer family choice *over* the opportunity to make our own choices in advance. The patient himself or herself may well judge the family's efforts less harshly than he or she would judge his or her own decisions made in advance or by the professional caregivers. I have had a number of seriously ill patients say that their next of kin will attend to some choice if it comes up. When challenged with the possibility that the next of kin might decide in a way that was not what the patient would have chosen, the patient would kindly calm my concern with the observation that such an error would not be very important. High[4] found that patients prefer family decision-making even if they have never discussed preferences with the family. Perhaps this is an important finding, one that should be enabled to find expression in advance directives if that is one mechanism that allows patients to express their views.

This is not the only way that the current focus on advance directives is troubling to a vigorous concept of family life. Families are those who grieve for the patient's suffering and death, who have a history of making decisions that account for the well-being of all concerned, and about whom the patient most likely would have had the most concern. Somehow to imagine that the society *could,* or *should* set up systems that remove the family from decision-making is almost outrageous. What if Nancy Cruzan had written a living will that stated that she wanted all treatment stopped if ever she were rendered unconscious for more than three days? Would the society really want caregivers to be obliged to stop treatment then, if her family vigorously objected?

Suppose that Justice Scalia, who wrote forcefully to encourage the requirement that life be sustained in the *Cruzan* case,[5] were afflicted with a terrible, lingering dying, relying upon all manner of medical torment to sustain life. Suppose also that his family claimed that they knew better what he would have wanted than do those who interpret his public writings and that they want treatment stopped. Should this society really establish systems of care that require that the family's voice be silenced? Surely not. While they might have to discuss their views at some length, surely the voice of a loving family should be prominent.

The idea of family decision-making is further constrained by the common requirement in durable powers of attorney and proxy statutes that there be one solo decision-maker designated. For many families, making a unitary designation is contrary to the family's history of making conjoint decisions and imposes the possibility of generating an unnecessary discord, as someone must be granted disproportionate authority.

The question at this point might well be "Why do I use advance directive at all?" rather than "Why do I not have one?" I have found four good uses for formal advance directives. First, for anyone for whom a legally-sanctioned surrogate either does not exist or might be controversial (e.g., should it be the mother or the long-term mate of an AIDS patient), a durable power of attorney is quite valuable. Provided that the person has at least one other person willing and capable of serving as surrogate, having that person properly designated can ease a great deal of administrative and legal concerns. In Virginia and the District of Columbia for persons whose next-of-kin are appropriate surrogates, they are automatically granted the authority.[6] However, in many jurisdictions, even patients with close family would be well-served by having a durable power of attorney.

For a much smaller number of people, I use [formal advance directives] to document unusually specific preferences or unusual preferences. Thus, a person who never wants to be in a particular hospital again, or to have a particular treatment again, or to be treated for pain, might well benefit by carefully documenting this preference.

For another group of patients and families, anxieties are best laid to rest by generating a formal advance directive. The formal document might be more weighty and enduring than any one surrogate or caregiver. Also, the discussion about priorities and preferences might most naturally and easily be organized around the task of writing a formal advance directive.

For patients and families that would use a next-of-kin surrogate (which is legally authorized without additional formalities in my jurisdiction), who have fairly conventional preferences about the goals and burdens of advanced illness, and who are most comfortable with informal agreements, I do not encourage formal advance directives. These criteria fit my situation.

What should I do? Clearly, I could not use a living will in any of its standard formats. What I should do is to write a durable power of attorney naming my husband as surrogate (if I were to become incompetent outside of Virginia and the District of Columbia) and asking that all concerned defer to his judgment, however he comes to it, unless they feel that his decision amounts to abuse. Specifically, I would not want any judge or other person to overrule my family's choice on the basis of anything I have written or said about medical treatment (including anything else that I have said in this article!). I believe I have a trustworthy family and a supportive circle of friends. I would prefer to endure the outcome if they "err" in predicting my preferences, or even if they choose to ignore my preferences other than the preference for family decision-making, rather than to remove from them the opportunity and the burden of making the choices. I do not want anyone else presuming to impose what are taken to be my desires as expressed elsewhere upon that family.

Once signed and witnessed, that last paragraph can serve as my advance directive.

REFERENCES

1 The Patient Self-Determination Act, Sections 4206, 4751, of the Omnibus Budget Reconciliation Act of 1990, P.L. 101–508 (Nov. 5, 1990).

2 President's Commission for the Study of Ethical Problems in Medicine and Biomedical and Behavioral Research, *Deciding to Forego Life-sustaining Treatment,* U.S. Government Printing Office, Washington, D.C., 1983; The Hastings Center, *Guidelines for the Termination of Treatment and the Care of the Dying,*

Indiana University Press, Bloomington, IN, 1987; L.L. Emanuel, E.J. Emanuel, "The Medical Directive. A new comprehensive advance care document." *J. Am. Med. Asso.* 2989; 261:3288–93; L.J. Schneiderman, J.D. Arras, "Counseling Patients to Counsel Physicians on Future Care in the Event of Patient Incompetence." *Ann Intern. Med.* 1985; 102:693–8; J.M. Gibson, National Values History Project. *Generations* 1990; XIV: 51–64; *Your Health Care Choices: A Guide to Preparing Advance Directives for Health Care Decisions in Arizona,* The Dorothy Garske Center and Arizona Health Decisions, 4250 East Camelback Road, Suite 185K, Phoenix, AZ 85018, October 1990.

3 *In re* O'Connor 72, N.Y.2d 517, 531 N.E.2d 607, 534 N.Y.S.2d 886 (1988); *Cruzan v Harmon,* 58 L.W. 4916, June 26, 1990; *In re* Christine Busalacchi, Missouri Court of Appeals No. 59582, March 5, 1991.

4 D.M. High, "All in the Family: Extended Autonomy and Expectations in Surrogate Health Care Decision-Making." *Gerontologist* 1988; 28 (Supplement):46–52.

5 *Cruzan v Harmon,* 58 L.W. 4916, at 4924, 6-26-90 (Scalia, J, concurring).

6 Health Care Decisions Act of 1988, The District of Columbia, 35 DCR 8653, D.C. Code Ann. Chap. 21-2210; VA Code Sections 54.1-2981 to -2992 (1988 and Supp. 1990).

My Annotated Living Will
Norman L. Cantor

Norman L. Cantor is professor of law and Justice Nathan L. Jacobs Scholar, Rutgers University School of Law, Newark, New Jersey. He has also served as advisor to the New Jersey Bioethics Commission. Widely published on the legal aspects of death and dying, Cantor is the author of *Legal Frontiers of Death and Dying* (1987) and *Advance Directives and the Pursuit of Death with Dignity* (1993).

Cantor provides an example of a highly personalized living will. Regarding the desirability of medical treatment in the event of a fatal condition, he presents a systematic account of the relative significance of various factors in a determination of his best interests. The factors he discusses are physical pain, indignity, mental deterioration, physical disability, economic considerations, and the interests of others. One of Cantor's principal concerns is to avoid life-preserving treatments should he be reduced to an existence that he (as a presently competent person) would consider clearly demeaning (degrading, undignified). This underlying concern is apparent in the specific instructions he gives with regard to permanent unconsciousness, progressive degenerative disease, and senility.

. . . The following personal "living will" is offered for publication for two reasons. First, by addressing various medical conditions and issues, it may encourage other people to consider a full spectrum of situations in advance and thus to provide better guidance than is currently offered in the abbreviated living will forms often used.[1] Further, to the extent that persons adopt positions identical or close to the instructions given here, they will be reinforcing one conception of what constitutes "humane" treatment for a previously vigorous adult who faces a life-threatening illness or condition. The annotations—the explanatory comments provided in brackets and boldface print—are unabashedly aimed at recruiting converts to the substantive provisions presented in the document.

Reprinted with permission of the author and the American Society of Law, Medicine & Ethics from *Law, Medicine & Health Care,* vol. 18, nos. 1–2 (1990), pp. 115–119.

MY LIVING WILL

I. INTRODUCTION

I hereby make this declaration before _____ witnesses in accordance with my state's living will legislation (or natural death act). Nonetheless, I understand that my instructions may extend beyond the classes of situations covered in such legislation. **[Conformity with the relevant state legislation—as to which each person should consult with a lawyer—helps reinforce the instructions. A living will statute usually provides some form of explicit legal sanction for medical failure to implement the patient's instructions, as well as explicit legal protection for physicians' good faith implementation of these instructions. Compliance with the formal statutory format (witnesses, etc.) assures that these elements will apply to the particular living will being drafted. Nonetheless, particular state statues may provide constraints which do not fit the wishes of persons like myself. For example, a statute may authorize discontinuance of life-preserving treatment only when death is imminent, or a statute may not include refusal of artificial nutrition within its range of rejectable medical interventions. My instructions are not drawn according to the substantive (as opposed to the procedural) bounds of the state legislation. My effort to fully describe my wishes, regardless of the ostensibly limited scope of a living will statute, is designed to invoke judicially developed, common law rights of self-determination and bodily integrity. Living Will Statutes generally preserve judicially developed rights of dying patients. Thus, even in a jurisdiction with a living will statute of limited scope, there is hope that medical care providers will adhere to the prior instructions of a currently incompetent patient even though those instructions appear to go beyond the statute's bounds.]**

I hereby designate _____ as my surrogate for purposes of implementing this document. I hereby authorize _____ [the designated surrogate] to act on my behalf with regard to all decisions regarding medical care after I have lost mental capacity to make my own medical decisions. This authorization includes, but is not limited to, authority to accept or refuse life-preserving measures, to hire and fire attending personnel, to admit and remove me from institutions, to gain access to relevant information, and to undertake litiga-tion on my behalf. I have consulted with _____ [the designated surrogate] and I have confidence that (s)he will implement my instructions with devotion to their letter and spirit. In the event that _____ [the designated surrogate] is not available to make determinations at the relevant moment, I request that my attending physician and any guardian involved in determining my care adhere to the contents of this document. **[In the absence of a designated agent or representative of an incompetent patient, the attending physician(s) would customarily consult with the patient's spouse or next of kin or other close relative willing to assume responsibility for medical decision-making. This may be a satisfactory arrangement, depending on the individual situation. I prefer to designate in advance a particularly trusted person who has expressed understanding of, and sympathy with, the instructions presented in this living will document. My hope and expectation is that my designated representative will be able to implement my instructions in a clear-headed fashion without the excessive emotional involvement which might affect some in my family. It may be advisable to designate an alternative surrogate who would function if the primary designated representative is unavailable at the appropriate time. Note also that in some states, legislation prescribes certain formalities for the appointment of such a representative, and care should be taken to adhere to those requirements.]**

This document applies to medical decisions on my behalf after I have become legally incompetent to make such decisions myself. **[Legal incompetence simply means that a patient no longer understands the nature and consequences of the particular medical decision in question. This is a judgment to be made by attending medical personnel in conjunction with the patient's representative(s). No formal process is ordinarily required in order to determine that decision-making competence is not present. My expectation is that my surrogate will strive to ensure that no premature determination of my incompetence is made, in addition to seeing that, once competence is lost, all medical decisions conform to my preferences as expressed in this document.]**

Before I turn to instructions relating to particular types of conditions, I mention certain guidelines which apply to all post-competence decisions on my behalf. First, while my instructions call for withholding of life-preserving medical care in various situations, palliative care is always to be provided. That is, pain relievers or sedatives should be provided to relieve intractable pain or extreme emotional upset insofar as the need for such palliative agents can be discerned. Also, I would always expect to be maintained in a clean, sheltered, and comfortable environment. Nursing care aimed at providing a clean and dignified environment should therefore always be furnished.

Second, the general criterion to be applied to decision-making on my behalf is my "best interests." In this document, I define various elements or factors to be considered in determining my best interests. According to these elements, it will sometimes be in my best interests to withhold life-preserving medical intervention and to permit me to die. In line with my normal preference and respect for life, any such terminal decision should be made only when that decision is clearly in my best interests.

Third, life-preserving medical treatment refers to all forms of medical intervention whether complex, like respirators, or simplistic, like blood transfusions or antibiotics. Different treatments may entail different consequences and side effects (e.g., the long term dependence on a dialysis machine), so that differentiations among types of treatment may have to be made in the course of actual decision-making. Yet there is no intention here to categorize certain treatments as ordinary and others as extraordinary for purposes of shaping my medical future. Best interests will have to be assessed on a case by case basis with regard to my specific condition and various proposed treatments.

II. SUBSTANTIVE INSTRUCTIONS ACCORDING TO HEALTH CONDITION

A. Permanent Unconsciousness

In the event that my capacity for sentient existence—consciousness or awareness of my environment—is permanently lost, I request that all life-extending medical intervention be ended. An existence devoid of all awareness is to my mind a demeaning state for a human being, and I don't wish to be maintained in such a status. I realize that the status of permanent unconsciousness can sometimes be artificially prolonged for long periods. This knowledge that death is not necessarily imminent merely reinforces my conviction to reject all life-extending medical intervention in such an instance.

I request only that the medical assessment of permanent unconsciousness be carefully made in accord with good medical practice and after consultation with a skilled neurologist other than the attending physician.

My rejection of medical intervention in the face of permanent unconsciousness is intended to be complete. It includes simplistic procedures such as blood transfusions, CPR, antibiotics, or other medicines, as well as more complicated procedures such as respirators or dialysis machines. In the event that my medical condition in the permanently unconscious state includes damage to the alimentary processes (inability to swallow or digest food), I request that artificial means of nutrition not be initiated or maintained. **[There are instances when a patient in permanent coma retains a swallowing reflex and can be fed manually. Some persons may desire to instruct that this feeding be ceased in order to permit the permanently unconscious being to expire. However, the legal status of such a request is uncertain. A patient is acknowledged to have a right to decline medical treatment, which has been understood by the courts to include artificial nutrition. There is no assurance that manual feeding will be included within declinable medical treatment. Moreover, there is some question whether medical ethics would permit personnel to cooperate with such a request.]**

B. A Fatal Organ Deficiency

At some point after I have become incompetent, disease or trauma will produce a fatal condition. By this I mean major dysfunction of a critical organ (such as the heart or kidneys) or an illness (such as cancer or pneumonia) which by its nature is life threatening. In the event that such a condition occurs, it is my desire that medical intervention be guided by my best interests as determined in accord with the following considerations.

1. *Physical Pain.* To the extent that analgesics still leave significant physical pain or produce prolonged stupor, this should be deemed a significant factor adverse to my best interests.

2. *Indignity.* There are certain conditions which for me, an independent person who has been extremely active in both intellectual and physical pursuits, would be demeaning and degrading. I understand that in my incompetent state I may not feel or sense the humiliation or degradation with which I am concerned. Nonetheless, it is important to me as a currently autonomous being to shape my medical future in accord

with my conception of indignity. It is important to me to be remembered as a person possessing certain characteristics, whose absence I consider undignified or demeaning. I direct that medical intervention in the face of a fatal organ deficiency be guided by my conception of personal dignity described herein. In other words, my best interests as an incompetent person should be judged with the following elements of indignity in mind.

A major element of indignity for me is helplessness. If, for example, I permanently lose the capacity to feed myself, this is a significant blow to my dignity. Inability to dress or bathe myself should also be considered a distasteful blow to my dignity. Similarly, if I lose control of my bodily evacuations, so that I must be diapered or otherwise attended, this constitutes a significant blow to my dignity.

Another aspect of helplessness is physical restraint. It may be that in my incompetence I will physically resist administration of medical treatment or otherwise act out so as to necessitate physical restraint in order to protect myself or others. Such conduct may be purely instinctive without any awareness or reason behind the actions. Nonetheless, it is demeaning to be trussed up or physically restrained for significant periods. If prolonged or repeated restraint (or, alternatively, prolonged or repeated sedation reducing me to a stupor) is necessary, this involuntary restraint is to be considered a significant blow to my dignity. . . .

3. *Mental Deterioration.* By definition, this living will is relevant only when I have lost competence to make my own medical decisions. While it is difficult for me to conceive of life without such mental capacity, I understand that persons lacking such capacity can still derive enjoyment and benefit from their existences. Therefore, while the prospect of mental incompetence is troubling to me, that fact, by itself, should not be deemed a basis for withholding or withdrawing medical treatment.

At the same time, there is a level of severe mental dysfunction which for me is demeaning and degrading. For example, permanent inability to recognize and/or interact with my relatives or friends would, by itself, constitute an undesirable, degrading status. Along these lines, total incapacity to read and understand a newspaper or magazine would reflect a level of dysfunction demeaning to me. If I am permanently reduced to such a level of dysfunction, this would at least constitute a significant blow to my dignity.

[Some persons might question my moral right to dictate an end to life-preserving care for my future self—particularly in a situation where that future self is not actually suffering from the undig- **nified state reached. Is this incompetent future self a different persona who deserves to be preserved unless shown to be suffering irremediably? My response is that my right to self-determination includes the prerogative of shaping my dying process even after competence has been lost.[2] Just as I have a legitimate right to shape handling of my future corpse, or to dispose of my property after death, I think I have a right to dictate my post-competence medical fate. In dictating the precise course to be followed, I have tried to be sensitive to how I am actually likely to feel (or not feel) in an advanced debilitated state.**

My preferences expressed in this document represent no disrespect for the mentally handicapped population. I understand that mentally handicapped individuals still deserve society's solicitous attention and care. I am simply defining my own preferences, as a mentally acute person, with regard to my own future incapacities and the personal indignity involved therein (See the section below relating to senility and chronic brain syndrome)].

4. *Physical Disability.* I have always been a vigorous person who loves participating in athletics and hiking. Thus, it is hard to imagine existence without capacity to engage in such pursuits. Nonetheless, I consider myself resilient enough and life-affirming enough to adjust to a significant degree of physical disability, including even blindness or inability to walk. Consequently, physical incapacity by itself should not be regarded in my case as a demeaning or degrading state. (This last statement is of course subject to the conditions which I have described above as depriving me of dignity—such as incontinence or inability to feed myself. I reiterate that such extreme debilities should be considered as significant blows to my dignity).

My degree of actual or prospective physical disability should be considered in conjunction with my level of mental dysfunction. That is, if my mental deterioration deprives me of the ability to cope with whatever physical disabilities are involved, that fact should be included in calculating my best interests. While severe physical disabilities would not by themselves be a basis for ending life-preserving care, such disabilities in combination with extreme mental deterioration might well prompt a determination that my best interests dictate the cessation of medical intervention in the face of a fatal organ deficiency.

5. *Economic Considerations.* In general, my best interests ought to be determined without reference to

the costs attributable to my care. So long as it is in my best interests to be medically maintained, I would expect care to continue. This is said with awareness that my assets are sufficient to cover even expensive medical care, and that I have no dependents whose economic well-being is threatened by the exhaustion of my estate. **[Were the financial situation otherwise, my instructions might well be different. If I were the head of a family of dependents, I would specify that the expense of prospective medical care be a factor to be considered in decision-making. I would instruct that if the decision regarding best interests is borderline, the extreme expense of prospective care should be considered as a factor weighing against initiation or continuation of the treatment. In addition, I would mention that financial dependence on loved ones would consti-tute a significant blow to my dignity. This means that if a decision regarding my best interests is otherwise borderline, financial dependence of this sort should be considered a significant factor dic-tating against further medical intervention.]**

6. *Interests of Others.* In general, my best interests ought to be determined without reference to the dis-comfort, inconvenience, anguish, or frustration of those surrounding me during the dying process. This is so whether those affected be medical staff or family and friends. It is not that I am indifferent to the interests of such persons. Rather, I have attempted in this docu-ment to design a dying process which would not be pro-longed beyond the point where I am no longer reaping some net benefit from existence. My assumption is that my instructions foreclose a protracted dying process in which I have declined to a level of indignity which would exact a serious toll upon those around me.

C. Progressive Degenerative Disease

I am aware that there are a number of incurable diseases which gradually and insidiously cause physical and/or mental deterioration over a prolonged period, before eventually leading to death. Alzheimer's disease and ALS (Lou Gehrig's disease) provide two examples known to me. If my incompetence coincides with such an affliction, I direct that medical intervention be shaped in accord with the best interests formula out-lined above. This directive means, *inter alia,* that when irreversible deterioration has reached a point which can be defined as clearly demeaning, life-preserving medical care should not be continued. I understand that as a

consequence death may be permitted much earlier than it would ensue if medical intervention were maintained until the most advanced stages of the disease process. My wish is to avoid those stages of the dying process in which my existence has clearly become degrading according to the standards described in this document.

A point may come in the degenerative disease process when my condition is clearly degrading, and medical intervention is either already in place or is being contemplated because the disease process has impacted on critical bodily systems. At that point, my wish is that life-preserving medical treatment be withheld or with-drawn. Again, this applies to all forms of treatment whether simplistic or complex, and includes artificial nutrition where normal alimentary processes have been incapacitated (whether by the underlying degenerative disease or any other pathology which has developed).

[The term "point" is used in this document advisedly. There will normally not be one magic moment (except perhaps for a lapse into perma-nent unconsciousness) when a degrading status is suddenly reached. Deterioration will more likely be gradual, both in physical and mental terms. Nonetheless, a stage will be reached when good faith application of the criteria presented here will prompt a conclusion that the patient's status is clearly degrading. The judgment of my represen-tative (or other decision-maker in the absence of my chosen surrogate) will determine when that stage has been reached.]

D. Senility and Organic Brain Syndrome

I understand that my mental faculties may become debilitated by these common afflictions of old age. There are obviously various degrees of mental incapac-ity connected with senility, and the condition may or may not be accompanied by serious physical afflictions. I address here senility serious enough so that compe-tence to make important medical decisions has been lost. If a fatal organ deficiency or serious malignant dis-ease coincides with senility or organic brain syndrome, I dictate that medical decisions be made according to the criteria listed above under "Fatal Organ Deficiencies." This means that my deteriorated mental status will be considered in accord with the approach described in the section on "mental deterioration."

A few words with regard to senility. As I have out-lined in the section on "mental deterioration," the fact of mental incompetence is not in itself to be deemed degrading or undignified so as to prompt withholding of life-preserving medical intervention. There is such a thing as "pleasantly senile," where an individual can still enjoy existence despite the loss of some mental faculties. Even though this persona is not the way I relish being remembered, I do not instruct that medical care be withheld solely because of this level of mental dysfunction. At the same time, the dysfunction may become so acute that my condition is clearly demeaning or degrading as I have defined it above. (For example, when I am in such a stupor that I no longer can recognize or relate to friends or relatives). At that stage, my best interests would dictate release from this demeaning status by withholding or withdrawing life-prolonging medical intervention.

The hardest issue for me in drafting this living will is how to deal with preventive or curative medical care once severe mental deterioration has set in, yet I am still physically healthy. I am referring to having reached a mental status that is clearly demeaning, yet my physical status entails no fatal organ deficiency or serious disease. I am concerned about treatment of pathological conditions which by themselves are not fatal, but which if not treated will develop into fatal conditions, such as minor infections which are treatable with antibiotics, or minor organ dysfunctions which are curable but which will lead to fatal dysfunctions if not treated. Should preventive and curative measures be withheld in order to facilitate onset of a dying process which will liberate me from my demeaning state?

My personal resolution of this issue is to say that such conditions should be treated during my incompetency up until the point when my mental status can be deemed clearly and permanently degrading under the criteria listed above. For example, existence in a semiconscious stupor, or existence without any recognition of relatives or friends, would trigger this instruction. Once such a status has been reached, even medical intervention for curable conditions should be withheld. Infections should not be treated with antibiotics unless the prospective pain and discomfort and indignity accompanying the ensuing dying process would outweigh the relief which death might offer from the currently degrading status. The same approach should be applied to minor kidney, heart, or other organ problems which would not normally be deemed fatal organ deficiencies. In short, once a clearly demeaning mental status has irreversibly set in, even minor medical problems should not be treated (except palliatively) unless the consequent dying process carries with it negative consequences for me which make continued maintenance in an albeit demeaning state consistent with my best interests.

There may be tension here between my preferences regarding preventive and curative care and the conscientious positions of some medical personnel. While I have no desire to force medical personnel to violate their conscientious scruples, I do want to have my instructions implemented. In the event that attending medical personnel (or the institutional host) cannot in good conscience honor my preferences, my representative(s) are instructed to seek alternative personnel who can, in good conscience, cooperate. Or, I should be transferred to another facility in which cooperation is available. . . .

REFERENCES

1 For another effort to assist in drafting medical directives, see L. Emmanuel & E. Emmanuel, "The Medical Directive," 261 *J.A.M.A.* 3288 (1989).
2 See Dworkin, "Autonomy and the Demented Self," 64:2 *Millbank Quarterly* (1986), pp. 4–16.

ANNOTATED BIBLIOGRAPHY: CHAPTER 6

Brody, Baruch: "Special Ethical Issues in the Management of PVS Patients," *Law, Medicine & Health Care* 20 (Spring–Summer 1992), pp. 104–115. Brody identifies and discusses a number of issues associated with the treatment of PVS patients.

Cantor, Norman L.: *Advance Directives and the Pursuit of Death with Dignity* (Bloomington: Indiana University Press, 1993). Cantor provides an accessible and broad-based discussion of advance directives.

Cranford, Ronald E.: "The Persistent Vegetative State: The Medical Reality (Getting the Facts Straight)," *Hastings Center Report* 18 (February/March 1988), pp. 27–32. Cranford clarifies the medical facts about persistent vegetative state and distinguishes a number of neurological conditions that may be confused with it.

Devettere, Raymond J.: "Neocortical Death and Human Death," *Law, Medicine & Health Care* 18 (Spring–Summer 1990), pp. 96–104. Devettere argues that neocortical death (i.e., permanent loss of consciousness) is compatible with our cultural understanding of death and that the capacity for making an accurate diagnosis of neocortical death is now emerging. However, he also argues that there are compelling public-policy reasons why neocortical death should not be accepted as a legal standard for human death.

Dresser, Rebecca S., and John A. Robertson: "Quality of Life and Non-Treatment Decisions for Incompetent Patients: A Critique of the Orthodox Approach," *Law, Medicine & Health Care* 17 (Fall 1989), pp. 234–244. The authors argue against the orthodox approach to surrogate decision making, which emphasizes the desirability of advance directives and the priority of the substituted-judgment standard. Their principal complaint is that the orthodox approach allows an incompetent patient's past wishes to take priority over his or her present interests.

Guidelines on the Termination of Life-Sustaining Treatment and the Care of the Dying: A Report by the Hastings Center (Bloomington: Indiana University Press, 1988). This document presents general guidelines on the decision-making process and then presents guidelines relevant to specific treatment modalities. Also included are guidelines on advance directives and the declaration of death.

Hardwig, John: "The Problem of Proxies with Interests of Their Own: Toward a Better Theory of Proxy Decisions," *The Journal of Clinical Ethics* 4 (Spring 1993), pp. 20–27. Hardwig challenges the appropriateness of exclusively patient-centered standards of surrogate decision making. In particular, he argues that it is morally unsound to expect proxy decision makers to disregard their own interests and those of other family members.

King, Nancy M. P.: *Making Sense of Advance Directives* (Boston: Kluwer Academic Publishers, 1991). King provides an overall account of advance directives. The book is primarily intended for health-care professionals but is entirely accessible to the general reader.

Lynn, Joanne, ed.: *By No Extraordinary Means: The Choice to Forgo Life-Sustaining Food and Water* (Bloomington: Indiana University Press, 1986). This anthology provides a wide range of material on the issue of forgoing artificial nutrition and hydration.

May, William E., et al.: "Feeding and Hydrating the Permanently Unconscious and Other Vulnerable Persons," *Issues in Law and Medicine* 3 (Winter 1987), pp. 203–217. A group of ten authors argues that it is morally wrong to withhold or withdraw artificial nutrition and hydration from the permanently unconscious or from those who are seriously debilitated but nondying.

Meisel, Alan: "Lessons from *Cruzan*," *The Journal of Clinical Ethics* 1 (Fall 1990), pp. 245–250. The *Cruzan* case is the first "right-to-die" case to reach the United States Supreme Court. Meisel explains the Court's holding as well as the many misperceptions of that holding.

———: "The Legal Consensus about Forgoing Life-Sustaining Treatment: Its Status and Its Prospects," *Kennedy Institute of Ethics Journal* 2 (December 1992), pp. 309–345. In this long and very useful article, Meisel articulates eight basic points as constitutive of the existing legal consensus.

President's Commission for the Study of Ethical Problems in Medicine and Biomedical and Behavioral Research: *Deciding to Forgo Life-Sustaining Treatment* (1983). This document is valuable in its entirety, but two chapters are especially noteworthy. Chapter 4 provides material on the determination of incapacity (incompetence), surrogate decision making, and advance directives. Chapter 5 deals with patients who have permanently lost consciousness but are not "brain-dead."

———: *Defining Death* (1981). In this document, the Commission provides an overall account of its deliberations leading to the recommendation that the Uniform Determination of Death Act be adopted in each of the states.

Schneiderman, Lawrence J., Nancy S. Jecker, and Albert R. Jonsen: "Medical Futility: Its Meaning and Ethical Implications," *Annals of Internal Medicine* 112 (June 15, 1990), pp. 949–954. The authors distinguish between a quantitative and a qualitative sense of futility, and they assign an operational meaning to each sense.

Tomlinson, Tom, and Howard Brody: "Futility and the Ethics of Resuscitation," *JAMA* 264 (September 12, 1990), pp. 1276–1280. The authors provide a further defense of their view that physicians can justifiably withhold CPR, without patient consent, on the basis of a futility judgment.

Truog, Robert D., Allan S. Brett, and Joel Frader: "The Problem with Futility," *New England Journal of Medicine* 326 (June 4, 1992), pp. 1560–1564. The authors emphasize ambiguities in the concept of futility and argue that it can seldom provide a sound basis for limiting life-sustaining treatment.

Youngner, Stuart J.: "Do-Not-Resuscitate Orders: No Longer Secret, but Still a Problem," *Hastings Center Report* 17 (February 1987), pp. 24–33. Youngner argues for the importance of (1) the improved documentation and specification of DNR orders; (2) the involvement of patient, family, and staff (including nurses) in DNR decisions; and (3) the regular (at least daily) review of a patient's DNR status. He also insists that DNR status does not entail medical or psychological abandonment.

Zaner, Richard M.: *Death: Beyond Whole-Brain Criteria* (Dordrecht, Netherlands: Kluwer Academic Publishers, 1988). Most of the authors in this collection of material defend a "higher-brain" approach to the definition of death.

CHAPTER 7

SUICIDE, ACTIVE EUTHANASIA, AND THE TREATMENT OF IMPAIRED INFANTS

INTRODUCTION

The mercy killing of patients, whether called "active euthanasia" (as it is here) or simply "euthanasia," is a topic of long-standing controversy in biomedical ethics. Can active euthanasia—especially in response to the request of a competent patient—be morally justified? Should it be legalized? Parallel questions can be raised about physician-assisted suicide, a closely related topic that has generated intense discussion in the 1990s. This chapter is designed in large part to deal with ethical questions about active euthanasia and physician-assisted suicide. Its point of departure, however, is a consideration of the morality of suicide, an issue whose relevance is not restricted to a medical context.

Most of the discussion in Chapters 6 and 7 centers on adult patients' confronting the problems of death and dying at the end of a long life. An important issue has been left for examination in the present chapter, and this issue is located at the other end of the spectrum of human life, where we are confronted with the severely impaired newborn child. Biomedical technology is sometimes sufficient to sustain or at least temporarily prolong the life of a severely impaired infant, depending on the particular nature of the child's medical condition, but we must ask under what conditions continued treatment is morally appropriate.

What Is Suicide?

It is unwise to discuss the morality of suicide without paying some attention to the concept of suicide. Consider two people, one saying that suicide is always immoral and the other saying that suicide is sometimes morally acceptable. It is possible that these two people are in substantive moral agreement and differ only with regard to an operating definition of suicide. One of them may hold that suicide is systematically immoral but say that a certain action is

368

not suicide and is therefore morally acceptable, whereas the other may consider the same action suicide but consider it a morally acceptable form of suicide. The following cases and the accompanying analysis are presented in order to shed some measure of light on the concept of suicide.

(1) A woman, having despaired of achieving a satisfying life, leaps to her death from the top of a city skyscraper. (2) An elderly man dies from a massive overdose of sleeping pills, leaving behind a note explaining that he is not bitter but that life seems to have passed him by. He has outlived his friends, he has no employment, he finds no enjoyment in his pastimes, and so forth. Both of these cases provide us with clear instances of suicide. In accordance with what might be called the standard definition of *suicide,* each of these cases is a suicide precisely because it features the *intentional termination of one's own life.* Consider a third case. (3) In time of war, a soldier is captured and subjected to torture. Feeling unable to resist any longer but determined not to yield any information that would endanger the lives of his comrades, he hangs himself. This third case is noteworthy, in contrast to the first two, in that it features an other-directed rather than a self-directed motivation. Still, it seems to be a clear case of the intentional termination of one's own life. It is sometimes said that the self-killing in such cases is sacrificial rather than suicidal, but to deny that case 3 is a case of suicide is surely to abandon the standard definition of suicide.

(4) A truck driver, foreseeing his own death, nevertheless steers his runaway truck into a concrete abutment in order to avoid hitting a schoolbus that has stopped on the roadway to discharge children. (5) In a somewhat similar and much discussed actual case, a certain Captain Oates fell ill and found himself physically unable to continue on with a party of explorers in the Antarctic. The explorers were struggling to find their way out of a blizzard. Captain Oates, determined not to further endanger his colleagues by hindering their progress but unable to convince them to leave him to die, simply walked off to meet his death in the blizzard. One may feel some puzzlement as to whether cases 4 and 5 are to be identified as cases of suicide. As in case 3, the notion of sacrificial death may come to mind. Presumably, neither the truck driver nor Captain Oates wanted to die; each sacrificed his own life so that the lives of others might be protected. In contrast to case 3, however, it is plausible to say, in accordance with the standard definition, that cases 4 and 5 are not cases of suicide. In this view, it would be said that neither the truck driver nor Captain Oates *intentionally terminated* his life. While each initiated a chain of events that was foreseen as leading to his own death, neither initiated the chain of events because he desired to die, but quite the contrary, because he desired to attain some other objective, that is, the protection of others. Thus the primary intention of the basic action (redirecting the truck, walking away from camp) was to protect others; one's own death, it is said, is foreseen but not intended. Still, many would insist, contrary to the line of thought just developed, that both the truck driver and Captain Oates did *intentionally terminate* their lives. It was in their power to avoid their deaths, but they chose (seemingly in noble fashion) not to do so.

There is one final case to be considered. (6) A Jehovah's Witness, as a matter of religious principle, refuses to consent to a blood transfusion and dies. Is this a case of suicide? This judgment turns, as does our judgment regarding cases 4 and 5, on the interpretation of the phrase *intentional termination.* The Jehovah's Witness, in many ways similar to the traditional Christian martyr, refuses to sacrifice religious principle and thereby brings about his or her own death. Those who say that case 6 is not a case of suicide point out that the Jehovah's Witness typically does not want to die. The Jehovah's Witness foresees but does not intend his or her own death. Those who say that case 6 is a case of suicide point out that, in effect, the avoidance of death is within the power of the Jehovah's Witness. Thus choosing to refuse the blood transfusion constitutes an intentional termination of life.

Notice, in certain circumstances, the refusal of life-sustaining treatment is undeniably suicide. Suppose a person in good health is accidentally injured and needs a routine surgical procedure in order to live (and fully recover). Suppose further that this person refuses medical intervention simply because he or she wants to die. In such a case, refusing life-sustaining treatment is simply a convenient way of committing suicide. The phrase *intentional termination,* however it is to be finally analyzed, clearly incorporates passive as well as active means. A person can commit suicide just as effectively by (passively) refusing to eat as by (actively) taking an overdose of drugs.

Ordinarily, the refusal of life-sustaining treatment by a terminally ill patient is not considered suicide—at least if the patient's death is reasonably imminent. Perhaps this is the case because the refusal of life-sustaining treatment in such cases is so naturally understood as a decision not to extend the dying process. On the other hand, consider a patient (not terminally ill) who is dissatisfied with the quality of life that has resulted from some incurable medical condition (e.g., paralysis) and refuses life-sustaining treatment for some treatable medical condition (e.g., pneumonia) that happens to arise. Is this not suicide?

The Morality of Suicide

Under what conditions, if at all, is suicide morally acceptable? Classical literature on the morality of suicide provides a number of sources who issue a strong moral condemnation of suicide. St. Augustine, St. Thomas Aquinas, and Immanuel Kant are prominent examples. Augustine's arguments are dominantly theological in character, but Aquinas and Kant advance philosophical as well as religiously based arguments against suicide. According to Aquinas, suicide is to be condemned not only because it violates our duty to God but also because it violates the natural law, and, moreover, because it injures the community. Kant, in the first selection of this chapter, argues that suicide degrades human worth and is therefore always immoral. R. B. Brandt, in a very different vein, critically analyzes the most influential of the classical arguments against suicide and vigorously defends the view that suicide is not always immoral. This more liberal viewpoint, it is important to note, is not unprecedented in the classical literature on suicide. The Roman Stoic Seneca and the eighteenth-century Scottish philosopher David Hume are quite notable in their articulation and defense of such a view.

The more liberal view on the morality of suicide might be explicated in general terms as follows. Suicide is morally acceptable to the extent that it does no substantial damage to the interests of other individuals. Moreover, even in cases where suicide has some significant negative impact on others, no person is morally obliged to undergo extreme distress to prevent others from undergoing some smaller measure of discomfort, sadness, and so forth.

In his discussion, Brandt considers not only the morality of suicide but also the rationality of suicide. It is sometimes asserted that a suicidal intention is necessarily irrational, thus a symptom of mental illness and incompetence. In other words, it is impossible for a competent adult to have a suicidal intention. Although this point seems to be built into some psychiatric theories, it is considered by many philosophers to be an implausible contention. Brandt, in particular, insists that suicide can be a rational choice, although he warns of the distorting effects that depression can exercise over human judgment.

The Morality of Active Euthanasia

There is both a narrow and a broad sense of *euthanasia,* and the difference between the two is best understood by reference to the categories of killing and allowing to die, although the distinction between killing and allowing to die is itself a controversial one. Understood in the narrow sense, the category of euthanasia is limited to mercy *killing.* Thus, if a physician administers a lethal dose of a drug to a terminally ill patient (on grounds of mercy), this act is a paradigm of euthanasia. On the other hand, if a physician *allows a patient to die* (e.g., by withholding or withdrawing a respirator), this does not count as euthanasia. Although the narrow sense of *euthanasia* is becoming increasingly common, many writers still use the word in the broad sense. Understood in the broad sense, the category of euthanasia encompasses both killing and allowing to die (on grounds of mercy). Those who employ the broad sense of *euthanasia* often distinguish between *active* euthanasia (i.e., killing) and *passive* euthanasia (i.e., allowing to die).

One other distinction is of central importance in discussions of euthanasia. *Voluntary* euthanasia proceeds in response to the (informed) request of a competent patient. *Nonvoluntary* euthanasia involves an individual who is incompetent to give consent. The possibility of nonvoluntary euthanasia might arise with regard to adults who have for any number of reasons (e.g., Alzheimer's disease) lost their decision-making capacity, and it might arise with regard to newborn infants or children. Both voluntary and nonvoluntary euthanasia may be further distinguished from *involuntary* euthanasia, which entails acting *against the will* or, at any rate, without the permission of a competent person. It is important to note, however, that many writers in biomedical ethics use the phrase *involuntary euthanasia* in referring to what has been identified here as *nonvoluntary euthanasia*.

If the voluntary/nonvoluntary distinction is combined with the active/passive distinction, four types of euthanasia can be distinguished: (1) voluntary active euthanasia, (2) nonvoluntary active euthanasia, (3) voluntary passive euthanasia, and (4) nonvoluntary passive euthanasia. Contemporary debate, however, focuses on the moral legitimacy of active euthanasia, especially voluntary active euthanasia. In a certain sense, there is no issue about the moral legitimacy of passive euthanasia, whether voluntary or nonvoluntary. The idea that it can be morally appropriate to withhold or withdraw life-sustaining treatment is firmly established, at least in the United States. This is not to say, of course, that there are no issues related to the specific conditions that must be satisfied in order for the withholding or withdrawing of life-sustaining treatment to be morally appropriate. (In this regard, see Chapter 6 and the last section of the present chapter, "The Treatment of Impaired Infants.")

James Rachels argues in this chapter for the moral legitimacy of active euthanasia. One of his central claims is that there is no morally significant distinction between killing and allowing to die. Daniel Callahan, by way of contrast, defends the coherence and moral importance of the distinction between killing and allowing to die. Callahan is opposed to active euthanasia and argues that killing patients is incompatible with the role of the physician in society. In his view, the power of the physician must be used "only to cure or comfort, never to kill." Dan W. Brock, in turn, rejects the idea that active euthanasia is incompatible with the fundamental professional commitments of a physician. Furthermore, in stating a case for the moral legitimacy of voluntary active euthanasia, Brock appeals to the centrality of two fundamental values—patient autonomy and patient well-being.

Those, like Rachels, who argue for the moral legitimacy of active euthanasia usually emphasize considerations of humaneness. When the intent is to provide an overall defense of *voluntary* active euthanasia, the humanitarian appeal is typically conjoined with an appeal to the primacy of individual autonomy. Thus the overall case for the moral legitimacy of voluntary active euthanasia incorporates two basic arguments. These arguments might be stated as follows: (1) It is cruel and inhumane to refuse the plea of a terminally ill person for his or her life to be mercifully ended in order to avoid future suffering and/or indignity. (2) Individual choice should be respected to the extent that it does not result in harm to others. Since no one is harmed by terminally ill patients' undergoing active euthanasia, a decision to have one's life ended in this fashion should be respected.

Those who argue against the moral legitimacy of active euthanasia typically rest their case on one or both of the following claims: (1) Killing an innocent person is intrinsically wrong. (2) Any systematic acceptance of active euthanasia would lead to detrimental social consequences (e.g., via a lessening of respect for human life). This second line of argument recurs in discussions of the legalization of active euthanasia.

Active Euthanasia and Social Policy

Should active euthanasia be legalized? If so, in what form or forms and with what safeguards? Although active euthanasia is presently illegal in all 50 states, proposals for its legalization have been recurrently advanced. Most commonly, it is the legalization of *voluntary* active euthanasia that has been proposed.

There are some who consider active euthanasia in any form intrinsically immoral (sometimes on overtly religious grounds) and for this reason are opposed to the legalization of voluntary active euthanasia. Others, such as Joan Teno and Joanne Lynn in this chapter, do not maintain that individual acts of voluntary active euthanasia are intrinsically immoral but still stand opposed to any social policy that would permit its practice. Teno and Lynn's concern is with the adverse social consequences of legalization: vulnerable persons will be subject to abuse, a disincentive for the availability of supportive services for the dying will be created, and public trust and confidence in physicians will be undermined. Another consequentialist concern is embodied in the frequently made "slippery-slope" argument: the legalization of *voluntary* active euthanasia would lead us down a slippery slope to the legalization of *nonvoluntary* (and perhaps *involuntary*) euthanasia. Those who support the legalization of voluntary active euthanasia recognize that some bad consequences may result from legalization. However, they typically seek to establish that potential dangers are either overstated or can be minimized with appropriate safeguards.

Consider, for a moment, some of the issues that might arise in specifying appropriate limits for a practice of voluntary active euthanasia. Would we want to restrict the practice to patients who are terminally ill (according to some definition), to patients who are experiencing unbearable suffering (according to some definition), or to patients who are *both* terminally ill and experiencing unbearable suffering? Would we want to insist that a patient be competent at the time he or she undergoes active euthanasia, or would we want to allow for the possibility of active euthanasia in accordance with an advance directive?

Voluntary active euthanasia is a well-established practice in the Netherlands (often referred to simply as "Holland"). One of the interesting aspects of the Dutch system is the fact that there is a requirement that active euthanasia be available only if the patient is experiencing unbearable (and unrelievable) suffering, but there is no requirement that the patient be terminally ill. Another interesting feature of the system as it actually operates is the apparent acceptance of an advance-directive principle. That is, active euthanasia is sometimes provided for patients who are now incompetent but who had clearly expressed their wishes while competent.[1] In one of this chapter's readings, Margaret P. Battin provides a discussion of the Dutch practice of voluntary active euthanasia. Although she believes that the practice is morally appropriate in relation to existing social conditions in Holland, she cites many important differences between the United States and Holland and ultimately concludes that "the United States is in many respects an untrustworthy candidate for practicing active euthanasia." In Battin's view, the United States is better suited for the practice of physician-assisted suicide.

Physician-Assisted Suicide and Social Policy

Physician-assisted suicide usually involves a physician in one or both of the following roles: (1) providing *information* to a patient about how to commit suicide in an effective manner;

(2) providing the *means* necessary for an effective suicide (most commonly, by writing a prescription for a lethal amount of medication). Other modes of physician assistance in suicide might include providing moral support for the patient's decision, "supervising" the actual suicide, and helping the patient carry out the necessary physical actions. For example, a very frail patient might need a certain amount of physical assistance just to take pills.

In both physician-assisted suicide and voluntary active euthanasia, a physician plays an active role in bringing about the death of a patient. However, at face value, there is this difference between the two. In voluntary active euthanasia, it is the physician who ultimately kills the patient. In physician-assisted suicide, it is the patient who ultimately kills himself or herself, albeit with the assistance of the physician. It is a controversial issue whether this difference in terms of ultimate causal agency can serve as a basis for the claim that there is a morally significant difference between physician-assisted suicide and voluntary active euthanasia.

Should the practice of physician-assisted suicide be permitted in our society?[2] Although many of the arguments advanced against the legalization of voluntary active euthanasia can also be advanced against the legalization of physician-assisted suicide, there may be good reason to believe that there is far less risk of abuse involved in the legalization of physician-assisted suicide. This point of view is embraced by Timothy E. Quill, Christine K. Cassel, and Diane E. Meier in one of this chapter's readings. These three physicians recommend the legalization of physician-assisted suicide in accordance with a set of conditions that they present. According to one other point of view, since terminally ill patients are already free to refuse hydration and nutrition, and thereby bring about death, there is no compelling need to legalize either voluntary active euthanasia or physician-assisted suicide.[3]

The Treatment of Impaired Infants

The selective nontreatment of severely impaired newborns, sometimes identified as the practice of *passive* euthanasia, is an issue that first made its way into the public consciousness in the early 1970s. In the 1980s, the issue gained an even higher profile. Media attention focused on a rash of "Baby Doe" cases, and the Reagan administration was conspicuous in its effort to activate the machinery of government via the introduction of "Baby Doe" regulations.[4] As a result, the practice of selective nontreatment of severely impaired newborns has been subjected to intense scrutiny, with regard to both its legality and its morality.

The central moral question with regard to the treatment of impaired newborns may be identified as follows: Under what conditions, if any, is it morally acceptable to allow a severely impaired newborn to die? Two other closely related issues are also worthy of mention. The first has to do with a procedural question: Who should make the decision to treat or not treat? It has sometimes been argued that the decision is a medical one, to be made by physicians. However, the more common view is that the parents are the appropriate decision makers, as informed by consultation with physicians and as limited by boundaries set by society at large. In this regard, it is often suggested that hospital ethics committees be assigned the responsibility of reviewing decisions to treat or not treat severely impaired newborns. The second issue worthy of mention has to do with the moral legitimacy of active euthanasia. If it is believed that a severely impaired newborn is better off dead, and thus it is believed that allowing the child to die is morally acceptable, would it not also be morally acceptable (perhaps morally preferable) to kill the child as painlessly as possible?

Broadly speaking, there are three different views on the moral acceptability of allowing severely impaired newborns to die.

(1) It is morally acceptable to allow a severely impaired newborn to die if and only if death would be in the infant's best interests, that is, if and only if the infant would be better off dead. Defenders of this view are firmly committed to so-called quality-of-life judgments,

but they systematically reject the contention that the cost (emotional and/or financial) of caring for severely impaired newborns is a relevant factor in the decision to treat or not to treat. A very similar but somewhat less restrictive view would endorse allowing a severely impaired newborn to die if and only if there is no significant potential for a meaningful human existence. In one of this chapter's selections, the members of The Hastings Center Research Project on the Care of Imperiled Newborns argue for the primacy of the best interests standard, but they also insist that in some cases a "relational potential" standard comes into play. According to this standard, treatment is optional for an infant who lacks the potential for human relationships.

(2) It is morally acceptable to allow a severely impaired newborn to die if at least one of the following conditions is satisfied: (*a*) there is no significant potential for a meaningful human existence; (*b*) the emotional and/or financial hardship of caring for the impaired child would constitute a grave burden for the family. It is the introduction of the cost factor that distinguishes view 2 from view 1. Defenders of this second view, such as H. Tristram Engelhardt, Jr., often emphasize that the newborn child does not have the status of personhood, thereby defending the legitimacy of the cost factor.

(3) It is never morally acceptable to allow a severely impaired newborn to die. To put it more exactly, it would never be morally acceptable to withhold treatment from a severely impaired newborn unless it would be morally acceptable to withhold such treatment from a normal infant. Although there is no requirement to prolong the life of a *dying* infant, whatever medical treatment is considered appropriate for an otherwise normal infant must be provided for the seriously impaired newborn as well. For example, if antibiotics are indicated for an otherwise normal infant with pneumonia, then antibiotics may not be withheld in a case where pneumonia arises for an infant whose central nervous system is severely compromised. In this view, it is usually presumed that a newborn child has the status of personhood and, however severely compromised, has a right to life. Defenders of this view, such as John A. Robertson in one of this chapter's selections, often make arguments against the validity of quality-of-life judgments (as featured in both of the aforementioned views) as well as the validity of the cost factor (as featured exclusively in the second view).

T.A.M.

NOTES

1 Norman L. Cantor, "Review Essay: *Regulating Death*," *Criminal Justice Ethics* 12 (Winter/Spring 1993), p. 73.
2 The legal status of physician-assisted suicide is very clouded and, at any rate, varies from state to state. Many states presently have statutes that ban assisted suicide, but these statutes may be subject to challenge on constitutional grounds. In November 1994, voters in Oregon approved a ballot initiative legalizing physician-assisted suicide in that state (see Appendix, Case 29). However, as this book goes to press, the Oregon law has not gone into effect because it is being challenged in federal court.
3 See, for example, James L. Bernat, Bernard Gert, and R. Peter Mogielnicki, "Patient Refusal of Hydration and Nutrition: An Alternative to Physician-Assisted Suicide or Voluntary Active Euthanasia," *Archives of Internal Medicine* 153 (December 27, 1993), pp. 2723–2728.
4 The so-called final Baby Doe rule was published by the Department of Health and Human Services on April 15, 1985. For one interpretation of this rule, see Thomas H. Murray, "The Final, Anticlimactic Rule on Baby Doe," *Hastings Center Report* 15 (June 1985), pp. 5–9. For an alternative interpretation, see John C. Moskop and Rita L. Saldanha, "The Baby Doe Rule: Still a Threat," *Hastings Center Report* 16 (April 1986), pp. 8–14.

The Morality of Suicide

Suicide
Immanuel Kant

Immanuel Kant (1724–1804), widely acknowledged as one of the most influential figures in the history of Western philosophy, was a native of East Prussia. Kant largely dedicated his life to academic philosophy and was eventually appointed to the chair of logic and metaphysics at the University of Königsberg. His works are voluminous and address a very wide range of philosophical issues. Kant's ethical theory, discussed in Chapter 1, is a landmark of deontological thought.

Kant issues a blanket moral condemnation of suicide: "Suicide is in no circumstances permissible." In his view, suicide is characterized by the intention to destroy oneself. Thus neither the "victim of fate" nor the person whose intemperance leads to a shortened life is guilty of suicide. Kant insists that suicide is self-contradictory, in the sense that the power of free will is used for its own destruction. In a related consideration, suicide is said to be a moral abomination because it degrades human worth. Kant also claims that suicide is rightly condemned on religious grounds.

DUTIES TOWARDS THE BODY IN REGARD TO LIFE

What are our powers of disposal over our life? Have we any authority of disposal over it in any shape or form? How far is it incumbent upon us to take care of it? These are questions which fall to be considered in connexion with our duties towards the body in regard to life. We must, however, by way of introduction, make the following observations. If the body were related to life not as a condition but as an accident or circumstance so that we could at will divest ourselves of it; if we could slip out of it and slip into another just as we leave one country for another, then the body would be subject to our free will and we could rightly have the disposal of it. This, however, would not imply that we could similarly dispose of our life, but only of our circumstances, of the movable goods, the furniture of life. In fact, however, our life is entirely conditioned by our body, so that we cannot conceive of a life not mediated by the body and we cannot make use of our freedom except through the body. It is, therefore, obvious that the body constitutes a part of ourselves. If a man

From Immanuel Kant, *Lectures on Ethics*, translated by Louis Infield (New York: Harper & Row, 1963), pp. 147–154. Reprinted by permission of Methuen & Co. Ltd.

destroys his body, and so his life, he does it by the use of his will, which is itself destroyed in the process. But to use the power of a free will for its own destruction is self-contradictory. If freedom is the condition of life it cannot be employed to abolish life and so to destroy and abolish itself. To use life for its own destruction, to use life for producing lifelessness, is self-contradictory. These preliminary remarks are sufficient to show that man cannot rightly have any power of disposal in regard to himself and his life, but only in regard to his circumstances. His body gives man power over his life; were he a spirit he could not destroy his life; life in the absolute has been invested by nature with indestructibility and is an end in itself; hence it follows that man cannot have the power to dispose of his life.

SUICIDE

Suicide can be regarded in various lights; it might be held to be reprehensible, or permissible, or even heroic. In the first place we have the specious view that suicide can be allowed and tolerated. Its advocates argue thus. So long as he does not violate the proprietary rights of others, man is a free agent. With regard to his body there are various things he can properly do; he can have a boil lanced or a limb amputated, and disregard a scar; he is, in fact, free to do whatever he may consider useful and advisable. If then he comes to the conclusion that the most useful and advisable thing that he can do is to put an end to his life, why should he not be entitled to do so? Why not, if he sees that he can no longer go on living and that he will be ridding himself of misfortune, torment and disgrace? To be sure he robs himself of a full life, but he escapes once and for all from calamity and misfortune. The argument sounds most plausible. But let us, leaving aside religious considerations, examine the act itself. We may treat our body as we please, provided our motives are those of self-preservation. If, for instance, his foot is a hindrance to life, a man might have it amputated. To preserve his person he has the right of disposal over his body. But in taking his life he does not preserve his person; he disposes of his person and not of its attendant circumstances; he robs himself of his person. This is contrary to the highest duty we have towards ourselves, for it annuls the condition of all other duties; it goes beyond the limits of the use of free will, for this use is possible only through the existence of the Subject.

There is another set of considerations which make suicide seem plausible. A man might find himself so placed that he can continue living only under circumstances which deprive life of all value; in which he can no longer live conformably to virtue and prudence, so that he must from noble motives put an end to his life. The advocates of this view quote in support of it the example of Cato. Cato knew that the entire Roman nation relied upon him in their resistance to Caesar, but he found that he could not prevent himself from falling into Caesar's hands. What was he to do? If he, the champion of freedom, submitted, every one would say, "If Cato himself submits, what else can we do?" If, on the other hand, he killed himself, his death might spur on the Romans to fight to the bitter end in defence of their freedom. So he killed himself. He thought that it was necessary for him to die. He thought that if he could not go on living as Cato, he could not go on living at all. It must certainly be admitted that in a case such as this, where suicide is a virtue, appearances are in its favour. But this is the only example which has given the world the opportunity of defending suicide. It is the only example of its kind and there has been no similar case since. Lucretia also killed herself, but on grounds of modesty and in a fury of vengeance. It is obviously our duty to preserve our honour, particularly in relation to the opposite sex, for whom it is a merit; but we must endeavour to save our honour only to this extent, that we ought not to surrender it for selfish and lustful purposes. To do what Lucretia did is to adopt a remedy which is not at our disposal; it would have been better had she defended her honour unto death; that would not have been suicide and would have been right; for it is no suicide to risk one's life against one's enemies, and even to sacrifice it, in order to observe one's duties towards oneself.

No one under the sun can bind me to commit suicide; no sovereign can do so. The sovereign can call upon his subjects to fight to the death for their country, and those who fall on the field of battle are not suicides, but the victims of fate. Not only is this not suicide, but the opposite; a faint heart and fear of the death which threatens by the necessity of fate, is no true self-preservation; for he who runs away to save his own life, and leaves his comrades in the lurch, is a coward; but he who defends himself and his fellows even unto death is no suicide, but noble and high-minded; for life is not to be highly regarded for its own sake. I should endeavor to preserve my own life only so far as I am worthy to live. We must draw a distinction between the suicide and the victim of fate. A man who shortens his life by intemperance is guilty of imprudence and indirectly of his own death; but his guilt is not direct; he did not intend to kill himself; his death was not premeditated. For all our offences are either *culpa* or *dolus*. There is certainly no *dolus* here, but there is *culpa;* and we can say of such a man that he was guilty of his own death, but we cannot say of him that he is a suicide. What constitutes suicide is the intention to destroy oneself. Intemperance and excess which shorten life ought not, therefore, to be called suicide; for if we raise intemperance to the level of suicide, we lower suicide to the level of intemperance. Imprudence, which does not imply a desire to cease to live, must, therefore, be distinguished from the intention to murder oneself. Serious violations of our duty towards ourselves produce an aversion accompanied either by horror or by disgust; suicide is of the horrible kind, *crimina carnis* of the disgusting. We shrink in horror from suicide because all nature seeks its own preservation; an injured tree, a living body, an animal does so; how then could man make of his freedom, which is the acme of life and constitutes its worth, a principle for his own destruction? Nothing more terrible can be imagined; for if man were on every occasion master of his own life, he would be master of the lives of others; and being ready to sacrifice his life at any and every time rather than be captured, he could perpetrate every conceivable crime and vice. We are, therefore, horrified at the very thought of suicide; by it man sinks lower than the beasts; we look upon a suicide as carrion, whilst our sympathy goes forth to the victim of fate.

Those who advocate suicide seek to give the widest interpretation to freedom. There is something flattering in the thought that we can take our own life if we are so minded; and so we find even right-thinking persons defining suicide in this respect. There are many circumstances under which life ought to be sacrificed. If I cannot preserve my life except by violating my duties towards myself, I am bound to sacrifice my life rather than violate these duties. But suicide is in no circumstances permissible. Humanity in one's own person is something inviolable; it is a holy trust; man is master of all else, but he must not lay hands upon himself. A being who existed of his own necessity could not possibly destroy himself; a being whose existence is not necessary must regard life as the condition of everything else, and in the consciousness that life is a trust reposed in him, such a being recoils at the thought of committing a breach of his holy trust by turning his life against himself. Man can only dispose over things; beasts are things in this sense; but man is not a thing, not a beast. If he disposes over himself, he treats his value as that of a beast. He who so behaves, who has no respect for human nature and makes a thing of himself, becomes for everyone an Object of freewill. We are free to treat him as a beast, as a thing, and to use him for our sport as we do a horse or a dog, for he is no longer a human being; he has made a thing of himself, and, having himself discarded his humanity, he cannot expect that others should respect humanity in him. Yet humanity is worthy of esteem. Even when a man is a bad man, humanity in his person is worthy of esteem. Suicide is not abominable and inadmissible because life should be highly prized; were it so, we could each have our own opinion of how highly we should prize it, and the rule of prudence would often indicate suicide as the best means. But the rule of morality does not admit of it under any condition because it degrades human nature below the level of animal nature and so destroys it. Yet there is much in the world far more important than life. To observe morality is far more important. It is better to sacrifice one's life than one's morality. To live is not a necessity; but to live honourably while life lasts is a necessity. We can at all times go on living and doing our duty towards ourselves without having to do violence to ourselves. But he who is prepared to take his own life is no longer worthy to live at all. The pragmatic ground of impulse to live is happiness. Can I then take my own life because I cannot live happily? No! It is not necessary that whilst I live I should live happily; but it is necessary that so long as I live I should live honourably. Misery gives no right to any man to take his own life, for then

we should all be entitled to take our lives for lack of pleasure. All our duties towards ourselves would then be directed towards pleasure; but the fulfillment of those duties may demand that we should even sacrifice our life.

Is suicide heroic or cowardly? Sophistication, even though well meant, is not a good thing. It is not good to defend either virtue or vice by splitting hairs. Even right-thinking people declaim against suicide on wrong lines. They say that it is arrant cowardice. But instances of suicide of great heroism exist. We cannot, for example, regard the suicides of Cato and Atticus as cowardly. Rage, passion and insanity are the most frequent causes of suicide, and that is why persons who attempt suicide and are saved from it are so terrified at their own act that they do not dare to repeat the attempt. There was a time in Roman and in Greek history when suicide was regarded as honourable, so much so that the Romans forbade their slaves to commit suicide because they did not belong to themselves but to their masters and so were regarded as things, like all other animals. The Stoics said that suicide is the sage's peaceful death; he leaves the world as he might leave a smoky room for another, because it no longer pleases him; he leaves the world, not because he is no longer happy in it, but because he disdains it. It has already been mentioned that man is greatly flattered by the idea that he is free to remove himself from this world, if he so wishes. He may not make use of this freedom, but the thought of possessing it pleases him. It seems even to have a moral aspect, for if man is capable of removing himself from the world at his own will, he need not submit to any one; he can retain his independence and tell the rudest truths to the cruellest of tyrants. Torture cannot bring him to heel, because he can leave the world at a moment's notice as a free man can leave the country, if and when he wills it. But this semblance of morality vanishes as soon as we see that man's freedom cannot subsist except on a condition which is immutable. This condition is that man may not use his freedom against himself to his own destruction, but that, on the contrary, he should allow nothing external to limit it. Freedom thus conditioned is noble. No chance or misfortune ought to make us afraid to live; we ought to go on living as long as we can do so as human beings and honourably. To bewail one's fate and misfortune is in itself dishonourable. Had Cato faced any torments which Caesar might have inflicted upon him with a resolute mind and remained steadfast, it would have been noble of him; to violate himself was not so. Those who advocate suicide and teach that there is authority for it necessarily do much harm in a republic of free men. Let us imagine a state in which men held as a general opinion that they were entitled to commit suicide, and that there was even merit and honour in so doing. How dreadful everyone would find them. For he who does not respect his life even in principle cannot be restrained from the most dreadful vices; he recks neither king nor torments.

But as soon as we examine suicide from the standpoint of religion we immediately see it in its true light. We have been placed in this world under certain conditions and for specific purposes. But a suicide opposes the purpose of his Creator; he arrives in the other world as one who has deserted his post; he must be looked upon as a rebel against God. So long as we remember the truth that it is God's intention to preserve life, we are bound to regulate our activities in conformity with it. We have no right to offer violence to our nature's powers of self-preservation and to upset the wisdom of her arrangements. This duty is upon us until the time comes when God expressly commands us to leave this life. Human beings are sentinels on earth and may not leave their posts until relieved by another beneficent hand. God is our owner; we are His property; His providence works for our good. A bondman in the care of a beneficent master deserves punishment if he opposes his master's wishes.

But suicide is not inadmissible and abominable because God has forbidden it; God has forbidden it because it is abominable in that it degrades man's inner worth below that of the animal creation. Moral philosophers must, therefore, first and foremost show that suicide is abominable. We find, as a rule, that those who labour for their happiness are more liable to suicide; having tasted the refinements of pleasure, and being deprived of them, they give way to grief, sorrow, and melancholy.

The Morality and Rationality of Suicide
R. B. Brandt

R. B. Brandt is professor emeritus of philosophy at the University of Michigan. He is the author of *Ethical Theory* (1959), *A Theory of the Good and the Right* (1979), and *Morality, Utilitarianism, & Rights* (1992). Brandt's article "Toward a Credible Form of Utilitarianism" is one prominent example of his many contributions to contemporary discussions of utilitarian theory.

Operating on the assumption that suicide is to be understood as the intentional termination of one's own life, Brandt sets himself firmly against the view that suicide is always immoral. He critically analyzes, and finds wanting, various classes of arguments that have been advanced to support the alleged immorality of suicide: (1) theological arguments, (2) arguments from natural law, and (3) arguments to the effect that suicide necessarily harms other persons or society in general. Brandt does acknowledge that there is some oblig-aion to refrain from committing suicide when that act would be injurious to others, but he insists that this obligation may often be overridden by other morally relevant considerations. Clearly, for Brandt, suicide is sometimes morally acceptable. He also insists that a person's decision to commit suicide may be quite rational, although he is careful to warn of potential errors in judgment. He concludes by analyzing the various factors that are relevant in establishing the moral obligation of other persons toward those who are contemplating suicide.

THE MORAL REASONS FOR AND AGAINST SUICIDE

[Assuming that there is suicide if and only if there is intentional termination of one's own life,] persons who say suicide is morally wrong must be asked which of two positions they are affirming: Are they saying that *every* act of suicide is wrong, *everything considered;* or are they merely saying that there is always *some* moral obligation—doubtless of serious weight—not to commit suicide, so that very often suicide is wrong, although it is possible that there are *countervailing considerations* which in particular situations make it right or even a moral duty? It is quite evident that the first position is absurd; only the second has a chance of being defensible.

In order to make clear what is wrong with the first view, we may begin with an example. Suppose an army pilot's single-seater plane goes out of control over a heavily populated area; he has the choice of staying in the plane and bringing it down where it will do little damage but at the cost of certain death for himself, and of bailing out and letting the plane fall where it will, very possibly killing a good many civilians. Suppose he chooses to do the former, and so, by our definition, commits suicide. Does anyone want to say that his action is morally wrong? Even Immanuel Kant, who opposed suicide in all circumstances, apparently would not wish to say that it is; he would, in fact, judge that this act is not one of suicide, for he says, "It is no suicide to risk one's life against one's enemies, and even to sacrifice it, in order to preserve one's duties toward oneself."[1] St. Thomas Aquinas, in his discussion of suicide, may seem to take the position that such an act would be wrong, for he says, "It is altogether unlawful to kill oneself," admitting as an exception only the case of being under special command of God. But I believe St. Thomas would, in fact, have concluded that the act is right because the basic intention of the pilot was to save the lives of civilians, and whether an act is right or wrong is a matter of basic intention.[2]

In general, we have to admit that there are things with some moral obligation to avoid which, on account of other morally relevant considerations, it is sometimes right or even morally obligatory to do. There may be some obligation to tell the truth on every occasion, but surely in many cases the consequences of telling the truth would be so dire that one is obligated to lie. The same goes for promises. There is some moral obligation to do what one has promised (with a few exceptions); but, if one can keep a trivial promise only at serious cost to another person (i.e., keep an appointment only by failing to give aid to someone injured in an accident), it is surely obligatory to break the promise.

The most that the moral critic of suicide could hold, then, is that there is *some* moral obligation not to do what one knows will cause one's death; but he surely cannot deny that circumstances exist in which there are obligations to do things which, in fact, will result in one's death. If so, then in principle it would be possible to argue, for instance, that in order to meet my obligation to my family, it might be right for me to take my own life as the only way to avoid catastrophic hospital expenses in a terminal illness. Possibly the main point that critics of suicide on moral grounds would wish to make is that it is never right to take one's own life *for reasons of one's own personal welfare,* of any kind whatsoever. Some of the arguments used to support the immorality of suicide, however, are so framed that if they were supportable at all, they would prove that suicide is *never* moral.

One well-known type of argument against suicide may be classified as *theological.* St. Augustine and others urged that the Sixth Commandment ("Thou shalt not kill") prohibits suicide, and that we are bound to obey a divine commandment. To this reasoning one might first reply that it is arbitrary exegesis of the Sixth Commandment to assert that it was intended to prohibit suicide. The second reply is that if there is not some consideration which shows on the merits of the case that suicide is morally wrong, God had no business prohibiting it. It is true that some will object to this point, and I must refer them elsewhere for my detailed comments on the divine-will theory of morality.[3]

Another theological argument with wide support was accepted by John Locke, who wrote: ". . . Men being all the workmanship of one omnipotent and infinitely wise Maker; all the servants of one sovereign Master, sent into the world by His order and about His business; they are His property, whose workmanship they are made to last during His, not one another's pleasure . . . Every one . . . is bound to preserve himself, and not to quit his station wilfully. . . ."[4] And Kant: "We have been placed in this world under certain conditions and for specific purposes. But a suicide opposes the purpose of his Creator; he arrives in the other world as one who has deserted his post; he must be looked upon as a rebel against God. So long as we remember the truth that it is God's intention to preserve life, we are bound to regulate our activities in conformity with it. This duty is upon us until the time comes when God expressly commands us to leave this life. Human beings are sentinels on earth and may not leave their posts until relieved by another beneficent hand."[5] Unfortunately, however, even if we grant that it is the duty of human beings to do what God commands or intends them to do, more argument is required to show that God does *not* permit human beings to quit this life when their own personal welfare would be maximized by so doing. How does one draw the requisite inference about the intentions of God? The difficulties and contradictions in arguments to reach such a conclusion are discussed at length and perspicaciously by David Hume in his essay "On Suicide," and in view of the unlikelihood that readers will need to be persuaded about these, I shall merely refer those interested to that essay.[6]

A second group of arguments may be classed as arguments *from natural law.* St. Thomas says: "It is altogether unlawful to kill oneself, for three reasons. First, because everything naturally loves itself, the result being that everything naturally keeps itself in being, and resists corruptions so far as it can. Wherefore suicide is contrary to the inclination of nature, and to charity whereby every man should love himself. Hence suicide is always a mortal sin, as being contrary to the natural law and to charity."[7] Here St. Thomas ignores two obvious points. First, it is not obvious why a human being is morally bound to do what he or she has some inclination to do. (St. Thomas did not criticize chastity.) Second, while it is true that most human beings do feel a strong urge to live, the human being who commits suicide obviously feels a stronger inclination to do something else. It is as natural for a human being to dislike, and to take steps to avoid, say, great pain, as it is to cling to life.

A somewhat similar argument by Immanuel Kant may seem better. In a famous passage Kant writes that the maxim of a person who commits suicide is "From self-love I make it my principle to shorten my life if its continuance threatens more evil than it promises pleasure. The only further question to ask is whether this principle of self-love can become a universal law of nature. It is then seen at once that a system of nature by whose law the very same feeling whose function is to stimulate the furtherance of life should actually destroy life would contradict itself and consequently could not subsist as a system of nature. Hence this maxim cannot possibly hold as a universal law of nature and is therefore entirely opposed to the supreme principle of all duty."[8] What Kant finds contradictory is that the motive of self-love (interest in one's own long-range welfare) should sometimes lead one to struggle to preserve one's

life, but at other times to end it. But where is the contradiction? One's circumstances change, and, if the argument of the following section in this [paper] is correct, one sometimes maximizes one's own long-range welfare by trying to stay alive, but at other times by bringing about one's demise.

A third group of arguments, a form of which goes back at least to Aristotle, has a more modern and convincing ring. These are arguments to show that, in one way or another, a suicide necessarily does harm to other persons, or to society at large. Aristotle says that the suicide treats the *state* unjustly.[9] Partly following Aristotle, St. Thomas says: "Every man is part of the community, and so, as such, he belongs to the community. Hence by killing himself he injures the community."[10] Blackstone held that a suicide is an offense against the king "who hath an interest in the preservation of all his subjects," perhaps following Judge Brown in 1563, who argued that suicide cost the king a subject—"he being the head has lost one of his mystical members."[11] The premise of such arguments is, as Hume pointed out, obviously mistaken in many instances. It is true that Freud would perhaps have injured society had he, instead of finishing his last book, committed suicide to escape the pain of throat cancer. But surely there have been many suicides whose demise was not a noticeable loss to society; an honest man could only say that in some instances society was better off without them.

It need not be denied that suicide is often injurious to other persons, especially the family of a suicide. Clearly it sometimes is. But, we should notice what this fact establishes. Suppose we admit, as generally would be done, that there is some obligation not to perform any action which will probably or certainly be injurious to other people, the strength of the obligation being dependent on various factors, notably the seriousness of the expected injury. Then there is *some* obligation not to commit suicide, when that act would probably or certainly be injurious to other people. But, as we have already seen, many cases of *some* obligation to do something nevertheless are *not* cases of a duty to do that thing, *everything considered.* So it could sometimes be morally justified to commit suicide, even if the act will harm someone. Must a man with a terminal illness undergo excruciating pain because his death will cause his wife sorrow—when she will be caused sorrow a month later anyway, when he is dead of natural causes? Moreover, to repeat, the fact that an individual has some obligation not to commit suicide when that act will probably injure other persons does not imply that, everything considered, it is wrong for him to do it, namely, that in all circumstances suicide *as such* is something there is some obligation to avoid.

Is there any sound argument, convincing to the modern mind, to establish that there is (or is not) *some moral obligation* to avoid suicide *as such,* an obligation, of course, which might be overridden by other obligations in some or many cases? (Captain Oates may have had a moral obligation not to commit suicide as such, but his obligation not to stand in the way of his comrades getting to safety might have been so strong that, everything considered, he was justified in leaving the polar camp and allowing himself to freeze to death.)

To present all the arguments necessary to answer this question convincingly would take a great deal of space. I shall, therefore, simply state one answer to it which seems plausible to some contemporary philosophers. Suppose it could be shown that it would maximize the long-run welfare of everybody affected if people were taught that there is a moral obligation to avoid suicide—so that people would be motivated to avoid suicide just because they thought it wrong (would have anticipatory guilt feelings at the very idea), and so that other people would be inclined to disapprove of persons who commit suicide unless there were some excuse. . . . One might ask: how could it maximize utility to mold the conceptual and motivational structure of persons in this way? To which the answer might be: feeling in this way might make persons who are impulsively inclined to commit suicide in a bad mood, or a fit of anger or jealousy, take more time to deliberate; hence, some suicides that have bad effects generally might be prevented. In other words, it might be a good thing in its effects for people to feel about suicide in the way they feel about breach of promise or injuring others, just as it might be a good thing for people to feel a moral obligation not to smoke, or to wear seat belts. However, it might be that negative moral feelings about suicide as such would stand in the way of action by those persons whose welfare really is best served by suicide and whose suicide is the best thing for everybody concerned.

WHEN A DECISION TO COMMIT SUICIDE IS RATIONAL FROM THE PERSON'S POINT OF VIEW

The person who is contemplating suicide is obviously making a choice between future world-courses; the world-course that includes his demise, say, an hour from now, and several possible ones that contain his demise at a later point. One cannot have precise knowledge about many features of the latter group of world-courses, but it is certain that they will all end with death some (possibly short) finite time from now.

Why do I say the choice is between *world*-courses and not just a choice between future life-courses of the prospective suicide, the one shorter than the other? The reason is that one's suicide has some impact on the world (and one's continued life has some impact on the world), and that conditions in the rest of the world will often make a difference in one's evaluation of the possibilities. One *is* interested in things in the world other than just oneself and one's own happiness.

The basic question a person must answer, in order to determine which world-course is best or rational for him to choose, is which he *would* choose under conditions of optimal use of information, when *all* of his desires are taken into account. It is not just a question of what we prefer *now,* with some clarification of all the possibilities being considered. Our preferences change, and the preferences of tomorrow (assuming we can know something about them) are just as legitimately taken into account in deciding what to do now as the preferences of today. Since any reason that can be given today for weighting heavily today's preference can be given tomorrow for weighting heavily tomorrow's preference, the preferences of any time-stretch have a rational claim to an equal vote. Now the importance of that fact is this: we often know quite well that our desires, aversions, and preferences may change after a short while. When a person is in a state of despair—perhaps brought about by a rejection in love or discharge from a long-held position—nothing but the thing he cannot have seems desirable; everything else is turned to ashes. Yet we know quite well that the passage of time is likely to reverse all this; replacements may be found or other types of things that are available to us may begin to look attractive. So, if we were to act on the preferences of today alone, when the emotion of despair seems more than we can stand, we might find death preferable to life; but, if we allow for the preferences of the weeks and years ahead, when many goals will be enjoyable and attractive, we might find life much preferable to death. So, if a choice of what is best is to be determined by what we want not only now but later (and later desires on an equal basis with the present ones)—as it should be—then what is the best or preferable world-course will often be quite different from what it would be if the choice, or what is best for one, were fixed by one's desires and preferences now.

Of course, if one commits suicide there are no future desires or aversions that may be compared with present ones and that should be allowed an equal vote in deciding what is best. In that respect the course of action that results in death is different from any other course of action we may undertake. I do not wish to suggest the rosy possibility that it is often or always reasonable to believe that next week "I shall be more interested in living than I am today, if today I take a dim view of continued existence." On the contrary, when a person is seriously ill, for instance, he may have no reason to think that the preference-order will be reversed—it may be that tomorrow he will prefer death to life more strongly.

The argument is often used that one can never be *certain* what is going to happen, and hence one is never rationally justified in doing anything as drastic as committing suicide. But we always have to live by probabilities and make our estimates as best we can. As soon as it is clear beyond reasonable doubt not only that death is now preferable to life, but also that it will be every day from now until the end, the rational thing is to act promptly.

Let us not pursue the question of whether it is rational for a person with a painful terminal illness to commit suicide; it is. However, the issue seldom arises, and few terminally ill patients do commit suicide. With such patients matters usually get worse slowly so that no particular time seems to call for action. They are often so heavily sedated that it is impossible for the mental processes of decision leading to action to occur; or else they are incapacitated in a hospital and the very physical possibility of ending their lives is not available. Let us leave this grim topic and turn to a practically more important problem: whether it is rational for persons to commit suicide for some reason other than painful terminal physical illness. Most persons who commit suicide do so, apparently, because they face a nonphysical problem that depresses them beyond their ability to bear.

Among the problems that have been regarded as good and sufficient reasons for ending life, we find (in addition to serious illness) the following: some event that has made a person feel ashamed or lose his prestige and status; reduction from affluence to poverty; the loss of a limb or of physical beauty; the loss of sexual capacity; some event that makes it seem impossible to achieve things by which one sets store; loss of a loved one; disappointment in love; the infirmities of increasing age. It is not to be denied that such things can be serious blows to a person's prospects of happiness.

Whatever the nature of an individual's problem, there are various plain errors to be avoided—errors to which a person is especially prone when he is depressed—in deciding whether, everything considered, he prefers a world-course containing his early demise to one in which his life continues to its natural terminus. Let us forget for a moment the relevance to the decision of preferences that he may have tomorrow, and concentrate on some errors that may infect his preference as of today, and for which correction or allowance must be made.

In the first place, depression, like any severe emotional experience, tends to primitivize one's intellectual processes. It restricts the range of one's survey of the possibilities. One thing that a rational person would do is compare the world-course containing his suicide with his *best* alternative. But his best alternative is precisely a possibility he may overlook if, in a depressed mood, he thinks only of how badly off he is and cannot imagine any way of improving his situation. If a person is disappointed in love, it is possible to adopt a vigorous plan of action that carries a good chance of acquainting him with someone he likes at least as well; and if old age prevents a person from continuing the tennis game with his favorite partner, it is possible to learn some other game that provides the joys of competition without the physical demands.

Depression has another insidious influence on one's planning; it seriously affects one's judgment about probabilities. A person disappointed in love is very likely to take a dim view of himself, his prospects, and his attractiveness; he thinks that because he has been rejected by one person he will probably be rejected by anyone who looks desirable to him. In a less gloomy frame of mind he would make different estimates. Part of the reason for such gloomy probability estimates is that depression tends to repress one's memory of evidence that supports a nongloomy prediction. Thus, a rejected lover tends to forget any cases in which he has elicited enthusiastic response from ladies in relation to whom he has been the one who has done the rejecting. Thus his pessimistic self-image is based upon a highly selected, and pessimistically selected, set of data. Even when he is reminded of the data, moreover, he is apt to resist an optimistic inference.

Another kind of distortion of the look of future prospects is not a result of depression, but is quite normal. Events distant in the future feel small, just as objects distant in space look small. Their prospect does not have the effect on motivational processes that it would have if it were of an event in the immediate future. Psychologists call this the "goal-gradient" phenomenon; a rat, for instance, will run faster toward a perceived food box than a distant unseen one. In the case of a person who has suffered some misfortune, and whose situation now is an unpleasant one, this reduction of the motivational influence of events distant in time has the effect that present unpleasant states weigh far more heavily than probable future pleasant ones in any choice of world-courses.

If we are trying to determine whether we now prefer, or shall later prefer, the outcome of one world-course to that of another (and this is leaving aside the questions of the weight of the votes of preferences at a later date), we must take into account these and other infirmities of our "sensing" machinery. Since knowing that the machinery is out of order will not tell us what results it would give if it were working, the best recourse might be to refrain from making any decision in a stressful frame of mind. If decisions have to be made, one must recall past reactions, in a normal frame of mind, to outcomes like those under assessment. But many suicides seem to occur in moments of despair. What should be clear from the above is that a moment of despair, if one is seriously contemplating suicide, ought to be a moment of reassessment of one's goals and values, a reassessment which the individual must realize is very difficult to make objectively, because of the very quality of his depressed frame of mind.

A decision to commit suicide may in certain circumstances be a rational one. But a person who wants to act rationally must take into account the various possible "errors" and make appropriate rectification of his initial evaluations.

THE ROLE OF OTHER PERSONS

What is the moral obligation of other persons toward those who are contemplating suicide? The question of their moral blameworthiness may be ignored and what is rational for them to do from the point of view of personal welfare may be considered as being of secondary concern. Laws make it dangerous to aid or encourage a suicide. The risk of running afoul of the law may partly determine moral obligation, since moral obligation to do something may be reduced by the fact that it is personally dangerous.

The moral obligation of other persons toward one who is contemplating suicide is an instance of a general obligation to render aid to those in serious distress, at least when this can be done at no great cost to one's self. I do not think this general principle is seriously questioned by anyone, whatever his moral theory; so I feel free to assume it as a premise. Obviously the person contemplating suicide is in great distress of some sort; if he were not, he would not be seriously considering terminating his life.

How great a person's obligation is to one in distress depends on a number of factors. Obviously family and friends have special obligations to devote time to helping the prospective suicide—which others do not have. But anyone in this kind of distress has a moral claim on the time of any person who knows the situation (unless there are others more responsible who are already doing what should be done).

What is the obligation? It depends, of course, on the situation, and how much the second person knows about the situation. If the individual has decided to terminate his life if he can, and it is clear that he is right in this decision, then, if he needs help in executing the decision, there is a moral obligation to give him help. On this matter a patient's physician has a special obligation, from which any talk about the Hippocratic oath does not absolve him. It is true that there are some damages one cannot be expected to absorb, and some risks which one cannot be expected to take, on account of the obligation to render aid.

On the other hand, if it is clear that the individual should not commit suicide, from the point of view of his own welfare, or if there is a presumption that he should not (when the only evidence is that a person is discovered unconscious, with the gas turned on), it would seem to be the individual's obligation to intervene, prevent the successful execution of the decision, and see to the availability of competent psychiatric advice and temporary hospitalization, if necessary. Whether one has a right to take such steps when a clearly sane person, after careful reflection over a period of time, comes to the conclusion that an end to his life is what is best for him and what he wants, is very doubtful, even when one thinks his conclusion a mistaken one; it would seem that a man's own considered decision about whether he wants to live must command respect, although one must concede that this could be debated.

The more interesting role in which a person may be cast, however, is that of adviser. It is often important to one who is contemplating suicide to go over his thinking with another, and to feel that a conclusion, one way or the other, has the support of a respected mind. One thing one can obviously do, in rendering the service of advice, is to discuss with the person the various types of issues discussed above, made more specific by the concrete circumstances of his case, and help him find whether, in view, say, of the damage his suicide would do to others, he has a moral obligation to refrain, and whether it is rational or best for him, from the point of view of his own welfare, to take this step or adopt some other plan instead.

To get a person to see what is the rational thing to do is no small job. Even to get a person, in a frame of mind when he is seriously contemplating (or perhaps has already unsuccessfully attempted) suicide, to recognize a plain truth of fact may be a major operation. If a man insists, "I am a complete failure," when it is obvious that by any reasonable standard he is far from that, it may be tremendously difficult to get him to see the fact. But there is another job beyond that of getting a person to see what is the rational thing to do; that is to help him *act* rationally, or *be* rational, when he has conceded what would be the rational thing.

How either of these tasks may be accomplished effectively may be discussed more competently by an experienced psychiatrist than by a philosopher. Loneliness and the absence of human affection are states which exacerbate any other problems; disappointment, reduction to poverty, and so forth, seem less impossible to bear in the presence of the affection of another. Hence simply to be a friend, or to find someone a friend, may be the largest contribution one can make either to helping a person be rational or see clearly what is rational for him to do; this service may make one who was contemplating suicide feel that there is a future for him which it is possible to face.

NOTES

1 Immanuel Kant, *Lectures on Ethics*, New York: Harper Torchbook (1963), p. 150.

2 See St. Thomas Aquinas, *Summa Theologica*, Second Part of the Second Part, Q. 64, Art. 5. In Article 7, he says: "Nothing hinders one act from having two effects, only one of which is intended, while the other is beside the intention. Now moral acts take their species according to what is intended, and not according to what is beside the intention, since this is accidental as explained above" (Q. 43, Art. 3: I-II, Q. 1, Art. 3, as 3). Mr. Norman St. John-Stevas, the most articulate contemporary defender of the Catholic view, writes as follows: "Christian thought allows certain exceptions to its general condemnation of suicide. That covered by a particular divine inspiration has already been noted. Another exception arises where suicide is the method imposed by the state for the execution of a just death penalty. A third exception is *altruistic* suicide, of which the best known example is Captain Oates. Such suicides are justified by invoking the principles of double effect. The act from which death results must be good or at least morally indifferent; some other good effect must result: The death must not be directly intended or the real means to the good effect, and a grave reason must exist for adopting the course of action" [*Life, Death and the Law*, Bloomington, Ind.: Indiana University Press (1961), pp. 250–51]. Presumably the Catholic doctrine is intended to allow suicide when this is required for meeting strong moral obligations; whether it can do so consistently depends partly on the interpretation given to "real means to the good effect." Readers interested in pursuing further the Catholic doctrine of double effect and its implications for our problem should read Philippa Foot, "The Problem of Abortion and the Doctrine of Double Effect," *The Oxford Review*, 5:5–15 (Trinity 1967).

3 R. B. Brandt, *Ethical Theory*, Englewood Cliffs, N.J.: Prentice-Hall (1959), pp. 61–82.

4 John Locke, *Two Treatises of Government*, Ch. 2.

5 Kant, *Lectures on Ethics*, p. 154.

6 This essay appears in collections of Hume's works.

7 For an argument similar to Kant's, see also St. Thomas Aquinas, *Summa Theologica*, II, II, Q. 64, Art. 5.

8 Immanuel Kant, *The Fundamental Principles of the Metaphysic of Morals*, trans H. J. Paton, London: The Hutchinson Group (1948), Ch. 2.

9 Aristotle, *Nicomachaean Ethics*, Bk. 5, Ch. 10., p. 1138a.

10 St. Thomas Aquinas, *Summa Theologica*, II, II, Q. 64, Art. 5.

11 Sir William Blackstone, *Commentaries*, 4:189; Brown in *Hales v. Petit*, I Plow. 253, 75 E.R. 387 (C. B. 1563). Both cited by Norman St. John-Stevas, *Life, Death and the Law*, p. 235.

The Morality of Active Euthanasia

Active and Passive Euthanasia
James Rachels

James Rachels is professor of philosophy at the University of Alabama at Birmingham. Specializing in ethics, he is the author of such articles as "Why Privacy Is Important" and "Can Ethics Provide Answers?" He is also the author of *The Elements of Moral Philosophy* (1986; 2d ed., 1993), *The End of Life: Euthanasia and Morality* (1986), and *Created from Animals: The Moral Implications of Darwinism* (1990).

In this classic article, Rachels identifies the "conventional doctrine" on the morality of euthanasia as the doctrine that allows passive euthanasia but does not allow active euthanasia. He then argues that the conventional doctrine may be challenged for four reasons. First, active euthanasia is in many cases more humane than passive euthanasia. Second, the conventional doctrine leads to decisions concerning life and death on irrelevant grounds. Third, the doctrine rests on a distinction between killing and letting die that itself has no moral importance. Fourth, the most common argument in favor of the doctrine is invalid.

The distinction between active and passive euthanasia is thought to be crucial for medical ethics. The idea is that it is permissible, at least in some cases, to withhold treatment and allow a patient to die, but it is never permissible to take any direct action designed to kill the patient. This doctrine seems to be accepted by most doctors, and it is endorsed in a statement adopted by the House of Delegates of the American Medical Association on December 4, 1973:

> The intentional termination of the life of one human being by another—mercy killing—is contrary to that for which the medical profession stands and is contrary to the policy of the American Medical Association.
>
> The cessation of the employment of extraordinary means to prolong the life of the body when there is irrefutable evidence that biological death is imminent is the decision of the patient and/or his immediate family. The advice and judgment of the physician should be freely available to the patient and/or his immediate family.

However, a strong case can be made against this doctrine. In what follows I will set out some of the relevant arguments, and urge doctors to reconsider their views on this matter.

To begin with a familiar type of situation, a patient who is dying of incurable cancer of the throat is in terrible pain, which can no longer be satisfactorily alleviated. He is certain to die within a few days, even if present treatment is continued, but he does not want to go on living for those days since the pain is unbearable. So he asks the doctor for an end to it, and his family joins in the request.

Suppose the doctor agrees to withhold treatment, as the conventional doctrine says he may. The justification for his doing so is that the patient is in terrible agony, and since he is going to die anyway, it would be wrong to prolong his suffering needlessly. But now notice this. If one simply withholds treatment, it may take the patient longer to die, and so he may suffer more than he would if more direct action were taken and a lethal injection given. This fact provides strong reason for thinking that, once the initial decision not to prolong his agony has been made, active euthanasia is actually preferable to passive euthanasia, rather than the reverse. To say otherwise is to endorse the option that leads to more suffering rather than less, and is contrary to the humanitarian impulse that prompts the decision not to prolong his life in the first place.

Part of my point is that the process of being "allowed to die" can be relatively slow and painful, whereas being given a lethal injection is relatively quick and painless. Let me give a different sort of example. In the United States about one in 600 babies is born with Down's syndrome. Most of these babies are otherwise

Reprinted by permission from the *New England Journal of Medicine*, vol. 292, no. 2 (January 9, 1975), pp. 78–80.

healthy—that is, with only the usual pediatric care, they will proceed to an otherwise normal infancy. Some, however, are born with congenital defects such as intestinal obstructions that require operations if they are to live. Sometimes, the parents and the doctor will decide not to operate, and let the infant die. Anthony Shaw describes what happens then:

> . . . When surgery is denied [the doctor] must try to keep the infant from suffering while natural forces sap the baby's life away. As a surgeon whose natural inclination is to use the scalpel to fight off death, standing by and watching a salvageable baby die is the most emotionally exhausting experience I know. It is easy at a conference, in a theoretical discussion, to decide that such infants should be allowed to die. It is altogether different to stand by in the nursery and watch as dehydration and infection wither a tiny being over hours and days. This is a terrible ordeal for me and the hospital staff—much more so than for the parents who never set foot in the nursery.[1]

I can understand why some people are opposed to all euthanasia, and insist that such infants must be allowed to live. I think I can also understand why other people favor destroying these babies quickly and painlessly. But why should anyone favor letting "dehydration and infection wither a tiny being over hours and days"? The doctrine that says that a baby may be allowed to dehydrate and wither, but may not be given an injection that would end its life without suffering, seems so patently cruel as to require no further refutation. The strong language is not intended to offend, but only to put the point in the clearest possible way.

My second argument is that the conventional doctrine leads to decisions concerning life and death made on irrelevant grounds.

Consider again the case of the infants with Down's syndrome who need operations for congenital defects unrelated to the syndrome to live. Sometimes, there is no operation, and the baby dies, but when there is no such defect, the baby lives on. Now, an operation such as that to remove an intestinal obstruction is not prohibitively difficult. The reason why such operations are not performed in these cases is, clearly, that the child has Down's syndrome and the parents and doctor judge that because of that fact it is better for the child to die.

But notice that this situation is absurd, no matter what view one takes of the lives and potentials of such babies. If the life of such an infant is worth preserving, what does it matter if it needs a simple operation? Or, if one thinks it better that such a baby should not live

on, what difference does it make that it happens to have an unobstructed intestinal tract? In either case, the matter of life and death is being decided on irrelevant grounds. It is the Down's syndrome, and not the intestines, that is the issue. The matter should be decided, if at all, on that basis, and not be allowed to depend on the essentially irrelevant question of whether the intestinal tract is blocked.

What makes this situation possible, of course, is the idea that when there is an intestinal blockage, one can "let the baby die," but when there is no such defect there is nothing that can be done, for one must not "kill" it. The fact that this idea leads to such results as deciding life or death on irrelevant grounds is another good reason why the doctrine should be rejected.

One reason why so many people think that there is an important moral difference between active and passive euthanasia is that they think killing someone is morally worse than letting someone die. But is it? Is killing, in itself, worse than letting die? To investigate this issue, two cases may be considered that are exactly alike except that one involves killing whereas the other involves letting someone die. Then, it can be asked whether this difference makes any difference to the moral assessments. It is important that the cases be exactly alike, except for this one difference, since otherwise one cannot be confident that it is this difference and not some other that accounts for any variation in the assessments of the two cases. So, let us consider this pair of cases:

In the first, Smith stands to gain a large inheritance if anything should happen to his six-year-old cousin. One evening while the child is taking his bath, Smith sneaks into the bathroom and drowns the child, and then arranges things so that it will look like an accident.

In the second, Jones also stands to gain if anything should happen to his six-year-old cousin. Like Smith, Jones sneaks in planning to drown the child in his bath. However, just as he enters the bathroom Jones sees the child slip and hit his head, and fall face down in the water. Jones is delighted; he stands by, ready to push the child's head back under if it is necessary, but it is not necessary. With only a little thrashing about, the child drowns all by himself, "accidentally," as Jones watches and does nothing.

Now Smith killed the child, whereas Jones "merely" let the child die. That is the only difference between them. Did either man behave better, from a moral point of view? If the difference between killing and letting die were in itself a morally important matter, one should say that Jones's behavior was less reprehensible than Smith's. But does one really want to say that? I think not. In the first place, both men acted from the same motive, personal gain, and both had exactly the same end in view when they acted. It may be inferred from Smith's conduct that he is a bad man, although that judgment may be withdrawn or modified if certain further facts are learned about him—for example, that he is mentally deranged. But would not the very same thing be inferred about Jones from his conduct? And would not the same further considerations also be relevant to any modification of this judgment? Moreover, suppose Jones pleaded, in his own defense, "After all, I didn't do anything except just stand there and watch the child drown. I didn't kill him; I only let him die." Again, if letting die were in itself less bad than killing, this defense should have at least some weight. But it does not. Such a "defense" can only be regarded as a grotesque perversion of moral reasoning. Morally speaking, it is no defense at all.

Now, it may be pointed out, quite properly, that the cases of euthanasia with which doctors are concerned are not like this at all. They do not involve personal gain or the destruction of normal, healthy children. Doctors are concerned only with cases in which the patient's life is of no further use to him, or in which the patient's life has become or will soon become a terrible burden. However, the point is the same in these cases: the bare difference between killing and letting die does not, in itself, make a moral difference. If a doctor lets a patient die, for humane reasons, he is in the same moral position as if he had given the patient a lethal injection for humane reasons. If his decision was wrong—if, for example, the patient's illness was in fact curable—the decision would be equally regrettable no matter which method was used to carry it out. And if the doctor's decision was the right one, the method used is not in itself important.

The AMA policy statement isolates the crucial issue very well; the crucial issue is "the intentional termination of the life of one human being by another." But after identifying this issue, and forbidding "mercy killing," the statement goes on to deny that the cessation of treatment is the intentional termination of life. This is where the mistake comes in, for what is the cessation of treatment, in these circumstances, if it is not "the intentional termination of the life of one human being by another"? Of course it is exactly that, and if it were not, there would be no point to it.

Many people will find this judgment hard to accept. One reason, I think, is that it is very easy to conflate the question of whether killing is, in itself, worse than letting die, with the very different question of whether most actual cases of killing are more reprehensible than most actual cases of letting die. Most actual cases of killing are clearly terrible (think, for example, of all the murders reported in the newspapers), and one hears of such cases every day. On the other hand, one hardly ever hears of a case of letting die, except for the actions of doctors who are motivated by humanitarian reasons. So one learns to think of killing in a much worse light than of letting die. But this does not mean that there is something about killing that makes it in itself worse than letting die, for it is not the bare difference between killing and letting die that makes the difference in these cases. Rather, the other factors—the murderer's motive of personal gain, for example, contrasted with the doctor's humanitarian motivation—account for different reactions to the different cases.

I have argued that killing is not in itself any worse than letting die; if my contention is right, it follows that active euthanasia is not any worse than passive euthanasia. What arguments can be given on the other side? The most common, I believe, is the following:

"The important difference between active and passive euthanasia is that, in passive euthanasia, the doctor does not do anything to bring about the patient's death. The doctor does nothing, and the patient dies of whatever ills already afflict him. In active euthanasia, however, the doctor does something to bring about the patient's death: he kills him. The doctor who gives the patient with cancer a lethal injection has himself caused his patient's death; whereas if he merely ceases treatment, the cancer is the cause of the death."

A number of points need to be made here. The first is that it is not exactly correct to say that in passive euthanasia the doctor does nothing, for he does do one thing that is very important: he lets the patient die. "Letting someone die" is certainly different, in some respects, from other types of action—mainly in that it is a kind of action that one may perform by way of not performing certain other actions. For example, one may let a patient die by way of not giving medication, just as one may insult someone by way of not shaking his hand. But for any purpose of moral assessment, it is a type of action nonetheless. The decision to let a patient die is subject to moral appraisal in the same way that a decision to kill him would be subject to moral appraisal: it may be assessed as wise or unwise, compassionate or sadistic, right or wrong. If a doctor deliberately let a patient die who was suffering from a routinely curable illness, the doctor would certainly be to blame for what he had done, just as he would be to blame if he had needlessly killed the patient. Charges against him would then be appropriate. If so, it would be no defense at all for him to insist that he didn't "do anything." He would have done something very serious indeed, for he let his patient die.

Fixing the cause of death may be very important from a legal point of view, for it may determine whether criminal charges are brought against the doctor. But I do not think that this notion can be used to show a moral difference between active and passive euthanasia. The reason why it is considered bad to be the cause of someone's death is that death is regarded as a great evil—and so it is. However, if it has been decided that euthanasia—even passive euthanasia—is desirable in a given case, it has also been decided that in this instance death is no greater an evil than the patient's continued existence. And if this is true, the usual reason for not wanting to be the cause of someone's death simply does not apply.

Finally, doctors may think that all of this is only of academic interest—the sort of thing that philosophers may worry about but that has no practical bearing on their own work. After all, doctors must be concerned about the legal consequences of what they do, and active euthanasia is clearly forbidden by the law. But even so, doctors should also be concerned with the fact that the law is forcing upon them a moral doctrine that may well be indefensible, and has a considerable effect on their practices. Of course, most doctors are not now in the position of being coerced in this matter, for they do not regard themselves as merely going along with what the law requires. Rather, in statements such as the AMA policy statement that I have quoted, they are endorsing this doctrine as a central point of medical ethics. In that statement, active euthanasia is condemned not merely as illegal but as "contrary to that for which the medical profession stands," whereas passive euthanasia is approved. However, the preceding considerations suggest that there is really no moral difference between the two, considered in themselves (there may be important moral differences in some cases in their *consequences,* but, as I pointed out, these differences may make active euthanasia, and not passive euthanasia, the morally preferable option). So, whereas doctors may have to discriminate between active and passive euthanasia to satisfy the law, they should not do any more than that. In particular, they should not give the distinction any added authority and weight by writing it into official statements of medical ethics.

NOTE

1 Shaw A.: "Doctor, Do We Have a Choice?" *The New York Times Magazine,* January 30, 1972, p. 54.

Killing and Allowing to Die
Daniel Callahan

Daniel Callahan, a philosopher, is president of The Hastings Center, which he cofounded in 1969. His numerous publications reflect an enduring concern with issues in biomedical ethics. He is, for example, the author of *Setting Limits: Medical Goals in an Aging Society* (1987), *What Kind of Life: The Limits of Medical Progress* (1990), and *The Troubled Dream of Life: Living with Mortality* (1993).

Callahan maintains that there is a valid distinction between killing and allowing to die, and he defends the distinction by reference to three overlapping perspectives—metaphysical, moral, and medical. In terms of a metaphysical perspective, Callahan emphasizes that the external world is distinct from the self and has its own causal dynamism. In terms of a moral

Reprinted with permission of the author and the publisher from *Hastings Center Report,* vol. 19 (January/February 1989), Special Supplement, pp. 5–6. © The Hastings Center.

perspective, he emphasizes the difference between *physical causality* and *moral culpability*. In conjunction with a medical perspective, he insists that killing patients is incompatible with the role of the physician in society.

. . . No valid distinction, many now argue, can be made between killing and allowing to die, or between an act of commission and one of omission. The standard distinction being challenged rests on the commonplace observation that lives can come to an end as the result of: (a) the direct action of another who becomes the cause of death (as in shooting a person), and (b) the result of impersonal forces where no human agent has acted (death by lightning, or by disease). The purpose of the distinction has been to separate those deaths caused by human action, and those caused by nonhuman events. It is, as a distinction, meant to say something about human beings and their relationship to the world. It is a way of articulating the difference between those actions for which human beings can be held rightly responsible, or blamed, and those of which they are innocent. At issue is the difference between physical causality, the realm of impersonal events, and moral culpability, the realm of human responsibility.

The challenges encompass two points. The first is that people can become equally dead by our omissions as well as our commissions. We can refrain from saving them when it is possible to do so, and they will be just as dead as if we shot them. It is our decision itself that is the reason for their death, not necessarily how we effectuate that decision. That fact establishes the basis of the second point: if we *intend* their death, it can be brought about as well by omitted acts as by those we commit. The crucial moral point is not how they die, but our intention about their death. We can, then, be responsible for the death of another by intending that they die and accomplish that end by standing aside and allowing them to die.

Despite these criticisms—resting upon ambiguities that can readily be acknowledged—the distinction between killing and allowing to die remains, I contend, perfectly valid. It not only has a logical validity but, no less importantly, a social validity whose place must be central in moral judgments. As a way of putting the distinction into perspective, I want to suggest that it is best understood as expressing three different, though overlapping, perspectives on nature and human action. I will call them the metaphysical, the moral, and the medical perspectives.

Metaphysical The first and most fundamental premise of the distinction between killing and allowing to die is that there is a sharp difference between the self and the external world. Unlike the childish fantasy that the world is nothing more than a projection of the self, or the neurotic person's fear that he or she is responsible for everything that goes wrong, the distinction is meant to uphold a simple notion: there is a world external to the self that has its own, and independent, causal dynamism. The mistake behind a conflation of killing and allowing to die is to assume that the self has become master of everything within and outside of the self. It is as if the conceit that modern man might ultimately control nature has been internalized: that, if the self might be able to influence nature by its actions, then the self and nature must be one.

Of course that is a fantasy. The fact that we can intervene in nature, and cure or control many diseases, does not erase the difference between the self and the external world. It is as "out there" as ever, even if more under our sway. That sway, however great, is always limited. We can cure disease, but not always the chronic illness that comes with the cure. We can forestall death with modern medicine, but death always wins in the long run because of the innate limitations of the body, inherently and stubbornly beyond final human control. And we can distinguish between a diseased body and an aging body, but in the end if we wait long enough they always become one and the same body. To attempt to deny the distinction between killing and allowing to die is, then, mistakenly to impute more power to human action than it actually has and to accept the conceit that nature has now fallen wholly within the realm of human control. Not so.

Moral At the center of the distinction between killing and allowing to die is the difference between physical causality and moral culpability. To bring the life of another to an end by an injection kills the other directly; our action is the physical cause of the death. To allow someone to die from a disease we cannot cure (and that we did not cause) is to permit the disease to act as the cause of death. The notion of physical causality in both cases rests on the difference between human agency and the action of external nature. The ambiguity arises precisely because we can be morally culpable for killing someone (if we have no moral right to do so, as we would in self-defense) and no less culpable for allowing someone to die (if we have both the possibility and the obligation of keeping that person alive). Thus there are cases where, morally speaking, it makes no difference whether we killed or allowed to die; we are equally responsible. In those instances, the lines of physical causality and moral culpability happen to cross. Yet the fact that they can cross in some cases in no way shows that they are always, or even usually, one and the same. We can normally find the difference in all but the most obscure cases. We should not, then, use the ambiguity of such cases to do away altogether with the distinction between killing and allowing to die. The ambiguity may obscure, but does not erase, the line between the two.

There is one group of ambiguous cases that is especially troublesome. Even if we grant the ordinary validity between killing and allowing to die, what about those cases that combine (a) an illness that renders a patient unable to carry out an ordinary biological function (to breathe or eat on his own, for example), and (b) our turning off a respirator or removing an artificial feeding tube? On the level of physical causality, have we killed the patient or allowed him to die? In one sense, it is our action that shortens his life, and yet in another sense his underlying disease brings his life to an end. I believe it reasonable to say that, since his life was being sustained by artificial means (respirator or feeding tube) made necessary because of the fact that he had an incapacitating disease, his disease is the ultimate reality behind his death. But for its reality, there would be no need for artificial sustenance in the first place and no moral issue at all. To lose sight of the paramount reality of the disease is to lose sight of the difference between our selves and the outer world.

I quickly add, and underscore, a moral point: the person who, without good moral reason, turns off a respirator or pulls a feeding tube, can be morally culpable; that the patient has been allowed to die of his underlying condition does not morally excuse him. The moral question is whether we are obliged to continue treating a life that is being artificially sustained. To cease treatment may or may not be morally acceptable; but it should be understood, in either case, that the physical cause of death was the underlying disease.

Medical   An important social purpose of the distinction between killing and allowing to die has been that of protecting the historical role of the physician as one who tries to cure or comfort patients rather than to kill patients. Physicians have been given special knowledge about the body, knowledge that can be used to kill or to cure. They are also given great privileges in making use of that knowledge. It is thus all the more important that physicians' social role and power be, and be seen to be, a limited power. It may be used only to cure or comfort, never to kill. They have not been given, nor should they be given, the power to use their knowledge and skills to bring life to an end. It would open the way for powerful misuse and, no less importantly, represent an intrinsic violation of what it has meant to be a physician.

Yet if it is possible for physicians to misuse their knowledge and power to kill people directly, are they thereby required to use that same knowledge always to keep people alive, always to resist a disease that can itself kill the patient? The traditional answer has been: not necessarily. For the physician's ultimate obligation is to the welfare of the patient, and excessive treatment can be as detrimental to that welfare as inadequate treatment. Put another way, the obligation to resist the lethal power of disease is limited—it ceases when the patient is unwilling to have it resisted, or where the resistance no longer serves the patient's welfare. Behind this moral premise is the recognition that disease (of some kind) ultimately triumphs and that death is both inevitable sooner or later and not, in any case, always the greatest human evil. To demand of the physician that he always struggle against disease, as if it was in his power always to conquer it, would be to fall into the same metaphysical trap mentioned above: that of assuming that no distinction can be drawn between natural and human agency.

A final word. I suggested [in an earlier discussion] that the most potent motive for active euthanasia and assisted suicide stems from a dread of the power of medicine. That power then seems to take on a drive of its own regardless of the welfare or wishes of patients. No one can easily say no—not physicians, not patients, not families. My guess is that happens because too many have already come to believe that it is their choice, and their choice alone, which brings about death; and they do not want to exercise that kind of authority. The solution is not to erase the distinction between killing and allowing to die, but to underscore its validity and importance. We can bring disease as a cause of death back into the care of the dying.

Voluntary Active Euthanasia
Dan W. Brock

A biographical sketch of Dan W. Brock is found on page 100.

In this excerpt from a much longer article, Brock argues that two fundamental ethical values support the ethical permissibility of voluntary active euthanasia. These values are individual self-determination (autonomy) and individual well-being, the same two values that support the consensus view that patients have a right to make decisions about life-sustaining treatment. Brock also argues that allowing physicians to perform euthanasia is not incompatible with the "moral center" of medicine.

. . . The central ethical argument for [voluntary active] euthanasia is familiar. It is that the very same two fundamental ethical values supporting the consensus on patient's rights to decide about life-sustaining treatment also support the ethical permissibility of euthanasia. These values are individual self-determination or autonomy and individual well-being. By self-determination as it bears on euthanasia, I mean people's interest in making important decisions about their lives for themselves according to their own values or conceptions of a good life, and in being left free to act on those decisions. Self-determination is valuable because it permits people to form and live in accordance with their own conception of a good life, at least within the bounds of justice and consistent with others doing so as well. In exercising self-determination people take responsibility for their lives and for the kinds of persons they become. A central aspect of human dignity lies in people's capacity to direct their lives in this way. The value of exercising self-determination presupposes some minimum of decision-making capacities or competence, which thus limits the scope of euthanasia supported by self-determination; it cannot justifiably be administered, for example, in cases of serious dementia or treatable clinical depression.

Does the value of individual self-determination extend to the time and manner of one's death? Most people are very concerned about the nature of the last stage of their lives. This reflects not just a fear of experiencing substantial suffering when dying, but also a desire to retain dignity and control during this last period of life. Death is today increasingly preceded by a long period of significant physical and mental decline, due in part to the technological interventions of modern medicine. Many people adjust to these disabilities and find meaning and value in new activities and ways. Others find the impairments and burdens in the last stage of their lives at some point sufficiently great to make life no longer worth living. For many patients near death, maintaining the quality of one's life, avoiding great suffering, maintaining one's dignity, and insuring that others remember us as we wish them to, become of paramount importance and outweigh merely extending one's life. But there is no single, objectively correct answer for everyone as to when, if at all, one's life becomes all things considered a burden and unwanted. If self-determination is a fundamental value, then the great variability among people on this question makes it especially important that individuals control the manner, circumstances, and timing of their dying and death.

The other main value that supports euthanasia is individual well-being. It might seem that individual well-being conflicts with a person's self-determination when the person requests euthanasia. Life itself is commonly taken to be a central good for persons, often valued for its own sake, as well as necessary for pursuit of all other goods within a life. But when a competent patient decides to forgo all further life-sustaining treatment then the patient, either explicitly or implicitly, commonly decides that the best life possible for him or her with treatment is of sufficiently poor quality that it is worse than no further life at all. Life is no longer considered a benefit by the patient, but has now become a burden. The same judgment underlies a request for euthanasia: continued life is seen by the patient as no longer a benefit, but now a burden. Especially in the often severely compromised and debilitated states of many critically ill or dying patients, there is no objective standard, but only the competent patient's judgment of whether continued life is no longer a benefit.

Of course, sometimes there are conditions, such as

Reprinted with permission of the author and the publisher from *Hastings Center Report*, vol. 22 (March/April 1992), pp. 16, 20. © The Hastings Center.

clinical depression, that call into question whether the patient has made a competent choice, either to forgo life-sustaining treatment or to seek euthanasia, and then the patient's choice need not be evidence that continued life is no longer a benefit for him or her. Just as with decisions about treatment, a determination of incompetence can warrant not honoring the patient's choice; in the case of treatment, we then transfer decisional authority to a surrogate, though in the case of voluntary active euthanasia a determination that the patient is incompetent means that choice is not possible.

The value or right of self-determination does not entitle patients to compel physicians to act contrary to their own moral or professional values. Physicians are moral and professional agents whose own self-determination or integrity should be respected as well. If performing euthanasia became legally permissible, but conflicted with a particular physician's reasonable understanding of his or her moral or professional responsibilities, the care of a patient who requested euthanasia should be transferred to another. . . .

. . . Permitting physicians to perform euthanasia, it is said, would be incompatible with their fundamental moral and professional commitment as healers to care for patients and to protect life. Moreover, if euthanasia by physicians became common, patients would come to fear that a medication was intended not to treat or care, but instead to kill, and would thus lose trust in their physicians. This position was forcefully stated in a paper by Willard Gaylin and his colleagues:

> The very soul of medicine is on trial . . . This issue touches medicine at its moral center; if this moral center collapses, if physicians become killers or are even licensed to kill, the profession—and, therewith, each physician—will never again be worthy of trust and respect as healer and comforter and protector of life in all its frailty.

These authors go on to make clear that, while they oppose permitting anyone to perform euthanasia, their special concern is with physicians doing so:

> We call on fellow physicians to say that they will not deliberately kill. We must also say to each of our fellow physicians that we will not tolerate killing of patients and that we shall take disciplinary action against doctors who kill. And we must say to the broader community that if it insists on tolerating or legalizing active euthanasia, it will have to find nonphysicians to do its killing.[1]

If permitting physicians to kill would undermine the very "moral center" of medicine, then almost certainly physicians should not be permitted to perform euthanasia. But how persuasive is this claim? Patients should not fear, as a consequence of permitting *voluntary* active euthanasia, that their physicians will substitute a lethal injection for what patients want and believe is part of their care. If active euthanasia is restricted to cases in which it is truly voluntary, then no patient should fear getting it unless she or he has voluntarily requested it. (The fear that we might in time also come to accept nonvoluntary, or even involuntary, active euthanasia is a slippery slope worry I address [in a later section].) Patients' trust of their physicians could be increased, not eroded, by knowledge that physicians will provide aid in dying when patients seek it.

Might Gaylin and his colleagues nevertheless be correct in their claim that the moral center of medicine would collapse if physicians were to become killers? This question raises what at the deepest level should be the guiding aims of medicine, a question that obviously cannot be fully explored here. But I do want to say enough to indicate the direction that I believe an appropriate response to this challenge should take. In spelling out above what I called the positive argument for voluntary active euthanasia, I suggested that two principal values—respecting patients' self-determination and promoting their well-being—underlie the consensus that competent patients, or the surrogates of incompetent patients, are entitled to refuse any life-sustaining treatment and to choose from among available alternative treatments. It is the commitment to these two values in guiding physicians' actions as healers, comforters, and protectors of their patients' lives that should be at the "moral center" of medicine, and these two values support physicians' administering euthanasia when their patients make competent requests for it.

What should not be at that moral center is a commitment to preserving patients' lives as such, without regard to whether those patients want their lives preserved or judge their preservation a benefit to them. . . .

REFERENCE

1 Willard Gaylin, Leon R. Kass, Edmund D. Pellegrino, and Mark Siegler, "Doctors Must Not Kill," *JAMA* 259 (1988): 2139–40.

Active Euthanasia, Physician-Assisted Suicide, and Social Policy

Euthanasia: The Way We Do It, The Way They Do It
Margaret P. Battin

Margaret P. Battin is professor of philosophy at the University of Utah. She is the author of *Ethical Issues in Suicide* (1982; 1995) and *Ethics in the Sanctuary: Examining the Practices of Organized Religion* (1990). Many of her published articles are collected in *The Least Worst Death: Essays in Bioethics on the End of Life* (1994).

Battin identifies three cultural models for dealing with dying. In the United States, there is an exclusive emphasis placed on the withholding or withdrawing of life-sustaining treatment. In the Netherlands (Holland), voluntary active euthanasia is an available option. In Germany, active euthanasia is prohibited, and physicians themselves are expected not to assist in a patient's suicide, but assisted suicide outside of a medical setting is an option that is legally available. Battin discusses various objections and problems associated with each of these cultural models. In the end, she argues, none of these models is well suited for the United States at this point in time. Taking into account the specific characteristics of contemporary life in the United States, she ultimately recommends the practice of permitting physician-assisted suicide.

Because we tend to be rather myopic in our discussions of death and dying, especially about the issues of active euthanasia and assisted suicide, it is valuable to place the question of how we go about dying in an international context. We do not always see that our own cultural norms may be quite different from those of other nations, and that our background assumptions and actual practices differ dramatically. Thus, I would like to examine the perspectives on end-of-life dilemmas in three countries, Holland, (West) Germany,* and the USA.

Holland, Germany, and the United States are all advanced industrial democracies. They all have sophisticated medical establishments and life expectancies over 70 years of age; their populations are all characterized by an increasing proportion of older persons. They are all in what has been called the fourth stage of the epidemiologic transition[1]—that stage of societal development in which it is no longer the case that most people die of acute parasitic or infectious diseases. In this stage, most people do not die of diseases with rapid, unpredictable onsets and sharp fatality curves; rather, the majority of the population—as much as

Reprinted, in a version slightly updated by the author, by permission of Elsevier Science Inc. from the *Journal of Pain and Symptom Management*, vol. 6, no. 5, pp. 298–305. Copyright 1991 by the U.S. Cancer Pain Relief Committee.

perhaps 70%–80%—dies of degenerative diseases, especially delayed degenerative diseases, that are characterized by late, slow onset and extended decline. Most people in highly industrialized countries die from cancer, atherosclerosis, heart disease (by no means always suddenly fatal), chronic obstructive pulmonary disease, liver, kidney or other organ disease, or degenerative neurological disorders. Thus, all three of these countries are alike in facing a common problem: how to deal with the characteristic new ways in which we die.

DEALING WITH DYING IN THE UNITED STATES

In the United States, we have come to recognize that the maximal extension of life-prolonging treatment in these late-life degenerative conditions is often inappropriate. Although we could keep the machines and tubes—the respirators, intravenous lines, feeding tubes—hooked up for extended periods, we recognize that this is inhumane, pointless, and financially impossible. Instead, as a society we have developed a number of mechanisms for dealing with these hopeless situations, all of which involve withholding or withdrawing various forms of treatment.

Some mechanisms for withholding or withdrawing

treatment are exercised by the patient who is confronted by such a situation or who anticipates it; these include refusal of treatment, the patient-executed DNR order, the Living Will, and the Durable Power of Attorney. Others are mechanisms for decision by second parties about a patient who is no longer competent or never was competent. The latter are reflected in a long series of court cases, including *Quinlan, Saikewicz, Spring, Eichner, Barber, Bartling, Conroy, Brophy,* the trio *Farrell, Peter* and *Jobes,* and *Cruzan.* These are cases that attempt to delineate the precise circumstances under which it is appropriate to withhold or withdraw various forms of therapy, including respiratory support, chemotherapy, antibiotics in intercurrent infections, and artificial nutrition and hydration. Thus, during the past 15 years or so, roughly since *Quinlan* (1976), we have developed an impressive body of case law and state statute that protects, permits, and facilitates our characteristic American strategy of dealing with end-of-life situations. These cases provide a framework for withholding or withdrawing treatment when we believe there is no medical or moral point in going on. This is sometimes termed *passive euthanasia;* more often, it is simply called *allowing to die,* and is ubiquitous in the United States.

For example, a recent study by Miles and Gomez indicates that some 85% of deaths in the United States occur in health-care institutions, including hospitals, nursing homes, and other facilities, and of these, about 70% involve electively withholding some form of life-sustaining treatment.[2] A 1989 study cited in the *Journal of the American Medical Association* claims that 85%–90% of critical care professionals state that they are withholding and withdrawing life-sustaining treatments from patients who are "deemed to have irreversible disease and are terminally ill."[3] Still another study identified some 115 patients in two intensive-care units from whom care was withheld or withdrawn; 110 were already incompetent by the time the decision to limit care was made. The 89 who died while still in the intensive-care unit accounted for 45% of all deaths there.[4] It is estimated that 1.3 million American deaths a year follow decisions to withhold life support;[5] this is a majority of the just over 2 million American deaths per year. Withholding and withdrawing treatment is the way we in the USA go about dealing with dying, and indeed "allowing to die" is the only legally protected alternative to maximal treatment recognized in the United States. We do not legally permit ourselves to actively cause death.

DEALING WITH DYING IN HOLLAND

In the Netherlands, voluntary active euthanasia is also an available response to end-of-life situations. Although active euthanasia remains prohibited by statutory law, it is protected by a series of lower and supreme court decisions and is widely regarded as legal, or, more precisely, *gedoeken,* legally "tolerated." These court decisions have the effect of protecting the physician who performs euthanasia from prosecution, provided the physician meets a rigorous set of guidelines.

These guidelines, variously stated, contain five central provisions:

1. that the patient's request be voluntary;

2. that the patient be undergoing intolerable suffering;

3. that all alternatives acceptable to the patient for relieving the suffering have been tried;

4. that the patient has full information;

5. that the physician has consulted with a second physician whose judgment can be expected to be independent.

Of these criteria, it is the first which is central: euthanasia may be performed only at the voluntary request of the patient. This criterion is also understood to require that the patient's request be a stable, enduring, reflective one—not the product of a transitory impulse. Every attempt is to be made to rule out depression, psychopathology, pressures from family members, unrealistic fears, and other factors compromising voluntariness. In general, pain is not the basis for euthanasia, since pain can, in most cases, be effectively treated; "intolerable suffering," understood to mean suffering that is in the patient's (rather than the physician's) view intolerable, may also include fear of or unwillingness to endure *entluisterung,* or that gradual effacement and loss of personal identity that characterizes the end stages of many terminal illnesses. It is also required that euthanasia be performed only by a physician; it may not be performed by a nurse, family member, or other party.

Until 1990, the physician who performed euthanasia was supposed to report it to the police or the Ministry of Justice, which would then decide if the case should be prosecuted. Not surprisingly, self-reports were comparatively few: just 454 in that year. With changes in the law, a physician now reports directly to the medical examiner, not the police, and the rate of reporting has been climbing. Although speculation concerning the actual number of cases had been rampant, ranging anywhere from 2,000 to 20,000 cases a year, a major empirical study published in 1991, the Remmelink Commission report, revealed that there are in fact around 2,300 cases of euthanasia per year (about 1.8% of the total annual mortality) and another 400 cases of physician-assisted suicide (0.3% of the annual mortality).[6] There are also about 1,000 cases (0.8% of the annual mortality) of what the Dutch call "life-terminating acts without explicit request," or LAWER, of which about 600 involved competent or incompetent patients who had previously made informal requests ("Doctor, please don't let me suffer too long") and about 400 involved patients, all incompetent, in severe suffering and very close to death.[7] Although a substantial proportion of patients, about 25,000 a year, seek their doctors' reassurance of assistance if their suffering becomes unbearable, only 9,000 explicit requests for euthanasia are made annually, and of these, fewer than one-third are honored. Euthanasia is performed in about 1:25 of deaths that occur at home, about 1:75 hospital deaths, and about 1:800 nursing home deaths.[8]

More than half (54%) of Dutch physicians report that they have performed euthanasia; 34% say they would be prepared to do so if the occasion arose; and 12% say they have not and would never do so. If euthanasia deaths were distributed equally (which they are not) among the Netherlands' 30,000 physicians, this would mean that only 1 in every 12 or 13 physicians would perform a case of euthanasia in a given year, or that a given physician would perform euthanasia once or at most twice in a decade of practice. But although euthanasia is comparatively rare, it is nevertheless a conspicuous alternative to terminal illness well known to both physicians and the general public. Surveys of public opinion have shown growing public support for a liberal euthanasia policy (increasing from 40% in 1966 to a high of 81% in 1988), and while there is a vocal minority opposed to the practice, including some physicians, both the majority of the population in the Netherlands and the majority of Dutch physicians support it.

In Holland, many hospitals now have protocols for the performance of euthanasia; these serve to ensure that the court-established guidelines have been met. However, most euthanasia is practiced in the patient's home, typically by the *huisarts* or general practitioner who is the patient's long-term family physician.

Euthanasia is usually performed after aggressive hospital treatment has failed to arrest the patient's terminal illness; the patient has come home to die, and the family physician is prepared to ease this passing. Whether practiced at home or in the hospital, euthanasia often takes place in the presence of the family members, perhaps the visiting nurse, and often, the patient's pastor or priest, with the doctor in continuous attendance. Many doctors say that performing euthanasia is never easy, but that it is something they believe a doctor ought to do for his or her patient, when nothing else can help.

Thus, in Holland a patient facing the end of life has an option not openly practiced in the United States: to ask the physician to bring his or her life to an end. Although not everyone does so—indeed, over 97% of people who die in a given year do not—it is a choice widely understood as available.

FACING DEATH IN GERMANY

In part because of its very painful history of Nazism, Germany appears to believe that doctors should have no role in causing death. Although societal generalizations are always risky, it is fair to say that there is vigorous and nearly universal opposition in Germany to the notion of active euthanasia. Euthanasia is viewed as always wrong, and the Germans view the Dutch as stepping out on a dangerously slippery slope.

However, although under German law killing on request, including active euthanasia, is illegal, German law has not prohibited assistance in suicide since the time of Frederick the Great (1751)—provided the person committing suicide is determined to do so, and is both competent and in control of his or her actions. Taking advantage of this situation, there has developed a private organization, the *Deutsche Gesellschaft für Humanes Sterben* (DGHS), or German Society for Humane Dying, which has openly provided support to its very extensive membership in choosing suicide as an alternative to terminal illness.[9] Although in the wake of a recent scandal concerning its former president and under the threat of more restrictive federal legislation the DGHS's activities are currently being redirected towards promoting living wills and other advance directives, the DGHS has for many years provided information about suicide, assisted its members in gaining access to the means for suicide, and, if requested, has provided *Sterbebegleitung* or "accompaniment in dying" for the person about to commit suicide, sending someone to be with the person who takes a fatal dose, especially if that person is alone or does not have a family supportive of such a choice. These practices all take place outside the medical system.

Furthermore, these practices are supported by a feature of German language that makes it possible to conceptualize them in more benign ways: while English, French, Spanish, and many other languages have just a single primary word for suicide, German has four: *Selbstmord, Selbstötung, Suizid,* and *Freitod,* of which the latter has comparatively positive, even somewhat heroic connotations. Thus Germans can think about the deliberate termination of their lives in a linguistic way not easily available to speakers of other languages, and the DGHS has consistently used *Freitod* rather than the language's other, more negative terms to describe the practice with which it provides assistance. No reliable figures are available about the number of suicides with which this organization has assisted, but it is fair to say, both because of the existence of this organization and the different conceptual horizons of German-speakers, that the option of self-produced death outside the medical system is more clearly open in Germany than it has been in the Netherlands or the United States.

OBJECTIONS TO THE THREE MODELS OF DYING

In response to the dilemmas raised by the new circumstances of death, in which the majority of the population in each of the advanced industrial nations dies of degenerative diseases after an extended period of terminal deterioration, different countries develop different practices. The United States legally permits only withholding and withdrawal of treatment, though of course active euthanasia and assisted suicide do occur. Holland also permits voluntary active euthanasia, and although Germany rejects euthanasia, it tolerates assisted suicide. But there are serious moral objections to be made to each of these practices, objections to be considered before resolving the issue of which practice our own culture ought to adopt.

Objections to the German Practice

German law does not prohibit assisting suicide, but postwar German culture discourages physicians from

taking any active role in death. This gives rise to distinctive moral problems. For one thing, it appears that there is little professional help or review provided for patients' choices about suicide; because the patient makes this choice essentially outside the medical establishment, medical professionals are not in a position to detect or treat impaired judgment on the part of the patient, especially judgment impaired by depression. Similarly, if the patient must commit suicide assisted only by persons outside the medical profession, there are risks that the patient's diagnosis and prognosis are inadequately confirmed, that the means chosen for suicide will be unreliable or inappropriately used, that the means used for suicide will fall into the hands of other persons, and that the patient will fail to recognize or be able to resist intrafamilial pressures and manipulation. The DGHS policy for providing assistance has required that the patient be terminally ill and have been a member of the DGHS for at least 1 year in order to make use of its services, the latter requirement intended to provide evidence of the stability of such a choice, but these minimal requirements are hardly sufficient to answer the charge that suicide decisions, which are made for medical reasons but must be made without medical help, may be rendered under less than ideally informed and voluntary conditions.

Objections to the Dutch Practice

The Dutch practice of physician-performed active voluntary euthanasia also raises a number of ethical issues, many of which have been discussed vigorously both in the Dutch press and in commentary on the Dutch practices from abroad. For one thing, it is sometimes said that the availability of physician-performed euthanasia creates a disincentive for providing good terminal care. I have seen no evidence that this is the case; on the contrary, Peter Admiraal, the anesthesiologist who is perhaps Holland's most vocal proponent of voluntary active euthanasia, insists that pain should rarely or never be the occasion for euthanasia, as pain (in contrast to suffering) is comparatively easily treated.[10] Instead, it is a refusal to endure the final stages of deterioration, both mental and physical, that motivates requests.

It is also sometimes said that active euthanasia violates the Hippocratic Oath. Indeed, it is true that the original Greek version of the Oath prohibits the physician from giving a deadly drug, even when asked for it;

but the original version also prohibits performing surgery and taking fees for teaching medicine, neither of which prohibitions has survived into contemporary medical practice. Dutch physicians often say that they see performing euthanasia—where it is genuinely requested by the patient and nothing else can be done to relieve the patient's condition—as part of their duty to the patient, not as a violation of it.

The Dutch are also often said to be at risk of starting down the slippery slope, that is, that the practice of voluntary active euthanasia for patients who meet the criteria will erode into practicing less-than-voluntary euthanasia on patients whose problems are not irremediable, and perhaps by gradual degrees develop into terminating the lives of people who are elderly, chronically ill, handicapped, mentally retarded, or otherwise regarded as undesirable. This risk is often expressed in vivid claims of widespread fear and wholesale slaughter, claims that are repeated in the Right-to-Life press in both Holland and the USA; however, these claims are simply not true. However, it is true that the Dutch are now beginning to agonize over the problems of the incompetent patient, the mentally ill patient, the newborn with serious deficits, and other patients who cannot make voluntary choices, though with some exceptions these are largely understood as issues about withholding or withdrawing treatment, not about direct termination.[11]

What is not often understood is that this new and acutely painful area of reflection for the Dutch—withholding and withdrawing treatment from incompetent patients—has already led in the United States to the development of a vast, highly developed body of law: namely, that series of cases just cited, beginning with *Quinlan* and culminating in *Cruzan*. Americans have been discussing these issues for a long time, and have developed a broad set of practices that are regarded as routine in withholding and withdrawing treatment. The Dutch see Americans as much further out on the slippery slope than they are, because Americans have already become accustomed to second-party choices about other people. Issues involving second-party choices are painful to the Dutch in a way they are not to us precisely because *voluntariness* is so central in the Dutch understanding of choices about dying. Concomitantly, the Dutch see the Americans' squeamishness about first-party choices—voluntary euthanasia, assisted suicide—as evidence that we are not genuinely committed to recognizing *voluntary* choice after all. For this reason, many Dutch commentators believe that the Amer-

icans are at a much greater risk of sliding down the slippery slope into involuntary killing than they are. I fear, I must add, that they are right about this.

Objections to the American Practice

There may be moral problems raised by the German and the Dutch practices, but there are also moral problems raised by the American practice of relying on withholding and withdrawal of treatment in end-of-life situations. The German, Dutch, and American practices all occur within similar conditions—in industrialized nations with highly developed medical systems, where a majority of the population dies of illnesses exhibiting characteristically extended downhill courses—but the issues raised by our own response to this situation may be even more disturbing than those of the Dutch or the Germans. We often assume that our approach is "safer" because it involves only letting someone die, not killing him or her; but it too raises very troubling questions.

The first of these issues is a function of the fact that withdrawing and especially withholding treatment are typically less conspicuous, less pronounced, less evident kinds of actions than direct killing, even though they can equally well lead to death. Decisions about nontreatment have an invisibility that decisions about directly causing death do not have, even though they may have the same result, and hence there is a much wider range of occasions in which such decisions can be made. One can decline to treat a patient in many different ways, at many different times—by not providing oxygen, by not instituting dialysis, by not correcting electrolyte imbalances, and so on—all of which will cause the patient's death; open medical killing also brings about death, but is a much more overt, conspicuous procedure. Consequently, letting die also invites many fewer protections. In contrast to the earlier slippery slope argument which sees killing as riskier than letting die, the slippery slope argument warns that because our culture relies primarily on decisions about nontreatment, grave decisions about living or dying are not as open to scrutiny as they are under more direct life-terminating practices, and hence, are more open to abuse.

Second, and closely related, reliance on withholding and withdrawal of treatment invites rationing in an extremely strong way, in part because of the comparative invisibility of these decisions. When a health-care provider does not offer a specific sort of care, it is not always possible to discern the motivation; the line between believing that it would not provide benefit to the patient and that it would not provide benefit worth the investment of resources in the patient can be very thin. This is a particular problem where health-care financing is highly decentralized, as in the United States, and where rationing decisions without benefit of principle are not always available for easy review.

Third, relying on withholding and withdrawal of treatment can often be cruel. It requires that the patient who is dying from one of the diseases that exhibits a characteristic extended, downhill course (as the majority of patients in Holland, Germany, and the US do) must in effect wait to die until the absence of a certain treatment will cause death. For instance, the cancer patient who forgoes chemotherapy or surgery does not simply die from this choice; he or she continues to endure the downhill course of the cancer until the tumor finally destroys some crucial bodily function or organ. The patient with amyotrophic lateral sclerosis who decides in advance to decline respiratory support does not die at the time this choice is made, but continues to endure increasing paralysis until breathing is impaired and suffocation occurs. We often try to ameliorate these situations by administering pain medication or symptom control at the same time we are withholding treatment, but these are all ways of disguising the fact that we are letting the disease kill the patient rather than directly bringing about death. But the ways diseases kill people are far more cruel than the ways physicians kill patients when performing euthanasia or assisting in suicide.

THE PROBLEM: A CHOICE OF CULTURES

Thus we see three similar cultures and countries and three similar sets of circumstances, but three quite different basic practices in approaching death. All three of these practices generate moral problems; none of them, nor any others we might devise, is free of moral difficulty. But the question that faces us is this: which of these practices is best?

It is not possible to answer this question in a less-than-ideal world without some attention to the specific characteristics and deficiencies of the society in question. In asking which of these practices is best, we must ask which is best *for us*. That we currently employ one set of these practices rather than others does not prove that it is best for us; the question is, would practices

developed in other cultures or those not yet widespread in any be better for our own culture than that which has developed here? Thus, it is necessary to consider the differences between our own society and these European cultures that have real bearing on which model of approach to dying we ought to adopt.

First, notice that different cultures exhibit different degrees of closeness between physicians and patients—different patterns of contact and involvement. The German physician is sometimes said to be more distant and more authoritarian than the American physician; on the other hand, the Dutch physician is sometimes said to be closer to his or her patients than either the American or the German is. In Holland, basic primary care is provided by the *huisarts,* the general practitioner or family physician, who typically lives in the neighborhood, makes house calls frequently, and maintains an office in his or her own home. The *huisarts* is usually the physician for the other members of the patient's family, and will remain the family's physician throughout his or her practice. Thus, the patient for whom euthanasia becomes an issue—say, the terminal cancer patient who has been hospitalized in the past but who has returned home to die—will be cared for by the trusted family physician on a regular basis. Indeed, for a patient in severe distress, the physician, supported by the visiting nurse, may make house calls as often as once a day, twice a day, or more (after all, it is right in the neighborhood), and is in continuous contact with the family. In contrast, the traditional American institution of the family doctor who makes house calls is rapidly becoming a thing of the past, and whereas some patients who die at home have access to hospice services and house calls from their long-term physician, many have no such long-term care and receive most of it from staff at a clinic or housestaff rotating through the services of a hospital. The degree of continuing contact the patient can have with a familiar, trusted physician clearly influences the nature of his or her dying, and also plays a role in whether physician-performed active euthanasia, assisted suicide, and/or withholding and withdrawing treatment is appropriate.

Second, the United States has a much more volatile legal climate than either Holland or Germany; our medical system is increasingly litigious, much more so than that of any other country in the world. Fears of malpractice action or criminal prosecution color much of what physicians do in managing the dying of their patients. We also tend to evolve public policy through court decisions, and to assume that the existence of a policy puts an end to any moral issue. A delicate legal and moral balance over the issue of euthanasia, as is the case in Holland, would not be possible here.

Third, we in the United States have a very different financial climate in which to do our dying. Both Holland and Germany, as well as every other industrialized nation except South Africa, have systems of national health insurance or national health care. Thus the patient is not directly responsible for the costs of treatment, and consequently the patient's choices about terminal care and/or euthanasia need not take personal financial considerations into account. Even for the patient who does have health insurance in the United States, many kinds of services are not covered, whereas the national health care or health insurance programs of many other countries variously provide many sorts of relevant services, including at-home physician care, home nursing care, home respite care, care in a nursing-home or other long-term facility, dietician care, rehabilitation care, physical therapy, psychological counseling, and so on. The patient in the United States needs to attend to the financial aspects of dying in a way that patients in many other countries do not, and in this country both the patient's choices and the recommendations of the physician are very often shaped by financial considerations.

There are many other differences between the USA on the one hand and Holland and Germany, with their different models of dying, on the other. There are differences in degrees of paternalism in the medical establishment and in racism, sexism, and ageism in the general culture, as well as awareness of a problematic historical past, especially Nazism. All of these and the previous factors influence the appropriateness or inappropriateness of practices such as active euthanasia and assisted suicide. For instance, Holland's tradition of close physician/patient contact, its absence of malpractice-motivated medicine, and its provision of comprehensive health insurance, together with its comparative lack of racism and ageism and its experience in resistance to Nazism, suggest that this culture is able to permit the practice of voluntary active euthanasia, performed by physicians, without risking abuse. On the other hand, it is sometimes said that Germany still does not trust its physicians, remembering the example of Nazi experimentation, and given a comparatively authoritarian medical climate in which the contact between physician and patient is quite distanced, the population could not be comfortable with the practice of active euthanasia. There, only a wholly patient-con-

trolled response to terminal situations, as in non-physician-assisted suicide, is a reasonable and prudent practice.

But what about the United States? This is a country where 1) sustained contact with a personal physician is decreasing, 2) the risk of malpractice action is increasing, 3) much medical care is not insured, 4) many medical decisions are financial as well, 5) racism is on the rise, and 6) the public is naive about direct contact with Nazism or similar totalitarian movements. Thus, the United States is in many respects an untrustworthy candidate for practicing active euthanasia. Given the pressures on individuals in an often atomized society, encouraging solo suicide, assisted if at all only by nonprofessionals, might well be open to considerable abuse too.

However, there is one additional difference between the United States and both Holland and Germany that may seem relevant here. At first, it appears to be a trivial, superficial difference—the apparent fact that we Americans are the biggest consumers of "pop psychology" in the world. While of course things are changing and our cultural tastes are widely exported, the fact remains that the ordinary American's cultural diet contains more in the way of do-it-yourself amateur psychology and self-analysis than anyone else's. This long tradition of pop psychology and self-analysis may put us in a better position for certain kinds of end-of-life practices than many other cultures—despite whatever other deficiencies we have, just because we live in a culture that encourages us to inspect our own motives, anticipate the impact of our actions on others, and scrutinize our own relationships with others, including our physicians. What, then, is appropriate for our own cultural situation? Physician-performed euthanasia, though not in itself morally wrong, is morally jeopardized where the legal, time allotment, and especially financial pressures on both patients and physicians are severe; thus, it is morally problematic in our culture in a way that it is not in Holland. Solo suicide outside the institution of medicine (as in Germany) is problematic in a culture (like the United States) that is increasingly alienated, offers deteriorating and uneven social services, is increasingly racist, and in other ways imposes unusual pressures on individuals. Reliance only on withholding and withdrawing treatment (as in the United States) can be, as we've seen, cruel, and its comparative invisibility invites erosion under cost containment and other pressures. These are the three principal alternatives we've considered; but none of them seems wholly suited to our actual situation for dealing with the new fact that most of us die of extended-decline, deteriorative diseases. However, permitting physicians to supply patients with the means for ending their own lives still grants physicians some control over the circumstances in which this can happen—only, for example, when the prognosis is genuinely grim and the alternatives for symptom control are poor—but leaves the fundamental decision about whether to use these means to the patient alone. It is up to the patient then, and his or her advisors, including family, clergy, physician, other health-care providers, and a raft of pop-psychology books, to be clear about whether he or she really wants to use these means or not. Thus, the physician is involved, but not directly; and it is the patient's choice, but the patient is not alone in making it. We live in a quite imperfect world, but, of the alternatives for facing death—which we all eventually must—I think that the practice of permitting physician-assisted suicide is the one most nearly suited to the current state of our own somewhat flawed society. This is a model not yet central in any of the three countries examined here—Holland, Germany, or the United States—but it is the one I think suits us best.

NOTE

*As the medical care system in the German Democratic Republic (East Germany) was structurally different and was faced with many unique problems, especially in terms of shortages in high-tech equipment, I will only be referring to what was known as the Federal Republic of (West) Germany up until 1990.

REFERENCES

1 Olshansky SJ, Ault AB. The fourth stage of the epidemiological transition: the age of delayed degenerative diseases. Milbank Memorial Fund Quarterly/Health and Society 1986;64:355–391.

2 Miles S, Gomez C. Protocols for elective use of life-sustaining treatment. New York: Springer-Verlag, 1988.

3 Sprung CL. Changing attitudes and practices in foregoing life-sustaining treatments. JAMA 1990;263:2213.

4 Smedira NG et al. Withholding and withdrawal of life support from the critically ill. N Engl J Med 1990;322:309–315.

5 New York Times, July 23, 1990, p. A13.

6 van der Mass PJ, van Delden JJM, and Pijnenborg L. Euthanasia and other medical decisions concerning the end of life: an investigation performed upon request of the Commission of Inquiry into the Medical Practice Concerning Euthanasia. Published in full in English as a special issue of Health Policy 1992; 22 (nos. 1 and 2), and, with Looman CWN, in summary in The Lancet 1991;338:669–74.

7 The LAWER cases are examined in Pijnenborg L, van der Maas PJ, van Delden JJM, and Looman CWN. Life-terminating acts without explicit request of patient. The Lancet 1993;341:1196–1199. This study finds just two cases, both from the early 1980s, in which a competent patient was euthanized without that patient's knowledge.

8 Dillmann RJM, van der Wal G, and van Delden JJM. Euthanasia in the Netherlands: the state of affairs. Manuscript in progress, Royal Dutch Medical Association, Utrecht.

9 Battin MP. Assisted suicide: can we learn from Germany? The Hastings Center Report, March-April 1992;41–51. Reprinted in Battin MP. The least worst death. New York: Oxford University Press, 1994:254–270.

10 Admiraal P. Euthanasia in a general hospital. Address to the Eighth World Congress of the International Federation of Right-To-Die Societies, Maastricht, Holland, June 8, 1990.

11 ten Have H. Coma: controversy and consensus. Newsletter of the European Society for Philosophy of Medicine and Health Care. May 1990;8:19–20.

Care of the Hopelessly Ill: Proposed Clinical Criteria for Physician-Assisted Suicide

Timothy E. Quill, Christine K. Cassel, and Diane E. Meier

Timothy E. Quill is associate professor of medicine and psychiatry at the University of Rochester and associate chief of medicine at Genesee Hospital, Rochester. He is the author of *Death and Dignity: Making Choices and Taking Charge* (1993). A biographical sketch of Christine K. Cassel is found on page 285. Diane E. Meier is associate professor of geriatrics and adult development and medicine, Mount Sinai School of Medicine. She is the author of articles such as "Physician-Assisted Dying: Theory and Reality."

The authors oppose the legalization of voluntary (active) euthanasia but endorse the legalization of physician-assisted suicide as "the policy best able to respond to patients' needs and to protect vulnerable people." In an effort to clarify the conditions under which physician-assisted suicide should be permitted, they introduce a set of relevant criteria. In their view, there are six conditions that must be satisfied, and there is also a documentation requirement.

. . . Although physician-assisted suicide and voluntary euthanasia both involve the active facilitation of a wished-for death, there are several important distinctions between them.[1] In assisted suicide, the final act is solely the patient's, and the risk of subtle coercion from doctors, family members, institutions, or other social forces is greatly reduced.[2] The balance of power between doctor and patient is more nearly equal in physician-assisted suicide than in euthanasia. The physician is counselor and witness and makes the means available, but ultimately the patient must be the one to act or not act. In voluntary euthanasia, the physician both provides the means and carries out the final act, with greatly amplified power over the patient and an increased risk of error, coercion, or abuse.

In view of these distinctions, we conclude that legalization of physician-assisted suicide, but not of voluntary euthanasia, is the policy best able to respond to patients' needs and to protect vulnerable people. From this perspective, physician-assisted suicide forms part of the continuum of options for comfort care, beginning with the forgoing of life-sustaining therapy, including more aggressive symptom-relieving measures, and permitting physician-assisted suicide only if all other alternatives have failed and all criteria have been met. Active voluntary euthanasia is excluded from this continuum

Reprinted with permission of the publisher from the *New England Journal of Medicine*, vol. 327 (November 5, 1992), pp. 1381–1383.

because of the risk of abuse it presents. We recognize that this exclusion is made at a cost to competent, incurably ill patients who cannot swallow or move and who therefore cannot be helped to die by assisted suicide. Such persons, who meet agreed-on criteria in other respects, must not be abandoned to their suffering; a combination of decisions to forgo life-sustaining treatments (including food and fluids) with aggressive comfort measures (such as analgesics and sedatives) could be offered, along with a commitment to search for creative alternatives. We acknowledge that this solution is less than ideal, but we also recognize that in the United States access to medical care is currently too inequitable, and many doctor–patient relationships too impersonal, for us to tolerate the risks of permitting active voluntary euthanasia. We must monitor any change in public policy in this domain to evaluate both its benefits and its burdens.

We propose the following clinical guidelines to contribute to serious discussion about physician-assisted suicide. Although we favor a reconsideration of the legal and professional prohibitions in the case of patients who meet carefully defined criteria, we do not wish to promote an easy or impersonal process.[3] If we are to consider allowing incurably ill patients more control over their deaths, it must be as an expression of our compassion and concern about their ultimate fate after all other alternatives have been exhausted. Such patients should not be held hostage to our reluctance or inability to forge policies in this difficult area.

PROPOSED CLINICAL CRITERIA FOR PHYSICIAN-ASSISTED SUICIDE

Because assisted suicide is extraordinary and irreversible treatment, the patient's primary physician must ensure that the following conditions are clearly satisfied before proceeding. First, the patient must have a condition that is incurable and associated with severe, unrelenting suffering. The patient must understand the condition, the prognosis, and the types of comfort care available as alternatives. Although most patients making this request will be near death, we acknowledge the inexactness of such prognostications[4-6] and do not want to exclude arbitrarily persons with incurable, but not imminently terminal, progressive illnesses, such as amyotrophic lateral sclerosis or multiple sclerosis. When there is considerable uncertainty about the patient's medical condition or prognosis, a second opinion or opinions should be sought and the uncertainty clarified as much as possible before a final decision about the patient's request is made.

Second, the physician must ensure that the patient's suffering and the request are not the result of inadequate comfort care. All reasonable comfort-oriented measures must at least have been considered, and preferably have been tried, before the means for a physician-assisted suicide are provided. Physician-assisted suicide must never be used to circumvent the struggle to provide comprehensive care or find acceptable alternatives. The physician's prospective willingness to provide assisted suicide is a legitimate and important subject to discuss if the patient raises the question, since many patients will probably find the possibility of an escape from suffering more important than the reality.

Third, the patient must clearly and repeatedly, of his or her own free will and initiative, request to die rather than continue suffering. The physician should understand thoroughly what continued life means to the patient and why death appears preferable. A physician's too-ready acceptance of a patient's request could be perceived as encouragement to commit suicide, yet it is important not to force the patient to "beg" for assistance. Understanding the patient's desire to die and being certain that the request is serious are critical steps in evaluating the patient's rationality and ensuring that all alternative means of relieving suffering have been adequately explored. Any sign of ambivalence or uncertainty on the part of the patient should abort the process, because a clear, convincing, and continuous desire for an end of suffering through death is a strict requirement to proceed. Requests for assisted suicide made in an advance directive or by a health care surrogate should not be honored.

Fourth, the physician must be sure that the patient's judgment is not distorted. The patient must be capable of understanding the decision and its implications. The presence of depression is relevant if it is distorting rational decision making and is reversible in a way that would substantially alter the situation. Expert psychiatric evaluation should be sought when the primary physician is inexperienced in the diagnosis and treatment of depression, or when there is uncertainty about the rationality of the request or the presence of a reversible mental disorder the treatment of which would substantially change the patient's perception of his or her condition.[7]

Fifth, physician-assisted suicide should be carried out only in the context of a meaningful doctor–patient relationship. Ideally, the physician should have witnessed the patient's previous illness and suffering. There may not always be a preexisting relationship, but the physician must get to know the patient personally in order to understand fully the reasons for the request. The physician must understand why the patient considers death to be the best of a limited number of very unfortunate options. The primary physician must personally confirm that each of the criteria has been met. The patient should have no doubt that the physician is committed to finding alternative solutions if at any moment the patient's mind changes. Rather than create a new subspecialty focused on death,[8] assistance in suicide should be given by the same physician who has been struggling with the patient to provide comfort care, and who will stand by the patient and provide care until the time of death, no matter what path is taken.[3]

No physician should be forced to assist a patient in suicide if it violates the physician's fundamental values, although the patient's personal physician should think seriously before turning down such a request. Should a transfer of care be necessary, the personal physician should help the patient find another, more receptive primary physician.

Sixth, consultation with another experienced physician is required to ensure that the patient's request is voluntary and rational, the diagnosis and prognosis accurate, and the exploration of comfort-oriented alternatives thorough. The consulting physician should review the supporting materials and should interview and examine the patient.

Finally, clear documentation to support each condition is required. A system must be developed for reporting, reviewing, and studying such deaths and clearly distinguishing them from other forms of suicide. The patient, the primary physician, and the consultant must each sign a consent form. A physician-assisted suicide must neither invalidate insurance policies nor lead to an investigation by the medical examiner or an unwanted autopsy. The primary physician, the medical consultant, and the family must be assured that if the conditions agreed on are satisfied in good faith, they will be free from criminal prosecution for having assisted the patient to die.

Informing family members is strongly recommended, but whom to involve and inform should be left to the discretion and control of the patient. Similarly, spiritual counseling should be offered, depending on the patient's background and beliefs. Ideally, close family members should be an integral part of the decision-making process and should understand and support the patient's decision. If there is a major dispute between the family and the patient about how to proceed, it may require the involvement of an ethics committee or even of the courts. It is to be hoped, however, that most of these painful decisions can be worked through directly by the patient, the family, and health care providers. Under no circumstances should the family's wishes and requests override those of a competent patient.

THE METHOD

In physician-assisted suicide, a lethal amount of medication is usually prescribed that the patient then ingests. Since this process has been largely covert and unstudied, little is known about which methods are the most humane and effective. If there is a change in policy, there must be an open sharing of information within the profession, and a careful analysis of effectiveness. The methods selected should be reliable and should not add to the patient's suffering. We must also provide support and careful monitoring for the patients, physicians, and families affected, since the emotional and social effects are largely unknown but are undoubtedly far-reaching.

Assistance with suicide is one of the most profound and meaningful requests a patient can make of a physician. If the patient and the physician agree that there are no acceptable alternatives and that all the required conditions have been met, the lethal medication should ideally be taken in the physician's presence. Unless the patient specifically requests it, he or she should not be left alone at the time of death. In addition to the personal physician, other health care providers and family members should be encouraged to be present, as the patient wishes. It is of the utmost importance not to abandon the patient at this critical moment. The time before a controlled death can provide an opportunity for a rich and meaningful goodbye between family members, health care providers, and the patient. For this reason, we must be sure that any policies and laws enacted to allow assisted suicide do not require that the patient be left alone at the moment of death in order for the assisters to be safe from prosecution. . . .

REFERENCES

1 Weir RF. The morality of physician-assisted suicide. Law Med Health Care 1992;20:116–26.

2 Glover J. Causing death and saving lives. New York: Penguin Books, 1977:182–9.

3 Jecker NS. Giving death a hand: when the dying and the doctor stand in a special relationship. J Am Geriatr Soc 1991;39:831–5.

4 Poses RM, Bekes C, Copare FJ, Scott WE. The answer to "What are my chances, doctor?" depends on whom is asked: prognostic disagreement and inaccuracy for critically ill patients. Crit Care Med 1989;17:827–33.

5 Charlson ME. Studies of prognosis: progress and pitfalls. J Gen Intern Med 1987;2:359–61.

6 Schonwetter RS, Teasdale TA, Storey P, Luchi RJ. Estimation of survival time in terminal cancer patients: an impedance to hospice admissions? Hospice J 1990;6:65–79.

7 Conwell Y, Caine ED. Rational suicide and the right to die—reality and myth. N Engl J Med 1991;325:1100–3.

8 Benrubi GI. Euthanasia—the need for procedural safeguards. N Engl J Med 1992;326:197–9.

Voluntary Active Euthanasia: The Individual Case and Public Policy
Joan Teno and Joanne Lynn

Joan Teno is assistant professor of medicine and of community and family medicine, Center for Evaluative Clinical Sciences, Dartmouth Medical School. She is the coauthor of articles such as "After the Patient Self-Determination Act: The Need for Empirical Research on Formal Advance Directives" and "The Use of Formal Advance Directives among Patients with HIV-Related Diseases." A biographical sketch of Joanne Lynn is found on page 355.

Teno and Lynn argue against the legalization of voluntary active euthanasia. (They also express opposition to the practice of physician-assisted suicide.) Their overall claim is that the potential adverse consequences of legalization significantly outweigh any potential benefits. In the view of the authors, legalization of voluntary active euthanasia would lead to the abuse of vulnerable persons in society, it would have a detrimental effect on the availability of supportive services for those who are dying, and it would have a negative impact on the practice of medicine, especially by undermining public trust and confidence in physicians.

In recent years, society has recognized patients' rights to use or forgo life-sustaining therapy. The American Geriatrics Society (A.G.S.) has supported this authority in a position statement, "Medical Treatment Decisions Concerning Elderly Persons."[1] Public debate has recently centered on whether this authority should be extended to requests for interventions whose purpose is directly and intentionally to cause the death of a patient (Voluntary Active Euthanasia, or V.A.E.). Recent events have again brought the debate regarding V.A.E. into national focus. The life of Mrs. Janet Adkins was taken with a "suicide machine" invented by Dr. Jack Kevorkian.[2] Dr. Timothy Quill published a thoughtful report of a case of assisted suicide.[3] In this latter case, the patient had the benefits of a compassionate and skillful physician, a resourceful and caring family, and the option of supportive care services provided by hospice. Yet, she apparently chose, with her physician's acquiescence, to take an overdose of a barbiturate. The voters in the state of Washington will vote this fall on Initiative 119 which would allow physicians to perform V.A.E. under specified circumstances.[4] One stimulus for this debate is the perceived peril of medical technology. Recent advances in technology not only may improve patient outcomes; they also can increase associated human suffering and the financial costs.[5] These events and developments have reopened

the debate on whether physicians should perform voluntary active euthanasia.

The outcome of this debate may have a profound impact on the lives of older persons. It will also impact upon the dying of all impoverished persons. The A.G.S. has addressed this issue with a position statement that is published in this issue.[6] In this position statement, the A.G.S. affirms that physicians should not participate in V.A.E., and the current legal prohibitions barring physician assistance in V.A.E. and suicide should not be changed.

The position statement recognizes that the greater good of the community requires that limits must be placed on patient's authority to obtain V.A.E. Limits on the patient's rights to choose are not uncommon. Patient autonomy may be limited by scarce resources, protection of the public health, and avoiding harm to others. Decisions to limit a patient's authority are, and should be, difficult. Especially in the case of euthanasia, health care providers are sometimes faced with the tension between compassion for a suffering individual and the policy implications of a general practice that would allow V.A.E.

POTENTIAL BENEFITS OF LEGALIZED EUTHANASIA

Arguments for V.A.E. are often based on the central theme of relieving the intolerable suffering of patients

Reprinted with permission from *Journal of the American Geriatrics Society,* vol. 39 (August 1991), pp. 827–830.

through the provision of a "merciful death." How many patients with intractable pain might benefit from legalization of V.A.E.? Saunders and other hospice providers have shown that the vast majority of patients with "intractable" pain can be made quite comfortable.[7] For the very small number who cannot avoid pain while awake, one could provide continuous anesthetic levels of pain-relieving medications.

A "weariness with life" may be a growing reason for requests of V.A.E. For dying patients, the mental anguish of facing another day just waiting to die may be more important than physical pain in choosing to request V.A.E. By legalizing euthanasia, patients could choose the exact circumstances and time of their death. This would potentially shorten the duration of psychological suffering for patients. Yet, little is known regarding the prevalence of "weariness with life" as a reason for requesting V.A.E.

Although mention of a welcoming of the end of life may be common, hospice physicians report only a small number of persistent or thoughtful requests for V.A.E.[8-10] Dr. Quill's recent case report illustrates that such patients do occur, but his obvious discomfort with and investment in this case illustrates that such cases are not commonplace.[3] One of us (JL) has cared for over 1,000 hospice patients, and only two of these patients seriously and repeatedly requested physician assistance in active euthanasia. Even these two patients did not seek another health care provider when it was explained that their requests could not be honored. New patients to hospice often state they want to "get it over with." At face value, this may seem a request for active euthanasia. However, these requests are often an expression of the patient's concerns regarding pain, suffering, and isolation, and their fears about whether their dying will be prolonged by technology. Furthermore, these requests may be attempts by the patient to see if anyone really cares whether he or she lives. Meeting such a request with ready acceptance could be disastrous for the patient who interprets the response as confirmation of his or her worthlessness. Future research should systematically document the number of patients who prefer V.A.E. even in the supportive environment of hospice.

An indirect benefit of legalization of V.A.E. might be the reassurance that some persons would feel knowing that dying need not be worse than being dead.[11] Honoring patient autonomy may be the strongest argument for the legalization of V.A.E. Deciding the timing and circumstances of one's death has been argued to be the fundamental decision where "individual interest is paramount."[11] This argument does have appeal. Most contrary claims rest on a particular moral or religious claim. This society is, with good cause, prone to allow wide variation when the issue is moral or religious. We would rather that persons make their own choices in these areas. Nevertheless, individual rights must sometimes be constrained within societal limits.[12] As noted previously, society has and must set limits on personal autonomy in health care decisions because of scarce resources, public health, and possible harm to others. Prudent public policy requires, in the A.G.S. view, that such constraints include prohibiting V.A.E. for the reasons given below.

POTENTIAL ADVERSE CONSEQUENCES OF LEGALIZED EUTHANASIA

Isolated cases of intolerable suffering unrelieved by available methods of pain control or dying patients with extreme mental anguish may present situations in which one is moved to accept voluntary active euthanasia or assisted suicide. However, legalization would not affect only the extraordinary case; it would be an allowable consideration generally. Beauchamp and Childress stated in summarizing an argument also put forth by Rawls, "it is one thing to justify an act; it is another to justify a general practice."[13-14] Legalizing V.A.E. would have serious adverse consequences including potential abuses against individual patients, a serious adverse impact on the availability of supportive services for dying persons, and a mistrust of physicians.

LEGALIZED VOLUNTARY ACTIVE EUTHANASIA: FAIRNESS AND EQUITY

The most feared consequence of V.A.E. is abuse affecting vulnerable persons in society. These abuses could be as subtle as the cultural manipulation of vulnerable persons so that they "request" euthanasia when doing so is more of a convenience to others than an affirmative choice for the patient.[15] In addition, active euthanasia could come to be accepted without the valid consent of the patients. Such a course would seem to be more likely to affect the frail and impoverished, not the affluent and outspoken.

One may cite the experience in the Netherlands as evidence that these abuses will not occur. However, the evidence from the Netherlands is ambiguous. Although euthanasia remains a criminal offense in the Netherlands, the current public policy is that physicians who perform V.A.E. within specified guidelines will not be prosecuted. The major protection ensuring that guidelines are followed is review by a coroner.[16] Estimates of the rate of V.A.E. in the Netherlands range from 2,000–10,000 deaths per year.[16,17] In 1987, coroners were notified of less than 200 cases of euthanasia.[18] If these estimates are accurate, legal safeguards that occur after the death of the patient are rarely employed in the Netherlands.

The degree of success of the Dutch experience with V.A.E. cannot be judged by available evidence. Furthermore, even if judged successful, it is doubtful that the Dutch safeguards and practice of euthanasia would be transferable to the United States. In the Netherlands, supportive services for the dying are uniformly available. There are no economic incentives to V.A.E.[19] Americans do not generally have this access to supportive care of the dying.

Cost containment is a driving force in the American health care system. A decision to legalize V.A.E. must be examined within the context of health care economics and supportive services available to the chronically ill and dying.[20] In the United States, access to comprehensive and effective supportive services, such as those provided by hospice, is uncommon. Families are faced with crippling costs for supportive services. Given these economic realities, if V.A.E. were a legal option, patients and families would choose euthanasia to escape family bankruptcy or to avoid wholly inadequate care. As noted in the A.G.S. position statement, legalized voluntary active euthanasia would reduce what little impetus now exists to provide supportive care for the dying.

IMPACT ON THE PRACTICE OF MEDICINE

Lifting the prohibition against V.A.E. may also change medical practice. The prohibition against V.A.E. has forced the clinician to focus on the humane care of the dying in which success depends upon meticulous attention to symptom control and each patient's psychosocial needs. Removing the prohibition could result in clinicians accepting euthanasia as an easier course of care.[21,22] The case report "It's Over, Debbie" illustrates this abuse of active euthanasia in a terminally ill patient.[23] While it is not clear whether this case was factual or fictional, the case illustrates how easy it might be for physicians to give less attentive care to the dying when they have the capacity to end the life of the sufferers instead.

Legalization of direct killing of patients would also have a negative impact on the way that society perceives the role of physicians. Traditionally, the goals of physicians have been to cure and comfort.[24] The implications of allowing "direct killing" as a way to comfort patients may result in the public no longer having the same degree of trust and confidence in physicians. The motives of physicians would increasingly be questioned. This may result in increasing judicial review of medical decisions which have traditionally been made privately at the patient's bedside.[21] The mandate not to kill does not imply that a "technological imperative" to preserve life is operative. Rather, health care providers must present patients with the potential outcomes with and without therapeutic interventions. Decisions are then made collaboratively, tailoring the care plan to the patient's values. Much of the public outcry for active euthanasia would be reduced if health care providers increasingly focused attention on better symptom control and on better communication with patients and families about decisions to employ or forgo life-sustaining technology.

REAPPRAISAL: BENEFITS AND ADVERSE CONSEQUENCES OF LEGALIZATION OF V.A.E.

The A.G.S. in its policy concludes that the potential adverse consequences of a public policy that would permit V.A.E. outweigh the benefits to patients. Cases such as the recent report by Dr. Quill of his patient named "Diana" are hard cases. While these cases are moving and difficult for the individual practitioner, policy must consider the potential adverse consequences of legalization of V.A.E. and assisted suicide.[3] Changes in policy based on hard cases risks making bad policy decisions. For the greater good of the community, active euthanasia should not be an available treatment option, and the laws that prohibit physician participation in V.A.E. and assisted suicide should not be changed. The position statement acknowledges that many would object to V.A.E. on the basis that it is morally wrong *per se*. Given the policy issues which were overwhelmingly against the legalization of V.A.E., the A.G.S. did not feel it had to address this issue.

Future debate regarding V.A.E. must address the degree to which supportive services are made available to dying persons and families. In these times of budgetary constraints, as noted in the position statement, ". . . our society should not make the adjustment in moral norms that would allow euthanasia as a means of cost savings".[6] The A.G.S. advocates commitment to improved access by dying patients to compassionate and supportive care.

For the individual health care practitioner faced with these difficult choices, the position statement calls for increased attentiveness and skill in the care of the dying. The position statement does not place any limit on aggressive treatment of symptoms, even if aggressive treatment of symptoms may hasten death. Much of the public outcry for V.A.E. is due to the perils of technology. Better understanding of medical outcomes will allow patients, families, and physicians to discuss when life-sustaining therapy is prolonging dying. At this juncture, health care providers must not withdraw from dying patients and their families. Rather, the focus should be on supportive and compassionate care of the dying. The A.G.S. has rightly chosen to urge public policy to focus on supportive and compassionate care of the dying, an effort that would be undercut in many ways if society were to legalize voluntary active euthanasia.

ACKNOWLEDGMENT

We would like to thank Donald J. Murphy, MD for review of the manuscript and insightful comments.

REFERENCES

1 AGS. Medical Treatment Decisions Concerning Elderly Persons. (AGS Position Statement, May, 1987.)

2 Cassel CK, Meier DE. Morals and moralism in the debate over euthanasia and assisted suicide. New Engl J Med 1990;323:750–752.

3 Quill TE. Death and dignity: A case for individualized decision making. N Engl J Med 1991;324:691–694.

4 Gianelli DM. A right to die: Debate intensifies over euthanasia and the doctor's role. American Medical News 1991; January 7:9–10.

5 Sprung CL: Changing attitudes and practices in forgoing life-sustaining treatments. JAMA 1990;263:2211–2215.

6 AGS. Voluntary active euthanasia. J Am Geriatr Soc 1991;39:826.

7 Saunders CM. The philosophy of terminal care. In: Saunders CM, ed. The Management of Terminal Disease. London: Edward Arnold Publishers, Ltd, 1978, p 194.

8 Parkes CM. Psychological aspects. In: Saunders CM, ed. The Management of Terminal Disease. London: Edward Arnold Publishers, Ltd, 1978, p 56.

9 Lynn J: Euthanasia—not in America. The Washington Post, April 19, 1990, p A-26.

10 Gillett G. Euthanasia, letting die and the pause. J Med Ethics 1988;14:61–68.

11 Brock DW, ed. Decisions about Life-Sustaining Treatment and Voluntary Active Euthanasia: Volume of Essays of American and Soviet Philosophers.

12 Carton RW. The road to euthanasia. JAMA 1990;263:2221.

13 Beauchamp TL, Childress JF. Principles of Biomedical Ethics, 3rd Ed. New York: Oxford University Press, 1989, p 138.

14 Rawls J. Two concepts of rules. Philosophical Rev 1955;64:3–32.

15 Singer PA, Siegler M. Euthanasia—a critique. N Engl J Med 1989;322(26):1881–1883.

16 de Wachter MA. Active euthanasia in the Netherlands. JAMA 1989;262(23):3316–3319.

17 Pence GE. Do not go slowly into that dark night: mercy killing in Holland. Am J Med 1988;84:139–141.

18 Gomez CF. Letter to the Editor. N Engl J Med 1989;321(14):977.

19 Rigter H. Euthanasia in the Netherlands: distinguishing facts from fiction. Hasting Center Rep 1989;19 [Special Supplement]: 31.

20 Lynn, J. Letter to the Editor. N Engl J Med 1989;321(14):978.

21 Wolf SM. Holding the line on euthanasia. Hastings Center Rep 1989;19 [Special Supplement]:13.

22 Vaux KL. Debbie's dying: Mercy killing and the good death. JAMA 1988;259(14):2140–2141.

23 It's Over Debbie. A piece of my mind. JAMA 1988;259(2):272.

24 Callahan D. Can we return death to disease? Hastings Center Rep 1989;19 [Special Supplement]:4.

The Treatment of Impaired Infants

Ethical Issues in Aiding the Death of Young Children
H. Tristram Engelhardt, Jr.

H. Tristram Engelhardt, Jr., is professor of medicine and community medicine at Baylor College of Medicine. He is the editor of the *Journal of Medicine and Philosophy* and the author of *The Foundations of Bioethics* (1986) and *Bioethics and Secular Humanism: The Search for a Common Morality* (1991). Engelhardt has also published numerous articles on issues in biomedical ethics and the philosophy of medicine.

After reviewing the differences between euthanasia in the case of adults and euthanasia in the case of children, Engelhardt focuses attention on the status of children. In his view, young children are not persons in a strict sense. Rather, they are persons only in "a social sense," by virtue of their role in a family and society. Since young children "belong" to their parents, it is the parents who are the proper decision makers with regard to the treatment or nontreatment of severely impaired newborns. Engelhardt finds it morally acceptable to allow a severely impaired newborn to die when (1) it is unlikely that the child can attain a "good quality of life" (i.e., a developed personal life) and/or (2) it seems clear that providing continued care for the child would constitute a "severe burden" for the family. Engelhardt goes on to develop the concept of "the injury of continued existence," arguing that a child has a right not to have its life prolonged in those cases where life would be painful and futile. Thus, he maintains, allowing a severely impaired newborn to die (in some cases) is not only *morally acceptable* but indeed *morally demanded*. In concluding, Engelhardt briefly discusses the justifiability of providing active euthanasia for severely impaired newborns.

Euthanasia in the pediatric age group involves a constellation of issues that are materially different from those of adult euthanasia.[1] The difference lies in the somewhat obvious fact that infants and young children are not able to decide about their own futures and thus are not persons in the same sense that normal adults are. While adults usually decide their own fate, others decide on behalf of young children. Although one can argue that euthanasia is or should be a personal right, the sense of such an argument is obscure with respect to children. Young children do not have any personal rights, at least none that they can exercise on their own behalf with regard to the manner of their life and death. As a result, euthanasia of young children raises special questions concerning the standing of the rights of children, the status of parental rights, the obligations of adults to prevent the suffering of children, and the possible effects on society of allowing or expediting the death of seriously defective infants.

What I will refer to as the euthanasia of infants and young children might be termed by others infanticide, while some cases might be termed the withholding of extraordinary life-prolonging treatment.[2] One needs a term that will encompass both death that results from active intervention and death that ensues when one simply ceases further therapy.[3] In using such a term, one must recognize that death is often not directly but only obliquely intended. That is, one often intends only to treat no further, not actually to have death follow, even though one knows death will follow.[4]

Finally, one must realize that deaths as the result of withholding treatment constitute a significant proportion of neonatal deaths. For example, as high as 14 percent of children in one hospital have been identified as dying after a decision was made not to treat further, the presumption being that the children would have lived longer had treatment been offered.[5]

Even popular magazines have presented accounts

of parental decisions not to pursue treatment.[6] These decisions often involve a choice between expensive treatment with little chance of achieving a full, normal life for the child and "letting nature take its course," with the child dying as a result of its defects. As this suggests, many of these problems are products of medical progress. Such children in the past would have died. The quandaries are in a sense an embarrassment of riches; now that one *can* treat such defective children, *must* one treat them? And, if one need not treat such defective children, may one expedite their death?

I will here briefly examine some of these issues. First, I will review differences that contrast the euthanasia of adults to euthanasia of children. Second, I will review the issue of the rights of parents and the status of children. Third, I will suggest a new notion, the concept of the "injury of continued existence," and draw out some of its implications with respect to a duty to prevent suffering. Finally, I will outline some important questions that remain unanswered even if the foregoing issues can be settled. In all, I hope more to display the issues involved in a difficult question than to advance a particular set of answers to particular dilemmas.

For the purpose of this paper, I will presume that adult euthanasia can be justified by an appeal to freedom. In the face of imminent death, one is usually choosing between a more painful and more protracted dying and a less painful or less protracted dying, in circumstances where either choice makes little difference with regard to the discharge of social duties and responsibilities. In the case of suicide, we might argue that, in general, social duties (for example, the duty to support one's family) restrain one from taking one's own life. But in the face of imminent death and in the presence of the pain and deterioration of a fatal disease, such duties are usually impossible to discharge and are thus rendered moot. One can, for example, picture an extreme case of an adult with a widely disseminated carcinoma, including metastases to the brain, who because of severe pain and debilitation is no longer capable of discharging any social duties. In these and similar circumstances, euthanasia becomes the issue of the right to control one's own body, even to the point of seeking assistance in suicide. Euthanasia is, as such, the issue of assisted suicide, the universalization of a maxim that all persons should be free, *in extremis,* to decide with regard to the circumstances of their death.

Further, the choice of positive euthanasia could be defended as the more rational choice: the choice of a less painful death and the affirmation of the value of a rational life. In so choosing, one would be acting to set limits to one's life in order not to live when pain and physical and mental deterioration make further rational life impossible. The choice to end one's life can be understood as a noncontradictory willing of a smaller set of states of existence for oneself, a set that would not include a painful death. As such, it would not involve a desire to destroy oneself. That is, adult euthanasia can be construed as an affirmation of the rationality and autonomy of the self.[7]

The remarks above focus on the active or positive euthanasia of adults. But they hold as well concerning what is often called passive or negative euthanasia, the refusal of life-prolonging therapy. In such cases, the patient's refusal of life-prolonging therapy is seen to be a right that derives from personal freedom, or at least from a zone of privacy into which there are no good grounds for social intervention.[8]

Again, none of these considerations apply directly to the euthanasia of young children, because they cannot participate in such decisions. Whatever else pediatric, in particular neonatal, euthanasia involves, it surely involves issues different from those of adult euthanasia. Since infants and small children cannot commit suicide, their right to assisted suicide is difficult to pose. The difference between the euthanasia of young children and that of adults resides in the difference between children and adults. The difference, in fact, raises the troublesome question of whether young children are persons, or at least whether they are persons in the sense in which adults are. Answering that question will resolve in part at least the right of others to decide whether a young child should live or die and whether he should receive life-prolonging treatment.

THE STATUS OF CHILDREN

Adults belong to themselves in the sense that they are rational and free and therefore responsible for their actions. Adults are *sui juris.* Young children, though, are neither self-possessed nor responsible. While adults exist in and for themselves, as self-directive and self-conscious beings, young children, especially newborn infants, exist for their families and those who love them. They are not, nor can they in any sense be, responsible for themselves. If being a person is to be a responsible agent, a bearer of rights and duties, children are not persons in a strict sense. They are, rather, persons in a social sense: others must act on their behalf and bear responsibility for them. They are, as it were, entities defined by their place in social roles (for example, mother-child, family-child) rather than beings that define themselves as persons, that is, in and through themselves. Young children live as persons in and through the care of those who are responsible for them, and those responsible for them exercise the children's rights on their behalf. In this sense children belong to families in ways that most adults do not. They exist in and through their family and society.

Treating young children with respect has, then, a sense different from treating adults with respect. One can respect neither a newborn infant's or very young child's wishes nor its freedom. In fact, a newborn infant or young child is more an entity that is valued highly because it will grow to be a person and because it plays a social role as if it were a person.[9] That is, a small child is treated as if it were a person in social roles such as mother-child and family-child relationships, though strictly speaking the child is in no way capable of claiming or being responsible for the rights imputed to it. All the rights and duties of the child are exercised and "held in trust" by others for a future time and for a person yet to develop.

Medical decisions to treat or not to treat a neonate or small child often turn on the probability and cost of achieving that future status—a developed personal life. The usual practice of letting anencephalic children (who congenitally lack all or most of the brain) die can be understood as a decision based on the absence of the possibility of achieving a personal life. The practice of refusing treatment to at least some children born with meninogomyelocele can be justified through a similar, but more utilitarian, calculus. In the case of anencephalic children one might argue that care for them as persons is futile since they will never be persons. In the case of a child with meningomyelocele, one might argue that when the cost of cure would likely be very high and the probable lifestyle open to attainment very truncated, there is not a positive duty to make a large investment of money and suffering. One should note that the cost here must include not only financial costs but also the anxiety and suffering that prolonged and uncertain treatment of the child would cause the parents.

This further raises the issue of the scope of positive duties not only when there is no person present in a strict sense, but when the likelihood of a full human life is also very uncertain. Clinical and parental judgment may and should be guided by the expected lifestyle and the cost (in parental and societal pain and money) of its attainment. The decision about treatment, however,

belongs properly to the parents because the child belongs to them in a sense that it does not belong to anyone else, even to itself. The care and raising of the child falls to the parents, and when considerable cost and little prospect of reasonable success are present, the parents may properly decide against life-prolonging treatment.

The physician's role is to present sufficient information in a usable form to the parents to aid them in making a decision. The accent is on the absence of a positive duty to treat in the presence of severe inconvenience (costs) to the parents; treatment that is very costly is not obligatory. What is suggested here is a general notion that there is never a duty to engage in extraordinary treatment and that "extraordinary" can be defined in terms of costs. This argument concerns children (1) whose future quality of life is likely to be seriously compromised and (2) whose present treatment would be very costly. The issue is that of the circumstances under which parents would not be obliged to take on severe burdens on behalf of their children or those circumstances under which society would not be so obliged. The argument should hold as well for those cases where the expected future life would surely be of normal quality, though its attainment would be extremely costly. The fact of little likelihood of success in attaining a normal life for the child makes decisions to do without treatment more plausible because the hope of success is even more remote and therefore the burden borne by parents or society becomes in that sense more extraordinary. But very high costs themselves could be a sufficient criterion, though in actual cases judgments in that regard would be very difficult when a normal life could be expected.[10]

The decisions in these matters correctly lie in the hands of the parents, because it is primarily in terms of the family that children exist and develop—until children become persons strictly, they are persons in virtue of their social roles. As long as parents do not unjustifiably neglect the humans in those roles so that the value and purpose of that role (that is, child) stands to be eroded (thus endangering other children), society need not intervene. In short, parents may decide for or against the treatment of their severely deformed children.

However, society has a right to intervene and protect children for whom parents refuse care (including treatment) when such care does not constitute a severe burden and when it is likely that the child could be brought to a good quality of life. Obviously, "severe burden" and "good quality of life" will be difficult to define and their meanings will vary, just as it is always difficult to say when grains of sand dropped on a table constitute a heap. At most, though, society need only intervene when the grains clearly do not constitute a heap, that is, when it is clear that the burden is light and the chance of a good quality of life for the child is high. A small child's dependence on his parents is so essential that society need intervene only when the absence of intervention would lead to the role "child" being undermined. Society must value mother-child and family-child relationships and should intervene only in cases where (1) neglect is unreasonable and therefore would undermine respect and care for children, or (2) where societal intervention would prevent children from suffering unnecessary pain.[11]

THE INJURY OF CONTINUED EXISTENCE

But there is another viewpoint that must be considered: that of the child or even the person that the child might become. It might be argued that the child has a right not to have its life prolonged. The idea that forcing existence on a child could be wrong is a difficult notion, which, if true, would serve to amplify the foregoing argument. Such an argument would allow the construal of the issue in terms of the perspective of the child, that is, in terms of a duty not to treat in circumstances where treatment would only prolong suffering. In particular, it would at least give a framework for a decision to stop treatment in cases where, though the costs of treatment are not high, the child's existence would be characterized by severe pain and deprivation.

A basis for speaking of continuing existence as an injury to the child is suggested by the proposed legal concept of "wrongful life." A number of suits have been initiated in the United States and in other countries on the grounds that life or existence itself is, under certain circumstances, a tort or injury to the living person.[12] Although thus far all such suits have ultimately failed, some have succeeded in their initial stages. Two examples may be instructive. In each case the ability to receive recompense for the injury (the tort) presupposed the existence of the individual, whose existence was itself the injury. In one case a suit was initiated on behalf of a child against his father alleging that his father's siring him out of wedlock was an injury to the child.[13] In another case a suit on behalf of a child born of an inmate of a state mental hospital impregnated by rape in that institution was brought against the state of New York.[14] The suit was brought on the grounds that being born

with such historical antecedents was itself an injury for which recovery was due. Both cases presupposed that nonexistence would have been preferable to the conditions under which the person born was forced to live.

The suits for tort for wrongful life raise the issue not only of when it would be preferable not to have been born but also of when it would be *wrong* to cause a person to be born. This implies that someone should have judged that it would have been preferable for the child never to have had existence, never to have been in the position to judge that the particular circumstances of life were intolerable.[15] Further, it implies that the person's existence under those circumstances should have been prevented and that, not having been prevented, life was not a gift but an injury. The concept of tort for wrongful life raises an issue concerning the responsibility for giving another person existence, namely, the notion that giving life is not always necessarily a good and justifiable action. Instead, in certain circumstances, so it has been argued, one may have a duty *not* to give existence to another person. This concept involves the claim that certain qualities of life have a negative value, making life an injury, not a gift; it involves, in short, a concept of human accountability and responsibility for human life. It contrasts with the notion that life is a gift of God and thus similar to other "acts of God" (that is, events for which no man is accountable). The concept thus signals the fact that humans can now control reproduction and that where rational control is possible humans are accountable. That is, the expansion of human capabilities has resulted in an expansion of human responsibilities such that one must now decide when and under what circumstances persons will come into existence.

The concept of tort for wrongful life is transferable in part to the painfully compromised existence of children who can only have their life prolonged for a short, painful, and marginal existence. The concept suggests that allowing life to be prolonged under such circumstances would itself be an injury of the person whose painful and severely compromised existence would be made to continue. In fact, it suggests that there is a duty not to prolong life if it can be determined to have a substantial negative value for the person involved.[16] Such issues are moot in the case of adults, who can and should decide for themselves. But small children cannot make such a choice. For them it is an issue of justifying prolonging life under circumstances of painful and compromised existence. Or, put differently, such cases indicate the need to develop social canons to allow a decent death for children for whom the only possibility is protracted, painful suffering.

I do not mean to imply that one should develop a new basis for civil damages. In the field of medicine, the need is to recognize an ethical category, a concept of wrongful continuance of existence, not a new legal right. The concept of injury for continuance of existence, the proposed analogue of the concept of tort for wrongful life, presupposes that life can be of a negative value such that the medical maxim *primum non nocere* ("first do no harm") would require not sustaining life.[17]

The idea of responsibility for acts that sustain or prolong life is cardinal to the notion that one should not under certain circumstances further prolong the life of a child. Unlike adults, children cannot decide with regard to euthanasia (positive or negative), and if more than a utilitarian justification is sought, it must be sought in a duty not to inflict life on another person in circumstances where that life would be painful and futile. This position must rest on the facts that (1) medicine now can cause the prolongation of the life of seriously deformed children who in the past would have died young and that (2) it is not clear that life so prolonged is a good for the child. Further, the choice is made not on the basis of costs to the parents or to society but on the basis of the child's suffering and compromised existence.

The difficulty lies in determining what makes life not worth living for a child. Answers could never be clear. It seems reasonable, however, that the life of children with diseases that involve pain and no hope of survival should not be prolonged. In the case of Tay-Sachs disease (a disease marked by a progressive increase in spasticity and dementia usually leading to death at age three or four), one can hardly imagine that the terminal stages of spastic reaction to stimuli and great difficulty in swallowing are at all pleasant to the child (even insofar as it can only minimally perceive its circumstances). If such a child develops aspiration pneumonia and is treated, it can reasonably be said that to prolong its life is to inflict suffering. Other diseases give fairly clear portraits of lives not worth living: for example, Lesch-Nyhan disease, which is marked by mental retardation and compulsive self-mutilation.

The issue is more difficult in the case of children with diseases for whom the prospects for normal intelligence and a fair lifestyle do exist, but where these chances are remote and their realization expensive. Children born with meningomyelocele present this dilemma. Imagine, for example, a child that falls within Lorber's fifth category (an IQ of sixty or less, sometimes blind, subject to fits, and always incontinent). Such a child has little prospect of anything approaching a normal life, and there is a good chance of its dying even with treatment.[18] But such judgments are statistical. And if one does not treat such children, some will still survive and, as John Freeman indicates, be worse off if not treated.[19] In such cases one is in a dilemma. If one always treats, one must justify extending the life of those who will ultimately die anyway and in the process subjecting them to the morbidity of multiple surgical procedures. How remote does the prospect of a good life have to be in order not to be worth great pain and expense?[20] It is probably best to decide, in the absence of a positive duty to treat, on the basis of the cost and suffering to parents and society. But, as Freeman argues, the prospect of prolonged or even increased suffering raises the issue of active euthanasia.[21]

If the child is not a person strictly, and if death is inevitable and expediting it would diminish the child's pain prior to death, then it would seem to follow that, all else being equal, a decision for active euthanasia would be permissible, even obligatory.[22] The difficulty lies with "all else being equal," for it is doubtful that active euthanasia could be established as a practice without eroding and endangering children generally, since, as John Lorber has pointed out, children cannot speak in their own behalf.[23] Thus, although there is no argument in principle against the active euthanasia of small children, there could be an argument against such practices based on questions of prudence. To put it another way, even though one might have a duty to hasten the death of a particular child, one's duty to protect children in general could override that first duty. The issue of active euthanasia turns in the end on whether it would have social consequences that refraining would not, on whether (1) it is possible to establish procedural safeguards for limited active euthanasia and (2) whether such practices would have a significant adverse effect on the treatment of small children in general. But since these are procedural issues dependent on sociological facts, they are not open to an answer within the confines of this article. In any event, the concept of the injury of continued existence provides a basis for the justification of the passive euthanasia of small children—a practice already widespread and somewhat established in our society—beyond the mere absence of a positive duty to treat.[24]

CONCLUSION

Though the lack of certainty concerning questions such as the prognosis of particular patients and the social consequence of active euthanasia of children prevents a clear answer to all the issues raised by the euthanasia of infants, it would seem that this much can be maintained: (1) Since children are not persons strictly but exist in and through their families, parents are the appropriate ones to decide whether or not to treat a deformed child when (*a*) there is not only little likelihood of full human life but also great likelihood of suffering if the life is prolonged, or (*b*) when the cost of prolonging life is very great. Such decisions must be made in consort with a physician who can accurately give estimates of cost and prognosis and who will be able to help the parents with the consequences of their decision. (2) It is reasonable to speak of a duty not to treat a small child when such treatment will only prolong a painful life or would in any event lead to a painful death. Though this does not by any means answer all the questions, it does point out an important fact—that medicine's duty is not always to prolong life doggedly but sometimes is quite the contrary.

NOTES

1 I am grateful to Laurence B. McCullough and James P. Morris for their critical discussion of this paper. They may be responsible for its virtues, but not for its shortcomings.

2 The concept of extraordinary treatment as it has been developed in Catholic moral theology is useful: treatment is extraordinary and therefore not obligatory if it involves great costs, pain, or inconvenience, and is a grave burden to oneself or others without a reasonable expectation that such treatment would be successful. See Gerald Kelly, S.J., *Medico-Moral Problems* (St. Louis: The Catholic Hospital Association Press, 1958), pp. 128–141. Difficulties are hidden in terms such as "great costs" and "reasonable expectation," as well as in terms such as "successful." Such ambiguity reflects the fact that precise operational definitions are not available. That is, the precise meaning of "great," "reasonable," and "successful" are inextricably bound to particular circumstances, especially particular societies.

3 I will use the term euthanasia in a broad sense to indicate a deliberately chosen course of action or inaction that is known at the time of decision to be such as will expedite death. This use of euthanasia will encompass not only positive or active euthanasia (acting in order to expedite death) and negative or passive euthanasia (refraining from action in order to expedite death), but acting and refraining in the absence of a direct intention that death occur more quickly (that is, those cases that fall under the concept of double effect). See note 4.

4 But, both active and passive euthanasia can be appreciated in terms of the Catholic moral notion of double effect. When the doctrine of double effect is invoked, one is strictly not intending euthanasia, but rather one intends something else. That concept allows actions or omissions that lead to death (1) because it is licit not to prolong life *in extremis* (allowing death is not an intrinsic evil), (2) if death is not actually willed or actively sought (that is, the evil is not directly willed), (3) if that which is willed is a major good (for example, avoiding useless major expenditure of resources or serious pain), and (4) if the good is not achieved by means of the evil (for example, one does not will to save resources or diminish pain *by* the death). With regard to euthanasia the doctrine of double effect means that one need not expend major resources in an endeavor that will not bring health but only prolong dying and that one may use drugs that decrease pain but hasten death. See Richard McCormick, *Ambiguity in Moral Choice* (Milwaukee: Marquette University Press, 1973). I exclude the issue of double effect from my discussion because I am interested in those cases in which the good may follow directly from the evil—the death of the child. In part, though, the second section of this paper is concerned with the concept of proportionate good.

5 Raymond S. Duff and A. G. M. Campbell, "Moral and Ethical Dilemmas in the Special-Care Nursery," *The New England Journal of Medicine*, 289 (Oct. 25, 1973), pp. 890–894.

6 Roger Pell, "The Agonizing Decision of Joanne and Roger Pell," *Good Housekeeping* (January 1972), pp. 76–77, 131–135.

7 This somewhat Kantian argument is obviously made in opposition to Kant's position that suicide involves a default of one's duty to oneself ". . . to preserve his life simply because he is a person and must therefore recognize a duty to himself (and a strict one at that)," as well as a contradictory volition: "that man ought to have the authorization to withdraw himself from all obligation, that is, to be free to act as if no authorization at all were required for this withdrawal, involves a contradiction. To destroy the subject of morality in his own person is tantamount to obliterating from the world . . ."

Immanuel Kant, *The Metaphysical Principles of Virtue: Part II of the Metaphysics of Morals,* trans. James Ellington (Indianapolis: Bobbs-Merrill, 1964), p. 83; Akademie Edition, VI, 422–423.

8 Norman L. Cantor, "A Patient's Decision to Decline Life-Saving Medical Treatment: Bodily Integrity Versus the Preservation of Life," *Rutgers Law Review,* 26 (Winter 1972), p. 239.

9 By "young child" I mean either an infant or child so young as not yet to be able to participate, in any sense, in a decision. A precise operational definition of "young child" would clearly be difficult to develop. It is also not clear how one would bring older children into such decisions. See, for example, Milton Viederman. "Saying 'No' to Hemodialysis: Exploring Adaptation," and Daniel Burke, "Saying 'No' to Hemodialysis: An Acceptable Decision," both in *The Hastings Center Report,* 4 (September 1974), pp. 8–10, and John E. Schowalter, Julian B. Ferholt, and Nancy M. Mann, "The Adolescent Patient's Decision to Die," *Pediatrics,* 51 (January 1973), pp. 97–103.

10 An appeal to high costs alone is probably hidden in judgments based on statistics: even though there is a chance for a normal life for certain children with apparently severe cases of meningomyelocele, one is not obliged to treat since that chance is small, and the pursuit of that chance is very expensive. Cases of the costs being low but the expected suffering of the child being high will be discussed under the concept of the injury of continued existence. It should be noted that none of the arguments in this paper bear on cases where neither the cost nor the suffering of the child is considerable. Cases in this last category probably include, for example, children born with mongolism complicated only by duodenal atresia.

11 I have in mind here the issue of physicians, hospital administrators, or others being morally compelled to seek an injunction to force treatment of the child in the absence of parental consent. In these circumstances, the physician, who is usually best acquainted with the facts of the case, is the natural advocate of the child.

12 G. Tedeschi, "On Tort Liability for 'Wrongful Life,' " *Israel Law Review,* 1 (1966), p. 513.

13 Zepeda v. Zepeda: 41 Ill. App. 2d 240, 190 N.E. 2d 849 (1963).

14 *Williams v. State of New York:* 46 Misc. 2d 824, 260 N.Y.S. 2d 953 (Ct. Cl., 1965).

15 Torts: "Illegitimate Child Denied Recovery against Father for 'Wrongful Life,' " *Iowa Law Review,* 49 (1969), p. 1009.

16 It is one thing to have a conceptual definition of the injury of continued existence (for example, causing a person to continue to live under circumstances of severe pain and deprivation when there are no alternatives but death) and another to have an operational definition of that concept (that is, deciding what counts as such severe pain and deprivation). This article has focused on the first, not the second, issue.

17 H. Tristram Engelhardt, Jr., "Euthanasia and Children: The Injury of Continued Existence," *The Journal of Pediatrics,* 83 (July 1973), pp. 170–171.

18 John Lorber, "Results of Treatment of Myelomeningocele," *Developmental Medicine and Child Neurology,* 13 (1971), p. 286.

19 John M. Freeman, "The Shortsighted Treatment of Myelomeningocele: A Long-Term Case Report," *Pediatrics,* 53 (March 1974), pp. 311–313.

20 John M. Freeman, "To Treat or Not to Treat," *Practical Management of Meningomyelocele,* ed. John Freeman (Baltimore: University Park Press, 1974), p. 21.

21 John Lorber, "Selective Treatment of Myelomeningocele: To Treat or Not to Treat," *Pediatrics,* 53 (March 1974), pp. 307–308.

22 I am presupposing that no intrinsic moral distinctions exist in cases such as these, between acting and refraining, between omitting care in the hope that death will ensue (that is, rather than the child living to be even more defective) and acting to ensure that death will ensue rather than having the child live under painful and seriously compromised circumstances. For a good discussion of the distinction between acting and refraining, see Jonathan Bennett, "Whatever the Consequences," *Analysis,* 26 (January 1966), pp. 83–102; P. J. Fitzgerald, "Acting and Refraining," *Analysis,* 27 (March 1967), pp. 133–139; Daniel Dinello, "On Killing and Letting Die," *Analysis,* 31 (April 1971), pp. 83–86.

23 Lorber, "Selective Treatment of Myelomeningocele," p. 308.

24 Positive duties involve a greater constraint than negative duties. Hence it is often easier to establish a duty not to do something (not to treat further) than a duty to do something (to actively hasten death). Even allowing a new practice to be permitted (for

example, active euthanasia) requires a greater attention to consequences than does establishing the absence of a positive duty. For example, at common law there is no basis for action against a person who watches another drown without giving aid; this reflects the difficulty of establishing a positive duty.

Involuntary Euthanasia of Defective Newborns
John A. Robertson

John A. Robertson is Thomas Watt Gregory Professor of Law, University of Texas at Austin. He is the author of *The Rights of the Critically Ill* (1983) and *Children of Choice: Freedom and the New Reproductive Technologies* (1994). His many published articles include "The Question of Human Cloning" and "Second Thoughts on Living Wills."

Robertson, in vivid contrast to Engelhardt, denies that the undesirable consequences of treating a severely impaired (defective) newborn can morally justify nontreatment. The consequentialist argument directly under attack by Robertson has two versions. One version is based on the suffering of the severely impaired newborn, whereas the other version is based on the suffering of others (principally the family but also health professionals and society as a whole). The first version of the consequentialist argument, identified by Robertson as the "quality-of-life argument," maintains that withholding treatment is morally justified because the severely impaired newborn is better off dead. Although Robertson insists that it is often false that death is a better fate than continued life for the severely impaired newborn, his fundamental objection to the quality-of-life argument stems from his reluctance to accept proxy assessments of quality of life. The second version of the consequentialist argument holds that withholding treatment is morally justified because of the emotional and financial burden falling on those who would have to provide the continued care for a severely impaired child. Robertson's central objection to this version of the consequentialist argument has to do with its utilitarian spirit, but he also argues that it is seldom plausible to think that the suffering of others is so grave as to outweigh the impaired newborn's interest in life.

One of the most perplexing dilemmas of modern medicine concerns whether "ordinary"[1] medical care justifiably can be withheld from defective newborns. Infants with malformations of the central nervous system[2] such as anencephaly,[3] hydrocephaly,[4] Down's syndrome,[5] spina bifida,[6] and myelomeningocele[7] often require routine surgical or medical attention[8] merely to stay alive. Until recent developments in surgery and pediatrics, these infants would have died of natural causes.

Reprinted with permission of the publisher from *Stanford Law Review*, vol. 27 (January 1975), pp. 213–214; 251–261. Copyright © 1975 by the Board of Trustees of the Leland Stanford Junior University.

Today with treatment many will survive for long periods, although some will be severely handicapped and limited in their potential for human satisfaction and interaction. Because in the case of some defective newborns, the chances are often slim that they will ever lead normal human lives, it is now common practice for parents to request, and for physicians to agree, not to treat such infants. Without treatment the infant usually dies. . . .

If we reject the argument that defective newborns are not persons, the question remains whether circumstances exist in which the consequences of treatment as compared with nontreatment are so undesirable that the omission of care is justified. . . .

. . . Many parents and physicians deeply committed to the loving care of the newborn think that treating severely defective infants causes more harm than good, thereby justifying the withholding of ordinary care. In their view the suffering and diminished quality of the child's life do not justify the social and economic costs of treatment. This claim has a growing commonsense appeal, but it assumes that the utility or quality of one's life can be measured and compared with other lives, and that health resources may legitimately be allocated to produce the greatest personal utility. This argument will now be analyzed from the perspective of the defective patient and others affected by his care.

A   THE QUALITY OF THE DEFECTIVE INFANT'S LIFE

Comparisons of relative worth among persons, or between persons and other interests, raise moral and methodological issues that make any argument that relies on such comparisons extremely vulnerable. Thus the strongest claim for not treating the defective newborn is that treatment seriously harms the infant's own interests, whatever may be the effects on others. When maintaining his life involves great physical and psychosocial suffering for the patient, a reasonable person might conclude that such a life is not worth living. Presumably the patient, if fully informed and able to communicate, would agree. One then would be morally justified in withholding lifesaving treatment if such action served to advance the best interests of the patient.

Congenital malformations impair development in several ways that lead to the judgment that deformed retarded infants are "a burden to themselves."[9] One is the severe physical pain, much of it resulting from repeated surgery that defective infants will suffer. Defective children also are likely to develop other pathological features, leading to repeated fractures, dislocations, surgery, malfunctions, and other sources of pain. The shunt, for example, inserted to relieve hydrocephalus, a common problem in defective children, often becomes clogged, necessitating frequent surgical interventions.

Pain, however, may be intermittent and manageable with analgesics. Since many infants and adults experience great pain, and many defective infants do not, pain alone, if not totally unmanageable, does not sufficiently show that a life is so worthless that death is preferable. More important are the psychosocial deficits resulting from the child's handicaps. Many defective children never can walk even with prosthesis, never interact with normal children, never appreciate growth, adolescence, or the fulfillment of education and employment, and seldom are even able to care for themselves. In cases of severe retardation, they may be left with a vegetative existence in a crib, incapable of choice or the most minimal response to stimuli. Parents or others may reject them, and much of their time will be spent in hospitals, in surgery, or fighting the many illnesses that beset them. Can it be said that such a life is worth living?

There are two possible responses to the quality-of-life argument. One is to accept its premises but to question the degree of suffering in particular cases, and thus restrict the justification for death to the most extreme cases. The absence of opportunities for schooling, career, and interaction may be the fault of social attitudes and the failings of healthy persons, rather than a necessary result of congenital malformations. Psychosocial suffering occurs because healthy, normal persons reject or refuse to relate to the defective, or hurry them to poorly funded institutions. Most nonambulatory, mentally retarded persons can be trained for satisfying roles. One cannot assume that a nonproductive existence is necessarily unhappy: even social rejection and nonacceptance can be mitigated. Moreover, the psychosocial ills of the handicapped often do not differ in kind from those experienced by many persons. With training and care, growth, development, and a full range of experiences are possible for most people with physical and mental handicaps. Thus, the claim that death is a far better fate than life cannot in most cases be sustained.

This response, however, avoids meeting the quality-of-life argument on its strongest grounds. Even if many defective infants can experience growth, interaction, and most human satisfactions if nurtured, treated, and trained, some infants are so severely retarded or grossly deformed that their response to love and care, in fact their capacity to be conscious, is always minimal. Although mongoloid and nonambulatory spina bifida children may experience an existence we would hesitate to adjudge worse than death, the profoundly retarded, nonambulatory, blind, deaf infant who will spend his few years in the back-ward cribs of a state institution is clearly a different matter.

To repudiate the quality-of-life argument, therefore, requires a defense of treatment in even these extreme cases. Such a defense would question the validity of any surrogate or proxy judgments of the worth or quality of life when the wishes of the person in question cannot be ascertained. The essence of the quality-of-life argument is a proxy's judgment that no reasonable person can prefer the pain, suffering, and loneliness of, for example, life in a crib at an IQ level of 20, to an immediate, painless death.

But in what sense can the proxy validly conclude that a person with different wants, needs, and interests, if able to speak, would agree that such a life were worse than death? At the start one must be skeptical of the proxy's claim to objective disinterestedness. If the proxy is also the parent or physician, as has been the case in pediatric euthanasia, the impact of treatment on the proxy's interests, rather than solely on those of the child, may influence his assessment. But even if the proxy were truly neutral and committed only to caring for the child, the problem of egocentricity and knowing another's mind remains. Compared with the situation and life prospects of a "reasonable man," the child's potential quality of life indeed appears dim. Yet a standard based on healthy, ordinary development may be entirely inappropriate to this situation. One who has never known the pleasures of mental operation, ambulation, and social interaction surely does not suffer from their loss as much as one who has. While one who has known these capacities may prefer death to a life without them, we have no assurance that the handicapped person, with no point of comparison, would agree. Life, and life alone, whatever its limitations, might be of sufficient worth to him.

One should also be hesitant to accept proxy assessments of quality of life because the margin of error in such predictions may be very great. For instance, while one expert argues that by a purely clinical assessment he can accurately forecast the minimum degree of future handicap an individual will experience, such forecasting is not infallible, and risks denying care to infants whose disability might otherwise permit a reasonably acceptable quality of life. Thus given the problems in ascertaining another's wishes, the proxy's bias to personal or culturally relative interests, and the unreliability of predictive criteria, the quality of life argument is open to serious question. Its strongest appeal arises in the case of a grossly deformed, retarded, institutionalied child, or one with incessant unmanageable pain, where continued life is itself torture. But these cases are few, and cast doubt on the utility of any such judgment. Even if the judgment occasionally may be defensible, the potential danger of quality-of-life assessments may be a compelling reason for rejecting this rationale for withholding treatment.

B   THE SUFFERING OF OTHERS

In addition to the infant's own suffering, one who argues that the harm of treatment justifies violation of the defective infant's right to life usually relies on the psychological, social, and economic costs of maintaining his existence to family and society. In their view the minimal benefit of treatment to persons incapable of full social and physical development does not justify the burdens that care of the defective infant imposes on parents, siblings, health professionals, and other patients. Matson, a noted pediatric neurosurgeon, states:

> [I]t is the doctor's and the community's responsibility to provide [custodial] care and to minimize suffering; but, at the same time, it is also their responsibility not to prolong such individual, familial, and community suffering unnecessarily, and not to carry out multiple procedures and prolonged, expensive, acute hospitalization in an infant whose chance for acceptable growth and development is negligible.[10]

Such a frankly utilitarian argument raises problems. It assumes that becuase of the greatly curtailed orbit of his existence, the costs or suffering of others is greater than the benefit of life to the child. This judgment, however, requires a coherent way of measuring and comparing interpersonal utilities, a logical-practical problem that utilitarianism has never surmounted. But even if such comparisons could reliably show a net loss from treatment, the fact remains that the child must sacrifice his life to benefit others. If the life of one individual, however useless, may be sacrificed for the benefit of any person, however useful, or for the benefit of any number of persons, then we have acknowledged the principle that rational utility may justify any outcome. As many philosophers have demonstrated, utilitarianism can always permit the sacrifice of one life for other interests, given the appropriate arrangement of utilities on the balance sheet. In the absence of principled grounds for such a decision, the social equation involved in mandating direct, involuntary euthanasia becomes a difference of degree, not kind, and we reach the point where protection of life depends solely on social judgments of utility.

These objections may well be determinative. But if we temporarily bracket them and examine the extent to which care of the defective infant subjects others to suffering, the claim that inordinate suffering outweighs the infant's interest in life is rarely plausible. In this regard we must examine the impact of caring for defective infants on the family, health professions, and society-at-large.

The Family

The psychological impact and crisis created by birth of a defective infant is devastating. Not only is the mother denied the normal tension release from the stresses of pregnancy, but both parents feel a crushing blow to their dignity, self-esteem and self-confidence. In a very short time, they feel grief for the loss of the normal expected child, anger at fate, numbness, disgust, waves of helplessness, and disbelief. Most feel personal blame for the defect, or blame their spouse. Adding to the shock is fear that social position and mobility are permanently endangered. The transformation of a "joyously awaited experience into one of catastrophe and profound psychological threat"[11] often will reactivate unresolved maturational conflicts. The chances for social pathology—divorce, somatic complaints, nervous and mental disorders—increase and hard-won adjustment patterns may be permanently damaged.

The initial reactions of guilt, grief, anger, and loss, however, cannot be the true measure of family suffering caused by care of a defective infant, because these costs are present whether or not the parents choose treatment. Rather, the question is to what degree treatment imposes psychic and other costs greater than would occur if the child were not treated. The claim that care is more costly rests largely on the view that parents and family suffer inordinately from nurturing such a child.

Indeed, if the child is treated and accepted at home, difficult and demanding adjustments must be made. Parents must learn how to care for a disabled child, confront financial and psychological uncertainty, meet the needs of other siblings, and work through their own conflicting feelings. Mothering demands are greater than with a normal child, particularly if medical care and hospitalization are frequently required. Counseling or professional support may be nonexistent or difficult to obtain. Younger siblings may react with hostility and guilt, older with shame and anger. Often the normal feedback of child growth that renders the turmoil of childrearing worthwhile develops more slowly or not at all. Family resources can be depleted (especially if medical care is needed), consumption patterns altered, or standards of living modified. Housing may have to be found closer to a hospital, and plans for further children changed. Finally, the anxieties, guilt, and grief present at birth may threaten to recur or become chronic.

Yet, although we must recognize the burdens and frustrations of raising a defective infant, it does not necessarily follow that these costs require nontreatment, or even institutionalization. Individual and group counseling can substantially alleviate anxiety, guilt, and frustration, and enable parents to cope with underlying conflicts triggered by the birth and the adaptations required. Counseling also can reduce psychological pressures on siblings, who can be taught to recognize and accept their own possibly hostile feelings and the difficult position of their parents. They may even be taught to help their parents care for the child.

The impact of increased financial costs also may vary. In families with high income or adequate health insurance, the financial costs are manageable. In others, state assistance may be available. If severe financial problems arise or pathological adjustments are likely, institutionalization, although undesirable for the child, remains an option. Finally, in many cases, the experience of living through a crisis is a deepening and enriching one, accelerating personality maturation, and giving one a new sensitivity to the needs of spouse, siblings, and others. As one parent of a defective child states: "In the last months I have come closer to people and can understand them more. I have met them more deeply. I did not know there were so many people with troubles in the world."[12]

Thus, while social attitudes regard the handicapped child as an unmitigated disaster, in reality the problem may not be insurmountable, and often may not differ from life's other vicissitudes. Suffering there is, but seldom is it so overwhelming or so imminent that the only alternative is death of the child.

Health Professionals

Physicians and nurses also suffer when parents give birth to a defective child, although, of course, not to the degree of the parents. To the obstetrician or general practitioner the defective birth may be a blow to his professional identity. He has the difficult task of informing the parents of the defects, explaining their causes, and dealing with the parents' resulting emotional shock. Often he feels guilty for failing to produce a normal baby. In addition, the parents may project anger or hostility on the physician, questioning his professional competence or seeking the services of other doctors. The physician also may feel that his expertise and training are misused when employed to maintain the life of an infant whose chances for a productive existence are so diminished. By neglecting other patients, he may feel that he is prolonging rather than alleviating suffering.

Nurses, too, suffer role strain from care of the defective newborn. Intensive-care-unit nurses may work with only one or two babies at a time. They face the daily ordeals of care—the progress and relapses—and often must deal with anxious parents who are themselves grieving or ambivalent toward the child. The situation may trigger a nurse's own ambivalence about death and mothering, in a context in which she is actively working to keep alive a child whose life prospects seem minimal.

Thus, the effects of care on physicians and nurses are not trivial, and must be intelligently confronted in medical education or in management of a pediatric unit. Yet to state them is to make clear that they can but weigh lightly in the decision of whether to treat a defective newborn. Compared with the situation of the parents, these burdens seem insignificant, are short term, and most likely do not evoke such profound emotions. In any case, these difficulties are hazards of the profession—caring for the sick and dying will always produce strain. Hence, on these grounds alone it is difficult to argue that a defective person may be denied the right to life.

Society

Care of the defective newborn also imposes societal costs, the utility of which is questioned when the infant's expected quality of life is so poor. Medical resources that can be used by infants with a better prognosis, or throughout the health-care system generally, are consumed in providing expensive surgical and intensive-care services to infants who may be severely retarded, never lead active lives, and die in a few months or years. Institutionalization imposes costs on taxpayers and reduces the resources available for those who might better benefit from it, while reducing further the quality of life experienced by the institutionalized defective.

One answer to these concerns is to question the impact of the costs of caring for defective newborns. Precise data showing the costs to taxpayers or the trade-offs with health and other expenditures do not exist. Nor would ceasing to care for the defective necessarily lead to a reallocation within the health budget that would produce net savings in suffering or life; in fact, the released resources might not be reallocated for health at all. In any case, the trade-offs within the health budget may well be small. With advances in prenatal diagnosis of genetic disorders many deformed infants who would formerly require care will be aborted beforehand. Then, too, it is not clear that the most technical and expensive procedures always constitute the best treatment for certain malformations. When compared with the almost seven percent of the GNP now spent on health, the money in the defense budget, or tax revenues generally, the public resources required to keep defective newborns alive seem marginal, and arguably worth the commitment to life that such expenditures reinforce. Moreover, as the Supreme Court recently recognized,[13] conservation of the taxpayer's purse does not justify serious infringement of fundamental rights. Given legal and ethical norms against sacrificing the lives of nonconsenting others, and the imprecisions in diagnosis and prediction concerning the eventual outcomes of medical care, the social cost argument does not compel nontreatment of defective newborns. . . .

NOTES

1 Few persons would argue that "extraordinary" care must be provided a defective newborn, or indeed, to any person. The difficult question, however, is to distinguish "ordinary" from "extraordinary" care. . . . In this Article "ordinary" care refers to those medical and surgical procedures that would normally be applied in situations not involving physically or mentally handicapped persons.

2 The need for ordinary treatment will also arise with noncentral nervous system malformations such as malformations of the cardiovascular, respiratory, orogastrointestinal, urogenital, muscular and skeletal systems, as well as deformities of the eye, ear, face, endocrine glands, and skin. *See generally* J. Warkany, CONGENITAL MALFORMATIONS (1971). Often these defects will accompany central nervous system malformations. The medical-ethical dilemma discussed in this Article has arisen chiefly with regard to central nervous system problems, perhaps because the presence of such defects seriously affects intelligence, social interaction, and the potential for development and growth, and will be discussed only in the context of the major central nervous system malformations. Parents of physically deformed infants with normal intelligence might face the same choice, but because of the child's capacity for development, pressure to withhold ordinary treatment will be less severe.

3 Anencephaly is partial or total absence of the brain. J. Warkany, *supra* note 2, at 189–99.

4 Hydrocephaly is characterized by an increase of free fluid in the cranial cavity which results in a marked enlargement of the head. *Id.* at 217. It is a symptom of many diverse disorders, and is associated with hereditary and chromosomal syndromes. *Id.* at 217–18. Warkany describes the symptoms as follows: "Bulging of the forehead, protrusion of the parietal areas and extension of the occipital region are characteristic changes. . . . The skin of the scalp is thin and stretched and its veins are dilated. . . . The head cannot be held up, and walking and talking are delayed. The legs are spastic, the tendon reflexes increased and convulsions may occur. Anorexia, vomiting and emaciation complicate severe cases. As a rule, hydrocephalic children are dull and lethargic. Blindness can develop, but hearing and the auditory memory may be good. Physical and mental development depend on several factors, such as rapidity of onset, intracranial pressure, compensatory growth of the head, nature of the basic malformations and progress or arrest of the process. Such variability makes the prognosis and evaluation of therapeutic measures difficult. Pressure on the hypothalamic area can cause obesity or precocious puberty in exceptional cases." *Id.* at 226–27.

5 Down's syndrome or mongolism is a chromosomal disorder producing mental retardation caused by the presence of 47 rather than 46 chromosomes in a patient's cells, and marked by a distinctively shaped head, neck, trunk, and abdomen. *Id.* at 311–12, 324. For summary of clinical and pathological characteristics, *see id.* at 324–31.

6 Spina bifida refers generally to midline defects of the osseous spine. The defect usually appears in the posterior aspects of the vertebral canal, and may be marked by an external saccular protrusion (spina bifida cystica). *Id.* at 272. Spina bifida is often seriously involved with urinary tract deficiency, hydro-

cephaly, and may involve paralysis of the lower extremities. *Id.* at 286–88. While there are important differences between spina bifida, meningoceles, and myelomeningocele, the terms will be used interchangeably in discussing and evaluating the duty to treat.

7 The saccular enlargements of spina bifida cystica protruding through osseous defects of the vertebral column that contain anomalous meninges and spinal fluid but do not have neural elements affixed to their walls are called meningoceles. If the spinal cord or nerves are included in the formation of the sac, the anomaly is called myelomeningocele. *Id.* at 272. As with spina bifida, myelomeningocele may substantially interfere with locomotion, sphincter and bladder control, and may be accompanied by kyphoscoliosis and hydrocephaly leading to mental retardation. For a description of symptoms and treatment alternatives, *see* Lorber, *Results of Treatment of Myelomeningocele*, 13 DEVELOP. MED. & CHILD NEUROL. 279–303 (1971).

8 The infant might suffer from duodenal atresia and need surgery to connect the stomach to the intestine; or need an appendectomy; or antibiotics to fight pneumonia; or suffer from Respirator Distress Syndrome and need breathing assistance. In some cases the question is whether to begin or continue feeding.

9 Smith & Smith, *Selection for Treatment in Spina Bifida Cystica*, 4 BRIT. MED. J. 189, 195 (1973).

10 Matson, *Surgical Treatment of Myelomeningocele*, 42 PEDIATRICS 225, 226 (1968).

11 Goodman, *Continuing Treatment of Parents with Congenitally Defective Infants*, SOCIAL WORK, Vol. 9, No. I, at 92 (1964).

12 *Quoted in* Johns, *Family Reactions to the Birth of a Child with a Congenital Abnormality*, 26 OBSTET. GYNECOL. SURVEY 635, 637 (1971).

13 *Memorial Hosp. v. Maricopa County*, 415 U.S. 250 (1974).

Standards of Judgment for Treatment of Imperiled Newborns
Members of The Hastings Center Research Project on the Care of Imperiled Newborns

In 1984 The Hastings Center initiated a research project dedicated to the problem of determining appropriate care for imperiled newborns. Philosophers, physicians, nurses, and lawyers were among the many project participants, and Arthur L. Caplan served as project director. A brief excerpt from the 1987 project report is reprinted here.

Concerned with the problem of selective nontreatment, the project group members first reject two distinctive sanctity-of-life positions—"vitalism" and "the medical indications policy." They then endorse the employment of quality-of-life standards, with the provision that quality must be measured by reference to the infant's own well-being and not in terms of social utility. In their view, two distinctive quality-of-life standards are relevant to the problem of selective nontreatment. In most cases, the relevant standard is the best interest of the infant, which would allow (and in fact mandate) nontreatment only when continued life would be worse for the infant than an early death. In some cases, however, the relevant standard is that of "relational potential," which would make treatment optional for an infant who lacks the potential for human relationships.

As parents and clinicians evaluate specific strategies for responding to uncertainty, it is essential to ask how they should determine whether treatment is *ethically right* for a particular infant. The ethical questions can only be resolved by establishing reasonable standards of judgment against which to measure strategies and procedures.

"SANCTITY OF LIFE" STANDARDS

Many critics of the practice of selective nontreatment argue that we must concentrate on the *sanctity* of life. But what does it mean to base our decisions on the sanctity of each child's life? Does it mean that caregivers may *never* forgo treatment, or that they may do so only for the most catastrophically afflicted newborns? Without further specification, the "sanctity of life" standard remains a vague slogan, rather than a meaningful guide to decisionmaking.

Vitalism

The most extreme sanctity of life position would hold that "where there is life, there is hope," and that so long as a child continues to cling to life, he or she must be

Reprinted with permission of the publisher from *Hastings Center Report*, vol. 17 (December 1987), pp. 13–16.

treated. According to this view, which we shall call "vitalism," the mere presence of a heartbeat, respiration, or brain activity is a compelling reason to sustain all efforts to save the child's life. Only the moment of death relieves caregivers of their duty to treat. An adherent of this vitalist philosophy would accordingly hold that, except in cases where the child has been declared dead, all withholding and withdrawal of treatment is ethically wrong.

This most extreme sanctity of life position has few advocates. Its major flaw is that it would insist upon aggressive treatments even for those children who are deemed to be in the process of dying. If responsible physicians have concluded that a particular child cannot be saved, that he will soon die, then it seems pointless and cruel to continue to treat the child with medical interventions that are by no means benign. By insisting on treatment even in such hopeless cases, the vitalist can justly be accused of worshipping an abstraction, "life," rather than focusing on the concrete good of the patient. As theologian Paul Ramsey has cogently argued, the appropriate response to a dying patient is not the futile imposition of painful medical treatments, but rather kind and respectful *care* designed to ease the child's passing.

The Medical Indications Policy

A more reasonable sanctity of life position has been proposed by Paul Ramsey and adopted (with some modifications) in various versions of the Department of Health and Human Services so-called "Baby Doe Rules." According to this standard, each child possesses equal dignity and intrinsic worth (i.e. "sanctity") and therefore no child should be denied life-sustaining medical treatments simply on the basis of his or her "handicap" or future quality of life. Such treatments must be provided to all infants, except (1) when the infant is judged to be in the process of dying, or (2) when the contemplated treatment is itself deemed to be "medically contraindicated." As Ramsey puts it, *treatments* may be compared in order to see which will be medically beneficial for a child, but abnormal *children* may not be compared with normal children in order to determine who shall live.

This policy is supported by two complementary ethical principles. First, the "nondiscrimination principle" states that children with impairments may not be selected for nontreatment solely on the basis of their "handicapping condition." If an otherwise normal child would receive a certain treatment—for example, surgery to repair an intestinal blockage—then a child with an abnormality must receive like treatment. Failure to do so discriminates unfairly against the child with impairments.

Second, the "medical benefit principle" states that caregivers are obliged to provide any and all treatments deemed, according to "reasonable medical judgment," to be "medically beneficial" to the patient. This means that if a certain medical or surgical procedure would be likely to bring about its intended result of avoiding infection or some other fatal consequence, then it must be provided to the child.

Although this medical indications policy was obviously well intended, insofar as it attempted to prevent instances of *unjust* discrimination against newborns with impairments, we believe that it is an overly rigid and inappropriate guide to decisionmaking. The first problem is that the nondiscrimination principle would have decisionmakers ignore, not just relatively mild handicaps of the sort encountered in most children with spina bifida and Down syndrome, but also impairments that are genuinely catastrophic.

Consider, for example, the child suffering from severe birth asphyxia who also happens to have a grave heart defect. Although surgeons would be willing to operate to fix the heart of an otherwise normal infant, the fact that this particular infant will never be sufficiently conscious to interact with his environment would appear to be a factor that the child's caretakers might permissibly take into consideration. Should the child be subjected to major and painful cardiac surgery only so that he might subsist in a permanently unconscious state? Even though treatment might be withheld from such a grievously afflicted infant "solely on the basis of his handicap," such a decision would in no way count as *unjust* discrimination precisely because the child's handicap is so severe that he can no longer meaningfully be compared to an "otherwise normal" infant.

The second problem with the medical indications policy lies in its "medical benefit" principle. Although this principle works well in many cases—for example, mild to moderate spina bifida—it does so because we think that the treatment confers a benefit, not merely upon the child's spine, but rather upon the whole child.

QUALITY OF LIFE STANDARDS

Although we conclude that quality of life judgments are ethically proper, and indeed inevitable, a great deal of care must be given to specifying why quality of life matters and what qualitative conditions might justify the denial of treatment. Merely invoking the phrase "quality of life" will get us no farther than invocations of the "sanctity of life."

The phrase "quality of life," as used in medical contexts, is ambiguous and frequently misunderstood. It is sometimes used to denote the social worth of an individual, the value that individual has for society. According to this interpretation, a person's quality of life is determined by utilitarian criteria, measured by balancing the burdens and benefits to others, especially family members. It is this meaning of the phrase that gives rise to the greatest worries about undertreatment of newborns with impairments.

This interpretation of quality of life has been defended on the grounds that external circumstances are crucially important in the outlook for certain newborns and because of the increased stress families undergo in raising children with disabilities. Despite the recognition that these external factors play a role in parental attitudes toward treatment, the consensus of this report is that "quality of life" should refer to the present or future characteristics of the infant, judged by standards of the infant's own well-being and not in terms of social utility.

Another way of understanding "quality of life" is as measured against a norm of "acceptable" life. Yet it is often noted that what would not be acceptable to some people, for themselves, is clearly acceptable to others. A danger lies in drawing the line too high, thereby ruling as "unacceptable" the life of a person with multiple handicaps or with mild-to-moderate mental retardation. When quality of life assessments are made for newborns with impairments, caution must be exercised to avoid this pitfall.

An example of drawing the line of "acceptable" life too high is "the ability to work or marry," a factor cited by the British pediatrician, John Lorber. An example of a very low standard is permanent coma, a criterion appearing in the 1984 Child Abuse Amendments. This threshold is so low as to be noncontroversial.

A subset of the quality of life standard and an alternative to a medical indications policy is the standard known as the "best interest of the child." Traditionally, this standard has been employed by courts in making child custody determinations and other decisions involving placement of an infant or child.

Unlike the medical indications policy, the "best interest" standard does incorporate quality of life considerations. This standard holds that infants should be treated with life-sustaining therapy except when (1) the infant is dying, (2) treatment is medically contraindicated (the two exceptions built into the medical indications policy), and (3) continued life would be worse for the infant than an early death. The third condition opens the door to quality of life considerations, but requires that such considerations be viewed from the infant's point of view. That is, certain states of being, marked by severe and intractable pain and suffering, can be viewed as worse than death. Thus, according to the best interest standard, there is room to consider the possibility that an infant's best interest can lie in withholding or withdrawing medical treatments, resulting in death.

Care must be taken, however, not to employ a standard based on the sensibilities of unimpaired adults; for example, one in which adult decisionmakers judge, from their own perspective, that they would not want to live a life with mental or physical disabilities. An infant-centered quality of life standard should be as objective as possible, in an attempt to determine whether continued life would be a benefit, from the child's point of view. An impaired child does not have the luxury of comparing his life to a "normal" existence; for such a child, it is a question of life with impairments versus no life at all.

The greatest merit of the best interest standard lies precisely in its child-centeredness. This focus on the individual child will aid decisionmakers in avoiding the twin evils of overtreatment, sanctioned by the medical indications policy, and undertreatment, which might result from allowing negative consequences for the family or society to determine what treatment is appropriate for the infant.

Although we believe the best interest of the infant should remain the primary standard for decisionmaking on behalf of newborns with impairments, it has limits. In addition to the undeniable problem of vagueness, there is the further question of the applicability of this standard to some of the most troubling dilemmas in the neonatal nursery. As one critic has noted about the standard suggested in the President's Commission report, *Deciding to Forgo Life-Sustaining Treatment:*

> The fact that the child-based best-interest standard would mandate treatment even in the face of a prognosis bereft of any distinctly human potentiality reveals a feature of that standard that has so far gone unnoticed. In such extreme cases, the best-interest standard tends to view the absence of pain as the only morally relevant consideration. No matter that the infant is doomed to a life of very short duration, and lacks the capacity for any distinctively human development or activity; so long as the child does not experience any severe burdens, interpreted from her point of view, the fact that she can anticipate no distinctly human benefits is of no moral consequence.

In an article published in 1974, Father Richard McCormick explained and defended a quality of life viewpoint that differs from the best interest standard. Noting that modern medicine can keep almost anyone alive, he posed the question: "Granted that we can easily save the life, what kind of life are we saving?" McCormick admits this is a quality of life judgment, and holds that we must face the possibility of answering this question when it arises.

McCormick's guideline is "the potential for human relationships associated with the infant's condition." Translated into the language of "best interests," an individual who lacks any present capacity or future potential for human relationships can be said to have no interests at all, except perhaps to be free from pain and discomfort.

Our conclusion is that there is a need for two different standards embodying relational potential considerations. The prevailing "best interest" notion presupposes that all infants have interests, but for some, the burdens of continued life can outweigh the benefits. The alternative "relational potential" standard focuses on the potential of the individual for human relationships, and presumes that some severely neurologically impaired children cannot be said to have interests to which a best interest standard might apply. In employing these two standards, decisionmakers should first determine whether the best interest standard applies to the case at hand. For the large majority of infants this standard is applicable, and should be used to determine whether life-sustaining treatment should be administered. However, if an infant is so severely neurologically impaired as to render the best interest standard inapplicable, then the alternative standard, lack of potential for human relationships, becomes the relevant criterion, placing decisionmaking within the realm of parental discretion.

When the best interest standard is applicable, because the infant's best interest can be determined, decisionmakers are obligated either to institute or to forgo life-sustaining treatment. In contrast, the relational potential standard is nonobligatory: it permits the withholding or withdrawing of therapy from infants who lack the potential for human relationships, but it does not require that treatment be forgone. Continued treatment would not benefit such infants, but neither would it harm them. An example might be an infant born with trisomy 13. Most such infants do not survive beyond the first year of life, are severely or profoundly mentally retarded, and have multiple malformations. Their chances of being able to experience human interactions are minimal. Unlike the best interest standard, which is infant-centered, the relational potential standard allows the interests of others—e.g., family or society—to weigh in the decision about whether to treat. . . .

ANNOTATED BIBLIOGRAPHY: CHAPTER 7

Battin, M. Pabst: *Ethical Issues in Suicide* (Englewood Cliffs, NJ: Prentice-Hall, 1982). In this very useful book, Battin provides a comprehensive discussion of the traditional arguments concerning suicide. She also suggests an analysis of the concept of rational suicide, discusses suicide intervention as well as suicide facilitation, and considers the notion of suicide as a right.

———, and David J. Mayo, eds.: *Suicide: The Philosophical Issues* (New York: St. Martin's Press, 1980). This valuable collection of articles includes material on the concept of suicide, the morality of suicide, and the rationality of suicide. There are also sections entitled "Suicide and Psychiatry" and "Suicide, Law, and Rights."

Beauchamp, Tom L.: "Suicide," in Tom Regan, ed., *Matters of Life and Death,* 3d ed. (New York: McGraw-Hill, 1993), pp. 69–120. In this long essay, Beauchamp provides both a conceptual analysis of suicide and an evaluation of various moral views. He also discusses suicide intervention and assisted suicide.

Beck, Robert N., and John B. Orr, eds.: *Ethical Choice: A Case Study Approach* (New York: Free Press, 1970). Section 2 of this work is entitled "Suicide" and conveniently reprints several classical sources on suicide: Seneca, St. Augustine, St. Thomas Aquinas, Hume, and Schopenhauer.

Caplan, Arthur L., Robert H. Blank, and Janna C. Merrick, eds.: *Compelled Compassion: Government Intervention in the Treatment of Critically Ill Newborns* (Totowa, NJ: Humana Press, 1992). This book provides an extensive collection of material on the federal "Baby Doe" legislation.

Gomez, Carlos F.: *Regulating Death: Euthanasia and the Case of the Netherlands* (New York: Free Press, 1991). Gomez describes and criticizes the practice of (active) euthanasia in the Netherlands. He argues that the Dutch system is plagued with inadequate controls.

Hastings Center Report 22 (March/April 1992). This issue provides a collection of articles under the heading "Dying Well? A Colloquy on Euthanasia and Assisted Suicide." Several of the articles deal specifically with the practice of (active) euthanasia in the Netherlands.

Also, Dan W. Brock offers an extensive defense of voluntary active euthanasia, which Daniel Callahan opposes in "When Self-Determination Runs Amok."

"Imperiled Newborns." Report of The Hastings Center Research Project on the Care of Imperiled Newborns. *Hastings Center Report* 17 (December 1987), pp. 5–32. This report is organized in seven sections and provides a wealth of factual information, conceptual clarification, and ethical analysis.

Journal of Pain and Symptom Management 6 (July 1991). This special issue provides a diverse collection of articles on physician-assisted suicide and (active) euthanasia.

King, Nancy M. P.: "Transparency in Neonatal Intensive Care," *Hastings Center Report* 22 (May/June 1992), pp. 18–25. Focusing on decision making for severely premature infants, King argues for the acceptance of a "transparency" model of informed consent. (See Howard Brody's discussion of this model in Chapter 2.)

McCormick, Richard A.: "To Save or Let Die: The Dilemma of Modern Medicine," *JAMA* 229 (July 8, 1974), pp. 172–176. In dealing with the problem of selective nontreatment of severely impaired newborns, McCormick argues that infants having no significant potential for human relationships may be allowed to die.

Pellegrino, Edmund D.: "Doctors Must Not Kill," *Journal of Clinical Ethics* 3 (Summer 1992), pp. 95–102. Pellegrino contends (1) that the moral arguments in favor of (active) euthanasia are flawed, (2) that killing by physicians would seriously distort the healing relationship, and (3) that the social consequences of allowing such killing would be very detrimental.

Prado, C. G.: *The Last Choice: Preemptive Suicide in Advanced Age* (Westport, CT: Greenwood Press, 1990). Prado's basic claim is that it is rational for an aging individual to commit suicide in order to avoid a demeaning decline.

Quill, Timothy E.: "Death and Dignity: A Case of Individualized Decision Making," *New England Journal of Medicine* 324 (March 7, 1991), pp. 691–694. Quill presents a brief account of a case—often referred to as "the case of Diane"—in which he assisted in the suicide of one of his patients.

Rachels, James: "Euthanasia," in Tom Regan, ed., *Matters of Life and Death,* 3d ed. (New York: McGraw-Hill, 1993), pp. 30–68. In this long essay, Rachels evaluates (1) arguments for and against the morality of active euthanasia and (2) arguments for and against legalizing it. He concludes that active euthanasia is morally acceptable and that it should be legalized.

Sherlock, Richard: "Selective Non-Treatment of Defective Newborns: A Critique," *Ethics in Science & Medicine* 7 (1980), pp. 111–117. Sherlock contends, against those who advocate nontreatment of newborns whose life "is not worth living anyway," that no one has succeeded in specifying reasonable, nonarbitrary criteria for the identification of such lives.

Steinbock, Bonnie, ed.: *Killing and Letting Die* (Englewood Cliffs, NJ: Prentice-Hall, 1980). This anthology provides a wealth of material on the distinction between killing and letting die.

Trammell Richard L.: "Euthanasia and the Law," *Journal of Social Philosophy* 9 (January 1978), pp. 14–18. Trammell contends that the legalization of voluntary positive (i.e., active) euthanasia would probably not "result in overall positive utility for the class of people eligible to choose." He emphasizes the unwelcome pressures that would be created by legalization.

Velasques, Manuel G.: "Defining Suicide," Issues in Law & Medicine 3 (1987), pp. 37–51.Velasquez criticizes some definitions of suicide as too broad, rejects others as too narrow, then advances his own proposal.

Weir, Robert F.: "The Morality of Physician-Assisted Suicide," *Law, Medicine & Health Care* 20 (Spring–Summer 1992), pp. 116–126. Weir surveys the ethical arguments for and against physician-assisted suicide. He believes that the practice is justified under certain conditions.

————: *Selective Nontreatment of Handicapped Newborns: Moral Dilemmas in Neonatal Medicine* (New York: Oxford University Press, 1984). Weir surveys and critically analyzes a wide range of views (advanced by various pediatricians, attorneys, and ethicists) on the subject of selective nontreatment. He then presents and defends an overall policy for the guidance of decision making in this area.

CHAPTER 8

ABORTION AND MATERNAL-FETAL CONFLICTS

INTRODUCTION

The first object of concern in this chapter is the issue of the ethical (moral) acceptability of abortion. Some attention is then given to the social policy aspects of abortion, especially in conjunction with developments in the United States Supreme Court. Finally, several ethical problems associated with maternal-fetal conflicts are identified and explored.

Abortion: The Ethical Issue

Discussions of the ethical acceptability of abortion often take for granted (1) an awareness of the various kinds of reasons that may be given for having an abortion and (2) a basic acquaintance with the biological development of a human fetus.

Reasons for Abortion Why would a woman have an abortion? The following catalog, not meant to provide an exhaustive survey, is sufficient to indicate that there is a wide range of potential reasons for abortion. (1) In certain extreme cases, if the fetus is allowed to develop normally and come to term, the pregnant woman herself will die. (2) In other cases it is not the woman's life but her health, physical or mental, that will be severely endangered if the pregnancy is allowed to continue. (3) There are also cases in which the pregnancy will probably, or surely, produce a severely impaired child,[1] and (4) there are others in which the pregnancy is the result of rape or incest.[2] (5) There are instances in which the pregnant woman is unmarried, and there will be the social stigma of illegitimacy. (6) There are other instances in which having a child, or having another child, will be an unbearable financial burden. (7) Certainly common, and perhaps most common of all, are those instances in which having a child will interfere with the happiness of the woman, the joint happiness of the parents, or even the joint happiness of a family unit that already includes children. Regarding this final category, there are almost endless possibilities. The woman may desire a professional career, a couple may be content and happy together and feel their relationship would be damaged by the intrusion of a child, parents may have older children and not feel up to raising another child, and so forth.

The Biological Development of a Human Fetus   During the course of a human pregnancy, in the nine-month period from conception to birth, the product of conception undergoes a continual process of change and development. *Conception* takes place when a male germ cell (the spermatozoon) combines with a female germ cell (the ovum), resulting in a single cell (the single-cell zygote), which embodies the full genetic code, twenty-three pairs of chromosomes. The single-cell zygote soon begins a process of cellular division. The resultant multicell zygote, while continuing to grow and beginning to take shape, proceeds to move through the fallopian tube and then to undergo gradual *implantation* at the uterine wall. The developing entity is formally designated a zygote up until the time that implantation is complete, almost two weeks after conception. Thereafter, until the end of the eighth week, the unborn entity is formally designated an embryo. It is in this embryonic period that organ systems and other human characteristics begin to undergo noticeable development; in particular, brain waves can be detected at the end of the sixth week. From the end of the eighth week until birth, the unborn entity is formally designated a *fetus*. (The term *fetus*, however, is commonly used as a general term to designate the developing entity, whatever its stage of development.) Two other points in the development of the fetus are especially noteworthy as relevant to discussions of abortion, but these points are usually identified by reference to gestational age as calculated not from conception but from the first day of the woman's last menstrual period. Accordingly, somewhere between the twelfth and the sixteenth week there usually occurs *quickening,* the point at which the woman begins to feel the movements of the fetus. And somewhere in the neighborhood of the twenty-fourth week, *viability* becomes a realistic possibility. Viability is the point at which the fetus is capable of surviving outside the womb.

With the facts of fetal development in view, it may be helpful to indicate the various medical techniques of abortion. Early (first trimester) abortions were at one time performed by *dilatation and curettage* (D&C) but are now commonly performed by *uterine aspiration,* also called "suction curettage." The D&C features the stretching (dilatation) of the cervix and the scraping (curettage) of the inner walls of the uterus. Uterine aspiration simply involves sucking the fetus out of the uterus by means of a tube connected to a suction pump. Later abortions require *dilatation and evacuation* (D&E), *induction techniques,* or *hysterotomy.* In the D&E, which is the abortion procedure commonly used in the early stages of the second trimester, a forceps is used to dismember the fetus within the uterus; the fetal remains are then withdrawn through the cervix. In one commonly employed induction technique, a saline solution injected into the amniotic cavity induces labor, thereby expelling the fetus. Another induction technique employs prostaglandins (hormonelike substances) to induce labor. Hysterotomy—in essence a miniature cesarean section—is a major surgical procedure and is uncommonly employed in the United States.

A brief discussion of fetal development together with a cursory survey of various reasons for abortion has prepared the way for a formulation of the ethical issue of abortion in its broadest terms. *Up to what point of fetal development, if any, and for what reasons, if any, is abortion ethically acceptable?* Some hold that abortion is *never* ethically acceptable, or at most that it is acceptable only when necessary to save the life of the pregnant woman. This view is frequently termed the "*conservative* view" on abortion. Others hold that abortion is *always* ethically acceptable—at any point of fetal development and for any of the standard reasons. This view is frequently termed the "*liberal* view" on abortion. Still others are anxious to defend perspectives that are termed "*moderate* views," holding that abortion is ethically acceptable up to a certain point of fetal development *and/or* holding that some reasons provide a sufficient justification for abortion whereas others do not.

The Conservative View and the Liberal View

The *moral status* of the fetus has been a pivotal issue in discussions of the ethical acceptability of abortion. To say that the fetus has *full moral status* is to say that it is entitled to the same degree of moral consideration that is deserved by more fully developed human beings, such as the writer and the reader of these words. In particular, assigning full moral status to the fetus entails that the fetus has a right to life that must be taken as seriously as the right to life of any other human being. On the other hand, to say that the fetus has *no (significant) moral status* is to say that it has no rights worth talking about. In particular, it does not possess a significant right to life. Conservatives typically claim that the fetus has full moral status, and liberals typically claim that the fetus has no significant moral status. (Some moderates argue that the fetus has a subsidiary or *partial moral status.*) Since the fetus has no significant moral status, the liberal is prone to argue, it has no more right to life than a piece of tissue such as an appendix and an abortion is no more morally objectionable than an appendectomy. Since the fetus has full moral status, the conservative is prone to argue, its right to life must be respected with the utmost seriousness and an abortion, except perhaps to save the life of a pregnant woman, is as morally objectionable as any other murder.

Discussions of the moral status of the fetus often refer directly to the biological development of the fetus and pose the question: At what point in the continuous development of the fetus does a human life exist? In the context of such discussions, *human* implies full moral status, *nonhuman* implies no (significant) moral status, and any notion of partial moral status is systematically excluded. To distinguish the human from the nonhuman, to "draw the line," and to do so in a nonarbitrary way, is the central matter of concern. The *conservative* on abortion typically holds that the line must be drawn at conception. Usually the conservative argues that conception is the only point at which the line can be nonarbitrarily drawn. Against attempts to draw the line at points such as implantation, quickening, viability, or birth, considerations of continuity in the development of the fetus are pressed. The conservative argues that a line cannot be securely drawn anywhere along the path of fetal development. It is said that the line will inescapably slide back to the point of conception in order to find objective support—by reference to the fact that the full genetic code is present subsequent to conception, whereas it is not present prior to conception.

With regard to drawing the line, the *liberal* typically contends that the fetus remains nonhuman even in its most advanced stages of development. The liberal, of course, does not mean to deny that a fetus is biologically a human fetus. Rather the claim is that the fetus is not human in any morally significant sense, that is, the fetus has no (significant) moral status. This point is often made in terms of the concept of personhood. Mary Anne Warren, who defends the liberal view on abortion in one of this chapter's selections, argues that the fetus is not a person. She also contends that the fetus bears so little resemblance to a person that it cannot be said to have a significant right to life. It is important to notice, as Warren analyzes the concept of personhood, that even a newborn baby is not a person. This conclusion, as might be expected, prompts Warren to a consideration of the moral justifiability of infanticide, an issue closely related to the problem of abortion.

Although the conservative view on abortion is most commonly predicated upon the straightforward contention that the fetus is a person from conception, there are at least two other lines of argument that have been advanced in its defense. One conservative, advancing what might be labeled "the presumption argument," writes:

> In being willing to kill the embryo, we accept responsibility for killing what we must admit *may* be a person. There is some reason to believe it is—namely the *fact* that it is a living, human individual and the inconclusiveness of arguments that try to exclude it from the protected circle of personhood.

To be willing to kill what for all we know could be a person is to be willing to kill it if it is a person. And since we cannot absolutely settle if it is a person except by a metaphysical postulate, for all practical purposes we must hold that to be willing to kill the embryo is to be willing to kill a person.[3]

In accordance with this line of argument, although it may not be possible to show conclusively that the fetus is a person from conception, we must presume that it is. Another line of argument that has been advanced by some conservatives emphasizes the potential rather than the actual personhood of the fetus. Even if the fetus is not a person, it is said, there can be no doubt that it is a potential person. Accordingly, by virtue of its potential personhood, the fetus must be accorded a right to life. Warren, in response to this line of argument, argues that the potential personhood of the fetus provides no basis for the claim that it has a significant right to life.

In one of the readings in this chapter, Don Marquis argues for a very conservative view on abortion, although he does not argue for what is commonly referred to as "the" conservative view on abortion. Whereas the standard conservative is committed to a "sanctity-of-life" viewpoint, according to which the lives of all biologically human beings (assuming their moral innocence) are considered immune from attack, Marquis bases his opposition to abortion on a distinctive theory about the wrongness of killing. Although Marquis claims that there is a strong moral presumption against abortion, and although he clearly believes that the vast majority of abortions are seriously immoral, he is not committed to the standard conservative contention that the only possible exception is the case in which abortion is necessary to save the life of the pregnant women.

Moderate Views

The conservative and liberal views, as explicated, constitute two extreme poles on the spectrum of ethical views of abortion. Each of the extreme views is marked by a formal simplicity. The conservative proclaims abortion to be immoral, irrespective of the stage of fetal development and irrespective of alleged justifying reasons. The one exception, admitted by some conservatives, is the case in which abortion is necessary to save the life of the pregnant woman.[4] The liberal proclaims abortion to be morally acceptable, irrespective of the stage of fetal development.[5] Moreover, there is no need to draw distinctions between those reasons that are sufficient to justify abortion and those that are not. No justification is needed. The moderate, in vivid contrast to both the conservative and the liberal, is unwilling either to condemn or condone abortion in sweeping terms. Some abortions are morally justifiable; some are morally objectionable. In some moderate views, the stage of fetal development is a relevant factor in the assessment of the moral acceptability of abortion. In other moderate views, the alleged justifying reason is a relevant factor in the assessment of the moral acceptability of abortion. In still other moderate views, both the stage of fetal development and the alleged justifying reason are relevant factors in the assessment of the moral acceptability of abortion.

Moderate views have been developed in accordance with the following clearly identifiable strategies:

1 Moderation of the Conservative View   One strategy for generating a moderate view presumes the typical conservative contention that the fetus is a person (i.e., has full moral status) from conception. What is denied, however, is that we must conclude to the moral impermissibility of abortion in *all* or nearly all cases. In a widely discussed article reprinted in this chapter, Judith Jarvis Thomson attempts to moderate the conservative view in just this way. For Thomson, even if it is presumed that the fetus is a person from conception, abortion is morally justified in a significant range of cases.

2 Moderation of the Liberal View   A second strategy for generating a moderate view presumes the liberal contention that the fetus has no (significant) moral status, even in the latest stages of pregnancy. What is denied, however, is that we must conclude to the moral permissibility of abortion in *all* cases. It might be said, in accordance with this line of thought, that abortion, even though it does not violate the rights of the fetus (which is presumed to have no rights), remains ethically problematic to the extent that negative social consequences flow from its practice. Such an argument seems especially forceful in the later stages of pregnancy, when the fetus increasingly resembles a newborn infant. It is argued that very late abortions have a brutalizing effect on those involved and, in various ways, lead to the breakdown of attitudes associated with respect for human life. Thus the conclusion is that very late abortions cannot be morally justified in the absence of very weighty reasons.

3 Moderation in Drawing the Line   A third strategy for generating a moderate view, in fact a whole range of moderate views, is associated with drawing-the-line discussions. Whereas the conservative typically draws the line between human (full moral status) and nonhuman (negligible moral status) at conception and the liberal typically draws that same line at birth (or sometime thereafter), a moderate view may be generated by drawing the line somewhere between these two extremes. For example, one might draw the line at implantation, at the point where brain activity begins, at quickening, at viability, and so forth. Whereas drawing the line at implantation would tend to generate a rather "conservative" moderate view, drawing the line at viability would tend to generate a rather "liberal" moderate view. Wherever the line is drawn, it is the burden of any such moderate view to show that the point specified is a nonarbitrary one. Once such a point has been specified, however, it might be argued that abortion is ethically acceptable before that point and ethically unacceptable after that point. Of course, further stipulations may be added in accordance with strategies 1 and 2.

4 Moderation in the Assignment of Moral Status   A fourth strategy for generating a moderate view is dependent upon assigning the fetus some sort of *partial moral status,* an approach taken by Daniel Callahan in one of this chapter's readings. It would seem that anyone who defends a moderate view based on the concept of partial moral status must first of all face the problem of explicating the nature of such partial moral status. Second, and closely related, there is the problem of showing how the interests of those with partial moral status are to be weighed against the interests of those with full moral status.

Abortion and Social Policy

In the United States, the Supreme Court's decision in *Roe v. Wade* (1973) has been the focal point of the social-policy debate over abortion. This case had the effect, for all practical purposes, of legalizing "abortion on request." The Court held that it was unconstitutional for a state to have laws prohibiting the abortion of a previable fetus. According to the *Roe* Court, a woman has a constitutionally guaranteed right to terminate a pregnancy (prior to viability), although a state, for reasons related to maternal health, may restrict the manner and circumstances in which abortions are performed subsequent to the end of the first trimester. The reasoning underlying the Court's holding in *Roe* can be found in the majority opinion reprinted in this chapter.

Since the action of the Court in *Roe* had the practical effect of establishing a woman's legal right to choose whether or not to abort, it was enthusiastically received by "right-to-choose" forces. On the other hand, "right-to-life" forces, committed to the conservative view on the morality of abortion, vehemently denounced the Court for "legalizing murder." In response to *Roe,* right-to-life forces adopted a number of political strategies, several of which are discussed here.

Right-to-life forces originally worked for the enactment of a constitutional amendment directly overruling *Roe.* The proposed "human life amendment"—declaring the personhood of the fetus—was calculated to achieve the legal prohibition of abortion, allowing an exception only for abortions necessary to save the life of a pregnant woman. Right-to-life support also emerged for the idea of a constitutional amendment allowing Congress and/or each state to decide whether to restrict abortion. (If this sort of amendment were enacted, it would undoubtedly have the effect of prohibiting abortion or at least severely restricting it in a number of states.) Right-to-choose forces reacted in strong opposition to these proposed constitutional amendments. In their view, any effort to achieve the legal prohibition of abortion represents an illicit attempt by one group (conservatives on abortion) to impose their moral views on those who have different views.

In 1980 right-to-life forces were notably successful in working toward a more limited political aim, the cutoff of Medicaid funding for abortion. Medicaid is a social program designed to provide public funds to pay for the medical care of impoverished people. At issue in *Harris v. McRae,* decided by the Supreme Court in 1980, was the constitutionality of the so-called Hyde amendment, legislation that had passed Congress with vigorous right-to-life support. The Hyde amendment, in the version considered by the Court, restricted federal Medicaid funding to (1) cases in which the pregnant woman's life is endangered and (2) cases of rape and incest. The Court, in a five-to-four decision, upheld the constitutionality of the Hyde amendment. According to the Court, a woman's right to an abortion does not entail *the right to have society fund the abortion.* However, if there is no constitutional obstacle to the cutoff of Medicaid funding for abortion, it must still be asked whether society's refusal to fund the abortions of poor women is an ethically sound social policy. Considerations of social justice are often pressed by those who argue that it is not.

With the decision of the Supreme Court in *Webster v. Reproductive Health Services* (1989), right-to-life forces celebrated a dramatic victory. Two crucial provisions of a Missouri statute were upheld. One provision bans the use of *public* facilities and *public* employees in the performance of abortions. Another requires physicians to perform tests to determine the viability of any fetus believed to be 20 weeks or older. From the perspective of right-to-life forces, the Court's holding in *Webster* represented the first benefits of a long-term strategy to undermine *Roe v. Wade* by controlling (through the political process) the appointment of new Supreme Court justices. More important than the actual holding of the case was the fact that the Court had apparently indicated its willingness to abandon *Roe.* In *Planned Parenthood of Southeastern Pennsylvania v. Casey, Governor of Pennsylvania* (1992), however, the Court once again reflected ongoing changes in its membership and reaffirmed the "essential holding" of *Roe.* The controlling opinion in *Casey,* written by Justices Sandra Day O'Connor, Anthony M. Kennedy, and David H. Souter, is reprinted in this chapter.

The recent emergence of RU 486 (mifepristone), a drug developed in France, has further complicated the social-policy debate over abortion in the United States. RU 486 can be taken as an "abortion pill" and effectively functions to terminate early pregnancies. Initial research in France indicated that the drug, when used within 49 days of a missed menstrual period, is 96 percent effective in inducing menses and thereby terminating pregnancy. Although minor side effects (e.g., heavier than normal bleeding, nausea, and fatigue) have sometimes been observed, there are no apparent long-term negative effects. Worries about safety aside, RU 486 has been warmly endorsed by right-to-choose forces. If the drug becomes legally available in the United States, women would have access to a very private, nonsurgical form of abortion. Of course, right-to-life forces are bitterly opposed to the legal availability of RU 486. They refer to the drug as a "human pesticide" and denounce its employment as "chemical warfare on the unborn."

Maternal-Fetal Conflicts

If a pregnant woman has made the decision to carry her fetus to term (i.e., if she has ruled out the possibility of an abortion), does she have a moral obligation to conduct her life so as to minimize the possibility that her child will be born unhealthy? Clearly, the lifestyle and behavior of a pregnant woman can have a negative impact on the well-being of a developing fetus. For example, the following behaviors are thought to create some likelihood of fetal harm: (1) maintaining an unhealthy diet, (2) smoking, (3) excessive consumption of alcohol, (4) recreational drug use. Moreover, if a pregnant woman suffers from certain medical conditions, additional complications arise. For example, if a diabetic woman does not exercise tight control over her blood sugar, it is likely that her fetus will be negatively affected.

If a woman should be prepared to endure inconvenience and lifestyle modification during pregnancy, should she also be prepared to accept invasive medical procedures in the name of fetal well-being? For example, if physicians tell her that a cesarean delivery is medically indicated for her child, is she morally obligated to undergo the pain and risks associated with the procedure? If physicians tell her that her fetus is suffering from a medical condition that can be treated in utero, is she morally obligated to undergo a procedure that would be identified as "fetal therapy"? Surely it makes a difference how well established and efficacious a certain medical procedure is, how risky it is for the pregnant woman, and how necessary it would seem to be for the fetus. However, suppose, in a certain case, that physicians form the view that a woman is acting in a morally irresponsible manner. If educational efforts fail to elicit a woman's consent to a medical procedure considered necessary for the well-being of her fetus, is persuasion in order? If efforts to persuade also fail, is coercion in order?

In one of this chapter's selections, Thomas H. Murray maintains that a pregnant woman has a moral duty to avoid harming her "not-yet-born child," but he emphasizes that this duty must be balanced against a multitude of other moral considerations, all of which have a rightful place within the overall moral context of her life. He also considers the dilemma faced by physicians who believe that a pregnant woman is failing to act in the best interests of her fetus. With regard to social policy in the area of maternal-fetal conflicts, Murray expresses strong reservations about the employment of coercion against a pregnant woman. In this chapter's final selection, Rosemarie Tong takes an even stronger stance against coercive intervention. Her distinctive contribution, however, is an analysis of "gestational conflicts" from the perspective of the ethics of care.

T.A.M.

NOTES

1 The first section of Chapter 9 provides an extensive discussion of prenatal diagnosis and selective abortion.

2 The expression *therapeutic abortion* suggests abortion for medical reasons. Accordingly, abortions corresponding to reasons 1, 2, and 3 are usually said to be therapeutic. More problematically, abortions corresponding to reason 4 have often been identified as therapeutic. Perhaps it is presumed that pregnancies resulting from rape or incest are traumatic, thus a threat to mental health. Alternatively, perhaps calling such an abortion "therapeutic" is just a way of indicating that it is thought to be justifiable.

3 Germain Grisez, *Abortion: The Myths, the Realities, and the Arguments* (New York: Corpus Books, 1970), p. 306.

4 One especially prominent conservative view is associated with the Roman Catholic Church. In accordance with Roman Catholic moral teaching, the *direct* killing of innocent human

life is forbidden. Hence, abortion is forbidden. Even if the pregnant woman's life is in danger, perhaps because her heart or kidney function is inadequate, abortion is impermissible. In two special cases, however, procedures resulting in the death of the fetus are allowable. In the case of an ectopic pregnancy, where the developing fetus is lodged in the fallopian tube, the fallopian tube may be removed. In the case of a pregnant woman with a cancerous uterus, the cancerous uterus may be removed. In these cases, the death of the fetus is construed as *indirect* killing, the foreseen but unintended by-product of a surgical procedure designed to protect the life of the woman. If the distinction between direct and indirect killing is a defensible one (and this is a controversial issue), it might still be suggested that the distinction is not rightly applied in the Roman Catholic view of abortion. For example, some critics contend that abortion may be construed as indirect killing, indeed an allowable form of indirect killing, in at least all cases in which it is necessary to save the life of the mother. For one helpful exposition and critical analysis of the Roman Catholic position on abortion, see Daniel Callahan, *Abortion: Law, Choice and Morality* (New York: Macmillan, 1970), chap. 12, pp. 409–447.

5 In considering the liberal contention that abortions are morally acceptable irrespective of the stage of fetal development, we should take note of an ambiguity in the concept of abortion. Does *abortion* refer merely to the termination of a pregnancy in the sense of detaching the fetus from the pregnant woman, or does *abortion* entail the death of the fetus as well? Whereas the abortion of a *previable* fetus entails its death, the "abortion" of a *viable* fetus, by means of hysterotomy (a miniature cesarean section), does not entail the death of the fetus and would seem to be tantamount to the birth of a baby. With regard to the "abortion" of a *viable* fetus, liberals can defend the woman's right to detach the fetus from her body without contending that the woman has the right to insist on the death of the child.

The Morality of Abortion

On the Moral and Legal Status of Abortion
Mary Anne Warren

Mary Anne Warren is associate professor of philosophy at San Francisco State University. Among her published articles are "The Moral Significance of Birth," "Do Potential People Have Moral Rights?" and "Is Androgyny the Answer to Sexual Stereotyping?" She is also the author of *The Nature of Woman: An Encyclopedia and Guide to the Literature* (1980) and *Gendercide: The Implications of Sex Selection* (1985).

Warren, defending the liberal view on abortion, promptly distinguishes two senses of the term *human*: (1) One is *human in the genetic sense* when one is a member of the biological species *Homo sapiens*. (2) One is *human in the moral sense* when one is a full-fledged member of the moral community. Warren attacks the presupposition underlying the standard conservative argument against abortion—that the fetus is human in the moral sense. She contends that the moral community, the set of beings with full and equal moral rights, consists of all and only people (persons). (Thus she takes the concept of personhood to be equivalent to the concept of humanity in the moral sense.) After analyzing the concept of a person, she concludes that there is no stage of fetal development at which a fetus resembles a person enough to have a significant right to life. She also argues that the fetus's *potential* for being a

Reprinted by permission from vol. 57, no. 1, of *The Monist*, LaSalle, Illinois 61301. "Postscript on Infanticide" reprinted with permission of the author from *The Problem of Abortion*, second edition, edited by Joel Feinberg (Belmont, Calif.: Wadsworth, 1984).

person does not provide a basis for the claim that it has a significant right to life. It follows, in her view, that a woman's right to obtain an abortion is absolute. Abortion is morally justified at any stage of fetal development, and no legal restrictions should be placed on a woman's right to abort. In a concluding postscript, Warren briefly assesses the moral justifiability of infanticide.

The question which we must answer in order to produce a satisfactory solution to the problem of the moral status of abortion is this: How are we to define the moral community, the set of beings with full and equal moral rights, such that we can decide whether a human fetus is a member of this community or not? What sort of entity, exactly, has the inalienable rights to life, liberty, and the pursuit of happiness? Jefferson attributed these rights to all *men,* and it may or may not be fair to suggest that he intended to attribute them *only* to men. Perhaps he ought to have attributed them to all human beings. If so, then we arrive, first, at [John] Noonan's problem of defining what makes a being human, and, second, at the equally vital question which Noonan does not consider, namely, What reason is there for identifying the moral community with the set of all human beings, in whatever way we have chosen to define that term?

1 ON THE DEFINITION OF "HUMAN"

One reason why this vital second question is so frequently overlooked in the debate over the moral status of abortion is that the term 'human' has two distinct, but not often distinguished, senses. This fact results in a slide of meaning, which serves to conceal the fallaciousness of the traditional argument that since (1) it is wrong to kill innocent human beings, and (2) fetuses are innocent human beings, then (3) it is wrong to kill fetuses. For if 'human' is used in the same sense in both (1) and (2) then, whichever of the two senses is meant, one of these premises is question-begging. And if it is used in two different senses then of course the conclusion doesn't follow.

Thus, (1) is a self-evident moral truth,[1] and avoids begging the question about abortion, only if 'human being' is used to mean something like 'a full-fledged member of the moral community.' (It may or may not also be meant to refer exclusively to members of the species *Homo sapiens.*) We may call this the *moral* sense of 'human.' It is not to be confused with what we call the *genetic* sense, i.e., the sense in which *any* member of

the species is a human being, and no member of any other species could be. If (1) is acceptable only if the moral sense is intended, (2) is non-question-begging only if what is intended is the genetic sense.

In "Deciding Who is Human," Noonan argues for the classification of fetuses with human beings by pointing to the presence of the full genetic code, and the potential capacity for rational thought.[2] It is clear that what he needs to show, for his version of the traditional argument to be valid, is that fetuses are human in the moral sense, the sense in which it is analytically true that all human beings have full moral rights. But, in the absence of any argument showing that whatever is genetically human is also morally human, and he gives none, nothing more than genetic humanity can be demonstrated by the presence of the human genetic code. And, as we will see, the *potential* capacity for rational thought can at most show that an entity has the potential for *becoming* human in the moral sense.

2 DEFINING THE MORAL COMMUNITY

Can it be established that genetic humanity is sufficient for moral humanity? I think that there are very good reasons for not defining the moral community in this way. I would like to suggest an alternative way of defining the moral community, which I will argue for only to the extent of explaining why it is, or should be, self-evident. The suggestion is simply that the moral community consists of all and only *people,* rather than all and only human beings,[3] and probably the best way of demonstrating its self-evidence is by considering the concept of personhood, to see what sorts of entity are and are not persons, and what the decision that a being is or is not a person implies about its moral rights.

What characteristics entitle an entity to be considered a person? This is obviously not the place to attempt a complete analysis of the concept of personhood, but we do not need such a fully adequate analysis just to determine whether and why a fetus is or isn't a person. All we need is a rough and approximate list of the most basic criteria of personhood, and some idea of which, or how many, of these an entity must satisfy in order to properly be considered a person.

In searching for such criteria, it is useful to look beyond the set of people with whom we are acquainted, and ask how we would decide whether a totally alien being was a person or not. (For we have no right to assume that genetic humanity is necessary for personhood.) Image a space traveler who lands on an unknown planet and encounters a race of beings utterly unlike any he has ever seen or heard of. If he wants to be sure of behaving morally toward these beings, he has to somehow decide whether they are people, and hence have full moral rights, or whether they are the sort of thing which he need not feel guilty about treating as, for example, a source of food.

How should he go about making this decision? If he has some anthropological background, he might look for such things as religion, art, and the manufacturing of tools, weapons, or shelters, since these factors have been used to distinguish our human from our prehuman ancestors, in what seems to be closer to the moral than the genetic sense of 'human.' And no doubt he would be right to consider the presence of such factors as good evidence that the alien beings were people, and morally human. It would, however, be overly anthropocentric of him to take the absence of these things as adequate evidence that they were not, since we can imagine people who have progressed beyond, or evolved without ever developing, these cultural characteristics.

I suggest that the traits which are most central to the concept of personhood, or humanity in the moral sense, are, very roughly, the following:

1. Consciousness (of objects and events external and/or internal to the being), and in particular the capacity to feel pain;

2. Reasoning (the *developed* capacity to solve new and relatively complex problems);

3. Self-motivated activity (activity which is relatively independent of either genetic or direct external control);

4. The capacity to communicate, by whatever means, messages of an indefinite variety of types, that is, not just with an indefinite number of possible contents, but on indefinitely many possible topics;

5. The presence of self-concepts, and self-awareness, either individual or racial, or both.

Admittedly, there are apt to be a great many problems involved in formulating precise definitions of these criteria, let alone in developing universally valid behavioral criteria for deciding when they apply. But I will assume that both we and our explorer know approximately what (1)–(5) mean, and that he is also able to determine whether or not they apply. How, then, should he use his findings to decide whether or not the alien beings are people? We needn't suppose that an entity must have *all* of these attributes to be properly considered a person; (1) and (2) alone may well be sufficient for personhood, and quite probably (1)–(3) are sufficient. Neither do we need to insist that any one of these criteria is *necessary* for personhood, although once again (1) and (2) look like fairly good candidates for necessary conditions, as does (3), if 'activity' is construed so as to include the activity of reasoning.

All we need to claim, to demonstrate that a fetus is not a person, is that any being which satisfies *none* of (1)–(5) is certainly not a person. I consider this claim to be so obvious that I think anyone who denied it, and claimed that a being which satisfied none of (1)–(5) was a person all the same, would thereby demonstrate that he had no notion at all of what a person is—perhaps because he had confused the concept of a person with that of genetic humanity. If the opponents of abortion were to deny the appropriateness of these five criteria, I do not know what further arguments would convince them. We would probably have to admit that our conceptual schemes were indeed irreconcilably different, and that our dispute could not be settled objectively.

I do not expect this to happen, however, since I think that the concept of a person is one which is very nearly universal (to people), and that it is common to both proabortionists and antiabortionists, even though neither group has fully realized the relevance of this concept to the resolution of their dispute. Furthermore, I think that on reflection even the antiabortionists ought to agree not only that (1)–(5) are central to the concept of personhood, but also that it is a part of this concept that all and only people have full moral rights. The concept of a person is in part a moral concept; once we have admitted that x is a person we have recognized, even if we have not agreed to respect, x's right to be treated as a member of the moral community. It is true that the claim that x is a *human being* is more commonly voiced as part of an appeal to treat x decently than is the claim that x is a person, but this is either because 'human being' is here used in the sense which implies personhood, or because the genetic and moral sense of 'human' have been confused.

Now if (1)–(5) are indeed the primary criteria of personhood, then it is clear that genetic humanity is neither necessary nor sufficient for establishing that an entity is a person. Some human beings are not people, and there may well be people who are not human beings. A man or woman whose consciousness has been permanently obliterated but who remains alive is a human being which is no longer a person; defective human beings, with no appreciable mental capacity, are not and presumably never will be people; and a fetus is a human being which is not yet a person, and which therefore cannot coherently be said to have full moral rights. Citizens of the next century should be prepared to recognize highly advanced, self-aware robots or computers, should such be developed, and intelligent inhabitants of other worlds, should such be found, as people in the fullest sense, and to respect their moral rights. But to ascribe full moral rights to an entity which is not a person is as absurd as to ascribe moral obligations and responsibilities to such an entity.

3 FETAL DEVELOPMENT AND THE RIGHT TO LIFE

Two problems arise in the application of these suggestions for the definition of the moral community to the determination of the precise moral status of a human fetus. Given that the paradigm example of a person is a normal adult human being, then (1) How like this paradigm, in particular how far advanced since conception, does a human being need to be before it begins to have a right to life by virtue, not of being fully a person as of yet, but of being *like* a person? and (2) To what extent, if any, does the fact that a fetus has the *potential* for becoming a person endow it with some of the same rights? Each of these questions requires some comment.

In answering the first question, we need not attempt a detailed consideration of the moral rights of organisms which are not developed enough, aware enough, intelligent enough, etc., to be considered people, but which resemble people in some respects. It does seem reasonable to suggest that the more like a person, in the relevant respects, a being is, the stronger is the case for regarding it as having a right to life, and indeed the stronger its right to life is. Thus we ought to take seriously the suggestion that, insofar as "the human individual develops biologically in a continuous fashion . . . the rights of a human person might develop in the same way."[4] But we must keep in mind that the attributes which are relevant in determining whether or not

an entity is enough like a person to be regarded as having some of the same moral rights are no different from those which are relevant to determining whether or not it is fully a person—i.e., are no different from (1)–(5)—and that being genetically human, or having recognizable human facial and other physical features, or detectable brain activity, or the capacity to survive outside the uterus, are simply not among these relevant attributes.

Thus it is clear that even though a seven- or eight-month fetus has features which make it apt to arouse in us almost the same powerful protective instinct as is commonly aroused by a small infant, nevertheless it is not significantly more personlike than is a very small embryo. It is *somewhat* more personlike; it can apparently feel and respond to pain, and it may even have a rudimentary form of consciousness, insofar as its brain is quite active. Nevertheless, it seems safe to say that it is not fully conscious, in the way that an infant of a few months is, and that it cannot reason, or communicate messages of indefinitely many sorts, does not engage in self-motivated activity, and has no self-awareness. Thus, in the *relevant* respects, a fetus, even a fully developed one, is considerably less personlike than is the average mature mammal, indeed the average fish. And I think that a rational person must conclude that if the right to life of a fetus is to be based upon its resemblance to a person, then it cannot be said to have any more right to life than, let us say, a newborn guppy (which also seems to be capable of feeling pain), and that a right of that magnitude could never override a woman's right to obtain an abortion, at any stage of her pregnancy.

There may, of course, be other arguments in favor of placing legal limits upon the stage of pregnancy in which an abortion may be performed. Given the relative safety of the new techniques of artificially inducing labor during the third trimester, the danger to the woman's life or health is no longer such an argument. Neither is the fact that people tend to respond to the thought of abortion in the later stages of pregnancy with emotional repulsion, since mere emotional responses cannot take the place of moral reasoning in determining what ought to be permitted. Nor, finally, is the frequently heard argument that legalizing abortion, especially late in the pregnancy, may erode the level of respect for human life, leading, perhaps, to an increase in unjustified euthanasia and other crimes. For this threat, if it is a threat, can be better met by educating people to the kinds of moral distinctions which we are making here than by limiting access to abortion (which limitation may, in its disregard for the rights of women, be just as damaging to the level of respect for human rights).

Thus, since the fact that even a fully developed fetus is not personlike enough to have any significant right to life on the basis of its personlikeness shows that no legal restrictions upon the stage of pregnancy in which an abortion may be performed can be justified on the grounds that we should protect the rights of the older fetus; and since there is no other apparent justification for such restrictions, we may conclude that they are entirely unjustified. Whether or not it would be *indecent* (whatever that means) for a woman in her seventh month to obtain an abortion just to avoid having to postpone a trip to Europe, it would not, in itself, be *immoral,* and therefore it ought to be permitted.

4 POTENTIAL PERSONHOOD AND THE RIGHT TO LIFE

We have seen that a fetus does not resemble a person in any way which can support the claim that it has even some of the same rights. But what about its *potential,* the fact that if nurtured and allowed to develop naturally it will very probably become a person? Doesn't that alone give it at least some right to life? It is hard to deny that the fact that an entity is a potential person is a strong prima facie reason for not destroying it; but we need not conclude from this that a potential person has a right to life, by virtue of that potential. It may be that our feeling that it is better, other things being equal, not to destroy a potential person is better explained by the fact that potential people are still (felt to be) an invaluable resource, not to be lightly squandered. Surely, if every speck of dust were a potential person, we would be much less apt to conclude that every potential person has a right to become actual.

Still, we do not need to insist that a potential person has no right to life whatever. There may well be something immoral, and not just imprudent, about wantonly destroying potential people, when doing so isn't necessary to protect anyone's rights. But even if a potential person does have some prima facie right to life, such a right could not possibly outweigh the right of a woman to obtain an abortion, since the rights of any actual person invariably outweigh those of any potential person, whenever the two conflict. Since this may not be immediately obvious in the case of a human fetus, let us look at another case.

Suppose that our space explorer falls into the hands of an alien culture, whose scientists decide to create a few hundred thousand or more human beings, by breaking his body into its component cells, and using these to create fully developed human beings, with, of course, his genetic code. We may imagine that each of these newly created men will have all of the original man's abilities, skills, knowledge, and so on, and also have an individual self-concept, in short that each of them will be a bona fide (though hardly unique) person. Imagine that the whole project will take only seconds, and that its chances of success are extremely high, and that our explorer knows all of this, and also knows that these people will be treated fairly. I maintain that in such a situation he would have every right to escape if he could, and thus to deprive all of these potential people of their potential lives; for his right to life outweighs all of theirs together, in spite of the fact that they are all genetically human, all innocent, and all have a very high probability of becoming people very soon, if only he refrains from acting.

Indeed, I think he would have a right to escape even if it were not his life which the alien scientists planned to take, but only a year of his freedom, or, indeed, only a day. Nor would he be obligated to stay if he had gotten captured (thus bringing all these people-potentials into existence) because of his own carelessness, or even if he had done so deliberately, knowing the consequences. Regardless of how he got captured, he is not morally obligated to remain in captivity for *any* period of time for the sake of permitting any number of potential people to come into actuality, so great is the margin by which one actual person's right to liberty outweighs whatever right to life even a hundred thousand potential people have. And it seems reasonable to conclude that the rights of a woman will outweigh by a similar margin whatever right to life a fetus may have by virtue of its potential personhood.

Thus, neither a fetus's resemblance to a person, nor its potential for becoming a person provides any basis whatever for the claim that it has any significant right to life. Consequently, a woman's right to protect her health, happiness, freedom, and even her life,[5] by terminating an unwanted pregnancy, will always override whatever right to life it may be appropriate to ascribe to a fetus, even a fully developed one. And thus, in the absence of any overwhelming social need for every possible child, the laws which restrict the right to obtain an abortion, or limit the period of pregnancy during which an abortion may be performed, are a wholly unjustified violation of a woman's most basic moral and constitutional rights.[6]

POSTSCRIPT ON INFANTICIDE, FEBRUARY 26, 1982

One of the most troubling objections to the argument presented in this article is that it may appear to justify not only abortion but infanticide as well. A newborn infant is not a great deal more personlike than a nine-month fetus, and thus it might seem that if late-term abortion is sometimes justified, then infanticide must also be sometimes justified. Yet most people consider that infanticide is a form of murder, and thus never justified.

While it is important to appreciate the emotional force of this objection, its logical force is far less than it may seem at first glance. There are many reasons why infanticide is much more difficult to justify than abortion, even though if my argument is correct neither constitutes the killing of a person. In this country, and in this period of history, the deliberate killing of viable newborns is virtually never justified. This is in part because neonates are so very *close* to being persons that to kill them requires a very strong moral justification—as does the killing of dolphins, whales, chimpanzees, and other highly personlike creatures. It is certainly wrong to kill such beings just for the sake of convenience, or financial profit, or "sport."

Another reason why infanticide is usually wrong, in our society, is that if the newborn's parents do not want it, or are unable to care for it, there are (in most cases) people who are able and eager to adopt it and to provide a good home for it. Many people wait years for the opportunity to adopt a child, and some are unable to do so even though there is every reason to believe that they would be good parents. The needless destruction of a viable infant inevitably deprives some person or persons of a source of great pleasure and satisfaction, perhaps severely impoverishing their lives. Furthermore, even if an infant is considered to be adoptable (e.g., because of some extremely severe mental or physical handicap) it is still wrong in most cases to kill it. For most of us value the lives of infants, and would prefer to pay taxes to support orphanages and state institutions for the handicapped rather than to allow unwanted infants to be killed. So long as most people feel this way, and so long as our society can afford to provide care for infants which are unwanted or which have special needs that preclude home care, it is wrong to destroy any infant which has a chance of living a reasonably satisfactory life.

If these arguments show that infanticide is wrong, at least in this society, then why don't they also show that late-term abortion is wrong? After all, third trimester fetuses are also highly personlike, and many people value them and would much prefer that they be preserved; even at some cost to themselves. As a potential source of pleasure to some family, a viable fetus is just as valuable as a viable infant. But there is an obvious and crucial difference between the two cases: once the infant is born, its continued life cannot (except, perhaps, in very exceptional cases) pose any serious threat to the woman's life or health, since she is free to put it up for adoption, or, where this is impossible, to place it in a state-supported institution. While she might prefer that it die, rather than being raised by others, it is not clear that such a preference would constitute a right on her part. True, she may suffer greatly from the knowledge that her child will be thrown into the lottery of the adoption system, and that she will be unable to ensure its well-being, or even to know whether it is healthy, happy, doing well in school, etc.: for the law generally does not permit natural parents to remain in contact with their children, once they are adopted by another family. But there are surely better ways of dealing with these problems than by permitting infanticide in such cases. (It might help, for instance, if the natural parents of adopted children could at least receive some information about their progress, without necessarily being informed of the identity of the adopting family.)

In contrast, a pregnant woman's right to protect her own life and health clearly outweighs other people's desire that the fetus be preserved—just as, when a person's life or limb is threatened by some wild animal, and when the threat cannot be removed without killing the animal, the person's right to self-protection outweighs the desires of those who would prefer that the animal not be harmed. Thus, while the moment of birth may not mark any sharp discontinuity in the degree to which an infant possesses a right to life, it does mark the end of the mother's absolute right to determine its fate. Indeed, if and when a late-term abortion could be safely performed without killing the fetus, she would have no absolute right to insist on its death (e.g., if others wish to adopt it or pay for its care), for the same reason that she does not have a right to insist that a viable infant be killed.

It remains true that according to my argument neither abortion nor the killing of neonates is properly considered a form of murder. Perhaps it is understandable that the law should classify infanticide as murder or homicide, since there is no other existing legal category which adequately or conveniently expresses the force of our society's disapproval of this action. But the moral distinction remains, and it has several important consequences.

In the first place, it implies that when an infant is born into a society which—unlike ours—is so impoverished that it simply cannot care for it adequately without endangering the survival of existing persons, killing it or allowing it to die is not necessarily wrong—provided that there is no *other* society which is willing and able to provide such care. Most human societies, from those at the hunting and gathering stage of economic development to the highly civilized Greeks and Romans, have permitted the practice of infanticide under such unfortunate circumstances, and I would argue that it shows a serious lack of understanding to condemn them as morally backward for this reason alone.

In the second place, the argument implies that when an infant is born with such severe physical anomalies that its life would predictably be a very short and/or very miserable one, even with the most heroic of medical treatment, and where its parents do not choose to bear the often crushing emotional, financial and other burdens attendant upon the artificial prolongation of such a tragic life, it is not morally wrong to cease or withhold treatment, thus allowing the infant a painless death. It is wrong (and sometimes a form of murder) to practice involuntary euthanasia on persons, since they have the right to decide for themselves whether or not they wish to continue to live. But terminally ill neonates cannot make this decision for themselves, and thus it is incumbent upon responsible persons to make the decision for them, as best they can. The mistaken belief that infanticide is always tantamount to murder is responsible for a great deal of unnecessary suffering, not just on the part of infants which are made to endure needlessly prolonged and painful deaths, but also on the part of parents, nurses, and other involved persons, who must watch infants suffering needlessly, helpless to end that suffering in the most humane way.

I am well aware that these conclusions, however modest and reasonable they may seem to some people, strike other people as morally monstrous, and that some people might even prefer to abandon their previous support for women's right to abortion rather than accept a theory which leads to such conclusions about infanticide. But all that these facts show is that abortion is not an isolated moral issue; to fully understand the moral status of abortion we may have to reconsider other moral issues as well, issues not just about infanticide and euthanasia, but also about the moral rights of women and of nonhuman animals. It is a philosopher's task to criticize mistaken beliefs which stand in the way of moral understanding, even when—perhaps especially when—those beliefs are popular and widespread. The belief that moral strictures against killing should apply equally to *all* genetically human entities, and *only* to genetically human entities, is such an error. The overcoming of this error will undoubtedly require long and often painful struggle; but it must be done.

NOTES

1 Of course, the principle that it is (always) wrong to kill innocent human beings is in need of many other modifications, e.g., that it may be permissible to do so to save a greater number of other innocent human beings, but we may safely ignore these complications here.

2 John Noonan, "Deciding Who is Human," *Natural Law Forum*, 13 (1968), 135.

3 From here on, we will use 'human' to mean genetically human, since the moral sense seems closely connected to, and perhaps derived from, the assumption that genetic humanity is sufficient for membership in the moral community.

4 Thomas L. Hayes, "A Biological View," *Commonweal*, 85 (March 17, 1967), 677–78; quoted by Daniel Callahan, in *Abortion: Law, Choice and Morality* (London: Macmillan & Co., 1970).

5 That is, insofar as the death rate, for the woman, is higher for childbirth than for early abortion.

6 My thanks to the following people, who were kind enough to read and criticize an earlier version of this paper: Herbert Gold, Gene Glass, Anne Lauterbach, Judith Thomson, Mary Mothersill, and Timothy Binkley.

Why Abortion Is Immoral
Don Marquis

Don Marquis is professor of philosophy at the University of Kansas. He specializes in applied ethics and medical ethics. His published articles include "Four Versions of Double Effect," "An Argument That All Prerandomized Clinical Trials Are Unethical," and "Harming the Dead."

Marquis argues that abortion, with rare exceptions, is seriously immoral. He bases this conclusion on a theory that he presents and defends about the wrongness of killing. In his view, killing another adult human being is wrong precisely because the victim is deprived of all the value—"activities, projects, experiences, and enjoyments"—of his or her future. Since abortion deprives a typical fetus of a "future like ours," he contends, the moral presumption against abortion is as strong as the presumption against killing another adult human being.

The view that abortion is, with rare exceptions, seriously immoral has received little support in the recent philosophical literature. No doubt most philosophers affiliated with secular institutions of higher education believe that the anti-abortion position is either a symptom of irrational religious dogma or a conclusion generated by seriously confused philosophical argument. The purpose of this essay is to undermine this general belief. This essay sets out an argument that purports to show, as well as any argument in ethics can show, that abortion is, except possibly in rare cases, seriously immoral, that it is in the same moral category as killing an innocent adult human being.

This argument is based on a major assumption: If fetuses are in the same category as adult human beings with respect to the moral value of their lives, then the *presumption* that any particular abortion is immoral is exceedingly strong. Such a presumption could be overridden only by considerations more compelling than a woman's right to privacy. The defense of this assumption is beyond the scope of this essay.[1]

Furthermore, this essay will neglect a discussion of whether there are any such compelling considerations and what they are. Plainly there are strong candidates: abortion before implantation, abortion when the life of a woman is threatened by a pregnancy or abortion after rape. The casuistry of these hard cases will not be explored in this essay. The purpose of this essay is to develop a general argument for the claim that, subject to the assumption above, the overwhelming majority of deliberate abortions are seriously immoral. . . .

. . . A necessary condition of resolving the abortion controversy is a . . . theoretical account of the wrongness of killing. After all, if we merely believe, but do not understand, why killing adult human beings such as ourselves is wrong, how could we conceivably show that abortion is either immoral or permissible? . . .

In order to develop such an account, we can start from the following unproblematic assumption concerning our own case: it is wrong to kill *us*. Why is it wrong? Some answers can be easily eliminated. It might be said that what makes killing us wrong is that a killing brutalizes the one who kills. But the brutalization consists of being inured to the performance of an act that is hideously immoral; hence, the brutalization does not explain the immorality. It might be said that what makes killing us wrong is the great loss others would experience due to our absence. Although such hubris is understandable, such an explanation does not account for the wrongness of killing hermits, or those whose lives are relatively independent and whose friends find it easy to make new friends.

A more obvious answer is better. What primarily makes killing wrong is neither its effect on the murderer nor its effect on the victim's friends and relatives, but its effect on the victim. The loss of one's life is one of the greatest losses one can suffer. The loss of one's life deprives one of all the experiences, activities, projects, and enjoyments that would otherwise have constituted one's future. Therefore, killing someone is wrong, pri-

Reprinted, as slightly modified by the author, with permission of the author and the publisher from the *Journal of Philosophy*, vol. 86 (April 1989).

marily because the killing inflicts (one of) the greatest possible losses on the victim. To describe this as the loss of life can be misleading, however. The change in my biological state does not by itself make killing me wrong. The effect of the loss of my biological life is the loss to me of all those activities, projects, experiences, and enjoyments which would otherwise have constituted my future personal life. These activities, projects, experiences, and enjoyments are either valuable for their own sakes or are means to something else that is valuable for its own sake. Some parts of my future are not valued by me now, but will come to be valued by me as I grow older and as my values and capacities change. When I am killed, I am deprived both of what I now value which would have been part of my future personal life, but also what I would come to value. Therefore, when I die, I am deprived of all of the value of my future. Inflicting this loss on me is ultimately what makes killing me wrong. This being the case, it would seem that what makes killing *any* adult human being prima facie seriously wrong is the loss of his or her future.[2]

How should this rudimentary theory of the wrongness of killing be evaluated? It cannot be faulted for deriving an 'ought' from an 'is', for it does not. The analysis assumes that killing me (or you, reader) is prima facie seriously wrong. The point of the analysis is to establish which natural property ultimately explains the wrongness of the killing, given that it is wrong. A natural property will ultimately explain the wrongness of killing, only if (1) the explanation fits with our intuitions about the matter and (2) there is no other natural property that provides the basis for a better explanation of the wrongness of killing. This analysis rests on the intuition that what makes killing a particular human or animal wrong is what it does to that particular human or animal. What makes killing wrong is some natural effect or other of the killing. Some would deny this. For instance, a divine-command theorist in ethics would deny it. Surely this denial is, however, one of those features of divine–command theory which renders it so implausible.

The claim that what makes killing wrong is the loss of the victim's future is directly supported by two considerations. In the first place, this theory explains why we regard killing as one of the worst of crimes. Killing is especially wrong, because it deprives the victim of more than perhaps any other crime. In the second place, people with AIDS or cancer who know they are dying believe, of course, that dying is a very bad thing for them. They believe that the loss of a future to them that they would otherwise have experienced is what makes their premature death a very bad thing for them.

A better theory of the wrongness of killing would require a different natural property associated with killing which better fits with the attitudes of the dying. What could it be?

The view that what makes killing wrong is the loss to the victim of the value of the victim's future gains additional support when some of its implications are examined. In the first place, it is incompatible with the view that it is wrong to kill only beings who are biologically human. It is possible that there exists a different species from another planet whose members have a future like ours. Since having a future like that is what makes killing someone wrong, this theory entails that it would be wrong to kill members of such a species. Hence, this theory is opposed to the claim that only life that is biologically human has great moral worth, a claim which many anti-abortionists have seemed to adopt. This opposition, which this theory has in common with personhood theories, seems to be a merit of the theory.

In the second place, the claim that the loss of one's future is the wrong-making feature of one's being killed entails the possibility that the futures of some actual nonhuman mammals on our own planet are sufficiently like ours that it is seriously wrong to kill them also. Whether some animals do have the same right to life as human beings depends on adding to the account of the wrongness of killing some additional account of just what it is about my future or the futures of other adult human beings which makes it wrong to kill us. No such additional account will be offered in this essay. Undoubtedly, the provision of such an account would be a very difficult matter. Undoubtedly, any such account would be quite controversial. Hence, it surely should not reflect badly on this sketch of an elementary theory of the wrongness of killing that it is indeterminate with respect to some very difficult issues regarding animal rights.

In the third place, the claim that the loss of one's future is the wrong-making feature of one's being killed does not entail, as sanctity of human life theories do, that active euthanasia is wrong. Persons who are severely and incurably ill, who face a future of pain and despair, and who wish to die will not have suffered a loss if they are killed. It is, strictly speaking, the value of a human's future which makes killing wrong in this theory. This being so, killing does not necessarily wrong some persons who are sick and dying. Of course, there may be other reasons for a prohibition of active euthanasia, but that is another matter. Sanctity-of-human-life theories seem to hold that active euthanasia is seriously wrong even in an individual case where there seems to be good reason for it independently of public policy considerations. This consequence is most implausible, and it is a plus for the claim that the loss of a future of value is what makes killing wrong that it does not share this consequence.

In the fourth place, the account of the wrongness of killing defended in this essay does straightforwardly entail that it is prima facie seriously wrong to kill children and infants, for we do presume that they have futures of value. Since we do believe that it is wrong to kill defenseless little babies, it is important that a theory of the wrongness of killing easily account for this. Personhood theories of the wrongness of killing, on the other hand, cannot straightforwardly account for the wrongness of killing infants and young children. Hence, such theories must add special ad hoc accounts of the wrongness of killing the young. The plausibility of such ad hoc theories seems to be a function of how desperately one wants such theories to work. The claim that the primary wrong-making feature of a killing is the loss to the victim of the value of its future accounts for the wrongness of killing young children and infants directly; it makes the wrongness of such acts as obvious as we actually think it is. This is a further merit of this theory. Accordingly, it seems that this value of a future-like-ours theory of the wrongness of killing shares strengths of both sanctity-of-life and personhood accounts while avoiding weaknesses of both. In addition, it meshes with a central intuition concerning what makes killing wrong.

The claim that the primary wrong-making feature of a killing is the loss to the victim of the value of its future has obvious consequences for the ethics of abortion. The future of a standard fetus includes a set of experiences, projects, activities, and such which are identical with the futures of adult human beings and are identical with the futures of young children. Since the reason that is sufficient to explain why it is wrong to kill human beings after the time of birth is a reason that also applies to fetuses, it follows that abortion is prima facie seriously morally wrong.

This argument does not rely on the invalid inference that, since it is wrong to kill persons, it is wrong to kill potential persons also. The category that is morally central to this analysis is the category of having a valuable future like ours; it is not the category of personhood. The argument to the conclusion that abortion is prima facie seriously morally wrong proceeded independently of the notion of person or potential person or any equivalent. Someone may wish to start with this analysis in terms of the value of a human future, conclude that abortion is, except perhaps in rare circumstances, seriously morally wrong, infer that fetuses have the right to life, and then call fetuses "persons" as a result of their having the right to life. Clearly, in this case, the category of person is being used to state the *conclusion* of the analysis rather than to generate the *argument* of the analysis.

The structure of this anti-abortion argument can be both illuminated and defended by comparing it to what appears to be the best argument for the wrongness of the wanton infliction of pain on animals. This latter argument is based on the assumption that it is prima facie wrong to inflict pain on me (or you, reader). What is the natural property associated with the infliction of pain which makes such infliction wrong? The obvious answer seems to be that the infliction of pain causes suffering and that suffering is a misfortune. The suffering caused by the infliction of pain is what makes the wanton infliction of pain on me wrong. The wanton infliction of pain on other adult humans causes suffering. The wanton infliction of pain on animals causes suffering. Since causing suffering is what makes the wanton infliction of pain wrong and since the wanton infliction of pain on animals causes suffering, it follows that the wanton infliction of pain on animals is wrong.

This argument for the wrongness of the wanton infliction of pain on animals shares a number of structural features with the argument for the serious prima facie wrongness of abortion. Both arguments start with an obvious assumption concerning what it is wrong to do to me (or you, reader). Both then look for the characteristic or the consequence of the wrong action which makes the action wrong. Both recognize that the wrong-making feature of these immoral actions is a property of actions sometimes directed at individuals other than postnatal human beings. If the structure of the argument for the wrongness of the wanton infliction of pain on animals is sound, then the structure of the argument for the prima facie serious wrongness of abortion is also sound, for the structure of the two arguments is the same. The structure common to both is the key to the explanation of how the wrongness of abortion can be demonstrated without recourse to the category of person. In neither argument is that category crucial. . . .

Of course, this value of a future-like-ours argument, if sound, shows only that abortion is prima facie wrong, not that it is wrong in any and all circumstances. Since the loss of the future to a standard fetus, if killed, is, however, at least as great a loss as the loss of the future to a standard adult human being who is killed, abortion, like ordinary killing, could be justified only by the most compelling reasons. The loss of one's life is almost the greatest misfortune that can happen to one. Presumably abortion could be justified in some circumstances, only if the loss consequent on failing to abort would be at least as great. Accordingly, morally permissible abortions will be rare indeed unless, perhaps, they occur so early in pregnancy that a fetus is not yet definitely an individual. Hence, this argument should be taken as showing that abortion is presumptively very seriously wrong, where the presumption is very strong—as strong as the presumption that killing another adult human being is wrong. . . .

In this essay, it has been argued that the correct ethic of the wrongness of killing can be extended to fetal life and used to show that there is a strong presumption that any abortion is morally impermissible. If the ethic of killing adopted here entails, however, that contraception is also seriously immoral, then there would appear to be a difficulty with the analysis of this essay.

But this analysis does not entail that contraception is wrong. Of course, contraception prevents the actualization of a possible future of value. Hence, it follows from the claim that futures of value should be maximized that contraception is prima facie immoral. This obligation to maximize does not exist, however; furthermore, nothing in the ethics of killing in this paper entails that it does. The ethics of killing in this essay would entail that contraception is wrong only if something were denied a human future of value by contraception. Nothing at all is denied such a future by contraception, however.

Candidates for a subject of harm by contraception fall into four categories: (1) some sperm or other, (2) some ovum or other, (3) a sperm and an ovum separately, and (4) a sperm and an ovum together. Assigning the harm to some sperm is utterly arbitrary, for no reason can be given for making a sperm the subject of harm rather than an ovum. Assigning the harm to some ovum is utterly arbitrary, for no reason can be given for making an ovum the subject of harm rather than a sperm. One might attempt to avoid these problems by insisting that contraception deprives both the sperm and the ovum separately of a valuable future like ours. On this alternative, too many futures are lost. Contraception was supposed to be wrong, because it deprived us of one future of value, not two. One might attempt to avoid this problem by holding that contraception deprives the combination of sperm and ovum of a valuable future like ours. But here the definite article misleads. At the time of contraception, there are hundreds of millions of sperm, one (released) ovum and millions of possible combinations of all of these. There is no

actual combination at all. Is the subject of the loss to be a merely possible combination? Which one? This alternative does not yield an actual subject of harm either. Accordingly, the immorality of contraception is not entailed by the loss of a future-like-ours argument simply because there is no nonarbitrarily identifiable subject of the loss in the case of contraception. . . .

The purpose of this essay has been to set out an argument for the serious presumptive wrongness of abortion subject to the assumption that the moral permissibility of abortion stands or falls on the moral status of the fetus. Since a fetus possesses a property, the possession of which in adult human beings is sufficient to make killing an adult human being wrong, abortion is wrong. This way of dealing with the problem of abortion seems superior to other approaches to the ethics of abortion, because it rests on an ethics of killing which is close to self-evident, because the crucial morally relevant property clearly applies to fetuses, and because the argument avoids the usual equivocations on 'human life', 'human being', or 'person'. The argument rests neither on religious claims nor on Papal dogma. It is not subject to the objection of "speciesism." Its soundness is compatible with the moral permissibility of euthanasia and contraception. It deals with our intuitions concerning young children.

Finally, this analysis can be viewed as resolving a standard problem—indeed, *the* standard problem—concerning the ethics of abortion. Clearly, it is wrong to kill adult human beings. Clearly, it is not wrong to end the life of some arbitrarily chosen single human cell. Fetuses seem to be like arbitrarily chosen human cells in some respects and like adult humans in other respects. The problem of the ethics of abortion is the problem of determining the fetal property that settles this moral controversy. The thesis of this essay is that the problem of the ethics of abortion, so understood, is solvable.

NOTES

1 Judith Jarvis Thomson has rejected this assumption in a famous essay, "A Defense of Abortion," *Philosophy and Public Affairs* 1, #1 (1971), 47–66.

2 I have been most influenced on this matter by Jonathan Glover, *Causing Death and Saving Lives* (New York: Penguin, 1977), ch. 3; and Robert Young, "What Is So Wrong with Killing People?" *Philosophy*, LIV, 210 (1979): 515–528.

A Defense of Abortion[1]
Judith Jarvis Thomson

Judith Jarvis Thomson is professor of philosophy at the Massachusetts Institute of Technology. She is the author of *Rights, Restitution, and Risk: Essays in Moral Theory* (1986) and *The Realm of Rights* (1990). "Self-Defense" and "Morality and Bad Luck" are two of her more recently published articles.

In an effort to moderate the conservative view, Thomson argues that the standard conservative claim about the moral impermissibility of abortion cannot be sustained even if (for the sake of argument) it is presumed that the fetus is a person from conception. Her central point is that the moral impermissibility of abortion does not follow simply from the admission that the fetus (as a person) has a right to life. In her view, the right to life is to be understood as the right not to be killed unjustly and does not entail the right to use another person's body. In cases where the pregnant woman has not extended to the fetus the right to use her body, most prominently in the case of rape, Thomson holds that abortion is not unjust killing and thus does not violate the fetus's right to life. Thomson acknowledges that there may be cases in which the fetus (presumed to be a person) has a right to the use of the pregnant woman's body and thus some cases where abortion would be unjust killing. She proceeds to distinguish between the moral demands of justice and the moral demands of decency. In some cases, she maintains, an abortion does no injustice (to the fetus) yet may be subject to moral criticism on the grounds that minimal standards of moral decency are transgressed.

Most opposition to abortion relies on the premise that the fetus is a human being, a person, from the moment of conception. The premise is argued for, but, as I think, not well. Take, for example, the most common argument. We are asked to notice that the development of a human being from conception through birth into childhood is continuous; then it is said that to draw a line, to choose a point in this development and say "before this point the thing is not a person, after this point it is a person" is to make an arbitrary choice, a choice for which in the nature of things no good reason can be given. It is concluded that the fetus is, or anyway that we had better say it is, a person from the moment of conception. But this conclusion does not follow. Similar things might be said about the development of an acorn into an oak tree, and it does not follow that acorns are oak trees, or that we had better say they are. Arguments of this form are sometimes called "slippery slope arguments"—the phrase is perhaps self-explanatory—

Philosophy and Public Affairs, vol. 1, no. 1 (1971), pp. 47–50, 54–66. © 1971 by Princeton University Press. Reprinted by permission of Princeton University Press.

and it is dismaying that opponents of abortion rely on them so heavily and uncritically.

I am inclined to agree, however, that the prospects for "drawing a line" in the development of the fetus look dim. I am inclined to think also that we shall probably have to agree that the fetus has already become a human person well before birth. Indeed, it comes as a surprise when one first learns how early in its life it begins to acquire human characteristics. By the tenth week, for example, it already has a face, arms and legs, fingers and toes; it has internal organs, and brain activity is detectable.[2] On the other hand, I think that the premise is false, that the fetus is not a person from the moment of conception. A newly fertilized ovum, a newly implanted clump of cells, is no more a person than an acorn is an oak tree. But I shall not discuss any of this. For it seems to me to be of great interest to ask what happens if, for the sake of argument, we allow the premise. How, precisely, are we supposed to get from there to the conclusion that abortion is morally impermissible? Opponents of abortion commonly spend most of their time establishing that the fetus is a person, and hardly any time explaining the step from there to the impermissibility of abortion. Perhaps they think the step too simple and obvious to require much comment. Or perhaps instead they are simply being economical in argument. Many of those who defend abortion rely on the premise that the fetus is not a person, but only a bit of tissue that will become a person at birth; and why pay out more arguments than you have to? Whatever the explanation, I suggest that the step they take is neither easy nor obvious, that it calls for closer examination than it is commonly given, and that when we do give it this closer examination we shall feel inclined to reject it.

I propose, then, that we grant that the fetus is a person from the moment of conception. How does the argument go from here? Something like this, I take it. Every person has a right to life. So the fetus has a right to life. No doubt the mother has a right to decide what shall happen in and to her body; everyone would grant that. But surely a person's right to life is stronger and more stringent than the mother's right to decide what happens in and to her body, and so outweighs it. So the fetus may not be killed; an abortion may not be performed.

It sounds plausible. But now let me ask you to imagine this. You wake up in the morning and find yourself back to back in bed with an unconscious violinist. A famous unconscious violinist. He has been found to have a fatal kidney ailment, and the Society of Music Lovers has canvassed all the available medical records and found that you alone have the right blood type to help. They have therefore kidnapped you, and last night the violinist's circulatory system was plugged into yours, so that your kidneys can be used to extract poisons from his blood as well as your own. The director of the hospital now tells you, "Look, we're sorry the Society of Music Lovers did this to you—we would never have permitted it if we had known. But still, they did it, and the violinist now is plugged into you. To unplug you would be to kill him. But never mind, it's only for nine months. By then he will have recovered from his ailment, and can safely be unplugged from you." Is it morally incumbent on you to accede to this situation? No doubt it would be very nice of you if you did, a great kindness. But do you *have* to accede to it? What if it were not nine months, but nine years? Or longer still? What if the director of the hospital says, "Tough luck, I agree, but you've now got to stay in bed, with the violinist plugged into you, for the rest of your life. Because remember this. All persons have a right to life, and violinists are persons. Granted you have a right to decide what happens in and to your body, but a person's right to life outweighs your right to decide what

happens in and to your body. So you cannot ever be unplugged from him." I imagine you would regard this as outrageous, which suggests that something really is wrong with that plausible-sounding argument I mentioned a moment ago.

In this case, of course, you were kidnapped; you didn't volunteer for the operation that plugged the violinist into your kidneys. Can those who oppose abortion on the ground I mentioned make an exception for a pregnancy due to rape? Certainly. They can say that persons have a right to life only if they didn't come into existence because of rape; or they can say that all persons have a right to life, but that some have less of a right to life than others, in particular, that those who came into existence because of rape have less. But these statements have a rather unpleasant sound. Surely the question of whether you have a right to life at all, or how much of it you have, shouldn't turn on the question of whether or not you are the product of a rape. And in fact the people who oppose abortion on the ground I mentioned do not make this distinction, and hence do not make an exception in case of rape.

Nor do they make an exception for a case in which the mother has to spend the nine months of her pregnancy in bed. They would agree that would be a great pity, and hard on the mother; but all the same, all persons have a right to life, the fetus is a person, and so on. I suspect, in fact, that they would not make an exception for a case in which, miraculously enough, the pregnancy went on for nine years, or even the rest of the mother's life.

Some won't even make an exception for a case in which continuation of the pregnancy is likely to shorten the mother's life; they regard abortion as impermissible even to save the mother's life. Such cases are nowadays very rare, and many opponents of abortion do not accept this extreme view. . . .

[1] Where the mother's life is not at stake, the argument I mentioned at the outset seems to have a much stronger pull. "Everyone has a right to life, so the unborn person has a right to life." And isn't the child's right to life weightier than anything other than the mother's own right to life, which she might put forward as ground for an abortion?

This argument treats the right to life as if it were unproblematic. It is not, and this seems to me to be precisely the source of the mistake.

For we should now, at long last, ask what it comes to, to have a right to life. In some views having a right to life includes having a right to be given at least the bare minimum one needs for continued life. But suppose that what in fact *is* the bare minimum a man needs for continued life is something he has no right at all to be given? If I am sick unto death, and the only thing that will save my life is the touch of Henry Fonda's cool hand on my fevered brow, then all the same, I have no right to be given the touch of Henry Fonda's cool hand on my fevered brow. It would be frightfully nice of him to fly in from the West Coast to provide it. It would be less nice, though no doubt well meant, if my friends flew out to the West Coast and carried Henry Fonda back with them. But I have no right at all against anybody that he should do this for me. Or again, to return to the story I told earlier, the fact that for continued life that violinist needs the continued use of your kidneys does not establish that he has a right to be given the continued use of your kidneys. He certainly has no right against you that *you* should give him continued use of your kidneys. For nobody has any right to use your kidneys unless you give him such a right; and nobody has the right against you that you shall give him this right—if you do allow him to go on using your kidneys, this is a kindness on your part, and not something he can claim from you as his due. Nor has he any right against anybody else that *they* should give him continued use of your kidneys. Certainly he had no right against the Society of Music Lovers that they should plug him into you in the first place. And if you now start to unplug yourself, having learned that you will otherwise have to spend nine years in bed with him, there is nobody in the world who must try to prevent you, in order to see to it that he is given something he has a right to be given.

Some people are rather stricter about the right to life. In their view, it does not include the right to be given anything, but amounts to, and only to, the right not to be killed by anybody. But here a related difficulty arises. If everybody is to refrain from killing that violinist, then everybody must refrain from doing a great many different sorts of things. Everybody must refrain from slitting his throat, everybody must refrain from shooting him—and everybody must refrain from unplugging you from him. But does he have a right against everybody that they shall refrain from unplugging you from him? To refrain from doing this is to allow him to continue to use your kidneys. It could be argued that he has a right against us that *we* should allow him to continue to use your kidneys. That is, while he had no right against us that we should give him the use of your kidneys, it might be argued that he anyway has a right against us that we shall not now intervene and deprive him of the use of your kidneys. I shall come back to third-party interventions later. But cer-

tainly the violinist has no right against you that *you* shall allow him to continue to use your kidneys. As I said, if you do allow him to use them, it is a kindness on your part, and not something you owe him.

The difficulty I point to here is not peculiar to the right to life. It reappears in connection with all the other natural rights; and it is something which an adequate account of rights must deal with. For present purposes it is enough just to draw attention to it. But I would stress that I am not arguing that people do not have a right to life—quite to the contrary, it seems to me that the primary control we must place on the acceptability of an account of rights is that it should turn out in that account to be a truth that all persons have a right to life. I am arguing only that having a right to life does not guarantee having either a right to be given the use of or a right to be allowed continued use of another person's body—even if one needs it for life itself. So the right to life will not serve the opponents of abortion in the very simple and clear way in which they seem to have thought it would.

[2] There is another way to bring out the difficulty. In the most ordinary sort of case, to deprive someone of what he has a right to is to treat him unjustly. Suppose a boy and his small brother are jointly given a box of chocolates for Christmas. If the older boy takes the box and refuses to give his brother any of the chocolates, he is unjust to him, for the brother has been given a right to half of them. But suppose that, having learned that otherwise it means nine years in bed with that violinist, you unplug yourself from him. You surely are not being unjust to him, for you gave him no right to use your kidneys, and no one else can have given him any such right. But we have to notice that in unplugging yourself, you are killing him; and violinists, like everybody else, have a right to life, and thus in the view we were considering just now, the right not to be killed. So here you do what he supposedly has a right you shall not do, but you do not act unjustly to him in doing it.

The emendation which may be made at this point is this: the right to life consists not in the right not to be killed, but rather in the right not to be killed unjustly. This runs a risk of circularity, but never mind: it would enable us to square the fact that the violinist has a right to life with the fact that you do not act unjustly toward him in unplugging yourself, thereby killing him. For if you do not kill him unjustly, you do not violate his right to life, and so it is no wonder you do him no injustice.

But if this emendation is accepted, the gap in the argument against abortion stares us plainly in the face: it is by no means enough to show that the fetus is a person, and to remind us that all persons have a right to life—we need to be shown also that killing the fetus violates its right to life, i.e., that abortion is unjust killing. And is it?

I suppose we may take it as a datum that in a case of pregnancy due to rape the mother has not given the unborn person a right to the use of her body for food and shelter. Indeed, in what pregnancy could it be supposed that the mother has given the unborn person such a right? It is not as if there were unborn persons drifting about the world, to whom a woman who wants a child says "I invite you in."

But it might be argued that there are other ways one can have acquired a right to the use of another person's body than by having been invited to use it by that person. Suppose a woman voluntarily indulges in intercourse, knowing of the chance it will issue in pregnancy, and then she does become pregnant; is she not in part responsible for the presence, in fact the very existence, of the unborn person inside her? No doubt she did not invite it in. But doesn't her partial responsibility for its being there itself give it a right to the use of her body?[3] If so, then her aborting it would be more like the boy's taking away the chocolates, and less like your unplugging yourself from the violinist—doing so would be depriving it of what it does have a right to, and thus would be doing it an injustice.

And then, too, it might be asked whether or not she can kill it even to save her own life: If she voluntarily called it into existence, how can she now kill it, even in self-defense?

The first thing to be said about this is that it is something new. Opponents of abortion have been so concerned to make out the independence of the fetus, in order to establish that it has a right to life, just as its mother does, that they have tended to overlook the possible support they might gain from making out that the fetus is *dependent* on the mother, in order to establish that she has a special kind of responsibility for it, a responsibility that gives it rights against her which are not possessed by any independent person—such as an ailing violinist who is a stranger to her.

On the other hand, this argument would give the unborn person a right to its mother's body only if her pregnancy resulted from a voluntary act, undertaken in full knowledge of the chance a pregnancy might result from it. It would leave out entirely the unborn person whose existence is due to rape. Pending the availability of some further argument, then, we would be left with the conclusion that unborn persons whose existence is due to rape have no right to the use of their mothers'

bodies, and thus that aborting them is not depriving them of anything they have a right to and hence is not unjust killing.

And we should also notice that it is not at all plain that this argument really does go even as far as it purports to. For there are cases and cases, and the details make a difference. If the room is stuffy, and I therefore open a window to air it, and a burglar climbs in, it would be absurd to say, "Ah, now he can stay, she's given him a right to the use of her house—for she is partially responsible for his presence there, having voluntarily done what enabled him to get in, in full knowledge that there are such things as burglars, and that burglars burgle." It would be still more absurd to say this if I had had bars installed outside my windows, precisely to prevent burglars from getting in, and a burglar got in only because of a defect in the bars. It remains equally absurd if we imagine it is not a burglar who climbs in, but an innocent person who blunders or falls in. Again, suppose it were like this: people-seeds drift about in the air like pollen, and if you open your windows, one may drift in and take root in your carpets or upholstery. You don't want children, so you fix up your windows with fine mesh screens, the very best you can buy. As can happen, however, and on very, very rare occasions does happen, one of the screens is defective; and a seed drifts in and takes root. Does the person-plant who now develops have a right to the use of your house? Surely not—despite the fact that you voluntarily opened your windows, you knowingly kept carpets and upholstered furniture, and you knew that screens were sometimes defective. Someone may argue that you are responsible for its rooting, that it does have a right to your house, because after all you *could* have lived out your life with bare floors and furniture, or with sealed windows and doors. But this won't do—for by the same token anyone can avoid a pregnancy due to rape by having a hysterectomy, or anyway by never leaving home without a (reliable!) army.

It seems to me that the argument we are looking at can establish at most that there are *some* cases in which the unborn person has a right to the use of its mother's body, and therefore *some* cases in which abortion is unjust killing. There is room for much discussion and argument as to precisely which, if any. But I think we should sidestep this issue and leave it open, for at any rate the argument certainly does not establish that all abortion is unjust killing.

[3] There is room for yet another argument here, however. We surely must all grant that there may be cases in which it would be morally indecent to detach a

person from your body at the cost of his life. Suppose you learn that what the violinist needs is not nine years of your life, but only one hour: all you need do to save his life is to spend one hour in that bed with him. Suppose also that letting him use your kidneys for that one hour would not affect your health in the slightest. Admittedly you were kidnapped. Admittedly you did not give anyone permission to plug him into you. Nevertheless it seems to me plain you *ought* to allow him to use your kidneys for that hour—it would be indecent to refuse.

Again, suppose pregnancy lasted only an hour, and constituted no threat to life or health. And suppose that a woman becomes pregnant as a result of rape. Admittedly she did not voluntarily do anything to bring about the existence of a child. Admittedly she did nothing at all which would give the unborn person a right to the use of her body. All the same it might well be said, as in the newly emended violinist story, that she *ought* to allow it to remain for that hour—that it would be indecent in her to refuse.

Now some people are inclined to use the term "right" in such a way that it follows from the fact that you ought to allow a person to use your body for the hour he needs, that he has a right to use your body for the hour he needs, even though he has not been given that right by any person or act. They may say that it follows also that if you refuse, you act unjustly toward him. This use of the term is perhaps so common that it cannot be called wrong; nevertheless it seems to me to be an unfortunate loosening of what we would do better to keep a tight rein on. Suppose that box of chocolates I mentioned earlier had not been given to both boys jointly, but was given only to the older boy. There he sits, stolidly eating his way through the box, his small brother watching enviously. Here we are likely to say "You ought not to be so mean. You ought to give your brother some of those chocolates." My own view is that it just does not follow from the truth of this that the brother has any right to any of the chocolates. If the boy refuses to give his brother any, he is greedy, stingy, callous—but not unjust. I suppose that the people I have in mind will say it does follow that the brother has a right to some of the chocolates, and thus that the boy does act unjustly if he refuses to give his brother any. But the effect of saying this is to obscure what we should keep distinct, namely the difference between the boy's refusal in this case and the boy's refusal in the earlier case, in which the box was given to both boys jointly, and in which the small brother thus had what was from any point of view clear title to half.

A further objection to so using the term "right" that from the fact that A ought to do a thing for B, it follows that B has a right against A that A do it for him, is that it is going to make the question of whether or not a man has a right to a thing turn on how easy it is to provide him with it; and this seems not merely unfortunate, but morally unacceptable. Take the case of Henry Fonda again. I said earlier that I had no right to the touch of his cool hand on my fevered brow, even though I needed it to save my life. I said it would be frightfully nice of him to fly in from the West Coast to provide me with it, but that I had no right against him that he should do so. But suppose he isn't on the West Coast. Suppose he has only to walk across the room, place a hand briefly on my brow—and lo, my life is saved. Then surely he ought to do it, it would be indecent to refuse. Is it to be said "Ah, well, it follows that in this case she has a right to the touch of his hand on her brow, and so it would be an injustice in him to refuse"? So that I have a right to it when it is easy for him to provide it, though no right when it's hard? It's rather a shocking idea that anyone's rights should fade away and disappear as it gets harder and harder to accord them to him.

So my own view is that even though you ought to let the violinist use your kidneys for the one hour he needs, we should not conclude that he has a right to do so—we would say that if you refuse, you are, like the boy who owns all the chocolates and will give none away, self-centered and callous, indecent in fact, but not unjust. And similarly, that even supposing a case in which a woman pregnant due to rape ought to allow the unborn person to use her body for the hour he needs, we should not conclude that he has a right to do so; we should conclude that she is self-centered, callous, indecent, but not unjust, if she refuses. The complaints are no less grave; they are just different. However, there is no need to insist on this point. If anyone does wish to deduce "he has a right" from "you ought," then all the same he must surely grant that there are cases in which it is not morally required of you that you allow that violinist to use your kidneys, and in which he does not have a right to use them, and in which you do not do him an injustice if you refuse. And so also for mother and unborn child. Except in such cases as the unborn person has a right to demand it—and we were leaving open the possibility that there may be such cases—nobody is morally *required* to make large sacrifices, of health, of all other interests and concerns, of all other duties and commitments, for nine years, or even for nine months, in order to keep another person alive.

[4] We have in fact to distinguish between two

kinds of Samaritan: the Good Samaritan and what we might call the Minimally Decent Samaritan. The story of the Good Samaritan, you will remember, goes like this:

> A certain man went down from Jerusalem to Jericho, and fell among thieves, which stripped him of his raiment, and wounded him, and departed, leaving him half dead.
>
> And by chance there came down a certain priest that way; and when he saw him, he passed by on the other side.
>
> And likewise a Levite, when he was at the place, came and looked on him, and passed by on the other side.
>
> But a certain Samaritan, as he journeyed, came where he was; and when he saw him he had compassion on him.
>
> And went to him, and bound up his wounds, pouring in oil and wine, and set him on his own beast, and brought him to an inn, and took care of him.
>
> And on the morrow, when he departed, he took out two pence, and gave them to the host, and said unto him, "Take care of him; and whatsoever thou spendest more, when I come again, I will repay thee."
>
> (Luke 10:30–35)

The Good Samaritan went out of his way, at some cost to himself, to help one in need of it. We are not told what the options were, that is, whether or not the priest and the Levite could have helped by doing less than the Good Samaritan did, but assuming they could have, then the fact they did nothing at all shows they were not even Minimally Decent Samaritans, not because they were not Samaritans, but because they were not even minimally decent.

These things are a matter of degree, of course, but there is a difference, and it comes out perhaps most clearly in the story of Kitty Genovese, who, as you will remember, was murdered while thirty-eight people watched or listened, and did nothing at all to help her. A Good Samaritan would have rushed out to give direct assistance against the murderer. Or perhaps we had better allow that it would have been a Splendid Samaritan who did this, on the ground that it would have involved a risk of death for himself. But the thirty-eight not only did not do this, they did not even trouble to pick up a phone to call the police. Minimally Decent Samaritanism would call for doing at least that, and their not having done it was monstrous.

After telling the story of the Good Samaritan, Jesus said "Go, and do thou likewise." Perhaps he meant that we are morally required to act as the Good Samaritan did. Perhaps he was urging people to do more than is morally required of them. At all events it seems plain that it was not morally required of any of the thirty-eight that he rush out to give direct assistance at the risk of his own life, and that it is not morally required of anyone that he give long stretches of his life—nine years or nine months—to sustaining the life of a person who has no special right (we were leaving open the possibility of this) to demand it.

Indeed, with one rather striking class of exceptions, no one in any country in the world is *legally* required to do anywhere near as much as this for anyone else. The class of exceptions is obvious. My main concern here is not the state of the law in respect to abortion, but it is worth drawing attention to the fact that in no state in this country is any man compelled by law to be even a Minimally Decent Samaritan to any person; there is no law under which charges could be brought against the thirty-eight who stood by while Kitty Genovese died. By contrast, in most states in this country women are compelled by law to be not merely Minimally Decent Samaritans, but Good Samaritans to unborn persons inside them. This doesn't by itself settle anything one way or the other, because it may well be argued that there should be laws in this country—as there are in many European countries—compelling at least Minimally Decent Samaritanism.[4] But it does show that there is a gross injustice in the existing state of the law. And it shows also that the groups currently working against liberalization of abortion laws, in fact working toward having it declared unconstitutional for a state to permit abortion, had better start working for the adoption of Good Samaritan laws generally, or earn the charge that they are acting in bad faith.

I should think, myself, that Minimally Decent Samaritan laws would be one thing, Good Samaritan laws quite another, and in fact highly improper. But we are not here concerned with the law. What we should ask is not whether anybody should be compelled by law to be a Good Samaritan, but whether we must accede to a situation in which somebody is being compelled—by nature, perhaps—to be a Good Samaritan. We have, in other words, to look now at third-party interventions. I have been arguing that no person is morally required to make large sacrifices to sustain the life of another who has no right to demand them, and this even where the sacrifices do not include life itself; we are not morally required to be Good Samaritans or anyway Very Good Samaritans to one another. But what if a man cannot extricate himself from such a situation? What if he appeals to us to extricate him? It seems to me plain that there are cases in which we can, cases in which a Good Samaritan would extricate him. There you are, you were kidnapped, and nine years in bed with that violinist lie ahead of you. You have your own life to lead. You are sorry, but you simply cannot see giving up so much of your life to the sustaining of his. You cannot extricate yourself, and ask us to do so. I should have thought that—in light of his having no right to the use of your body—it was obvious that we do not have to accede to your being forced to give up so much. We can do what you ask. There is no injustice to the violinist in our doing so.

[5] Following the lead of the opponents of abortion, I have throughout been speaking of the fetus merely as a person, and what I have been asking is whether or not the argument we began with, which proceeds only from the fetus' being a person, really does establish its conclusion. I have argued that it does not.

But of course there are arguments and arguments, and it may be said that I have simply fastened on the wrong one. It may be said that what is important is not merely the fact that the fetus is a person, but that it is a person for whom the woman has a special kind of responsibility issuing from the fact that she is its mother. And it might be argued that all my analogies are therefore irrelevant—for you do not have that special kind of responsibility for that violinist, Henry Fonda does not have that special kind of responsibility for me. And our attention might be drawn to the fact that men and women both *are* compelled by law to provide support for their children.

I have in effect dealt (briefly) with this argument in section [2] above; but a (still briefer) recapitulation now may be in order. Surely we do not have any such "special responsibility" for a person unless we have assumed it, explicitly or implicitly. If a set of parents do not try to prevent pregnancy, do not obtain an abortion, and then at the time of birth of the child do not put it out for adoption, but rather take it home with them, then they have assumed responsibility for it, they have given it rights, and they cannot *now* withdraw support from it at the cost of its life because they now find it difficult to go on providing for it. But if they have taken all reasonable precautions against having a child, they do not simply by virtue of their biological relationship to the child who comes into existence have a special responsibility for it. They may wish to assume responsibility for it, or they may not wish to. And I am suggesting that if assuming responsibility for it would require large sacrifices, then they may refuse. A Good Samaritan would not refuse—or anyway, a Splendid Samaritan, if the sacrifices that

had to be made were enormous. But then so would a Good Samaritan assume responsibility for that violinist; so would Henry Fonda, if he is a Good Samaritan, fly in from the West Coast and assume responsibility for me.

[6] My argument will be found unsatisfactory on two counts by many of those who want to regard abortion as morally permissible. First, while I do argue that abortion is not impermissible, I do not argue that it is always permissible. There may well be cases in which carrying the child to term requires only Minimally Decent Samaritanism of the mother, and this is a standard we must not fall below. I am inclined to think it a merit of my account precisely that it does *not* give a general yes or a general no. It allows for and supports our sense that, for example, a sick and desperately frightened fourteen-year-old schoolgirl, pregnant due to rape, may *of course* choose abortion, and that any law which rules this out is an insane law. And it also allows for and supports our sense that in other cases resort to abortion is even positively indecent. It would be indecent in the woman to request an abortion, and indecent in a doctor to perform it, if she is in her seventh month, and wants the abortion just to avoid the nuisance of postponing a trip abroad. The very fact that the arguments I have been drawing attention to treat all cases of abortion, or even all cases of abortion in which the mother's life is not at stake, as morally on a par ought to have made them suspect at the outset.

Secondly, while I am arguing for the permissibility of abortion in some cases, I am not arguing for the right to secure the death of the unborn child. It is easy to confuse these two things in that up to a certain point in the life of the fetus it is not able to survive outside the mother's body; hence removing it from her body guarantees its death. But they are importantly different. I have argued that you are not morally required to spend nine months in bed, sustaining the life of that violinist; but to say this is by no means to say that if, when you unplug yourself, there is a miracle and he survives, you then have a right to turn round and slit his throat. You may detach yourself even if this costs him his life; you have no right to be guaranteed his death, by some other means, if unplugging yourself does not kill him. There are some people who will feel dissatisfied by this feature of my argument. A woman may be utterly devastated by the thought of a child, a bit of herself, put out for adoption and never seen or heard of again. She may therefore want not merely that the child be detached from her, but more, that it die. Some opponents of abortion are inclined to regard this as beneath contempt—thereby showing insensitivity to what is surely a powerful source of despair. All the same, I agree that the desire for the child's death is not one which anybody may gratify, should it turn out to be possible to detach the child alive.

At this place, however, it should be remembered that we have only been pretending throughout that the fetus is a human being from the moment of conception. A very early abortion is surely not the killing of a person, and so is not dealt with by anything I have said here.

NOTES

1 I am very much indebted to James Thomson for discussion, criticism, and many helpful suggestions.
2 Daniel Callahan, *Abortion: Law, Choice and Morality* (New York, 1970), p. 373. This book gives a fascinating survey of the available information on abortion. The Jewish tradition is surveyed in David M. Feldman, *Birth Control in Jewish Law* (New York, 1968), Part 5, the Catholic tradition in John T. Noonan, Jr., "An Almost Absolute Value in History," in *The Morality of Abortion*, ed. John T. Noonan, Jr. (Cambridge, Mass., 1970).
3 The need for a discussion of this argument was brought home to me by members of the Society for Ethical and Legal Philosophy, to whom this paper was originally presented.
4 For a discussion of the difficulties involved, and a survey of the European experience with such laws, see *The Good Samaritan and the Law*, ed. James M. Ratcliffe (New York, 1966).

Abortion Decisions: Personal Morality
Daniel Callahan

A biographical sketch of Daniel Callahan is found on page 388.

Callahan defends one kind of moderate view on the problem of the ethical acceptability of abortion. On the issue of the moral status of the fetus, he steers a middle course. He rejects the "tissue" theory, the view that the fetus has negligible moral status, on the grounds that such a theory is out of tune with both the biological evidence and a respect for the sanctity of human life. On the other hand, he contends that the fetus does not qualify as a person and thus rejects the view that the fetus has full moral status. His contention that the fetus is nevertheless an "important and valuable form of human life" can be understood as implying that the fetus has some kind of *partial* moral status. In Callahan's view, a respect for the sanctity of human life should incline every woman to a strong initial (moral) bias against abortion. Yet, he argues, since a woman has duties to herself, her family, and her society, there may be circumstances in which such duties would override the prima facie duty not to abort.

. . . To press the problem to a finer point, what ought [women] to think about as they try to work out their own views on abortion?

Only a few suggestions will be made here, taking the form of arguing for an ethic of personal responsibility which tries, in the process of decision-making, to make itself aware of a number of things. The biological evidence should be considered, just as the problem of methodology must be considered; the philosophical assumptions implicit in different uses of the word "human" need to be considered; a philosophical theory of biological analysis is required; the social consequences of different kinds of analyses and different meanings of the word "human" should be thought through; consistency of meaning and use should be sought to avoid *ad hoc* and arbitrary solutions.

It is my own conviction that the "developmental school" offers the most helpful and illuminating approach to the problem of the beginning of human life, avoiding, on the one hand, a too narrow genetic criterion of human life and, on the other, a too broad and socially dangerous social definition of the "human." Yet the kinds of problems which appear in any attempt to decide upon the beginning of life suggest that no one position can be either proved or disproved from biological evidence alone. It becomes a question of trying to do justice to the evidence while, at the same time, realizing that how the evidence is approached and used will be a function of one's way of looking at reality, one's moral policy, the values and rights one believes need balancing, and the type of questions one thinks need to be asked. At the very least, however, the genetic evidence for the uniqueness of zygotes and embryos (a uniqueness of a different kind than that of the uniqueness of sperm and ova), their potentiality for development into a human person, their early development of human characteristics, their genetic and organic distinctness from the organism of the mother, appear to rule out a treatment even of zygotes, much less the more developed stages of the conceptus, as mere pieces of "tissue," of no human significance or value. The "tissue" theory of the significance of the conceptus can only be made plausible by a systematic disregard of the biological evidence. Moreover, though one may conclude that a conceptus is only potential human life, in the process of continually actualizing its potential through growth and development, a respect for the sanctity of life, with its bias in favor even of undeveloped life, is enough to make the taking of such life a moral problem. There is a choice to be made and it is a moral choice. . . .

It is possible to imagine a huge number of situations where a woman could, in good and sensitive conscience, choose abortion as a moral solution to her personal or social difficulties. But, at the very least, the bounds of morality are overstepped when either through a systematic intellectual negligence or a willful choosing of that moral solution most personally convenient, personal choice is deliberately made easy and problem-free. . . .

. . . Abortion is *one* way to solve the problem of an unwanted or hazardous pregnancy (physically, psychologically, economically or socially), but it is rarely the only way, at least in affluent societies (I would be considerably less certain about making the same statement about poor societies). Even in the most extreme cases—rape, incest, psychosis, for instance—alternatives will usually be available and different choices, open. It is not necessarily the end of every woman's chance for a happy, meaningful life to bear an illegitimate child. It is not necessarily the automatic destruction of a family to have a seriously defective child born into it. It is not necessarily the ruination of every family living in overcrowded housing to have still another child. It is not inevitable that every immature woman would become even more so if she bore a child or another child. It is not inevitable that a gravely handicapped child can hope for nothing from life. It is not inevitable that every unwanted child is doomed to misery. It is not written in the essence of things, as a fixed law of human nature, that a woman cannot come to accept, love and be a good mother to a child who was initially unwanted. Nor is it a fixed law that she could not come to cherish a grossly deformed child. Naturally, these are only generalizations. The point is only that human beings are as a rule flexible, capable of doing more than they sometimes think they can, able to surmount serious dangers and challenges, able to grow and mature, able to transform inauspicious beginnings into satisfactory conclusions. Everything in life, even in procreative and family life, is not fixed in advance; the future is never wholly unalterable. . . .

Assuming . . . that most women would seek a broader ethical horizon than that of their exclusively personal self-interest, what might they think about when faced with an abortion decision? A respect for the sanctity of human life should, I believe, incline them toward a general and strong bias against abortion. Abortion is an act of killing, the violent, direct destruction of potential human life, already in the process of development. That fact should not be disguised, or glossed over by euphemism and circumlocution. It is not the destruction of a human person—for at no stage of its development does the conceptus fulfill the definition of a person, which implies a developed capacity for reasoning, willing, desiring and relating to others—but it is the destruction of an important and valuable form of human life. Its value and its potentiality are not dependent upon the attitude of the woman toward it; it grows by its own biological dynamism and has a genetic and morphological potential distinct from that of the woman. It has its own distinctive and individual future. If contraception and abortion are both seen as forms of birth limitation, they are distinctly different acts; the former precludes the possibility of a conceptus being formed, while the latter stops a conceptus already in existence from developing. The bias implied by the principle of the sanctity of human life is toward the protection of all forms of human life, especially, in ordinary circumstances, the protection of the right to life. That right should be accorded even to doubtful life; its existence should not be wholly dependent upon the personal self-interest of the woman.

Yet she has her own rights as well, and her own set of responsibilities to those around her; that is why she may have to choose abortion. In extreme situations of overpopulation, she may also have a responsibility for the survival of the species or of a people. In many circumstances, then, a decision in favor of abortion—one which overrides the right to life of that potential human being she carries within—can be a responsible moral decision, worthy neither of the condemnation of others nor of self-condemnation. But the bias of the principle of the sanctity of life is against a routine, unthinking employment of abortion; it bends over backwards not to take life and gives the benefit of the doubt to life. It does not seek to diminish the range of responsibility toward life—potential or actual—but to extend it. It does not seek the narrowest definition of life, but the widest and the richest. It is mindful of individual possibility, on the one hand, and of a destructive human tendency, on the other, to exclude from the category of "the human" or deny rights to those beings whose existence is or could prove burdensome to others. . . .

. . . Moral seriousness presupposes one is concerned with the protection and furthering of life. This means that, out of respect for human life, one bends over backwards not to eliminate human life, not to desensitize oneself to the meaning and value of potential life, not to seek definitions of the "human" which serve one's self-interest only. A desire to respect human life in all of its forms means, therefore, that one voluntarily imposes upon oneself a pressure against the taking of life; that one demands of oneself serious reasons for doing so, even in the case of a very early embryo; that one use not only the mind but also the imagination when a decision is being made; that one seeks not to

evade the moral issues but to face them; that one searches out the alternatives and conscientiously entertains them before turning to abortion. A bias in favor of the sanctity of human life in all of its forms would include a bias against abortion on the part of women; it would be the last rather than the first choice when unwanted pregnancies occurred. It would be an act to be avoided if at all possible.

A bias of this kind, voluntarily imposed by a woman upon herself, would not trap her; for it is also part of a respect for the dignity of life to leave the way open for an abortion when other reasonable choices are not available. For she also has duties toward herself, her family and her society. There can be good reasons for taking the life even of a very late fetus; once that also is seen and seen as a counterpoise in particular cases to the general bias against the taking of potential life, the way is open to choose abortion. The bias of the moral policy implies the need for moral rules which seek to preserve life. But, as a policy which leaves room for choice—rather than entailing a fixed set of rules—it is open to flexible interpretation when the circumstances point to the wisdom of taking exception to the normal ordering of the rules in particular cases. Yet, in that case, one is not genuinely taking exception to the rules. More accurately, one would be deciding that, for the preservation or furtherance of other values or rights—species-rights, person-rights—a choice in favor of abortion would be serving the sanctity of life. That there would be, in that case, conflict between rights, with one set of rights set aside (reluctantly) to serve another set, goes without saying. A subversion of the principle occurs when it is made out that there is no conflict and thus nothing to decide.

Abortion and Social Policy

Majority Opinion in *Roe v. Wade*
Justice Harry Blackmun

Harry Blackmun, a graduate of Harvard Law School, was associate justice of the United States Supreme Court from 1970 to 1994. After some 15 years in private practice, he became legal counsel to the Mayo Clinic (1950–1959). Justice Blackmun also served as United States circuit judge (1959–1970) before his appointment to the Supreme Court.

In this case, a pregnant single woman, suing under the fictitious name of Jane Roe, challenged the constitutionality of the existing Texas criminal abortion law. According to the

United States Supreme Court; January 22, 1973. 410 U.S. 113, 93 S.Ct. 705.

Texas Penal Code, the performance of an abortion, except to save the life of the pregnant woman, constituted a crime that was punishable by a prison sentence of two to five years. At the time this case was finally resolved by the Supreme Court, abortion legislation varied widely from state to state. Some states, principally New York, had already legalized abortion on demand. Most other states, however, had legalized various forms of therapeutic abortion but had retained some measure of restrictive abortion legislation.

Justice Blackmun, writing an opinion concurred in by six other justices, argues that a woman's decision to terminate a pregnancy is encompassed by a *right to privacy*—but only up to a certain point in the development of the fetus. As the right to privacy is not an absolute right, it must yield at some point to the state's legitimate interests. Justice Blackmun contends that the state has a legitimate interest in protecting the health of the mother and that this interest becomes compelling at approximately the end of the first trimester in the development of the fetus. He also contends that the state has a legitimate interest in protecting potential life and that this interest becomes compelling at the point of viability.

It is . . . apparent that at common law, at the time of the adoption of our Constitution, and throughout the major portion of the 19th century, abortion was viewed with less disfavor than under most American statutes currently in effect. Phrasing it another way, a woman enjoyed a substantially broader right to terminate a pregnancy than she does in most States today. At least with respect to the early stage of pregnancy, and very possibly without such a limitation, the opportunity to make this choice was present in this country well into the 19th century. Even later, the law continued for some time to treat less punitively an abortion procured in early pregnancy. . . .

Three reasons have been advanced to explain historically the enactment of criminal abortion laws in the 19th century and to justify their continued existence.

It has been argued occasionally that these laws were the product of a Victorian social concern to discourage illicit sexual conduct. Texas, however, does not advance this justification in the present case, and it appears that no court or commentator has taken the argument seriously. . . .

A second reason is concerned with abortion as a medical procedure. When most criminal abortion laws were first enacted, the procedure was a hazardous one for the woman. This was particularly true prior to the development of antisepsis. Antiseptic techniques, of course, were based on discoveries by Lister, Pasteur, and others first announced in 1867, but were not generally accepted and employed until about the turn of the century. Abortion mortality was high. Even after 1900, and perhaps until as late as the development of antibi-

otics in the 1940's, standard modern techniques such as dilation and curettage were not nearly so safe as they are today. Thus it has been argued that a State's real concern in enacting a criminal abortion law was to protect the pregnant woman, that is, to restrain her from submitting to a procedure that placed her life in serious jeopardy.

Modern medical techniques have altered this situation. Appellants and various *amici* refer to medical data indicating that abortion in early pregnancy, that is, prior to the end of first trimester, although not without its risk, is now relatively safe. Mortality rates for women undergoing early abortions, where the procedure is legal, appear to be as low as or lower than the rates for normal childbirth. Consequently, any interest of the State in protecting the woman from an inherently hazardous procedure, except when it would be equally dangerous for her to forego it, has largely disappeared. Of course, important state interests in the area of health and medical standards do remain. The State has a legitimate interest in seeing to it that abortion, like any other medical procedure, is performed under circumstances that insure maximum safety for the patient. This interest obviously extends at least to the performing physician and his staff, to the facilities involved, to the availability of after-care, and to adequate provision for any complication or emergency that might arise. The prevalence of high mortality rates at illegal "abortion mills" strengthens, rather than weakens, the State's interest in regulating the conditions under which abortions are performed. Moreover, the risk to the woman increases as her pregnancy continues. Thus the State retains a definite interest in protecting the woman's own health and safety when an abortion is performed at a late stage of pregnancy.

The third reason is the State's interest—some phrase it in terms of duty—in protecting prenatal life. Some of the argument for this justification rests on the theory that a new human life is present from the moment of conception. The State's interest and general obligation to protect life then extends, it is argued, to prenatal life. Only when the life of the pregnant mother herself is at stake, balanced against the life she carries within her, should the interest of the embryo or fetus not prevail. Logically, of course, a legitimate state interest in this area need not stand or fall on acceptance of the belief that life begins at conception or at some other point prior to live birth. In assessing the State's interest, recognition may be given to the less rigid claim that as long as at least *potential* life is involved, the State may assert interests beyond the protection of the pregnant woman alone.

Parties challenging state abortion laws have sharply disputed in some courts the contention that a purpose of these laws, when enacted, was to protect prenatal life. Pointing to the absence of legislative history to support the contention, they claim that most state laws were designed solely to protect the woman. Because medical advances have lessened this concern, at least with respect to abortion in early pregnancy, they argue that with respect to such abortions the laws can no longer be justified by any state interest. There is some scholarly support for this view of original purpose. The few state courts called upon to interpret their laws in the late 19th and early 20th centuries did focus on the State's interest in protecting the woman's health rather than in preserving the embryo and fetus. . . .

The Constitution does not explicitly mention any right of privacy. In a line of decisions, however, going back perhaps as far as *Union Pacific R. Co. v. Botsford* (1891), the Court has recognized that a right of personal privacy, or a guarantee of certain areas or zones of privacy, does exist under the constitution. In varying contexts the Court or individual Justices have indeed found at least the roots of that right in the First Amendment, . . . in the Fourth and Fifth Amendments . . . in the penumbras of the Bill of Rights . . . in the Ninth Amendment . . . or in the concept of liberty guaranteed by the first section of the Fourteenth Amendment. . . . These decisions make it clear that only personal rights that can be deemed "fundamental" or "implicit in the concept of ordered liberty," . . . are included in this guarantee of personal privacy. They also make it clear that the right has some extension to activities relating to marriage, . . . procreation, . . . contraception, . . . family relationships, . . . and child rearing and education, . . .

This right of privacy, whether it be founded in the Fourteenth Amendment's concept of personal liberty and restrictions upon state action, as we feel it is, or, as the District Court determined, in the Ninth Amendment's reservation of rights to the people, is broad enough to encompass a woman's decision whether or not to terminate her pregnancy. . . .

. . . [A]ppellants and some *amici* argue that the woman's right is absolute and that she is entitled to terminate her pregnancy at whatever time, in whatever way, and for whatever reason she alone chooses. With this we do not agree. Appellants' arguments that Texas either has no valid interest at all in regulating the abortion decision, or no interest strong enough to support any limitation upon the woman's sole determination, is unpersuasive. The Court's decisions recognizing a right of privacy also acknowledges that some state regulation in areas protected by that right is appropriate. As noted above, a state may properly assert important interests in safe-guarding health, in maintaining medical standards, and in protecting potential life. At some point in pregnancy, these respective interests become sufficiently compelling to sustain regulation of the factors that govern the abortion decision. The privacy right involved, therefore, cannot be said to be absolute. . . .

We therefore conclude that the right of personal privacy includes the abortion decision, but that this right is not unqualified and must be considered against important state interests in regulation.

We note that those federal and state courts that have recently considered abortion law challenges have reached the same conclusion. . . .

Although the results are divided, most of these courts have agreed that the right of privacy, however based, is broad enough to cover the abortion decision; that the right, nonetheless, is not absolute and is subject to some limitations; and that at some point the state interests as to protection of health, medical standards, and prenatal life, become dominant. We agree with this approach. . . .

The appellee and certain *amici* argue that the fetus is a "person" within the language and meaning of the Fourteenth Amendment. In support of this they outline at length and in detail the well-known facts of fetal development. If this suggestion of personhood is established, the appellant's case, of course, collapses, for the fetus' right to life is then guaranteed specifically by the Amendment. The appellant conceded as much on reargument. On the other hand, the appellee conceded on reargument that no case could be cited that holds that a fetus is a person within the meaning of the Fourteenth Amendment. . . .

All this, together with our observation, *supra,* that throughout the major portion of the 19th century prevailing legal abortion practices were far freer than they are today, persuades us that the word "person," as used in the Fourteenth Amendment, does not include the unborn. . . . Indeed, our decision in *United States v. Vuitch* (1971) inferentially is to the same effect, for we there would not have indulged in statutory interpretation favorable to abortion in specified circumstances if the necessary consequence was the termination of life entitled to Fourteenth Amendment protection.

. . . As we have intimated above, it is reasonable and appropriate for a State to decide that at some point in time another interest, that of health of the mother or that of potential human life, becomes significantly involved. The woman's privacy is no longer sole and any right of privacy she possesses must be measured accordingly.

Texas urges that, apart from the Fourteenth Amendment, life begins at conception and is present throughout pregnancy, and that, therefore, the State has a compelling interest in protecting that life from and after conception. We need not resolve the difficult question of when life begins. When those trained in the respective disciplines of medicine, philosophy, and theology are unable to arrive at any consensus, the judiciary, at this point in the development of man's knowledge, is not in a position to speculate as to the answer.

It should be sufficient to note briefly the wide divergence of thinking on this most sensitive and difficult question. There has always been strong support for the view that life does not begin until live birth. This was the belief of the Stoics. It appears to be the predominant, though not the unanimous, attitude of the Jewish faith. It may be taken to represent also the position of a large segment of the Protestant community, insofar as that can be ascertained; organized groups that have taken a formal position on the abortion issu have generally regarded abortion as a matter for theconscience of the individual and her family. As we have noted, the common law found greater significance in quickening. Physicians and their scientific colleagues have regarded that event with less interest and have tended to focus either upon conception or upon live birth or upon the interim point at which the fetus becomes "viable," that is, potentially able to live outside the mother's womb, albeit with artificial aid. Viability is usually placed at about seven months (28 weeks) but may occur earlier, even at 24 weeks. . . .

In areas other than criminal abortion the law has been reluctant to endorse any theory that life, as we recognize it, begins before live birth or to accord legal rights to the unborn except in narrowly defined situations and except when the rights are contingent upon live birth. . . . In short, the unborn have never been recognized in the law as persons in the whole sense.

In view of all this, we do not agree that, by adopting one theory of life, Texas may override the rights of the pregnant woman that are at stake. We repeat, however, that the State does have an important and legitimate interest in preserving and protecting the health of the pregnant woman, whether she be a resident of the State or a nonresident who seeks medical consultation and treatment there, and that it has still *another* important and legitimate interest in protecting the potentiality of human life. These interests are separate and distinct. Each grows in substantiality as the woman approaches term and, at a point during pregnancy, each becomes "compelling."

With respect to the State's important and legitimate interest in the health of the mother, the "compelling" point, in the light of present medical knowledge, is at approximately the end of the first trimester. This is so because of the now established medical fact . . . that until the end of the first trimester mortality in abortion is less than mortality in normal childbirth. It follows that, from and after this point, a State may regulate the abortion procedure to the extent that the regulation reasonably relates to the preservation and protection of maternal health. Examples of permissible state regulation in this area are requirements as to the qualifications of the person who is to perform the abortion; as to the licensure of that person; as to the facility in which the procedure is to be performed, that is, whether it must be a hospital or may be a clinic or some other place of less-than-hospital status; as to the licensing of the facility; and the like.

This means, on the other hand, that, for the period of pregnancy prior to this "compelling" point, the attending physician, in consultation with his patient, is free to determine, without regulation by the State, that in his medical judgment the patient's pregnancy should be terminated. If that decision is reached, the judgment may be effectuated by an abortion free of interference by the State.

With respect to the State's important and legitimate interest in potential life, the "compelling" point is at viability. This is so because the fetus then presumably has the capability of meaningful life outside the mother's womb. State regulation protective of fetal life after viability thus has both logical and biological justifications. If the State is interested in protecting fetal life after viability, it may go so far as to proscribe abortion during that period except when it is necessary to preserve the life or health of the mother. . . .

To summarize and repeat:

1 A state criminal abortion statute of the current Texas type, that excepts from criminality only a *life saving* procedure on behalf of the mother, without regard to pregnancy stage and without recognition of the other interests involved, is violative of the Due Process Clause of the Fourteenth Amendment.

a For the stage prior to approximately the end of the first trimester, the abortion decision and its effectuation must be left to the medical judgment of the pregnant woman's attending physician.

b For the stage subsequent to approximately the end of the first trimester, the State, in promoting its interest in the health of the mother, may, if it chooses, regulate the abortion procedure in ways that are reasonably related to maternal health.

c For the stage subsequent to viability the State, in promoting its interest in the potentiality of human life, may, if it chooses, regulate, and even proscribe, abortion except where it is necessary, in appropriate medical judgment, for the preservation of the life or health of the mother.

2 The State may define the term "physician," as it has been employed [here], to mean only a physician currently licensed by the State, and may proscribe any abortion by a person who is not a physician as so defined.

. . . The decision leaves the State free to place increasing restrictions on abortion as the period of pregnancy lengthens, so long as those restrictions are tailored to the recognized state interests. The decision vindicates the right of the physician to administer medical treatment according to his professional judgment up to the points where important state interests provide compelling justifications for intervention. Up to those points the abortion decision in all its aspects is inherently, and primarily, a medical decision, and basic responsibility for it must rest with the physician. If an individual practitioner abuses the privilege of exercising proper medical judgment, the usual remedies, judicial and intraprofessional, are available. . . .

Opinion in *Planned Parenthood of Southeastern Pennsylvania v. Casey, Governor of Pennsylvania*
Justices Sandra Day O'Connor, Anthony M. Kennedy, and David H. Souter

Sandra Day O'Connor, Anthony M. Kennedy, and David H. Souter are associate justices of the United States Supreme Court. Justice O'Connor was serving on the Arizona Court of Appeals when, in 1981, she became the first woman ever appointed to the Supreme Court. She had earlier served as Arizona assistant attorney general (1965–1969) and Arizona state senator (1969–1975). Justice Kennedy was appointed to the Court in 1988. He had previously spent a number of years in private practice and also served as judge, United States Court of Appeals, Ninth Circuit (1976–1988). Justice Souter received his appointment to the Court in 1990. He had earlier served as attorney general of New Hampshire (1976–1978), associate justice of the New Hampshire Superior Court (1978–1983), and associate justice of the New Hampshire Supreme Court (1983–1990).

United States Supreme Court. 112 S.Ct. 2791 (1992).

At issue in this case is the constitutionality of the various provisions of the Pennsylvania Abortion Control Act. Of principal concern are (1) the informed consent provision, which includes a specification of a 24-hour waiting period, (2) the spousal notification provision, and (3) the parental consent provision. In announcing the judgment of a Court that is deeply divided on the fundamental issues, Justices O'Connor, Kennedy, and Souter reaffirm the "essential holding" of *Roe v. Wade* while at the same time rejecting the trimester framework so closely identified with that landmark ruling. Committed instead to an "undue burden analysis," the three Justices conclude that the informed consent and parental consent provisions are constitutional but the spousal notification provision is not.

I

Liberty finds no refuge in a jurisprudence of doubt. Yet 19 years after our holding that the Constitution protects a woman's right to terminate her pregnancy in its early stages, *Roe* v. *Wade* (1973), that definition of liberty is still questioned. Joining the respondents as *amicus curiae*, the United States, as it has done in five other cases in the last decade, again asks us to overrule *Roe*.

At issue . . . are five provisions of the Pennsylvania Abortion Control Act of 1982 as amended in 1988 and 1989. . . . The Act requires that a woman seeking an abortion give her informed consent prior to the abortion procedure, and specifies that she be provided with certain information at least 24 hours before the abortion is performed. §3205. For a minor to obtain an abortion, the Act requires the informed consent of one of her parents, but provides for a judicial bypass option if the minor does not wish to or cannot obtain a parent's consent. §3206. Another provision of the Act requires that, unless certain exceptions apply, a married woman seeking an abortion must sign a statement indicating that she has notified her husband of her intended abortion. §3209. The Act exempts compliance with these three requirements in the event of a "medical emergency," which is defined in §3203 of the Act. In addition to the above provisions regulating the performance of abortions, the Act imposes certain reporting requirements on facilities that provide abortion services.

Before any of these provisions took effect, the petitioners, who are five abortion clinics and one physician representing himself as well as a class of physicians who provide abortion services, brought this suit seeking declaratory and injunctive relief. Each provision was challenged as unconstitutional on its face. The District Court entered a preliminary injunction against the enforcement of the regulations, and, after a 3-day bench trial, held all the provisions at issue here unconstitutional, entering a permanent injunction against Pennsylvania's enforcement of them. The Court of Appeals for the Third Circuit affirmed in part and reversed in part, upholding all of the regulations except for the husband notification requirement. . . .

. . . [W]e find it imperative to review once more the principles that define the rights of the woman and the legitimate authority of the State respecting the termination of pregnancies by abortion procedures.

After considering the fundamental constitutional questions resolved by *Roe*, principles of institutional integrity, and the rule of *stare decisis*, we are led to conclude this: the essential holding of *Roe* v. *Wade* should be retained and once again reaffirmed.

It must be stated at the outset and with clarity that *Roe*'s essential holding, the holding we reaffirm, has three parts. First is a recognition of the right of the woman to choose to have an abortion before viability and to obtain it without undue interference from the State. Before viability, the State's interests are not strong enough to support a prohibition of abortion or the imposition of a substantial obstacle to the woman's effective right to elect the procedure. Second is a confirmation of the State's power to restrict abortions after fetal viability, if the law contains exceptions for pregnancies which endanger a woman's life or health. And third is the principle that the State has legitimate interests from the outset of the pregnancy in protecting the health of the woman and the life of the fetus that may become a child. These principles do not contradict one another; and we adhere to each.

II

Constitutional protection of the woman's decision to terminate her pregnancy derives from the Due Process Clause of the Fourteenth Amendment. It declares that no State shall "deprive any person of life, liberty, or property, without due process of law." The controlling word in the case before us is "liberty." . . .

. . . It is a promise of the Constitution that there is a realm of personal liberty which the government may not enter. We have vindicated this principle before. Marriage is mentioned nowhere in the Bill of Rights and interracial marriage was illegal in most States in the 19th century, but the Court was no doubt correct in finding it to be an aspect of liberty protected against state interference by the substantive component of the Due Process Clause. . . .

Neither the Bill of Rights nor the specific practices of States at the time of the adoption of the Fourteenth Amendment marks the outer limits of the substantive sphere of liberty which the Fourteenth Amendment protects. . . . It is settled now, as it was when the Court heard arguments in *Roe* v. *Wade,* that the Constitution places limits on a State's right to interfere with a person's most basic decisions about family and parenthood, as well as bodily integrity.

The inescapable fact is that adjudication of substantive due process claims may call upon the Court in interpreting the Constitution to exercise that same capacity which by tradition courts always have exercised: reasoned judgment. . . .

III

. . . No evolution of legal principle has left *Roe*'s doctrinal footings weaker than they were in 1973. No development of constitutional law since the case was decided has implicitly or explicitly left *Roe* behind as a mere survivor of obsolete constitutional thinking. . . .

We have seen how time has overtaken some of *Roe*'s factual assumptions: advances in maternal health care allow for abortions safe to the mother later in pregnancy than was true in 1973, and advances in neonatal care have advanced viability to a point somewhat earlier. But these facts go only to the scheme of time limits on the realization of competing interests, and the divergences from the factual premises of 1973 have no bearing on the validity of *Roe*'s central holding, that viability marks the earliest point at which the State's interest in fetal life is constitutionally adequate to justify a legislative ban on nontherapeutic abortions. The soundness or unsoundness of that constitutional judgment in no sense turns on whether viability occurs at approximately 28 weeks, as was usual at the time of *Roe*, at 23 to 24 weeks, as it sometimes does today, or at some moment

even slightly earlier in pregnancy, as it may if fetal respiratory capacity can somehow be enhanced in the future. Whenever it may occur, the attainment of viability may continue to serve as the critical fact, just as it has done since *Roe* was decided; which is to say that no change in *Roe*'s factual underpinning has left its central holding obsolete, and none supports an argument for overruling it. . . .

The Court's duty in the present case is clear. In 1973, it confronted the already-divisive issue of governmental power to limit personal choice to undergo abortion, for which it provided a new resolution based on the due process guaranteed by the Fourteenth Amendment. Whether or not a new social consensus is developing on that issue, its divisiveness is no less today than in 1973, and pressure to overrule the decision, like pressure to retain it, has grown only more intense. A decision to overrule *Roe*'s essential holding under the existing circumstances would address error, if error there was, at the cost of both profound and unnecessary damage to the Court's legitimacy, and to the Nation's commitment to the rule of law. It is therefore imperative to adhere to the essence of *Roe*'s original decision, and we do so today.

IV

From what we have said so far it follows that it is a constitutional liberty of the woman to have some freedom to terminate her pregnancy. . . .

. . . Liberty must not be extinguished for want of a line that is clear. And it falls to us to give some real substance to the woman's liberty to determine whether to carry her pregnancy to full term.

We conclude the line should be drawn at viability, so that before that time the woman has a right to choose to terminate her pregnancy. We adhere to this principle for two reasons. First . . . is the doctrine of *stare decisis.* Any judicial act of line-drawing may seem somewhat arbitrary, but *Roe* was a reasoned statement, elaborated with great care. We have twice reaffirmed it in the face of great opposition. . . .

The second reason is that the concept of viability, as we noted in *Roe*, is the time at which there is a realistic possibility of maintaining and nourishing a life outside the womb, so that the independent existence of the second life can in reason and all fairness be the object of state protection that now overrides the rights of the woman. . . . We must justify the lines we draw. And there is no line other than viability which is more workable. To be sure, as we have said, there may be some medical developments that affect the precise point of viability, but this is an imprecision within tolerable limits given that the medical community and all those who must apply its discoveries will continue to explore the matter. The viability line also has, as a practical matter, an element of fairness. In some broad sense it might be said that a woman who fails to act before viability has consented to the State's intervention on behalf of the developing child.

The woman's right to terminate her pregnancy before viability is the most central principle of *Roe* v. *Wade*. It is a rule of law and a component of liberty we cannot renounce. . . .

Yet it must be remembered that *Roe* v. *Wade* speaks with clarity in establishing not only the woman's liberty but also the State's "important and legitimate interest in potential life." That portion of the decision in *Roe* has been given too little acknowledgement and implementation by the Court in its subsequent cases. . . .

Roe established a trimester framework to govern abortion regulations. Under this elaborate but rigid construct, almost no regulation at all is permitted during the first trimester of pregnancy; regulations designed to protect the woman's health, but not to further the State's interest in potential life, are permitted during the second trimester; and during the third trimester, when the fetus is viable, prohibitions are permitted provided the life or health of the mother is not at stake. Most of our cases since *Roe* have involved the application of rules derived from the trimester framework.

The trimester framework no doubt was erected to ensure that the woman's right to choose not become so subordinate to the State's interest in promoting fetal life that her choice exists in theory but not in fact. We do not agree, however, that the trimester approach is necessary to accomplish this objective. . . .

Though the woman has a right to choose to terminate or continue her pregnancy before viability, it does not at all follow that the State is prohibited from taking steps to ensure that this choice is thoughtful and informed. Even in the earliest stages of pregnancy, the State may enact rules and regulations designed to encourage her to know that there are philosophic and social arguments of great weight that can be brought to bear in favor of continuing the pregnancy to full term and that there are procedures and institutions to allow adoption of unwanted children as well as a certain degree of state assistance if the mother chooses to raise the child herself. . . .

. . . Numerous forms of state regulation might have the incidental effect of increasing the cost or decreasing the availability of medical care, whether for abortion or any other medical procedure. The fact that a law which serves a valid purpose, one not designed to strike at the right itself, has the incidental effect of making it more difficult or more expensive to procure an abortion cannot be enough to invalidate it. Only where state regulation imposes an undue burden on a woman's ability to make this decision does the power of the State reach into the heart of the liberty protected by the Due Process Clause. . . .

. . . Before viability, *Roe* and subsequent cases treat all governmental attempts to influence a woman's decision on behalf of the potential life within her as unwarranted. This treatment is, in our judgment, incompatible with the recognition that there is a substantial state interest in potential life throughout pregnancy.

The very notion that the State has a substantial interest in potential life leads to the conclusion that not all regulations must be deemed unwarranted. Not all burdens on the right to decide whether to terminate a pregnancy will be undue. In our view, the undue burden standard is the appropriate means of reconciling the State's interest with the woman's constitutionally protected liberty. . . .

. . . We give this summary:

(a) To protect the central right recognized by *Roe* v. *Wade* while at the same time accommodating the State's profound interest in potential life, we will employ the undue burden analysis as explained in this opinion. An undue burden exists, and therefore a provision of law is invalid, if its purpose or effect is to place a substantial obstacle in the path of a woman seeking an abortion before the fetus attains viability.

(b) We reject the rigid trimester framework of *Roe* v. *Wade*. To promote the State's profound interest in potential life, throughout pregnancy the State may take measures to ensure that the woman's choice is informed, and measures designed to advance this interest will not be invalidated as long as their purpose is to persuade the woman to choose childbirth over abortion. These measures must not be an undue burden on the right.

(c) As with any medical procedure, the State may enact regulations to further the health or safety of a woman seeking an abortion. Unnecessary health regulations that have the purpose or effect of presenting a substantial obstacle to a woman seeking an abortion impose an undue burden on the right.

(d) Our adoption of the undue burden analysis

does not disturb the central holding of *Roe* v. *Wade,* and we reaffirm that holding. Regardless of whether exceptions are made for particular circumstances, a State may not prohibit any woman from making the ultimate decision to terminate her pregnancy before viability.

(e) We also reaffirm *Roe*'s holding that "subsequent to viability, the State in promoting its interest in the potentiality of human life may, if it chooses, regulate, and even proscribe, abortion except where it is necessary, in appropriate medical judgment, for the preservation of the life or health of the mother."

These principles control our assessment of the Pennsylvania statute, and we now turn to the issue of the validity of its challenged provisions.

V

The Court of Appeals applied what it believed to be the undue burden standard and upheld each of the provisions except for the husband notification requirement. We agree generally with this conclusion, but refine the undue burden analysis in accordance with the principles articulated above. We now consider the separate statutory sections at issue.

[A]

We [now] consider the informed consent requirement. §3205. Except in a medical emergency, the statute requires that at least 24 hours before performing an abortion a physician inform the woman of the nature of the procedure, the health risks of the abortion and of childbirth, and the "probable gestational age of the unborn child." The physician or a qualified nonphysician must inform the woman of the availability of printed materials published by the State describing the fetus and providing information about medical assistance for childbirth, information about child support from the father, and a list of agencies which provide adoption and other services as alternatives to abortion. An abortion may not be performed unless the woman certifies in writing that she has been informed of the availability of these printed materials and has been provided them if she chooses to view them.

Our prior decisions establish that as with any medical procedure, the State may require a woman to give her written informed consent to an abortion. . . .

In *Akron* v. *Akron Center for Reproductive Health, Inc.* (1983) *(Akron I),* we invalidated an ordinance which required that a woman seeking an abortion be provided by her physician with specific information "designed to influence the woman's informed choice between abortion or childbirth." As we later described the *Akron I* holding in *Thornburgh* v. *American College of Obstetricians and Gynecologists* (1986), there were two purported flaws in the Akron ordinance: the information was designed to dissuade the woman from having an abortion and the ordinance imposed "a rigid requirement that a specific body of information be given in all cases, irrespective of the particular needs of the patient. . . ."

. . . It cannot be questioned that psychological well-being is a facet of health. Nor can it be doubted that most women considering an abortion would deem the impact on the fetus relevant, if not dispositive, to the decision. In attempting to ensure that a woman apprehend the full consequences of her decision, the State furthers the legitimate purpose of reducing the risk that a woman may elect an abortion, only to discover later, with devastating psychological consequences, that her decision was not fully informed. If the information the State requires to be made available to the woman is truthful and not misleading, the requirement may be permissible.

We also see no reason why the State may not require doctors to inform a woman seeking an abortion of the availability of materials relating to the consequences to the fetus, even when those consequences have no direct relation to her health. An example illustrates the point. We would think it constitutional for the State to require that in order for there to be informed consent to a kidney transplant operation the recipient must be supplied with information about risks to the donor as well as risks to himself or herself. A requirement that the physician make available information similar to that mandated by the statute here was described in *Thornburgh* as "an outright attempt to wedge the Commonwealth's message discouraging abortion into the privacy of the informed-consent dialogue between the woman and her physician." We conclude, however, that informed choice need not be defined in such narrow terms that all considerations of the effect on the fetus are made irrelevant. As we have made clear, we depart from the holdings of *Akron I* and *Thornburgh* to the extent that we permit a State to further its legitimate goal of protecting the life of the unborn by enacting legislation aimed at ensuring a decision that is mature and informed, even when in so doing the State expresses a preference for childbirth over abortion. In short, requiring that the woman be informed of the availability of information relating to fetal development and the assistance available should she decide to carry the pregnancy to full term is a reasonable measure to insure an informed choice, one which might cause the woman to choose childbirth over abortion. This requirement cannot be considered a substantial obstacle to obtaining an abortion, and, it follows, there is no undue burden. . . .

The Pennsylvania statute also requires us to reconsider the holding in *Akron I* that the State may not require that a physician, as opposed to a qualified assistant, provide information relevant to a woman's informed consent. Since there is no evidence on this record that requiring a doctor to give the information as provided by the statute would amount in practical terms to a substantial obstacle to a woman seeking an abortion, we conclude that it is not an undue burden. . . .

Our analysis of Pennsylvania's 24-hour waiting period between the provision of the information deemed necessary to informed consent and the performance of an abortion under the undue burden standard requires us to reconsider the premise behind the decision in *Akron I* invalidating a parallel requirement. In *Akron I* we said: "Nor are we convinced that the State's legitimate concern that the woman's decision be informed is reasonably served by requiring a 24-hour delay as a matter of course." We consider that conclusion to be wrong. The idea that important decisions will be more informed and deliberate if they follow some period of reflection does not strike us as unreasonable, particularly where the statute directs that important information become part of the background of the decision. The statute, as construed by the Court of Appeals, permits avoidance of the waiting period in the event of a medical emergency and the record evidence shows that in the vast majority of cases, a 24-hour delay does not create any appreciable health risk. In theory, at least, the waiting period is a reasonable measure to implement the State's interest in protecting the life of the unborn, a measure that does not amount to an undue burden.

Whether the mandatory 24-hour waiting period is nonetheless invalid because in practice it is a substantial obstacle to a woman's choice to terminate her pregnancy is a closer question. The findings of fact by the District Court indicate that because of the distances many women must travel to reach an abortion provider, the practical effect will often be a delay of much more than a day because the waiting period requires that a woman seeking an abortion make at least two visits to the doctor. The District Court also found that in many

instances this will increase the exposure of women seeking abortions to "the harassment and hostility of anti-abortion protestors demonstrating outside a clinic." As a result, the District Court found that for those women who have the fewest financial resources, those who must travel long distances, and those who have difficulty explaining their whereabouts to husbands, employers, or others, the 24-hour waiting period will be "particularly burdensome."

These findings are troubling in some respects, but they do not demonstrate that the waiting period constitutes an undue burden. . . .

[B]

Section 3209 of Pennsylvania's abortion law provides, except in cases of medical emergency, that no physician shall perform an abortion on a married woman without receiving a signed statement from the woman that she has notified her spouse that she is about to undergo an abortion. The woman has the option of providing an alternative signed statement certifying that her husband is not the man who impregnated her; that her husband could not be located; that the pregnancy is the result of spousal sexual assault which she has reported; or that the woman believes that notifying her husband will cause him or someone else to inflict bodily injury upon her. A physician who performs an abortion on a married woman without receiving the appropriate signed statement will have his or her license revoked, and is liable to the husband for damages. . . .

. . . In well-functioning marriages, spouses discuss important intimate decisions such as whether to bear a child. But there are millions of women in this country who are the victims of regular physical and psychological abuse at the hands of their husbands. Should these women become pregnant, they may have very good reasons for not wishing to inform their husbands of their decision to obtain an abortion. Many may have justifiable fears of physical abuse, but may be no less fearful of the consequences of reporting prior abuse to the Commonwealth of Pennsylvania. Many may have a reasonable fear that notifying their husbands will provoke further instances of child abuse; these women are not exempt from §3209's notification requirement. Many may fear devastating forms of psychological abuse from their husbands, including verbal harassment, threats of future violence, the destruction of possessions, physical confinement to the home, the withdrawal of financial support, or the disclosure of the abortion to family and friends. These methods of psychological abuse may act as even more of a deterrent to notification than the possibility of physical violence, but women who are the victims of the abuse are not exempt from §3209's notification requirement. And many women who are pregnant as a result of sexual assaults by their husbands will be unable to avail themselves of the exception for spousal sexual assault, because the exception requires that the woman have notified law enforcement authorities within 90 days of the assault, and her husband will be notified of her report once an investigation begins. If anything in this field is certain, it is that victims of spousal sexual assault are extremely reluctant to report the abuse to the government; hence, a great many spousal rape victims will not be exempt from the notification requirement imposed by §3209.

The spousal notification requirement is thus likely to prevent a significant number of women from obtaining an abortion. It does not merely make abortions a little more difficult or expensive to obtain; for many women, it will impose a substantial obstacle. We must not blind ourselves to the fact that the significant number of women who fear for their safety and the safety of their children are likely to be deterred from procuring

an abortion as surely as if the Commonwealth had outlawed abortion in all cases. . . .

[C]

We next consider the parental consent provision. Except in a medical emergency, an unemancipated young woman under 18 may not obtain an abortion unless she and one of her parents (or guardian) provides informed consent as defined above. If neither a parent nor a guardian provides consent, a court may authorize the performance of an abortion upon a determination that the young woman is mature and capable of giving informed consent and has in fact given her informed consent, or that an abortion would be in her best interests.

We have been over most of this ground before. Our cases establish, and we reaffirm today, that a State may require a minor seeking an abortion to obtain the consent of a parent or guardian, provided that there is an adequate judicial bypass procedure. Under these precedents, in our view, the one-parent consent requirement and judicial bypass procedure are constitutional. . . .

Maternal-Fetal Conflicts

Moral Obligations to the Not-Yet Born: The Fetus as Patient
Thomas H. Murray

Thomas H. Murray is professor and director, Center for Biomedical Ethics, Case Western Reserve University. He is the coeditor of *Feeling Good and Doing Better: Ethics and Nontherapeutic Drug Use* (1984) and *Which Babies Shall Live?* (1985). His published articles include "The Poisoned Gift: AIDS and Blood" and "Genetics and the Moral Mission of Health Insurance."

Murray distinguishes between fetuses who will be aborted and fetuses who will be brought to live birth. He calls the latter "not-yet-born" children and argues that we have moral obligations to them. In his view, even if it is morally permissible to abort a fetus prior to viability, it does not follow that it is permissible to harm a not-yet-born child prior to viability; the timing of harm is morally irrelevant. In exploring the scope and magnitude of a woman's obligation to avoid harming a not-yet-born child, Murray warns against losing track of the overall moral context of a woman's life. In typical cases, he argues, a woman's duty to avoid harming her not-yet-born child must be balanced against a multitude of other moral considerations. Murray also provides a brief analysis of an obstetrician's duty to ensure that the fetus-patient is being protected. With regard to public policy, he maintains that "the

Reprinted with permission of the author and the publisher from *Clinics in Perinatology,* vol. 14 (June 1987), pp. 329–343.

state must be very cautious in using its power to enforce particular notions of maternal duties."

The health of the not-yet-born child—the fetus intended to be brought to live birth—periodically emerges as a subject of concern. From dramatic interventions such as fetal surgery through drugs and special diets on to efforts to get pregnant women to abstain from alcohol and tobacco or to bar them from workplaces possibly toxic to developing fetuses, there has been a recent surge of ideas on how to prevent, ameliorate, or remedy damage to the not-yet-born.

Many things might be done *with,* *by* or *to* a pregnant woman to benefit her not-yet-born child. They range from the most physically intrusive to the least, from the most technologically sophisticated to mundane efforts at education and persuasion, from those with clearly established benefit to the fetus to those of highly uncertain benefit. The ethical issues raised by interventions of all kinds designed to aid a fetus share essential features. Once some form of fetal surgery becomes established, the case of a woman who refuses it will raise many of the same moral questions as that of a woman whose alcoholism threatens her fetus's health to a point where incarceration or institutionalization are being considered. Although different in several respects, both of the cases require asking how far the state—and physicians as agents of the state—ought to go in coercively intervening in the life of a woman in order to benefit her fetus. And both presume at least a tentative answer to a difficult ethical question: What is the moral status of a fetus?

To answer such a question sensibly and with a modicum of wisdom is our ultimate goal. A burgeoning literature on fetal therapies, fetal surgery, fetal rights, and maternal-fetal conflicts has enlivened the argument. While technologically sophisticated interventions like fetal surgery are receiving the most attention, they will probably be relevant to only a minute proportion of all pregnancies. Yet most of the ethical questions raised by fetal surgery are equally pertinent to a host of other, less glamorous means to the same end. Some sample questions include the following:

How far should we go in getting diabetic women to manage their disease during pregnancy? Should we inform them of the consequences to their fetus? Should we try to persuade them gently? Browbeat them? If they refuse to cooperate should we initiate civil or criminal proceedings to try and coerce them? Should we try to institutionalize them as has been done in some cases of drug addicted mothers, and then perhaps strip them of their children once they are born?

What about a mother suspected of using drugs—legal or illegal—that might deleteriously affect the fetus? What of the mother who smokes or drinks? How hard do we try to discourage her smoking or drinking during pregnancy? If she continues to do either or both heavily, at what point if any do we move beyond persuasion to coercion?

If we think that low levels of a potentially embryotoxic or fetotoxic substance are present in a workplace, should all pregnant women be kept out? What about "potentially pregnant," that is, nonsterile women? Many United States companies have "Fetal Protection Policies" that do just that.[25]

KEY ISSUES

Given the present, chaotic state of the debate over fundamental issues of ethics, law, and public policy regarding the fetus, offering simple answers to questions such as the ones just asked would require ignoring even more important questions. It is more valuable in the long run to clarify some of the fundamental issues now. Five are discussed in this article.

1. Whether there are any moral duties to a fetus.

2. Whether viability affects those duties.

3. How the concept of duties to a fetus is frequently misused.

4. What pitfalls must be avoided in moving from moral judgments to public policy.

5. The importance of the social and historical context of the current debate.

DO WE HAVE MORAL DUTIES TO A FETUS?

The moral status of those fetuses who will never be born alive is problematic. Right-to-life advocates claim that even the fertilized ovum is a person, entitled to all the protections and respect due every person. Many other people, including many of those with qualms about abortion, believe that the fetus, especially in its early stages of development, has a lesser moral stature than adults, infants, or even late-term fetuses. No consensus exists on such fetuses. Fortunately, we can discuss the fetus as patient without becoming bogged down in the mire of the abortion debate. All we need is a simple distinction between those fetuses destined to be brought to live birth, and those who will not know extrauterine life.

The Not-Yet-Born Child

The situation is quite different for fetuses who will be born alive. A few theorists argue that the fetus, or even the infant and young child, has no moral status, or else an inferior one.[24] Some writers, while not directly addressing the question, argue that whatever moral claims the fetus might have are always secondary to those of the woman in whose body the fetus lies.[2] Nonetheless, there is good reason to believe that we have moral obligations to the fetus destined to be born, who we will call the not-yet-born child to distinguish it from both the already-born child and from the fetus who will not be born alive. Further, this view has considerable popular support, as evidenced by the efforts aimed at preserving fetal health through antenatal medical care, public health education of pregnant women, and the like.

The Timing of a Harm Is Irrelevant

Imagine two different cases. In the first, a man assaults a woman with the intention of inflicting grave harm on her fetus. He succeeds, causing permanent, irreparable—but not fatal—damage to the fetus's spinal cord, resulting in paralysis. In the second case, all the circumstances are identical, except that the man attacks an infant rather than a fetus, with the same result—permanent, irreparable paralysis. Was the first act any less wrong than the second? In both cases, lifelong harm was done to humans who, whatever your beliefs about when personhood begins, would eventually cross that line and attain full moral status.

My thesis, in short, is that the timing of a harm, in itself, is not morally relevant. An act resulting in harm to a not-yet-born person (who will eventually be a full-fledged person according to everyone's moral theory) is as great a harm as if it were done later. The morally relevant factors are the usual ones: the actor's intentions; excuses; mitigating circumstances, and so on. In practice, a fetus is rarely harmed intentionally; typically, harm to a fetus occurs as a result of intentional or unintentional harm to its mother. The lack of intention to harm then is what affects our judgment about the wrongness of the act, and not the fact that it was a not-yet-born person who was harmed. We would judge unintended harm to a child or adult in a similar manner. The debate over the ethics of abortion aside, then, we can talk sensibly and without inherent contradiction about moral duties to the fetus destined to become a person—to the not-yet-born person. There will be duties to avoid harm, and there may be duties to render aid.

We can discuss moral duties to not-yet-born persons without becoming hopelessly trapped in the abortion debate. Before moving on to discuss the scope of our duties to the fetus, we need to consider whether viability affects these duties.

THE MORAL RELEVANCE OF VIABILITY

Viability is, at best, a slippery concept. For one thing it is a moving front. As our ability to save younger and smaller newborns improves, the so-called age of viability is reached earlier. Physicians frequently use viability as a statistical concept: the age at which some unspecified percentage of newborns will survive. Sometimes the concept is used with reference to specific infants. We could describe survival possibilities as a probabilistic function of weight or gestational age. For example, the BW or GA 10 would be the birthweight or gestational age at which 10 per cent of infants survive. The GA 50 would be the level at which 50 per cent live, and so on. These numbers would change as our ability to save these infants changes.

Viability and Abortion

The central question is whether our moral obligations to the fetus change as a function of viability. Viability as a determinant of our duties to a fetus was given great importance by its inclusion in the well-known Supreme Court abortion decision, *Roe v. Wade*.[19] The complex ruling says in its summary: "For the stage subsequent to viability, the State in promoting its interest in the potentiality of human life may, if it chooses, regulate, and even proscribe, abortion except where it is necessary, in appropriate medical judgment, for the preservation of the life or health of the mother."[19]

Viability serves as a threshhold in *Roe v. Wade.* Even though the Court uses the ambiguous phrase "potentiality of human life," behind their decision must lie some notion of the fetus growing in legal and presumably moral stature as it approaches term. Otherwise, there would be no justification for linking the State's interest in protecting that potential life with viability which, at the time of that decision (1973), roughly coincided with the end of the second trimester for most fetuses.

Attempting to uncover the moral reasoning underlying a legal decision can be perilous because one may simply be wrong and because it may encourage the unfortunate tendency to see moral disapproval as a sufficient reason for taking legal action, something we will take up later. Bearing that caution in mind, we nonetheless must try to determine what moral ideas underlie the legal reasoning in *Roe v. Wade.* The court appears to believe that, prior to viability, whatever claim the fetus may have not to be killed is outweighed by a woman's right to choose whether or not to bear and give birth to a child, with all that those activities bring in their wake. After viability, the fetus's increasing nearness to actual rather than merely potential life strengthens its moral claim against being killed to the point where it overrides the mother's right to choose not to bear a child, though not so far as to force her to risk her own life in doing so.

Viability Is Irrelevant for Nonfatal Harms

In other words, for the problem of deciding whether a woman can abort her fetus, it may be important to know what the fetus's moral status is *at that particular moment:* whether or not it is a person or how close it is to becoming a full-fledged person may be important in this context. In stark contrast, the fetus's moral standing at that moment in its development is not relevant to judging our duties to avoid or avert nonfatal harms, since, as far as we know, the fetus will some day be a full person, and the timing of such nonlethal harms is not pertinent to determining their wrongfulness. Interestingly, the law itself seems to agree.

Until 1946, a child injured prenatally then born alive but impaired rarely found a court willing to sustain a suit for damages. But in that year began what Prosser, who wrote the standard reference work on tort law, called "the most spectacular abrupt reversal of a well settled rule in the whole history of the law of torts. The child, provided that he is born alive, is permitted to maintain an action for the consequences of prenatal injuries, and if he dies of such injuries after birth an action will lie for his wrongful death."[16] Prosser believed that the earlier denials of claims on behalf of children injured while they were still fetuses were based on invalid reasoning, and he approved of the reversal.

With the concept of prenatal injuries established as a valid one, does it matter whether the fetus was viable at the time of injury? Some courts have required that the fetus have been viable, or at least "quickened" at the time of injury.[16] But many courts have rejected viability as a relevant factor in determining whether the born child may recover for prenatal injury.[9] One critic of the concept of fetal rights says pointedly: "[V]iability is a meaningless distinction in the fetal rights context because the state's interest in the health of its future citizens is equally strong throughout pregnancy."[8] Prosser himself says: "[c]ertainly the [previable] infant may be no less injured; and all logic is in favor of ignoring the stage at which it occurs." Acknowledging that proving injury early in pregnancy might be difficult, he concludes "[t]his, however, goes to proof rather than principle; and if, as is undoubtedly the case there are injuries as to which reliable medical proof is possible, it makes no sense to deny recovery on any such arbitrary basis."[16] The moral principle, that is, does not depend on the arbitrary criterion of viability.

While most cases have focused on recovering damages for harms already done, a number of recent cases attempt to prevent harm by affecting the pregnant woman's behavior, even to the point of outright coercion. . . . [F]orced caesarean cases . . . are one sort of example.[23] In another case (reported by a newspaper) a physician accused a woman, seven months pregnant, of endangering her fetus's development by abusing drugs. The woman was ordered to enter a drug rehabilitation program and undergo regular urinalyses until the child was born.[21] Whether this is a reasonable response to the problem is the subject of the next section.

MISUSING THE IDEA OF DUTIES TO A FETUS

A recurrent theme in this essay is the danger of making moral judgments or public policy without sufficient regard for context. Just this sort of misuse of the concept of duties to a fetus occurs with unsettling frequency.

The Dangers of Oversimplifying Moral Decisions

The moral world we inhabit is one marked by a multiplicity of interests and duties. We are certainly entitled to give good moral weight to our own interests. Then there are duties to those with whom we have special relationships, relationships that prescribe even strenuous moral duties in certain domains. Finally, we have duties to "strangers"—those with whom no special moral relationship exists. Most significant moral decisions have implications for many of these interests and relationships simultaneously. For example, a woman who must decide whether to place her fetus at risk of harm by working in a factory with low levels of a suspected fetotoxin must weigh her own interests in having a job with the psychological and material benefits that may bring against the risks imposed on herself as well as her fetus. She must also consider possible benefits to her fetus that the job makes possible, such as improved nutrition for herself and prenatal care facilitated by health insurance. Then there may be others dependent on her working: a spouse, other children, perhaps elderly parents. When we portray the ethical dimensions of her decision as beginning and ending with the question of whether or not she has duties to avoid exposing her fetus to risks, we rip such a complex decision out of its moral, as well as its social and political, context. Yet, this is commonly done. Or, not much better, the woman's "right" to do whatever she desires is counterposed to the fetus's right to protection from harm. Once the problem is framed this way, giving a nuanced answer becomes impossible. A more complex view of the moral life, one that encompasses a multiplicity of legitimate moral concerns, of interests and duties, of roles and relationships, allows us to frame the question in a way that can be answered, if not more easily, at least more satisfactorily.

Warnings of Fearful Consequences

In a clash of rights, complex issues can become stripped of their nuances and turned into simplistic all-or-none contests. On either extreme, we can imagine bleak consequences. If, on the one hand, we give pre-eminence to the fetus's right to avoid being harmed, then must pregnant women structure every detail of their lives in order to avoid all suspected risks to their not-yet-born child? Such an attitude appears to have influenced some companies to adopt so-called "Fetal Protection Policies," or FPPs, that deny employment opportunities to women.[25] Fears of what would happen should fetal rights gain the upper hand generate a litany of nightmarish possibilities:

> A woman could be held civilly or criminally liable for fetal injuries caused by accidents resulting from maternal negligence, such as automobile or household accidents. She could also be held liable for any behavior during her pregnancy having potentially adverse effects on her fetus, including failure to eat properly, using prescription, nonprescription and illegal drugs, smoking, drinking alcohol, exposing herself to infectious disease or to any workplace hazards, engaging in immoderate exercise or sexual intercourse, residing at high altitudes for prolonged periods, or using a general anesthetic or drugs to induce rapid labor during delivery. If the current trend in fetal rights continues, pregnant women would live in constant fear that any accident or "error" in judgment could be deemed "unacceptable" and become the basis for a criminal prosecution by the state or a civil suit . . .[8]

On the other hand, if we give full sway to the woman's right to control her body, can we even level moral criticism against a case such as the one of a woman who at 40 weeks gestation, in labor with abruptio placenta with fetal distress, refused a caesarean section? After the infant was delivered stillborn, she explained to a nurse that "the death of the fetus solved complicated personal problems."[12] The language of rights in conflict may not permit us to give full and weighty consideration to a host of factors that we believe are important in making moral judgments. Examining relationships, legitimate interests, and duties may give us a more adequate picture of the moral choices people face.

Obligations to the Not-Yet-Born Are Not All or None

Take, for example, the case of the woman who must decide whether to accept a job that might pose some risk to her fetus. Let us suppose that she intends to bring the child to birth, so we do not have to worry about the ethics of abortion. As far as we know, this is a not-yet-born child; therefore the woman has some obligation to avoid harming it while it is still a fetus. What is the scope and intensity of this obligation? Must she refuse the job?

Because of the link between most discussions of the fetus's moral status and abortion, there is an unfortunate tendency to think of our obligations to the fetus as all-or-none. But there are other creatures dependent on us, to whom we have obligations, but where those duties do not unequivocally overwhelm all other considerations—our children for example. We certainly have a duty to do what is reasonable to protect our young children from harm. That requires keeping them from known and probable dangers. But we are not required to sacrifice everything else to this task. We should teach them not to play in busy streets, and offer them a protected play-area. But must we build crash-proof barriers around their playground, strong enough to stop a cement truck run wild? Obviously not. That would be beyond "reasonable" responsibility. Anytime we take them in a car, there is a risk of injury or death. Responsible parents should provide a secure carseat for their infant or toddler. But we are not forbidden from going for a drive, even though no matter how carefully we drive there is always the distinct possibility of an accident.

What is it that makes certain risks reasonable, and others the kind that responsible parents would not take? The probability of harm and its severity should it occur are certainly relevant. Also significant is the importance of the purpose for which the risk is run and the avoidability of the risk. If we want the children to see their grandparents, a long car ride may be unavoidable. And exposing our child to the considerable risks of cytotoxic drugs is clearly justifiable if and only if our purpose is to treat them for cancer.

My purpose here is to put us on more familiar ground than the exotic situations in which questions of fetal status typically arise. Two points come out of the discussion. First, whatever moral duties we might have to a fetus—a not-yet-born child—they may equal but not exceed our duties to already-born children. The circumstances of a fetus's physical enclosure within and link to its mother's body confuses many discussions. This linkage may mean that a broader range of actions might affect the fetus, and the facts of the case will be accordingly affected. But the same moral considerations apply equally to both the not-yet-born and the already-born—considerations such as intentions, probability and severity of risk, and duties to others. Second, duties to the not-yet-born, like duties to the already-born, are usually just one of many factors to be considered in judging the moral acceptability of an act.

Another advantage of discussing our obligations to the not-yet-born and already-born together is that it enables us to talk about fathers and not just mothers. To the extent that cultural blinders distort our view of a mother's responsibility to her fetus, then looking at a case with comparable morally relevant features, but one that asks about a father's responsibility to his child, may restore some moral clarity.

A Father-Child Analogy

Take the plausible case of a man who lost his job in the oil fields of west Texas. He has two children counting on him for support; his wife is also out of work. An offer comes of a job in a petrochemical plant near Houston. Taking that job will mean moving his family to a part of Texas crawling with petrochemical complexes where toxic releases into the air, ground, and water are not unknown, and where the risk of cancer is somewhat, though not drastically, higher than in their current community. There are a number of good reasons to take the job. He will be able to afford better food, clothing, and housing for his family and himself. Being unemployed threatens his sense of self-worth, which depresses him and incidentally also makes him a less thoughtful parent and spouse. Like most unemployed Americans, when he lost his job he also lost his health insurance; the new job will assure better access to health care for himself and his family. Perhaps the schools are better in the new community. Suppose he accepts the job even though he knows and regrets the increased risk that will mean for his children. Decisions such as this are all-things-considered choices: by their nature they involve weighing and balancing many things. Would we say that this man's choice was immoral? That he should not have exposed his children to the slightly increased risk of cancer whatever else was involved? It would make better sense to say that he made a responsible, morally defensible decision, even if we share his regret about the increased risk to which his children as well as his wife and himself will be exposed.

How was this man's decision any different from that of a woman who chooses to accept a job, knowing that her fetus will be exposed to some low but nonetheless increased risk of harm because of exposures there? Perhaps she too is without health insurance. Perhaps having a job is important to her sense of self-worth. Perhaps there are other children and a spouse at home who are dependent on her. The fact that she carries a fetus within her, a not-yet-born child, that she has moral duties to protect that fetus from harm, and that the workplace increases slightly the probability of harm does not make her decision immoral. Exactly the same considerations were relevant to the man's decision. To the

extent that the morally relevant factors are comparable—and in this case they might well be identical—the
decisions are equally justified. And if the circumstances
vary, at least we know the kinds of morally significant
considerations that will influence our judgments.[15]
Whether it is a man or a woman is not relevant. Nor, I
have argued, does it matter whether it is a not-yet-born
or already-born child.

FROM ETHICAL JUDGMENTS TO PUBLIC POLICY

We do not ban all conduct we regard as morally suspect, nor do we compel people to carry out every moral
duty. Many things are left to personal conscience, to
moral suasion, or to social pressure. For good reasons,
including moral ones, we are reluctant to allow the state
to force its view of correct conduct on individuals unless
the harm to be avoided is grave, especially when doing
so requires coercion, bodily invasion, or incarceration.
These means are among the most repugnant and are
reserved for extreme circumstances. If we conclude then
that a woman morally ought to quit smoking during
pregnancy, moderate or eliminate her consumption of
alcohol, and do likewise with caffeine, this does not
automatically justify heavy-handed state intervention to
assure that she does these things. Some wrongs are minimally so. The state should not exercise its often great
power on such things. Sometimes the effort to correct a
wrong itself creates new moral problems. The moral
and other costs of enforcement may outweigh the good
that might be done.

The fetus becomes a "patient" when its welfare
becomes the physician's concern. The obstetrician caring for a mother and not-yet-born child has two
patients. In much the way that a pediatrician advises
parents about their newborn's diet, monitors the infant's
health, and prescribes needed medication or other therapeutic interventions, an obstetrician routinely does the
same for the mother and the fetus-patient. How extensive is the obstetrician's duty to assure that the fetus-
patient's welfare is being protected?

The "Child-as-Maximum" Principle

One useful guideline might be called the "child-as-maximum" principle. The principle says that our obligations
to ensure the fetus's welfare can equal but not exceed
our obligations to a born child. If a pediatrician would

not be obliged to do more than try to persuade parents
to do a certain thing—say observe a special diet—then
under conditions of comparable burdens and benefits,
obstetricians cannot be obliged to do more to protect a
fetus, although they may be required to do less.

One inescapable difference between the obstetrician's and the pediatrician's case is of course that the
former's second patient, the fetus, is encased in the
body of the first patient, the mother. All interventions
directed at the fetus literally must go through its mother.
The burdens created, therefore, generally will be much
greater, as will be the potential for morally wronging one
person in the effort to aid another. This is why the
child-as-maximum principle emphasizes that our duties
to a born child constitute an upper-bound for our duties
to a not-yet-born child rather than a strict equivalence.
A drug that might benefit a fetus but that will be harmful to the mother can be refused. That same drug for
that same being, now born, should probably be administered. The pediatrician in the latter instance is justified in pushing harder for consent from the parents than
was the obstetrician.

A Variety of Needs, a Range of Interventions

One study shows that women who smoke a pack of cigarettes or more a day have babies on average about 180
gm smaller at birth than women who do not smoke.
The same study found that women who drank twenty
or more beers per month sacrificed roughly 100 gm of
birthweight, while those who consumed 300 or more
grams of caffeine daily (three or four cups of coffee or
seven cola beverages) had babies 40 to 50 gm smaller
on average.[11] What should physicians do? When the
risks are small, we usually employ education and persuasion. That is the typical and appropriate response to
maternal smoking, diet, nutritional supplements, and
the like. These anchor one end of a continuum of possible "interventions." We can move to stronger measures,
such as New York City has done, by requiring that signs
be posted in public places serving alcohol warning pregnant women that alcohol may endanger their fetus's
health. This is a public policy that relies as much on
shame as on the educative effect of the signs.

Beyond this is a broad range of more traditionally
"medical" interventions: managing maternal diabetes in
pregnancy[4]; placing women with PKU on low-phenylalanine diets when they wish to become pregnant[18];
treating fetal methylmelonic acidemia by giving Vitamin
B-12 to the mother[20]; treating congenital hypothy-

roidism by injections into the amniotic fluid[26]; drug therapy for fetal ventricular tachycardia,[10] and other possibilities.

There are surgical routes as well. In addition to the familiar exchange transfusions for erythroblastosis fetalis, a variety of still-experimental fetal surgeries are under development. They include procedures responding to urinary tract obstruction,[5] ventriculomegaly,[1] diaphragmatic hernia,[7] and hematopoietic stem cell transplantation for severe immunologic deficiencies.[22] (The law and ethics of fetal surgery have been amply discussed elsewhere.[3, 14, 17])

Our ethical analysis of any proposed interventions to benefit a fetus intended to be brought to birth should include at least the following considerations:

1. How certain is the benefit to the fetus? (Is the intervention experimental? Is it well-established? Does it carry substantial risks to the fetus?)

2. How great are the benefits? (Will a successful intervention make a large or small difference in the fetus's prognosis?)

3. How intrusive, coercive, or harmful will it be to the mother?

4. Will anything be lost or gained by waiting until after the child is born?

Even if we are convinced that the mother has a moral responsibility to agree to the intervention, the question of how far we should go in attempting to persuade or coerce her raises an entirely new set of issues at the intersection of ethics and public policy. Once we move to the level of policy, political and historical considerations become very important. At this point, a brief look at another era's concern for the health of the not-yet-born is appropriate.

ALCOHOL AND "RACE-DECAY" IN EDWARDIAN ENGLAND

This is not the first time that parental behavior has been held responsible for harm to the not-yet-born or the already-born. The oldest prenatal health advice of which I am aware is in the Old Testament. In Judges 13:7 the mother of Samson is told "Behold, thou shalt conceive and bear a son: and drink no wine or strong drink."

Many women today are fearful and suspicious of the movement towards ascribing moral status to the fetus. For women who aspire to compete in the economic marketplace on an equal footing with men, those fears and suspicions have substantial historical validity. Past social movements to protect helpless infants and not-yet-born children have had something less than pure and altruistic motives. One illuminating example comes from England at the turn of the century—the Edwardian era.

In the first decade of this century, England found itself losing its empire abroad and awash with immigrants at home: immigrants, moreover, whose children were more likely to survive infancy than their British neighbors. A number of laypeople and physicians believed they understood the problem—alcohol. A campaign to arouse public ire against parents who drank flourished in the first decade of the 1900s. While it was directed largely against women who drank, men came in for their share of the blame as well. Indeed, one highly influential Swiss study reported that 78 per cent of women unable to breastfeed had fathers who drank heavily. But for the most part, women were faulted.

In 1906, a British physician wrote:

Undoubtedly much of the high infant mortality is due to alcoholism, and conditions directly . . . or indirectly arising from this morbid condition. The widespread prevalence of alcoholism among women, especially during the reproductive period of life, is one of the most important factors making for racial-decay.[6]

"Race-decay" is but one of many dubious reasons given for worrying about women and drink. George Sims, a prominent journalist of the time, had a related concern: "What can be the future of our Empire, if on a falling birth rate 120,000 infants continue to die annually in the first year of their lives . . . !"[6] And he knew the cause: "Bad motherhood is the first great cause of our appalling infant mortality."[6] No less an examplar of success than Andrew Carnegie, the American industrialist, pointed to the drunken worker as a central threat to British productivity.[6]

For the most part, this was a campaign waged by the upper classes, including a number of male physicians, against working class women. They were not doing their national duty by outreproducing the immigrants—Jews, Italians, Scots, and Irish. Theophilus Hyslop, a physician active in the anti-drink movement, referred to immigrants derogatorily and declared that if the British worker would give up alcohol, he could "drive the foreigner from our midst."[6]

Perhaps Dr. Robert Jones best expressed the sentiment feared by contemporary women: "Women are now the companions of men in . . . industrial pursuits, and the freedom to work on equal terms with men has caused . . . the same depressing physical and mental influences . . . , for which stimulants offer a temporary relief."[6] Women, that is, as vessels of reproduction, as the assurers of racial integrity, as the saviors of the empire, as the protectors of the innocent must be made to look after their offspring, and not be contaminated in the labor marketplace.

Many women understand any contemporary movement emphasizing their biologic role as bearers of children to be a threat to their economic liberty and equality—"fetal rights" being no exception. The need to control reproduction so that they could compete in the job market emerged as a major theme among pro-choice activists in Kristin Luker's study of anti- and pro-abortion activists. Conversely, having and raising children were crucial sources of self-value for many who worked against abortion.[13] Because it focuses attention on women's reproductive capacities, it is not surprising that the trend toward regarding the fetus as a patient has evoked concern and controversy. And with the long history of efforts to keep women in roles defined by and in the interests of men, it is no less surprising that women regard the current trend with suspicion. Legitimate concerns for fetal rights can also be carried along by other, questionable, motives and may carry with them other destructive social consequences.

CONCLUSIONS

Five points emerge from this analysis. First, we can discuss moral duties to the fetus destined to be born—to the not-yet-born child—without logical contradiction and without becoming hopelessly mired in debate over abortion.

Second, whether the fetus is viable may be regarded as morally significant in the context of abortion decisions, but it is not directly relevant to our duties to not-yet-born children. This is so because of the irrelevance of the timing of a harm.

Third, that we do have moral duties to fetuses, viable and previable alike, may not have the horrendous consequences for women that is typically thought. Our common error has been to focus exclusively on a pregnant woman's duty to avoid harming her fetus, without regard for the multitude of other moral considerations she ought to include in her decision. A more complex and adequate view of the moral life understands that in such decisions a host of factors may be relevant such as promises made, the woman's own interests, her obligations to other family members, and the welfare of her not-yet-born child. Seeing the mother's moral relationship to the fetus as morally analogous to a father's relationship to his child will help avoid oversimplification.

Fourth, establishing that women have moral duties to their not-yet-born children does not justify automatically coercive public policies to force them to fulfill those obligations. Again, the analogy to fathers and children may be helpful. The state must be very cautious in using its power to enforce particular notions of maternal duties. Effective enforcement might necessitate forcible invasion of a woman's body or prolonged incarceration. These are usually "last resorts" used only under very restricted circumstances. We must be careful to assure that they are not used more casually against pregnant women.

Fifth, women have ample reason to be suspicious of the growing tendency to focus on the welfare of the fetus-as-patient and, by implication, on the woman's role as bearer of children. Historically, movements allegedly directed toward aiding fetuses and children have often been motivated as much by other, less praiseworthy concerns, including racism, and especially by men's fear of women's political, social, and economic equality.

Rather than arguing over "fetal rights," let us use the less heated language of moral obligations to not-yet-born children. We must not oversimplify complex moral decisions, especially our tendency to focus on a pregnant woman's obligations to her not-yet-born child as the *only* morally important factor in her decisions. We would not tolerate such oversimplification when discussing parents' duties toward their children, and we must not tolerate it in the difficult decisions we now face regarding the welfare of the not-yet-born. History provides forceful reminders of the dangers of thinking of women as mere "vessels of reproduction." Finally, we must continue the work of clarifying our obligations toward both the fetus destined to be born and the mother who retains her full moral individuality and interests, and in whose body that developing person exists for a time.

REFERENCES

1 Clewell WH, Meier PR, Manchester DK, et al: Ventriculomegaly: Evaluation and management. Sem Perinatol 9:98–102, 1985

2 Engelhardt HT: The Foundations of Bioethics. New York, Oxford, 1986

3 Fletcher JC: Ethical considerations in and beyond experimental fetal therapy. Sem Perinatol 9:130–135, 1985

4 Gabbe SG: Management of diabetes mellitus in pregnancy. Am J Obstet Gynecol 153:824–827, 1985

5 Golbus MS, Filly RA, Callen PW, et al: Fetal urinary tract obstruction: Management and selection for treatment. Sem Perinatol 9:91–97, 1985

6 Gutzke DW: "The cry of the children": The Edwardian medical campaign against maternal drinking. Br J Addiction 79:71–84, 1984

7 Harrison MR, Adzick NS, Nakayama DK, et al: Fetal diaphragmatic hernia: Fatal but fixable. Sem Perinatol 9:103–112, 1985

8 Johnsen DE: The creation of fetal rights: Conflicts with women's constitutional rights to liberty, privacy, and equal protection. Yale Law J 95:599–625, 1986

9 Keeton WP, Dobbs D, Keeton R, et al: Prosser and Keeton on the Law of Torts. Edition 5. Mineola, NY, West Publishing Co, 1984

10 Kleinman CS, Copel JA, Weinstein EM, et al: In utero diagnosis and treatment of fetal supraventricular tachycardia. Sem Perinatol 9:113–129, 1985

11 Kuzma JW, Sokol RJ: Maternal drinking behavior and decreased intrauterine growth. Alcohol Clin Exp Res 6:396–402, 1982

12 Leiberman JR, Mazor M, Chaim W, et al: The fetal right to live. Obstet Gynecol 53:515–517, 1979

13 Luker K: Abortion and the Politics of Motherhood. University of California, Berkeley, 1984

14 Murray TH: Ethical issues in fetal surgery. Bull Am Col Surg 70(6):6–10, 1985

15 Murray TH: Who do fetal protection policies really protect? Tech Rev 88(7):12–13, 20, 1985

16 Prosser WL: Handbook of the Law of Torts. Edition 3. St Paul, MN, West Publishing Co, 1964

17 Robertson JA: Legal issues in fetal therapy. Sem Perinatol 9:136–142, 1985

18 Robertson JA, Schulman JD: PKU women and pregnancy: The limits of reproductive autonomy. Unpublished manuscript

19 Roe v Wade. 410 U.S. 113, 1973

20 Schulman JD: Prenatal treatment of biochemical disorders. Sem Perinatol 9:75–78, 1985

21 Shaw MW: Conditional prospective rights of the fetus. J Leg Med 5:63–116, 1984

22 Simpson TJ, Golbus MS: In utero fetal hematopoietic stem cell transplantation. Sem Perinatol 9:68–74, 1985

23 Strong C: Ethical conflicts between mother and fetus in obstetrics. Clin Perinatol 14:313–327, 1987

24 Tooley M: Abortion and Infanticide. New York, Oxford University Press, 1983

25 US Congress, Office of Technology Assessment: Reproductive Health Hazards in the Workplace. US Government Printing Office: Washington, DC, 1985

26 Weiner S, Scharf JF, Bolognese PJ, et al: Antenatal diagnosis and treatment of fetal goiter. J Reprod Med 24:39–42, 1980

Blessed Are the Peacemakers: Commentary on Making Peace in Gestational Conflicts

Rosemarie Tong

Rosemarie Tong is Thatcher Professor in Medical Humanities and Philosophy at Davidson College. She is the author of *Women, Sex, and the Law* (1984), *Feminist Thought: A Comprehensive Introduction* (1989), and *Feminine and Feminist Ethics* (1993). She is also coeditor of *Feminist Philosophies: Problems, Theories, and Applications* (1992).

Tong analyzes two representative attempts to use the language of rights to deal with the problem of gestational conflicts (understood as conflicts between the interests of a pregnant

Theoretical Medicine, vol. 13 (1992), pp. 329–335. © 1992 Kluwer Academic Publishers. Reprinted by permission of Kluwer Academic Publishers.

woman and the interests of the fetus she is carrying). Ultimately, she concludes, the language of care is more appropriate than the language of rights for "making peace in gestational conflicts." (See Chapter 1 for a discussion of the ethics of care.) One of Tong's principal points is that a pregnant woman's ability to care for her fetus is largely dependent on the pregnant woman herself being cared for by the community.

In his provocative article on gestational pregnancies, James Nelson [1] invites us to answer some of the Solomonic questions involving women and fetuses that have been raised over the past fifteen years. Since these questions concern crucial issues about women's reproductive freedom, I feel compelled to comment upon the weak as well as the strong points of Nelson's analysis. So-called "interventionists" reason that if it is permissible for the State to ban or otherwise regulate a post-viability abortion, then it is also permissible for the State to monitor or otherwise control a post-viability and perhaps also a previability pregnancy. If a third- or even second-trimester fetus's right to life is sometimes sufficiently strong to trump its mother's right to bodily integrity and/or privacy, then this fact obtains whether the mother wants or does not want to carry her fetus to term. Indeed, "interventionists" sometimes argue that the State has a greater rather than lesser interest in fetal life that is destined for birth rather than extinction. As they see it, since healthy babies are simply less burdensome to the State than unhealthy babies are, it makes sense for the State to intervene in a woman's pregnancy if her actions are jeopardizing the health and/or life of the fetus.

Some United States jurisdictions have already held mothers criminally responsible for using illegal drugs—especially cocaine—during pregnancy and for subsequently giving birth to "cocaine" babies. Other jurisdictions have jailed pregnant women to force them to care for themselves properly and/or to keep them away from their drug, alcohol, and cigarette suppliers. Still other jurisdictions have forced unwilling mothers to undergo Caesarean sections because their physicians saw this invasive procedure as being in the best interests of the fetus. There has even been talk about legislation that would punish, as fetal abusers, women who drink and smoke during their pregnancies [2]. The step from such legislation to requiring a woman to do everything in her power to produce the healthiest baby possible would be a relatively small one. Women who gave birth to less than perfect babies would be liable to moral condemnation even if the district attorney decided not

to prosecute them for prenatal child negligence or abuse.

In the context of such developments, I can only agree with Nelson [1] that pregnancy is rapidly becoming a nine-month-long war between a fetus and its mother. As he sees it, within a rights paradigm, it is not only the woman who refuses a Caesarean section, or who shoots cocaine that is at war with her fetus, but the woman who fails to take her iron supplement. Similarly, whether a fetus is the source of its mother's nausea or toxemia, it is not to be trusted—encroacher that it is. But clearly this *is* the wrong way to view pregnancy. A woman would be ill-advised to get pregnant unless she were willing to give her life over to that of her fetus. All of her actions would have to be conceived and executed in terms of her fetus's ever-increasing rights, as if she had no rights of her own. The law would call pregnant women to a level of other-directedness and self-sacrifice that it has imposed on no other group in society.

But even though the language of rights is largely a discourse of conflict, it is, for many people, the mother tongue. Indeed, feminists are quite fluent in this language. We have used it to obtain the vote, to gain access to jobs and educational institutions, and to secure a modicum of reproductive freedom. Before we abandon the rhetoric of rights, then, and start speaking in a "different voice" we had best be sure that the rights paradigm is indeed unable to make peace in gestational conflicts. I suggest, therefore, that we look at two representative attempts to use "rights-talk" for the purpose of adjudicating between a mother's and a fetus's interest. The two accounts I have in mind are those of lawyers John Robertson and George Annas.

I

John Robertson [3] argues that it is reasonable to regard mothers as having a moral duty to the babies they choose to deliver. If mothers (and fathers) have moral obligations to refrain from harming their children *after* they are born, then they have these obligations to their children *before* they are born. If it is wrong to neglect or abuse a child *ex utero,* then it is wrong to neglect or abuse a child *in utero.* Whatever legal rights a woman has to abort her fetus, if she chooses not to exercise those rights, she is morally obligated not to harm her fetus *in utero.* Presumably, she is so obligated because her fetus has an interest in being born as healthy as possible. As Robertson sees it, however, the fetus's interest in health does not automatically override all of its mother's interests. He observes that:

> Ethical analysis must balance the mother's interest in freedom and bodily integrity against the offspring's interest in being born healthy. This balance will vary with the burdens of altering the mother's conduct and the risk of prenatally caused harm to offspring. Depending on the balance of risk, benefits, and burdens, prenatal conduct may be morally discretionary, advisable, prudent, or even obligatory. The evaluation depends upon the reasonableness (as viewed by reasonable persons) of avoiding the harm, in light of its severity, certainty, and the difficulty of avoiding it ([3], p. 261).

Although I am not certain exactly what moral judgement Robertson would make in a case like that of Mrs. Pamela Monson, my best guess is that he would judge her morally at fault for what happened to her child. In this case, Mrs. Monson's physician advised her not to take amphetamines. As he saw it, her drug addiction was the primary cause of her seeming disinterest in the course of her pregnancy. Appealing to the best interests of the fetus, he advised Mrs. Monson not to engage in sexual intercourse, to stay off her feet, and to go to the hospital immediately should she start to hemorrhage. Allegedly, Mrs. Monson did not follow any of her physician's advice, including his advice about the amphetamines. Her son was born with massive brain damage and died about six weeks later—arguably, the victim of "fetal neglect." Criminal charges, which were later dismissed, were brought against Mrs. Monson [4].

But even *if* the morally prudent, or even obligatory thing for Mrs. Monson to have done was to follow her physician's advice, was it good policy for the district attorney to press criminal charges against her? Robertson considers three ways to influence pregnant women's behavior: (1) education, (2) post-birth civil and criminal sanctions, and (3) pre-birth seizure. Although he thinks that education is the best way to influence preg-

nant women's behavior, he is willing to consider option (2) or even option (3) when education fails. Criminal and/or civil courts may sanction new mothers, says Robertson, if the injuries to their children prenatally "would not be tolerated if caused after birth, or if caused prenatally by third parties" ([3], p. 264). These same courts, however, should refrain from incarcerating still pregnant women or treating them against their wills unless "the intrusion or seizure is minimal in length and the harm to be prevented is certain and substantial" ([3], p. 265). Even then, concludes Robertson, these courts should think long and hard. Since uncertainty is the rule rather than the exception in medicine, Robertson's final view on pre-birth seizure is that it is better to err on the side of maternal freedom than on the side of fetal well-being.

II

In contrast to Robertson, George Annas [5] does not engage the moral issues in a case like that of Mrs. Monson. He is concerned only about the policy implications of the case. Interestingly, his main fear about "fetal neglect" statutes, for example, is the fear most feminists have; namely, that they pave the way for treating women like "fetal containers." If the state has a compelling interest in healthy fetuses, and education is unable to influence the behavior of pregnant women, then, logically, the state should favor (contra Robertson) a policy of pre-birth seizure over a policy of post-birth civil and criminal sanctions. After all, sending a woman like Mrs. Monson to jail after she gives birth to a harmed baby will not benefit it. But if the best way to maximize a fetus's well-being is to minimize its mother's freedom so that she is unable to harm it, then, asks Annas, why not confine her for nine-months to an environment in which her behavior can be effectively controlled? Annas's answer to his own question is, I think, that any such confinement would be the result of not taking a pregnant woman's rights to bodily integrity and privacy seriously enough. Specifically, he comments that:

> To have a legal rule that there are no restrictions on a woman's decision to have an abortion, but if she elects childbirth instead, then the state will require her to surrender her basic rights of bodily integrity and privacy, creates a state-erected penalty on her exercise of her right to bear a child . . . Such a penalty would (or at least should) be unconstitutional ([5], p. 14).

Fortunately, insists Annas, the state does not have to *abrogate* women's rights in order to serve the interests of the fetus. On the contrary, the best way for the state to serve the interests of the fetus may be for it to enhance women's rights "by fostering reasonable pay for the work they do and equal employment opportunities, and providing a reasonable social safety net, quality prenatal services, and day care programs" ([5], p. 14).

III

As much as I support Annas's policy recommendations, they are won primarily by minimizing *fetuses'* rights. Similarly, as much as someone else may support Robertson's policy recommendations, they are won primarily by minimizing *mothers'* rights. Apparently, Annas and Robertson resolve gestational conflicts by deciding *in advance* which of the two contending parties should win the *really* hard cases. Whereas the fetus wins in Robertson's world, the mother wins in Annas's world. What is more, as I mentioned above, Annas tells us nothing, and Robertson very little about pregnant women's *moral* obligations to their fetuses. The fact that I do not think the state should lay a hand on someone like Mrs. Monson before *or* after she delivers her harmed baby does not mean that I am prepared to morally justify or even morally excuse her conduct. Robertson tells us that such conduct is morally wrong because women who intend to carry their fetuses to term have moral obligations to their fetuses—obligations that are presumably rooted in their fetuses' interests (rights) in being born healthy. But is the best way to understand a mother's (or father's) moral obligations to her/his fetus in terms of its moral *rights?*

Like Nelson, I think the language of rights (and correlative obligations) cannot adequately motivate or guide women's (or men's) moral conduct *vis-à-vis* their fetuses (or children); and like Nelson, I am looking to the language of care (and correlative responsibilities) to "make peace" in "gestational conflicts." Unfortunately, I do not speak the language of care nearly as well as the language of rights. I find myself stuttering and stammering as I try to explain the moral wrongness of certain actions without explicitly or implicitly appealing to a notion of moral rights. Perhaps my newness to "care speak" partly explains why I had to read Nelson's article several times before it occurred to me that *partiality* has little to do with fetal-maternal conflicts. If partiality was the crucial moral concept in such cases, we would expect a moral argument on behalf of the obvious;

namely, that pregnant women are morally permitted (indeed required) to care more about their *own* fetuses than the fetuses of other mothers. But there is no need to belabor the obvious since the crucial moral concept in gestational conflicts is not partiality but another concept to which Nelson alludes; namely, *particularity*. What makes the conduct of someone like Mrs. Monson morally wrong or not depends on the "particulars" of her life—especially on her network of human relationships.

As someone who carried two baby boys to term, and who followed her physicians' recommendations (well, most of them), I kept wondering *why* Mrs. Monson failed to follow her physician's recommendations. Was it really because she did not *care* enough about her fetus? Then it occurred to me that an individual's ability to care is, in large measure, a function of whether the community is demonstrating care with respect to him or her. Had my physician given me the recommendations that Mrs. Monson's physician gave to her, the Dean of my college would have arranged a sabbatical leave for me; my husband would have figured out ways to sexually satisfy himself and me that did not involve the act of sexual intercourse; and my family and friends would have knocked each other over in their rush to drive me to the hospital at the first sign of fetal and/or maternal distress. Enmeshed in this community of care-givers, it would have been easy for me to care about my fetus.

But I suspect that it was not all that easy for Mrs. Monson to care about her fetus. Admittedly, I do not know the particulars of Mrs. Monson's circumstances, but it is conceivable to me that, even if she had wanted to get over her drug addiction, there may have been no available slot in the local drug rehabilitation program. It is also conceivable to me that Mrs. Monson's decisions to have sexual intercourse were the result of spousal badgering, bullying, pleading, cajoling, or even rape. Finally, it is conceivable to me that Mrs. Monson did not have time to put her feet up while on the job, and that neither she nor her immediate neighbors owned a car for quick transport to the hospital. Under this set of circumstances, I am prepared to say that if anyone is to blame for the sad shape Mrs. Monson's baby boy was born in, it is not only or mostly Mrs. Monson.

IV

My purpose in contrasting a plausible tale about me with a plausible tale about Mrs. Monson is to make three points about the ethics of care [6, 7].

First, an ethics of care forces us to reconsider the role of excuses in the moral life. An ethics of rights accepts only two sorts of excuses: those based on ignorance ("I didn't really understand the risks my conduct posed to the fetus"), and those based on lack of control ("Because of some physical and/or psychological impediment I had, I couldn't take care of my fetus"). Excuses that seek to "pin the blame" on other people are regarded as bad form, as a threat to the notion of the solitary moral agent who has no one to blame but himself/herself for his/her actions. In contrast, an ethics of care accepts excuses that pin at least some of the blame on other people because sometimes that is where the blame needs to be pinned.

Second, an ethics of care invites us to base public policy on meeting people's *needs* rather than simply on acknowledging people's *rights*. An ethics of care proceeds from inclination and not from duty. It is about people *wanting* to be good to each other, and not about people *having* to be good to each other; and in order to want to be good to each other, people need to have the positive experience of not being harmed by others.

Third, and finally, an ethics of care is precisely suited for making peace in gestational conflicts that exist less in reality than in the thoughts of some philosphers. Mothers and their wanted fetuses—and it is wanted fetuses of which we speak—are symbiotically related. Unless a mother thinks her physician's recommendations are wrongheaded or ill-advised for any number of reasons, she is going to want to follow them (even if she like I, "cheats" a bit here and there). After all, it is in her own best interest as well as that of her fetus that it be born healthy. And so, if the private and public worlds in which a mother lives give her the means to act upon her pro-fetal wants, she will.

An ethics of care is not a reformist ethic; it is a revolutionary ethic. Sartre was half right when he claimed that when we choose for ourselves, we choose for others [8]. He should have remembered what an ethics of care cannot forget; namely, that in choosing for others, we choose for ourselves. If we want pregnant women to take good care of their fetuses, then we ourselves should also want to take good care of pregnant women. It is a "package deal"—the only kind of deal an ethics of care makes.

REFERENCES

1 Nelson JL. Making peace in gestational conflicts. *Theor Med* 1992;13:319–28.

2 Gallagher J. Fetus as patient. In: Cohen S, Taub N, eds. *Reproductive Laws for the 1990s*. Clifton: Humana Press, 1989:185–235.

3 Robertson J. Reconciling offspring and maternal interests during pregnancy. In: Cohen S, Taub N, eds. *Reproductive Laws for the 1990s*. Clifton: Humana Press, 1989:259–76.

4 Anonymous. Doctors aren't policemen. *San Diego Union* 1987 March 7:A3.

5 Annas G. Pregnant women as fetal containers. *Hastings Cent Rep* 1986;16:13–14.

6 Gilligan C. *In a Different Voice*. Cambridge: Harvard University Press, 1982.

7 Noddings N. *Caring*. Berkeley: University of California Press, 1984.

8 Warnock H. *Existentialist Ethics*. London: St Martin's Press, 1967.

ANNOTATED BIBLIOGRAPHY: CHAPTER 8

Bolton, Martha Brandt: "Responsible Women and Abortion Decisions," in Onora O'Neill and William Ruddick, eds., *Having Children: Philosophical and Legal Reflections on Parenthood* (New York: Oxford University Press, 1979), pp. 40–51. In defending a moderate view on the morality of abortion, Bolton emphasizes the importance of contextual features in the life of a pregnant woman. She argues that the decision to bear a child must "fit" into a woman's life and make sense in terms of her responsibilities to her family and to the larger society.

Brody, Baruch: "On the Humanity of the Foetus," in Robert L. Perkins, ed., *Abortion: Pro and Con* (Cambridge, MA: Schenkman, 1974), pp. 69–90. Brody critically examines various proposals for "drawing the line" on the humanity of the fetus, ultimately suggesting that the most defensible view would draw the line at the point where fetal brain activity begins.

Chervenak, Frank A., and Laurence B. McCullough: "Justified Limits on Refusing Intervention," *Hastings Center Report* 21 (March/April 1991), pp. 12–18. The authors argue that court orders compelling cesarean delivery can be justified in the case of "well-documented, complete placenta previa."

Engelhardt, H. Tristram, Jr.: "The Ontology of Abortion," *Ethics* 84 (April 1974), pp. 217–234. Engelhardt focuses attention on the issue of "whether or to what extent the fetus is a person." He argues that, strictly speaking, a human person is not present until the later stages of infancy. However, he finds the point of viability significant in that, with viability, an infant can play the social role of "child" and thus be treated "as if it were a person."

English, Jane: "Abortion and the Concept of a Person," *Canadian Journal of Philosophy* 5 (October 1975), pp. 233–243. English advances one line of argument calculated to moderate the conservative view on the morality of abortion and another line of argument calculated to moderate the liberal view.

Feinberg, Joel, ed.: *The Problem of Abortion,* 2d ed. (Belmont, CA: Wadsworth, 1984). This excellent anthology features a wide range of articles on the moral justifiability of abortion.

Humber, James M.: "Abortion: The Avoidable Moral Dilemma," *Journal of Value Inquiry* 9 (Winter 1975), pp. 282–302. Humber, defending the conservative view on the morality of abortion, examines and rejects what he identifies as the major defenses of abortion. He also contends that proabortion arguments are typically so poor that they can only be viewed as "after-the-fact-rationalizations."

Johnsen, Dawn: "A New Threat to Pregnant Women's Autonomy," *Hastings Center Report* 17 (August 1987), pp. 33–40. Johnsen argues that the power of the state should not be used to coerce pregnant women to behave in ways considered to be best for their fetuses. In her view, the assertion of "fetal rights" against a pregnant woman is not an effective way of promoting a healthy fetal environment.

King, Patricia: "Should Mom Be Constrained in the Best Interests of the Fetus?" *Nova Law Review* 13 (Spring 1989), pp. 393–404. King emphasizes equity concerns and privacy concerns in arguing that the law should not be employed to constrain a pregnant woman to act in ways perceived to be in the best interests of her fetus.

Langerak, Edward A.: "Abortion: Listening to the Middle," *Hastings Center Report* 9 (October 1979), pp. 24–28. Langerak suggests a theoretical framework for a moderate view that incorporates two "widely shared beliefs": (1) that there is something about the fetus *itself* that makes abortion morally problematic and (2) that late abortions are significantly more problematic than early abortions.

Noonan, John T., Jr.: "An Almost Absolute Value in History." In John T. Noonan, ed., *The Morality of Abortion: Legal and Historical Perspectives* (Cambridge, MA: Harvard University Press, 1970), pp. 51–59. In this well-known statement of the conservative view on the morality of abortion, Noonan argues that conception is the only objectively based and nonarbitrary point at which to "draw the line" between the nonhuman and the human.

Pojman, Louis P., and Francis J. Beckwith: *The Abortion Controversy: A Reader* (Boston: Jones and Bartlett, 1994). The articles in this long anthology are organized under eight headings, including "Evaluations of *Roe v. Wade,*" "Personhood Arguments on Abortion," and "Feminist Arguments on Abortion."

Rhoden, Nancy K.: "The New Neonatal Dilemma: Live Births from Late Abortions." *Georgetown Law Journal* 72 (June 1984), pp. 1451–1509. Rhoden reviews the various medical techniques employed for second-trimester abortions and considers the dilemma that arises when a late second-trimester abortion results in live birth. She also discusses the future of second-trimester abortions in the light of technological developments and constitutional considerations.

Ross, Steven L.: "Abortion and the Death of the Fetus, " *Philosophy and Public Affairs* 11 (summer 1982), pp. 232-245. Ross draws a distinction between abortion as the termination of pregnancy and abortion as the termination of the life of the fetus. He proceeds to defend abortion in the latter sense, insisting that it is justifiable for a woman to desire not only the termination of pregnancy but also the death of the fetus.

Sherwin, Susan: *No Longer Patient: Feminist Ethics and Health Care* (Philadelphia: Temple University Press, 1992). In Chapter 5 of this book (pp. 99–116), Sherwin presents an analysis of abortion from the perspective of feminist ethics.

Strong, Carson: "Ethical Conflicts between Mother and Fetus in Obstetrics," *Clinics in Perinatology* 14 (June 1987), pp. 313–327. Strong argues that it is sometimes ethical for physicians to override the decision of a pregnant woman who refuses treatment considered necessary for the fetus. He considered in particular the maternal-fetal conflict that arises in conjunction with cesarean deliveries.

Tooley, Michael: *Abortion and Infanticide* (New York: Oxford University Press, 1983). In this long book, Tooley defends the liberal view on the morality of abortion. He insists that the question of the morality of abortion cannot be satisfactorily resolved "in isolation from the questions of the morally of infanticide and of the killing of nonhuman animals."

CHAPTER 9

GENETICS AND HUMAN REPRODUCTION

INTRODUCTION

With the rapid advance of knowledge and techniques in human genetics and the biology of human reproduction, a number of complex and troubling ethical issues have arisen. This chapter is designed to address some of the most important of these issues.

Genetic Disease and the Language of Genetics

Tay-Sachs disease is one prominent example of a genetic disease. This disease, which most commonly affects Jewish children of Eastern European heritage, is characterized by progressive neurological degeneration and death in early childhood. Although a child afflicted with Tay-Sachs disease has the disease by virtue of his or her genetic inheritance, the child's parents do not have the disease. (Those afflicted with Tay-Sachs disease do not survive to reproduce.) The parents are *carriers*. Tay-Sachs carriers are those persons who have one normal gene and one variant, or defective, gene (the Tay-Sachs gene) at the same location on paired chromosomes. The Tay-Sachs gene is a *recessive* gene. When it is paired with a normal gene, as is the case with the carrier, the normal gene is dominant. As a result, the carrier does not manifest the disease. However, if a child inherits the Tay-Sachs gene from both parents, then the child will be afflicted with Tay-Sachs disease.

Since Tay-Sachs disease is traceable to a recessive gene, it is said to be a recessive disease. Moreover, it is said to be an *autosomal* recessive disease, where the word *autosomal* simply indicates that the defective genes are located on some pair of chromosomes other than the sex chromosomes. Furthermore, in the language of genetics, Tay-Sachs carriers are said to be in the *heterozygous* state, whereas a child afflicted with Tay-Sachs disease is said to be in the *homozygous* state, with regard to the Tay-Sachs gene. Carriers, having the Tay-Sachs gene paired with a different (normal) gene, are heterozygous with regard to the Tay-Sachs gene. The afflicted child, having two identical Tay-Sachs genes, is homozygous with regard to the Tay-Sachs gene. The carrier is sometimes termed a "heterozygote"; the afflicted child, a "homozygote."

According to the laws of heredity, when two carriers of a trait associated with an autosomal recessive disease produce offspring, there is 1 chance in 4 (25 percent) that their child will be afflicted with the genetic disease in question. There are 2 chances in 4 (50 percent) that their child will be, like them, a carrier. Finally, there is 1 chance in 4 (25 percent) that their child will be free both of the disease and of the carrier status.

The genetic disease usually called "sickle-cell anemia" is, like Tay-Sachs disease, a well-known autosomal recessive disease. Most commonly affecting blacks, sickle-cell anemia is characterized by acute attacks of abdominal pain and exhibits a range of severity. It is estimated that 10 to 12 percent of blacks in the United States carry the sickle-cell trait. As is typical of autosomal recessive diseases, if two carriers of the sickle-cell trait produce offspring, there is 1 chance in 4 (25 percent) that their child will be afflicted with sickle-cell anemia.

Cystic fibrosis provides one further example of an autosomal recessive disease. In the United States, since about 1 in 20 Caucasians carries the cystic fibrosis gene, about 1 in 400 Caucasian couples will be a carrier-carrier pairing and thus be at risk (1 chance in 4) of producing offspring with the disease. At present, although hopes are high for therapeutic advances, most victims of cystic fibrosis die before the age of 30. The disease is primarily characterized by a dysfunction of the exocrine glands. This dysfunction results in abnormal amounts of mucus that can obstruct organ passages and produce intense pulmonary and digestive distress.

Huntington's disease provides a leading example of a genetic disease in the category of autosomal *dominant* diseases. Typically, the symptoms of Huntington's disease emerge only in the prime of life, between the ages of 35 and 50. It is characterized by mental and physical deterioration, leading to death within several years. The defective gene responsible for Huntington's disease is a dominant one. If a person has the defective gene, that person will eventually fall victim to the disease. Moreover, there is 1 chance in 2 (50 percent) that the person carrying the defective gene will pass it on to each of his or her children.

In contrast to autosomal genetic diseases, some genetic diseases are linked to mutant genes located on the sex chromosomes. Prominent among the genetic diseases in this latter category are the so-called X-linked diseases. Hemophilia, a well-known disease characterized by uncontrollable bleeding, is a leading example of an X-linked disease. Of the 46 chromosomes that constitute the normal complement of genetic material in human beings, there are two sex chromosomes. A female has two X chromosomes and a male has one X and one Y chromosome. In human reproduction, if the sperm fertilizing the egg provides an X chromosome, the child will be female. If the sperm fertilizing the egg provides a Y chromosome, the child will be male. (The egg always provides an X chromosome.) Hemophilia is a *recessive* X-linked disease. A female, therefore, will have the disease of hemophilia only if she has the mutant gene on both of her X chromosomes. If a female has one normal gene and one mutant gene, however, she will be a carrier. Since a male has only one X chromosome, if he has the mutant gene associated with hemophilia, he will have the disease. On the assumption that a female carrier mates with a male who is free of the disease, there is no risk that their female children will have the disease. Female children will inherit a normal gene from their father and thus themselves be free of the disease, although there is 1 chance in 2 (50 percent) that they will inherit their mother's mutant gene and be, like her, a carrier. In contrast, there is 1 chance in 2 (50 percent) that male children will have the disease of hemophilia.

Prenatal Diagnosis and Selective Abortion

A number of techniques are presently employed for the detection of chromosomal abnormalities, many genetic diseases, and certain serious anatomical abnormalities in the fetus in utero. Among these techniques, amniocentesis and chorionic villi sampling (CVS) are the most prominent, although ultrasound is also of great importance. Ultrasound is a noninvasive technique that produces a visual representation of the developing fetus, thereby allowing the detection of many anatomical abnormalities.

In amniocentesis, a needle is inserted through a pregnant woman's abdomen, and a sample of the amniotic fluid surrounding the fetus is withdrawn. There are fetal cells in the amniotic fluid, and a continually increasing number of genetic diseases in the fetus can be detected through biochemical studies and recombinant DNA techniques. Also detectable, via chromosomal analysis, are conditions associated with an abnormal number of chromosomes or an abnormal arrangement of chromosomes. Down's syndrome, for example, is associated with the presence of an extra chromosome, namely, three instead of two number 21 chromosomes. Amniocentesis can also be employed for the detection of neural-tube defects (anencephaly and spina bifida). In this case, a positive diagnosis rests on the presence of increased levels of alphafetoprotein in the amniotic fluid.

Amniocentesis, first introduced in the late 1960s, has achieved wide acceptance among physicians as a relatively low-risk medical procedure. However, it is not ordinarily performed prior to the 15th to the 16th week of gestation, and selective abortion must await the results of diagnostic testing, usually available around the 20th week. Since second-trimester abortions are in many ways more problematic than first-trimester abortions, a procedure capable of combining the prenatal diagnostic value of amniocentesis with the possibility of first-trimester abortion is much to be preferred, assuming, of course, that risk factors are within acceptable limits. Chorionic villi sampling, a procedure developed in Europe and first introduced in the United States in 1983, has now emerged as a clear alternative to amniocentesis in the detection of genetic diseases and chromosomal abnormalities. In CVS, a procedure that can be performed in the first trimester, usually around the 10th week, a small amount of tissue is extracted from the placenta. Although CVS may be largely comparable to amniocentesis in terms of various risk factors (e.g., the possibilities of miscarriage and maternal infection), some research has suggested a link between CVS and missing or shortened fingers and toes.

Since prenatal diagnosis is ordinarily undertaken with an eye toward selective abortion, the practice of prenatal diagnosis clearly confronts us with one particular aspect of the more general problem of abortion, as discussed in Chapter 8. (There is also a close link with the problem of the treatment of impaired newborns, as discussed in Chapter 7.) Is the practice of selective abortion, on grounds of genetic defect, ethically acceptable? Leon R. Kass, in one of this chapter's selections, abstracts from the problem of abortion in general and argues specifically against the practice of selective (genetic) abortion. Although many ethicists, in opposition to Kass, would defend the practice of selective abortion on grounds of genetic defect, far fewer are willing to endorse the employment of prenatal diagnosis for purposes of sex selection.

Morality and Reproductive Risk

One important ethical issue associated with human genetics has to do with the morality of reproduction under circumstances of genetic risk. Laura M. Purdy argues in this chapter that it is morally wrong to reproduce in those cases where there is a high risk of serious genetic disease. She considers in particular the case of Huntington's disease. If it is justifiable to maintain that there is a moral obligation of the sort that Purdy outlines, we may find ourselves once more faced with the problem of prenatal diagnosis and selective abortion. Clearly, in those cases where prenatal diagnosis is available (e.g., Huntington's disease, Tay-Sachs disease, sickle-cell anemia, cystic fibrosis), abortion offers a means of sidestepping the risk of serious genetic disease.

Closely associated with the issue of the morality of reproduction under circumstances of genetic risk is another ethical issue, the justifiability of the use of coercive measures to achieve social control over individual reproductive decisions. It is one thing to say that certain reproductive choices are immoral and quite another to say that coercive measures for the control of reproductive choices are justified. Such coercive controls as compulsory sterilization and mandatory amniocentesis followed by forced abortion are widely rejected as invasive of fundamental rights. Mandatory screening programs for the identification of carriers, while surely less intrusive than other coercive measures, are also widely opposed as unjustifiable. Those who argue in support of coercive measures sometimes introduce claims, difficult to assess, about the dangers of uncontrolled reproduction leading to a deterioration of the human gene pool. Thus, proposals for coercive measures often reflect a "negative eugenics" rationale.[1] Such proposals are rejected by those who maintain that there is no clear and present danger of genetic deterioration.[2]

Reproductive Technologies and the Treatment of Infertility

Human reproduction, as it naturally occurs, is characterized by sexual intercourse, tubal fertilization, implantation in the uterus, and subsequent in utero gestation. The expression *reproductive technologies* can be understood as applicable to an array of technical procedures that would replace the various steps in the natural process of reproduction, to a lesser or greater extent.

Artificial insemination is a procedure that replaces sexual intercourse as a means of achieving tubal fertilization. Artificial insemination has long been available, primarily as a means of overcoming infertility on the part of a male, usually a husband. It is sometimes possible that the husband's infertility may be overcome by AIH, artificial insemination with the sperm of the *husband*. More often, the couple must turn to AID, artificial insemination with the sperm of a *donor*. AID can also be employed when it has been established that the husband carries a mutant gene that would place a couple's offspring at genetic risk. Moreover, it has been suggested, most prominently in the work of the well-known geneticist Hermann J. Muller, that AID be voluntarily employed as a way of achieving the aims of positive eugenics.[3] Muller recommended the formation of sperm banks, which would collect and store the sperm of men judged to be "outstanding" in various ways. His idea was that any "enlightened" couple desiring a child would have recourse to one of these banks in order to arrange for the wife's artificial insemination. Another controversial use of AID is its employment by unmarried women. Probably even more controversial is the employment of artificial insemination within the context of a surrogacy arrangement. In the most typical case, a wife's infertility motivates a couple to seek out a so-called surrogate mother. The surrogate agrees to be artificially inseminated with the husband's sperm, in order to bear a child for the couple.

In vitro fertilization (IVF) literally means "fertilization in glass." The sperm of a husband (or a donor) is united, in a laboratory, with the ovum of a wife (or a donor). Whereas artificial insemination is a technically simple procedure, in vitro fertilization followed by embryo transfer (to the uterus for implantation) is a system of reproductive technology that features a high degree of technical sophistication. The first documented "test-tube baby," Louise Brown, was born in England in July 1978. Her birth was the culmination of years of collaboration between a gynecologist, Patrick Steptoe, and an embryologist, Robert Edwards. This pioneering team developed methods for obtaining mature eggs from a woman's ovaries (via a minor surgical procedure called a laparoscopy), effectively fertilizing eggs in the laboratory, cultivating them to the eight-cell stage, and then transferring a developing embryo to the uterus for implantation.

Reproductive centers throughout the United States now provide in vitro procedures for the treatment of infertility. Although success rates continue to be somewhat disappointing, it is expected that they will improve as techniques are further refined. An important development in this regard is the achievement of the first frozen-embryo birth by an Australian team in 1984. Since it is now also possible, with the use of fertility drugs, to harvest a crop of mature eggs (perhaps ten or so) from a woman's ovaries, embryos frozen at the eight-cell stage can be thawed over a period of several months in an effort to achieve a successful implantation. Of course, the freezing of embryos is a technique that seems to suggest a number of ominous possibilities. However, the freezing of unfertilized eggs, which at face value seems preferable to the freezing of embryos, has proven to be technically more difficult.

In vitro fertilization followed by embryo transfer is a system of reproductive technology that replaces not only sexual intercourse but also tubal fertilization in the natural process of reproduction. But consider also the future possibility of dispensing with implantation and in utero gestation as well. There seems to be no theoretical obstacle to totally artificial gestation, which would take place within the confines of an artificial womb. If *ectogenesis,* the process of artificial gestation, becomes a reality, then the combination of in vitro fertilization and ectogenesis would provide us with a system of reproductive technology in which each element in the natural process of reproduction has been effectively replaced. At the present time, however, in vitro fertilization (accompanied by embryo transfer) is seen primarily as a means of overcoming infertility, especially infertility due to obstruction of the fallopian tubes.

One important spinoff of IVF technology is a procedure known as GIFT, that is, gamete intrafallopian transfer. In this procedure, eggs are obtained as they would be for IVF, but instead of fertilization in vitro, the eggs are placed together with sperm in the fallopian tube (or tubes) where it is hoped that fertilization will take place in vivo (i.e., in the living situation). Although there is some risk of ectopic pregnancy in GIFT, the success rates reported for this procedure are somewhat higher than the success rates for IVF in combination with embryo transfer. Higher success rates have also been reported with a closely related procedure, ZIFT (i.e., zygote intrafallopian transfer). In ZIFT, a single-cell zygote, which is the product of in vitro fertilization, is transferred to the fallopian tube.

In contrast to a woman whose infertility can be traced to fallopian tube obstruction, consider a woman whose ovaries are either absent or nonfunctional. Since she has no ova, she cannot produce genetic offspring. If her uterus is functional, however, there is no biological obstacle to her bearing a child. Let us suppose that she very much wants to bear a child that is her husband's genetic offspring. Her problem can be addressed by some form of *egg dona-tion,* including the following possibilities:[4] (1) In vitro fertilization of a donor egg with the husband's sperm, followed by embryo transfer to the wife. (2) Artificial insemination of an egg donor with the husband's sperm, producing in vivo fertilization; nonsurgical removal of the embryo via lavage (a washing out) of the donor's uterus; recovery of the embryo and transfer to the uterus of the wife.[5] (3) Transfer of a donor egg together with the husband's sperm to the wife's fallopian tube, thus employing GIFT in an effort to achieve tubal fertilization and subsequent implantation. Since both the first and second procedures, in contrast to the third, entail embryo transfers that involve a donated egg, the expressions *surrogate embryo transfer* and *prenatal adoption* are sometimes used to describe them.

In the case just discussed, a woman has a functional uterus but nonfunctional ovaries. Consider now the converse case—a woman has functional ovaries but a nonfunctional uterus. Perhaps she has had a hysterectomy. She is capable of becoming the *genetic* but not the *gesta-tional* mother of a child. Now, suppose that she and her husband desire a child "of their own." This situation gives rise to the possibility of a surrogacy arrangement somewhat different from the kind predicated upon artificial insemination. In this case, in vitro fertilization could be employed to fertilize the wife's egg with the husband's sperm. The embryo could then be transferred to the uterus of a surrogate who would agree to bear the child for the couple. The surrogate would then be the gestational but not the genetic mother of the child.

One other proposed scheme of reproductive technology is based on cloning. Some scientists believe that successful human cloning could become a realistic possibility in the not-too-distant future.[6] Accordingly, the following sequence of events can be imagined. A mature human egg will be obtained from a woman and enucleated in a laboratory—that is, the nucleus of the egg cell will be removed. Meanwhile, a body cell from a donor (who might be anyone including the woman who has provided the egg) will be obtained and enucleated. The extracted nucleus, which contains the donor's heretofore unique genotype, will undergo a process calculated to activate its dormant genes and then be inserted into the egg cell. From this point, the renucleated egg will develop in the way that a newly fertilized egg ordinarily develops. Embryo transfer (not necessarily into the uterus of the woman from whom the original egg was obtained) and subsequent in utero gestation will then lead to the birth of a human "clone." In contrast to offspring resulting from sexual reproduction, where the resultant genotype is the result of contributions by two parents, the "clone" will have the same genotype as his or her "parent."

Reproductive Technologies: Ethical Concerns

To what extent, if at all, is it ethically acceptable to employ the various reproductive technologies just discussed? A host of ethical concerns have been expressed about these technologies, and a brief survey of the most prominent of these concerns should prove helpful.

Most of the ethical opposition to artificial insemination derives from religious views. AID especially has been attacked on the grounds that it illicitly separates procreation from the marriage relationship. Inasmuch as AID introduces a third party (the sperm donor) into a marriage relationship, it has been called a form of adultery. Even AIH, which cannot be accused of separating procreation from the marriage relationship, has not uniformly escaped attack. Some religious ethicists have gone so far as to contend that procreation is morally illicit whenever it is not the product of personal lovemaking. Although these sorts of objections frequently recur in discussions of in vitro fertilization (and related procedures), the various forms of egg donation, and cloning, they seem to have little force for those who do not share the basic worldview from which they proceed.

In one of this chapter's selections, Paul Lauritzen raises objections to the secrecy that is often associated with the practice of AID (which he refers to as "donor insemination"). He is not opposed to the employment of donor insemination but argues that responsible parenthood requires not hiding from a child the fact that he or she has been conceived in this way.

Much of the ethical opposition to surrogate motherhood can be traced to (1) concerns about psychosocial problems likely to arise for the child who is born as a result of a surrogacy arrangement and (2) concerns that the practice will have a negative impact on family structure. Another frequently expressed concern relates especially to *commercial* surrogacy contracts, which provide for a fee to be paid to the surrogate. The worry here is that the practice of commercial surrogacy will encourage society to think of children as commodities.

Several selections in this chapter deal with the controversial practice of surrogate motherhood. In one, excerpted from the New Jersey Supreme Court's opinion in the celebrated Baby M case, *commercial* surrogacy contracts are held to be invalid and unenforceable in the state of New Jersey. At present, however, the legal status of commercial surrogacy contracts varies from state to state, and legislatures continue to struggle with the social policy aspects of surrogacy. One option is for a state simply to recognize commercial surrogacy contracts as valid and legally enforceable. Another option is for the state to prohibit commercial surrogacy contracts altogether. Bonnie Steinbock argues in this chapter against the legal prohibition of surrogacy contracts, although she insists on the importance of state regulation. In her view, commercial surrogacy contracts should be permitted only if provision is made for a "waiting period" subsequent to birth. During this period, the surrogate would have the opportunity to change her mind about surrendering her parental rights.

In the Baby M case, the "surrogate" was both the genetic and the gestational mother of a child. Other cases involve purely gestational surrogates, that is, women who have agreed to carry a child for a couple each of whom is a genetic parent. Here the surrogate is the gestational but not the genetic mother of a child. If this type of surrogacy agreement breaks down, the following issue arises: Should we identify the genetic mother or the gestational mother as the child's legal mother? In one of this chapter's selections, Ruth Macklin explores this and related questions. In a companion selection, Barbara Katz Rothman argues that the gestational mother should be recognized as the child's legal mother.

Some of the ethical opposition to in vitro fertilization (and related procedures) is based on the perceived "unnaturalness" of the procedure. Closely related is the charge that the procedure depersonalizes or dehumanizes procreation. Other opponents of in vitro fertilization have argued that we must abstain from any intervention that inflicts unknown risks on developing offspring. Another recurrent argument against in vitro fertilization is that its acceptance by society will lead to the acceptance of more and more objectionable developments in reproductive technology (e.g., ectogenesis).

In addition to arguments advanced in support of a wholesale rejection of in vitro fertilization, a number of concerns having a more limited scope can be identified. Some commentators have been quite willing to endorse the employment of in vitro fertilization and embryo transfer within the framework of a marital relationship but find any third-party involvement, such as egg donation or surrogate motherhood, objectionable. Other critics object primarily to a frequent concomitant of in vitro procedures, the discarding of embryos considered unneeded or unsuitable for implantation. (Those who consider even an early embryo a person are especially vocal on this score.) Although the practice of freezing embryos offers a partial solution to the problem of surplus embryos, some would argue that, in this case, the "solution" creates more problems than it solves.

Two readings in this chapter focus directly on the ethics of IVF. In providing an overall defense of IVF, Peter Singer rejects many of the standard arguments against it. He also contends that there is no ethical problem with freezing *early* embryos, discarding them, or using them for research purposes. Susan Sherwin, in a very different spirit, works out a critique of IVF based on her commitment to feminist ethics. From a feminist point of view, she maintains, IVF is morally problematic for a number of closely related reasons. Although there is a diversity of views in the feminist community about the ethics of IVF, many feminists believe that the availability of IVF (and other reproductive technologies) is at best a mixed blessing for women.

In terms of ethical acceptability, cloning would seem to be the most problematic of all the reproductive technologies.[7] Whereas the fundamental value of the other reproductive technologies under discussion can be located in the relief of infertility, the connection between cloning and the relief of infertility is more tenuous. Related to this consideration is the argument that cloning is the reproductive technology most likely to be misused, to the detriment of society. Of course, the stock charges against reproductive technology—that it is "unnatural" and depersonalizes reproduction—are also raised against cloning. But probably the most important arguments against cloning are those that emphasize psychological and social difficulties associated with a clone's manner of origin and lack of genetic uniqueness.

Genetic Engineering and the Human Genome Project

Two important distinctions are involved in discussions of the ethics of genetic engineering (intervention, manipulation). *Therapeutic* genetic engineering, commonly called "gene therapy," involves interventions directed at the cure of disease. *Nontherapeutic* genetic engineering, often called "enhancement engineering," involves interventions directed at the enhancement of human capabilities (e.g., memory). *Somatic-cell* genetic interventions involve introducing modifications into nonreproductive cells (e.g., blood cells), so that the resultant changes are not passed on to future generations. *Germ-line* genetic interventions involve introducing modifications into sperm, ova, or embryos, so that the resultant changes are passed on to future generations. By reference to these two distinctions, four categories of genetic engineering are commonly distinguished: (1) somatic-cell gene therapy, (2) germ-line gene therapy, (3) somatic-cell enhancement (nontherapeutic) engineering, (4) germ-line enhancement (nontherapeutic) engineering.

It may be possible in the foreseeable future to cure a wide range of genetic diseases (e.g., cystic fibrosis) by the genetic manipulation of somatic cells. Despite the complaint that any employment of genetic engineering places human beings in the role of "playing God," the continued development and employment of somatic-cell gene therapy is widely endorsed and relatively uncontroversial. On the other hand, there is extensive debate about the ethical acceptability of both germ-line gene therapy and enhancement engineering. In one of this chapter's selections, a position paper representing the views of the Council for Responsible Genetics, it is argued that no germ-line manipulations (including therapeutic ones) should be permitted. In another selection, W. French Anderson argues against any employment of enhancement engineering. A contrasting view of the ethics of enhancement engineering can be found in a brief discussion at the end of the selection by Singer on the ethics of IVF.

Two fundamental goals underlie the Human Genome Project. The first is to "map" the human genome, which entails determining on which chromosome and at what location each of the estimated 50,000 to 100,000 human genes can be found. The second is to "sequence" the human genome, which entails determining the order of occurrence of the estimated 3 billion base pairs in human DNA. The project involves extensive international cooperation, was funded by the U.S. government beginning in 1990, and was originally projected to last for 15 years.

Numerous ethical questions have been raised about the Human Genome Project and about the explosion of genetic information that is expected to be available as a result. Thomas H. Murray deals with some of these questions in this chapter's last reading.

T.A.M.

NOTES

1 Roughly, positive eugenics aims at enhancing the genetic heritage of the species, whereas negative eugenics aims at preventing deterioration of the gene pool.

2 This view is defended by Marc Lappe, "Moral Obligations and the Fallacies of 'Genetic Control,'" *Theological Studies* 33 (September 1972), pp. 411–427.

3 See, for example, Hermann J. Muller, "Means and Aims in Human Genetic Betterment," in T. M. Sonneborn, ed., *The Control of Human Heredity and Evolution* (New York: Macmillan, 1965), pp. 100–122.

4 Some form of egg donation might also be considered when a woman's own ova would place her offspring at risk for genetic disease.

5 To date, the success rates for this technique have not been impressive. There is also a risk of unwanted pregnancy on the part of the donor, because lavage might fail to wash out the embryo.

6 The type of cloning under discussion here involves nuclear transplantation from a somatic cell. A less dramatic form of cloning involves the splitting of a very early embryo (e.g., at

the four-cell stage) and thus the formation of duplicate embryos. The embryo-splitting type of cloning is already technically feasible.

7 This brief discussion of the ethics of cloning is restricted to the type of cloning that involves nuclear transplantation from a somatic cell. A collection of articles on the ethical issues raised by the embryo-splitting type of cloning can be found in *Kennedy Institute of Ethics Journal* 4 (September 1994).

Reproductive Risk, Prenatal Diagnosis, and Selective Abortion

Implications of Prenatal Diagnosis for the Human Right to Life
Leon R. Kass

Leon R. Kass, a biologist as well as a medical doctor, is Addie Clark Harding Professor, The College and the Committee on Social Thought, University of Chicago. He is the author of *Toward a More Natural Science: Biology and Human Affairs* (1985). Among the more prominent of his many articles on issues in biomedical ethics are "Regarding the End of Medicine and the Pursuit of Health," "Making Babies—The New Biology and the 'Old' Morality," and "Is There a Right to Die?"

Setting aside a discussion of the moral problem of abortion in general, Kass focuses on some of the ethical difficulties associated with the abortion of fetuses known by amniocentesis to be genetically defective. He maintains that the practice of *genetic* abortion, inasmuch as it involves a qualitative assessment of fetuses, represents a threat to the "radical moral equality of all human beings." As a result of the practice of genetic abortion, Kass suggests, we will be inclined to take a more negative view of those who are genetically defective or otherwise "abnormal." Thus we will be inclined to treat them in a second-class manner. Moreover, he contends, to commit ourselves to the practice of genetic abortion is to reflect acceptance of a very dangerous principle, that "defectives should not be born."

It is especially fitting on this occasion to begin by acknowledging how privileged I feel and how pleased I am to be a participant in this symposium. I suspect that I am not alone among the assembled in considering myself fortunate to be here. For I was conceived after antibiotics yet before amniocentesis, late enough to have benefited from medicine's ability to prevent and control fatal infectious diseases, yet early enough to have escaped from medicine's ability to prevent me from living to suffer from my genetic diseases. To be sure, my genetic vices are, as far as I know them, rather modest, taken individually—myopia, asthma and other allergies, bilateral forefoot adduction, bowleggedness, loqua-

Reprinted by permission of the author and Plenum Publishing Corporation from *Ethical Issues in Human Genetics,* edited by Bruce Hilton et al., 1973.

ciousness, and pessimism, plus some four to eight as yet undiagnosed recessive lethal genes in the heterozygous condition—but, taken together, and if diagnosable prenatally, I might never have made it.

Just as I am happy to be here, so am I unhappy with what I shall have to say. Little did I realize when I first conceived the topic, "Implications of Prenatal Diagnosis for the Human Right to Life," what a painful and difficult labor it would lead to. More than once while this paper was gestating, I considered obtaining permission to abort it, on the grounds that, by prenatal diagnosis, I knew it to be defective. My lawyer told me that I was legally in the clear, but my conscience reminded me that I had made a commitment to deliver myself of this paper, flawed or not. Next time, I shall practice better contraception.

Any discussion of the ethical issues of genetic counseling and prenatal diagnosis is unavoidably haunted by a ghost called the morality of abortion. This ghost I shall not vex. More precisely, I shall not vex the reader by telling ghost stories. However, I would be neither surprised nor disappointed if my discussion of an admittedly related matter, the ethics of aborting the genetically defective, summons that hovering spirit to the reader's mind. For the morality of abortion is a matter not easily laid to rest, recent efforts to do so notwithstanding. A vote by the legislature of the State of New York can indeed legitimatize the disposal of fetuses, but not of the moral questions. But though the questions remain, there is likely to be little new that can be said about them, and certainly not by me.

Yet before leaving the general question of abortion, let me pause to drop some anchors for the discussion that follows. Despite great differences of opinion both as to what to think and how to reason about abortion, nearly everyone agrees that abortion is a moral issue.[1] What does this mean? Formally, it means that a woman seeking or refusing an abortion can expect to be asked to justify her action. And we can expect that she should be able to give reasons for her choice other than "I like it" or "I don't like it." Substantively, it means that, in the absence of good reasons for intervention, there is some presumption in favor of allowing the pregnancy to continue once it has begun. A common way of expressing this presumption is to say that "the fetus has a right to continued life."[2] In this context, disagreement concerning the moral permissibility of abortion concerns what rights (or interests or needs), and whose, override (take precedence over, or outweigh) this fetal "right." Even most of the "opponents" of abortion agree that the mother's right to live takes precedence, and that abortion to save her life is permissible, perhaps obligatory. Some believe that a woman's right to determine the number and spacing of her children takes precedence, while yet others argue that the need to curb population growth is, at least at this time, overriding.

Hopefully, this brief analysis of what it means to say that abortion is a moral issue is sufficient to establish two points. First, that the fetus is a living thing with some moral claim on us not to do it violence, and therefore, second, that justification must be given for destroying it.

Turning now from the general questions of the ethics of abortion, I wish to focus on the special ethical issues raised by the abortion of "defective" fetuses (so-called "abortion for fetal indications"). I shall consider only the cleanest cases, those cases where well-characterized genetic diseases are diagnosed with a high degree

of certainty by means of amniocentesis, in order to side-step the added moral dilemmas posed when the diagnosis is suspected or possible, but unconfirmed. However, many of the questions I shall discuss could also be raised about cases where genetic analysis gives only a statistical prediction about the genotype of the fetus, and also about cases where the defect has an infectious or chemical rather than a genetic cause (e.g., rubella, thalidomide).

My first and possibly most difficult task is to show that there is anything left to discuss once we have agreed not to discuss the morality of abortion in general. There is a sense in which abortion for genetic defect is, after abortion to save the life of the mother, perhaps the most defensible kind of abortion. Certainly, it is a serious and not a frivolous reason for abortion, defended by its proponents in sober and rational speech—unlike justifications based upon the false notion that a fetus is a mere part of a woman's body, to be used and abused at her pleasure. Standing behind genetic abortion are serious and well-intentioned people, with reasonable ends in view: the prevention of genetic diseases, the elimination of suffering in families, the preservation of precious financial and medical resources, the protection of our genetic heritage. No profiteers, no sex-ploiters, no racists. No arguments about the connection of abortion with promiscuity and licentiousness, no perjured testimony about the mental health of the mother, no arguments about the seriousness of the population problem. In short, clear objective data, a worthy cause, decent men and women. If abortion, what better reason for it?

Yet if genetic abortion is but a happily wagging tail on the dog of abortion, it is simultaneously the nose of a camel protruding under a rather different tent. Precisely because the quality of the fetus is central to the decision to abort, the practice of genetic abortion has implications which go beyond those raised by abortion in general. What may be at stake here is the belief in the radical moral equality of all human beings, the belief that all human beings possess equally and independent of merit certain fundamental rights, one among which is, of course, the right to life.

To be sure, the belief that fundamental human rights belong equally to all human beings has been but an ideal, never realized, often ignored, sometimes shamelessly. Yet it has been perhaps the most powerful moral idea at work in the world for at least two centuries. It is this idea and ideal that animates most of the current political and social criticism around the globe. It is ironic that we should acquire the power to detect and eliminate the genetically unequal at a time when we have finally succeeded in removing much of the stigma and disgrace previously attached to victims of congenital illness, in providing them with improved care and support, and in preventing, by means of education, feelings of guilt on the part of their parents. One might even wonder whether the development of amniocentesis and prenatal diagnosis may represent a backlash against these same humanitarian and egalitarian tendencies in the practice of medicine, which, by helping to sustain to the age of reproduction persons with genetic disease has itself contributed to the increasing incidence of genetic disease, and with it, to increased pressures for genetic screening, genetic counseling, and genetic abortion.

No doubt our humanitatian and egalitarian principles and practices have caused us some new difficulties, but if we mean to weaken or turn our backs on them, we should do so consciously and thoughtfully. If, as I believe, the idea and practice of genetic abortion points in that direction, we should make ourselves aware of it. . . .

GENETIC ABORTION AND THE LIVING DEFECTIVE

The practice of abortion of the genetically defective will no doubt affect our view of and our behavior toward those abnormals who escape the net of detection and abortion. A child with Down's syndrome or with hemophilia or with muscular dystrophy born at a time when most of his (potential) fellow sufferers were destroyed prenatally is liable to be looked upon by the community as one unfit to be alive, as a second-class (or even lower) human type. He may be seen as a person who need not have been, and who would not have been, if only someone had gotten to him in time.

The parents of such children are also likely to treat them differently, especially if the mother would have wished but failed to get an amniocentesis because of ignorance, poverty, or distance from the testing station, or if the prenatal diagnosis was in error. In such cases, parents are especially likely to resent the child. They may be disinclined to give it the kind of care they might have before the advent of amniocentesis and genetic abortion, rationalizing that a second-class specimen is not entitled to first-class treatment. If pressed to do so, say by physicians, the parents might refuse, and the courts may become involved. This has already begun to happen.

In Maryland, parents of a child with Down's syn-

drome refused permission to have the child operated on for an intestinal obstruction present at birth. The physicians and the hospital sought an injunction to require the parents to allow surgery. The judge ruled in favor of the parents, despite what I understand to be the weight of precedent to the contrary, on the grounds that the child was Mongoloid, that is, had the child been "normal," the decision would have gone the other way. Although the decision was not appealed to and hence not affirmed by a higher court, we can see through the prism of this case the possibility that the new powers of human genetics will strip the blindfold from the lady of justice and will make official the dangerous doctrine that some men are more equal than others.

The abnormal child may also feel resentful. A child with Down's syndrome or Tay-Sachs disease will probably never know or care, but what about a child with hemophilia or with Turner's syndrome? In the past decade, with medical knowledge and power over the prenatal child increasing and with parental authority over the postnatal child decreasing, we have seen the appearance of a new type of legal action, suits for wrongful life. Children have brought suit against their parents (and others) seeking to recover damages for physical and social handicaps inextricably tied to their birth (e.g., congenital deformities, congenital syphilis, illegitimacy). In some of the American cases, the courts have recognized the justice of the child's claim (that he was injured due to parental negligence), although they have so far refused to award damages, due to policy considerations. In other countries, e.g., in Germany, judgments with compensation have gone for the plaintiffs. With the spread of amniocentesis and genetic abortion, we can only expect such cases to increase. And here it will be the soft-hearted rather than the hard-hearted judges who will establish the doctrine of second-class human beings, out of compassion for the mutants who escaped the traps set out for them.

It may be argued that I am dealing with a problem which, even if it is real, will affect very few people. It may be suggested that very few will escape the traps once we have set them properly and widely, once people are informed about amniocentesis, once the power to detect prenatally grows to its full capacity, and once our "superstitious" opposition to abortion dies out or is extirpated. But in order even to come close to this vision of success, amniocentesis will have to become part of every pregnancy—either by making it mandatory, like the test for syphilis, or by making it "routine medical practice," like the Pap smear. Leaving aside the other problems with universal amniocentesis, we could expect that the problem for the few who escape is likely to be even worse precisely because they will be few.

The point, however, should be generalized. How will we come to view and act toward the many "abnormals" that will remain among us—the retarded, the crippled, the senile, the deformed, and the true mutants—once we embark on a program to root out genetic abnormality? For it must be remembered that we shall always have abnormals—some who escape detection or whose disease is undetectable *in utero*, others as a result of new mutations, birth injuries, accidents, maltreatment, or disease—who will require our care and protection. The existence of "defectives" cannot be fully prevented, not even by totalitarian breeding and weeding programs. Is it not likely that our principle with respect to these people will change from "We try harder" to "Why accept second best?" The idea of "the unwanted because abnormal child" may become a self-fulfilling prophecy, whose consequences may be worse than those of the abnormality itself.

GENETIC AND OTHER DEFECTIVES

The mention of other abnormals points to a second danger of the practice of genetic abortion. Genetic abortion may come to be seen not so much as the prevention of genetic disease, but as the prevention of birth of defective or abnormal children—and, in a way, understandably so. For in the case of what other diseases does preventive medicine consist in the elimination of the patient-at-risk? Moreover, the very language used to discuss genetic disease leads us to the easy but wrong conclusion that the afflicted fetus or person is rather than has a disease. True, one is partly defined by his genotype, but only partly. A person is more than his disease. And yet we slide easily from the language of possession to the language of identity, from "He has hemophilia" to "He is a hemophiliac," from "She has diabetes" through "She is diabetic" to "She is a diabetic," from "The fetus has Down's syndrome" to "The fetus is a Down's." This way of speaking supports the belief that it is defective persons (or potential persons) that are being eliminated, rather than diseases.

If this is so, then it becomes simply accidental that the defect has a genetic cause. Surely, it is only because of the high regard for medicine and science, and for the accuracy of genetic diagnosis, that genotypic defectives are likely to be the first to go. But once the principle, "Defectives should not be born," is established, grounds other than cytological and biochemical may

very well be sought. Even ignoring racialists and others equally misguided—of course, they cannot be ignored—we should know that there are social scientists, for example, who believe that one can predict with a high degree of accuracy how a child will turn out from a careful, systematic study of the socio-economic and psycho-dynamic environment into which he is born and in which he grows up. They might press for the prevention of socio-psychological disease, even of "criminality," by means of prenatal environmental diagnosis and abortion. I have heard rumor that a crude, unscientific form of eliminating potential "phenotypic defectives" is already being practiced in some cities, in that submission to abortion is allegedly being made a condition for the receipt of welfare payments. "Defectives should not be born" is a principle without limits. We can ill-afford to have it established.

Up to this point, I have been discussing the possible implications of the practice of genetic abortion for our belief in and adherence to the idea that, at least in fundamental human matters such as life and liberty, all men are to be considered as equals, that for these matters we should ignore as irrelevant the real qualitative differences amongst men, however important these differences may be for other purposes. Those who are concerned about abortion fear that the permissible time of eliminating the unwanted will be moved forward along the time continuum, against newborns, infants, and children. Similarly, I suggest that we should be concerned lest the attack on gross genetic inequality in fetuses be advanced along the continuum of quality and into the later stages of life.

I am not engaged in predicting the future; I am not saying that amniocentesis and genetic abortion will lead down the road to Nazi Germany. Rather, I am suggesting that the principles underlying genetic abortion simultaneously justify many further steps down that road. The point was very well made by Abraham Lincoln:

> If A can prove, however conclusively, that he may, of right, enslave B—Why may not B snatch the same argument and prove equally, that he may enslave A?
>
> You say A is white, and B is black. It is color, then; the lighter having the right to enslave the darker? Take care. By this rule, you are to be slave to the first man you meet with a fairer skin than your own.
>
> You do not mean color exactly? You mean the whites are intellectually the superiors of the blacks, and, therefore have the right to enslave them? Take care again. By this rule, you are to be slave to the first man you meet with an intellect superior to your own.

But, say you, it is a question of interest; and, if you can make it your interest, you have the right to enslave another. Very well. And if he can make it his interest, he has the right to enslave you.[3]

Perhaps I have exaggerated the dangers; perhaps we will not abandon our inexplicable preference for generous humanitarianism over consistency. But we should indeed be cautious and move slowly as we give serious consideration to the question "What price the perfect baby?"[4] . . .

NOTES

1 This strikes me as by far the most important inference to be drawn from the fact that men in different times and cultures have answered the abortion question differently. Seen in this light, the differing and changing answers themselves suggest that it is a question not easily put under, at least not for very long.

2 Other ways include: one should not do violence to living or growing things; life is sacred; respect nature; fetal life has value; refrain from taking innocent life; protect and preserve life. As some have pointed out, the terms chosen are of different weight, and would require reasons of different weight to tip the balance in favor of abortion. My choice of the "rights" terminology is not meant to beg the questions of whether such rights really exist, or of where they come from. However, the notion of a "fetal right to life" presents only a little more difficulty in this regard than does the notion of a "human right to life," since the former does not depend on a claim that the human fetus is already "human." In my sense of terms "right" and "life," we might even say that a dog or fetal dog has a "right to life," and that it would be cruel and immoral for a man to go around performing abortions even on dogs for no good reason.

3 Lincoln, A. (1854). In *The Collected Works of Abraham Lincoln,* R. P. Basler, editor. New Brunswick, New Jersey, Rutgers University Press, Vol. II, p. 222.

4 For a discussion of the possible biological rather than moral price of attempts to prevent the birth of defective children see Motulsky, A. G., G. R. Fraser, and J. Felsenstein (1971). In Symposium on Intra-uterine Diagnosis, D. Bergsma, editor. *Birth Defects: Original Article Series,* Vol. 7, No. 5. Also see Neel, J. (1972). In *Early Diagnosis of Human Genetic Defects: Scientific and Ethical Considerations,* M. Harris, editor. Washington, D.C., U.S. Government Printing Office, pp. 366–380.

Genetics and Reproductive Risk: Can Having Children Be Immoral?

Laura M. Purdy

Laura M. Purdy is professor of philosophy at Wells College, Aurora, New York. She is coeditor of *Feminist Perspectives in Medical Ethics* (1992) and the author of *In Their Best Interest? The Case Against Equal Rights for Children* (1992). Her many published articles include "The Morality of New Reproductive Technologies" and "Surrogate Mothering: Exploitation or Empowerment?"

Purdy argues that it can be morally wrong to reproduce in circumstances of genetic risk, most clearly in cases where there is a high risk of serious genetic disease. In developing her overall argument, she is committed to the view that we have a duty to try to provide a *minimally satisfying life* for our children. Much of Purdy's analysis focuses on Huntington's disease, and she emphasizes how the emergence of reliable genetic testing has opened up new possibilities for those at risk of passing on the disease.

Is it morally permissible for me to have children?[1] A decision to procreate is surely one of the most significant decisions a person can make. So it would seem that it ought not to be made without some moral soul-searching.

There are many reasons why one might hesitate to bring children into this world if one is concerned about their welfare. Some are rather general, like the deteriorating environment or the prospect of poverty. Others have a narrower focus, like continuing civil war in Ireland, or the lack of essential social support for child rearing persons in the United States. Still others may be relevant only to individuals at risk of passing harmful diseases to their offspring.

There are many causes of misery in this world, and most of them are unrelated to genetic disease. In the general scheme of things, human misery is most efficiently reduced by concentrating on noxious social and political arrangements. Nonetheless, we shouldn't ignore preventable harm just because it is confined to a relatively small corner of life. So the question arises: can it be wrong to have a child because of genetic risk factors?[2]

Unsurprisingly, most of the debate about this issue has focused on prenatal screening and abortion: much useful information about a given fetus can be made available by recourse to prenatal testing. This fact has meant that moral questions about reproduction have become entwined with abortion politics, to the detriment of both. The abortion connection has made it especially difficult to think about whether it is wrong to prevent a child from coming into being since doing so might involve what many people see as wrongful killing; yet there is no necessary link between the two. Clearly, the existence of genetically compromised children can be prevented not only by aborting already existing fetuses but also by preventing conception in the first place.

Worse yet, many discussions simply assume a particular view of abortion, without any recognition of other possible positions and the difference they make in how people understand the issues. For example, those who object to aborting fetuses with genetic problems often argue that doing so would undermine our conviction that all humans are in some important sense equal.[3] However, this position rests on the assumption that conception marks the point at which humans are endowed with a right to life. So aborting fetuses with genetic problems looks morally the same as killing "imperfect" people without their consent.

This position raises two separate issues. One pertains to the legitimacy of different views on abortion. Despite the conviction of many abortion activists to the contrary, I believe that ethically respectable views can be found on different sides of the debate, including one that sees fetuses as developing humans without any serious moral claim on continued life. There is no space here to address the details, and doing so would be once again to fall into the trap of letting the abortion question swallow up all others. Fortunately, this issue need not be resolved here. However, opponents of abortion need to face the fact that many thoughtful individuals do not *see* fetuses as moral persons. It follows that their reasoning process and hence the implications of their decisions are radically different from those envisioned by opponents of prenatal screening and abortion. So where the latter see genetic abortion as murdering people who just don't measure up, the former see it as a way to prevent the development of persons who are more likely to live miserable lives. This is consistent with a world view that values persons equally and holds that each deserves high quality life. Some of those who object to genetic abortion appear to be oblivious to these psychological and logical facts. It follows that the nightmare scenarios they paint for us are beside the point: many people simply do not share the assumptions that make them plausible.

How are these points relevant to my discussion? My primary concern here is to argue that conception can sometimes be morally wrong on grounds of genetic risk, although this judgment will not apply to those who accept the moral legitimacy of abortion and are willing to employ prenatal screening and selective abortion. If my case is solid, then those who oppose abortion must be especially careful not to conceive in certain cases, as they are, of course, free to follow their conscience about abortion. Those like myself who do not see abortion as murder have more ways to prevent birth.

HUNTINGTON'S DISEASE

There is always some possibility that reproduction will result in a child with a serious disease or handicap. Genetic counselors can help individuals determine whether they are at unusual risk and, as the Human Genome Project rolls on, their knowledge will increase by quantum leaps. As this knowledge becomes available, I believe we ought to use it to determine whether possible children are at risk *before* they are conceived.

I want in this paper to defend the thesis that it is morally wrong to reproduce when we know there is a high risk of transmitting a serious disease or defect. This thesis holds that some reproductive acts are wrong, and my argument puts the burden of proof on those who disagree with it to show why its conclusions can be overridden. Hence it denies that people should be free to reproduce mindless of the consequences.[4] However, as moral argument, it should be taken as a proposal for further debate and discussion. It is not, by itself, an argument in favor of legal prohibitions of reproduction.[5]

There is a huge range of genetic diseases. Some are quickly lethal; others kill more slowly, if at all. Some are mainly physical, some mainly mental; others impair both kinds of function. Some interfere tremendously with normal functioning, others less. Some are painful, some are not. There seems to be considerable agreement that rapidly lethal diseases, especially those, like Tay-Sachs, accompanied by painful deterioration, should be prevented even at the cost of abortion. Conversely, there seems to be substantial agreement that relatively trivial problems, especially cosmetic ones, would not be legitimate grounds for abortion.[6] In short, there are cases ranging from low risk of mild disease or disability to high risk of serious disease or disability. Although it is difficult to decide where the duty to refrain from procreation becomes compelling, I believe that there are some clear cases. I have chosen to focus on Huntington's Disease to illustrate the kinds of concrete issues such decisions entail. However, the arguments presented here are also relevant to many other genetic diseases.[7]

The symptoms of Huntington's Disease usually begin between the ages of thirty and fifty. It happens this way:

> Onset is insidious. Personality changes (obstinacy, moodiness, lack of initiative) frequently antedate or accompany the involuntary choreic movements. These usually appear first in the face, neck, and arms, and are jerky, irregular, and stretching in character. Contractions of the facial muscles result in grimaces; those of the respiratory muscles, lips, and tongue lead to hesitating, explosive speech. Irregular movements of the trunk are present; the gait is shuffling and dancing. Tendon reflexes are increased. . . . Some patients display a fatuous euphoria; others are spiteful, irascible, destructive, and violent. Paranoid reactions are common. Poverty of thought and impairment of attention, memory, and judgment occur. As the disease progresses, walking becomes impossible, swallowing difficult, and dementia profound. Suicide is not uncommon.[8]

The illness lasts about fifteen years, terminating in death.

Huntington's Disease is an autosomal dominant disease, meaning that it is caused by a single defective gene located on a non-sex chromosome. It is passed from one generation to the next via affected individuals. Each child of such an affected person has a fifty percent risk of inheriting the gene and thus of eventually developing the disease, even if he or she was born before the parent's disease was evident.[9]

Until recently, Huntington's Disease was especially problematic because most affected individuals did not know whether they had the gene for the disease until well into their childbearing years. So they had to decide about childbearing before knowing whether they could transmit the disease or not. If, in time, they did not develop symptoms of the disease, then their children could know they were not at risk for the disease. If unfortunately they did develop symptoms, then each of their children could know there was a fifty percent chance that they, too, had inherited the gene. In both cases, the children faced a period of prolonged anxiety as to whether they would develop the disease. Then, in the 1980s, thanks in part to an energetic campaign by Nancy Wexler, a genetic marker was found that, in certain circumstances, could tell people with a relatively high degree of probability whether or not they had the gene for the disease.[10] Finally, in March 1993, the defective gene itself was discovered.[11] Now individuals can find out whether they carry the gene for the disease, and prenatal screening can tell us whether a given fetus has inherited it. These technological developments change the moral scene substantially.

How serious are the risks involved in Huntington's Disease? Geneticists often think a ten percent risk is high.[12] But risk assessment also depends on what is at stake: the worse the possible outcome the more undesirable an otherwise small risk seems. In medicine, as elsewhere, people may regard the same result quite differently. But for devastating diseases like Huntington's this part of the judgment should be unproblematic: no one wants a loved one to suffer in this way.[13]

There may still be considerable disagreement about the acceptability of a given risk. So it would be difficult in many circumstances to say how we should respond to a particular risk. Nevertheless, there are good grounds for a conservative approach, for it is reasonable to take special precautions to avoid very bad consequences, even if the risk is small. But the possible consequences here *are* very bad: a child who may inherit Huntington's Disease has a much greater than average chance of being subjected to severe and prolonged suffering. And it is one thing to risk one's own welfare, but quite another to do so for others and without their consent.

Is this judgment about Huntington's Disease really defensible? People appear to have quite different opinions. Optimists argue that a child born into a family afflicted with Huntington's Disease has a reasonable chance of living a satisfactory life. After all, even children born of an afflicted parent still have a fifty percent chance of escaping the disease. And even if afflicted themselves, such people will probably enjoy some thirty years of healthy life before symptoms appear. It is also possible, although not at all likely, that some might not mind the symptoms caused by the disease. Optimists can point to diseased persons who have lived fruitful lives, as well as those who seem genuinely glad to be alive. One is Rick Donohue, a sufferer from the Joseph family disease: "You know, if my mom hadn't had me, I wouldn't be here for the life I have had. So there is a good possibility I will have children."[14] Optimists therefore conclude that it would be a shame if these persons had not lived.

Pessimists concede some of these facts, but take a less sanguine view of them. They think a fifty percent risk of serious disease like Huntington's appallingly high. They suspect that many children born into afflicted families are liable to spend their youth in dreadful anticipation and fear of the disease. They expect that the disease, if it appears, will be perceived as a tragic and painful end to a blighted life. They point out that Rick Donohue is still young, and has not experienced the full horror of his sickness. It is also well-known that some young persons have such a dilated sense of time that they can hardly envision themselves at thirty or forty, so the prospect of pain at that age is unreal to them.[15]

More empirical research on the psychology and life history of sufferers and potential sufferers is clearly needed to decide whether optimists or pessimists have a more accurate picture of the experiences of individuals at risk. But given that some will surely realize pessimists' worst fears, it seems unfair to conclude that the pleasures of those who deal best with the situation simply cancel out the suffering of those others when that suffering could be avoided altogether.

I think that these points indicate that the morality of procreation in situations like this demands further investigation. I propose to do this by looking first at the position of the possible child, then at that of the potential parent.

POSSIBLE CHILDREN AND POTENTIAL PARENTS

The first task in treating the problem from the child's point of view is to find a way of referring to possible future offspring without seeming to confer some sort of morally significant existence upon them. I will follow the convention of calling children who might be born in the future but who are not now conceived "possible" children, offspring, individuals, or persons.

Now, what claims about children or possible children are relevant to the morality of childbearing in the circumstances being considered? Of primary importance is the judgment that we ought to try to provide every child with something like a minimally satisfying life. I am not altogether sure how best to formulate this standard but I want clearly to reject the view that it is morally permissible to conceive individuals so long as we do not expect them to be so miserable that they wish they were dead.[16] I believe that this kind of moral minimalism is thoroughly unsatisfactory and that not many people would really want to live in a world where it was the prevailing standard. Its lure is that it puts few demands on us, but its price is the scant attention it pays to human well-being.

How might the judgment that we have a duty to try to provide a minimally satisfying life for our children be justified? It could, I think, be derived fairly straightforwardly from either utilitarian or contractarian theories of justice, although there is no space here for discussion of the details. The net result of such analysis would be the conclusion that neglecting this duty would create unnecessary unhappiness or unfair disadvantage for some persons.

Of course, this line of reasoning confronts us with the need to spell out what is meant by "minimally satisfying" and what a standard based on this concept would require of us. Conceptions of a minimally satisfying life vary tremendously among societies and also within them. *De Rigueur* in some circles are private music lessons and trips to Europe, while in others providing eight years of schooling is a major accomplishment. But there is no need to consider this complication at length here since we are concerned only with health as a prerequisite for a minimally satisfying life. Thus, as we draw out what such a standard might require of us, it seems reasonable to retreat to the more limited claim that parents should try to ensure something like normal health for their children. It might be thought that even this moderate claim is unsatisfactory since in some places debilitating conditions are the norm, but one could circumvent this objection by saying that parents ought to try to provide for their children health normal for that culture, even though it may be inadequate if measured by some outside standard.[17] This conservative position would still justify efforts to avoid the birth of children at risk for Huntington's Disease and other serious genetic diseases in virtually all societies.[18]

This view is reinforced by the following considerations. Given that possible children do not presently exist as actual individuals, they do not have a right to be brought into existence, and hence no one is maltreated by measures to avoid the conception of a possible person. Therefore, the conservative course that avoids the conception of those who would not be expected to enjoy a minimally satisfying life is at present the only fair course of action. The alternative is a laissez-faire approach which brings into existence the lucky, but only at the expense of the unlucky. Notice that attempting to avoid the creation of the unlucky does not necessarily lead to *fewer* people being brought into being; the question boils down to taking steps to bring those with better prospects into existence, instead of those with worse ones.

I have so far argued that if people with Huntington's Disease are unlikely to live minimally satisfying lives, then those who might pass it on should not have genetically related children. This is consonant with the principle that the greater the danger of serious problems, the stronger the duty to avoid them. But this principle is in conflict with what people think of as the right to reproduce. How might one decide which should take precedence?

Expecting people to forego having genetically related children might seem to demand too great a sacrifice of them. But before reaching that conclusion we need to ask what is really at stake. One reason for wanting children is to experience family life, including love, companionship, watching kids grow, sharing their pains and triumphs, and helping to form members of the next generation. Other reasons emphasize the validation of parents as individuals within a continuous family line, children as a source of immortality, or perhaps even the gratification of producing partial replicas of oneself. Children may also be desired in an effort to prove that one is an adult, to try to cement a marriage or to benefit parents economically.

Are there alternative ways of satisfying these desires? Adoption or new reproductive technologies can fulfil many of them without passing on known genetic defects. Replacements for sperm have been available for many years via artificial insemination by donor. More recently, egg donation, sometimes in combination with contract pregnancy,[19] has been used to provide eggs for women who prefer not to use their own. Eventually it may be possible to clone individual humans, although that now seems a long way off. All of these approaches to avoiding the use of particular genetic material are controversial and have generated much debate. I believe that tenable moral versions of each do exist.[20]

None of these methods permits people to extend both genetic lines, or realize the desire for immortality or for children who resemble both parents; nor is it clear that such alternatives will necessarily succeed in proving that one is an adult, cementing a marriage, or providing economic benefits. Yet, many people feel these desires strongly. Now, I am sympathetic to William James's dictum regarding desires: "Take any demand, however slight, which any creature, however weak, may make. Ought it not, for its own sole sake be satisfied? If not, prove why not."[21] Thus a world where more desires are satisfied is generally better than one where fewer are. However, not all desires can be legitimately satisfied since, as James suggests, there may be good reasons—such as the conflict of duty and desire—why some should be overruled.

Fortunately, further scrutiny of the situation reveals that there are good reasons why people should attempt—with appropriate social support—to talk themselves out of the desires in question or to consider novel ways of fulfilling them. Wanting to see the genetic line continued is not particularly rational when it brings a sinister legacy of illness and death. The desire for immortality cannot really be satisfied anyway, and people need to face the fact that what really matters is how they behave in their own lifetime. And finally, the desire for children who physically resemble one is understandable, but basically narcissistic, and its fulfillment cannot be guaranteed even by normal reproduction. There are other ways of proving one is an adult, and other ways of cementing marriages—and children don't necessarily do either. Children, especially prematurely ill children, may not provide the expected economic benefits anyway. Nongenetically related children may also provide benefits similar to those that would have been provided by genetically related ones, and expected economic benefit is, in many cases, a morally questionable reason for having children.

Before the advent of reliable genetic testing, the options of people in Huntington's families were cruelly limited. On the one hand, they could have children, but at the risk of eventual crippling illness and death for them. On the other, they could refrain from childbearing, sparing their possible children from significant risk of inheriting this disease, perhaps frustrating intense desires to procreate—only to discover, in some cases, that their sacrifice was unnecessary because they did not develop the disease. Or they could attempt to adopt or try new reproductive approaches.

Reliable genetic testing has opened up new possibilities. Those at risk who wish to have children can get tested. If they test positive, they know their possible children are at risk. Those who are opposed to abortion must be especially careful to avoid conception if they are to behave responsibly. Those not opposed to abortion can responsibly conceive children, but only if they are willing to test each fetus and abort those who carry the gene. If individuals at risk test negative, they are home free.

What about those who cannot face the test for themselves? They can do prenatal testing and abort fetuses who carry the defective gene. A clearly positive test also implies that the parent is affected, although negative tests do not rule out that possibility. Prenatal testing can thus bring knowledge that enables one to avoid passing the disease to others, but only, in some cases, at the cost of coming to know with certainty that one will indeed develop the disease. This situation raises with peculiar force the question of whether parental responsibility requires people to get tested.

Some people think that we should recognize a right "not to know." It seems to me that such a right could be defended only where ignorance does not put others at serious risk. So if people are prepared to forego genetically related children, they need not get tested. But if they want genetically related children then they must do whatever is necessary to ensure that affected babies are not the result. There is, after all, something inconsistent about the claim that one has a right to be shielded from the truth, even if the price is to risk inflicting on one's children the same dread disease one cannot even face in oneself.

In sum, until we can be assured that Huntington's Disease does not prevent people from living a minimally satisfying life, individuals at risk for the disease have a moral duty to try not to bring affected babies into this world. There are now enough options available so that this duty needn't frustrate their reasonable desires. Society has a corresponding duty to facilitate moral behavior on the part of individuals. Such support ranges from the narrow and concrete (like making sure that medical testing and counseling is available to all) to the more general social environment that guarantees that all pregnancies are voluntary, that pronatalism is eradicated, and that women are treated with respect regardless of the reproductive options they choose.

NOTES

1 This paper is loosely based on "Genetic Diseases: Can Having Children Be Immoral?" originally published in *Genetics Now,* ed. John L. Buckley (Wash-

ington, DC: University Press of America, 1978) and subsequently anthologized in a number of medical ethics texts. Thanks to Thomas Mappes and David DeGrazia for their helpful suggestions about updating the paper.

2 I focus on genetic considerations, although with the advent of AIDS the scope of the general question here could be expanded. There are two reasons for sticking to this relatively narrow formulation. One is that dealing with a smaller chunk of the problem may help us think more clearly, while realizing that some conclusions may nonetheless be relevant to the larger problem. The other is the peculiar capacity of some genetic problems to affect ever more individuals in the future.

3 For example, see Leon Kass, "Implications of Prenatal Diagnosis for the Human Right to Life," *Ethical Issues in Human Genetics,* eds. Bruce Hilton et al. (New York: Plenum Press, 1973).

4 This is, of course, a very broad thesis. I defend an even broader version in "Loving Future People," *Reproduction, Ethics and the Law,* ed. Joan Callahan (Bloomington: Indiana University Press, forthcoming).

5 Why would we want to resist legal enforcement of every moral conclusion? First, legal action has many costs, costs not necessarily worth paying in particular cases. Second, legal enforcement would tend to take the matter in question out of the realm of debate and treat it as settled. But in many cases, especially where mores or technology are rapidly evolving, we don't want that to happen. Third, legal enforcement would undermine individual freedom and decision-making capacity. In some cases, the ends envisioned are important enough to warrant putting up with these disadvantages, but that remains to be shown in each case.

6 Those who do not see fetuses as moral persons with a right to life may nonetheless hold that abortion is justifiable in these cases. I argue at some length elsewhere that lesser defects can cause great suffering. Once we are clear that there is nothing discriminatory about failing to conceive particular possible individuals, it makes sense, other things being equal, to avoid the prospect of such pain if we can. Naturally, other things rarely are equal. In the first place, many problems go undiscovered until a baby is born. Secondly, there are often substantial costs associated with screening programs. Thirdly, although women should be encouraged to consider the moral dimensions of routine pregnancy, we do

not want it to be so fraught with tension that it becomes a miserable experience. (See "Loving Future People.")

7 It should be noted that failing to conceive a single individual can affect many lives: in 1916, nine hundred and sixty-two cases could be traced from six seventeenth-century arrivals in America. See Gordon Rattray Taylor, *The Biological Time Bomb* (New York, 1968), p. 176.

8 *The Merck Manual* (Rahway, NJ: Merck, 1972), pp. 1363, 1346. We now know that the age of onset and severity of the disease is related to the number of abnormal replications of the glutamine code on the abnormal gene. See Andrew Revkin, "Hunting Down Huntington's," *Discover,* December 1993, p. 108.

9 Hymie Gordon, "Genetic Counseling," *JAMA,* Vol. 217, n. 9 (August 30, 1971), p. 1346.

10 See Revkin, "Hunting Down Huntington's," pp. 99–108.

11 "Gene for Huntington's Disease Discovered," *Human Genome News,* Vol. 5, n. 1 (May 1993), p. 5.

12 Charles Smith, Susan Holloway, and Alan E. H. Emery, "Individuals at Risk in Families—Genetic Disease," *Journal of Medical Genetics,* Vol. 8 (1971), p. 453.

13 To try to separate the issue of the gravity of the disease from the existence of a given individual, compare this situation with how we would assess a parent who neglected to vaccinate an existing child against a hypothetical viral version of Huntington's.

14 *The New York Times,* September 30, 1975, p. 1, col. 6. The Joseph family disease is similar to Huntington's Disease except that symptoms start appearing in the twenties. Rick Donohue was in his early twenties at the time he made this statement.

15 I have talked to college students who believe that they will have lived fully and be ready to die at those ages. It is astonishing how one's perspective changes over time, and how ages that one once associated with senility and physical collapse come to seem the prime of human life.

16 The view I am rejecting has been forcefully articulated by Derek Parfit, *Reasons and Persons* (Oxford: Oxford University Press, 1984). For more discussion, see "Loving Future People."

17 I have some qualms about this response since I fear that some human groups are so badly off that it might still be wrong for them to procreate, even if that would mean great changes in their cultures. But this is a complicated issue that needs its own investigation.

18 Again, a troubling exception might be the isolated Venezuelan group Nancy Wexler found where, because of in-breeding, a large proportion of the population is affected by Huntington's. See Revkin, "Hunting Down Huntington's."

19 Or surrogacy, as it has been popularly known. I think that "contract pregnancy" is more accurate and more respectful of women. Eggs can be provided either by a woman who also gestates the fetus or by a third party.

20 The most powerful objections to new reproductive technologies and arrangements concern possible bad consequences for women. However, I do not think that the arguments against them on these grounds have yet shown the dangers to be as great as some believe. So although it is perhaps true that new reproductive technologies and arrangements shouldn't be used lightly, avoiding the conceptions discussed here is well worth the risk. For a series of viewpoints on this issue, including my own "Another Look at Contract Pregnancy," see Helen B. Holmes, *Issues in Reproductive Technology I: An Anthology* (New York: Garland Press, 1992).

21 *Essays in Pragmatism,* ed. A. Castell (New York, 1948), p. 73.

Opinion in the *Matter of Baby M*
Justice Robert N. Wilentz

Robert N. Wilentz is chief justice of the New Jersey Supreme Court. A graduate of Columbia University Law School, he was admitted to the New Jersey bar in 1952 and appointed chief justice in 1979.

This case developed when Mary Beth Whitehead entered into a commercial surrogacy agreement with a married couple (Elizabeth and William Stern) and subsequently decided not to surrender the child to them. The original trial court in New Jersey ruled that the surrogacy contract was valid. It also ordered termination of Whitehead's parental rights, awarded sole custody of the child to Mr. Stern, and authorized adoption by Mrs. Stern.

Chief Justice Wilentz, writing for a unanimous New Jersey Supreme Court, argues that the surrogacy contract is invalid and unenforceable in New Jersey because it conflicts with both the statutes and public policies of that state. Although consideration of the best interests of the child leads him to award primary custody to the Sterns, he finds no basis for the termination of Whitehead's parental rights and therefore holds that she is entitled to visitation.

In this matter the Court is asked to determine the validity of a contract that purports to provide a new way of bringing children into a family. For a fee of $10,000, a woman agrees to be artificially inseminated with the semen of another woman's husband; she is to conceive a child, carry it to term, and after its birth surrender it to the natural father and his wife. The intent of the contract is that the child's natural mother will thereafter be forever separated from her child. The wife is to adopt the child, and she and the natural father are to be regarded as its parents for all purposes. The contract providing for this is called a "surrogacy contract," the natural mother inappropriately called the "surrogate mother."

We invalidate the surrogacy contract because it conflicts with the law and public policy of this State. While we recognize the depth of the yearning of infertile couples to have their own children, we find the payment of money to a "surrogate" mother illegal, perhaps criminal, and potentially degrading to women. Although in this case we grant custody to the natural father, the evidence having clearly proved such custody to be in the best interests of the infant, we void both the termination of the surrogate mother's parental rights and the adoption of the child by the wife/stepparent. We thus restore

New Jersey Supreme Court (1988). Reprinted with permission from 109 N.J. 396. Copyright © 1988 by West Publishing Co.

the "surrogate" as the mother of the child. We remand the issue of the natural mother's visitation rights to the trial court, since that issue was not reached below and the record before us is not sufficient to permit us to decide it *de novo*.

We find no offense to our present laws where a woman voluntarily and without payment agrees to act as a "surrogate" mother, provided that she is not subject to a binding agreement to surrender her child. Moreover, our holding today does not preclude the Legislature from altering the current statutory scheme, within constitutional limits, so as to permit surrogacy contracts. Under current law, however, the surrogacy agreement before us is illegal and invalid.

FACTS

In February 1985, William Stern and Mary Beth Whitehead entered into a surrogacy contract. It recited that Stern's wife, Elizabeth, was infertile, that they wanted a child, and that Mrs. Whitehead was willing to provide that child as the mother with Mr. Stern as the father.

The contract provided that through artificial insemination using Mr. Stern's sperm, Mrs. Whitehead would become pregnant, carry the child to term, bear it, deliver it to the Sterns, and thereafter do whatever was necessary to terminate her maternal rights so that Mrs.

Stern could thereafter adopt the child. Mrs. White-head's husband, Richard,[1] was also a party to the contract; Mrs. Stern was not. Mr. Whitehead promised to do all acts necessary to rebut the presumption of paternity under the Parentage Act. Although Mrs. Stern was not a party to the surrogacy agreement, the contract gave her sole custody of the child in the event of Mr. Stern's death. Mrs. Stern's status as a nonparty to the surrogate parenting agreement presumably was to avoid the application of the baby-selling statute to this arrangement.

Mr. Stern, on his part, agreed to attempt the artificial insemination and to pay Mrs. Whitehead $10,000 after the child's birth, on its delivery to him. In a separate contract, Mr. Stern agreed to pay $7,500 to the Infertility Center of New York ("ICNY"). The Center's advertising campaigns solicit surrogate mothers and encourage infertile couples to consider surrogacy. ICNY arranged for the surrogacy contract by bringing the parties together, explaining the process to them, furnishing the contractual form, and providing legal counsel.

The history of the parties' involvement in this arrangement suggests their good faith. William and Elizabeth Stern were married in July 1974, having met at the University of Michigan, where both were Ph.D. candidates. Due to financial considerations and Mrs. Stern's pursuit of a medical degree and residency, they decided to defer starting a family until 1981. Before then, however, Mrs. Stern learned that she might have multiple sclerosis and that the disease in some cases renders pregnancy a serious health risk. Her anxiety appears to have exceeded the actual risk, which current medical authorities assess as minimal. Nonetheless that anxiety was evidently quite real, Mrs. Stern fearing that pregnancy might precipitate blindness, paraplegia, or other forms of debilitation. Based on the perceived risk, the Sterns decided to forego having their own children. The decision had special significance for Mr. Stern. Most of his family had been destroyed in the Holocaust. As the family's only survivor, he very much wanted to continue his bloodline.

Initially the Sterns considered adoption, but were discouraged by the substantial delay apparently involved and by the potential problem they saw arising from their age and their differing religious backgrounds. They were most eager for some other means to start a family.

The paths of Mrs. Whitehead and the Sterns to surrogacy were similar. Both responded to advertising by ICNY. The Sterns' response, following their inquiries into adoption, was the result of their long-standing decision to have a child. Mrs. Whitehead's response apparently resulted from her sympathy with family members and others who could have no children (she stated that she wanted to give another couple the "gift of life"); she also wanted the $10,000 to help her family. . . .

. . . The two couples met to discuss the surrogacy arrangement and decided to go forward. On February 6, 1985, Mr. Stern and Mr. and Mrs. Whitehead executed the surrogate parenting agreement. After several artificial inseminations over a period of months, Mrs. Whitehead became pregnant. The pregnancy was uneventful and on March 27, 1986, Baby M was born.

Not wishing anyone at the hospital to be aware of the surrogacy arrangement, Mr. and Mrs. Whitehead appeared to all as the proud parents of a healthy female child. Her birth certificate indicated her name to be Sara Elizabeth Whitehead and her father to be Richard Whitehead. In accordance with Mrs. Whitehead's request, the Sterns visited the hospital unobtrusively to see the newborn child.

Mrs. Whitehead realized, almost from the moment of birth, that she could not part with this child. She had felt a bond with it even during pregnancy. Some indication of the attachment was conveyed to the Sterns at the hospital when they told Mrs. Whitehead what they were going to name the baby. She apparently broke into tears and indicated that she did not know if she could give up the child. She talked about how the baby looked like her other daughter, and made it clear that she was experiencing great difficulty with the decision.

Nonetheless, Mrs. Whitehead was, for the moment, true to her word. Despite powerful inclinations to the contrary, she turned her child over to the Sterns on March 30 at the Whiteheads' home.

The Sterns were thrilled with their new child. They had planned extensively for its arrival, far beyond the practical furnishing of a room for her. It was a time of joyful celebration—not just for them but for their friends as well. The Sterns looked forward to raising their daughter, whom they named Melissa. While aware by then that Mrs. Whitehead was undergoing an emotional crisis, they were as yet not cognizant of the depth of that crisis and its implications for their newly-enlarged family.

Later in the evening of March 30, Mrs. Whitehead became deeply disturbed, disconsolate, stricken with unbearable sadness. She had to have her child. She could not eat, sleep, or concentrate on anything other than her need for her baby. The next day she went to the Sterns' home and told them how much she was suffering.

The depth of Mrs. Whitehead's despair surprised

and frightened the Sterns. She told them that she could not live without her baby, that she must have her, even if only for one week, that thereafter she would surrender her child. The Sterns, concerned that Mrs. Whitehead might indeed commit suicide, not wanting under any circumstances to risk that, and in any event believing that Mrs. Whitehead would keep her word, turned the child over to her. It was not until four months later, after a series of attempts to regain possession of the child, that Melissa was returned to the Sterns, having been forcibly removed from the home where she was then living with Mr. and Mrs. Whitehead, the home in Florida owned by Mary Beth Whitehead's parents.

The struggle over Baby M began when it became apparent that Mrs. Whitehead could not return the child to Mr. Stern. Due to Mrs. Whitehead's refusal to relinquish the baby, Mr. Stern filed a complaint seeking enforcement of the surrogacy contract. He alleged, accurately, that Mrs. Whitehead had not only refused to comply with the surrogacy contract but had threatened to flee from New Jersey with the child in order to avoid even the possibility of his obtaining custody. The court papers asserted that if Mrs. Whitehead were to be given notice of the application for an order requiring her to relinquish custody, she would, prior to the hearing, leave the state with the baby. And that is precisely what she did. After the order was entered, *ex parte,* the process server, aided by the police, in the presence of the Sterns, entered Mrs. Whitehead's home to execute the order. Mr. Whitehead fled with the child, who had been handed to him through a window while those who came to enforce the order were thrown off balance by a dispute over the child's current name.

The Whiteheads immediately fled to Florida with Baby M. They stayed initially with Mrs. Whitehead's parents, where one of Mrs. Whitehead's children had been living. For the next three months, the Whiteheads and Melissa lived at roughly twenty different hotels, motels, and homes in order to avoid apprehension. From time to time Mrs. Whitehead would call Mr. Stern to discuss the matter; the conversations, recorded by Mr. Stern on advice of counsel, show an escalating dispute about rights, morality, and power, accompanied by threats of Mrs. Whitehead to kill herself, to kill the child, and falsely to accuse Mr. Stern of sexually molesting Mrs. Whitehead's other daughter.

Eventually the Sterns discovered where the Whiteheads were staying, commenced supplementary proceedings in Florida, and obtained an order requiring the Whiteheads to turn over the child. Police in Florida enforced the order, forcibly removing the child from her grandparents' home. She was soon thereafter brought to New Jersey and turned over to the Sterns. The prior order of the court, issued *ex parte,* awarding custody of the child to the Sterns *pendente lite,* was reaffirmed by the trial court after consideration of the certified representations of the parties (both represented by counsel) concerning the unusual sequence of events that had unfolded. Pending final judgment, Mrs. Whitehead was awarded limited visitation with Baby M.

The Sterns' complaint, in addition to seeking possession and ultimately custody of the child, sought enforcement of the surrogacy contract. Pursuant to the contract, it asked that the child be permanently placed in their custody, that Mrs. Whitehead's parental rights be terminated, and that Mrs. Stern be allowed to adopt the child, *i.e.,* that, for all purposes, Melissa become the Sterns' child.

The trial took thirty-two days over a period of more than two months. . . . Soon after the conclusion of the trial, the trial court announced its opinion from the bench. 217 *N.J.Super.* 313 (1987). It held that the surrogacy contract was valid; ordered that Mrs. Whitehead's parental rights be terminated and that sole custody of the child be granted to Mr. Stern; and, after hearing brief testimony from Mrs. Stern, immediately entered an order allowing the adoption of Melissa by Mrs. Stern, all in accordance with the surrogacy contract. Pending the outcome of the appeal, we granted a continuation of visitation to Mrs. Whitehead, although slightly more limited than the visitation allowed during the trial.

Although clearly expressing its view that the surrogacy contract was valid, the trial court devoted the major portion of its opinion to the question of the baby's best interests. . . .

On the question of best interests . . . the court's analysis of the testimony was perceptive, demonstrating both its understanding of the case and its considerable experience in these matters. We agree substantially with both its analysis and conclusions on the matter of custody.

The court's review and analysis of the surrogacy contract, however, is not at all in accord with ours. . . .

INVALIDITY AND UNENFORCEABILITY OF SURROGACY CONTRACT

We have concluded that this surrogacy contract is invalid. Our conclusion has two bases: direct conflict with existing statutes and conflict with the public policies of this State, as expressed in its statutory and decisional law.

One of the surrogacy contract's basic purposes, to achieve the adoption of a child through private placement, though permitted in New Jersey "is very much disfavored." Its use of money for this purpose—and we have no doubt whatsoever that the money is being paid to obtain an adoption and not, as the Sterns argue, for the personal services of Mary Beth Whitehead—is illegal and perhaps criminal. In addition to the inducement of money, there is the coercion of contract: the natural mother's irrevocable agreement, prior to birth, even prior to conception, to surrender the child to the adoptive couple. Such an agreement is totally unenforceable in private placement adoption. Even where the adoption is through an approved agency, the formal agreement to surrender occurs only *after* birth . . . , and then, by regulation, only after the birth mother has been offered counseling. Integral to these invalid provisions of the surrogacy contract is the related agreement, equally invalid, on the part of the natural mother to cooperate with, and not to contest, proceedings to terminate her parental rights, as well as her contractual concession, in aid of the adoption, that the child's best interests would be served by awarding custody to the natural father and his wife—all of this before she has even conceived, and, in some cases, before she has the slightest idea of what the natural father and adoptive mother are like.

The foregoing provisions not only directly conflict with New Jersey statutes, but also offend long-established State policies. These critical terms, which are at the heart of the contract, are invalid and unenforceable; the conclusion therefore follows, without more, that the entire contract is unenforceable.

A Conflict with Statutory Provisions

The surrogacy contract conflicts with: (1) laws prohibiting the use of money in connection with adoptions; (2) laws requiring proof of parental unfitness or abandonment before termination of parental rights is ordered or an adoption is granted; and (3) laws that make surrender of custody and consent to adoption revocable in private placement adoptions. . . .

B Public Policy Considerations

The surrogacy contract's invalidity, resulting from its direct conflict with the above statutory provisions, is further underlined when its goals and means are measured against New Jersey's public policy. The contract's basic premise, that the natural parents can decide in advance of birth which one is to have custody of the child, bears no relationship to the settled law that the child's best interests shall determine custody. . . . The surrogacy contract guarantees permanent separation of the child from one of its natural parents. Our policy, however, has long been that to the extent possible, children should remain with and be brought up by both of their natural parents. . . .

The surrogacy contract violates the policy of this State that the rights of natural parents are equal concerning their child, the father's right no greater than the mother's. . . . The whole purpose and effect of the surrogacy contract was to give the father the exclusive right to the child by destroying the rights of the mother.

The policies expressed in our comprehensive laws governing consent to the surrender of a child stand in stark contrast to the surrogacy contract and what it implies. . . .

Under the contract, the natural mother is irrevocably committed before she knows the strength of her bond with her child. She never makes a totally voluntary, informed decision, for quite clearly any decision prior to the baby's birth is, in the most important sense, uninformed, and any decision after that, compelled by a preexisting contractual commitment, the threat of a lawsuit, and the inducement of a $10,000 payment, is less than totally voluntary. Her interests are of little concern to those who controlled this transaction. . . .

Worst of all, however, is the contract's total disregard of the best interests of the child. There is not the slightest suggestion that any inquiry will be made at any time to determine the fitness of the Sterns as custodial parents, of Mrs. Stern as an adoptive parent, their superiority to Mrs. Whitehead, or the effect on the child of not living with her natural mother.

This is the sale of a child, or, at the very least, the sale of a mother's right to her child, the only mitigating factor being that one of the purchasers is the father. Almost every evil that prompted the prohibition on the payment of money in connection with adoptions exists here. . . .

The main difference [between an adoption and a surrogacy contract], that the unwanted pregnancy is unintended while the situation of the surrogate mother is voluntary and intended, is really not significant. Initially, it produces stronger reactions of sympathy for the mother whose pregnancy was unwanted than for the surrogate mother, who "went into this with her eyes wide open." On reflection, however, it appears that the essential evil is the same, taking advantage of a woman's circumstances (the unwanted pregnancy or the need for money) in order to take away her child, the difference being one of degree.

In the scheme contemplated by the surrogacy contract in this case, a middle man, propelled by profit, promotes the sale. Whatever idealism may have motivated any of the participants, the profit motive predominates, permeates, and ultimately governs the transaction. The demand for children is great and the supply small. The availability of contraception, abortion, and the greater willingness of single mothers to bring up their children has led to a shortage of babies offered for adoption. The situation is ripe for the entry of the middleman who will bring some equilibrium into the market by increasing the supply through the use of money.

Intimated, but disputed, is the assertion that surrogacy will be used for the benefit of the rich at the expense of the poor. In response it is noted that the Sterns are not rich and the Whiteheads not poor. Nevertheless, it is clear to us that it is unlikely that surrogate mothers will be as proportionately numerous among those women in the top twenty percent income bracket as among those in the bottom twenty percent. Put differently, we doubt that infertile couples in the low-income bracket will find upper income surrogates.

In any event, even in this case one should not pretend that disparate wealth does not play a part simply because the contrast is not the dramatic "rich versus poor." At the time of trial, the Whiteheads' net assets were probably negative—Mrs. Whitehead's own sister was foreclosing on a second mortgage. Their income derived from Mr. Whitehead's labors. Mrs. Whitehead is a homemaker, having previously held part-time jobs. The Sterns are both professionals, she a medical doctor, he a biochemist. Their combined income when both were working was about $89,500 a year and their assets sufficient to pay for the surrogacy contract arrangements.

The point is made that Mrs. Whitehead *agreed* to the surrogacy arrangement, supposedly fully understanding the consequences. Putting aside the issue of how compelling her need for money may have been, and how significant her understanding of the consequences, we suggest that her consent is irrelevant. There are, in a civilized society, some things that money cannot buy. In America, we decided long ago that merely because conduct purchased by money was "voluntary" did not mean that it was good or beyond regulation and prohibition. Employers can no longer buy labor at the lowest price they can bargain for, even though that labor is "voluntary," or buy women's labor for less money than paid to men for the same job, or purchase the agreement of children to perform oppressive labor, or purchase the agreement of workers to subject themselves to unsafe or unhealthful working conditions. There are, in short, values that society deems more important than granting to wealth whatever it can buy, be it labor, love, or life. Whether this principle recommends prohibition of surrogacy, which presumably sometimes results in great satisfaction to all of the parties, is not for us to say. We note here only that, under existing law, the fact that Mrs. Whitehead "agreed" to the arrangement is not dispositive.

The long-term effects of surrogacy contracts are not known, but feared—the impact on the child who learns her life was bought, that she is the offspring of someone who gave birth to her only to obtain money; the impact on the natural mother as the full weight of her isolation is felt along with the full reality of the sale of her body and her child; the impact on the natural father and adoptive mother once they realize the consequences of their conduct. Literature in related areas suggests these are substantial considerations, although, given the newness of surrogacy, there is little information.

The surrogacy contract is based on principles that are directly contrary to the objectives of our laws. It guarantees the separation of a child from its mother; it looks to adoption regardless of suitability; it totally ignores the child; it takes the child from the mother regardless of her wishes and her maternal fitness; and it does all of this, it accomplishes all of its goals, through the use of money.

Beyond that is the potential degradation of some women that may result from this arrangement. In many cases, of course, surrogacy may bring satisfaction, not only to the infertile couple, but to the surrogate mother herself. The fact, however, that many women may not perceive surrogacy negatively but rather see it as an opportunity does not diminish its potential for devastation to other women.

In sum, the harmful consequences of this surrogacy arrangement appear to us all too palpable. In New Jersey the surrogate mother's agreement to sell her child is void. Its irrevocability infects the entire contract, as does the money that purports to buy it.

TERMINATION

We have already noted that under our laws termination of parental rights cannot be based on contract, but may be granted only on proof of the statutory requirements. That conclusion was one of the bases for invalidating the surrogacy contract. Although excluding the contract as a basis for parental termination, we did not explicitly deal with the question of whether the statutory bases for termination existed. We do so here.

As noted before, if termination of Mrs. Whitehead's parental rights is justified, Mrs. Whitehead will have no further claim either to custody or to visitation, and adoption by Mrs. Stern may proceed pursuant to the private placement adoption statute. If termination is not justified, Mrs. Whitehead remains the legal mother, and even if not entitled to custody, she would ordinarily be expected to have some rights of visitation. . . .

Nothing in this record justifies a finding that would allow a court to terminate Mary Beth Whitehead's parental rights under the statutory standard. It is not simply that obviously there was no "intentional abandonment or very substantial neglect of parental duties without a reasonable expectation of reversal of that conduct in the future," quite the contrary, but furthermore that the trial court never found Mrs. Whitehead an unfit mother and indeed affirmatively stated that Mary Beth Whitehead had been a good mother to her other children. . . .

CUSTODY

Having decided that the surrogacy contract is illegal and unenforceable, we now must decide the custody question without regard to the provisions of the surrogacy contract that would give Mr. Stern sole and permanent custody. . . .

. . . The question of custody in this case, as in practically all cases, assumes the fitness of both parents, and no serious contention is made in this case that either is unfit. The issue here is which life would be *better* for Baby M, one with primary custody in the Whiteheads or one with primary custody in the Sterns.

The circumstances of this custody dispute are unusual and they have provoked some unusual contentions. The Whiteheads claim that even if the child's best interests would be served by our awarding custody to the Sterns, we should not do so, since that will encourage surrogacy contracts—contracts claimed by the Whiteheads, and we agree, to be violative of important legislatively-stated public policies. Their position is that in order that surrogacy contracts be deterred, custody should remain in the surrogate mother unless she is unfit, regardless of the best interests of the child. We disagree. Our declaration that this surrogacy contract is unenforceable and illegal is sufficient to deter similar agreements. We need not sacrifice the child's interests in order to make that point sharper. . . .

Our custody conclusion is based on strongly persuasive testimony contrasting both the family life of the Whiteheads and the Sterns and the personalities and characters of the individuals. The stability of the Whitehead family life was doubtful at the time of trial. Their finances were in serious trouble (foreclosure by Mrs. Whitehead's sister on a second mortgage was in process). Mr. Whitehead's employment, though relatively steady, was always at risk because of his alcoholism, a condition that he seems not to have been able to confront effectively. Mrs. Whitehead had not worked for quite some time, her last two employments having been part-time. One of the Whiteheads' positive attributes was their ability to bring up two children, and apparently well, even in so vulnerable a household. Yet substantial question was raised even about that aspect of their home life. The expert testimony contained criticism of Mrs. Whitehead's handling of her son's educational difficulties. Certain of the experts noted that Mrs. Whitehead perceived herself as omnipotent and omniscient concerning her children. She knew what they were thinking, what they wanted, and she spoke for them. As to Melissa, Mrs. Whitehead expressed the view that she alone knew what that child's cries and sounds meant. Her inconsistent stories about various things engendered grave doubts about her ability to explain honestly and sensitively to Baby M—and at the right time—the nature of her origin. Although faith in professional counseling is not a *sine qua non* of parenting, several experts believed that Mrs. Whitehead's contempt for professional help, especially professional psychological help, coincided with her feelings of omnipotence in a way that could be devastating to a child who most likely will need such help. In short, while love and affection there would be, Baby M's life with the Whiteheads promised to be too closely controlled by Mrs. Whitehead. The prospects for wholesome, independent psychological growth and development would be at serious risk.

The Sterns have no other children, but all indications are that their household and their personalities promise a much more likely foundation for Melissa to grow and thrive. There *is* a track record of sorts—during the one-and-a-half years of custody Baby M has done very well, and the relationship between both Mr. and Mrs. Stern and the baby has become very strong. The household is stable, and likely to remain so. Their finances are more than adequate, their circle of friends supportive, and their marriage happy. Most important, they are loving, giving, nurturing, and open-minded people. They have demonstrated the wish and ability to nurture and protect Melissa, yet at the same time to encourage her independence. Their lack of experience is more than made up for by a willingness to learn and to listen, a willingness that is enhanced by their professional training, especially Mrs. Stern's experience as a pediatrician. They are honest; they can recognize error, deal with it, and learn from it. They will try to determine rationally the best way to cope with problems in their relationship with Melissa. When the time comes to tell her about her origins, they will probably have found a means of doing so that accords with the best interests of Baby M. All in all, Melissa's future appears solid, happy, and promising with them.

Based on all of this we have concluded, independent of the trial court's identical conclusion, that Melissa's best interests call for custody in the Sterns. . . .

VISITATION

The trial court's decision to terminate Mrs. Whitehead's parental rights precluded it from making any determination on visitation. Our reversal of the trial court's order, however, requires delineation of Mrs. Whitehead's rights to visitation. It is apparent to us that this factually sensitive issue, which was never addressed below, should not be determined *de novo* by this Court. We therefore remand the visitation issue to the trial court for an abbreviated hearing and determination. . . .

We have decided that Mrs. Whitehead is entitled to visitation at some point, and that question is not open

to the trial court on this remand. The trial court will determine what kind of visitation shall be granted to her, with or without conditions, and when and under what circumstances it should commence. . . .

CONCLUSION

. . . We have found that our present laws do not permit the surrogacy contract used in this case. Nowhere, however, do we find any legal prohibition against surrogacy when the surrogate mother volunteers, without any payment, to act as a surrogate and is given the right to change her mind and to assert her parental rights. Moreover, the Legislature remains free to deal with this most sensitive issue as it sees fit, subject only to constitutional constraints. . . .

NOTE

1 Subsequent to the trial court proceedings, Mr. and Mrs. Whitehead were divorced, and soon thereafter Mrs. Whitehead remarried. Nevertheless, in the course of this opinion we will make reference almost exclusively to the facts as they existed at the time of trial, the facts on which the decision we now review was reached. We note moreover that Mr. Whitehead remains a party to this dispute. For these reasons, we continue to refer to appellants as Mr. and Mrs. Whitehead.

Surrogate Motherhood as Prenatal Adoption
Bonnie Steinbock

Bonnie Steinbock is professor of philosophy at the State University of New York, Albany. She is the editor of *Killing and Letting Die* (1980), the coeditor of *Ethical Issues in Modern Medicine* (4th ed., 1995), and the author of *Life Before Birth* (1992). Her published articles include "Prenatal Wrongful Death" and "Drunk Driving."

Steinbock maintains that commercial surrogacy contracts should not be prohibited by the state. She argues that it is unjustifiably paternalistic for the state to ban surrogacy in an effort to protect the potential surrogate from a choice that may later be regretted. She also

From *Law, Medicine, and Health Care*, vol. 16 (Spring 1988). Reprinted with permission of the author and the publisher (American Society of Law, Medicine & Ethics).

argues that concerns about a negative psychological impact on potential offspring are insufficient to warrant an outright ban. Moreover, in her view, commercial surrogacy is neither inherently exploitive nor inconsistent with human dignity. In dealing with the charge that commercial surrogacy amounts to baby selling, she insists that payment to the surrogate can be understood as compensation for "the risks, sacrifice, and discomfort the surrogate undergoes during pregnancy." Although Steinbock considers the legal prohibition of surrogacy contracts to be incompatible with a proper regard for the value of individual freedom, she believes that the practice of surrogacy should be regulated by the state. In particular, she would insist that surrogacy contracts be structured so as to allow the surrogate a postnatal waiting period during which she would be free to change her mind and keep the child.

The recent case of "Baby M" has brought surrogate motherhood to the forefront of American attention. Ultimately, whether we permit or prohibit surrogacy depends on what we take to be good reasons for preventing people from acting as they wish. A growing number of people want to be, or hire, surrogates; are there legitimate reasons to prevent them? Apart from its intrinsic interest, the issue of surrogate motherhood provides us with an opportunity to examine different justifications for limiting individual freedom.

. . . I examine claims that surrogacy is ethically unacceptable because it is exploitive, inconsistent with human dignity, or harmful to the children born of such arrangements. I conclude that these reasons justify restrictions on surrogate contracts, rather than an outright ban. . . .

SHOULD SURROGACY BE PROHIBITED?

On June 27, 1988, Michigan became the first state to outlaw commercial contracts for women to bear children for others.[1] Yet making a practice illegal does not necessarily make it go away: witness black-market adoption. The legitimate concerns that support a ban on surrogacy might be better served by careful regulation. However, some practices, such as slavery, are ethically unacceptable, regardless of how carefully regulated they are. Let us consider the arguments that surrogacy is intrinsically unacceptable.

Paternalistic Arguments

These arguments against surrogacy take the form of protecting a potential surrogate from a choice she may later regret. As an argument for banning surrogacy, as opposed to providing safeguards to ensure that contracts are freely and knowledgeably undertaken, this is a form of paternalism.

At one time, the characterization of a prohibition as paternalistic was a sufficient reason to reject it. The pendulum has swung back, and many people are willing to accept at least some paternalistic restrictions on freedom. Gerald Dworkin points out that even Mill made one exception to his otherwise absolute rejection of paternalism: he thought that no one should be allowed to sell himself into slavery, because to do so would be to destroy his future autonomy.

This provides a narrow principle to justify some paternalistic interventions. To preserve freedom in the long run, we give up the freedom to make certain choices, those that have results that are "far-reaching, potentially dangerous and irreversible."[2] An example would be a ban on the sale of crack. Virtually everyone who uses crack becomes addicted and, once addicted, a slave to its use. We reasonably and willingly give up our freedom to buy the drug, to protect our ability to make free decisions in the future.

Can a Dworkinian argument be made to rule out surrogacy agreements? Admittedly, the decision to give up a child is permanent, and may have disastrous effects on the surrogate mother. However, many decisions may have long-term, disastrous effects (e.g., postponing childbirth for a career, having an abortion, giving a child up for adoption). Clearly we do not want the state to make decisions for us in all these matters. Dworkin's argument is rightly restricted to paternalistic interferences that protect the individual's autonomy or ability to make decisions in the future. Surrogacy does not involve giving up one's autonomy, which distinguishes it from both the crack and selling-oneself-into-slavery examples. Respect for individual freedom requires us to permit people to make choices they may later regret.

Moral Objections

. . . We must all agree that a practice that exploits people or violates human dignity is immoral. However, it is not clear that surrogacy is guilty on either count.

Exploitation The mere fact that pregnancy is *risky* does not make surrogate agreements exploitive, and therefore morally wrong. People often do risky things for money; why should the line be drawn at undergoing pregnancy? The usual response is to compare surrogacy and kidney-selling. The selling of organs is prohibited because of the potential for coercion and exploitation. But why should kidney-selling be viewed as intrinsically coercive? A possible explanation is that no one would do it, unless driven by poverty. The choice is both forced and dangerous, and hence coercive.

The situation is quite different in the case of the race-car driver or stuntman. We do not think that they are *forced* to perform risky activities for money: they freely choose to do so. Unlike selling one's kidneys, these are activities that we can understand (intellectually, anyway) someone choosing to do. Movie stuntmen, for example, often enjoy their work, and derive satisfaction from doing it well. Of course they "do it for the money," in the sense that they would not do it without compensation; few people are willing to work "for free." The element of coercion is missing, however, because they enjoy the job, despite the risks, and could do something else if they chose.

The same is apparently true of most surrogates. "They choose the surrogate role primarily because the fee provides a better economic opportunity than alternative occupations, but also because they enjoy being pregnant and the respect and attention that it draws."[3] Some may derive a feeling of self-worth from an act they regard as highly altruistic: providing a couple with a child they could not otherwise have. If these motives are present, it is far from clear that the surrogate is being exploited. Indeed, it seems objectionally paternalistic to insist that she is.

Human Dignity It may be argued that even if womb-leasing is not necessarily exploitive, it should still be rejected as inconsistent with human dignity. But why? As John Harris points out, hair, blood, and other tissue is often donated or sold; what is so special about the uterus?[4]

Human dignity is more plausibly invoked in the strongest argument against surrogacy, namely, that it is the sale of a child. Children are not property, nor can they be bought or sold. It could be argued that surrogacy is wrong because it is analogous to slavery, and so is inconsistent with human dignity.

However, there are important differences between slavery and a surrogate agreement. The child born of a surrogate is not treated cruelly or deprived of freedom or resold; none of the things that make slavery so awful are part of surrogacy. Still, it may be thought that simply putting a market value on a child is wrong. Human life has intrinsic value; it is literally priceless. Arrangements that ignore this violate our deepest notions of the value of human life. It is profoundly disturbing to hear in a television documentary on surrogacy the boyfriend of a surrogate say, quite candidly, "We're in it for the money."

[The trial court judge in the Baby M case] accepted the premise that producing a child for money denigrates human dignity, but he denied that this happens in a surrogate agreement. Ms. Whitehead was not paid for the surrender of the child to the father: she was paid for her willingness to be impregnated and carry Mr. Stern's child to term. The child, once born, is his biological child. "He cannot purchase what is already his."[5]

This is misleading, and not merely because Baby M is as much Ms. Whitehead's child as Mr. Stern's. It is misleading because it glosses over the fact that the surrender of the child was part—indeed, the whole point—of the agreement. If the surrogate were paid merely for being willing to be impregnated and carrying the child to term, then she would fulfill the contract upon giving birth. She could take the money *and* the child. Mr. Stern did not agree to pay Ms. Whitehead merely to *have* his child, but to provide him with a child. The New Jersey Supreme Court held that this violated New Jersey's laws prohibiting the payment or acceptance of money in connection with adoption.

One way to remove the taint of baby-selling would be to limit payment to medical expenses associated with the birth or incurred by the surrogate during pregnancy (as is allowed in many jurisdictions, including New Jersey, in ordinary adoptions). Surrogacy could be seen, not as baby-selling, but as a form of adoption. Nowhere did the Supreme Court find any legal prohibition against surrogacy when there is no payment, and when the surrogate has the right to change her mind and keep the child. However, this solution effectively prohibits surrogacy, since few women would become surrogates solely for self-fulfillment or reasons of altruism.

The question, then, is whether we can reconcile paying the surrogate, beyond her medical expenses, with the idea of surrogacy as prenatal adoption. We can do this by separating the terms of the agreement, which include surrendering the infant at birth to the biological father, from the justification for payment. The payment should be seen as compensation for the risks, sacrifice, and discomfort the surrogate undergoes during pregnancy. This means that if, through no fault on the part of the surrogate, the baby is stillborn, she should still be paid in full, since she has kept her part of the bargain. (By contrast, in the Stern-Whitehead agreement, Ms. Whitehead was to receive only $1,000 for a stillbirth).[6] If, on the other hand, the surrogate changes her mind and decides to keep the child, she would break the agreement, and would not be entitled to any fee or to compensation for expenses incurred during pregnancy. . . .

. . . There are sound moral and policy . . . reasons to provide a postnatal waiting period in surrogate agreements. As the Baby M case makes painfully clear, the surrogate may underestimate the bond created by gestation and the emotional trauma caused by relinquishing the baby. Compassion requires that we acknowledge these findings, and not deprive a woman of the baby she has carried because, before conception, she underestimated the strength of her feelings for it. Providing a waiting period, as in ordinary postnatal adoptions, will help protect women from making irrevocable mistakes, without banning the practice.

Some may object that this gives too little protection to the prospective adoptive parents. They cannot be sure that the baby is theirs until the waiting period is over. While this is hard on them, a similar burden is placed on other adoptive parents. If the absence of a guarantee serves to discourage people from entering surrogacy agreements, that is not necessarily a bad thing, given all the risks inherent in such contracts. In addition, this requirement would make stricter screening and counseling of surrogates essential, a desirable side-effect.

Harm to Others

Paternalistic and moral objections to surrogacy do not seem to justify an outright ban. What about the effect on the offspring of such contracts? We do not yet have solid data on the effects of being a "surrogate child." Any claim that surrogacy creates psychological problems in the children is purely speculative. But what if we did discover that such children have deep feelings of worthlessness from learning that their natural mothers deliberately created them with the intention of giving them away? Might we ban surrogacy as posing an unacceptable risk of psychological harm to the resulting children?

Feelings of worthlessness are harmful. They can prevent people from living happy, fulfilling lives. However, a surrogate child, even one whose life is miserable because of these feelings, cannot claim to have been harmed by the surrogate agreement. Without the agreement, the child would never have existed. Unless she is willing to say that her life is not worth living because of these feelings, that she would be better off never having been born, she cannot claim to have been harmed by being born of a surrogate mother.

Elsewhere I have argued that children can be *wronged* by being brought into existence, even if they are not, strictly speaking, *harmed*.[7] They are wronged if they are deprived of the minimally decent existence to which all citizens are entitled. We owe it to our children to see that they are not born with such serious impairments that their most basic interests will be doomed in advance. If being born to a surrogate is a handicap of this magnitude, comparable to being born blind or deaf or severely mentally retarded, then surrogacy can be seen as wronging the offspring. This would be a strong reason against permitting such contracts. However, it does not seem likely. Probably the problems arising from surrogacy will be like those faced by adopted children and children whose parents divorce. Such problems are not trivial, but neither are they so serious that the child's very existence can be seen as wrongful.

If surrogate children are neither harmed nor wronged by surrogacy, it may seem that the argument for banning surrogacy on grounds of its harmfulness to the offspring evaporates. After all, if the children themselves have no cause for complaint, how can anyone else claim to reject it on their behalf? Yet it seems extremely counter-intuitive to suggest that the risk of emotional damage to the children born of such arrangements is not even relevant to our deliberations. It seems quite reasonable and proper—even morally obligatory—for policy-makers to think about the possible detrimental effects of new reproductive technologies, and to reject those likely to create physically or emotionally damaged people. The explanation for this must involve the idea that it is wrong to bring people into the world in a harmful condition, even if they are not, strictly speaking, harmed by having been brought into existence. Should evidence emerge that surrogacy produces children with serious psychological problems, that would be a strong reason for banning the practice.

There is some evidence on the effect of surrogacy on the other children of the surrogate mother. One woman reported that her daughter, now seventeen, who was eleven at the time of the surrogate birth, "is still having problems with what I did, and as a result she is still angry with me." She explains: "Nobody told me that a child could bond with a baby while you're still pregnant. I didn't realize then that all the times she listened to his heartbeat and felt his legs kick that she was becoming attached to him."[8]

A less sentimental explanation is possible. It seems likely that her daughter, seeing one child given away, was fearful that the same might be done to her. We can expect anxiety and resentment on the part of children whose mothers give away a brother or sister. The psychological harm to these children is clearly relevant to a determination of whether surrogacy is contrary to public policy. At the same time, it should be remembered that many things, including divorce, remarriage, and even moving to a new neighborhood, create anxiety and resentment in children. We should not use the effect on children as an excuse for banning a practice we find bizarre or offensive.

CONCLUSION

There are many reasons to be extremely cautious of surrogacy. I cannot imagine becoming a surrogate, nor would I advise anyone else to enter into a contract so fraught with peril. But the fact that a practice is risky,

foolish, or even morally distasteful is not sufficient reason to outlaw it. It would be better for the state to regulate the practice, and minimize the potential for harm, without infringing on the liberty of citizens.

NOTES

1 *New York Times,* June 28, 1988, A20.
2 Gerald Dworkin, "Paternalism," in R. A. Wasserstrom, ed., *Morality and the Law* (Belmont, Cal.: Wadsworth, 1971); reprinted in J. Feinberg and H. Gross, eds., *Philosophy of Law,* 3d ed. (Belmont, Cal.: Wadsworth, 1986), 265.
3 John Robertson, "Surrogate Mothers: Not So Novel after All," *Hastings Center Report,* 13, no. 5 (1983): 29; citing P. Parker, "Surrogate Mother's Motivations: Initial Findings," *American Journal of Psychiatry,* 140 (1983): 1.
4 J. Harris, *The Value of Life* (London: Routledge & Kegan Paul, 1985), 144.
5 In re Baby "M," 217 N.J. Super. 372, 525 A.2d 1157 (1987).
6 George Annas, "Baby M: Babies (and Justice) for Sale," *Hastings Center Report,* 17, no. 3 (1987): 14.
7 Bonnie Steinbock, "The Logical Case for 'Wrongful Life'," *Hastings Center Report,* 16, no. 2 (1986): 15.
8 "Baby M Case Stirs Feelings of Surrogate Mothers," *New York Times,* March 2, 1987, B1.

Artificial Means of Reproduction and Our Understanding of the Family
Ruth Macklin

A biographical sketch of Ruth Macklin is found on page 327.

Macklin explores the impact of artificial means of reproduction, especially surrogacy arrangements, on our understanding of the family. In addition to the biological meaning of *family,* she identifies three other determinants of meaning—law, custom, and subjective intentions. Macklin also discusses the problem of whether a child's *genetic* mother or *gestational* mother has a greater claim on the child. With reference to cases in which a surrogate is unwilling to give up a child after its birth, Macklin identifies three main options for identifying who is the "primary mother" (i.e., the woman presumed to have a greater claim on the child). One alternative is to say that gestation is the key factor, another alternative is to say that genet-

Reprinted with permission of the author and the publisher from *Hastings Center Report* 21 (January/February 1991), pp. 5–11. © The Hastings Center.

ics is the key factor, and a third alternative is to say that both gestation and genetics are significant factors. The third alternative provides a resolution for cases in which the surrogate provides both womb and egg, but it does not provide a resolution for cases in which the surrogate provides only the womb. Macklin further identifies three "supplementary views," all of which incorporate a consideration of the contribution of the genetic father.

It is an obvious truth that scientific and technologic innovations produce changes in our traditional way of perceiving the world around us. We have only to think of the telescope, the microscope, and space travel to recall that heretofore unimagined perceptions of the macrocosm and the microcosm have become commonplace. Yet it is not only perceptions, but also conceptions of the familiar that become altered by advances in science and technology. As a beginning student of philosophy, I first encountered problems in epistemology generated by scientific knowledge: If physical objects are really composed of molecules in motion, how is it that we perceive them as solid? Why is it that objects placed on a table don't slip through the empty spaces between the molecules? If the mind is nothing but electrical processes occurring in the brain, how can we explain Einstein's ability to create the special theory of relativity or Bach's ability to compose the Brandenburg Concertos?

Now questions are being raised about how a variety of modes of artificial means of reproduction might alter our conception of the family. George Annas has observed:

> Dependable birth control made sex without reproduction possible. . . . Now medicine is closing the circle . . . by offering methods of reproduction without sex; including artificial insemination by donor (AID), in vitro fertilization (IVF), and surrogate embryo transfer (SET). As with birth control, artificial reproduction is defended as life-affirming and loving by its proponents, and denounced as unnatural by its detractors.[1]

Opponents of artificial reproduction have expressed concerns about its effects on the family. This concern has centered largely but not entirely on surrogacy arrangements. Among the objections to surrogacy made by the Roman Catholic Church is the charge that "the practice of surrogate motherhood is a threat to the stability of the family."[2] But before the consequences for the family of surrogacy arrangements or other new reproductive practices can be assessed, we need to inquire into our understanding of the family. Is there a single, incontrovertible conception of the family? And

who are the "we" presupposed in the phrase, "our understanding"? To begin, I offer three brief anecdotes.

The first is a remark made by a long-married, middle-aged man at a wedding. The wedding couple were both about forty. The bride had been married and divorced once, the groom twice. During a light-hearted discussion about marriage and divorce, the middle-aged man remarked: "I could never divorce my wife. She's family!"

The second is a remark made by a four-year-old boy. I had just moved to the neighborhood and was getting to know the children. The four-year-old, named Mikey, was being tormented by a five-year-old named Timmy. I asked Mikey, "Is Timmy your brother?" Mikey replied: "Not any more. Not the way he acts!"

The third story appears in a case study presented as part of a bioethics project on everyday dilemmas in nursing home life. A resident, Mrs. Finch, is a constant complainer who seeks more choices and independence than the nursing home allows. A social worker at the home talked to Mrs. Finch about her adaptation, suggesting that she think of the residents and staff group as a large family where "we all make allowances for each other" and "we all pull our weight." Mrs. Finch responded that she is in the nursing home because she needs health care. She already has a family and does not want another one.

In my commentary on the case of Mrs. Finch, I gave an analysis that suggests some of the complexities in understanding the concept of the family. I wrote:

> Mrs. Finch is quite right to reject the social worker's suggestion that the nursing home be viewed as "a large family." A family is a well-defined social and cultural institution. People may choose to "adopt" unrelated persons into their own family, and biologically related family members may choose to "disown" one of their members (which doesn't sever the kinship ties, though it may sever relations). But an organization or institution does not become a "family" because members or residents are exhorted to treat each other in the way family members should. The social worker's well-intended chat with Mrs. Finch is an exhortation to virtue rather than a proper reminder about the resident's obligations to her new "family."[3]

THE BIOLOGICAL CONCEPT
OF FAMILY

It is possible, of course, to settle these conceptual matters simply and objectively by adopting a biological criterion for determining what counts as a family. According to this criterion, people who are genetically related to one another would constitute a family, with the type and degree of relatedness described in the manner of a family tree. This sense of *family* is important and interesting for many purposes, but it does not and cannot encompass everything that is actually meant by *family*, nor does it reflect the broader cultural customs and kinship systems that also define family ties.

What makes the first anecdote amusing is the speaker's deliberate use of the biological sense of *family* in a nonbiological context, that is, the context of being related by marriage. In saying that he could never divorce his wife because "she's family," he was conjuring up the associations normally connected with biologically related family and transferring those associations to a person related by the convention of marriage. In a society in which the divorce rate hovers around 50 percent, being a family member related by marriage is often a temporary state of affairs.

What makes the second anecdote amusing is Mikey's denial, based solely on Timmy's behavior, that his biologically related sibling was his brother. When two people are biologically related, they cannot wave away that kinship relation on grounds of their dislike of the other's character or conduct. They can sever their relationship, but not their genetic relatedness. Whether family members ought to remain loyal to one another, regardless of how they act, is an ethical question, not a conceptual one.

The third story also relies on the biological notion of family. Mrs. Finch construed the concept literally when she insisted that she already had a family and "didn't need another one." When I observed in my commentary that a family is a well-defined social and cultural institution, I meant to rebut the social worker's implication that anything one wants to call a family can thereby become a family. Yet considered from a moral perspective, our conception of the family does draw on notions of what members owe to one another in a functional understanding of the family:

> Families should be broadly defined to include, besides the traditional biological relationships, those committed relationships between individuals which fulfill the functions of family.[4]

It seems clear that we need a richer concept than that of biological relatedness to flesh out our understanding of the family. Although the biological concept is accurate in its delineation of one set of factors that determine what is a family, it fails to capture other significant determinants.

Newly developed artificial means of reproduction have rendered the term *biological* inadequate for making some critical conceptual distinctions, along with consequent moral decisions. The capability of separating the process of producing eggs from the act of gestation renders obsolete the use of the word *biological* to modify the word *mother*. The techniques of egg retrieval, in vitro fertilization (IVF), and gamete intrafallopian transfer (GIFT) now make it possible for two different women to make a biological contribution to the creation of a new life. It would be a prescriptive rather than a descriptive definition to maintain that the egg donor should properly be called the biological mother. The woman who contributes her womb during gestation—whether she is acting as a surrogate or is the intended rearing mother—is also a biological mother. We have only to reflect on the many ways that the intrauterine environment and maternal behavior during pregnancy can influence fetal and later child development to acknowledge that a gestating woman is also a biological mother. I will return to this issue later in considering how much genetic contributions should count in disputed surrogacy arrangements.

ADDITIONAL DETERMINANTS
OF THE MEANING OF *FAMILY*

In addition to the biological meaning, there appear to be three chief determinants of what is meant by *family*. These are law, custom, and what I shall call subjective intentions. All three contribute to our understanding of the family. The effect of artificial means of reproduction on our understanding of the family will vary, depending on which of these three determinants is chosen to have priority. There is no way to assign a priori precedence to any one of the three. Let me illustrate each briefly.

Law as a Determinant of Family Legal scholars can elaborate with precision and detail the categories and provisions of family law. This area of law encompasses legal rules governing adoption, artificial insemination by donor, foster placement, custody arrangements, and removal of children from a home in which they have been abused or neglected. For present purposes, it will suffice to summarize the relevant areas in which legal definitions or decisions have determined what is to count as a family.

Laws governing adoption and donor insemination stipulate what counts as a family. In the case of adoption, a person or couple genetically unrelated to a child is deemed that child's legal parent or parents. By this legal rule, a new family is created. The biological parent or parents of the child never cease to be genetically related, of course. But by virtue of law, custom, and usually emotional ties, the adoptive parents become the child's family.

The Uniform Parentage Act holds that a husband who consents to artificial insemination by donor (AID) of his wife by a physician is the legal father of the child. Many states have enacted laws in conformity with this legal rule. I am not aware of any laws that have been enacted making an analogous stipulation in the case of egg donation, but it is reasonable to assume that there will be symmetry of reasoning and legislation.

Commenting on the bearing of family law on the practice of surrogacy, Alexander M. Capron and Margaret J. Radin contend that the "legal rules of greatest immediate relevance" to surrogacy are those on adoption. These authors identify a number of provisions of state laws on adoption that should apply in the case of surrogacy. The provisions include allowing time for a "change of heart" period after the agreement to release a child, and prohibition of agreements to relinquish parental rights prior to the child's birth.[5]

Capron and Radin observe that in the context of adoption, "permitting the birth mother to reclaim a child manifests society's traditional respect for biological ties."[6] But how does this observation bear on artificial reproduction where the biological tie can be either genetic or gestational?

Consider first the case of the gestational surrogate who is genetically unrelated to the child. Does society's traditional respect for biological ties give her or the genetic mother the right to "reclaim" (or claim in the first place) the child? Society's traditional respect is more likely a concern for genetic inheritance than a recognition of the depth of the bond a woman may feel toward a child she has given birth to.

Secondly, consider the case of egg donation and embryo transfer to the wife of the man whose sperm was used in IVF. If the sperm donor and egg recipient were known to the egg donor, could the donor base her claim to the child on "society's traditional respect for biological ties"? As I surmised earlier, it seems reasonable to assume that any laws enacted for egg donation will be similar to those now in place for donor insemination. In the latter context, society's traditional respect for biological ties gave way to other considerations arising out of the desire of couples to have a child who is genetically related to at least one of the parents.

Custom as a Determinant of Family   The most telling examples of custom as a determinant of family are drawn from cultural anthropology. Kinship systems and incest taboos dictated by folkways and mores differ so radically that few generalizations are possible.

Ruth Benedict writes: "No known people regard all women as possible mates. This is not in an effort, as is so often supposed, to prevent inbreeding in our sense, for over great parts of the world it is an own cousin, often the daughter of one's mother's brother, who is the predestined spouse."[7] In contrast, Benedict notes, some incest taboos are

> extended by a social fiction to include vast numbers of individuals who have no traceable ancestors in common. . . . This social fiction receives unequivocal expression in the terms of relationship which are used. Instead of distinguishing lineal from collateral kin as we do in the distinction between father and uncle, brother and cousin, one term means literally "man of my father's group (relationship, locality, etc.) or his generation." . . . Certain tribes of eastern Australia use an extreme form of this so-called classificatory kinship system. Those whom they call brothers and sisters are all those of their generation with whom they recognize any relationship.[8]

One anthropologist notes that "the family in all societies is distinguished by a stability that arises out of the fact that it is based on marriage, that is to say, on socially sanctioned mating entered into with the assumption of permanency."[9] If we extend the notion of socially sanctioned mating to embrace socially sanctioned procreation, it is evident that the new artificial means of reproduction call for careful thought about what should be socially sanctioned before policy decisions are made.

Subjective Intention as a Determinant of Family   This category is most heterogeneous and amorphous. It includes a variety of ways in which individuals—singly, in pairs, or as a group—consider themselves a family even if their arrangement is not recognized by law or custom. Without an accompanying analysis, I list here an array of examples, based on real people and their situations.

- A homosexual couple decides to solidify their relationship by taking matrimonial vows. Despite the fact that their marriage is not recognized by civil law, they find an ordained minister who is willing to perform the marriage ceremony. Later they apply to be foster parents of children with AIDS whose biological parents have died or abandoned them. The foster agency accepts the couple. Two children are placed in foster care with them. They are now a family.

- A variation on this case: A lesbian couple has a long-term monogamous relationship. They decide they want to rear a child. Using "turkey-baster" technology, one of the women is inseminated, conceives, and gives birth to a baby. The three are now a family, with one parent genetically related to the child.

- Pat Anthony, a forty-seven-year-old grandmother in South Africa, agreed to serve as gestational surrogate for her own daughter. The daughter had had her uterus removed, but could still produce eggs and wanted more children. The daughter's eggs were inseminated with her husband's sperm, and the resulting embryos implanted in her own mother. Mrs. Anthony gave birth to triplets when she was forty-eight. She was the gestational mother and the genetic grandmother of the triplets.

- Linda Kirkman was the gestational mother of a baby conceived with a sister's egg and destined to live with the infertile sister and her husband. Linda Kirkman said, "I always considered myself her aunt." Carol Chan donated eggs so that her sister Susie could bear and raise a child. Carol Chan said: "I could never regard the twins as anything but my nephews." The two births occurred in Melbourne within weeks of each other.[10]

My point in elucidating this category of heterogeneous examples is to suggest that there may be entirely subjective yet valid elements that contribute to our understanding of the family, family membership, or family relationships. I believe it would be arbitrary and narrow to rule out all such examples by fiat. The open texture of our language leaves room for conceptions of family not recognized by law or preexisting custom.

Posing the question, Who counts as family? Carol Levine replies: "The answer to this apparently simple question is by no means easy. It depends on why the question is being asked and who is giving the answer."[11]

Levine's observation, made in the context of AIDS, applies equally well to the context of artificial means of reproduction.

THE GESTATIONAL VERSUS THE GENETIC MOTHER

One critical notion rendered problematic by the new technological capabilities of artificial reproduction is the once-simple concept of a mother. The traditional concept is complicated by the possibility that a woman can gestate a fetus genetically unrelated to her. This prospect has implications both for public policy and our understanding of the family. The central policy question is, How much should genetic relatedness count in disputed surrogacy arrangements?

A Matter of Discovery or Decision?   Which criterion—genetic or gestational—should be used to determine who is the "real" mother? I contend that this question is poorly formulated. Referring to the "real" mother implies that it is a matter of discovery, rather than one calling for a decision. To speak of "the real x" is to assume that there is an underlying metaphysical structure to be probed by philosophical inquiry. But now that medical technology has separated the two biological contributions to motherhood, in place of the single conjoint role provided by nature, some decisions will have to be made.

One decision is conceptual, and a second is moral. The conceptual question is: Should a woman whose contribution is solely gestational be termed a mother of the baby? We may assume, by analogy with our concept of paternity, that the woman who makes the genetic contribution in a surrogacy arrangement can properly be termed a mother of the baby. So it must be decided whether there can be only one mother, conceptually speaking, or whether this technological advance calls for new terminology.

Conceptual decisions often have implications beyond mere terminology. A decision not to use the term *mother* (even when modified by the adjective *gestational*) to refer to a woman who acts in this capacity can have important consequences for ethics and public policy. As a case in point, the Wayne County Circuit Court in Michigan issued an interim order declaring a gamete donor couple to be the biological parents of a fetus being carried to term by a woman hired to be the gestational mother. Upon birth, the court entered an order that the names of the ovum and sperm donors be listed on the birth certificate, rather than that of the woman who gave birth, who was termed by the court a "human incubator."[12]

The ethical question posed by the separation of biological motherhood into genetic and gestational components is, Which role should entitle a woman to a greater claim on the baby, in case of dispute? Since the answer to this question cannot be reached by discovery, but is, like the prior conceptual question, a matter for decision, we need to determine which factors are morally relevant and which have the greatest moral weight. To avoid begging any ethical questions by a choice of terminology, I use the terms *genetic mother* and *gestational mother* to refer to the women who make those respective contributions. And instead of speaking of the "real" mother, I'll use the phrase *primary mother* when referring to the woman presumed to have a greater claim on the child.

Morally Relevant Factors   The possibilities outlined below are premised on the notion that surrogacy contracts are voidable. I take this to mean that no legal presumption is set up by the fact that there has been a prior contract between the surrogate and the intended rearing parents. From an ethical perspective, that premise must be argued for independently, and convincing arguments have been advanced by a number of authors.[13] If we accept the premise that a contractual provision to relinquish a child born of a surrogacy agreement has no legal force, the question then becomes, Is there a morally relevant distinction between the two forms of surrogacy with respect to a claim on the child? Who has the weightiest moral claim when a surrogate is unwilling to give the baby up after its birth? Where should the moral presumption lie? The question may be answered in one of three ways.

1. Gestation. According to this position, whether a woman is merely the gestational surrogate, or also contributes her genetic material, makes no difference in determining moral priorities. In either case, the surrogate is the primary mother because the criterion is gestation.

The gestational position is adopted by George Annas and others who have argued that the gestational mother should be legally presumed to have the right and responsibility to rear the child. One reason given in support of this presumption is "the greater biological and psychological investment of the gestational mother in the child."[14] This is referred to as "sweat equity." A related yet distinct reason is "the biological reality that

the mother at this point has contributed more to the child's development, and that she will of necessity be present at birth and immediately thereafter to care for the child."[15]

The first reason focuses on what the gestational mother deserves, based on her investment in the child, while the second reason, though mentioning her contribution, also focuses on the interests of the child during and immediately after birth. Annas adds that "to designate the gestational mother, rather than the genetic mother, the legal or 'natural mother' would be protective of children."[16]

2. Genetics. In surrogacy arrangements, it is the inseminating male who is seen as the father, not the husband of the woman who acts as a surrogate. This is because the genetic contribution is viewed as determinative for fatherhood. By analogy, the woman who makes the genetic contribution is the primary mother. This position sharply distinguishes between the claim to the child made by the two different types of surrogate. It makes the surrogate who contributes her egg as well as her womb the primary (or sole) mother. But now recall the fact that in AID, the law recognizes the husband of the inseminated woman as the father—proof that laws can be made to go either way.

This position was supported by the court in *Smith & Smith v. Jones & Jones,* on grounds of the analogy with paternity. The court said: "The donor of the ovum, the biological mother, is to be deemed, in fact, the natural mother of this infant, as is the biological father to be deemed the natural father of this child."[17]

Legal precedents aside, is there a moral reason that could be invoked in support of this position? One possibility is "ownership" of one's genetic products. Since each individual has a unique set of genes, people might be said to have a claim on what develops from their own genes, unless they have explicitly relinquished any such claims. This may be a metaphorical sense of ownership, but it reflects the felt desire to have genetically related children—the primary motivation behind all forms of assisted reproduction.

Another possible reason for assigning greater weight to the genetic contribution is the child-centered position. Here it is argued that it is in children's best interest to be reared by parents to whom they are genetically related. Something like this position is taken by Sidney Callahan. She writes:

The most serious ethical problems in using third-party donors in alternative reproduction concern the well-being of the potential child. . . . A child who has donor(s) intruded into its parentage will be cut off from its genetic heritage and part of its kinship relations in new ways. Even if there is no danger of transmitting unknown genetic disease or causing physiological harm to the child, the psychological relationship of the child to its parents is endangered—with or without the practice of deception and secrecy about its origins.[18]

Additional considerations lending plausibility to this view derive from data concerning adopted children who have conducted searches for their biological parents, and similar experiences of children whose birth was a result of donor insemination and who have sought out their biological fathers. In the case of gestational surrogacy, the child is genetically related to both of the intended rearing parents. However, there is no data to suggest whether children born of gestational mothers might someday begin to seek out those women in a quest for their "natural" or "real" mothers.

3. Gestation and genetics. According to this position, the surrogate who contributes both egg and womb has more of a claim to being the primary mother than does the surrogate who contributes only her womb. Since the first type of surrogate makes both a genetic and a gestational contribution, in case of a dispute she gets to keep the baby instead of the biological father, who has made only one contribution. But this does not yet settle the question of who has a greater moral claim to the infant in cases where the merely gestational surrogate does not wish to give up the baby to the genetic parents. To determine that, greater weight must be given either to the gestational component or the genetic component.

Subsidiary Views   One may reject the notion that the only morally relevant considerations are the respective contributions of each type of surrogate. Another possible criterion draws on the biological conception of family, and thus takes into account the contribution of the genetic father. According to this position, two genetic contributions count more than none. This leads to three subsidiary views, in addition to the three main positions outlined above.

4. Gestational surrogates have less of a moral claim to the infant than the intended parents, both of whom have made a genetic contribution. This is because two (genetic) contributions count more than one (gestational) contribution. This view, derived from "society's traditional respect for biological ties," gives greatest weight to the concept of family based on genetic inheritance.

5. A woman who contributes both egg and womb has a claim equal to that of the biological father, since both have made genetic contributions. If genetic contribution is what determines both "true" motherhood and fatherhood, the policy implications of this view are that each case in which a surrogate who is both genetic and gestational mother wishes to keep the baby would have to go to court and be settled in the manner of custody disputes.

As a practical suggestion, this model is of little value. It throws every case of this type of surrogacy—the more common variety—open to this possibility, which is to move backwards in public policy regarding surrogacy.

6. However, if genetic and gestational contributions are given equal weight, but it is simply the number of contributions that counts, the artificially inseminated surrogate has the greater moral claim since she has made two contributions—genetic and gestational—while the father has made only one, the genetic contribution.

What can we conclude from all this about the effects of artificial means of reproduction on the family and on our conception of the family? Several conclusions emerge, although each requires a more extended elaboration and defense than will be given here.

A broad definition of *family* is preferable to a narrow one. A good candidate is the working definition proposed by Carol Levine: "Family members are individuals who by birth, adoption, marriage, or declared commitment share deep personal connections and are mutually entitled to receive and obligated to provide support of various kinds to the extent possible, especially in times of need."[19]

Some of the effects of the new reproductive technologies on the family call for the development of public policy, while others remain private, personal matters to be decided within a given family. An example of the former is the determination of where the presumptions should lie in disputed surrogacy arrangements, whose rights and interests are paramount, and what procedures should be followed to safeguard those rights and interests. An example of the latter is disclosure to a child of the facts surrounding genetic paternity or maternity in cases of donor insemination or egg donation, including the identity of the donor when that is known. These are profound moral decisions, about which many people have strong feelings, but they are not issues to be addressed by public policy. . . .

REFERENCES

1 George J. Annas, "Redefining Parenthood and Protecting Embryos," in *Judging Medicine* (Clifton, N.J.: Humana Press, 1988), p. 59. Reprinted from the *Hastings Center Report* 14, no. 5 (1984).

2 William F. Bolan, Jr., Executive Director, New Jersey Catholic Conference, "Statement of New Jersey Catholic Conference in Connection with Public Hearing on Surrogate Mothering," Commission on Legal and Ethical Problems in the Delivery of Health Care, Newark, N.J., 11 May 1988.

3 Ruth Macklin, "Good Citizen, Bad Citizen: Case Commentary," in *Everyday Ethics: Resolving Dilemmas in Nursing Home Life,* ed. Rosalie A. Kane and Arthur L. Caplan (New York: Springer, 1990), p. 65.

4 Cited in Carol Levine, "AIDS and Changing Concepts of Family," *Milbank Quarterly* 68, supp. 1 (1990): 37.

5 Alexander M. Capron and Margaret J. Radin, "Choosing Family Law over Contract Law as a Paradigm for Surrogate Motherhood," *Law, Medicine & Health Care* 16 (Spring–Summer 1988): 35.

6 Capron and Radin, "Choosing Family Law over Contract Law," p. 35.

7 Ruth Benedict, *Patterns of Culture* (New York: Mentor Books, 1934), p. 29.

8 Benedict, *Patterns of Culture,* p. 30.

9 Melville J. Herskovits, *Cultural Anthropology* (New York: Alfred A. Knopf, 1955), p. 171.

10 R. Alta Charo, "Legislative Approaches to Surrogate Motherhood," *Law, Medicine & Health Care* 16 (Spring–Summer 1988): 104.

11 Levine, "AIDS and Changing Concepts of Family," p. 35.

12 O.T.A. report, "Infertility: Medical and Social Choices," p. 284; case cited *Smith & Smith v. Jones & Jones,* 85-532014 DZ, Detroit MI, 3rd Dist. (15 March 1986), as reported in *BioLaw,* ed. James F. Childress, Patricia King, Karen H. Rothenberg, et al. (Frederick, Md.: University Publishers of America, 1986). See also George J. Annas, "The Baby Broker Boom," *Hastings Center Report* 16, no. 3 (1986): 30–31.

13 See, e.g., George J. Annas, "Death without Dignity for Commercial Surrogacy: The Case of Baby M," *Hastings Center Report,* 18, no. 2 (1988): 21–24; and Bonnie Steinbock, "Surrogate Motherhood as Prenatal Adoption," in *Surrogate Motherhood: Politics and Privacy,* ed. Larry Gostin (Bloomington: Indiana University Press, 1990), pp. 123–35.

14 Sherman Elias and George J. Annas, "Noncoital Reproduction," *JAMA* 255 (3 January 1986): 67.

15 Annas, "Death without Dignity," p. 23.

16 Annas, "Death without Dignity," p. 24.

17 Annas, "The Baby Broker Boom," p. 31.

18 "The Ethical Challenge of the New Reproductive Technology," presentation before the Task Force on New Reproductive Practices; published in John F. Monagle and David C. Thomasma, eds., *Medical Ethics: A Guide for Health Care Professionals* (Frederick, Md.: Aspen Publishers, 1987).

19 Levine, "AIDS and Changing Concepts of Family," p. 36.

Motherhood: Beyond Patriarchy
Barbara Katz Rothman

Barbara Katz Rothman is professor of sociology at Baruch College and the Graduate Center, City University of New York. She is the author of *The Tentative Pregnancy: Prenatal Diagnosis and the Future of Motherhood (1986)* and *Recreating Motherhood: Ideology and Technology in a Patriarchal Society* (1989). She is also the editor of *Encyclopedia of Childbearing: Critical Perspectives* (1993).

Reprinted with permission of the publisher from *Nova Law Review* 13 (Spring 1989), pp. 481–486. Parts of this article are drawn from the author's book, *Recreating Motherhood* (W. W. Norton & Co., 1989).

Rothman maintains that our contemporary societal thinking about procreation still reflects the historical origin of our society as a patriarchal system. Although the genetic parenthood of women is now recognized as equivalent to the genetic parenthood of men, the unique significance of gestation as constitutive of motherhood goes unrecognized. Rothman is critical of the fact that American society sometimes determines legal motherhood by reference to a woman's relationship with the father. In her view, our society and its legal system must recognize that "every woman is the mother of the child she bears, regardless of the source of the sperm, and regardless of the source of the egg."

INTRODUCTION

Law works by precedent and by analogy. While that has shown extraordinary advantages in maintaining an orderly system and avoiding capriciousness, it has its limitations. The law has a hard time confronting something new. New things can be incorporated only by stressing their points of similarity to old things, to concepts already embedded in the law.

The "something new" to which I refer here is not so much surrogacy arrangements and new reproductive technology per se, as it is the issues and concerns, the *interests,* of women where those are not the same as, or analogous to, those of men.

American law has, since the time of the constitution, continually if haltingly expanded the definition of citizen, of individual entitled to full legal rights. The rights and privileges of the white men framers of the constitution have thus been extended to men of color, to native American men, and eventually to women. In the areas of employment, housing, education—all of the areas of what we think of as the "public sphere"—this has been an effective technique to achieve a more just society.

As new concerns arise around family and procreation—the areas we think of in America as "private life"—the limitations of the workings of the law become apparent. It is these limitations which I address here.

PATRIARCHY, PATERNITY AND MATERNITY

Legal definitions of the family are reflections not of biological relationships, but rather of cultural values and ideology. The law reifies the values and beliefs of the law-makers. American family law has its roots in patriarchy, and in men's view of family relationships.

The term "patriarchy" is often used loosely as a synonym for "sexism," or to refer to any social system where men rule. The term has a more specific, technical meaning, however: the rule of fathers. It is in that specific sense that I am using it here.

Patriarchal kinship is the core of what is meant by patriarchy: the idea that paternity is the definitive social relationship. A very clear statement of patriarchal kinship is found in the book of Genesis, in the "begats." Each man, from Adam onward, is described as having begot a son in his likeness, after his image. After the birth of this firstborn son, the men are described as having lived so many years, and having begot sons and daughters. The text then turns to that firstborn son, and in turn his firstborn son after him. Women appear as "the daughters of men who bore them offspring." In a patriarchal kinship system, children are reckoned as being born to men, out of women. Women, in this system of patriarchy, bear the children of men.

The central concept here is the "seed," that part of men that grows into the children of their likeness within the bodies of women. Such a system is inevitably male dominated, but it is a particular kind of male domination. Men control women as daughters, much as they control their sons, but they also control women as the mothers of men's children. It is women's motherhood that men must control to maintain patriarchy. In a patriarchy, because what is valued is the relationship of a man to his sons, women are a vulnerability that men have: to beget these sons, men must pass their seed through the body of a woman.

While all societies appear to be male dominated to some degree, not all societies are patriarchal. In some, the line of descent is not from father to son, but along the lines of the women. These are called "matrilineal" societies: it is a shared woman that makes for shared lineage of the family group. Men still rule in these groups, but they do not rule as fathers. They rule the women and children who are related to them through their mother's line. In such a system, people are not men's children coming through the bodies of women, but the children of women.

Our society developed out of a patriarchal system, in which paternity was the fundamentally important relationship. Some of our social customs and traditions, as well as such laws as those defining "illegitimacy," reflected men's concern for maintaining paternity. But the modern American society's kinship system is not classically patriarchal. It is what anthropologists call a bilateral system, in that individuals are considered to be equally related to both their mother's and their father's "sides" of the family.

We carry our history with us, though. Out of the patriarchal focus on the seed as the source of being, on the male production of children from men's seed, has grown our current thinking about procreation.

Modern procreative technology has been forced to go beyond the sperm as seed, to recognize the egg as seed also. But the central concept of patriarchy, the importance of the seed, was retained by extending the concept to women. Women too have seed, and women too can be said to have their "own" children, just as men do. In this modified system based on the older ideology of patriarchy, women's "rights" to their children are not based on the unique relationship of pregnancy, the long months of gestation and nurturance, the intimate connections of birth and suckling, but on women's status as producers of seed. Women gain their control over their children not as mothers, but as father-equivalents. Thus the rights and privileges of men are extended to women. But there are costs, as we are increasingly coming to see.

REDEFINING MOTHERHOOD AND FATHERHOOD

When biological paternity could only be assumed and never proved, the legal relationship between men and women in marriage gave men control over the children of women: any child of a man's wife was legally a child of the man. Motherhood was obvious; and fatherhood was reckoned by the relationship of the man to the mother.

Now that biological paternity can be brought under the control of science, with doctors both controlling paternity by moving insemination from the bed to the operating table or petri dish, and by proving paternity with newly definitive paternity testing, the legal relationship between men, women and their children has begun to shift.

A man's paternity need no longer be reckoned through his legal relationship with the mother of the child, but can now be ascertained directly. In consequence, we occasionally find ourselves reckoning maternity through a woman's legal relationship with the father. Consider here the newly available technology which permits a woman to carry to term a fetus not conceived of her ovum. There is nothing in *in vitro* technology that requires the fertilized ovum to be placed in the uterus of the same woman from whom the ovum was originally retrieved. We have, to put it simply, a technology that takes Susan's egg and puts it in Mary's body. And so who, we ask, is the mother? Is Mary substituting for Susan's body, growing Susan's baby for Susan? Or is Susan's egg substituting for Mary's, growing into Mary's baby in Mary's body?

The way American society has been answering that question depends on which woman is married to the baby's father. If Mary's husband is the father, then Mary is the mother, and Susan considered an "ovum donor," comparable to a sperm donor, with no recognized claim to the child. But if Susan's husband is the father, then Susan is the mother, and Mary the surrogate, the hired uterus, the incubator. There exist now in the U.S., birth certificates that list as the mother the ovum donor, and the name of the woman who carried the pregnancy and birthed the baby is nowhere on the birth certificate. Just as there exist birth certificates that list as the mother, the woman who carried the baby, and not the name of the woman who donated the egg. Legal motherhood is being determined by the relationship of the woman to the father.

Thus, while we have moved beyond traditional patriarchal definitions, we have not moved beyond the focus on seeds and genetics, and sperm and paternity specifically. This focus on the genetic connection between parents and their children is not a simple reflection of biological reality. The parent-child relationship is invested with social and legal rights and claims that are not recognized, in this society, in any other genetic relationship. And that is not because it is a uniquely close relationship. If an individual carries a certain gene, the chances that a sibling will carry the same gene are fifty-fifty, the same as the parent-child relationship. Genetically, "there is nothing special about the parent-offspring relationship except its close degree and a certain fundamental asymmetry. The full-sib relationship is just as close."[1]

The significance we claim for the parent-child relationship is rooted in our social heritage of patriarchy: that genetic connection was the basis for men's control over the children of women. The contemporary modification of traditional patriarchy has been to recognize the genetic parenthood of women as being equivalent to the genetic parenthood of men. Genetic parenthood is the only parenthood men could have biologically; and thus in our legal system, the only parenthood that is recognized for women. The significance of gestation, having no analogy to the experience of men's parenthood, is dismissed.

SURROGACY: BEYOND BABY M

It is in this context, in which genetic parenthood is acknowledged and pregnancy ignored, that the marketing of mothering services, commercial surrogacy, has developed.

Surrogacy, some people tell us, is not new; it is as old as the bible, as old as the story of Abraham, Sarah and Hagar. But Hagar was not a surrogate mother for Ishmael. She was unquestionably the mother of that child. Sarah was not Ishmael's adoptive, foster, rearing, or social mother. She was Abraham's wife, and Hagar was the mother of the child, *his* child, the child of Abraham. If Hagar served as a surrogate, it was as a surrogate wife, bearing a child for Abraham, the child of his seed, in her body.

Abraham and Hagar were living in a true patriarchy; William Stern and Mary Beth Whitehead do not. Our society, recognizing the genetic tie between mother and child, understood Baby M to be "half his, half hers." But the child might just as well have grown in the backyard. The unique relationship of pregnancy, the motherhood experience, received no recognition. Even without a legal contract for a surrogacy arrangement, Stern had as much right to the child, in our modified patriarchy, as did Whitehead. Abraham claimed his child but acknowledged the mother. Stern claimed his child but recognized no mother, only a rented uterus, a human incubator. The court ultimately rejected his argument, but only to the extent of recognizing Whitehead's *genetic* tie to the child, not the significance of her mothering of that child through pregnancy and birth.

The "Baby M" case simply highlighted what is true for all mothers in this system: we are only recognized as half owners of the children of our bodies. Women have gained recognition of our genetic ties to our children, but we have lost recognition of our nurturance, our motherhood. In a sense, we have gained paternity rights at the cost of maternity rights.

And now that women's genetic parenthood can be split off from gestational parenthood, the costs of equating our parenthood with that of men comes clear. If parenthood is understood as a genetic relationship, divided equally between sperm and ovum donors, then where is the place for pregnancy?

The new reproductive technology permits the development of surrogacy arrangements quite different from that of the Baby M situation. What will happen as the new technology allows brokers to hire women who are not related genetically to the babies that are to be sold? Like the poor and non-white women who are hired to do other kinds of nurturing and caretaking tasks, these mothers can be paid very little, with few benefits, and no long-term commitment. The same women who are pushing white babies in strollers, white old folks in wheelchairs, can be carrying white babies in their bellies. Poor, uneducated, third world women and women of color from the United States and elsewhere, with fewer economic alternatives, can be hired more cheaply. They can also be controlled more tightly. With a legally supported surrogate motherhood contract, and with new technology, the marketing possibilities are enormous—and terrifying. Just as Perdue and Holly Farms advertise their chickens based on superior breeding and feeding, the baby brokers could begin to advertise their babies: brand-name, state-of-the-art babies, produced from the "finest" of genetic materials and an all-natural, vitamin-enriched diet.

IN SUM: BEYOND PATERNITY

We cannot allow the law to inch along, extending to women some of the privileges of patriarchy, but understanding the experiences of women only as they are analogous to those of men. What is needed is to move beyond the principles of patriarchy and beyond its modifications, to an explicit recognition of *mother-hood*. Women are not, and must not be thought of as, incubators, bearing the children of others—not the children of men, and not the children of other women. Every woman is the mother of the child she bears, regardless of the source of the sperm, and regardless of the source of the egg. The law must come to such an explicit recognition of the maternity relationship.

NOTE

1 Hamilton, *The Genetic Evolution of Social Behavior,* in THE SOCIOBIOLOGY DEBATE: READINGS ON ETHICAL AND SCIENTIFIC ISSUES 191 (A. Caplan, ed. 1978).

Donor Insemination and Responsible Parenting
Paul Lauritzen

Paul Lauritzen is associate professor of religious studies at John Carroll University. He is the author of *Religious Belief and Emotional Transformation* (1992) and *Pursuing Parenthood: Ethical Issues in Assisted Reproduction* (1993). Among his published articles is "Reflections on the Nether World: Some Problems for a Feminist Ethic of Care and Compassion."

Lauritzen identifies two problems confronting the practice of donor insemination—the problem of secrecy and the problem of asymmetry. He believes that the employment of donor insemination can be morally acceptable but is sharply critical of the secrecy that is typically associated with the practice. He emphasizes the negative consequences of secrecy and maintains that responsible parenthood is incompatible with hiding from a child the truth that he or she has been conceived via donor insemination. The problem of asymmetry arises in donor insemination because the child's mother is both a social and a biological parent but the child's father is a social but not a biological parent. Lauritzen recognizes that this asymmetry can be the basis of significant conflict but argues that the problem of asymmetry does not constitute an overwhelming obstacle for responsible parenthood.

. . . Just as we should expect a couple who are contemplating parenthood, but who do not require assisted reproduction, to consider whether they can properly care for a child at that particular point in time and under some particular set of circumstances, so we should expect a couple considering donor insemination to consider whether they can properly care for a child conceived in this particular way. So is there something about conceiving a child through donor insemination that poses a threat to that child's future well-being?

I want to focus on two such dangers that donor insemination poses for responsible parenthood. The first arises from the secrecy that now typically surrounds donor insemination. The second emerges from the asymmetry that donor insemination creates between the mother of the donor child, who is both the biological and the social mother, and the father of the child, who is the social but not the biological father. The first obstacle is a function of the current practice of donor insemination, and I will argue that practice can and should be changed. The second obstacle is less tractable, but it is not, I will argue, an insuperable barrier to responsible parenthood.

Reprinted with permission of Indiana University Press from Paul Lauritzen, *Pursuing Parenthood: Ethical Issues in Assisted Reproduction* (1993), pp. 83–91.

THE PROBLEM OF SECRECY

One of the most striking features of donor insemination as it is currently practiced is the secrecy that surrounds it. Although the Office of Technology Assessment estimates that approximately 30,000 children are born every year of donor insemination in the United States, very little is known about these children, their parents, or the donors. There are a number of reasons for this lack of information. Because no formal process exists for screening prospective donor parents such as exists with adoption and because the husband of the child's mother is typically listed as the child's father on the birth certificate there is little public information available even about general trends associated with donor insemination; specific information is even harder to obtain. According to the OTA, only about half of the physicians doing donor inseminations keep records sufficiently specific to permit them to identify a particular donor for a particular pregnancy, and a majority would not release recorded information to anyone, even if all identifying information were removed.[1]

The fact that so little public information is available on donor insemination, however, does not necessarily mean that donor insemination is typically undertaken in secret. There is a difference between privacy and secrecy, and physicians may protect the confidentiality of the physician-patient relationship as indeed they may protect the privacy of sperm donors by assuring anonymity without counseling or sanctioning secrecy.[2] Nevertheless, it appears that most physicians counsel prospective donor parents to keep the truth about donor insemination not simply private but secret, that is, hidden from immediate family and the child. The view of the Royal College of Obstetricians and Gynecologists appears to be the norm. "Unless you [the parents] decide to tell the child," they write, "there is no reason for him (or her) ever to know that he (or she) was conceived by AID."[3] The clear implication is that if there is no reason to know, there is no reason for the couple to decide to tell the child. Add to this the fact that the few studies that have queried prospective donor parents have found that the majority either decided not to tell the child the truth about his or her conception or were undecided about whether to tell the truth as they actually began donor insemination, and we can safely conclude that donor insemination is most frequently undertaken in secrecy and that the lack of detailed record-keeping is often a form of collusion in the maintenance of the secret.[4] My experience certainly bears this out. When donor insemination was offered to my wife and me as a possible form of treatment, we were advised by the head of the donor program not to tell the child because the child did not need to know. Can such secrecy be justified morally?

My own view is that it cannot. Indeed, I believe that the secrecy in which donor insemination is now typically undertaken is a serious obstacle to responsible parenthood and thus a reason to oppose this form of assisted reproduction in many cases. To keep the truth about a child's conception hidden from him is, at least in theory if not always in practice, to plant at the heart of the parent-child relationship the seed of its undoing and the potential for serious psychological and emotional harm to the child.

That secrecy cannot be justified in relation to donor insemination can be seen by examining the reasons for and against maintaining the secrecy and exploring the likely consequences of keeping this information hidden. As Ken Daniels has pointed out, a variety of explanations have been offered to account for the secrecy surrounding donor insemination.[5] Three of the suggested explanations appear to be plausible reasons to which parents might appeal to justify secrecy. First, it might be argued that the truth should be concealed to protect the child from any stigma or disapprobation that is associated with donor insemination. Since donor insemination is not particularly common, and since

donor insemination is still controversial, to tell the child that he or she was conceived through DI is to put the child at risk of feeling, or being treated as, marginal. So one reason is to protect the child.

A second reason is to protect the donor. George Annas has suggested that this is the primary reason donor insemination is conducted in secret.[6] Because so few states have, until recently, addressed the issue surrounding the legal rights and responsibilities of parenthood in DI cases, secrecy protected the donor from liability for child support for any children produced through DI or from claims of inheritance from such offspring. Since the legal situation was uncertain, secrecy protected the donor from legal responsibility and thus ensured a reliable pool of donors, who might otherwise refuse to participate. Physicians who counsel secrecy may thus be understood as acting to protect the anonymity of donors in order to ensure a continued supply of sperm, and parents who embrace secrecy may be understood as acting to protect the donor in order to protect themselves from an unwelcome and unexpected assertion of parental rights on the part of the donor as biological father.

If the first argument for secrecy is to protect the child and the second is to protect the donor, the third is to protect the infertile husband. In their study of donor insemination, for example, Baran and Pannor found that many of the infertile men who consented to donor insemination to overcome childlessness did so "because it would permit them to appear fertile in the eyes of the outside world."[7] Indeed, Baran and Pannor suggest that one of the reasons donor insemination may be so popular as a form of treatment for male infertility is that it offers an infertile man the hope that he may feel fertile if he appears fertile. Secrecy, however, is necessary to protect the appearance of fertility, and so secrecy protects an infertile husband by allowing him to avoid the pain and embarrassment of public recognition of his inability to father a child. Baran and Pannor are not alone in suggesting this explanation. Drawing on in-depth interviews with sixty couples who are parents of DI children, Snowden also concluded that the main reason for secrecy was to protect an infertile husband from public disclosure of his problem.[8]

What reasons weigh against secrecy? The primary reason is that to hide the truth about a child's conception from him is to build the parent-child relationship on a foundation of deception. I [reject] the claim that the parent-child bond requires a biological base, but this is not to say that we may put a fiction in its place. Indeed, to reject the necessity of biological connection to relational bonds is to reject the necessity of lying about biological connection to ensure those bonds. Notice that in rejecting secrecy here I am not saying that a child has a right to know his or her biological parents; this is a stronger and more controversial claim.[9] Nor am I saying that a parent-child bond depends upon complete or total honesty. Rather, I am suggesting that there must not be deception at the core of the parent-child relationship. Such a relationship depends on truth telling, and it creates expectations of truthfulness that will be violated when a child is misled about such a basic matter as the identity of the biological father. At the very least, not telling the child the truth about donor insemination will be deceptive. Even if the child never asks directly about his origins, even if the parents do not have to lie about the conception, they will be intentionally deceiving the child, who will reasonably assume that he is the biological offspring of his parents.

Unfortunately, the deception is unlikely to end with merely withholding the truth. As Sisela Bok has noted, lies are particularly corrosive and contagious within families. "The need to shore up lies, [to] keep them in good repair," she writes, "the anxieties relating to possible discovery, the entanglements and threats to integrity—are greatest in a close relationship where it is rare that one lie will suffice."[10] The truth of what Bok says here is even more striking when we extend her reasoning to cover, not one isolated incident of lying in a close relationship, but a whole relationship built on a lie. Indeed, the notion of "living a lie" seems particularly apt to capture a father's relation to a donor child from whom he has kept the truth. The pattern of deceit that such a life involves is simply incompatible with the commitments that responsible parenthood entails.

Deceit is incompatible with responsible parenthood, not simply in theory but in practice as well. The effort to "live a lie" will be accompanied by a sense of shame and guilt that will do nothing to foster the parent-child relationship. On the contrary, the anxiety that comes from persistent evasiveness and from the constant fear of disclosure will be a significant barrier between parent and child. Where trust should be paramount, we can expect fear and suspicion: the father's fear of being discovered, the child's suspicion that all is not what it seems. This is precisely what Baran and Pannor found in their study of seventy donor insemination families and nineteen donor offspring, and the picture they draw of the consequences of keeping donor insemination secret is so disturbing, it is worth looking briefly at their findings.

According to Baran and Pannor, the destructive dynamic of secrecy is readily discerned. When donor insemination is used to circumvent male infertility, secrecy is attractive because it allows an infertile male to hide his problem from everyone, save his spouse. Unfortunately, to mask a problem is not to resolve it, and secrecy only serves to delay an acknowledgment of the emotional and psychological effects of sterility. Infertile individuals need to mourn and grieve the children they will not produce, they need to resolve any feelings of inadequacies that sterility may engender, and secrecy is an obstacle to meeting both needs. The upshot of undertaking donor insemination without resolving these difficulties, however, is that the relationship of the parents to each other and to any children they may raise together is fundamentally altered. The man's spouse knows the truth about his inadequacy and becomes more powerful; the child is a constant reminder of that inadequacy and may be treated accordingly.

Baran and Pannor summarize their findings as follows:

> For most of the men we interviewed, the choice of donor insemination had been an acute response to the pain they were experiencing. They never permitted themselves the time and opportunity to explore their feelings about the devastating ego blow. They prevented themselves from becoming comfortable with and accepting of their handicap. Instead, they cast the handicap in concrete, and their feelings of inadequacy were continuously reinforced by visual proof: their donor offspring.
>
> With this enormous deficit in place, the relationship between the husband and wife had to be realigned. The husband became weaker and more passive; the wife became stronger and more powerful. The wife was the real mother of the children, and this message, although never spoken, was clearly given to the husband in many ways. The husband could be devoted and caring toward the children, while at the same time recognizing the difference between his parental role and his wife's.[11]

Moreover, according to Baran and Pannor, the children in donor insemination families are generally aware of the difference in roles played by their parents and are often suspicious that something is not right with their family. Further, however hard the parents work at maintaining the secret, disclosure is only an angry word away. Many children will thus learn the truth ultimately in any event, often under the worst possible circumstances. This was true of the donor children Baran and Pannor interviewed, almost all of whom "had learned the truth of their origins in a punitive manner, when their parents' relationship began to disintegrate."[12] It will not be surprising to learn that discovery of the truth under these circumstances was deeply traumatic. Baran and Pannor concluded that, for all the parties involved, secrecy is destructive. It is destructive of the parents' relationship to one another because it reinforces a sense of failure that will interfere with truly equal and cooperative parenting. It is destructive of the parents' relationship to a child because it is grounded on an unstable foundation. When secrecy is the norm, a donor child may become an unwelcome reminder of unresolved failure or a potential weapon in a power struggle between the parents or both.

In my terminology, secrecy is a serious obstacle to responsible parenting. If I am right that responsible parenting should be both the goal we seek to promote and the standard by which we judge assisted reproduction, then at the very least we should be skeptical about the legitimacy of donor insemination as it is currently practiced. When we further consider the reasons given for secrecy in light of the reasons given against it, we cannot but conclude that donor insemination undertaken in secret is morally unacceptable. Recall the reasons for maintaining secrecy. The first was that secrecy protects the child from harm. Given the impact that secrecy is likely to have on the parent-child relationship, we may well ask whether secrecy causes more harm than it could possibly prevent. Moreover, even if it were the case that harm came to the child as the result of being conceived in a way not fully accepted by everyone in our society, it does not follow that donor insemination should then be undertaken in secret. Rather than hide the truth, the appropriate response would be to combat the fear and prejudice that causes donor insemination to be stigmatized or to avoid donor insemination altogether in order to avoid possible harm.

The second and third reasons to maintain secrecy fare no better. As we have seen, secrecy to hide the embarrassment of infertility hides, too, the pain and suffering that accompany it. Secrecy thus protects the infertile from embarrassment, but at a very high price. When pain and anger cannot be acknowledged, they cannot be resolved either. Behind the mask of apparent fertility, there is likely to be the clenched jaw of resentment. So secrecy to protect an infertile man from embarrassment appears problematic even as a measure to protect a husband from harm. Is protection of the donor any more compelling a reason to keep donor insemination a secret?

In one sense, of course, this question supervenes upon the question of whether donor insemination, with or without secrecy, is morally acceptable. If the concern in protecting donors is to ensure a pool of available donors in order to maintain the practice of donor insemination, then we first need to know whether the practice is worth saving. Yet even if we reach the conclusion, as I have, that donor insemination in general is morally acceptable, it does not follow that secrecy is justified to maintain the practice or even that it is necessary. I have already suggested implicitly why I think truthfulness is not incompatible with donor anonymity, at least for a considerable period of time. If we draw a distinction between secrecy and privacy, then it makes sense to affirm openness while nevertheless guarding privacy and anonymity, constrained only by concern for the well-being of the child.

THE PROBLEM OF ASYMMETRY

We began our discussion of secrecy in donor insemination in response to the question of whether there is anything about conceiving a child through DI that stands as an obstacle to discharging the core commitments of responsible parenthood. I suggested that although secrecy is not a constitutive feature of donor insemination, it is a pervasive part of current DI practice and is in fact a barrier to the development of a healthy parent-child relationship. I now consider an aspect of donor insemination that is a constitutive feature of the practice and that many think is an obstacle to responsible parenthood, namely, the asymmetry between the mother's relation to the child and the father's. The difference between the two relations is clear: the mother is both a biological and social parent to the child, whereas the father is only a social parent. Will this difference impede responsible parenting?

I have already suggested that the mere absence of genetic connection does not bar the development of a caring nurturing relationship of a social parent to a child. The evidence from adoption is clear on this point. It is important to notice, however, that donor insemination is here quite different from adoption. In the case of adoption, a couple is in the same position vis-à-vis the child: neither is a biological parent, both are social parents. With donor insemination, this is not the case. The mother is the biological parent, and the father is not. We have seen from the study undertaken by Baran and Pannor that when this discrepancy in relation is kept secret, it easily contributes to a power struggle between the parents that has a deleterious effect on the father's relation to the child. At the very least, then, donor insemination is different from adoption in that we can expect the absence of a genetic relation to have greater significance in donor insemination than in adoption. Even if the asymmetry is not kept secret, it may contribute to stress in the marriage that would not exist in the case of adoption. For there is a difference between the mother's relation to the child and the father's that is ineradicable; it can be overcome but it cannot be eliminated.

Overcoming this difference, however, may prove extremely difficult. When the child is young, there will be the inevitable speculation by others about whom the child resembles. For the father this is likely to be painful and to frustrate rather than further the parent-child bond. If the child develops in a way or with interests unlike the father, or if the child is particularly close to the mother, the father may feel left out. If the child is told about the conception, he is likely at some point to wield this information like a blunt instrument to inflict pain. He may shout in anger that he hates his mother, but it is only to his father that he will say that he is not his real parent. So the absence of genetic relation is likely to be painful and isolating, and this is a pain and isolation that the mother cannot fully share. . . .

. . . Conceiving a child through donor insemination may introduce a series of important life experiences into a marriage that cannot be fully shared, however committed a couple is to one another. This lack of mutuality may interfere with the couple's ability to care for and to love the child that is created.

The question, of course, is whether the disunity that donor insemination may introduce into a relationship is an overwhelming obstacle to responsible parenthood. The answer, it seems to me, is that it is not. To be sure, we must not dismiss this concern too quickly. The potential for significant conflict exists, and this conflict could lead to serious harm to the child. Yet we must also acknowledge that the potential for conflict or disunity exists whenever a child is created, and the circumstances that increase the potential for conflict in this instance are not so different from those in other cases that we currently accept. So-called blended families in which children are raised by a biological parent and a nonbiological parent experience many of the same difficulties raised by donor insemination. Nevertheless, in the case of blended families we believe that a committed relation based on honesty, trust, and respect can over-

come the difficulties that everyone acknowledges. The same can be said of donor insemination. No one should be deceived about the difficulties that may arise when parenthood is pursued in this way, but neither should the pitfalls be exaggerated. . . .

NOTES

1 U.S. Congress, Office of Technology Assessment, *Artificial Insemination Practice in the United States: Summary of a 1987 Survey* (Washington: Government Printing Office, 1988), p. 10.

2 They would, however, be sanctioning secrecy, in my view, if they withheld nonidentifying information about donors.

3 As quoted in Ken R. Daniels, "Artificial Insemination Using Donor Semen and the Issue of Secrecy: The Views of Donors and Recipient Couples," *Social Science and Medicine* 27/4 (1988): 379.

4 We can see how the absence of record-keeping can serve to support secrecy by noting that one justification for not telling a child about his or her conception could well be that, in the absence of available records, such information could not be put to any use by the child. He could not seek out his biological father, nor could he even obtain useful medical information.

5 Daniels, "Artificial Insemination Using Donor Semen," p. 378.

6 George J. Annas, "Fathers Anonymous: Beyond the Best Interests of the Sperm Donor," *Family Law Quarterly* 14 (1980): 1–13.

7 Annette Baran and Reuben Pannor, *Lethal Secrets: The Shocking Consequences and Unsolved Problems of Artificial Insemination* (New York: Warner Books, 1989), p. 50.

8 See Daniels, "Artificial Insemination Using Donor Semen," p. 378.

9 Although I would resist using the language of "rights" here, I believe that children conceived through DI should be able to learn the identity of their genetic parents, if they so choose.

10 Sisela Bok, *Lying: Moral Choice in Public and Private Life* (New York: Vintage Books, 1978), p. 224.

11 Baran and Pannor, *Lethal Secrets,* p. 51.

12 Ibid., p. 153.

Creating Embryos
Peter Singer

A biographical sketch of Peter Singer is found on page 235.

Singer identifies seven distinct objections that have been made to the use of in vitro fertilization (IVF) even in the "simple case"—a case in which a married couple is infertile, only eggs and sperm provided by the couple are involved, and all resulting embryos are transferred to the uterus of the wife. He takes some of these objections more seriously than others but ultimately concludes that none should "count against going ahead" with IVF in the simple case. Singer then considers a number of variations on the simple case, and he identifies the moral status of the embryo as an underlying issue of great importance. In his view, early embryos have no moral status because they are incapable of feeling pain or pleasure. Accordingly, he finds no ethical problem with freezing early embryos, discarding them, or using them for research purposes. Singer concludes with a brief discussion of future possibilities associated with IVF technology. In particular, he considers genetic engineering.

The treatment of human embryos became a matter of public controversy in July 1978. That month saw the birth of Louise Brown, the first human being to have developed from an embryo which at some point in its existence was outside a human body. This marked the beginning of what can properly be called a revolution in human reproduction. The point is not that *in vitro* fertilization (the technique used to make possible the birth of Louise Brown) is itself so extraordinary. On the contrary, *in vitro* fertilization, or IVF, can be seen as simply a way of overcoming certain forms of infertility, such as blocked fallopian tubes. In this sense, IVF is no more revolutionary than a microsurgical operation to remove the blockage in the tubes. But IVF is revolutionary because it brings the embryo out of the human body. Once the embryo is in the open, human beings can observe it, manipulate it, and make life-or-death decisions about it. These possibilities make IVF, and its future applications, a subject of the utmost moral importance.

Consider what has already happened, all within the first decade after Brown. Women who do not produce eggs have been given eggs by other women who do; they

From *Ethical Issues at the Outset of Life* (1987), edited by William B. Weil, Jr., and Martin Benjamin, pp. 43–51, 57–59, 60–62. Based on work done together with Deane Wells and previously published in *Making Babies* (1985). Reprinted with permission of Scribner's, an imprint of Simon & Schuster. Copyright © 1984, 1985 Peter Singer and Deane Wells.

have then given birth to babies to whom they are genetically entirely unrelated (1).

Embryos have been frozen in liquid nitrogen, stored for more than a year, thawed, and then transferred to women who have given birth to normal children. In one case, two "twins"—that is, children conceived from eggs produced by a single ovulatory cycle—were born 16 months apart. Another case illustrated the pitfalls of embryo freezing: two embryos, in storage in a Melbourne laboratory, were orphaned when their parents were killed in a plane crash, apparently leaving no instructions regarding the disposition of their embryos (1).

Scientists have begun to speculate on the medical purposes to which embryos might be put. Dr. Robert Edwards, the scientist who, together with Patrick Steptoe, made it possible for Louise Brown to be born, has suggested that if embryos could be grown for about 17 days, we could take from them developing blood cells which would have the potential to overcome such fatal diseases as sickle cell anemia and perhaps leukemia (2).

There was a time when our ethical codes could slowly adapt to changing circumstances. Those days are gone. We have to decide, right now, whether the moral status of embryos is such that it is wrong to freeze them or experiment upon them. We have also to make an immediate decision on whether there is any objection to allowing some women to carry and bring to birth embryos to which they have no genetic link. We have, at most, until the end of the century to decide how to handle new technologies for selecting and manipulating embryos, technologies that will force us to ask which human qualities are most desirable. We must start by acquainting ourselves with the new techniques and deciding which of them should form part of the society in which we live.

IVF: THE SIMPLE CASE

The so-called simple case of IVF is that in which a married, infertile couple use an egg taken from the wife and sperm taken from the husband, and all embryos created are inserted into the womb of the wife. This case allows us to consider the ethics of IVF in itself, without the complications of the many other issues that can arise in different circumstances. Then we can go on to look at these complications separately.

The Technique

The technique itself is now well known and is fast becoming a routine part of infertility treatment in many countries. The infertile woman is given a hormone treatment to induce her ovaries to produce more than one egg in her next cycle. Her hormone levels are carefully monitored to detect the precise moment at which the eggs are ripening. At this time the eggs are removed. This is usually done by laparoscopy, a minor operation in which a fine tube is inserted into the woman's abdomen and the egg is sucked out up the tube. A laparoscope, a kind of periscope illuminated by fiber optics, is also inserted into the abdomen so that the surgeon can locate the place where the ripe egg is to be found. Instead of laparoscopy, some IVF teams are now using ultrasound techniques, which eliminate the need for a general anesthetic.

Once the eggs have been collected they are placed in culture in small glass dishes known as petri dishes, not in test tubes despite the popular label of "test-tube babies." Sperm is then obtained from the male partner by means of masturbation and placed with the egg. Fertilization follows in at least 80 percent of the ripe eggs. The resulting embryos are allowed to cleave once or twice and are usually transferred to the woman some 48 to 72 hours after fertilization. The actual transfer is done via the vagina and is a simple procedure.

It is after the transfer, when the embryo is back in the uterus and beyond the scrutiny of medical science, that things are most likely to go wrong. Even with the most experienced IVF teams, the majority of embryos transferred fail to implant in the uterus. One pregnancy for every five transfers is currently considered to be a good working average for a competent IVF team. Many of the newer teams fail to achieve anything like this rate. Nevertheless, there are so many units around the world now practicing IVF that thousands of babies have been produced as a result of the technique. IVF has ceased to be experimental and is now a routine, if still "last resort" method of treating some forms of infertility.

Objections to the Simple Case

There is some opposition to IVF even in the simple case. The most frequently heard objections are as follows:

1. IVF is unnatural.
2. IVF is risky for the offspring.
3. IVF separates the procreative and the conjugal aspects of marriage and so damages the marital relationship.
4. IVF is illicit because it involves masturbation.
5. Adoption is a better solution to the problem of childlessness.
6. IVF is an expensive luxury and the resources would be better spent elsewhere.
7. IVF allows increased male control over reproduction and hence threatens the status of women in the community.

We can deal swiftly with the first four of these objections. If we were to reject medical advances on the grounds that they are "unnatural" we would be rejecting modern medicine as a whole, for the very purpose of the medical enterprise is to resist the ravages of nature which would otherwise shorten our lives and make them much less pleasant. If anything is in accordance with the nature of our species, it is the application of our intelligence to overcome adverse situations in which we find ourselves. The application of IVF to infertile couples is a classic example of this application of human intelligence.

The claim that IVF is risky for the offspring is one that was argued with great force before IVF became a widely used technique. It is sufficient to note that the results of IVF so far have happily refuted these fears. The most recent Australian figures, for example, based on 934 births, indicate that the rate of abnormality was 2.7%, which is very close to the national average of 1.5%. When we take into account the greater average age of women seeking IVF, as compared with the child-bearing population as a whole, it does not seem that the *in vitro* technique itself adds to the risk of an abnormal offspring. This view is reinforced by the fact that the abnormalities were all ones that arise with the ordinary method of reproduction; there have been no new "monsters" produced by IVF (3). Perhaps we still cannot claim with statistical certainty that the risk of defect is no higher with IVF than with the more common method of conception; but if the risk is higher at all, it would appear to be only very slightly higher, and still within limits which may be considered acceptable.

The third and fourth objections have been urged by spokesmen for certain religious groups, but they are difficult to defend outside the confines of particular religions. Few infertile couples will take seriously the view that their marital relationship will be damaged if they use the technique which offers them the best chance of having their own child. It is in any case extraordinarily paternalistic for anyone else to tell a couple that they should not use IVF because it will harm their marriage. That, surely, is for them to decide.

The objection to masturbation comes from a similar source and can be even more swiftly dismissed. Religious prohibitions on masturbation are taboos from past times which even religious spokesmen are beginning to consider outdated. Moreover, even if one could defend a prohibition on masturbation for sexual pleasure—perhaps on the (very tenuous) ground that sexual activity is wrong unless it is directed either toward procreation or toward the strengthening of the bond between marriage partners—it would be absurd to extend a prohibition with that kind of rationale to a case in which masturbation is being used in the context of a marriage and precisely in order to make reproduction possible. (The fact that some religions do persist in regarding masturbation as wrong, even in these circumstances, is indicative of the folly of an ethical system based on absolute rules, irrespective of the circumstances in which those rules are being applied, or the consequences of their application.)

Overpopulation and the Allocation of Resources

The next two objections, however, deserve more careful consideration. In an overpopulated world in which there are so many children who cannot be properly fed and cared for, there is something incongruous about using all the ingenuity of modern medicine to create more children. And similarly, when there are so many deaths caused by preventable diseases, is there not something wrong with the priorities which lead us to develop expensive techniques for overcoming the relatively less serious problem of infertility?

These objections are sound to the following extent: in an ideal world we would find loving families for unwanted children before we created additional children; and in an ideal world we would clear up all the preventable ill-health and malnutrition-related diseases before we went on to tackle the problem of infertility. But is it appropriate to ask, of IVF alone, whether it can stand the test of measurement against what we would do in an ideal world? In an ideal world, none of us would consume more than our fair share of resources. We would not drive expensive cars while others die for the lack of drugs costing a few cents. We would not eat a diet rich in wastefully produced animal products while others cannot get enough to nourish their bodies. We cannot demand more of infertile couples than we are ready to demand of ourselves. If fertile couples are free to have large families of their own, rather than adopt destitute children from overseas, infertile couples must also be free to do what they can to have their own families. In both cases, overseas adoption, or perhaps the adoption of local children who are unwanted because of some impairment, should be considered; but if we are not going to make this compulsory in the former case, it should not be made compulsory in the latter.

There is a further question: to what extent do infertile couples have a right to assistance from community medical resources? Again, however, we must not single out IVF for harsher treatment than we give to other medical techniques. If tubal surgery is available and covered by one's health insurance, or is offered as part of a national health scheme, then why should IVF be treated any differently? And if infertile couples can get free or subsidized psychiatry to help them overcome the psychological problems of infertility, there is something absurd about denying them free or subsidized treatment which could overcome the root of the problem, rather than the symptoms. By today's standards, after all, IVF is not an inordinately expensive medical technique; and there is no country, as far as I know, which limits its provision of free or subsidized health care to those cases in which the patient's life is in danger. Once we extend medical care to cover cases of injury, incapacity, and psychological distress, IVF has a strong claim to be included among the range of free or subsidized treatments available.

The Effect on Women

The final objection is one that has come from some feminists. In a recently published collection of essays by women titled *Test-Tube Women: What Future for Motherhood?*, several contributors are suspicious of the new reproductive technology. None is more hostile than Robyn Rowland, an Australian sociologist, who writes:

> Ultimately the new technology will be used for the benefit of men and to the detriment of women. Although technology itself is not always a negative development, the real question has always been—who controls it? Biological technology is in the hands of men (4).

And Rowland concludes with a warning as dire as any uttered by the most conservative opponents of IVF:

> What may be happening is the last battle in the long war of men against women. Women's position is most precarious . . . we may find ourselves without a product of any kind with which to bargain. For the history of "mankind" women have been seen in terms of their value as childbearers. We have to ask, if that last power is taken and controlled by men, what role is envisaged for women in the new world? Will women become obsolete? Will we be fighting to retain or reclaim the right to bear children—has patriarchy conned us once again? I urge you sisters to be vigilant (4).

I can see little basis for such claims. For a start, women have figured quite prominently in the leading IVF teams in Britain, Australia, and the United States: Jean Purdy was an early colleague of Edwards and Steptoe in the research that led to the birth of Louise Brown; Linda Mohr has directed the development of embryo freezing at the Queen Victoria Medical Centre in Melbourne; and in the United States Georgeanna Jones and Joyce Vargyas have played leading roles in the groundbreaking clinics in Norfolk, Virginia, and at the University of Southern California, respectively. It seems odd for a feminist to neglect the contributions these women have made.

Even if one were to grant, however, that the technology remains predominantly in male hands, it has to be remembered that it was developed in response to the needs of infertile couples. From interviews I have conducted and meetings I have attended, my impression is that while both partners are often very concerned about their childlessness, in those cases in which one partner is more distressed than the other by this situation, that partner is usually the woman. Feminists usually accept

that this is so, attributing it to the power of social conditioning in a patriarchal society; but the origin of the strong female desire for children is not really what is in question here. The question is: in what sense is the new technology an instrument of male domination over women? If it is true that the technology was developed at least as much in response to the needs of women as in response to the needs of men, then it is hard to see why a feminist should condemn it.

It might be objected that whatever the origins of IVF and no matter how benign it may be when used to help infertile couples, the further development of techniques such as ectogenesis—the growth of the embryo from conception totally outside the body, in an artificial womb—will reduce the status of women. Again, it is not easy to see why this should be so. Ectogenesis will, if it is ever successful, provide a choice for women. Shulamith Firestone argued several years ago in her influential feminist work *The Dialectic of Sex* (5) that this choice will remove the fundamental biological barrier to complete equality. Hence Firestone welcomed the prospect of ectogenesis and condemned the low priority given by our male-dominated society to research in this area.

Firestone's view is surely more in line with the drive to sexual equality than the position taken by Rowland. If we argue that to break the link between women and childbearing would be to undermine the status of women in our society, what are we saying about the ability of women to obtain true equality in other spheres of life? I am not so pessimistic about the abilities of women to achieve equality with men across the broad range of human endeavor. For that reason I think women will be helped, rather than harmed, by the development of a technology which makes it possible for them to have children without being pregnant. As Nancy Breeze, a very differently inclined contributor to the same collection of essays, puts it:

> Two thousand years of morning sickness and stretch marks have not resulted in liberation for women or children. If you should run into a Petri dish, it could turn out to be your best friend. So rock it; don't knock it! (6)

So to sum up this discussion of the ethics of the simple case of IVF: the ethical objections urged against IVF under these conditions are not strong. They should not count against going ahead with IVF when it is the best way of overcoming infertility and when the infertile couple are not prepared to consider adoption as a means of overcoming their problem. There is, admittedly, a serious question about how much of the national health budget should be allocated to this area. But then, there are serious questions about the allocation of resources in other areas of medicine as well.

IVF: OTHER CASES

IVF can be used in circumstances that differ from those of the simple case in the following respects:

1. The couple may not be legally married; or there may be no couple at all, the patient being a single woman.

2. The couple may not be infertile but may wish to use IVF for some other reason, for instance because the woman carries a genetic defect.

3. The sperm, or the egg, or both, may come from another person, not from the couple themselves.

4. Some of the embryos created may not be inserted into the womb of the wife; instead they may be frozen and stored for later use, or donated to others, or used for research, or simply discarded.

All of these variations on the simple case raise potentially difficult issues. I say "potentially difficult" because in some cases the difficulties arise only once we consider the more extreme instances. For instance, there are no good grounds for discriminating against couples who are not legally married but have a long-standing de facto relationship; on the other hand one would need to consider more carefully whether to allow a single woman to make use of IVF. It is true that single fertile women are entirely free to procreate as irresponsibly as they like; yet the doctor who assists an infertile woman to do the same must take some care that the child in whose creation he or she is assisting will grow up in circumstances that are compatible with a good start in life. A single mother may well be able to provide such circumstances, but it is at least appropriate for the doctor to make some inquiries before going ahead.

IVF for fertile couples when the woman carries a serious genetic defect is scarcely problematic; if we would allow artificial insemination when the man has a similar defect, we should also allow IVF when the woman is the carrier. Here too, however, there is a question about how far we should go. What if the defect is a very minor one? What if there is no defect at all, but the woman wants a donor egg from a friend whose intelligence or beauty she considers superior to her own? A California sperm bank is already offering selected women the sperm of Nobel Prize-winning scientists. It is only a matter of time before eggs are offered in the same manner. Nevertheless it seems clear that as long as IVF is in short supply, those who are infertile or who carry a serious genetic defect should have the first claim upon it. (The issue of genetic selection itself will be touched upon in the final section of this [essay].)

The use of donor sperm, eggs, and embryos raises further questions. There is a precedent in the use of donor sperm in artificial insemination. The lesson that has been learned here is that there is a great need for counseling the couple because there may be psychological problems when one parent is not the genetic parent of the child. There is also the question of whether the child is to be told of her or his genetic origins. Many adopted persons now consider that they have a right to full information about their genetic parents. There is a strong case for saying that the same applies to people born as a result of the use of donor sperm or eggs, and that nonidentifying data about the donor should be released to the parents, with a view to the child being informed at a later stage.

The most controversial of these issues is that of the moral status of the embryo; this is the question at stake when we consider whether to create more embryos than we are willing to put back into the womb at one time. Disposing of the embryos, or using them for research purposes, runs counter to the view held by some that the embryo is a human being with the same right to life as any other human being. Even embryo freezing does little to placate those who take this view, since on present indications the chances of a frozen embryo surviving to become a living child are not high. But, religious doctrines apart, is it plausible to hold that the embryo has a right to life? The moral status of the embryo is perhaps the most fundamental of all the moral issues raised by the reproduction revolution. Many people believe it to be an insoluble philosophical problem, one on which we just have to take our stand, more or less arbitrarily, without hope of persuading those of a different view. I believe, on the contrary, that the issue is amenable to rational discussion. . . .

THE MORAL STATUS OF THE EMBRYO

. . . [A]ttempts to argue that the early embryo has a right to life [can be shown to be inadequate]. It remains only to say something positive about when in its development the embryo may acquire rights.

The answer must depend on the actual characteristics of the embryo. The minimal characteristic which is needed to give the embryo a claim to consideration is sentience, or the capacity to feel pain or pleasure. Until the embryo reaches that point, there is nothing we can do to the embryo which causes harm to *it*. We can, of course, damage it in such a way as to cause harm to the person it will become, if it lives, but if it never becomes a person, the embryo has not been harmed, because its total lack of awareness means that it can have no interest in becoming a person.

Once an embryo may be capable of feeling pain, there is a clear case for very strict controls over the experimentation which can be done with it. At this point the embryo ranks, morally, with other creatures who are conscious but not self-conscious. Many nonhuman animals come into this category, and in my view they have often been unjustifiably made to suffer in scientific research. We should have stringent controls over research to ensure that this cannot happen to embryos, just as we should have stringent controls to ensure that it cannot happen to animals.

Practical Implications of the Moral Status of Embryos

The conclusion to draw from this is that as long as the parents give their consent, there is no ethical objection to discarding a very early embryo. If the early embryo can be used for significant research, so much the better. What is crucial is that the embryo not be kept beyond the point at which it has formed a brain and a nervous system, and might be capable of suffering. Two government committees—the Warnock Committee in Britain (7) and the Waller Committee in Victoria, Australia (8)—have recently recommended that research on embryos should be allowed, but only up to 14 days after fertilization. This is the period at which the so-called "primitive streak," the first indication of the development of a nervous system, begins to form, and up to this stage there is certainly no possibility of the embryo feeling anything at all. In fact, the 14-day limit is unnecessarily conservative. A limit of, say, 28 days would still be very much on the safe side of the best estimates of when the embryo may be able to feel pain; but such a limit would, in contrast to the 14-day limit, allow research on embryos at the stage at which some of the more specialized cells have begun to form. As we saw earlier, this research would, according to Robert Edwards, have the potential to cure such terrible diseases as sickle cell anemia and leukemia (2).

As for freezing the embryo with a view to later implantation, the question here is essentially one of risk. If freezing carries no special risk of abnormality, there seems to be nothing objectionable about it. With embryo freezing, this appears to be the case. The ethical objections some people have to freezing embryos has led to the suggestion that it would be better to freeze eggs (7); for this and other reasons there has been a considerable research effort directed at freezing eggs. Human eggs are more difficult to freeze than human embryos, and until recently it had not proved possible to freeze them in a manner which allowed fertilization after thawing. In December 1985, however, an IVF team at Flinders University, in Adelaide, South Australia, announced that it had succeeded in obtaining a pregnancy from an egg which had been frozen and thawed before being fertilized (9). The technique used involved stripping away a protective outer layer from the egg, so that it would take up a chemical which would protect it during the freezing process. This technique does overcome the ethical problems some find in freezing embryos, but it does so at the cost of introducing a new potential cause of risk to the offspring, the risk that the chemicals absorbed by the egg may have some harmful effect (10). Whether or not this risk proves to be a real one, from the point of view of ethics, one may doubt whether the risk is worth running, if the primary reason for running it is to avoid objections, which we have now seen to be ill-founded, to the freezing of embryos.

Going beyond the simple case does bring us into a more ethically controversial area, but there is no overall case against applying IVF outside the restricted ambit of the simple case. The essential point is to consider each additional step carefully before it is taken. Some steps will prove unwise, but others will be beneficial and not open to any well-grounded objections.

THE FUTURE OF THE REPRODUCTION REVOLUTION

What lies ahead? IVF has opened the door to a wide range of further possibilities. In the near future we shall have to consider which of these possibilities to pursue, and which to reject. Here are some of the possibilities:

1. A surrogate could bear a child for another couple; the child would be the genetic child of the other couple, and would be returned to the genetic parents after birth. The genetic parents might be unable to conceive in the normal way,

or they might simply find the surrogate arrangement more convenient. The surrogate might be paid for her services, or—in the case of otherwise infertile couples—she may have more altruistic motives.

2. Embryos may be used in order to provide "spare parts" for people who through accident or illness need some kind of transplant. It has been suggested that embryonic tissue could restore nerve function to paraplegics. Embryos might be grown to the point at which the organs begin to form, and then the organs could be separated and grown in culture until they were large enough to be used.

3. Several embryos could be produced, and some of their genetic characteristics identified; the one considered most desirable could then be implanted, and the remainder discarded; alternatively it will eventually be possible to modify the genetic properties of an embryo so as to eliminate defects and to build in desirable genetic qualities. . . .

The proposal that embryos be used for "spare parts" has already caused howls of protest from those who regard embryos as having the same rights as normal human beings. [This view, however,] cannot be defended by rational argument. As long as there are adequate safeguards to ensure that the embryo is at all times incapable of suffering in any way, it is difficult to find sound ethical reason against this proposal—and it is obvious that the possible benefits are considerable.

Of all the possible applications of IVF, however, it is genetic selection and genetic engineering which raise the most far-reaching questions. Should we tinker with the human genetic pool? If so, in what way? Here I will limit myself to pointing out that we already tinker with the genetic pool when we offer genetic counseling, amniocentesis, and abortion to those who are at special risk of producing genetically defective offspring. And this is nothing new, at least insofar as its impact on the genetic pool is concerned: other societies have practiced infanticide to the same end, and of course in the past, even if one tried to rear the defective child, in most cases nature used its own brutal methods to ensure that the genes were eliminated from the gene pool.

So genetic engineering differs only in its techniques from what is now going on, and has gone on for a long time. But this difference is a significant one, because the new techniques are so much more powerful, and because they would, in principle, allow us to select for desirable traits as well as to select against undesirable ones. Many fear that these techniques will place too much power in the hands of governments, who will not be able to resist the temptation of designing future generations to be docile and to vote for the governing party at every election.

The fear that genetic engineering will produce the ultimate in entrenched dictatorship is exaggerated. Most political leaders want quick results, and it would take at least 18 years for genetic engineering to have any effect at the polls. If we have succeeded in keeping our freedom in the age of television and state education, we should be able to cling to it in the age of genetic engineering as well.

But should we allow positive modifications, as distinct from the elimination of defects, at all? In time we might come to accept the desirability of positive modifications. One reason for accepting this is that, looking around us, there is reason to think that natural selection has left ample room for improvement. Another reason is that the distinction between eliminating a defect and making a positive modification is a difficult one to draw. If we learn how to eliminate a wide range of defects which predispose us to common diseases, we will have created an abnormally healthy person. If we learn how to affect intelligence, should we stop short at eliminating mental ability below the above-average range? If we eliminate abnormally depressive personalities, would it be wrong to try to produce people who tend to be a little more cheerful than most of us are now? If we eliminate tendencies toward criminal violence, might we not build just a little more kindness into the human constitution? If the risks of such an enterprise are great, so too are the potential rewards for us all.

REFERENCES

1 Singer P, Wells D. Making babies. New York: Scribner's, 1985.

2 Edwards RG. Paper presented at the Fourth World Congress on IVF. Melbourne, Australia, Nov 22, 1985.

3 Abstract. Proceedings of the Fifth Scientific Meeting of the Fertility Society of Australia, Adelaide, Dec 2–6, 1986.

4 Rowland R. Reproductive technologies: the final solution to the woman question? In: Arditti R, Klein RD, Minden S, eds, Test-tube women: what future for motherhood? London: Pandora, 1984.

5 Firestone S. The dialectic of sex. New York: Bantam, 1971.

6 Breeze N. Who is going to rock the petri dish? In: Arditti R, Klein RD, Minden S, eds, Test-tube women: what future for motherhood? London: Pandora, 1984.

7 Warnock M (Chairperson). Report of the Committee of Inquiry into Human Fertilisation and Embryology. London: Her Majesty's Stationery Office, 1984, p 66.

8 Waller L (Chairman). Victorian Government Committee to Consider the Social, Ethical and Legal Issues Arising from In Vitro Fertilization. Report on the disposition of embryos produced by in vitro fertilization. Melbourne: Victorian Government Printer, 1984, p 47.

9 The Australian, Dec 19, 1985.

10 Trounson A. Paper presented at the Fourth World Congress on IVF, Melbourne, Australia, Nov 22, 1985.

Feminist Ethics and In Vitro Fertilization
Susan Sherwin

Susan Sherwin is professor of philosophy at Dalhousie University, Halifax, Nova Scotia. She is coeditor of *Moral Problems in Medicine* (1976; 2d ed., 1983) and the author of *No Longer Patient: Feminist Ethics and Health Care* (1992). Her published articles include "The Concept of a Person in the Context of Abortion" and "Feminist and Medical Ethics: Two Different Approaches to Contextual Ethics."

Sherwin outlines the nature of feminist ethics and provides a feminist critique of in vitro fertilization (IVF). She maintains that IVF is morally problematic for a number of closely related reasons, including the following: (1) Although the desires of infertile couples for access to IVF are understandable and worthy of sympathetic regard, such desires themselves emerge from social arrangements and cultural values that are deeply oppressive to women; (2) IVF technology gives the appearance of providing women with increased reproductive freedom but in reality threatens women with a significant decrease of reproductive freedom. Sherwin also insists that those who find themselves in moral opposition to IVF have a responsibility to support medical and social developments that would reduce the perceived need of couples for IVF.

Many authors from all traditions consider it necessary to ask why it is that some couples seek [IVF] technology so desperately. Why is it so important to so many people to produce their 'own' child? On this question, theorists in the analytic tradition seem to shift to previously rejected ground and suggest that this is a natural, or at least a proper, desire. Englehardt, for example, says, 'The use of technology in the fashioning of children is integral to the goal of rendering the world congenial to persons.'[1] Bayles more cautiously observes that

Reprinted with permission of the author and the publisher from *Canadian Journal of Philosophy*, Supplementary Volume 13 (1987), pp. 276–284.

'A desire to beget for its own sake . . . is probably irrational'; nonetheless, he immediately concludes, 'these techniques for fulfilling that desire have been found ethically permissible.'[2] R. G. Edwards and David Sharpe state the case most strongly: 'the desire to have children must be among the most basic of human instincts, and denying it can lead to considerable psychological and social difficulties.'[3] Interestingly, although the recent pronouncement of the Catholic Church assumes that 'the desire for a child is natural,'[4] it denies that a couple has a right to a child: 'The child is not an object to which one has a right.'[5]

Here, I believe, it becomes clear why we need a deeper sort of feminist analysis. We must look at the sort of social arrangements and cultural values that underlie the drive to assume such risks for the sake of biological parenthood. We find that the capitalism, racism, sexism, and elitism of our culture have combined to create a set of attitudes which views children as commodities whose value is derived from their possession of parental chromosomes. Children are valued as privatized commodities, reflecting the virility and heredity of their parents. They are also viewed as the responsibility of their parents and are not seen as the social treasure and burden that they are. Parents must tend their needs on pain of prosecution, and, in return, they get to keep complete control over them. Other adults are inhibited from having warm, stable interactions with the children of others—it is as suspect to try to hug and talk regularly with a child who is not one's own as it is to fondle and hang longingly about a car or a bicycle which belongs to someone else—so those who wish to know children well often find they must have their own.

Women are persuaded that their most important purpose in life is to bear and raise children; they are told repeatedly that their life is incomplete, that they are lacking in fulfillment if they do not have children. And, in fact, many women do face a barren existence without children. Few women have access to meaningful, satisfying jobs. Most do not find themselves in the centre of the romantic personal relationships which the culture pretends is the norm for heterosexual couples. And they have been socialized to be fearful of close friendships with others—they are taught to distrust other women, and to avoid the danger of friendship with men other than their husbands. Children remain the one hope for real intimacy and for the sense of accomplishment which comes from doing work one judges to be valuable.

To be sure, children can provide that sense of self worth, although for many women (and probably for all mothers at some times) motherhood is not the romanticized satisfaction they are led to expect. But there is something very wrong with a culture where childrearing is the only outlet available to most women in which to pursue fulfillment. Moreover, there is something wrong with the ownership theory of children that keeps other adults at a distance from children. There ought to be a variety of close relationships possible between children and adults so that we all recognize that we have a stake in the well-being of the young, and we all benefit from contact with their view of the world.

In such a world, it would not be necessary to spend the huge sums on designer children which IVF requires while millions of other children starve to death each year. Adults who enjoyed children could be involved in caring for them whether or not they produced them biologically. And, if the institution of marriage survives, women and men would marry because they wished to share their lives together, not because the men needed someone to produce heirs for them and women needed financial support for their children. That would be a world in which we might have reproductive freedom of choice. The world we now live in has so limited women's options and self-esteem, it is legitimate to question the freedom behind women's demand for this technology, for it may well be largely a reflection of constraining social perspectives.

Nonetheless, I must acknowledge that some couples today genuinely mourn their incapacity to produce children without IVF and there are very significant and unique joys which can be found in producing and raising one's own children which are not accessible to persons in infertile relationships. We must sympathize with these people. None of us shall live to see the implementation of the ideal cultural values outlined above which would make the demand for IVF less severe. It is with real concern that some feminists suggest that the personal wishes of couples with fertility difficulties may not be compatible with the overall interests of women and children.

Feminist thought, then, helps us to focus on different dimensions of the problem than do other sorts of approaches. But, with this perspective, we still have difficulty in reaching a final conclusion on whether to encourage, tolerate, modify, or restrict this sort of reproductive technology. I suggest that we turn to the developing theories of feminist ethics for guidance in resolving this question.[6]

In my view, a feminist ethics is a moral theory that focusses on relations among persons as well as on individuals. It has as a model an inter-connected social fabric, rather than the familiar one of isolated, independent atoms; and it gives primacy to bonds among people rather than to rights to independence. It is a theory that focusses on concrete situations and persons and not on free-floating abstract actions.[7] Although many details have yet to be worked out, we can see some of its implications in particular problem areas such as this.

It is a theory that is explicitly conscious of the social, political, and economic relations that exist among persons; in particular, as a feminist theory, it attends to the implications of actions or policies on the status of women. Hence, it is necessary to ask questions from the perspective of feminist ethics in addition to those which are normally asked from the perspective of mainstream ethical theories. We must view issues such as this one in the context of the social and political realities in which they arise, and resist the attempt to evaluate actions or practices in isolation (as traditional responses in biomedical ethics often do). Thus, we cannot just address the question of IVF per se without asking how IVF contributes to general patterns of women's oppression. As Kathryn Pyne Addelson has argued about abortion,[8] a feminist perspective raises questions that are inadmissible within the traditional ethical frameworks, and yet, for women in a patriarchal society, they are value questions of greater urgency. In particular, a feminist ethics, in contrast to other approaches in biomedical ethics, would take seriously the concerns just reviewed which are part of the debate in the feminist literature.

A feminist ethics would also include components of theories that have been developed as 'feminine ethics,' as sketched out by the empirical work of Carol Gilligan.[9] (The best example of such a theory is the work of Nel Noddings in her influential book *Caring*.)[10] In other words, it would be a theory that gives primacy to interpersonal relationships and woman-centered values such as nurturing, empathy, and co-operation. Hence, in the case of IVF, we must care for the women and men who are so despairing about their infertility as to want to spend the vast sums and risk the associated physical and emotional costs of the treatment, in pursuit of 'their own children.' That is, we should, in Noddings' terms, see their reality as our own and address their very real sense of loss. In so doing, however, we must also consider the implications of this sort of solution to their difficulty. While meeting the perceived desires of some women—desires which are problematic in themselves, since they are so compatible with the values of a culture deeply oppressive to women—this technology threatens to further entrench those values which are responsible for that oppression. A larger vision suggests that the technology offered may, in reality, reduce women's freedom and, if so, it should be avoided.

A feminist ethics will not support a wholly negative response, however, for that would not address our obligation to care for those suffering from infertility; it is the responsibility of those who oppose further implementation of this technology to work towards the changes in the social arrangements that will lead to a reduction of the sense of need for this sort of solution. On the medical front, research and treatment ought to be stepped up to reduce the rates of peral sepsis and gonorrhea which often result in tubal blockage, more attention should be directed at the causes and possible cures for male infertility, and we should pursue techniques that will permit safe reversible sterilization providing women with better alternatives to tubal ligation as a means of fertility control; these sorts of technology would increase the control of many women over their own fertility and would be compatible with feminist objectives. On the social front, we must continue the social pressure to change the status of women and children in our society from that of breeder and possession respectively; hence, we must develop a vision of society as community where all participants are valued members, regardless of age or gender. And we must challenge the notion that having one's wife produce a child with his own genes is sufficient cause for the wives of men with low sperm counts to be expected to undergo the physical and emotional assault such technology involves.

Further, a feminist ethics will attend to the nature of the relationships among those concerned. Annette Baier has eloquently argued for the importance of developing an ethics of trust,[11] and I believe a feminist ethics must address the question of the degree of trust appropriate to the relationships involved. Feminists have noted that women have little reason to trust the medical specialists who offer to respond to their reproductive desires, for, commonly women's interests have not come first from the medical point of view.[12] In fact, it is accurate to perceive feminist attacks on reproductive technology as expressions of the lack of trust feminists have in those who control the technology. Few feminists object to reproductive technology per se; rather they express concern about who controls it and how it can be used to further exploit women. The problem with reproductive technology is that it concentrates power in reproductive matters in the hands of those who are not directly involved in the actual bearing and rearing of the child; i.e., in men who relate to their clients in a technical, professional, authoritarian manner. It is a further step in the medicalization of pregnancy and birth which, in North America, is marked by relationships between pregnant women and their doctors which are very different from the traditional relationships between pregnant women and midwives. The latter relationships fostered an atmosphere of mutual trust which is impossible to replicate in hospital deliveries today. In fact, current approaches to pregnancy, labour, and birth tend to view the mother as a threat to the fetus who must be coerced to comply with medical procedures designed to ensure delivery of healthy babies at whatever cost necessary to the mother. Frequently, the fetus-mother relationship is medically characterized as adversarial and the physicians choose to foster a sense of alienation and passivity in the role they permit the mother. However well IVF may serve the interests of the few women with access to it, it more clearly serves the interests (be they commercial, professional, scholarly, or purely patriarchal) of those who control it.

Questions such as these are a puzzle to those engaged in the traditional approaches to ethics, for they always urge us to separate the question of evaluating the morality of various forms of reproductive technology in themselves, from questions about particular uses of that technology. From the perspective of a feminist ethics, however, no such distinction can be meaningfully made. Reproductive technology is not an abstract activity, it is an activity done in particular contexts and it is those contexts which must be addressed.

Feminist concerns [make] clear the difficulties we have with some of our traditional ethical concepts; hence, feminist ethics directs us to rethink our basic ethical notions. Autonomy, or freedom of choice, is not a matter to be determined in isolated instances, as is commonly assumed in many approaches to applied ethics. Rather it is a matter that involves reflection on one's whole life situation. The freedom of choice feminists appeal to in the abortion situation is freedom to define one's status as childbearer, given the social, economic, and political significance of reproduction for women. A feminist perspective permits us to understand that reproductive freedom includes control of one's sexuality, protection against coerced sterilization (or iatrogenic sterilization, e.g. as caused by the Dalkon Shield), and the existence of a social and economic network of support for the children we may choose to bear. It is the freedom to redefine our roles in society according to our concerns and needs as women.

In contrast, the consumer freedom to purchase technology, allowed only to a few couples of the privileged classes (in traditionally approved relationships), seems to entrench further the patriarchal notions of woman's role as childbearer and of heterosexual monogamy as the only acceptable intimate relationship. In other words, this sort of choice does not seem to foster autonomy for women on the broad scale. IVF is a practice which seems to reinforce sexist, classist, and often racist assumptions of our culture; therefore, on our revised understanding of freedom, the contribution of this technology to the general autonomy of women is largely negative.

We can now see the advantage of a feminist ethics over mainstream ethical theories, for a feminist analysis explicitly accepts the need for a political component to our understanding of ethical issues. In this, it differs from traditional ethical theories and it also differs from a simply feminine ethics approach, such as the one Noddings offers, for Noddings seems to rely on individual relations exclusively and is deeply suspicious of political alliances as potential threats to the pure relation of caring. Yet, a full understanding of both the threat of IVF, and the alternative action necessary should we decide to reject IVF, is possible only if it includes a political dimension reflecting on the role of women in society.

From the point of view of feminist ethics, the primary question to consider is whether this and other forms of reproductive technology threaten to reinforce the lack of autonomy which women now experience in our culture—even as they appear, in the short run, to be increasing freedom. We must recognize that the interconnections among the social forces oppressive to women underlie feminists' mistrust of this technology which advertises itself as increasing women's autonomy.[13] The political perspective which directs us to look at how this technology fits in with general patterns of treatment for women is not readily accessible to traditional moral theories, for it involves categories of concern not accounted for in those theories—e.g. the complexity of issues which makes it inappropriate to study them in isolation from one another, the role of oppression in shaping individual desires, and potential differences in moral status which are connected with differences in treatment.

It is the set of connections constituting women's continued oppression in our society which inspires feminists to resurrect the old slippery slope arguments to warn against IVF. We must recognize that women's existing lack of control in reproductive matters begins the debate on a pretty steep incline. Technology with the potential to further remove control of reproduction from women makes the slope very slippery indeed. This new technology, though offered under the guise of increasing reproductive freedom, threatens to result, in fact, in a significant decrease in freedom, especially since it is a technology that will always include the active involvement of designated specialists and will not ever be a private matter for the couple or women concerned.

Ethics ought not to direct us to evaluate individual cases without also looking at the implications of our decisions from a wide perspective. My argument is that a theory of feminist ethics provides that wider perspective, for its different sort of methodology is sensitive to both the personal and the social dimensions of issues. For that reason, I believe it is the only ethical perspective suitable for evaluating issues of this sort.

NOTES

1 H. Tristram Englehardt, *The Foundations of Bioethics* (Oxford: Oxford University Press 1986), 239

2 Michael Bayles, *Reproductive Ethics* (Englewood Cliffs, NJ: Prentice-Hall 1984) 31

3 Robert G. Edwards and David J. Sharpe, 'Social Values and Research in Human Embryology,' *Nature* 231 (May 14, 1971), 87

4 Joseph Card Ratzinger and Alberto Bovone, 'Instruction on Respect for Human Life in its Origin and on the Dignity of Procreation: Replies to Certain Questions of the Day' (Vatican City: Vatican Polyglot Press 1987), 33

5 Ibid., 34

6 Many authors are now working on an understanding of what feminist ethics entail. Among the Canadian papers I am familiar with, are Kathryn Morgan's 'Women and Moral Madness,' Sheila Mullett's 'Only Connect: The Place of Self-Knowledge in Ethics,' both in this volume, and Leslie Wilson's 'Is a Feminine Ethics Enough?' *Atlantis* (forthcoming).

7 Susan Sherwin, 'A Feminist Approach to Ethics,'

Dalhousie Review 64, 4 (Winter 1984–85) 704–13

8 Kathryn Pyne Addelson, 'Moral Revolution,' in Marilyn Pearsall, ed., *Women and Values* (Belmont, CA: Wadsworth 1986), 291–309

9 Carol Gilligan, *In a Different Voice* (Cambridge, MA: Harvard University Press 1982)

10 Nel Noddings, *Caring* (Berkeley: University of California Press 1984)

11 Annette Baier, 'What Do Women Want in a Moral Theory?' *Nous* 19 (March 1985) 53–64, and 'Trust and Antitrust,' *Ethics* 96 (January 1986) 231–60

12 Linda Williams presents this position particularly clearly in her invaluable work 'But What Will They Mean for Women? Feminist Concerns about the New Reproductive Technologies,' No. 6 in the *Feminist Perspective* Series, CRIAW.

13 Marilyn Frye vividly describes the phenomenon of inter-relatedness which supports sexist oppression by appeal to the metaphor of a bird cage composed of thin wires, each relatively harmless in itself, but, collectively, the wires constitute an overwhelming barrier to the inhabitant of the cage. Marilyn Frye, *The Politics of Reality: Essays in Feminist Theory* (Trumansburg, NY: The Crossing Press 1983), 4–7

Genetic Engineering and the Human Genome Project

Genetics and Human Malleability
W. French Anderson

W. French Anderson is professor of biochemistry and pediatrics at the University of Southern California School of Medicine. A pioneer in gene therapy research, he is also editor-in-chief of *Human Gene Therapy*. Anderson's many articles on gene therapy include "Human Gene Therapy: Scientific and Ethical Considerations," and "Human Gene Therapy: Why Draw a Line?"

Anderson's principal concern is to reject the employment of *enhancement* genetic engineering. He endorses the use of somatic-cell gene therapy (and is not opposed to germ-line gene therapy—as he makes clear in other published work), but he insists that gene transfer techniques must be restricted to the treatment of *serious disease*. They must not be employed for the purpose of producing improved human characteristics (e.g., increased memory capacity). Anderson argues that somatic-cell enhancement engineering should be rejected for two basic reasons: (1) it could be medically hazardous and (2) it would be morally precarious.

Reprinted with permission of the author and the publisher from *Hastings Center Report*, vol. 20 (January/February 1990), pp. 21–24. © The Hastings Center.

Just how much can, and should we change human nature . . . by genetic engineering? Our response to that hinges on the answers to three further questions: (1) What *can* we do now? Or more precisely, what *are* we doing now in the area of human genetic engineering? (2) What *will* we be able to do? In other words, what technical advances are we likely to achieve over the next five to ten years? (3) What *should* we do? I will argue that a line can be drawn and should be drawn to use gene transfer only for the treatment of serious disease, and not for any other purpose. Gene transfer should never be undertaken in an attempt to enhance or "improve" human beings.

WHAT CAN WE DO?

In 1980 John Fletcher and I published a paper in the *New England Journal of Medicine* in which we delineated what would be necessary before it would be ethical to carry out human gene therapy.[1] As with any other new therapeutic procedure, the fundamental principle is that it should be determined in advance that the probable benefits outweigh the probable risks. We analyzed the risk/benefit determination for somatic cell gene therapy and proposed three questions that need to have been answered from prior animal experimentation: Can the new gene be inserted stably into the correct target cells? Will the new gene be expressed (that is, function) in the cells at an appropriate level? Will the new gene harm the cell or the animal? These criteria are very similar to those required before use of any new therapeutic procedure, surgical operation, or drug. They simply require that the new treatment should get to the area of disease, correct it, and do more good than harm.

A great deal of scientific progress has occurred in the nine years since that paper was published. The technology does now exist for inserting genes into some types of target cells.[2] The procedure being used is called "retroviral-mediated gene transfer." In brief, a disabled murine retrovirus serves as a delivery vehicle for transporting a gene into a population of cells that have been removed from a patient. The gene-engineered cells are then returned to the patient. . . .

WHAT WILL WE BE ABLE TO DO?

. . . Many genetic diseases that are caused by a defect in a single gene should be treatable, such as ADA deficiency (a severe immune deficiency disease of children),

sickle cell anemia, hemophilia, and Gaucher disease. Some types of cancer, viral diseases such as AIDS, and some forms of cardiovascular disease are targets for treatment by gene therapy. In addition, germline gene therapy, that is, the insertion of a gene into the reproductive cells of a patient, will probably be technically possible in the foreseeable future. My position on the ethics of germline gene therapy is published elsewhere.[3]

But successful somatic cell gene therapy also opens the door for enhancement genetic engineering, that is, for supplying a specific characteristic that individuals might want for themselves (somatic cell engineering) or their children (germ-line engineering) which would not involve the treatment of a disease. The most obvious example at the moment would be the insertion of a growth hormone gene into a normal child in the hope that this would make the child grow larger. Should parents be allowed to choose (if the science should ever make it possible) whatever useful characteristics they wish for their children?

WHAT SHOULD WE DO?

A line can and should be drawn between somatic cell gene therapy and enhancement genetic engineering.[4] Our society has repeatedly demonstrated that it can draw a line in biomedical research when necessary. The Belmont Report illustrates how guidelines were formulated to delineate ethical from unethical clinical research and to distinguish clinical research from clinical practice. Our responsibility is to determine how and where to draw lines with respect to genetic engineering.

Somatic cell gene therapy for the treatment of severe disease is considered ethical because it can be supported by the fundamental moral principle of beneficence: It would relieve human suffering. Gene therapy would be, therefore, a moral good. Under what circumstances would human genetic engineering not be a moral good? In the broadest sense, when it detracts from, rather than contributes to, the dignity of man. Whether viewed from a theological perspective or a secular humanist one, the justification for drawing a line is founded on the argument that, beyond the line, human values that our society considers important for the dignity of man would be significantly threatened.

Somatic cell enhancement engineering would threaten important human values in two ways: It could be medically hazardous, in that the risks could exceed the potential benefits and the procedure therefore cause harm. And it would be morally precarious, in that it would require moral decisions our society is not now prepared to make, and it could lead to an increase in inequality and discriminatory practices.

Medicine is a very inexact science. We understand roughly how a simple gene works and that there are many thousands of housekeeping genes, that is, genes that do the job of running a cell. We predict that there are genes which make regulatory messages that are involved in the overall control and regulation of the many housekeeping genes. Yet we have only limited understanding of how a body organ develops into the size and shape it does. We know many things about how the central nervous system works—for example, we are beginning to comprehend how molecules are involved in electric circuits, in memory storage, in transmission of signals. But we are a long way from understanding thought and consciousness. And we are even further from understanding the spiritual side of our existence.

Even though we do not understand how a thinking, loving, interacting organism can be derived from its molecules, we are approaching the time when we can change some of those molecules. Might there be genes that influence the brain's organization or structure or metabolism or circuitry in some way so as to allow abstract thinking, contemplation of good and evil, fear of death, awe of a 'God'? What if in our innocent attempts to improve our genetic make-up we alter one or more of those genes? Could we test for the alteration? Certainly not at present. If we caused a problem that would affect the individual or his or her offspring, could we repair the damage? Certainly not at present. Every parent who has several children knows that some babies accept and give more affection than others, in the same environment. Do genes control this? What if these genes were accidentally altered? How would we even know if such a gene were altered?

My concern is that, at this point in the development of our culture's scientific expertise, we might be like the young boy who loves to take things apart. He is bright enough to disassemble a watch, and maybe even bright enough to get it back together again so that it works. But what if he tries to "improve" it? Maybe put on bigger hands so that the time can be read more easily. But if the hands are too heavy for the mechanism, the watch will run slowly, erratically, or not at all. The boy can understand what is visible, but he cannot comprehend the precise engineering calculations that determined exactly how strong each spring should be, why the gears interact in the ways that they do, etc. Attempts on his part to improve the watch will probably only

harm it. We are now able to provide a new gene so that a property involved in a human life would be changed, for example, a growth hormone gene. If we were to do so simply because we could, I fear we would be like that young boy who changed the watch's hands. We, too, do not really understand what makes the object we are tinkering with tick.

In summary, it could be harmful to insert a gene into humans. In somatic cell gene therapy for an already existing disease the potential benefits could outweigh the risks. In enhancement engineering, however, the risks would be greater while the benefits would be considerably less clear.

Yet even aside from the medical risks, somatic cell enhancement engineering should not be performed because it would be morally precarious. Let us assume that there were no medical risks at all from somatic cell enhancement engineering. There would still be reasons for objecting to this procedure. To illustrate, let us consider some examples. What if a human gene were cloned that could produce a brain chemical resulting in markedly increased memory capacity in monkeys after gene transfer? Should a person be allowed to receive such a gene on request? Should a pubescent adolescent whose parents are both five feet tall be provided with a growth hormone gene on request? Should a worker who is continually exposed to an industrial toxin receive a gene to give him resistance on his, or his employer's request?

These scenarios suggest three problems that would be difficult to resolve: What genes should be provided; who should receive a gene; and, how to prevent discrimination against individuals who do or do not receive a gene.

We allow that it would be ethically appropriate to use somatic cell gene therapy for treatment of serious disease. But what distinguishes a serious disease from a "minor" disease from cultural "discomfort"? What is suffering? What is significant suffering? Does the absence of growth hormone that results in a growth limitation to two feet in height represent a genetic disease? What about a limitation to a height of four feet, to five feet? Each observer might draw the lines between serious disease, minor disease, and genetic variation differently. But all can agree that there are extreme cases that produce significant suffering and premature death. Here then is where an initial line should be drawn for determining what genes should be provided: treatment of serious disease.

If the position is established that only patients suffering from serious diseases are candidates for gene insertion, then the issues of patient selection are no different than in other medical situations: the determination is based on medical need within a supply and demand framework. But if the use of gene transfer extends to allow a normal individual to acquire, for example, a memory-enhancing gene, profound problems would result. On what basis is the decision made to allow one individual to receive the gene but not another: Should it go to those best able to benefit society (the smartest already)? To those most in need (those with low intelligence? But how low? Will enhancing memory help a mentally retarded child?)? To those chosen by a lottery? To those who can afford to pay? As long as our society lacks a significant consensus about these answers, the best way to make equitable decisions in this case should be to base them on the seriousness of the objective medical need, rather than on the personal wishes or resources of an individual.

Discrimination can occur in many forms. If individuals are carriers of a disease (for example, sickle cell anemia), would they be pressured to be treated? Would they have difficulty in obtaining health insurance unless they agreed to be treated? These are ethical issues raised also by genetic screening and by the Human Genome project. But the concerns would become even more troublesome if there were the possibility for "correction" by the use of human genetic engineering.

Finally, we must face the issue of eugenics, the attempt to make hereditary "improvements." The abuse of power that societies have historically demonstrated in the pursuit of eugenic goals is well documented.[5] Might we slide into a new age of eugenic thinking by starting with small "improvements"? It would be difficult, if not impossible, to determine where to draw a line once enhancement engineering had begun. Therefore, gene transfer should be used only for the treatment of serious disease and not for putative improvements.

Our society is comfortable with the use of genetic engineering to treat individuals with serious disease. On medical and ethical grounds we should draw a line excluding any form of enhancement engineering. We should not step over the line that delineates treatment from enhancement.

REFERENCES

1 W. French Anderson and John C. Fletcher, "Gene Therapy in Human Beings: When Is It Ethical to Begin?," *New England Journal of Medicine* 303:22 (1980), 1293–97.

2 See also W. French Anderson, "Prospects for Human Gene Therapy," *Science,* 26 October 1984, 401–409; T. Friedman, "Progress towards Human Gene Therapy," *Science,* 16 June 1989, 1275–81.

3 W. French Anderson, "Human Gene Therapy: Scientific and Ethical Considerations," *Journal of Medicine and Philosophy* 10 (1985): 275–91.

4 W. French Anderson, "Human Gene Therapy: Why Draw a Line?," *Journal of Medicine and Philosophy* 14 (1989), 681–93.

5 See, for example, Kenneth M. Ludmerer, *Genetics and American Society* (Baltimore, MD: The Johns Hopkins University Press, 1972), and Daniel J. Kevles, *In the Name of Eugenics* (New York: Alfred A. Knopf, 1985).

Position Paper on Human Germ Line Manipulation
Council for Responsible Genetics, Human Genetics Committee

The Council for Responsible Genetics is a national organization (based in Cambridge, Massachusetts) whose membership wants to ensure that biotechnology is developed safely and in the public interest. This document was written in 1992 by the council's Human Genetics Committee, a 14-member committee chaired by Abby Lippman, professor of epidemiology, McGill University.

The Council for Responsible Genetics is unconditionally opposed to germ-line gene modification (manipulation) in humans. The position paper clarifies the nature of germ-line modification, inquires into the purposes that might be served by germ-line modification in humans, and briefly considers the feasibility and technical pitfalls of germ-line modification in humans. The unpredictability of germ-line modifications is emphasized throughout, and a set of ethical arguments is explicitly formulated at the end of the paper.

THE POSITION OF THE COUNCIL FOR RESPONSIBLE GENETICS

The Council for Responsible Genetics (CRG) strongly opposes the use of germ line gene modification in humans. This position is based on scientific, ethical, and social concerns.

Proponents of germ line manipulation assume that once a gene implicated in a particular condition is identified, it might be appropriate and relatively easy to change, supplement or otherwise modify the gene by some form of therapy. However, biological characteristics or traits usually depend on interactions among many genes, and these genes are themselves affected by processes that occur both inside the organism and in its surroundings. This means that scientists cannot predict the full effect that any gene modification will have on the traits of people or other organisms. In purely biological terms, the relationship between genes and traits is not well enough understood to guarantee that by eliminating or changing genes associated with traits one might want to avoid, we may not simultaneously alter or eliminate traits we would like to preserve. Even genes that are associated with diseases that may cause problems in one context can be beneficial in another context.

Two frequently destructive aspects of contemporary culture are linked together in an unprecedented fashion in germ line gene modification. The first is the notion that the value of a human being is dependent on the degree to which he or she approximates some ideal of biological perfection. The second is the ideology that all limitations imposed by nature can and should be overcome by technology. To make intentional changes in the genes that people will pass on to their descendants would require that we, as a society, agree on how to identify 'good' and 'bad' genes. We do not have such criteria, nor are there mechanisms for establishing them. Any formulation of such criteria would necessarily reflect current social biases.

Moreover, the definition of the standards and the technological means for implementing them would largely be determined by the economically and socially privileged. By implementing a program of germ line manipulation these groups would exercise unwarranted influence over the common biological heritage of humanity.

WHAT IS "GERM LINE MANIPULATION"?

The undifferentiated cells of an early embryo develop into either germ cells or somatic cells. *Germ* cells, or reproductive cells, are those that develop into the egg or sperm of a developing organism and transmit all its heritable characteristics. *Somatic* cells, or body cells, refer to all other cells of the body. While both types of cells contain chromosomes, only the chromosomes of germ cells are passed on to future generations.

Techniques are now available to change chromosomes of animal cells by inserting new segments of DNA into them. If this insertion is performed on specialized or *differentiated* body tissues, such as liver, muscle, or blood cells, it is referred to as *somatic cell* gene modification, and the changes do not go beyond the individual organism. If it is performed on sperm or eggs before fertilization, or on the undifferentiated cells of an early embryo, it is called *germ cell* or *germ line* gene modification, and the changes are not limited to the individual organism. For when DNA is incorporated into an embryo's germ cells, or undifferentiated cells that give rise to germ cells, the introduced gene or genes will be passed on to future generations and may become a permanent part of the gene pool.

Deliberate gene alterations in humans are often referred to as 'gene therapy'. The Council for Responsible Genetics (CRG) prefers to use the terms 'gene modification' and 'gene manipulation' because the word 'therapy' promises health benefits, and it is not yet clear that gene manipulations are beneficial.

WHY MIGHT GERM LINE MODIFICATION BE ATTEMPTED IN HUMANS?

If one or both partners carry a version of a gene that could predispose their offspring to inherit a condition they want to avoid, genetic manipulation may appear to be a potential way to prevent the undesired outcome. The earlier during embryonic development the targeted gene or genes are replaced, the less likely is the resulting individual to be affected by the unwanted gene. But while the immediate goal of such a modification might be to alter the genetic constitution of a single individual, modifications made at the early embryonic stages would incidentally result in germ line modification, and so all the offspring of this person would have and pass on the modification.

Alternatively, germ line modification may be the intended consequence of the procedure. One goal might be to 'cleanse' the gene pool of 'deleterious' genes. For example, Daniel E. Koshland, Jr., a molecular biologist, and the editor-in-chief of *Science*, has written, "keeping diabetics alive with insulin, which increases the propagation of an inherited disease, seems justified only if one ultimately is willing to do genetic engineering to remove diabetes from the germ line and thus save the anguish and cost to millions of diabetics." (1) Another goal of germ line manipulation may be to avoid multiple treatments of somatic gene modification that would be required under proposed treatment protocols for certain conditions such as cystic fibrosis.

Some people may also look forward to the possibility of introducing genes into the germ line that can 'enhance' certain characteristics desired by parents or other custodians of the resulting offspring. In the article referred to above, Koshland raises the possibility that germ line alterations could be perceived to meet future 'needs' to design individuals "better at computers, better as musicians, better physically."

The attempt to improve the human species biologically is known as *eugenics,* and was the basis of a popular movement in Europe and North America during the first half of this century. Eugenics was advocated by prominent scientists across the entire political spectrum, who represented it as the logical consequence of the most advanced biological thinking of the period. In the U.S., eugenic thinking resulted in social policies that called for forced sterilization of individuals regarded as inferior because they were 'feeble minded or paupers.' In Europe, the Nazis took up these ideas, and their attempts at implementation led to widespread revulsion against the concept of eugenics. Today public discussion in favor of influencing the genetic constitution of future generations has gained new respectability with the increased possibility for intervention presented by in-vitro fertilization and embryo implantation technologies. Although it is once again espoused by individuals with a variety of political perspectives, the doctrine of social advancement through biological perfectibility underlying the new eugenics is almost indistinguishable from the older version so avidly embraced by the Nazis.

It is important to recognize that the dream of eliminating 'harmful' genes (such as those associated with cystic fibrosis or Duchenne muscular dystrophy) from the entire human gene pool could be realized only over time scales of thousands of years, and then only with massive, coercive programs of germ line manipulation. Such a program would be neither feasible nor morally acceptable. As a practical matter then, any presumed beneficial effects of germ line modification would pertain to individual families, not to the human population as a whole. This is in contrast to harmful effects, which would be widely disseminated.

Furthermore, parents who carry a gene which they would not want a child of theirs to inherit could arrange to have unaffected, biologically-related offspring *without* germ line modification. If a gene is well enough characterized to consider gene manipulation, there will always be a diagnostic test available to identify a fetus that carries that gene and parents, if they choose, may then terminate the pregnancy. Given that there are alternatives for avoiding the inheritance of unwanted genes, the main selling point of germ line modification techniques over the long term would appear to be the prospect of enhancement of desired traits.

WHAT IS THE FEASIBILITY OF MODIFYING THE GERM LINE OF HUMANS?

Both somatic and germ line modification are widely performed on laboratory animals for research purposes. Somatic gene modifications have already been performed on humans and additional experimental protocols are being approved by the National Institutes of Health in increasing numbers.

No published reports have yet appeared on germ line modification in humans, but there appear to be no technical obstacles to such experiments, and articles proposing these procedures are becoming more and more common in the literature (2,3,4). Germ line gene modification has actually proved technically easier than somatic modification in mice and other vertebrate animals which have been employed as 'models' for human biology in the past, because the cells of early embryos incorporate foreign DNA and synthesize corresponding functional proteins more readily than most differentiated somatic cells. A widely-reported example of the successful experimental use of the germ line technique was the introduction of an extra gene that specified growth hormone into fertilized mouse eggs. In the presence of the high levels of growth hormone produced, the mice grew to double their normal size. Germ line techniques are also being used in attempts to modify farm animals, with stated goals of increasing yields or enhancing nutritional quality of meat and other animal products.

Given what has been accomplished in animals, the only remaining technical requirements for germ line gene modification in humans are procedures for collecting a woman's eggs, fertilizing them outside her body, and implanting them in the uterus of the same or another woman, where they can be brought to term. These are already well established procedures for humans and are widely used in in-vitro fertilization clinics.

WHAT ARE THE TECHNICAL PITFALLS?

Current methods for germ line gene modification of mammals are inefficient, requiring the microinjection of numerous eggs with foreign DNA before an egg is successfully modified. Moreover, introduction of a foreign gene (even if there is a copy of one already present) into an inappropriate location in an embryo's chromosomes can have unexpected consequences. For example, the offspring of a mouse that received an extra copy of the normally present myc gene developed cancer at 40 times the rate of the unmodified strain of mice. (5)

Techniques to introduce foreign DNA into eggs, however, are constantly being improved and eventually will be portrayed as efficient and reliable enough for human applications. It may soon be possible to place a gene into a specified location on a chromosome while simultaneously removing the unwanted gene. This will increase the accuracy of the procedures, but does not eliminate the possibility that gene combinations will be created that will be harmful to the modified embryo, and its descendants in future generations. Such inadvertent damage could be caused by technical error, or

more importantly, by biologists' inability to predict how genes or their products interact with one another and with the organism's environment to give rise to biological traits. It would have been impossible to predict, a priori, for example, that someone who has even one copy of the gene for a blood protein known as hemoglobin-S would be protected against malaria, whereas a person who has two copies of this gene would have sickle cell disease.

This unpredictability applies with equal force to genetic modifications introduced to 'correct' presumed disorders and to those introduced to enhance characteristics. Inserting new segments of DNA into the germ line could have major, unpredictable consequences for both the individual and the future of the species that include the introduction of susceptibilities to cancer and other diseases into the human gene pool.

WHAT ARE THE SOCIAL AND ETHICAL IMPLICATIONS OF GERM LINE MODIFICATION?

Clinical trials in humans to treat Adenosine Deaminase Deficiency—a life threatening immune disorder—and terminal cancer with somatic gene modification are already in progress and experiments to treat diabetes and hypertension are under development. It is important to distinguish the ethical problems raised by these protocols from the additional, and more profound questions raised by germ line modification. While the biological effects of somatic manipulations reside entirely in the individual in which they are attempted, such treatments are not strictly analogous to other therapies with individual risk. Radiation, chemical or drug treatment can be withdrawn if they prove harmful to the patient, while some forms of somatic modification cannot. Thus, somatic gene modification requires a person to forfeit his/her rights to withdraw from a research study because the intervention cannot be stopped, whether harmful or not. Valid objections have also been raised to the fact that the first somatic gene modification experiments, involving Adenosine Deaminase Deficiency, were carried out on young children who were not themselves in a position to give informed consent. While it appears that somatic gene modification techniques will be used increasingly in the future, the CRG urges that they be used with greatest caution, and only for clearly life-threatening conditions.

Germ line modification, in contrast, has not yet been attempted in humans. The Council for Responsible Genetics opposes it unconditionally. Ethical arguments against germ line modification include many of those that pertain to somatic cell modification, as well as the following:

- Germ line modification is not needed in order to save the lives or alleviate suffering of existing people. Its target population are 'future people' who have not yet even been conceived.
- The cultural impact of treating humans as biologically perfectible artifacts would be entirely negative. People who fall short of some technically achievable ideal would increasingly be seen as 'damaged goods.' And it is clear that the standards for what is genetically desirable will be those of the society's economically and politically dominant groups. This will only reinforce prejudices and discrimination in a society where they already exist.
- Accountability to individuals of future generations who are harmed or stigmatized by wrongful or unsuccessful germ line modifications of their ancestors is unlikely.

In conclusion, the Council calls for a ban on germ line modification.

REFERENCES

1 Koshland Jr., Daniel E., "The Future of Biological Research: What Is Possible and What Is Ethical?", *MBL Science*, v. 3, no. 2, pps. 11–15, 1988.

2 Walters, Leroy, "Human Gene Therapy: Ethics and Public Policy", *Human Gene Therapy*, v. 2, pp. 115–122, 1991.

3 Working Group on Genetic Screening and Testing, *Report of Discussions in Genetics, Ethics and Human Values*, XXIVth CIOMS Conference, Tokyo and Inuyama, Japan, 24–26 July 1990.

4 Buster, John E. and Carson, Sandra A., "Genetic Diagnosis of the Preimplantation Embryo", *American Journal of Medical Centers*, v. 34, pp. 211–216, 1989.

5 Leder, A. et al, "Consequences of Widespread Deregulation of the c-myc Gene in Transgenic Mice: Multiple Neoplasms and Normal Development," *Cell*, v. 42, p. 485, 1986.

Unnatural Selection
Jerry E. Bishop

Jerry E. Bishop is deputy news editor for *The Wall Street Journal*. A science writer who has won many awards for his articles, he is also coauthor of *Genome: The Story of the Most Astonishing Scientific Adventure of Our Time—The Attempt to Map All the Genes in the Human Body* (1990).

Bishop describes the procedure of preimplantation embryo genetic testing and identifies some of the emerging possibilities and problems associated with its employment. Not only will preimplantation diagnosis be employed to avoid the implantation of embryos carrying genetic diseases, but it will also make it possible—increasingly so as the Human Genome Project advances—for prospective parents to select the traits (e.g., height, musical ability, intelligence) of their children. Moreover, Bishop points out, widespread use of preimplantation genetic selection might function to weaken ethical objections to the genetic modification of embryos. Bishop's discussion is not intended to provide an ethical analysis, but numerous ethical questions can and should be raised about the possibilities he identifies.

In 1990 a married couple in Walnut, California, Abe and Mary Ayala, set off a national controversy by conceiving a child. It was not the fact that Mrs. Ayala became pregnant by Mr. Ayala that sparked the uproar; it was the reason she became pregnant.

The Ayalas' seventeen-year-old daughter, Anissa, was suffering from chronic myelogenous leukemia, an ultimately fatal cancer of the blood. To cure her, cancer specialists at the City of Hope Medical Center in Duarte, California, wanted to destroy her native blood-forming bone marrow and replace it with marrow donated by a healthy person. Unable to find a donor whose tissues "matched" Anissa's, the Ayalas decided to have a second child. They hoped the new sibling would share enough genes with Anissa to permit a successful bone-marrow transplant.

While most of the public debated the morality of bearing a child for the purpose of saving the life of another child, a handful of molecular geneticists were acutely aware that the Ayala case put a new light on experiments then getting underway in some of the world's biological laboratories.

The Ayala case suggested a new use for "preimplantation embryo genetic testing," that is, genetic testing of an embryo before it becomes implanted in the womb to produce a pregnancy. The problem that the Ayalas faced was the possibility that the second child might be born in vain. Each conception involves a new roll of the genetic dice, and there was no guarantee that the second child would inherit a combination of the parents' genes that would be compatible with the genes of the cancer-stricken daughter. If the two siblings were too different genetically, the marrow transplant was certain to fail.

Preimplantation diagnosis begins with the test-tube conception technique widely used to treat infertility. An ovum, or egg, is removed from the female, fertilized in the test tube with sperm, and allowed to divide three times. This creates a microscopic cluster of eight identical cells, a test-tube embryo. Then the geneticist teases a single cell out of the test-tube embryo and, aided by a new technology, analyzes its genetic makeup. Since at this stage of development, the cells are still exact duplicates of each other, the results tell the geneticist whether the remaining seven cells are genetically healthy or defective.

As the publicity about the Ayala case broke, some molecular geneticists realized that preimplantation testing, with only minor development, could dramatically increase the odds that the California couple's second child would be genetically compatible with the older daughter. With six to eight ova fertilized simultaneously in the test tube, the genetic tests could then identify the embryo whose genes most closely matched those of the potential recipient. This embryo would be selected for producing a pregnancy and ultimately a sibling whose bone marrow would be most likely to lead to a successful transplant.

As it was, Anissa and her parents lucked out with the birth of Marissa Eve Ayala; the infant's bone marrow was ideally matched to her older sister's. In 1991, when Marissa was 14 months old, a thin hollow needle was used to withdraw a small vial of bone marrow from her hip bone and inject it into Anissa. Today Anissa is alive, cured of her leukemia and leading a normal life, as is her little sister.

But the case is a deceptively innocuous example of a situation in which a couple could, if they desired, select the genetic traits of a child before the pregnancy even occurs. The same choice is now being offered to hundreds of other young couples, albeit under considerably different circumstances. And in the near future, the choice will be expanded to thousands of others.

The implications of such widespread availability of preimplantation diagnosis are just beginning to surface, and they are among the most far-reaching and the least discussed issues to arise from the newfound ability to identify and manipulate human genes. The implications range from a subtle variation of the controversy over abortion to the question of whether one day soon society may have to step in and determine which human genetic traits are desirable and permissible.

Development of this diagnostic technology is proceeding far more rapidly than the efforts at gene therapy—and with far less notice. The first preimplantation diagnosis was carried out on a set of test-tube mouse embryos in mid-1989 by two British molecular biologists. Within weeks, a team of Americans reported that they had taken several ova from a woman who suffered a genetic defect and had been able to distinguish, before fertilization, which of the ova had inherited the defect.

A year later, my fellow science reporter, Michael Waldholz, and I published a book, *Genome*, in which we took note of these developments and daringly (we thought) predicted that embryo selection "for genetic disorders, genetic susceptibilities, and sex will be available to young couples within a decade or two." We added that "in a generation or two, young couples, should they so desire, will be able to make choices about the nature of their children that today seem to lie in the realm of science fiction."

We were far too cautious. Instead of a decade or

two, it was less than two years before preimplantation diagnosis was being offered to young couples who were worried about genetic disorders in their offspring. In the fall of 1992, Waldholz reported in *The Wall Street Journal* that "doctors in Britain reported the birth of a healthy test-tube baby who was examined for cystic fibrosis as an eight-cell embryo two days after conception."

The British report prompted the director of the Prenatal Genetics Center at the Baylor Medical School in Houston to declare, "the success with this first family means it is possible to test for a number of genetic diseases before a pregnancy occurs."

A Virginia fertility clinic not far from Washington, D.C., told Waldholz in the fall of 1992 that it had begun offering preimplantation diagnosis for cystic fibrosis to young couples six months earlier; and about 100 couples had inquired about the testing.

However, none of the couples who inquired about preimplantation diagnosis were able or willing to pay the $12,000 such testing would cost. Most of this cost is associated with the test-tube fertilization procedure, and the genetic diagnosis of the test-tube embryos is a minor part of it. The cost, however, is bound to come down rapidly as the practice of preimplantation diagnosis spreads. Molecular biologist Walter Gilbert, Nobel laureate from Harvard University, predicted recently that by the year 2000 genetic testing for any of fifty or so genetic diseases will cost $300 to $500. And the cost will drop rapidly in succeeding years, he believes. By 2020 or 2030, gene testing will be so cheap that a customer could give a few drops of blood to his neighborhood pharmacy and receive his complete genome encoded on a compact disc, Gilbert ventures.

As of this writing, the diseases that can be detected within genes by preimplantation diagnosis include cystic fibrosis; muscular dystrophy; Huntington's disease; a common type of mental retardation called the fragile X syndrome; some types of blindness; and, some inheritable nerve and heart disorders. Molecular geneticists say that they are on the verge of identifying a variety of genes that render individuals susceptible to later developing cancer of the breast, colon, ovaries, and possibly other organs, as well as genes for abnormally high cholesterol levels that render a person susceptible to heart attacks in mid or late life.

As the Human Genome Project rushes to its goal of identifying all human genes, the potential use of preimplantation diagnosis could easily go beyond distinguishing which test-tube embryos are free of genetic disease. Besides the genes for such physical characteristics as sex, height, and eye and hair color, the project will reveal the genes that protect against future illness and that contribute to longevity. The genes for musical, artistic, and athletic ability will become known, as will also the complex of genes for the traits and abilities that comprise intelligence.

The rapidity with which young couples will begin using preimplantation genetic diagnoses should not be underestimated. It was only a generation ago that prenatal diagnosis by withdrawing amniotic fluid—a procedure called amniocentesis—was considered novel and strictly a research tool that would never be widely used. After all, amniocentesis was pointless unless the woman were willing to undergo an abortion should the test show that the fetus was defective; and abortion not only was illegal but was socially unacceptable. Today, abortion is legal; 300,000 American women a year also undergo amniocentesis, each of whom presumably has few objections to abortion.

Although preimplantation diagnosis involves a somewhat uncomfortable procedure for removing ova from the woman, it avoids an abortion, and this fact is likely to appeal to a fairly large segment of prospective parents. Most of the couples inquiring about the procedure at the Virginia clinic, the clinic physician explained, had relatives with cystic fibrosis and were worried that they themselves might bear a child with the disorder. They wanted to avoid becoming pregnant and discovering at the sixteenth week of pregnancy, when a prenatal test can diagnose cystic fibrosis in the fetus, that they faced a decision about an abortion.

Even young couples who have moral qualms about abortion may not object to preimplantation diagnosis. Unlike abortion, this procedure is aimed at achieving pregnancy and birth. Discarding the microscopic clumps of cells that are left over after the prospective parents have made their selection may not have the same psychological impact as the abortion of a sixteen-week-old fetus might, particularly if one adheres to the dictionary definition of an embryo as "the developing human individual *from the time of implantation* (emphasis added) to the end of the eighth week after conception."

There is evidence, such as the growth of prenatal testing via amniocentesis, that suggests that young couples today are increasingly willing to use whatever technology is available to reduce the risks of bearing a defective child. As more couples resort to preimplantation diagnosis to avoid genetic diseases, there will be a growing tendency to redefine certain traits as "disorders." For example, throughout history short stature has been considered normal, albeit unfortunate. However, the advent of genetically engineered hormones that can spur a child's growth has made shortness a treatable medical condition. Thus, it seems highly likely that preimplantation selection will be used by at least some couples to avoid bearing a short child—and that this will be a socially acceptable use.

In sum, it is quite likely that in the near future young couples will begin taking advantage of preimplantation diagnosis to select the traits of their children.

At present, there are no attempts to insert new genes into human test-tube embryos. Thus, the test-tube embryos can inherit only the genes of the two parents. A couple who lacks a gene for "tallness" cannot produce a six-and-a-half-foot basketball player.

But this prohibition is largely a social bar. The technology for adding genes to a test-tube embryo is already perfected in the case of laboratory mice and is being rapidly extended to large mammals, notably cattle and swine. The fact that it is not being done in human embryos is not for any lack of technology but the result only of general agreement that this would be unethical. The advent and use of preimplantation genetic selection, however, may well weaken any ethical or moral objections to altering the genetic endowment of a test-tube embryo. There is not much difference between selecting an embryo to avoid having a short child and inserting a gene into the embryo to make sure the child will be of normal height.

As genetic selection becomes more widely used, society will have to begin making decisions that it has not faced since the turn of the century, when the eugenics movement was at the peak of its influence. As the number of genes that can be detected expands, clinics that perform the preimplantation diagnoses will likely be the first to face a decision on which genetic traits are "worthy." Some clinics, for instance, may well limit their services to diagnoses of the genetic disorders and turn away couples who want to select the sex of their child, or its stature, or who may want to make sure they pick the embryo that carries the mother's gene for perfect pitch. But other clinics may not have any qualms at all about carrying out embryo selections for nondisease traits. Ultimately, competition among the clinics may lead all to offer embryo selection for any trait that is diagnosable and that the prospective parents want.

Almost certainly, medical-care plans will have to cover the cost of preimplantation genetic diagnoses and selections. It would be cost-effective to pay for selecting a test-tube embryo and thus avoid the bearing of a child with a genetic disease who would need medical care for years or decades. The plans then will have to stipulate whether they will cover the cost of all such diagnoses or just certain ones. In the case of employer-financed health-insurance plans, insurance carriers have been willing to cover the cost of any test the employer is willing to pay for. Therefore, employers may well have to decide whether embryo selection for certain nondisease traits is desirable for their employees and, if so, which traits.

And as the federal government takes on the burden of covering the medical cost of the impoverished, a bureaucracy will begin making decisions about which genetic traits are "coverable" and which are not.

There are many potential scenarios, of course. If the cost of preimplantation diagnosis and selection is to be borne only by the prospective parents, then the use of the procedure will be limited largely to the middle- and upper-income groups and denied to the poor. As it becomes possible to select an embryo for its intelligence, the poor could rightly claim overt discrimination. After all, they could argue, in a democracy the poor, above all, should be given every chance to improve the prospects for their children. Such an argument could lead the federal government to begin paying for preimplantation diagnoses and selection for the traits that comprise intelligence. Given the ferocity of the debate in the Congress and the courts over abortion, it is impossible to imagine the uproar that would accompany any attempt by the government to determine who will benefit from embryo selection, what traits the government will finance, and which traits it will determine to be socially nonuseful.

Until now, the selection of human genetic traits has been a process beyond human control. Nature has had three billion years to experiment with such genetic selection and has devised a technology that discards undesirable and harmful traits as they develop while preserving the desirable.

Humans, who have been present for less than one million years, are now acquiring the ability to select the genetic traits of their own species. They have absolutely no experience to guide them in determining which traits they should preserve and which are simply innocuous.

How humans might wield the power of unnatural selection that science is placing in their hands is frightening—and exciting.

Ethical Issues in Human Genome Research
Thomas H. Murray

A biographical sketch of Thomas H. Murray is found on page 464.

Murray explores some of the ethical issues associated with the Human Genome Project. One of the principal issues he addresses is genetic testing in the workplace. Murray argues that genetic screening for susceptibility to workplace-related diseases is ethically permissible, provided the testing is voluntary and the worker is allowed to decide whether to accept an increased risk of disease. In his view, it is ethically problematic for employers to exclude workers from jobs based on genetic susceptibility to workplace-related diseases, and it is even more problematic for employers to exclude workers based on genetic susceptibility to non-workplace-related diseases (i.e., common diseases). In a closely related discussion, Murray briefly considers the issue of insurance companies' discriminating on the basis of genetic predisposition to disease. "Challenges to Our Self-Understanding" is the heading he chooses for one other major area of concern.

Scientific research into human genetics has been a continuing source of intriguing, and at times formidable, ethical issues. The recent worldwide interest in a project to map and ultimately sequence the estimated three billion base pairs of the human genome has generated controversy over the effect such knowledge might have on us, as well as about the wisdom of investing so much research funding—an estimated $3 billion over 15 years in the United States alone—on such a targeted effort.

The latter question is largely a matter of science policy rather than ethics. As an investment of scarce resources, the genome initiative may not be the wisest at this time. Respectable arguments have been made on both sides of the question. But even if it is not the wisest way to spend research resources, that would not make it unethical. . . .

From the standpoint of bioethics, research on the human genome presents no completely novel ethical questions, at least for now. That is partly because of the nature of new ethical questions, which typically are variants of ethical questions that scholars and others have wrestled with before. This embeddedness of questions in experience with analogous questions means that we do not have to invent every response totally anew, but rather can draw on the history of scholarly analysis that has come before. The acceleration of knowledge about human genetics promised by genome research assures

Reprinted with permission of the author and the publisher from *The FASEB Journal*, vol. 5 (January 1991), pp. 55–60.

that the ethical questions presented will be plentiful and significant. They may be grouped into three categories: *1)* the possibility of greatly increased genetic information about individuals and populations; *2)* the manipulation of human genotypes and phenotypes; and *3)* challenges to our understanding of ourselves, individually and collectively.

USES AND MISUSES OF GENETIC INFORMATION

Genome research will allow us to learn a great deal about the genetic makeup of individuals, especially their propensities toward diseases. In many instances, our powers to predict the likelihood (or in some cases certainty) of disease will come years or decades before any effective treatment for the disease is available. . . .

Genetic testing for presymptomatic disease and carrier screening are only two of the uses to which knowledge gained in the Human Genome Initiative might be put. Prenatal screening for genetic disease is another; it stirs controversy because one of the choices upon finding that a fetus is afflicted with genetic disease is abortion. Much scholarship has been devoted to the ethics of abortion, with no resolution of the political battle (1, 2).

These three forms of screening are done, at least purportedly, for the benefit of the individual being screened. New uses of genetic tests are evoking controversy. In these proposed uses, the test is being done not for the good of the person being tested, but rather for some organization—for example, a prospective employer or insurer.

Genetic Testing in the Workplace

In 1938, the geneticist J. B. S. Haldane observed that not all workers exposed to a particular occupational hazard became symptomatic. He postulated that the difference in response to toxic exposures was at least in part genetically determined. If we could assure that individuals who were genetically susceptible to the disease were steered to other occupations, Haldane reasoned, we could reduce the number of people who became ill (3). Workplace genetic screening was justified by its consequences for public health. In Haldane's time, the technology to do genetic screening was not available. But his rationale for workplace genetic screening was revivified in the 1960s and 1970s with suggestions that new screening techniques might make it possible to put his idea into practice (4).

The early proponents of workplace genetic screening did not foresee the political, economic, and ethical complexities their idea would later reveal. The first publicized case of such screening was by a U.S. corporation. A plant owned by this company [was] screening for sickle cell trait among its black workers. The company maintains that the screening was purely voluntary, initiated at the request of an organization of black employees, and that the results were not used in hiring or placement decisions. The journalist who reported the story claims otherwise (5).

Debate about the ethics of workplace genetic testing has focused on the purposes for which such tests might be used. Four purposes have been identified: diagnosis, research, information, and exclusion (6). Genetic tests, like many other procedures, can be helpful in diagnosis and research. Their use in those contexts are governed by the ethics of medical diagnosis and treatment and the ethics of research with human subjects. No novel moral dilemmas attend the use of genetic tests for those purposes.

Genetic tests may also be used before hiring or placing a particular worker to uncover a genetic susceptibility believed to put the individual at greater risk of occupational disease associated with hazards in that workplace. The crucial distinction here is between giving the tests voluntarily, with the information given to the worker who then decides whether to accept any additional risk, or compelling workers to take the tests and using the results to exclude workers who may have genetic susceptibilities.

A program of voluntary testing to inform workers of their risks is ethically defensible. In general, we believe that the individuals affected are the ones with the greatest ethical right to decide whether or not to accept risks. There are some risks that are so nearly certain to occur and cause grievous harm that we do limit choices for individuals. Except for such circumstances we usually allow competent adults to decide for themselves what risks are acceptable to them.

With presymptomatic genetic testing, a program of workplace genetic testing should include effective education and counseling to prevent misunderstanding of the results and to deal with emotional responses to learning that one has genetic risks. A carefully designed program of workplace genetic testing to inform workers, leaving the choice up to individual workers about whether to accept risks, does not confront any insurmountable ethical barriers. The same cannot be said for compelled genetic testing.

Compulsory genetic testing, leading to possible exclusion from jobs, has been controversial. Critics argue that it violates deeply held notions of individual autonomy and could be used in socially undesirable ways. For example, testing for sickle cell anemia followed by exclusion of those with the trait would effectively exclude one of every eight black job candidates in the U.S. Where workers are plentiful, employers might prefer to screen out susceptible workers rather than invest in equipment to reduce exposure to hazards. The prospect of such undesirable effects, along with our respect for individual liberty and choice, make compulsory workplace genetic testing ethically problematic.

The U.S. Congress Office of Technology Assessment (OTA) studied workplace genetic screening in the early 1980s (7). The OTA report concluded that the present state of genetic testing and knowledge about genetic contributions to workplace disease did not justify screening employees for genetic susceptibility. A survey reported in the same study shows some use of genetic tests by U.S. employers, but ambiguities in the report make it impossible to know if the tests were used for legitimate and unproblematic purposes, such as diagnosing the illness of an employee or for the controversial purpose of excluding so-called hypersusceptibles. The OTA is writing another report on genetic testing in the workplace to be released in the fall of 1990.

From Reducing Illness to Reducing Cost

The most important movement in the ethics of workplace genetic testing has been away from the original vision of a public health measure to screening as a way of reducing illness-related costs with no effect on the overall incidence of disease.

Although there is still little evidence that workplace genetic screening could identify individuals with increased risks of workplace-related disease, there is increasing reason to believe that genetic screening for common diseases such as arterial disease (including coronary disease), stroke, and cancer may soon be possible. Other disabling diseases, including mental diseases such as depression and schizophrenia, might also become the targets of genetic screening. Employers might find such tests attractive ways to save money by screening prospective employees and hiring those without evidence of genetic susceptibilities to disease.

Employee illness, at least in the U.S., costs employers money. With health insurance costs becoming an increasingly larger proportion of employer's expenses, employers are looking for ways to diminish health-related costs including health insurance, disability insurance, the cost of lost productivity from ill workers, and the cost of training replacement workers for skilled positions.

The combination of increased employer concerns about the costs of illness and the prospect of genetic tests for predisposition to common, costly diseases are fertile ground for the use of such tests to screen workers.

The ethics of genetic screening for non-workplace-related disease differ in part from genetic screening for workplace-related disease. Working in the particular workplace does not put the worker at an increased risk; the disease to which the person may be susceptible is not related to the workplace. The information to be gained from such tests is not relevant to the individual's choice of whether to work in that environment, although it might be relevant to other life choices, such as diet, exercise, and other health-related behavior. Being denied a job because of predisposition to a non-workplace-related disease is as great an affront to an individual's liberty as a denial for predisposition to a workplace-related disease. But here there is no compensating reduction in risk to the individuals denied employment nor is there any public health benefit; those who will die from heart disease or cancer will still die from it—unemployed and possibly unemployable.

Employers are not the only ones likely to be interested in people's predisposition to common disabling and killing diseases. Companies selling life, disability, or health insurance are also interested in genetic tests.

Genetic Testing in Insurance

Insurance works on the principle of sharing risk. When the risk is equally uncertain to all, then all can be asked to contribute equally to the insurance pool. Not all individuals have the same risk of dying, for example. The older one is (beyond early childhood), the greater the risk of death. Older people are charged more for the same amount of life insurance than younger people. Some occupations are riskier than others. Test pilots pay more for life insurance than accountants. None of this seems unfair. The ethics of discriminating according to genetic predisposition, on the other hand, seems much more ethically complex.

Insurance companies have begun to think about what to do with tests for genetic predisposition to disease (8). As the authors of an industry-sponsored report see it, two factors may force insurers to use genetic tests. First, once such tests become available in medical practice, individuals can be tested privately to learn whether they have enhanced risks of disease. People who learn they have higher risks are more likely to buy insurance and are more likely to buy larger amounts. In the insurance industry, this phenomenon is known as adverse selection—the tendency to purchase insurance when one expects to file a claim. Second, competition among insurance companies will tend to drive companies toward screening for predisposition. If one company begins using such tests, it would be able to offer lower rates to individuals who do not have genetic predisposition to disease and higher rates to those with such predispositions. Individuals offered the lower rates are more likely to purchase insurance from that company, whereas the ones with genetic predisposition to disease will seek insurance from another company that does not do genetic testing. The latter company will either have to raise its rates (to avoid bankruptcy) or it will also have to use genetic tests.

GENETIC MANIPULATION

Probably the most widely discussed and fear-inspiring use of genetic science is genetic manipulation, especially gene therapy. Other uses of genetics to manipulate human physique, physiology, or behavior may be equally significant and raise important ethical issues of their own. . . .

CHALLENGES TO OUR SELF-UNDERSTANDING

There is a tendency in bioethics, as in other fields, to focus on the immediate, practical dilemmas posed by new developments. It may be that the most important challenges posed by the human genome project will not be the pragmatic concerns discussed thus far, but will have to do with the way we understand ourselves, our nature and significance, and our connections with our ancestors and descendants.

One manifestation of the genome initiative will be increased understanding of our genetic similarity with other species. Scientists have tried to estimate DNA homology between humans and other primates to clarify evolutionary relationships among primate species (9). These early efforts to gauge genetic similarity seem to indicate that human DNA is strikingly similar to that of chimpanzees, at least as assessed by the relatively crude measures thus far available. Human DNA appears to be related to more distant species as well. Comparisons of synteny between mouse and human chromosomes show a substantial degree of correspondence, which suggests an evolutionary relationship, coincidentally giving researchers clues to where in the genome to search for a particular gene if its homolog has been found in mice (or humans) (10).

Evidence of our genetic relationship with other species is nothing more than additional confirmation of the theory of evolution. On the other hand, if more and more sophisticated tests of similarity continue to show how much like other species we are, genetically speaking, we may reevaluate not only our molecular but also our moral relationship with nonhuman forms of life.

Genetics as Explanation/Excuse?

One of the most common ethical and legal questions is whether and to what extent a person is responsible for something. We ask if the individual who committed a violent act was responsible for his behavior—morally blameworthy, legally culpable. We ask if the inventor was responsible for the new device (credit rather than blame being at stake here), the scientist for the discovery, the author for the idea, style, and specific words.

We also ask about responsibility for larger issues than discrete acts or inventions. We question whether the overweight person is responsible for his or her obesity, and by extension, for the illnesses to which obesity is a contributing factor, and perhaps for the expense of caring for those illnesses. We ask whether alcoholics are responsible for their addiction and for the consequences of acts committed while they were inebriated.

On an even broader level, we ask whether groups who do especially well (or especially poorly) in various social and economic realms experience the outcomes they do because of some intrinsic traits and abilities or because of lack of opportunity.

Genetics frequently provides an explanation or excuse for individual behaviors or traits, as well as for group differences. The genome project will enhance the tendency to give genetic explanations for individual and group differences in two ways. First, research will suggest genetic correlates for a wide range of human traits and behavior. Some may prove to be spurious, but others will withstand scrutiny. Whenever such a genetic correlate is suggested for some ethically, legally, or economically consequential outcome, there will be a temptation to explain it as fundamentally—that is exclusively or exhaustively—genetic, and hence outside the individual's responsibility or capacity to control. Researchers have recently reported a link between a dopamine receptor gene and alcoholism (11). Others have warned against attributing too much significance to this finding (12).

Second, in the initial rush of findings of genetic connections to important human traits and behavior, both scientists and the public may become too eager to embrace genetic explanations for a vast range of ethically significant phenomena. The phenomena in question may range from illness, including mental illness, addiction, occupational and environmental illness, to the educational and occupational attainments of different racial and ethnic groups.

History is rich with examples of scientific perspectives used inappropriately for political purposes. Frequently, genetic or earlier hereditarian theories have been the subject of such misuse. The first large-scale intelligence testing program in the U.S. was the Army alpha program, which was designed to screen incoming recruits according to their intellectual capacities. Certain groups did not fare well on the test, including immigrants from southern Europe. Because the results conveniently fit the beliefs of those overseeing the testing, they accepted the tests as valid measures of intrinsic ability rather than as the profoundly culture-bound instruments they were. They also overlooked the fact that many of these immigrants spoke English poorly or not at all; the test was in English.

In recent decades the debate has been over the heritability of intelligence and the reason for disparities in IQ test scores among racial and ethnic groups (13). The political consequences of such debates are clear: if educational and economic inequalities are caused by social inequities, then society has an obligation to remedy those inequities; if, on the other hand, the inequalities in outcome are a function of (which in political debate can rapidly be translated into determined by) inherited differences, then we do not have to be so troubled, or worry about our own unjust actions.

The questions raised here also have important, in some instances profoundly important, legal ramifications that must be thoroughly explored. As George Annas has written:

> Although we are utterly unprepared to deal with issues of mandatory screening, confidentiality, privacy, and discrimination, we will likely tell ourselves that we have already dealt with them well . . . (p. 20) (14).

The point here is not that we should ignore the influence of genetics on human affairs. Scientists should be the last people to abandon evidence in favor of sentimental, comforting illusion. Lucidity demands that we confront the truth as it is. Rather, we must learn not to overinterpret what we find. We must learn how to communicate effectively among ourselves and with the public about the limits of our knowledge.

Last, we must acknowledge the limited ethical and political significance of our genetic knowledge. When the founders of the United States wrote that all men (all people) are created equal, they did not mean this as a statement of biological fact, but as an ethical, legal, and political proclamation: before the collectivity of the state, all persons must be regarded as equal—each due equal respect, equal liberty, and equal protection, among other fundamental rights. The sciences of inequality, with genetics at the forefront, will force us to reinterpret what equal treatment and equal regard mean in an enormous range of contexts. But they need not threaten the ethical core of that commitment.

REFERENCES

1 Callahan, D. (1970) *Abortion: Law, Choice and Morality.* Macmillan, New York
2 Luker, K. (1984) *Abortion and the Politics of Motherhood.* University of California, Berkeley
3 Haldane, J. B. S. (1938) *Heredity and Politics.* Allen and Unwin, London
4 Stokinger, H. E., and Mountain, J. T. (1963) Tests for hypersusceptibility to hemolytic chemicals. *Arch. Environ. Hlth.* 6, 57–64
5 Severo, R. (1980) Screening of blacks by DuPont sharpens debate on genetic tests. *New York Times.* 4 February, p. 1
6 Murray, T. H. (1983) Warning: screening workers for genetic risk. *Hastings Center Rep.* 13, (Feb.) 5–8
7 United States Congress Office of Technology Assessment. (1983) *The role of genetic testing in the prevention of occupational disease.* U.S. Government Printing Office, Washington, D.C.
8 Genetic Testing Committee to the Medical Section of the American Council of Life Insurance. (1989) *The potential role of genetic testing in risk classification.* American Council of Life Insurance, Washington, D.C.
9 Koop, B. F., Goodman, M., Xu, P., Chan, K., and Slightom, J. L. (1986) Primate n-globin DNA sequences and man's place among the great apes. *Nature (London)* 319, 234–238
10 McKusick, V. A. (1990) *Mendelian Inheritance in Man,* 8th Ed. Johns Hopkins University Press, Baltimore
11 Blum, K., Noble, E. P., Sheridan, P. J., Montgomery, A., Ritchie, T., Jagadeeswaran, P., Nogami, H., Briggs, A. H., and Cohn, J. B. (1990) Allelic association of human dopamine D_2 receptor gene in alcoholism. *JAMA* 263, 2055–2060
12 Gordis, E., Tabakoff, B., Goldman, D., and Berg, K. (1990) Finding the gene(s) for alcoholism. *JAMA* 263, 2094–2095
13 Jensen, A. R. (1973) *Educability and Group Differences.* Harper and Row, New York
14 Annas, G. (1989) Who's afraid of the human genome? *Hastings Center Rep.* 19, (July/August) 19–21

ANNOTATED BIBLIOGRAPHY: CHAPTER 9

Alpern, Kenneth D.: *The Ethics of Reproductive Technology* (New York: Oxford University Press, 1992). This anthology is designed to address both normative and conceptual questions associated with innovations—both technological (e.g., IVF) and social (e.g., surrogate motherhood)—in human reproduction.

Annas, George J., and Sherman Elias: *Gene Mapping: Using Law and Ethics as Guides* (New York: Oxford University Press, 1992). This collection of articles addresses ethical and legal issues raised by the Human Genome Project.

Boone, C. Keith: "Bad Axioms in Genetic Engineering," *Hastings Center Report* 18 (August/September 1988), pp. 9–13. Boone warns against reliance on simplistic axioms (e.g., we must not "play God" or "interfere with nature") in making ethical judgments in the area of genetic engineering. He emphasizes the need for balanced judgment and attempts to identify in the case of each simplistic axiom a partial truth wrongly represented as the whole truth.

Boss, Judith A.: *The Birth Lottery: Prenatal Diagnosis and Selective Abortion* (Chicago: Loyola University Press, 1993). The first two chapters of this book provide very useful factual information on genetic disorders and prenatal diagnostic procedures. In later chapters, Boss examines various proposed justifications for selective abortion and ultimately concludes that the practice cannot be justified.

Chadwick, Ruth F.: "Cloning," *Philosophy* 57 (April 1982), pp. 201–210. Chadwick contends, on utilitarian grounds, that cloning could be morally justified in some circumstances.

Council on Ethical and Judicial Affairs, American Medical Association: "Use of Genetic Testing by Employers," *JAMA* 266 (October 2, 1991), pp. 1827–1830. The council provides an analysis of the issues involved in the use of genetic testing by employers for the purpose of identifying employees or potential employees at risk for various diseases.

Glover, Jonathan: *What Sort of People Should There Be?* (New York: Penguin Books, 1984). Part One of this book (pp. 23–56) deals with genetic engineering. Glover argues in defense of using genetic engineering to enhance desirable human characteristics.

Holmes, Helen Bequaert: "In Vitro Fertilization: Reflections on the State of the Art," *Birth* 15 (September 1988), pp. 134–145. Holmes provides an account of the various steps involved in the clinical practice of IVF and embryo transfer. She calls attention to a wide array of risks, clinical problems, and ethical issues.

Hull, Richard T., ed.: *Ethical Issues in the New Reproductive Technologies* (Belmont, CA: Wadsworth, 1990). This anthology provides useful material on artificial insemination, IVF, and surrogate motherhood.

Journal of Medicine and Philosophy 16 (December 1991). This issue features a series of articles under the general title of "Human Germ-Line Engineering." A wide range of arguments for and against germ-line gene therapy can be found in the various articles.

Lauritzen, Paul: *Pursuing Parenthood: Ethical Issues in Assisted Reproduction* (Bloomington: Indiana University Press, 1993). Lauritzen considers the ethics of AIH, IVF, donor insemination (AID), and surrogate motherhood. His final chapter is entitled, "The Myth and Reality of Current Adoption Practice."

Law, Medicine & Health Care 16 (Spring/Summer 1988). This special issue is entirely dedicated to surrogate motherhood. Articles are organized under the headings of (1) civil liberties, (2) ethics, and (3) women's autonomy. Material is also provided on the case of Baby M.

Munson, Ronald, and Lawrence H. Davis: "Germ-Line Gene Therapy and the Medical Imperative," *Kennedy Institute of Ethics Journal* 2 (June 1992), pp. 137–158. The authors argue that moral objections to germ-line gene therapy cannot be sustained. They also argue that medicine has a prima facie moral obligation to develop and employ germ-line gene therapy.

National Forum 73 (Spring 1993). This issue features a collection of articles under the heading of "The Human Genome Project." The scientific goals of the project are discussed, as are various social and ethical issues.

Overall, Christine: *Ethics and Human Reproduction: A Feminist Analysis* (Boston: Allen & Unwin, 1987). Overall embraces a feminist perspective on reproductive ethics and contrasts a feminist approach with nonfeminist and antifeminist approaches. Chapter 2 deals with sex preselection, Chapter 6 deals with surrogate motherhood, and Chapter 7 deals with artificial reproduction.

Purdy, Laura M.: "Surrogate Mothering: Exploitation or Empowerment?" *Bioethics* 3 (January 1989), pp. 18–34. Purdy argues against the view that surrogate mothering is necessarily immoral. She acknowledges the danger that surrogate mothering could deepen the exploitation of women but also insists that surrogacy has the potential to empower women.

Robertson, John A.: *Children of Choice: Freedom and the New Reproductive Technologies* (Princeton, NJ: Princeton University Press, 1994). Emphasizing the importance of procreative freedom, Robertson provides an analysis of the ethical, legal, and social issues associated with various reproductive technologies. Chapter 5 deals with IVF; Chapter 6 deals with sperm donation, egg donation, and gestational surrogacy; and Chapter 7 deals with the selection and shaping of offspring characteristics.

Rothman, Barbara Katz: *The Tentative Pregnancy: Prenatal Diagnosis and the Future of Motherhood* (New York: Viking Penguin, 1986). Rothman raises a host of concerns about the social impact of prenatal diagnosis.

Tiefel, Hans O.: "Human *In Vitro* Fertilization: A Conservative View," *JAMA* 247 (June 18, 1982), pp. 3235–3242. Tiefel contends that "the decisive objection to clinical uses of [IVF] lies in the possible and even likely risk of greater than normal harm to offspring." He also argues that nonclinical (purely experimental) uses of IVF are morally unjustifiable, because such uses fail to accord due respect to human embryos.

Walters, LeRoy: "Ethical Issues in Human Gene Therapy," *Journal of Clinical Ethics* 2 (Winter 1991), pp. 267–274. Walters discusses the creation and development of a review process in the United States for somatic-cell gene therapy in humans. He also discusses the ethics of germ-line gene therapy.

Warren, Mary Anne: "IVF and Women's Interests: An Analysis of Feminist Concerns," *Bioethics* 2 (January 1988), pp. 37–57. Warren argues that, although IVF (and other reproductive technologies) "pose some significant dangers for women, it would be wrong to conclude that women's interests demand an end to IVF and other reproductive research." In an effort to guard against a possible negative impact on the interests of women, she insists that IVF is not an adequate overall societal response to the problem of involuntary infertility.

Wertz, Dorothy C., and John C. Fletcher: "Fatal Knowledge? Prenatal Diagnosis and Sex Selection," *Hastings Center Report* 19 (May/June 1989), pp. 21–27. The authors argue against the employment of prenatal diagnosis for the purpose of sex selection.

CHAPTER 10

SOCIAL JUSTICE AND HEALTH-CARE POLICY

INTRODUCTION

No honest discussion of American health care can deny that our system is in crisis. In a reading reprinted in this chapter, Dan E. Beauchamp tersely conveys some of the leading reasons for concern:

> The middle class has joined the nation's poor in doubting its protection against unpaid medical bills. Never-ending increases in insurance costs crowd out wage increases. Employees fear changing jobs and losing their insurance while employers edgily seek to shift coverage costs to workers' shoulders. . . .
>
> Defending against rising costs often adds more costs. Private insurers routinely require doctors and hospitals to justify their use of costly procedures, adding red tape to the system. Medicare's prospective payment system of price controls, called diagnostic-related groups, adds a new layer of administrative personnel to the nation's hospitals. Today, the United States spends well over twice what Canada does on administration. . . .
>
> Rising costs are shredding the private insurance market. As waves of new cost increases hit every year, insurers seek ingenious ways to avoid sick people. Entire trades are "redlined" as too costly to insure; insurance for small business is drying up.
>
> Public programs are permanently destabilized. The urban poor, living where no doctor ever goes, crowd hospital emergency rooms and out-patient clinics. Hospitals respond with costly, often long-delayed care. Medicaid and other payers are hit with a new round of hospital increases. The increases doom legislative plans to fund more primary care for poor neighborhoods, in part to ease hospital crowding. . . .

Unfortunately, the major problems plaguing the American health-care system appear to be worsening. In 1986 the United States spent 10.9 percent of its gross national product (GNP) on health care. In 1994 the figure was about 14 percent. If health-care costs continue to rise at present levels, the United States will devote a staggering 20 percent of its GNP to health care by the year 2003. Somewhat paradoxically, increased expenditures have not been associated with progress on the major goal of expanded access to health care. The United States and South Africa are the only industrial nations not to provide health-care coverage to all of their citizens. In 1986, 37 million Americans were without health insurance; this number rose to 39 million in 1994. If present trends continue, 43 million Americans will lack coverage in 2003.

Because most Americans are disadvantaged by these trends, it is not surprising that, as reflected in public-opinion polls, the American public has largely favored health-care reform for many years. Specifically, most Americans support the goals of (1) universal access to health care and (2) controlling health-care costs. However, the public's preferences are not the only ones that carry weight. Special-interest groups with a financial stake in the shape of health-care delivery exerted extraordinary political muscle in opposing major reform in 1993 and 1994—as the Clinton administration developed and proposed a comprehensive health-care plan and various other plans were sponsored by members of Congress. In particular, the insurance industry, drug companies, to some extent even the American Medical Association (which has resisted major reform several times this century), and other interest groups invested millions of dollars in an effort to preserve the status quo or something relatively close to it.

What does justice require in the way of health-care reform? Is rationing morally defensible, and, if so, what kinds of rationing? What sort of health-care-delivery system would satisfy the demands of justice as well as more practical demands? This chapter explores these and related questions.

Justice, Rights, and Societal Obligations

Does society have a moral obligation to ensure that everyone has access to at least some level of health care? If so, what level of care is the appropriate standard? For example, should society ensure universal access to all needed services, including the most exotic hospital care? Should only basic care be guaranteed? Answering such questions requires an understanding of various conceptions of justice as well as other possible grounds for establishing societal obligations regarding health care.

Justice, Liberty, Equality, and the Right to Health Care   Three broad *conceptions*, or *visions*, of justice dominate in contemporary sociopolitical theory: libertarian, socialist, and liberal. These conceptions, or visions, are sometimes sharpened into specific *theories* of justice. Two moral values, liberty and equality, are of key importance. (Utility also plays a role insofar as everyone agrees that efficiency and practicality are important values, but utility does not unambiguously favor one of the three basic conceptions.) The *libertarian* conception of justice holds liberty to be the ultimate moral ideal; the *socialist* conception of justice takes social equality to be the ultimate moral ideal; and the *liberal* conception tries to combine equality and liberty into one moral ideal.

The Libertarian Conception of Justice   From a libertarian view, individuals have moral rights to life, liberty, and property, which any just society must recognize and respect. These are conceived as negative rights, or rights of noninterference: If *A* has a right to *X*, no one should prevent *A* from pursuing *X* or deprive *A* of *X*. According to libertarians, the sole function of government is to protect the individual's life, liberty, and property against force and fraud. Everything else in society is a matter of individual responsibility and action. Providing for the welfare of those who cannot or will not provide for themselves is not a morally justifiable function of government. To make such provisions, the government would have to take from some against their will in order to give to others. This is perceived as an unjustifiable

limitation on individual liberty. Individuals own their own bodies and, therefore, the labor they exert. It follows, for the libertarian, that individuals have the right to whatever income or wealth their labor can earn in a free marketplace, and no one has the right to take part of that income to provide health care for others.

The Socialist Conception of Justice   A direct challenge to libertarians comes from those who defend the socialist conception of justice. Although socialist views differ in many respects, one common element is a commitment to social equality and to government or collective measures furthering that equality. Since social equality is the ultimate value, limitations on individual liberty that are necessary to promote equality are seen as justified. Socialists attack the libertarian views on the primacy of liberty in at least two ways. First, they defend their ideal of social equality. Their arguments take various forms and need not concern us here. Second, they point out the meaninglessness of rights of noninterference to those who lack adequate food, health care, and so forth. For those who lack the money to buy food and health care needed to sustain life, the libertarian right to life is an empty sham. The rights of liberty, such as the right to exchange goods freely, are meaningless to those who cannot exercise such rights because of economic limitations. Where libertarians stress freedom from governmental interference, socialists stress the government's obligation to promote the welfare of its citizens by ensuring that their most important needs are met. Where libertarians stress *negative rights*, socialists stress *positive rights*, that is, rights to be provided with certain things. Where libertarians criticize socialism for the limitations it imposes on liberty, socialists criticize libertarianism for allowing gross inequalities among those who are "equally human."

The Liberal Conception of Justice   Liberals reject the libertarian conception of justice for failing to include what liberals perceive as a fundamental moral concern: the requirement that those who have more than enough must help those in need. Like the socialist, the liberal recognizes the extent to which economic constraints in an industrial society actually limit the exercise of negative rights by those lacking economic means. Unlike the socialist, the liberal sees some of the negative rights of the libertarian as extremely important but advocates institutions that will function to ensure certain basic liberties (e.g., freedom of speech) while providing for the basic needs of disadvantaged members of society. Liberals are not opposed to all social and economic inequalities, but they disagree concerning both the morally acceptable extent of those inequalities and their justification. A utilitarian liberal, for example, might hold that inequalities are justified to the extent that they increase the total amount of good in society. A different approach is taken by a contemporary philosopher, John Rawls, who maintains that the only justified inequalities in the distribution of primary social goods (e.g., income, opportunities) are those that will benefit everyone in society, especially the least advantaged.[1] The primary concern here is not with the total amount of good in a society but with the good of the least advantaged.

Theories of Justice and a Right to Health Care   What, if anything, can be inferred from theories of justice regarding the existence of a moral right to health care? In one of this chapter's readings, Allen Buchanan asks this question in regard to both a libertarian and a liberal theory of justice. After discussing the libertarian approach as exemplified in the work of Robert Nozick, Buchanan points out that for the libertarian, there is no moral right to health care and no societal obligation to provide it. Citing Rawls's views as an example of a liberal position, Buchanan explains Rawls's central principles of justice before speculating about their implications regarding what constitutes justice in health care. According to Buchanan, the implications of Rawls's theory for a right to health care are far from clear.[2]

Buchanan also discusses the stance a utilitarian might take regarding a right to health care. He has in mind rule-utilitarianism, which (as noted in chapter 1) can support the assertion of certain rights. In rule-utilitarianism, the correct conception of justice and of related moral rights is the one whose application maximizes the net amount of good in society. Buchanan examines some of the implications of a utilitarian approach for a right to health care and the scope of any such right. Buchanan does not discuss the socialist position on justice. In another reading in this chapter, however, Kai Nielsen implicitly argues from a socialist position in defending a right to health care based on a view of justice whose fundamental principle is that of moral equality. Nielsen argues that this principle means that everyone's life matters equally. On his account, any society committed to moral equality must make publicly funded medical treatment of the same quality and extent available to all.

Societal Obligations or Commitments to Provide Health Care   Some arguments supporting a societal obligation to provide health care do not involve the claim that individuals have a *right* to health care. These arguments often appeal to considerations of beneficence as well as considerations of the special nature of health-care needs, a strategy adopted by the President's Commission for the Study of Ethical Problems in Medicine and Biomedical and Behavioral Research.[3] In its influential report, the Commission asserts that society has an obligation to ensure that each of its members has access to adequate care without being subject to excessive burdens. The claim is based on (1) the special moral significance of some health care, (2) the fact that many health-care needs are undeserved, and (3) the implausibility of expecting everyone to be able to meet their health-care needs using their own resources when these needs are so unpredictable, costly, and unevenly distributed among people. Unlike Nielsen, who holds that the same quality and extent of care must be available to everyone, the Commission contends that society has an obligation to ensure universal access to an adequate level of care. This view is consistent with a two-tier medical system in which those who are better off can purchase additional services beyond what is available to everyone.

Other arguments can be developed to support a societal obligation to provide health care without assuming a right to health care. One approach would focus on what universal access to health care (or lack thereof) expresses about a society's character. It might be argued that no decent and compassionate society could fail to provide health care to its members when it has the financial resources to do so. This argument amounts to an appeal to *virtue;* someone advancing such an argument might not even use the term *societal obligation* (since virtue ethics downplays the concept of obligation), preferring instead to speak of *appropriate societal commitments.* A similar argument could be developed from the perspective of *the ethics of care:* A caring society would commit itself to guaranteeing adequate health care to its people, thereby strengthening the social bonds among them. (See Chapter 1 for discussions of virtue ethics and the ethics of care.)

Macroallocation Decisions and the Problem of Rationing

In our society, policy decisions about the allocation of health-care resources are made every day by Congress, state legislatures, health organizations, private foundations, health insurance companies, and federal, state, and local agencies. The allocation decisions made by such groups about health-care expenditures and the distribution of health-care resources are usually called *macroallocation decisions.* They are contrasted with *microallocation decisions,* those made by particular hospital staffs and individual professionals about the allocation of scarce health-care resources (e.g., transplantable organs) to particular patients.

Two of the most important questions concerning macroallocation decisions are the following: (1) How much of our total economic resources should go for health care?; (2) how should this total be divided among specific areas, such as preventive measures, "crisis care," and the production of new equipment used in treatment and diagnosis? Regarding the first, further questions must be asked about the importance of health care vis-à-vis other goods. For example, current biomedical technology is making it possible to save and prolong lives that could not have been saved before. Is the value of prolonging these lives so great that we should adopt public policies that encourage life-prolonging measures no matter what the costs? Should other social goods, such as education, receive less funding in order to prolong individual lives as long as possible? Regarding the second, further questions must be asked concerning both the correct method for making macroallocation decisions and the values that should guide those decisions.

Though the term *rationing* is used in several ways, rationing may be broadly understood, for our purposes, as relating to the second question above and involving choices within a particular area of biomedicine concerning the relative weight to be given to competing needs. For example, concerning the allocation of public funds, should the funding of prenatal care take precedence over the funding of heart transplants? One sense of *rationing* is that of *denying* individuals services they need or want because of limited resources. It is in this sense of *rationing* that we may say that the American health-care system presently rations *by the ability to pay;* persons lacking health insurance or sufficient funds are often denied health care they need or want. In this age of soaring health-care costs, a question receiving increasing attention is whether more *explicit* forms of rationing should be accepted.

If it is necessary or desirable to ration health care explicitly, what are the morally appropriate criteria to use? One suggested criterion is that of *age.* Daniel Callahan, who in a reading in this chapter advocates age-based rationing, points out that in 1986 those older than 65 consumed 31 percent of the total of 450 billion dollars spent on health care in the United States. Demographers predict that by the year 2040, 21 percent of the United States population will be older than 65 and will consume 45 percent of all health-care expenditures. In light of such projections, it is not surprising that some individuals defend the use of advanced age as a criterion for denying public funding for certain kinds of medical care. Two other articles in this chapter—those by Amitai Etzioni and Nora Kizer Bell—respond specifically to Callahan's proposals and condemn age-based rationing, though for different reasons.

The state of Oregon has directly confronted the problems of access to health care and rising costs by developing an explicit rationing plan, whose goal is to ensure that all Oregonians have access to basic health care. A state commission appointed in 1989 was assigned the task of ranking medical services available through Medicaid. Rankings—from most important to least important—were to take into account both the costs of services and their likely effects on patients' quality of life. The plan called for funding as many of the services as possible within the limits of the state budget, provided that all Oregonians at or below the federal poverty line would be covered. The state commission's long list of ranked medical services, presented in 1990, stirred ethical and political debate about particular rankings, criteria used for ranking, and the list's consequences for particular groups of patients. This debate continues as Oregon makes explicit rationing decisions in accordance with its plan, which was revised several times in the face of political and legal pressures and was finally given federal approval in 1993. In a reading reprinted in this chapter, Norman Daniels explores the question of whether the Oregon rationing plan is fair or just. His analysis considers such aspects of the plan as (1) extending health-care coverage to those who had lacked it, (2) removing coverage of some (relatively low-ranked) services for persons who had been covered by Medicaid, and (3) attempting to base health-care priorities on values expressed in public meetings.

Debates over what criteria to use for rationing and how to implement a rationing plan are fueled by the assumption that rationing is in some sense inevitable or necessary. At least when taken to mean some harsh limitation or denial of services, rationing is typically thought to be ethical *only because* it is necessary. However, a sensible discussion of whether rationing really is necessary requires clarity about what precisely is meant by *rationing.* In one of this chapter's articles, Daniel Wikler distinguishes senses of the term that are particularly useful in this context. "Trimming," the limiting or exclusion of services that few people want and no one needs (e.g., ineffective treatments), is not really controversial; indeed, it would be irresponsible not to engage in this form of rationing, he argues. Truly painful rationing decisions concern "cutting" or "hard rationing," the limiting or exclusion of services that are clearly both wanted and needed. (Wikler also considers an intermediate form of rationing that we need not consider here.) Wikler challenges the common assumption that even cutting is necessary. In reply to the common view that cutting is necessitated by exploding medical costs, Wikler argues that we must seek to understand what is driving up costs and ask whether some alternative to cutting could relieve this financial pressure in a morally preferable way. He strongly suspects that there are alternatives:

> International comparisons suggest that the choices that are so unwelcome are not necessary ones; given the right kind of reforms in our health care system, we could exchange [our] ethical dilemmas for the more acceptable problems which other countries face.

Thus the question of whether the most painful form of rationing is necessary leads to the question of what is possible in the way of health-care reform.

Health-Care-Delivery Systems

In considering what sort of health-care-delivery system we should have, we need to know our starting point. The American health-care system is presently a mix of private and public elements. A large percentage of the United States population has some form of private health insurance, often paid for largely or partly by employers. Federal funds provide government-financed insurance to people older than 65 (Medicare) and to those below a certain income level (Medicaid), though income thresholds vary greatly from state to state. In addition, special groups, such as veterans and those suffering from certain diseases, such as cancer or tuberculosis, are directly cared for in hospitals operated by the government. Veterans' hospitals, for example, are operated by the federal government; other hospitals are supported by federal, state, and local funds. In 1994 about 85 percent of the U.S. population was covered by private or public health insurance. However, about 39 million Americans were not covered by either public or private health insurance.

Assuming some type of health-care reform in the United States is morally imperative, the question arises as to what sorts of reforms should be sought. What kind of health-care-delivery system should we have? Plausible answers—which tend to agree on the goals of universal access and controlling costs—can be divided into two groups: (1) those that favor retaining a mix of private and public elements; (2) those that favor moving to an entirely publicly funded or "single-payer" system.

"Mixed" Health-Care-Delivery Systems   Advocates of reform within a "mixed" system generally seek to restructure both public and private elements of our health-care system to make them more effective in extending access and containing costs. An example of public-sector inefficiency would be a state whose eligibility criteria for Medicaid are so strict that they exclude many indigent persons. A common effect of leaving poor persons uncovered for even basic care is that preventable health problems eventually take them to the most expensive places of health-care delivery—emergency rooms—where law requires that people be treated regardless of ability to pay. A major source of private-sector inefficiency is a fee-for-service system in which (1) physicians and hospitals are reimbursed by insurance companies for particular services rendered, and (2) neither patients nor physicians have any incentive to be cost-conscious. In such a system, only the insurance companies have an incentive to reduce costs. Yet, for insurance companies to review treatment decisions in an effort to prevent unnecessary treatment (and therefore unnecessary costs), they must engage in a highly intensive form of micromanagement, adding a deep, expensive layer of administration to the health-care system. Because our system makes extensive use of fee-for-service reimbursement by insurance companies, realistic health-care reform that retains a public-private framework must include measures that alleviate the cost pressures just described.

A leading model for containing costs within a public-private framework has been called *managed competition.* As explained by its proponents Alain C. Enthoven and Richard Kronick in an article reprinted in this chapter, the major idea of this model is that restructuring our system so as to correct the financial incentives will eventually lead to a system in which costs are under control and everyone has access to *managed care.* An example of managed care is the care provided by health maintenance organizations (HMOs). In contrast to fee-for-service reimbursement by insurance companies, HMOs provide needed care to individuals for a lump sum per month. Since HMOs are paid a lump sum, and not paid each time a service is provided, they have an incentive to be cost-conscious; they therefore emphasize preventive and basic care over "crisis" and specialty care. The authors' proposal seeks to make available to everyone a choice of managed-care plans that compete with each other within certain restrictions designed to set the right financial incentives (managed competition), with state "Public Sponsors" providing subsidized care to those who would otherwise lack insurance. A crucial part of the proposal is an *employer mandate:* Employers must cover employees with plans meeting federal requirements or else pay a payroll tax that helps fund the system.

The Single-Payer Option   Concerns about controlling the costs of health care while achieving universal access have led many Americans to prefer the administratively simpler single-payer option. Canada is one of numerous industrial nations with single-payer systems affording universal access to health care. While spending considerably less per capita on health care than the United States does, Canada provides high-quality care and achieves health indexes that are at least comparable to those of the United States. Significantly, Canada provides a *complete* package of health-care services for all its citizens; it is not as if certain clearly essential services are cut out of the budget due to projected costs (as in cutting).

Financing Canada's single-payer system is made possible by the administrative savings that result from a streamlined finance system. For a point of comparison, while the United States spends about 25 cents of every health-care dollar on administration, Canada spends about 13 cents. The United States has more than 1,500 different payers. Most of them, as part of the private sector, must advertise, determine patient eligibility, elaborate restrictions on coverage, conduct patient-by-patient utilization reviews, try to collect on bad debts, and so on, while seeking a profit. In contrast, Canada funds all health care through provincial governments. No patient is billed. Physicians and hospitals submit simple, standardized forms and get paid on a fee-for-service basis.

Despite its record of success on several counts, the Canadian system has its critics (including the American Medical Association). It is commonly argued that any government-run system would be highly bureaucratic and inefficient. Supporters of the Canadian system, however, contend that precisely because it is *less* bureaucratic—cutting out the wasteful insurance-companies component—it is more efficient. Interestingly, of the numerous plans submitted to Congress and studied by the U.S. Congressional Budget Office (CBO), the single-payer plan was the only one the CBO projected to achieve universal coverage while saving money (billions of dollars per year). The Canadian system is also criticized for making patients wait in line for needed services. However, these waits (which have been greatly exaggerated by some special-interest groups) are generally for elective services; seriously ill persons are prioritized. That does not mean the waits that do exist are not inconvenient, however.

While the vast majority of Canadians would not trade their health-care system for the American system (according to polls), some wealthy Canadians have sought high-technology services in the United States rather than wait for them in Canada.

In an article reprinted in this chapter, Steffie Woolhandler and David U. Himmelstein argue that only a single-payer system will enable the United States to achieve universal coverage while controlling costs. Citing extensive data on the American and Canadian health-care systems, the authors outline the publicly funded national health plan that they propose. In this chapter's final reading, Dan E. Beauchamp tries to reconcile the administrative advantages of a single-payer system with American political values. He concludes that the best resolution might be what he calls a "single-fund" health-care system that retains a place for insurance companies.

D.D.

NOTES

1 John Rawls, *A Theory of Justice* (Cambridge, MA: Harvard University Press, 1971).
2 Philosophers have, in fact, emphasized different elements in Rawls's theory of justice in spelling out consequences for health-care allocation. See, e.g., Ronald M. Green, "Health Care and Justice in Contract Theory Perspective," in Robert M. Veatch and Roy Branson, eds., *Ethics and Health Policy* (Cambridge, MA: Ballinger, 1976), pp. 111–126; Norman Daniels, "Health Care Needs and Distributive Justice," *Philosophy and Public Affairs* 10 (Spring 1981), pp. 146–179; and David DeGrazia, "Grounding a Right to Health Care in Self-Respect and Self-Esteem," *Public Affairs Quarterly* 5 (October 1991), pp. 301–318.
3 President's Commission for the Study of Ethical Problems in Medicine and Biomedical and Behavioral Research, *Securing Access to Health Care* (Washington, DC: Government Printing Office, 1983).

Justice, Rights, and Societal Obligations

Justice: A Philosophical Review
Allen Buchanan

A biographical sketch of Allen Buchanan is found on pages 100–101.

Buchanan begins by setting out three theoretical approaches to justice: (1) a utilitarian approach, (2) Rawls's theory of justice as fairness, and (3) Nozick's libertarian theory. He confronts each position with several questions about health care. These questions deal with a right to health care, the relative importance of health care or health-care needs vis-à-vis other goods or needs, the relative importance of various forms of health care, and the compatibility of our current health-care system with the demands of justice. Buchanan concludes that none of the three theoretical approaches provides unambiguous answers to all the questions raised and that the application of each depends on numerous unavailable empirical premises. This leaves a great deal of work to be done in developing an account of justice in health care.

From *Justice and Health Care,* edited by Earl Shelp, pp. 3–21. Copyright © 1981 by D. Reidel Publishing Company, Dordrecht, Holland. Reprinted by permission of Kluwer Academic Publishers.

INTRODUCTION

The past decade has seen the burgeoning of bioethics and the resurgence of theorizing about justice. Yet until now these two developments have not been as mutually enriching as one might have hoped. Bioethicists have tended to concentrate on micro issues (moral problems of individual or small group decisionmaking), ignoring fundamental moral questions about the macro structure within which the micro issues arise. Theorists of justice have advanced very general principles but have typically neglected to show how they can illuminate the particular problems we face in health care and other urgent areas.

Micro problems do not exist in an institutional vacuum. The parents of a severely impaired newborn and the attending neonatologist are faced with the decision of whether to treat the infant aggressively or to allow it to die because neonatal intensive care units now exist which make it possible to preserve the lives of infants who previously would have died. Neonatal intensive care units exist because certain policy decisions have been made which allocated certain social resources to the development of technology for sustaining defective newborns rather than for preventing birth defects. Limiting moral inquiry to the micro issues supports an unreasoned conservatism by failing to examine the health care institutions within which micro problems arise and by not investigating the larger array of institutions of which the health care sector is only one part. Since not only particular actions but also policies and institutions may be just or unjust, serious theorizing about justice forces us to expand the narrow focus of the micro approach by raising fundamental queries about the background social, economic, and political institutions from which micro problems emerge.

On the other hand, the attention to individual cases which dominates contemporary bioethics can provide a much needed concrete focus for refining and assessing competing theories of justice. The adequacy or inadequacy of a moral theory cannot be determined by inspecting the principles which constitute it. Instead, rational assessment requires an on-going process in which general principles are revised and refined through confrontation with the rich complexity of our considered judgments about particular cases, while our judgments about particular cases are gradually structured and modified by our provisional acceptance of general principles. Since our considered judgments about particular cases may often be more sensitive and sure than our assessments of abstract principles, careful attention to accurately described, concrete moral situations is essential for theorizing about justice.

Further, it is not just that the problems of bioethics provide one class of test cases for theories of justice among others: the problems of bioethics are among the most difficult and pressing issues with which a theory of justice must cope. It appears, then, that the continued development of both bioethics and of theorizing about justice in general requires us to explore the problems of justice in health care. In this essay I hope to contribute to that enterprise by first providing a sketch of three major theories of justice and by then attempting to ascertain some of their implications for moral problems in health care.

THEORIES OF JUSTICE

Utilitarianism

Utilitarianism purports to be a comprehensive moral theory, of which a utilitarian theory of justice is only one part. There are two main types of comprehensive utilitarian theory: Act and Rule Utilitarianism. Act Utilitarianism defines rightness with respect to particular acts: an act is right if and only if it maximizes utility. Rule Utilitarianism defines rights with respect to rules of action and makes the rightness of particular acts depend upon the rules under which those acts fall. A rule is right if and only if general compliance with that rule (or with a set of rules of which it is an element) maximizes utility, and a particular action is right if and only if it falls under such a rule.

Both Act and Rule Utilitarianism may be versions of either Classic or Average Utilitarianism. Classic Utilitarianism defines the rightness of acts or rules as maximization of *aggregate* utility; Average Utilitarianism defines rightness as maximization of utility *per capita*. The aggregate utility produced by an act or by general compliance with a rule is the sum of the utility produced for each individual affected. Average utility is the aggregate utility divided by the number of individuals affected. 'Utility' is defined as pleasure, satisfaction, happiness, or as the realization of preferences, as the latter are revealed through individuals' choices.

The distinction between Act and Rule Utilitarianism is important for a utilitarian theory of justice, since the latter must include an account of when *institutions* are just. Thus, institutional rules may maximize utility even though those rules do not direct individuals as individuals or as occupants of institutional positions to maximize utility in a case by case fashion. For example, it may be that a judicial system which maximizes utility will do so by including rules which prohibit judges from deciding a case according to their estimates of what would maximize utility in that particular case. Thus the utilitarian justification of a particular action or decision may not be that it maximizes utility, but rather that it falls under some rule of an institution or set of institutions which maximizes utility.[1]

Some utilitarians, such as John Stuart Mill, hold that principles of justice are the most basic moral principles because the utility of adherence to them is especially great. According to this view, utilitarian principles of justice are those utilitarian moral principles which are of such importance that they may be *enforced*, if necessary. Some utilitarians, including Mill perhaps, also hold that among the utilitarian principles of justice are principles specifying individual rights, whether the latter are thought of as enforceable claims which take precedence over appeals to what would maximize utility in the particular case. Indeed, some contemporary rights theorists such as Ronald Dworkin define a (justified) right claim as one which takes precedence over mere appeals to what would maximize utility.

A utilitarian moral theory, then, can include rights principles which themselves prohibit appeals to utility maximization, so long as the justification of those principles is that they are part of an institutional system which maximizes utility. In cases where two or more rights principles conflict, considerations of utility may be invoked to determine which rights principles are to be given priority. Utilitarianism is incompatible with rights only if rights exclude appeals to utility maximization at all levels of justification, including the most basic institutional level. Rights founded ultimately on considerations of utility may be called *derivative*, to distinguish them from rights in the *strict* sense.

Utilitarianism is the most influential version of teleological moral theory. A moral theory is teleological if and only if it defines the good independently of the right and defines the right as that which maximizes the good. Utilitarianism defines the good as happiness (satisfaction, etc.), independently of any account of what is morally right, and then defines the right as that which maximizes the good (either in the particular case or at the institutional level). A moral theory is *deontological* if and only if it is not a teleological theory, i.e., if and only if it either does not define the good independently of the right or does not define the right as that which maximizes the good. Both the second and third theories of justice we shall consider are deontological theories.

John Rawls's Theory: Justice as Fairness

In *A Theory of Justice* Rawls pursues two main goals. The first is to set out a small but powerful set of principles of justice which underlie and explain the considered moral judgments we make about particular actions, policies, laws, and institutions. The second is to offer a theory of justice superior to Utilitarianism. These two goals are intimately related for Rawls because he believes that the theory which does a better job of supporting and accounting for our considered judgments is the better theory, other things being equal. The principles of justice Rawls offers are as follows:

1. The principle of greatest equal liberty: Each person is to have an equal right to the most extensive system of equal basic liberties compatible with a similar system of liberty for all ([6], pp. 60, 201–205).

2. The principle of equality of fair opportunity: Offices and positions are to be open to all under conditions of equality of fair opportunity—persons with similar abilities and skills are to have equal access to offices and positions. ([6], pp. 60, 73, 83–89).[2]

3. The difference principle: Social and economic institutions are to be arranged so as to benefit maximally the worst off ([6], pp. 60, 75–83).[3]

The basic liberties referred to in (1) include freedom of speech, freedom of conscience, freedom from arbitrary arrest, the right to hold personal property, and freedom of political participation (the right to vote, to run for office, etc.).

Since the demands of these principles may conflict, some way of ordering them is needed. According to Rawls, (1) is *lexically prior* to (2) and (2) is *lexically prior* to (3). A principle 'P' is lexically prior to a principle 'Q' if and only if we are first to satisfy all the requirements of 'P' before going on to satisfy the requirements of 'Q.' Lexical priority allows no trade-offs between the demands of conflicting principles: the lexically prior principle takes absolute priority.

Rawls notes that "many kinds of things are said to be just or unjust: not only laws, institutions, and social systems, but also particular actions . . . decisions, judgments and imputations. . . ." ([6], p. 7). But he insists that the primary subject of justice is the *basic structure* of society because it exerts a pervasive and profound influence on individuals' life prospects. The basic structure is the entire set of major political, legal, economic, and social institutions. In our society the basic structure includes the Constitution, private ownership of the means of production, competitive markets, and the monogamous family. The basic structure plays a large role in distributing the burdens and benefits of cooperation among members of society.

If the primary subject of justice is the basic structure, then the primary problem of justice is to formulate and justify a set of principles which a just basic structure must satisfy. These principles will specify how the basic structure is to distribute prospects of what Rawls calls *primary goods*. They include the basic liberties (listed above under (2)), as well as powers, authority, opportunities, income, and wealth. Rawls says that primary goods are things that every rational person is presumed to want, because they normally have a use, whatever a person's rational plan of life ([6], p. 62). Principle (1) regulates the distribution of prospects of basic liberties; (2) regulates the distribution of prospects of powers and authority, so far as these are attached to institutional offices and positions, and (3) regulates the distribution of prospects of the other primary goods, including wealth and income. Though the first and second principles require equality, the difference principle allows inequalities so long as the total system of institutions of which they are a part maximizes the prospects of the worst off to the primary goods in question.

Rawls advances three distinct types of justification for his principles of justice. Two appeal to our considered judgments, while the third is based on what he calls the Kantian interpretation of his theory.

The first type of justification rests on the idea, mentioned earlier, that if a set of principles provides the best account of our considered judgments about what is just or unjust, then that is a reason for accepting those principles. A set of principles accounts for our judgments only if those judgments can be derived from the principles, granted the relevant facts for their application.

Rawls's second type of justification maintains that if a set of principles would be chosen under conditions which, according to our considered judgments, are appropriate conditions for choosing principles of justice, then this is a reason for accepting those principles. The second type of justification includes three parts: (1) A set of conditions for choosing principles of justice must be specified. Rawls labels the complete set of conditions the 'original position.' (2) It must be shown that the conditions specified are (according to our considered judgments) the appropriate conditions of choice. (3) It must be shown that Rawls's principles are indeed the

principles which would be chosen under those conditions.

Rawls construes the choice of principles of justice as an ideal social contract. "The principles of justice for the basic structure of society are the principles that free and rational persons . . . would accept in an initial situation of equality as defining the fundamental terms of their association" ([6], p. 11). The idea of a social contract has several advantages. First, it allows us to view principles of justice as the object of a *rational collective choice*. Second, the idea of *contractual obligation* is used to emphasize that the choice expresses a basic commitment and that the principles agreed on may be rightly enforced. Third, the idea of a contract as a *voluntary agreement* which set terms for mutual advantage suggests that the principles of justice should be "such as to draw forth the willing cooperation" ([6], p. 15) of all members of society, including those who are worse off.

The most important elements of the original position for our purposes are a) the characterization of the parties to the contract as individuals who desire to pursue their own life plans effectively and who "have a highest-order interest in how . . . their interests . . . are shaped and regulated by social institutions" ([8], p. 64); b) the 'veil of ignorance,' which is a constraint on the information the parties are able to utilize in choosing principles of justice; and c) the requirement that the principles are to be chosen on the assumption that they will be complied with by all (the universalizability condition) ([6], p. 132).

The parties are characterized as desiring to maximize their shares of primary goods, because these goods enable one to implement effectively the widest range of life plans and because at least some of them, such as freedom of speech and of conscience, facilitate one's freedom to choose and revise one's life plan or conception of the good. The parties are to choose "from behind a veil of ignorance" so that information about their own particular characteristics or social positions will not lead to bias in the choice of principles. Thus they are described as not knowing their race, sex, socioeconomic, or political status, or even the nature of their particular conceptions of the good. The informational restriction also helps to insure that the principles chosen will not place avoidable restrictions on the individual's freedom to choose and revise his or her life plan.[4]

Though Rawls offers several arguments to show that his principles would be chosen in the original position, the most striking is the maximin argument. According to this argument, the rational strategy in the original position is to choose that set of principles whose implementation will maximize the minimum share of primary goods which one can receive as a member of society, and principles (1), (2), and (3) will insure the greatest minimal share. Rawls's claim is that because these principles protect one's basic liberties and opportunities and insure an adequate minimum of goods such as wealth and income (even if one should turn out to be among the worst off) the rational thing is to choose them, rather than to gamble with one's life prospects by opting for alternative principles. In particular, Rawls contends that it would be irrational to reject his principles and allow one's life prospect to be determined by what would maximize utility, since utility maximization might allow severe deprivation or even slavery for some, so long as this contributed sufficiently to the welfare of others.

Rawls raises an important question about this second mode of justification when he notes that this original position is purely hypothetical. Granted that the agreement is never actually entered into, why should we regard the principles as binding? The answer, according to Rawls, is that we do in fact accept the conditions embodied in the original position ([6], p. 21). The following qualification, which Rawls adds immediately after claiming that the conditions which constitute the original position are appropriate for the choice of principles of justice according to our considered judgments, introduces his third type of justification: "Or if we do not [accept the conditions of the original position as appropriate for choosing principles of justice] *then perhaps we can be persuaded to do so by the philosophical reflections*" (emphasis added [6], p. 21). In the Kantian interpretation section of *A Theory of Justice*, Rawls sketches a certain kind of philosophical justification for the conditions which make up the original position (based on Kant's conception of the 'noumenal self' or autonomous agent).

For Kant an autonomous agent's will is determined by rational principles and rational principles are those which can serve as principles for all rational beings, not just for this or that agent, depending upon whether or not he has some particular desire which other rational beings may not have. Rawls invites us to think of the original position as the perspective from which autonomous agents see the world. The original position provides a "procedural interpretation" of Kant's idea of a Realm of Ends or community of "free and equal rational beings." We express our nature as autonomous agents when we act from principles that would be chosen in conditions which reflect that nature ([6], p. 252). Rawls concludes that, when persons such as you

and I accept those principles that would be chosen in the original position, we express our nature as autonomous agents, i.e., we act autonomously. There are three main grounds for this thesis, corresponding to the three features of the original position cited earlier. First, since the veil of ignorance excludes information about any particular desires which a rational agent may or may not have, the choice of principles is not determined by any particular desire. Second, since the parties strive to maximize their share of primary goods, and since primary goods are attractive to them because they facilitate freedom in choosing and revising life plans and because they are flexible means not tied to any particular ends, this is another respect in which their choice is not determined by particular desires. Third, the original position includes the requirement that they will be principles of rational agents in general and not just for agents who happen to have this or that particular desire.

In the *Foundation of the Metaphysics of Morals* Kant advances a moral philosophy which identifies autonomy with rationality [4]. Hence for Kant the question "Why should one express our nature as autonomous agents?" is answered by the thesis that rationality requires it. Thus if Rawls's third type of justification succeeds in showing that we best express our autonomy when we accept those principles in the belief that they would be chosen from the original position, and if Kant's identification of autonomy with rationality is successful, the result will be a justification of Rawls's principles which is distinct from both the first and second modes of justification. So far as this third type of justification does not make the acceptance of Rawls's principles hinge on whether the principles themselves or the conditions from which they would be chosen match our considered judgments, it is not directly vulnerable either to the charge that Rawls has misconstrued our considered judgments or that congruence with considered judgments, like the appeal to mere consensus, has no justificatory force.

It is important to see that Rawls understands his principles of justice as principles which generate *rights* in what I have called the strict sense. Claims based upon the three principles are to take precedence over considerations of utility and the principles themselves are not justified on the grounds that a basic structure which satisfies them will maximize utility. Moreover, Rawls's theory is not a teleological theory of any kind because it does not define the right as that which maximizes the good, where the good is defined independently of the right. Instead it is perhaps the most influential current instance of a deontological theory.

Nozick's Libertarian Theory

There are many versions of libertarian theory, but their characteristic doctrine is that coercion may only be used to prevent or punish physical harm, theft, and fraud, and to enforce contracts. Perhaps the most influential and systematic recent instance of Libertarianism is the theory presented by Robert Nozick in *Anarchy, State, and Utopia* [5]. In Nozick's theory of justice, as in libertarian theories generally, the right to private property is fundamental and determines both the legitimate role of the state and the most basic principles of individual conduct.

Nozick contends that individuals have a property right in their persons and in whatever 'holdings' they come to have through actions which conform to (1) "the principle of justice in [initial] acquisition" and (2) "the principle of justice in transfer" ([5], p. 151). The first principle specifies the ways in which an individual may come to own hitherto unowned things without violating anyone else's rights. Here Nozick largely follows John Locke's famous account of how one makes natural objects one's own by "mixing one's labor" with them or improving them through one's labor. Though Nozick does not actually formulate a principle of justice in (initial) acquisition, he does argue that whatever the appropriate formulation is it must include a 'Lockean Proviso,' which places a constraint on the holdings which one may acquire through one's labor. Nozick maintains that one may appropriate as much of an unowned item as one desires so long as (a) one's appropriation does not worsen the conditions of others in a special way, namely, by creating a situation in which others are "no longer . . . able to use freely [without exclusively appropriating] what [they] . . . previously could" or (b) one properly compensates those whose condition is worsened by one's appropriation in the way specified in (a) ([5], pp. 178–179). Nozick emphasizes that the Proviso only picks out one way in which one's appropriation may worsen the condition of others; it does not forbid appropriation or require compensation in cases in which one's appropriation of an unowned thing worsens another's condition merely by limiting his opportunities to appropriate (rather than merely use) that thing, i.e., to make it his property.

The second principle states that one may justly transfer one's legitimate holdings to another through sale, trade, gift or bequest and that one is entitled to whatever one receives in any of these ways, so long as the person from whom one receives it was entitled to that which he transferred to you. The right to property

which Nozick advances is the right to exclusive control over anything one can get through initial appropriation (subject to the Lockean Proviso) or through voluntary exchanges with others entitled to what they transfer. Nozick concludes that a distribution is just if and only if it arose from another just distribution by legitimate means. The principle of justice in initial acquisition specifies the legitimate 'first moves,' while the principle of justice in transfers specifies the legitimate ways of moving from one distribution to another: "Whatever arises from a just situation by just steps is itself just" ([5], p. 151).

Since not all existing holdings arose through the 'just steps' specified by the principles of justice in acquisition and transfer, there will be a need for a *principle of rectification* of past injustices. Though Nozick does not attempt to formulate such a principle he thinks that it might well require significant redistribution of holdings.

Apart from the case of rectifying past violations of the principles of acquisition and transfer, however, Nozick's theory is strikingly anti-redistributive. Nozick contends that attempts to force anyone to contribute any part of his legitimate holdings to the welfare of others is a violation of that person's property rights, whether it is undertaken by private individuals or the state. On this view, coercively backed taxation to raise funds for welfare programs of any kind is literally theft. Thus, a large proportion of the activities now engaged in by the government involve gross injustices.

After stating his theory of rights, Nozick tries to show that the state is legitimate so long as it limits its activities to the enforcement of these rights and eschews redistributive functions. To do this he employs an 'invisible hand explanation,' which purports to show how the minimal state could arise as an unintended consequence of a series of voluntary transactions which violate no one's rights. The phrase 'invisible hand explanation' is chosen to stress that the process by which the minimal state could emerge fits Adam Smith's famous account of how individuals freely pursuing their own private ends in the market collectively produce benefits which are not the aim of anyone.

The process by which the minimal state could arise without violating anyone's rights is said to include four main steps ([5], pp. 10–25).[5] First, individuals in a 'state of nature' in which (Libertarian) moral principles are generally respected would form a plurality of 'protective agencies' to enforce their libertarian rights, since individual efforts at enforcement would be inefficient and liable to abuse. Second, through competition for clients, a 'dominant protective agency' would eventually emerge in given geographical area. Third, such an agency would eventually become a 'minimal state' by asserting a claim of monopoly over protective services in order to prevent less reliable efforts at enforcement which might endanger its clients: it would forbid 'independents' (those who refused to purchase its services) from seeking other forms of enforcement. Fourth, again assuming that correct moral principles are generally followed, those belonging to the dominant protective agency would compensate the 'independents,' presumably by providing them with free or partially subsidized protection services. With the exception of taxing its clients to provide compensation for the independents, the minimal state would act only to protect persons against physical injury, theft, fraud, and violations of contracts.

It is striking that Nozick does not attempt to provide any systematic *justification* for the Lockean rights principles he advocates. In this respect he departs radically from Rawls. Instead, Nozick assumes the correctness of the Lockean principles and then, on the basis of that assumption, argues that the minimal state and only the minimal state is compatible with the rights those principles specify.

He does, however, offer some arguments against the more-than-minimal state which purport to be independent of that particular theory of property rights which he assumes. These arguments may provide indirect support for his principles insofar as they are designed to make alternative principles, such as Rawls's, unattractive. Perhaps most important of these is an argument designed to show that any principle of justice which demands a certain distributive end state or pattern of holdings will require frequent and gross disruptions of individuals' holdings for the sake of maintaining that end state or pattern. Nozick supports this general conclusion by a vivid example. He asks us to suppose that there is some distribution of holdings 'D$_1$' which is required by some end-state or patterned theory of justice and that 'D$_1$' is achieved at time 'T.' Now suppose that Wilt Chamberlain, the renowned basketball player, signs a contract stipulating that he is to receive twenty-five cents from the price of each ticket to the home games in which he performs, and suppose that he nets $250,000, from this arrangement. We now have a new distribution 'D$_2$.' Is 'D$_2$' unjust? Notice that by hypothesis those who paid the price of admission were entitled to control over the resources they held in 'D$_1$' (as were Chamberlain and the team's owners). The new distribution arose through *voluntary exchanges of legitimate holdings,* so it is difficult to see how it could be unjust, even if it does diverge from 'D$_1$.' From this and

like examples, Nozick concludes that attempts to maintain any end-state or patterned distributive principle would require continuous interference in peoples' lives ([5], pp. 161–163).

As in the cases of Utilitarianism and Rawls's theory, Nozick and libertarians generally do not limit morality to justice. Thus, Nozick and others emphasize that a libertarian theory of individual rights is to be supplemented by a libertarian theory of virtues which recognizes that not all moral principles are suitable objects of enforcement and that moral life includes more than the nonviolation of rights. Libertarians invoke the distinction between justice and charity to reply to those who complain that a Lockean theory of property rights legitimizes crushing poverty for millions. They stress that while justice demands that we not be *forced* to contribute to the well-being of others, charity requires that we help even those who have no *right* to our aid.[6]

IMPLICATIONS FOR HEALTH CARE

Now that we have a grasp of the main ideas of three major theories of justice, we can explore briefly some of their implications for health care. To do this we may confront the theories with four questions:

1. Is there a right to health care? (If so, what is its basis and what is its content?)

2. How, in order of priority, is health care related to other goods, or how are health care needs related to other needs? (If there is a right to health care, how is it related to other rights?)

3. How, in order of priority, are various forms of health care related to one another?

4. What can we conclude about the justice or injustice of the current health care system?

In some cases, as we shall see, the theories will provide opposing answers to the same question; in others, the theories may be unhelpfully silent.

We have already seen that the Utilitarian position on rights in general is complex. If by a right we mean a right in the strict sense, i.e., a claim which takes precedence over mere appeals to utility at all levels, including the most basic institutional level, then Utilitarianism denies the existence of rights in general, including the right to health care. If, on the other hand, we mean by right a claim that takes precedence over mere appeals to utility at the level of particular actions or at some institutional level short of the most basic, but which is justified ultimately by appeal to the utility of the total set of institutions, then Utilitarianism does not exclude, and indeed may even require rights, including a right to health care. Whether or not the total institutional array which maximizes utility will include a right to health care will depend upon a wealth of *empirical facts* not deducible from the principle of utility itself. The nature and complexity of the relevant facts can best be appreciated by considering briefly the bearing of Utilitarianism on questions (2) and (3). A utilitarian system of (derivative) rights will pick out certain goods as those which make an especially large contribution to the maximization of utility. It is reasonable to assume, on the basis of empirical data, that health care, or at least certain forms of health care, is among them. Consider, for example, prenatal care, broadly conceived as including genetic screening and counseling (at least for special risk groups), prenatal nutritional care and medical examinations for expectant mothers, medical care during delivery, and basic pediatric services in the crucial months after birth. If empirical research indicates (1) that a system of institutional arrangements which maximizes utility would include such services and (2) that such services can best be assured if they are accorded the status of a right, with all that this implies, including the use of coercive sanctions where necessary, then according to Utilitarianism there is such a (derivative) right. The strength and content of this right relative to other (derivative) rights will be determined by the utility of health care as compared with other kinds of goods.

It is crucial to note that, for the utilitarian, empirical research must determine not only whether certain health care services are to be provided as a matter of right, but also whether the right in question is to be an equal right enjoyed by all persons. No commitment to equality of rights is included in the utilitarian principle itself, nor is there any commitment to equal distribution of any kind. Utilitarianism is egalitarian only in the sense that in calculating what will maximize utility each person's welfare is to be included.

Utilitarian arguments, sometimes based on empirical data, have been advanced to show that providing health care free of charge as a matter of right would encourage wasteful use of scarce and costly resources because the individual would have no incentive to restrain his 'consumption' of health care. The cumulative result, it is said, would be quite disutilitarian: a breakdown of the health care system or a disastrous curtailment of other basic services to cover the spiraling costs of health care. In contrast (proponents of this

argument continue) a *market* in health care encourages 'consumers' to use resources wisely because the costs of the services an individual receives are borne by that individual.

On the other side of the utilitarian ledger, empirical evidence may be marshalled to show that the benefits of a right to health care outweigh the costs, including the costs of possible over-use, and that a market in health care would not maximize utility because those who need health care the most may not be able to afford it.

Similarly, even if there is a utilitarian justification for a right to health care, empirical evidence must again be presented to show that it should be an equal right. For it is certainly conceivable that, under certain circumstances at least, utility could be maximized by providing extensive health care only for some groups, perhaps even a minority, rather than for all persons.

Utilitarians who advocate a right to health care often argue that this right, like other basic rights, should be equal, on the basis of the assumption of diminishing marginal utility. The idea, roughly, is that with respect to many goods, including health care, there is a finite upper bound to the satisfaction a person can gain from being provided with additional amounts of the goods in question. Hence, if in general we are all subject to the phenomenon of diminishing marginal utility in the case of health care and if the threshold of diminishing marginal utility is in general sufficiently low, then there are sound utilitarian reasons for distributing health care equally.

Finally, it should be clear that for the utilitarian the issue of priorities within health care, as well as that of priorities between health care and other goods, must again be settled by empirical research. If, as seems likely, utility maximization requires more resources for prevention and health maintenance rather than for curative intervention after pathology has already developed, then this will be reflected in the content of the utilitarian right to health care. If, as many writers have contended, the current emphasis in the U.S. on high technology intervention produces less utility than would a system which stresses prevention and health maintenance (for example through stricter control of pollution and other environmental determinants of disease), then the utilitarian may conclude that the current system is unjust in this respect. Empirical data would also be needed to ascertain whether more social resources should be devoted to high- or low-technology intervention: for example, neonatal intensive care units versus 'well-baby clinics.' These examples are intended merely to illustrate the breadth and complexity of the empirical research needed to apply Utilitarianism to crucial issues in health care.

Libertarian theories such as Nozick's rely much less heavily upon empirical premises for answers to questions (1)–(4). Since the libertarian is interested only in preventing violations of libertarian rights, and since the latter are rights against certain sorts of interferences rather than rights to be provided with anything, the question of what will maximize utility is irrelevant. Further, any effort to implement any right to health care whatsoever is an injustice, according to the libertarian.

There are only two points at which empirical data are relevant for Nozick. First, whether or not any current case of appropriation of hitherto unheld things satisfies the Lockean Proviso is a matter of fact to be ascertained by empirical methods. Second, empirical historical research is needed to determine what sort of redistribution for the sake of rectifying past injustices is necessary. If, for example, physicians' higher incomes are due in part to government policies which violate libertarian rights, then rectificatory redistribution may be required. And indeed libertarians have argued that two basic features of the current health care system do involve gross violations of libertarian rights. First, compulsory taxation to provide equipment, hospital facilities, research funds, and educational subsidies for medical personnel is literally theft. Second, some argue that government enforced occupational licensing laws which prohibit all but the established forms of medical practice violate the right to freedom of contract [3]. Those who raise this second objection also usually argue that the function of such laws is to secure a monopoly for the medical establishment while sharply limiting the supply of doctors so as to keep medical fees artificially high. Whether or not such arguments are sound it is important to note that Libertarianism is not to be confused with Conservatism. A theory which would institute a free market in medical services, abolish government subsidies, and reduce government regulation of medical practice to the prevention of injury and fraud and the enforcement of contracts has radical implications for changing the current system.

Libertarianism offers straightforward answers to questions (2) and (3). Even if it can be shown that health care in general, and certain forms of health care more than others, are especially important for the happiness or even the freedom of most persons, this fact is quite irrelevant from the perspective of a libertarian theory of justice, though it is no doubt significant for the libertarian concerned with charity or other virtues which exceed the requirements of justice. Nozick and other libertarians recognize that a free market in medical services may in fact produce severe inequalities and that there is no assurance that all or even most will be able to afford adequate medical care. Though the humane libertarian will find this condition unfortunate and will aid those in need and encourage others to do likewise voluntarily, he remains adamant that no one has a right to health care and that hence none may rightly be forced to aid another.

According to Rawls, the most basic questions about health care are not to be decided either by consideration of utility or by market processes. Instead they are to be settled ultimately by appeal to those principles of justice which would be chosen in the original position. As we shall see, however, the implications of Rawls's principles for health care are far from clear.[7]

No principle explicitly specifying a right to health care is included among Rawls's principles of justice. Further, since those principles are intended to regulate the basic structure of society as a whole, they are not themselves intended to guide the decisions individuals make in particular health care situations, nor are they themselves to be applied directly to health care institutions. We are not to assume that either individual physicians or administrators of particular policies or programs are to attempt to allocate health care so as to maximize the prospects of the worst off. In Rawls's theory, as in Utilitarianism, the rightness or wrongness of particular actions or policies depends ultimately upon the nature of the entire institutional structure within which they exist. Hence, Rawls's theory can provide us with fruitful answers at the micro level only if its implications at the macro level are adequately developed.

If Rawls's theory includes a right to health care, it must be a right which is in some way derivative upon the basic rights laid down by the Principle of Greatest Equal Liberty, the Principle of Equality of Fair Opportunity, and the Difference Principle. And if there is to be such a derivative right to health care, then health care must either be among the primary goods covered by the three principles or it must be importantly connected with some of those goods. Now at least some forms of health care (such as broad services for prevention and health maintenance, including mental health) seem to share the earmarks of Rawlsian primary goods: they facilitate the effective pursuit of ends in general and may also enhance our ability to criticize and revise our conceptions of the good. Nonetheless, Rawls does not explicitly list health care among the social primary goods included under the three principles. However, he does include wealth under the Difference Principle and defines it so broadly that it might be thought to include access to health care services. In "Fairness to Goodness" Rawls defines wealth as virtually any legally exchangeable social asset; this would cover health care 'vouchers' if they could be cashed or exchanged for other goods ([7], p. 540).

Let us suppose that health care is either itself a primary good covered by the Difference Principle or that health care may be purchased with income or some other form of wealth which is included under the Difference Principle. In the former case, depending upon various empirical conditions, it might turn out that the best way to insure that the basic structure satisfies the Difference Principle is to establish a state-enforced right to health care. But whether maximizing the prospects of the worst off will require such a right and what the content of the right will be will depend upon what weight is to be assigned to health care relative to other primary goods included under the Difference Principle. Similarly, a weighting must also be assigned if we are to determine whether the share of wealth one receives under the Difference Principle would be sufficient both for health care needs and for other ends. Unfortunately, though Rawls acknowledges that a weighted index of primary goods is needed if we are to be able to determine what would maximize the prospects of the worst off, he offers no account of how the weighting is to be achieved.

The problem is especially acute in the case of health care, because some forms of health care are so costly that an unrestrained commitment to them would undercut any serious commitment to providing other important goods. Thus, it appears that until we have some solution to the weighting problem Rawls's theory can shed only a limited light upon the question of priority relations between health care and other goods and among various forms of health care. Rawls's conception of primary goods may explain what distinguishes health care from those things that are not primary goods, but this is clearly not sufficient.

Perhaps because he is aware of the exorbitant demands which certain health care needs may place upon social resources, Rawls stipulates that the parties in the original position are to choose principles of justice on the assumption that their needs fall within the 'normal range' ([9], pp. 9–10). His ideal may be that the satisfaction of extremely costly special needs for health care may not be a matter of justice but rather of *charity*. If some reasonable way of drawing the line between 'normal' needs which fall within the gambit of princi-

ples of justice and 'special' needs which are the proper object of the virtue of charity could be developed, then this would be a step towards solving the priority problems mentioned above.

It has been suggested that the Principle of Equality of Fair Opportunity, rather than the Difference Principle, might provide the basis for a Rawlsian right to health care ([2], pp. 16–18). While I cannot accord this proposal the consideration it deserves here, I wish to point out that there are four difficulties which make it problematic. First, priority problems still remain. For now we are faced with the task of assigning a weight to health care relative to those other factors (such as education) which are also determinants of opportunity. Further, since the Principle of Equality of Fair Opportunity is lexically prior to the Difference Principle, we must again face the prospect that commitment to the former principle might swallow up social resources needed for providing important goods included under the latter.

Second, because it refers only to opportunities for occupying social *positions* and *offices*, rather than to opportunities in general, the Principle of Equality of Fair Opportunity might be thought too narrow to provide an adequate foundation for a right to health care. Rawls might respond either by defining 'position' rather broadly or by arguing that opportunities for attaining positions and offices are related to opportunities in general in such a way that equality in the former insures equality in the latter.

Third, and more importantly, Rawls's Principle of Equality of Fair Opportunity takes 'abilities' and 'skills' as given, requiring only that persons with equal or similar abilities and skills are to have equal prospects of attaining social positions and offices. Yet clearly inequalities in health care can produce severe inequalities in abilities and skills. For example, poor nutrition and medical care during gestation can result in mental retardation, and many health problems hinder the development of skills and abilities. Hence it might be argued that if the Principle of Opportunity is to provide an adequate basis for a right to health care it must be reformulated to capture the crucial influence of health care or the lack of it upon individual development.

Each of the theories of justice under consideration offers a theoretical basis for answering some basic questions concerning justice in health care. We have seen, however, that none of them provides unambiguous answers to all of the questions and that each depends for its application upon a wealth of empirical premises, many of which may not now be available. Each theory does at least rule out some answers and each supplies us with a perspective from which to pursue issues which we cannot ignore. Nonetheless, almost all of the work in developing an account of justice in health care remains to be done.[8]

NOTES

1 In this essay I shall be concerned for the most part with utilitarianism at the institutional level, and I shall proceed on the assumption that a set of institutions which maximizes utility will include rules which bar other direct applications of the principle of utility itself. Consequently, I will mainly be concerned with Rule Utilitarianism, rather than Act Utilitarianism (the latter being the view that the rightness or wrongness of a given act depends solely upon whether it maximizes utility). For an original and interesting attempt to show that Act Utilitarianism is compatible with social norms that bar direct appeals to utility, see [10].

2 Rawls sometimes refers to the "Principle of Equality of Fair Opportunity" and sometimes to the "Principle of Fair Equality of Opportunity." For convenience I will stay with the former label.

3 The phrase "worst off" refers to those who are worst off with respect to prospects of the social primary goods regulated by the Difference Principle.

4 For a detailed elaboration of this point, see [1].

5 For a fundamental objection to Nozick's invisible hand explanation, see [11].

6 P. Singer [12], expanding an argument developed earlier by R. Titmuss, argues that the existence of markets for certain goods may in fact undermine the motivation for charity.

7 See [2].

8 I would like to thank Earl Shelp and William Hanson for their very helpful comments on an earlier draft of this paper.

REFERENCES

1 Buchanan, A. "Revisability and Rational Choice." *Canadian Journal of Philosophy* 5:395–408, 1975.

2 Daniels, N. "Rights to Health Care and Distributive Justice: Programmatic Worries." *Journal of Medicine and Philosophy* 4:174–191, 1979.

3 Friedman, M. *Capitalism and Freedom.* Chicago: University of Chicago Press, 1962, pp. 137–160.

4 Kant, I. *Foundations of the Metaphysics of Morals* (transl. by L. W. Beck), New York: Bobbs-Merrill, 1959, Part III.

5 Nozick, R. *Anarchy, State and Utopia.* New York: Basic Books, 1974.

6 Rawls, J. *A Theory of Justice.* Cambridge, Mass.: Harvard University Press, 1971.

7 Rawls, J. "Fairness to Goodness." *Philosophical Review* 84:536–554, 1975.

8 Rawls, J. "Reply to Alexander and Musgrave." *Quarterly Journal of Economics* 88:633–655, November 1974.

9 Rawls, J. "Responsibility for Ends." Stanford University, Unpublished Lecture, 1979.

10 Sartorius, R. *Individual Conduct and Social Norms.* Encino, Calif.: Dickenson Publishing, 1975.

11 Sartorius, R. "The Limits of Libertarianism." In *Liberty and the Rule of Law,* edited by R. L. Cunningham, 87–131. College Station, Texas: Texas A and M University Press, 1979.

12 Singer, P. "Rights and the Market." In *Justice and Economic Distribution,* edited by J. Arthur and W. Shaw, pp. 207–221. Englewood Cliffs, N.J.: Prentice-Hall, 1978.

Autonomy, Equality and a Just Health Care System
Kai Nielsen

Kai Nielsen is professor emeritus of philosophy at the University of Calgary. He is the author of *Equality and Liberty: A Defense of Radical Egalitarianism* (1985), *Marxism and the Moral Point of View* (1988), and *Ethics Without God* (1990).

According to Nielsen, justice requires social institutions that work on the premise of moral equality—the life of everyone matters and matters equally. Beginning with this premise and an analysis of basic needs, Nielsen argues that individuals have a moral right to have their health-care needs met. Furthermore, on his account, a commitment to egalitarianism is incompatible with a two- or three-tier system of medical care. Moral equality requires the open and free provision of medical treatment of the same extent and quality to everyone in society. In his view, a system intended to achieve this end would have to take medicine out of the private sector altogether and place both the ownership and control of medicine in the public sector.

I

Autonomy and equality are both fundamental values in our firmament of values, and they are frequently thought to be in conflict. Indeed the standard liberal view is that we must make difficult and often morally ambiguous trade-offs between them.[1] I shall argue that this common view is mistaken and that autonomy cannot be widespread or secure in a society which is not egalitarian: where, that is, equality is not also a very fundamental value which has an operative role within society.[2] I shall further argue that, given human needs and a commitment to an autonomy respecting egalitarianism, a very different health care system would come into being than that which exists at present in the United States.

I shall first turn to a discussion of autonomy and equality and then, in terms of those conceptions, to a conception of justice. In modernizing societies of Western Europe, a perfectly just society will be a society of equals and in such societies there will be a belief held across the political spectrum in what has been called *moral* equality. That is to say, when viewed with the impartiality required by morality, the life of everyone matters and matters equally.[3] Individuals will, of course, and rightly so, have their local attachments but they will

Reprinted with permission of the publisher from *The International Journal of Applied Philosophy*, vol. 4 (Spring 1989), pp. 39–44.

acknowledge that justice requires that the social institutions of the society should be such that they work on the premise that the life of everyone matters and matters equally. Some privileged elite or other group cannot be given special treatment simply because they are that group. Moreover, for there to be a society of equals there must be a rough equality of condition in the society. Power must be sufficiently equally shared for it to be securely the case that no group or class or gender can dominate others through the social structures either by means of their frequently thoroughly unacknowledged latent functions or more explicitly and manifestly by institutional arrangements sanctioned by law or custom. Roughly equal material resources or power are not things which are desirable in themselves, but they are essential instrumentalities for the very possibility of equal well-being and for as many people as possible having as thorough and as complete a control over their own lives as is compatible with this being true for everyone alike. Liberty cannot flourish without something approaching this equality of condition, and people without autonomous lives will surely live impoverished lives. These are mere commonplaces. In fine, a commitment to achieving equality of condition, far from undermining liberty and autonomy, is essential for their extensive flourishing.

If we genuinely believe in moral equality, we will want to see come into existence a world in which all people capable of self-direction have, and have as nearly as is feasible equally, control over their own lives and can, as far as the institutional arrangements for it obtaining are concerned, all live flourishing lives where their needs and desires as individuals are met as fully as possible and as fully and extensively as is compatible with that possibility being open to everyone alike. The thing is to provide institutional arrangements that are conducive to that.

People, we need to remind ourselves, plainly have different capacities and sensibilities. However, even in the extreme case of people for whom little in the way of human flourishing is possible, their needs and desires, as far as possible, should still also be satisfied in the way I have just described. Everyone in this respect at least has equal moral standing. No preference or pride of place should be given to those capable, in varying degrees, of rational self-direction. The more rational, or, for that matter, the more loveable, among us should not be given preference. No one should. Our needs should determine what is to be done.

People committed to achieving and sustaining a society of equals will seek to bring into stable existence conditions such that it would be possible for everyone, if they were personally capable of it, to enjoy an equally worthwhile and satisfying life or at least a life in which, for all of them, their needs, starting with and giving priority to their more urgent needs, were met and met as equally and as fully as possible, even where their needs are not entirely the same needs. This, at least, is the heuristic, though we might, to gain something more nearly feasible, have to scale down talk of meeting needs to providing conditions propitious for the equal satisfaction for everyone of their *basic* needs. Believers in equality want to see a world in which everyone, as far as this is possible, have equal whole life prospects. This requires an equal consideration of their needs and interests and a refusal to just override anyone's interests: to just regard anyone's interests as something which comes to naught, which can simply be set aside as expendable. Minimally, an egalitarian must believe that taking the moral point of view requires that each person's good is afforded equal consideration. Moreover, this is not just a bit of egalitarian ideology but is a deeply embedded considered judgment in modern Western culture capable of being put into wide reflective equilibrium.[4]

II

What is a need, how do we identify needs and what are our really basic needs, needs that are presumptively universal? Do these basic needs in most circumstances at least trump our other needs and our reflective considered preferences?

Let us start this examination by asking if we can come up with a list of universal needs correctly ascribable to all human beings in all cultures. In doing this we should, as David Braybrooke has, distinguish *adventitious* and *course-of-life* needs.[5] Moreover, it is the latter that it is essential to focus on. Adventitious needs, like the need for a really good fly rod or computer, come and go with particular projects. Course-of-life needs, such as the need for exercise, sleep or food, are such that every human being may be expected to have them all at least at some stage of life.

Still, we need to step back a bit and ask: how do we determine what is a need, course-of-life need or otherwise? We need a relational formula to spot needs. We say, where we are speaking of needs, B needs x in order to y, as in Janet needs milk or some other form of calcium in order to protect her bone structure. With course-of-life needs the relation comes out platitudinously as in 'People need food and water in order to live' or 'People need exercise in order to function normally or well'. This, in the very identification of the need, refers to human flourishing or to human well-being, thereby giving to understand that they are basic needs. Perhaps it is better to say instead that this is to specify in part what it is for something to be a basic need. Be that as it may, there are these basic needs we *must* have to live well. If this is really so, then, where they are things we as individuals can have without jeopardy to others, no further question arises, or can arise, about the desirability of satisfying them. They are just things that in such circumstances ought to be met in our lives if they can. The satisfying of such needs is an unequivocally good thing. The questions 'Does Janet need to live?' and 'Does Sven need to function well?' are at best otiose.

In this context David Braybrooke has quite properly remarked that being "essential to living or to functioning normally may be taken as a criterion for being a basic need. Questions about whether needs are genuine, or well-founded, come to an end of the line when the needs have been connected with life or health."[6] Certainly to flourish we must have these things and in some instances they must be met at least to a certain extent even to survive. This being so, we can quite properly call them basic needs. Where these needs do not clash or the satisfying of them by one person does not conflict with the satisfying of the equally basic needs of another no question about justifying the meeting of them arises.

By linking the identification of needs with what we

must have to function well and linking course-of-life and basic needs with what all people, or at least almost all people, must have to function well, a list of basic needs can readily be set out. I shall give such a list, though surely the list is incomplete. However, what will be added is the same sort of thing similarly identified. First there are needs connected closely to our physical functioning, namely the need for food and water, the need for excretion, for exercise, for rest (including sleep), for a life supporting relation to the environment, and the need for whatever is indispensable to preserve the body intact. Similarly there are basic needs connected with our function as social beings. We have needs for companionship, education, social acceptance and recognition, for sexual activity, freedom from harassment, freedom from domination, for some meaningful work, for recreation and relaxation and the like.[7]

The list, as I remarked initially, is surely incomplete. But it does catch many of the basic things which are in fact necessary for us to live or to function well. Now an autonomy respecting egalitarian society with an interest in the well-being of its citizens—something moral beings could hardly be without—would (trivially) be a society of equals, and as a society of equals it would be committed to (a) *moral* equality and (b) an equality of *condition* which would, under conditions of moderate abundance, in turn expect the equality of condition to be rough and to be principally understood (cashed in) in terms of providing the conditions (as far as that is possible) for meeting the needs (including most centrally the basic needs) of everyone and meeting them equally, as far as either of these things is feasible.

III

What kind of health care system would such an autonomy respecting egalitarian society have under conditions of moderate abundance such as we find in Canada and the United States?

The following are health care needs which are also basic needs: being healthy and having conditions treated which impede one's functioning well or which adversely affect one's well-being or cause suffering. These are plainly things we need. Where societies have the economic and technical capacity to do so, as these societies plainly do, without undermining other equally urgent or more urgent needs, these health needs, as basic needs, must be met, and the right to have such medical care is a right for everyone in the society regardless of her capacity to pay. This just follows from a commitment to

moral equality and to an equality of condition. Where we have the belief, a belief which is very basic in non-fascistic modernizing societies, that each person's good is to be given equal consideration, it is hard not to go in that way, given a plausible conception of needs and reasonable list of needs based on that conception.[8] If there is the need for some particular regime of care and the society has the resources to meet that need, without undermining structures protecting other at least equally urgent needs, then, *ceteris paribus,* the society, if it is a decent society, must do so. The commitment to more equality—the commitment to the belief that the life of each person matters and matters equally—entails, given a few plausible empirical premises, that each person's health needs will be the object of an equal regard. Each has an equal claim, *prima facie,* to have her needs satisfied where this is possible. That does not, of course, mean that people should all be treated alike in the sense of their all getting the same thing. Not everyone needs flu shots, braces, a dialysis machine, a psychiatrist, or a triple bypass. What should be equal is that each person's health needs should be the object of equal societal concern since each person's good should be given equal consideration.[9] This does not mean that equal energy should be directed to Hans's rash as to Frank's cancer. Here one person's need for a cure is much greater than the other, and the greater need clearly takes precedence. Both should be met where possible, but where they both cannot then the greater need has pride of place. But what should not count in the treatment of Hans and Frank is that Hans is wealthy or prestigious or creative and Frank is not. Everyone should have their health needs met where possible. Moreover, where the need is the same, they should have (where possible), and where other at least equally urgent needs are not thereby undermined, the same quality treatment. No differentiation should be made between them on the basis of their ability to pay or on the basis of their being (one more so than the other) important people. There should, in short, where this is possible, be open and free medical treatment of the same quality and extent available to everyone in the society. And no two- or three-tier system should be allowed to obtain, and treatment should only vary (subject to the above qualification) on the basis of variable needs and unavoidable differences in different places in supply and personnel, e.g., differences between town and country. Furthermore, these latter differences should be remedied where technically and economically feasible. The underlying aim should be to meet the health care needs of everyone and meet them, in the sense explicated, equally: everybody's needs here should be met as fully as possible; different treatment is only justified where the need is different or where both needs cannot be met. Special treatment for one person rather than another is only justified where, as I remarked, both needs cannot be met or cannot as adequately be met. Constrained by ought implies can, where these circumstances obtain, priority should be given to the greater need that can feasibly be met. A moral system or a social policy, plainly, cannot be reasonably asked to do the impossible. But my account does not ask that.

To have such a health care system would, I think, involve taking medicine out of the private sector altogether including, of course, out of private entrepreneurship where the governing rationale has to be profit and where supply and demand rules the roost. Instead there must be a health care system firmly in the public sector (publicly owned and controlled) where the rationale of the system is to meet as efficiently and as fully as possible the health care needs of everyone in the society in question. The health care system should not be viewed as a business anymore than a university should be viewed as a business—compare a university and a large hospital—but as a set of institutions and practices designed to meet urgent human needs.

I do not mean that we should ignore costs or efficiency. The state-run railroad system in Switzerland, to argue by analogy, is very efficient. The state cannot, of course, ignore costs in running it. But the aim is not to make a profit. The aim is to produce the most rapid, safe, efficient and comfortable service meeting travellers' needs within the parameters of the overall socio-economic priorities of the state and the society. Moreover, since the state in question is a democracy, if its citizens do not like the policies of the government here (or elsewhere) they can replace it with a government with different priorities and policies. Indeed the option is there (probably never to be exercised) to shift the railroad into the private sector.

Governments, understandably, worry with aging populations about mounting health care costs. This is slightly ludicrous in the United States, given its military and space exploration budgets, but is also a reality in Canada and even in Iceland where there is no military or space budget at all. There should, of course, be concern about containing health costs, but this can be done effectively with a state-run system. Modern societies need systems of socialized medicine, something that obtains in almost all civilized modernizing societies. The United States and South Africa are, I believe, the only exceptions. But, as is evident from my own country

(Canada), socialized health care systems often need altering, and their costs need monitoring. As a cost-cutting and as an efficiency measure that would at the same time improve health care, doctors, like university professors and government bureaucrats, should be put on salaries and they should work in medical units. They should, I hasten to add, have good salaries but salaries all the same; the last vestiges of petty entrepreneurship should be taken from the medical profession. This measure would save the state-run health care system a considerable amount of money, would improve the quality of medical care with greater cooperation and consultation resulting from economies of scale and a more extensive division of labor with larger and better equipped medical units. (There would also be less duplication of equipment.) The overall quality of care would also improve with a better balance between health care in the country and in the large cities, with doctors being systematically and rationally deployed throughout the society. In such a system doctors, no more than university professors or state bureaucrats, could not just set up a practice anywhere. They would no more be free to do this than university professors or state bureaucrats. In the altered system there would be no cultural space for it. Placing doctors on salary, though not at a piece work rate, would also result in its being the case that the financial need to see as many patients as possible as quickly as possible would be removed. This would plainly enhance the quality of medical care. It would also be the case that a different sort of person would go into the medical profession. People would go into it more frequently because they were actually interested in medicine and less frequently because this is a rather good way (though hardly the best way) of building a stock portfolio.

There should also be a rethinking of the respective roles of nurses (in all their variety), paramedics and doctors. Much more of the routine work done in medicine—taking the trout fly out of my ear for example—can be done by nurses or paramedics. Doctors, with their more extensive training, could be freed up for other more demanding tasks worthy of their expertise. This would require somewhat different training for all of these different medical personnel and a rethinking of the authority structure in the health care system. But doing this in a reasonable way would improve the teamwork in hospitals, make morale all around a lot better, improve medical treatment and save a very considerable amount of money. (It is no secret that the relations between doctors and nurses are not good.) Finally, a far greater emphasis should be placed on preventive medicine than is done now. This, if really extensively done, utilizing the considerable educational and fiscal powers of the state, would result in very considerable health care savings and a very much healthier and perhaps even happier population. (Whether with the states we actually have we are likely to get anything like that is—to understate it—questionable. I wouldn't hold my breath in the United States. Still, Finland and Sweden are very different places from the United States and South Africa.)

IV

It is moves of this *general* sort that an egalitarian and autonomy loving society under conditions of moderate scarcity should implement. (I say 'general sort' for I am more likely to be wrong about some of the specifics than about the general thrust of my argument.) It would, if in place, limit the freedom of some people, including some doctors and some patients, to do what they want to do. That is obvious enough. But any society, any society at all, as long as it had norms (legal and otherwise) will limit freedom in some way.[10] There is no living in society without some limitation on the freedom to do some things. Indeed a society without norms and thus without any limitation on freedom is a contradiction in terms. Such a mass of people wouldn't be a society. They, without norms, would just be a mass of people. (If these are 'grammatical remarks,' make the most of them.) In our societies I am not free to go for a spin in your car without your permission, to practice law or medicine without a license, to marry your wife while she is still your wife and the like. Many restrictions on our liberties, because they are so common, so widely accepted and thought by most of us to be so reasonable, hardly *seem* like restrictions on our liberty. But they are all the same. No doubt some members of the medical profession would feel quite reined in if the measures I propose were adopted. (These measures are not part of conventional wisdom.) But the restrictions on the freedom of the medical profession and on patients I am proposing would make for both a greater liberty all around, everything considered, and, as well, for greater well-being in the society. Sometimes we have to restrict certain liberties in order to enhance the overall system of liberty. Not speaking out of turn in parliamentary debate is a familiar example. Many people who now have a rather limited access to medical treatment would come to have it and have it in a more adequate way with such a socialized system in place. Often we have to choose between a greater or lesser liberty in a society,

and, at least under conditions of abundance, the answer almost always should be 'Choose the greater liberty'. If we really prize human autonomy, if, that is, we want a world in which as many people as possible have as full as is possible control over their own lives, then we will be egalitarians. Our very egalitarianism will commit us to something like the health care system I described, but so will the realization that, without reasonable health on the part of the population, autonomy can hardly flourish or be very extensive. Without the kind of equitability and increased coverage in health care that goes with a properly administered socialized medicine, the number of healthy people will be far less than could otherwise feasibly be the case. With that being the case, autonomy and well-being as well will be neither as extensive nor so thorough as it could otherwise be. Autonomy, like everything else, has its material conditions. And to will the end is to will the necessary means to the end.

To take—to sum up—what since the Enlightenment has come to be seen as the moral point of view, and to take morality seriously, is to take it as axiomatic that each person's good be given equal consideration.[11] I have argued that (a) where that is accepted, and (b) where we are tolerably clear about the facts (including facts about human needs), and (c) where we live under conditions of moderate abundance, a health care system bearing at least a family resemblance to the one I have gestured at will be put in place. It is a health care system befitting an autonomy respecting democracy committed to the democratic and egalitarian belief that the life of everyone matters and matters equally.

NOTES

1 Isaiah Berlin, "On the Pursuit of the Ideal," *The New York Review of Books* XXXV (March 1987), pp. 11–18. See also his "Equality" in his *Concepts and Categories* (Oxford, England: Oxford University Press, 1980), pp. 81–102. I have criticized that latter paper in my "Formulating Egalitarianism: Animadversions on Berlin," *Philosophia* 13:3–4 (October 1983), pp. 299–315.

2 For three defenses of such a view see Kai Nielsen, *Equality and Liberty* (Totowa, New Jersey: Rowman and Allanheld, 1985), Richard Norman, *Free and Equal* (Oxford, England: Oxford University Press, 1987), and John Baker, *Arguing for Equality* (London: Verso Press, 1987).

3 Will Kymlicka, "Rawls on Teleology and Deontology," *Philosophy and Public Affairs* 17:3 (Summer

1988), pp. 173–190 and John Rawls, "The Priority of Right and Ideas of the Good," *Philosophy and Public Affairs* 17:4 (Fall 1988), pp. 251–276.

4 Kai Nielsen, "Searching for an Emancipatory Perspective: Wide Reflective Equilibrium and the Hermeneutical Circle" in Evan Simpson (ed.), *Anti-Foundationalism and Practical Reasoning* (Edmonton, Alberta: Academic Printing and Publishing, 1987), pp. 143–164 and Kai Nielsen, "In Defense of Wide Reflective Equilibrium" in Douglas Odegard (ed.) *Ethics and Justification* (Edmonton, Alberta: Academic Printing and Publishing, 1988), pp. 19–37.

5 David Braybrooke, *Meeting Needs* (Princeton, New Jersey: Princeton University Press, 1987), p. 29.
6 *Ibid.*, p. 31.
7 *Ibid.*, p. 37.
8 Will Kymlicka, *op cit.*, p. 190.
9 *Ibid.*
10 Ralf Dahrendorf, *Essays in the Theory of Society* (Stanford, California: Stanford University Press, 1968), pp. 151–78 and G. A. Cohen, "The Structure of Proletarian Unfreedom," *Philosophy and Public Affairs* 12 (1983), pp. 2–33.
11 Will Kymlicka, *op cit.*, p. 190.

Rationing

Aging and the Ends of Medicine
Daniel Callahan

A biographical sketch of Daniel Callahan is found on page 388.

Callahan maintains that since health-care resources are scarce, elderly individuals who have lived a natural life span should be offered care that relieves suffering but should be denied expensive life-prolonging technologies. In arguing for his position, Callahan stresses the need to reexamine questions about aging and the proper ends of medicine as well as the concept of a natural life span. He concludes that medicine should have two goals as it confronts aging: (1) averting premature death, that is, death prior to the completion of a natural life span and (2) the relief of suffering, rather than the extension of life, after that natural span has been completed.

In October of 1986, Dr. Thomas Starzl of the Presbyterian-University Hospital in Pittsburgh successfully transplanted a liver into a 76-year-old woman. The typical cost of such an operation is over $200,000. He thereby accelerated the extension to the elderly of the most expensive and most demanding form of high-technology medicine. Not long after that, Congress brought organ transplantation under Medicare coverage, thus guaranteeing an even greater extension of this form of life-saving care to older age groups.

This is, on the face of it, the kind of medical progress we have long grown to hail, a triumph of med-

Reprinted with permission of the author and the publisher from *Annals of the New York Academy of Sciences*, vol. 530 (June 15, 1988), pp. 125–132.

ical technology and a new-found benefit to be provided by an established entitlement program. But now an oddity. At the same time those events were taking place, a parallel government campaign for cost containment was under way, with a special targeting of health care to the aged under the Medicare program.

It was not hard to understand why. In 1980, the 11% of the population over age 65 consumed some 29% of the total American health care expenditures of $219.4 billion. By 1986, the percentage of consumption by the elderly had increased to 31% and total expenditures to $450 billion. Medicare costs are projected to rise from $75 billion in 1986 to $114 billion in the year 2000, and in real not inflated dollars.

There is every incentive for politicians, for those who care for the aged, and for those of us on the way to becoming old to avert our eyes from figures of that kind. We have tried as a society to see if we can simply muddle our way through. That, however, is no longer sufficient. The time has come, I am convinced, for a full and open reconsideration of our future direction. We can not for much longer continue on our present course. Even if we could find a way to radically increase the proportion of our health care dollar going to the elderly, it is not clear that that would be a good social investment.

Is it sensible, in the face of a rapidly increasing burden of health care costs for the elderly, to press forward with new and expensive ways of extending their lives? Is it possible to even hope to control costs while, simultaneously, supporting the innovative research that generates ever-new ways to spend money? These are now unavoidable questions. Medicare costs rise at an extraordinary pace, fueled by an ever-increasing number and proportion of the elderly. The fastest-growing age group in the United States are those over the age of 85, increasing at a rate of about 10% every two years. By the year 2040, it has been projected that the elderly will represent 21% of the population and consume 45% of all health care expenditures. Could costs of that magnitude be borne?

Yet even as this intimidating trend reveals itself, anyone who works closely with the elderly recognizes that the present Medicare and Medicaid programs are grossly inadequate in meeting the real and full needs of the elderly. They fail, most notably, in providing decent long-term care and medical care that does not constitute a heavy out-of-pocket drain. Members of minority groups, and single or widowed women, are particularly disadvantaged. How will it be possible, then, to keep pace with the growing number of elderly in even providing present levels of care, much less in ridding the system of its present inadequacies and inequities—and, at the same time, furiously adding expensive new technologies?

The straight answer is that it will not be possible to do all of those things and that, worse still, it may be harmful to even try. It may be harmful because of the economic burdens it will impose on younger age groups, and because of the skewing of national social priorities too heavily toward health care that it is coming to require. But it may also be harmful because it suggests to both the young and the old that the key to a happy old age is good health care. That may not be true.

It is not pleasant to raise possibilities of that kind. The struggle against what Dr. Robert Butler aptly and brilliantly called "ageism" in 1968 has been a difficult one. It has meant trying to persuade the public that not all the elderly are sick and senile. It has meant trying to convince Congress and state legislatures to provide more help for the old. It has meant trying to educate the elderly themselves to look upon their old age as a time of new, open possibilities. That campaign has met with only partial success. Despite great progress, the elderly are still subject to discrimination and stereotyping. The struggle against ageism is hardly over.

Three major concerns have, nonetheless, surfaced over the past few years. They are symptoms that a new era has arrived. The first is that an increasingly large share of health care is going to the elderly in comparison with benefits for children. The federal government, for instance, spends six times as much on health care for those over 65 as for those under 18. As the demographer Samuel Preston observed in a provocative 1984 presidential address to the Population Association of America:

> There is surely something to be said for a system in which things get better as we pass through life rather than worse. The great leveling off of age curves of psychological distress, suicide and income in the past two decades might simply reflect the fact that we have decided in some fundamental sense that we don't want to face futures that become continually bleaker. But let's be clear that the transfers from the working-age population to the elderly are also transfers away from children, since the working ages bear far more responsibility for childrearing than do the elderly.[1]

Preston's address had an immediate impact. The mainline aging advocacy groups responded with pained indignation, accusing Preston of fomenting a war between the generations. But led by Dave Durenberger, Republican Senator from Minnesota, it also stimulated the formation of Americans for Generational Equity (AGE), an organization created to promote debate on the burden to future generations, but particularly the Baby Boom generation, of "our major social insurance programs."[2] These two developments signalled the outburst of a struggle over what has come to be called "Intergenerational equity" that is only now gaining momentum.

The second concern is that the elderly dying consume a disproportionate share of health care costs. Stanford economist Victor Fuchs has noted:

> At present, the United States spends about 1 percent of the gross national product on health care for elderly persons who are in their last year of life. . . . One of the

biggest challenges facing policy makers for the rest of this century will be how to strike an appropriate balance between care of the [elderly] dying and health services for the rest of the population.[3]

The third concern is summed up in an observation by Jerome L. Avorn, M.D., of the Harvard Medical School:

With the exception of the birth-control pill, each of the medical-technology interventions developed since the 1950s has its most widespread impact on people who are past their fifties—the further past their fifties, the greater the impact.[4]

Many of these interventions were not intended for the elderly. Kidney dialysis, for example, was originally developed for those between the ages of 15 and 45. Now some 30% of its recipients are over 65.

These three concerns have not gone unchallenged. They have, on the contrary, been strongly resisted, as has the more general assertion that some form of rationing of health care for the elderly might become necessary. To the charge that the elderly receive a disproportionate share of resources, the response has been that what helps the elderly helps every other age group. It both relieves the young of the burden of care for elderly parents they would otherwise have to bear and, since they too will eventually become old, promises them similar care when they come to need it. There is no guarantee, moreover, that any cutback in health care for the elderly would result in a transfer of the savings directly to the young. Our system is not that rational or that organized. And why, others ask, should we contemplate restricting care for the elderly when we wastefully spend hundreds of millions of dollars on an inflated defense budget?

The charge that the elderly dying receive a large share of funds hardly proves that it is an unjust or unreasonable amount. They are, after all, the most in need. As some important studies have shown, moreover, it is exceedingly difficult to know that someone is dying; the most expensive patients, it turns out, are those who are expected to live but who actually die. That most new technologies benefit the old more than the young is perfectly sensible: most of the killer diseases of the young have now been conquered.

These are reasonable responses. It would no doubt be possible to ignore the symptoms that the raising of such concerns represents, and to put off for at least a few more years any full confrontation with the over-powering tide of elderly now on the way. There is little incentive for politicians to think about, much less talk about, limits of any kind on health care for the aged; it is a politically hazardous topic. Perhaps also, as Dean Guido Calabresi of the Yale Law School and his colleague Philip Bobbitt observed in their thoughtful 1978 book *Tragic Choices,* when we are forced to make painful allocation choices, "Evasion, disguise, temporizing . . . [and] averting our eyes enables us to save some lives even when we will not save all."[5]

Yet however slight the incentives to take on this highly troubling issue, I believe it is inevitable that we must. Already rationing of health care under Medicare is a fact of life, though rarely labeled as such. The requirement that Medicare recipients pay the first $500 of the costs of hospital care, that there is a cutoff of reimbursement of care beyond 60 days, and a failure to cover long-term care, are nothing other than allocation and cost-saving devices. As sensitive as it is to the votes of the elderly, the Reagan administration only grudgingly agreed to support catastrophic health care costs of the elderly (a benefit that will not, in any event, help many of the aged). It is bound to be far more resistant to long-term care coverage, as will any administration.

But there are other reasons than economics to think about health care for the elderly. The coming economic crisis provides a much-needed opportunity to ask some deeper questions. Just what is it that we want medicine to do for us as we age? Earlier cultures believed that aging should be accepted, and that it should be in part a time of preparation for death. Our culture seems increasingly to reject that view, preferring instead, it often seems, to think of aging as hardly more than another disease, to be fought and rejected. Which view is correct? To ask that question is only to note that disturbing puzzles about the ends of medicine and the ends of aging lie behind the more immediate financing worries. Without some kind of answer to them, there is no hope of finding a reasonable, and possibly even a humane, solution to the growing problem of health care for the elderly.

Let me put my own view directly. The future goal of medicine in the care of the aged should be that of improving the quality of their life, not in seeking ways to extend that life. In its long-standing ambition to forestall death, medicine has in the care of the aged reached its last frontier. That is hardly because death is absent elsewhere—children and young adults obviously still die of maladies that are open to potential cure—but because the largest number of deaths (some 70%) now occur among those over the age of 65, with the highest proportion in those over 85. If death is ever to be humbled, that is where the essentially endless work remains to be done. But however tempting that challenge, medicine should now restrain its ambition at that frontier. To do otherwise will, I believe, be to court harm to the needs of other age groups and to the old themselves.

Yet to ask medicine to restrain itself in the face of aging and death is to ask more than it, or the public that sustains it, is likely to find agreeable. Only a fresh understanding of the ends and meaning of aging, encompassing two conditions, are likely to make that a plausible stance. The first is that we—both young and old—need to understand that it is possible to live out a meaningful old age that is limited in time, one that does not require a compulsive effort to turn to medicine for more life to make it bearable. The second condition is that, as a culture, we need a more supportive context for aging and death, one that cherishes and respects the elderly while at the same time recognizing that their primary orientation should be to the young and the generations to come, not to their own age group. It will be no less necessary to recognize that in the passing of the generations lies the constant reinvigoration of biological life.

Neither of these conditions will be easy to realize. Our culture has, for one thing, worked hard to redefine old age as a time of liberation, not decline. The terms "modern maturity" or "prime time" have, after all, come to connote a time of travel, new ventures in education and self-discovery, the ever-accessible tennis court or golf course, and delightfully periodic but gratefully brief visits from well-behaved grandchildren.

This is, to be sure, an idealized picture. Its attraction lies not in its literal truth but as a widely-accepted utopian reference point. It projects the vision of an old age to which more and more believe they can aspire and which its proponents think an affluent country can afford if it so chooses. That it requires a medicine that is singleminded in its aggressiveness against the infirmities of old age is of a piece with its hopes. But as we have come to discover, the costs of that kind of war are prohibitive. No matter how much is spent the ultimate problem will still remain: people age and die. Worse still, by pretending that old age can be turned into a kind of endless middle age, we rob it of meaning and significance for the elderly themselves. It is a way of saying that old age can be acceptable only to the extent that it can mimic the vitality of the younger years.

There is a plausible alternative: that of a fresh vision of what it means to live a decently long and adequate life, what might be called a natural life span. Earlier generations accepted the idea that there was a nat-

ural life span—the biblical norm of three score years and ten captures that notion (even though, in fact, that was a much longer life span than was then typically the case). It is an idea well worth reconsidering, and would provide us with a meaningful and realizable goal. Modern medicine and biology have done much, however, to wean us away from that kind of thinking. They have insinuated the belief that the average life span is not a natural fact at all, but instead one that is strictly dependent upon the state of medical knowledge and skill. And there is much to that belief as a statistical fact: the average life expectancy continues to increase, with no end in sight.

But that is not what I think we ought to mean by a natural life span. We need a notion of a full life that is based on some deeper understanding of human need and sensible possibility, not the latest state of medical technology or medical possibility. We should instead think of a natural life span as the achievement of a life long enough to accomplish for the most part those opportunities that life typically affords people and which we ordinarily take to be the prime benefits of enjoying a life at all—that of loving and living, of raising a family, of finding and carrying out work that is satisfying, of reading and thinking, and of cherishing our friends and families.

If we envisioned a natural life span that way, then we could begin to intensify the devising of ways to get people to that stage of life, and to work to make certain they do so in good health and social dignity. People will differ on what they might count as a natural life span; determining its appropriate range for social policy purposes would need extended thought and debate. My own view is that it can now be achieved by the late 70s or early 80s.

That many of the elderly discover new interests and new facets of themselves late in life—my mother took up painting in her seventies and was selling her paintings up until her death at 86—does not mean that we should necessarily encourage a kind of medicine that would make that the norm. Nor does it mean that we should base social and welfare policy on possibilities of that kind. A more reasonable approach is to ask how medicine can help most people live out a decently long life, and how that life can be enhanced along the way.

A longer life does not guarantee a better life—there is no inherent connection between the two. No matter how long medicine enabled people to live, death at any time—at age 90, or 100, or 110—would frustrate some possibility, some as-yet-unrealized goal. There is sadness in that realization, but not tragedy. An easily preventable death of a young child is an outrage. The death from an incurable disease of someone in the prime of young adulthood is a tragedy. But death at an old age, after a long and full life, is simply sad, a part of life itself.

As it confronts aging, medicine should have as its specific goal that of averting premature death, understood as death prior to a natural life span, and the relief of suffering thereafter. It should pursue those goals in order that the elderly can finish out their years with as little needless pain as possible, and with as much vigor as can be generated in contributing to the welfare of younger age groups and to the community of which they are a part. Above all, the elderly need to have a sense of the meaning and significance of their stage in life, one that is not dependent for its human value on economic productivity or physical vigor.

What would a medicine oriented toward the relief of suffering rather than the deliberate extension of life be like? We do not yet have a clear and ready answer to that question, so long-standing, central, and persistent has been the struggle against death as part of the self-conception of medicine. But the Hospice movement is providing us with much helpful evidence. It knows how to distinguish between the relief of suffering and the extension of life. A greater control by the elderly over their dying—and particularly a more readily respected and enforceable right to deny aggressive life-extending treatment—is a long-sought, minimally necessary goal.

What does this have to do with the rising cost of health care for the elderly? Everything. The indefinite extension of life combined with a never-satisfied improvement in the health of the elderly is a recipe for monomania and limitless spending. It fails to put health in its proper place as only one among many human goods. It fails to accept aging and death as part of the human condition. It fails to present to younger generations a model of wise stewardship.

How might we devise a plan to limit health care for the aged under public entitlement programs that is fair, humane, and sensitive to their special requirements and dignity? Let me suggest three principles to undergird a quest for limits. First, government has a duty, based on our collective social obligations to each other, to help people live out a natural life span, but not actively to help medically extend life beyond that point. Second, government is obliged to develop under its research subsidies, and pay for, under its entitlement programs, only that kind and degree of life-extending technology necessary for medicine to achieve and serve the end of a natural life span. The question is not whether a technology is available that can save the life of someone who

has lived out a natural life span, but whether there is an obligation for society to provide them with that technology. I think not. Third, beyond the point of natural life span, government should provide only the means necessary for the relief of suffering, not life-extending technology. By proposing that we use age as a specific criterion for the limitation of life-extending health care, I am challenging one of the most revered norms of contemporary geriatrics: that medical need and not age should be the standard of care. Yet the use of age as a principle for the allocation of resources can be perfectly valid, both a necessary and legitimate basis for providing health care to the elderly. There is not likely to be any better or less arbitrary criterion for the limiting of resources in the face of the open-ended possibilities of medical advancement in therapy for the aged.

Medical "need," in particular, can no longer work as an allocation principle. It is too elastic a concept, too much a function of the state of medical art. A person of 100 dying from congestive heart failure "needs" a heart transplant no less than someone who is 30. Are we to treat both needs as equal? That is not economically feasible or, I would argue, a sensible way to allocate scarce resources. But it would be required by a strict need-based standard.

Age is also a legitimate basis for allocation because it is a meaningful and universal category. It can be understood at the level of common sense. It is concrete enough to be employed for policy purposes. It can also, most importantly, be of value to the aged themselves if combined with an ideal of old age that focuses on its quality rather than its indefinite extension.

I have become impressed with the philosophy underlying the British health care system and the way it meets the needs of the old and the chronically ill. It has, to begin with, a tacit allocation policy. It emphasizes improving the quality of life through primary care medicine and well-subsidized home care and institutional programs for the elderly rather than through life-extending acute care medicine. The well-known difficulty in getting dialysis after 55 is matched by like restrictions on access to open heart surgery, intensive care units, and other forms of expensive technology. An undergirding skepticism toward technology makes that a viable option. That attitude, together with a powerful drive for equity, "explains," as two commentators have noted, "why most British put a higher value on primary care for the population as a whole than on an abundance of sophisticated technology for the few who may benefit from it."[6]

That the British spend a significantly smaller proportion of their GNP (6.2%) on health care than Americans (10.8%) for an almost identical outcome in health status is itself a good advertisement for its priorities. Life expectancies are, for men, 70.0 years in the U.S. and 70.4 years in Great Britain; and, for women, 77.8 in the U.S. and 76.7 in Great Britain. There is, of course, a great difference in the ethos of the U.S. and Britain, and our individualism and love of technology stand in the way of a quick shift of priorities.

Yet our present American expectations about aging and death, it turns out, may not be all that reassuring. How many of us are really so certain that high-technology American medicine promises us all that much better an aging and death, even if some features appear improved and the process begins later than in earlier times? Between the widespread fear of death in an impersonal ICU, cozened about machines and invaded by tubes, on the one hand, or wasting away in the back ward of a nursing home, on the other, not many of us seem comforted.

Once we have reflected on those fears, it is not impossible that most people could be persuaded that a different, more limited set of expectations for health care could be made tolerable. That would be all the more possible if there was a greater assurance than at present that one could live out a full life span, that one's chronic illnesses would be better supported, and that long-term care and home care would be given a more powerful societal backing than is now the case. Though they would face a denial of life-extending medical care beyond a certain age, the old would not necessarily fear their aging anymore than they now do. They would, on the contrary, know that a better balance had been struck between making our later years as good as possible rather than simply trying to add more years.

This direction would not immediately bring down the costs of care of the elderly; it would add new costs. But it would set in place the beginning of a new understanding of old age, one that would admit of eventual stabilization and limits. The time has come to admit we can not go on much longer on the present course of open-ended health care for the elderly. Neither confident assertions about American affluence, nor tinkering with entitlement provisions and cost-containment strategies will work for more than a few more years. It is time for the dream that old age can be an infinite and open frontier to end, and for the unflagging, but self-deceptive, optimism that we can do anything we want with our economic system to be put aside.

The elderly will not be served by a belief that only a lack of resources, or better financing mechanisms, or political power, stand between them and the limitations of their bodies. The good of younger age groups will not be served by inspiring in them a desire to live to an old age that will simply extend the vitality of youth indefinitely, as if old age is nothing but a sign that medicine has failed in its mission. The future of our society will not be served by allowing expenditures on health care for the elderly endlessly and uncontrollably to escalate, fueled by a false altruism that thinks anything less is to deny the elderly their dignity. Nor will it be served by that pervasive kind of self-serving that urges the young to support such a crusade because they will eventually benefit from it also.

We require instead an understanding of the process of aging and death that looks to our obligation to the young and to the future, that recognizes the necessity of limits and the acceptance of decline and death, and that values the old for their age and not for their continuing youthful vitality. In the name of accepting the elderly and repudiating discrimination against them, we have mainly succeeded in pretending that, with enough will and money, the unpleasant part of old age can be abolished. In the name of medical progress we have carried out a relentless war against death and decline, failing to ask in any probing way if that will give us a better society for all age groups.

The proper question is not whether we are succeeding in giving a longer life to the aged. It is whether we are making of old age a decent and honorable time of life. Neither a longer lifetime nor more life-extending technology are the way to that goal. The elderly themselves ask for greater financial security, for as much self-determination and independence as possible, for a decent quality of life and not just more life, and for a respected place in society.

The best way to achieve those goals is not simply to say more money and better programs are needed, however much they have their important place. We would do better to begin with a sense of limits, of the meaning of the human life cycle, and of the necessary coming and going of the generations. From that kind of starting point, we could devise a new understanding of old age.

REFERENCES

1 Preston, S. H. 1984. Children and the elderly: divergent paths for America's dependents. Demography 21: 491–495.

2 Americans for Generational Equity. Case Statement. May 1986.

3 Fuchs, V. R. 1984. Though much is taken: reflections on aging, health, and medical care. Milbank Mem. Fund Q. 62: 464–465.

4 Avorn, J. L. 1986. Medicine, health, and the geriatric transformation. Daedalus 115: 211–225.

5 Calabresi, G. & P. Bobbit. 1978. Tragic Choices. W. W. Norton. New York, NY.

6 Miller, F. H. & G. A. H. Miller. 1986. The painful prescription: a procrustean perspective. N. Engl. J. Med. 314: 1385.

Spare the Old, Save the Young

Amitai Etzioni

Amitai Etzioni, a sociologist, is University Professor at George Washington University. He is the author of *Capital Corruption: The New Attack on American Democracy* (1984), *The Moral Dimension: Toward a New Economics* (1988), and *The Spirit of Community: Rights, Responsibilities, and the Communitarian Agenda* (1993).

Etzioni rejects age-based rationing of health care and criticizes Callahan's position. In his view, such rationing would encourage intergenerational conflict. Furthermore, he argues, adopting Callahan's recommendations would start us on a slippery slope leading to growing restrictions on health care for other groups. Etzioni also suggests several ways in which funds required to avoid age-based health-care rationing might be raised.

In the coming years, Daniel Callahan's call to ration health care for the elderly, put forth in his book *Setting Limits*, is likely to have a growing appeal. Practically all economic observers expect the United States to go through a difficult time as it attempts to work its way out of its domestic (budgetary) and international (trade) deficits. Practically every serious analyst realizes that such an endeavor will initially entail slower growth, if not an outright cut in our standard of living, in order to release resources to these priorities. When the national economic "pie" grows more slowly, let alone contracts, the fight over how to divide it up intensifies. The elderly make an especially inviting target because they have been taking a growing slice of the resources (at least those dedicated to health care) and are expected to take even more in the future. Old people are widely held to be "nonproductive" and to constitute a growing "burden" on an ever-smaller proportion of society that is young and working. Also, the elderly are viewed as politically well-organized and powerful; hence "their"

programs, especially Social Security and Medicare, have largely escaped the Reagan attempts to scale back social expenditures, while those aimed at other groups—especially the young, but even more so future generations—have been generally curtailed. There are now some signs that a backlash may be forming.

If a war between the generations, like that between the races and between the genders, does break out, historians may accord former Governor Richard Lamm of Colorado the dubious honor of having fired the opening shot in his statement that the elderly ill have "got a duty to die and get out of the way." Phillip Longman, in his book *Born to Pay*, sounded an early alarm. However, the historians may well say, it was left to Daniel Callahan, a social philosopher and ethicist, to provide a detailed rationale and blueprint for limiting the care to the elderly, explicitly in order to free resources for the young [see Daniel Callahan, "Limiting Health Care for the Old," *The Nation*, August 15/22, 1987]. Callahan's thesis deserves close examination because he attempts to deal with the numerous objections his approach raises. If his thesis does not hold, the champions of limiting funds available to the old may have a long wait before they will find a new set of arguments on their behalf.

In order to free up economic resources for the young, Callahan offers the older generation a deal: Trade quantity for quality; the elderly should not be given life-*extending* services but better years while alive. Instead of the relentless attempt to push death to an older age, Callahan would stop all development of life-extending technologies and prohibit the use of ones at hand for those who outlive their "natural" life span, say, the age of 75. At the same time, the old would be granted more palliative medicine (e.g., pain killers) and more nursing-home and home-health care, to make their natural years more comfortable.

Callahan's call to break an existing ethical taboo and replace it with another raises the problem known among ethicists and sociologists as the "slippery slope." Once the precept that one should do "all one can" to avert death is given up, and attempts are made to fix a specific age for a full life, why stop there? If, for instance, the American economy experiences hard times in the 1990s, should the "maximum" age be reduced to 72, 65—or lower? And should the care for other so-called unproductive groups be cut off, even if they are even younger? Should countries that are economically worse off than the United States set their limit, say, at 55?

This is not an idle thought, because the idea of limiting the care the elderly receive in itself represents a partial slide down such a slope. Originally, Callahan, the Hastings Center (which he directs) and other think tanks played an important role in redefining the concept of death. Death used to be seen by the public at large as occurring when the lungs stopped functioning and, above all, the heart stopped beating. In numerous old movies and novels, those attending the dying would hold a mirror to their faces to see if it fogged over, or put an ear to their chests to see if the heart had stopped. However, high technology made these criteria obsolete by mechanically ventilating people and keeping their hearts pumping. Hastings et al. led the way to provide a new technological definition of death: brain death. Increasingly this has been accepted, both in the medical community and by the public at large, as the point of demise, the point at which care should stop even if it means turning off life-extending machines, because people who are brain dead do not regain consciousness. At the same time, most doctors and a majority of the public as well continue strongly to oppose terminating care to people who are conscious, even if there is little prospect for recovery, despite considerable debate about certain special cases.

Callahan now suggests turning off life-extending technology for all those above a certain age, even if they could recover their full human capacity if treated. It is instructive to look at the list of technologies he would withhold: mechanical ventilation, artificial resuscitation, antibiotics and artificial nutrition and hydration. Note that while several of these are used to maintain brain-dead bodies, they are also used for individuals who are temporarily incapacitated but able to recover fully; indeed, they are used to save young lives, say, after a car accident. But there is no way to stop the development of such new technologies and the improvement of existing ones without depriving the young of benefit as well. (Antibiotics are on the list because of an imminent "high cost" technological advance—administering them with a pump implanted in the body, which makes their introduction more reliable and better distributes dosages.)

One may say that this is Callahan's particular list; other lists may well be drawn. But any of them would start us down the slope, because the savings that are achieved by turning off the machines that keep brain-dead people alive are minimal compared with those that would result from the measures sought by the people calling for new equity between the generations. And any significant foray into deliberately withholding medical care for those who can recover does raise the question, Once society has embarked on such a slope, where will it stop?

Those opposed to Callahan, Lamm and the other advocates of limiting care to the old, but who also favor extending the frontier of life, must answer the question, Where will the resources come from? One answer is found in the realization that defining people as old at the age of 65 is obsolescent. That age limit was set generations ago, before changes in life styles and medicines much extended not only life but also the number and quality of productive years. One might recognize that many of the "elderly" can contribute to society not merely by providing love, companionship and wisdom to the young but also by continuing to work, in the traditional sense of the term. Indeed, many already work in the underground economy because of the large penalty—a cut in Social Security benefits—exacted from them if they hold a job "on the books."

Allowing elderly people to retain their Social Security benefits while working, typically part-time, would immediately raise significant tax revenues, dramatically change the much-feared dependency-to-dependent ratio, provide a much-needed source of child-care workers and increase contributions to Social Security (under the assumption that anybody who will continue to work will continue to contribute to the program). There is also evidence that people who continue to have meaningful work will live longer and healthier lives, without requiring more health care, because psychic well-being in our society is so deeply associated with meaningful work. Other policy changes, such as deferring retirement, modifying Social Security benefits by a small, gradual stretching out of the age of full-benefit entitlement, plus some other shifts under way, could be used readily to gain more resources. Such changes might be justified prima facie because as we extend life and its quality, the payouts to the old may also be stretched out.

Beyond the question of whether to cut care or stretch out Social Security payouts, policies that seek to promote intergenerational equity must be assessed as to how they deal with another matter of equity: that between the poor and the rich. A policy that would stop Federal support for certain kinds of care, as Callahan and others propose, would halt treatment for the aged, poor, the near-poor and even the less-well-off segment of the middle class (although for the latter at a later point), while the rich would continue to buy all the care they wished to. Callahan's suggestion that a consensus of doctors would stop certain kinds of care for all elderly people is quite impractical; for it to work, most if not all doctors would have to agree to participate. Even if this somehow happened, the rich would buy their services overseas either by going there or by importing the services. There is little enough we can do to significantly enhance economic equality. Do we want to exacerbate the inequalities that already exist by completely eliminating access to major categories of health care services for those who cannot afford to pay for them?

In addition to concern about slipping down the slope of less (and less) care, the *way* the limitations are to be introduced raises a serious question. The advocates of changing the intergenerational allocation of resources favor rationing health care for the elderly but nothing else. This is a major intellectual weakness of their argument. There are other major targets to consider within health care, as well as other areas, which seem, at least by some criteria, much more inviting than terminating care to those above a certain age. Within the medical sector, for example, why not stop all interventions for which there is no hard evidence that they are beneficial? Say, public financing of psychotherapy and coronary bypass operations? Why not take the $2 billion or so from plastic surgery dedicated to face lifts, reducing behinds and the like? Or require that all burials be done by low-cost cremations rather than using high-cost coffins?

Once we extend our reach beyond medical care to health care, if we cannot stop people from blowing $25 billion per year on cigarettes and convince them to use the money to serve the young, shouldn't we at least cut out public subsidies to tobacco growers before we save funds by denying antibiotics to old people? And there is the matter of profits. The high-technology medicine Callahan targets for savings is actually a minor cause of the increase in health care costs for the elderly or for anyone—about 4 percent. A major factor is the very high standard of living American doctors have, compared to those of many other nations. Indeed, many doctors tell interviewers that they love their work and would do it for half their current income as long as the incomes of their fellow practitioners were also cut. Another important area of saving is the exorbitant profits made by the nondoctor owners of dialysis units and nursing homes. If we dare ask how many years of life are enough, should we not also be able to ask how much profit is "enough"? This profit, by the way, is largely set not by the market but by public policy.

Last but not least, as the United States enters a time of economic constraints, should we draw new lines of conflict or should we focus on matters that sustain our societal fabric? During the 1960s numerous groups gained in political consciousness and actively sought to address injustices done to them. The result has been some redress and an increase in the level of societal stress (witness the deeply troubled relationships between the genders). But these conflicts occurred in an affluent society and redressed deeply felt grievances. Are the young like blacks and women, except that they have not yet discovered their oppressors—a group whose consciousness should be raised, so it will rally and gain its due share?

The answer is in the eye of the beholder. There are no objective criteria that can be used here the way they can be used between the races or between the genders. While women and minorities have the same rights to the same jobs at the same pay as white males, the needs of the young and the aged are so different that no simple criteria of equity come to mind. Thus, no one would argue that the teen-agers and those above 75 have the same need for schooling or nursing homes.

At the same time, it is easy to see that those who try to mobilize the young—led by a new Washington research group, Americans for Generational Equity (AGE), formed to fight for the needs of the younger generation—offer many arguments that do not hold. For instance, they often argue that today's young, age 35 or less, will pay for old people's Social Security, but by the time that they come of age they will not be able to collect, because Social Security will be bankrupt. However, this argument is based on extremely far-fetched assumptions about the future. In effect, Social Security is now and for the foreseeable future overprovided, and its surplus is used to reduce deficits caused by other expenditures, such as Star Wars, in what is still an integrated budget. And, if Social Security runs into the red again somewhere after the year 2020, relatively small adjustments in premiums and payouts would restore it to financial health.

Above all, it is a dubious sociological achievement to foment conflict between the generations, because, unlike the minorities and the white majority, or men and women, many millions of Americans are neither young nor old but of intermediate ages. We should not avoid issues just because we face stressing times in an already strained society; but maybe we should declare a moratorium on raising new conflicts until more compelling arguments can be found in their favor, and more evidence that this particular line of divisiveness is called for.

If Age Becomes a Standard for Rationing Health Care . . .
Nora Kizer Bell

Nora Kizer Bell is dean, college of arts and sciences, University of North Texas. She is the author of such articles as "Ethical Dilemmas in Trauma Nursing," "Treatment Decisions: Autonomy, Beneficence, and the Patient's Best Interests," and "AIDS and Women: Remaining Ethical Issues."

Bell contests Callahan's thesis that society may justifiably place an age limit on expensive, publicly funded, life-extending health care. Such age-based rationing, she argues, would affect elderly women more drastically than elderly men. In her view, there are several major reasons for this differential impact. (1) Women, on average, live longer than men, and there are more elderly women than elderly men. (2) Because elderly women are typically poorer, more likely to live alone, and less likely to have supports of various kinds than are elderly men, elderly women are more in need of the sorts of health-care services that would be rationed. Yet their consumption of such services will encourage the perception that, if services should be limited for any group, they should be limited for elderly women.

In two recent and controversial books, *Setting Limits* (1987) and *What Kind of Life: The Limits of Medical Progress* (1990), Daniel Callahan of the Hastings Center has put forth a provocative thesis: that "intergenerational equity" might require us to rethink some of the traditional goals of medicine as they affect care that is provided to the elderly. Specifically, Callahan suggests that the increasing numbers of the elderly, coupled with medicine's increased technological capabilities, create

Reprinted with permission of Indiana University Press from Helen Bequaert Holmes and Laura M. Purdy, eds., *Feminist Perspectives in Medical Ethics* (1992), pp. 82–90.

the potential within medicine for "an unending medical struggle against aging and death" that is, perhaps, not properly one of medicine's "deepest ends" or goals.

In his view, we have reached a crisis in medicine—about the meaning and nature of health, as well as about the proper role that an open-ended pursuit of health should play in the future. "We have come ever more to desire what we cannot any longer have in unlimited measure—a healthier, extended life—and cannot even afford to pursue much longer without harm to our personal lives and our social institutions" (Callahan 1990, 11).

Others advance a similar claim: put bluntly, society is going to have to make some hard choices. Many believe that one of those choices should be to limit the public provision of expensive, life-extending medical treatment for persons beyond age seventy or eighty. The claim is that in an era of scarce resources and spiraling health care costs—when important social goods are competing with expanding health care needs—persons can no longer expect to pursue medical advances "wherever they lead us."

On its face, this thesis is one for which I have a great deal of sympathy. I have been present in the ICU when a ninety-two-year-old woman with terminal metastatic cancer is intubated repeatedly each time she extubates herself. I have argued in favor of the "validity" of giving effect to a living will that was executed in a state other than the one in which the elderly patient finds herself hospitalized. I, myself, have argued that the prolongation of life, or the forestalling of death, can be a "false goal" of medicine. I agree that one's quality of life is not necessarily a function of the length of one's life, and I, too, worry about "creeping medical immortality."

But I am more worried about society's setting *involuntary* limits. If age becomes a limiting factor in the provision of medical treatment, apart from the obvious consequences to which many before me have taken objection, there is yet another consequence that I feel must not be overlooked. The limits that will be set will be limits that affect women more drastically than they affect men because the so-called "frontier" of old age extends indefinitely for many more women than it does men.

My objective in writing this essay, therefore, is to examine the implications of such a thesis for elderly women.

RECONSTRUCTING THE ENDS OF AGING

To propose using age as a specific criterion for the allocation and limitation of health care is to suggest that upon reaching the end of a "natural life span" further medical intervention should be acknowledged as inappropriate.

This, however, seems to imply a conception of life and the natural end of one's life in old age different from what we have normally taken it to be, a conception that focuses on the fact that one's life *on the whole* has had numerous and bountiful experiences whose richness in old age now suggests completeness. Such a conception of life makes no evaluative claims about the experiences by which one's life is so defined. Rather, on this so-called *biographical* definition of life there simply

comes a time when the biography is complete, even though there might be many more pages one could write.

> For the lifelong reader there will still be many old books not read, and a constant stream of new books to be read. For the painter, there will be an infinite number of further possibilities, as there will be for one who enjoys investing in the stock market, understanding nature, watching scientific and other knowledge being discovered, growing a garden, observing the sunset, enjoying music, and taking walks. In that sense, however, life's possibilities will never be exhausted. . . . Yet even if we will lose such possibilities by death in old age, we will on the whole already have had ample time to know the pleasures of such things. (Callahan 1987, 67)

As Callahan argues in *What Kind of Life,* recognizing the necessity of setting limits on the provision of health care acknowledges acceptance of a full ("but not necessarily biologically maximum") life span, the appropriateness of death from "conditions whose eradication would require an unreasonable expenditure of resources, and a circumscribed place for the pursuit of health as a societal good" (Callahan 1990, 151).

On such a view, the end of the aging process is not properly spent, therefore, "warring" against the diseases that accompany longevity. Rather, death at the end of a long and full life is fitting and orderly. Furthermore, the natural end to a long and full life is a "tolerable death": (a) a death that occurs when one has accomplished most of what life has to offer, (2) a death that occurs when one has fulfilled one's obligations to all those to whom one has responsibilities, and (3) a death that no longer offends or engenders rage and despair at human finitude (Callahan 1987, 66).

The goal of geriatric medicine, therefore, is not to seek new ways to predict or prevent late-onset genetic disease, it is not to define "premature" death as a function of state-of-the-art medicine at any given moment, it is not to seek "just a little longer life," it is not to practice opportunistic medicine or to imagine medicine as providing the fountain of youth. Rather, so that one may experience the natural end of life, the goal is to put aside the allures that medicine offers for staving off old age. Hence, society should seek to impose limits on health care for the elderly so that the richness and fullness of old age aren't lost, and so that old age isn't vilified by our fight against it.

> It is a tragedy when life ends prematurely even though it is possible to save that life, and when old age is

full of burdens even though resources are available to relieve them. It is an outrage when, through selfishness, discrimination, or culpable indifference, the elderly are denied what they need and deserve. But it is only a sadness, an ineradicable part of life itself, when after a long and full life a person ages and dies. . . . It is wise to want to banish the tragedy and the outrage, but not the sadness. (Callahan 1987, 204)

In fact, Callahan acknowledges that the notion of a decent biographical life span may be different for different persons and that we may have obligations to have helped with preventive medicine early in an individual's life—with immunizations and with decent primary care. Yet, he argues, we are not obliged "to follow the culture of modernized aging wherever it might lead, especially when we come to know what it will cost, and how little in improved happiness we might get anyway" (Callahan 1990, 153). Society, he concludes, would be perfectly justified in setting an age limit on the public provision of expensive, life-extending, *curative* health care.

TOLERABLE OR TRAGIC DEATHS?

The elderly are currently the heaviest users of health services, and the great bulk of those services is spent in "forestalling death" and in "warehousing" persons until their deaths. These facts represent part of the challenge society would face in setting limits. When one looks closely at the data, however, what one very quickly discovers is that there are many more elderly women than there are elderly men, and these older women are poorer, more apt to live alone, and less likely to have informal social and personal supports than their male counterparts. Furthermore, a disproportionate number of nursing home patients are women. Older *women,* therefore, are more likely to make the heaviest demand on health care resources.[1]

What would it mean in practice, then, to have a health policy for the aged of the kind outlined above?

Unfortunately, serious problems underlie using age as a criterion for rationing health care, problems that, despite the insistence that the elderly would never be denied compassionate and thoughtful care, redound negatively against such a thesis. I want to argue that setting limits according to the rationale outlined above may in some cases still be properly described as a "tragedy" and an "outrage."

None of the arguments for rationing by age take note of the implications for women of employing such a criterion, or of the special plight of women among the aged (except to mention that women are burdened more than men in being caregivers for sick and aging parents). None of the arguments about the limits of society's obligations to the aged acknowledges historical failures of the health care system to note gender differences in medical research, diagnosis, and treatment. None of the arguments addresses the question of whether there might be differences in the definition of "natural life span" or one's perception of a "tolerable death" that are gender-relative. None of the arguments takes note of the fact that the limits they suggest imposing may have tragic consequences for women.

In my view, however, these are the very consequences of age-based rationing that need to be examined more carefully. In what follows, I would like to offer such an examination by looking more closely at Callahan's three-part definition of what counts as a tolerable death.

First: *A tolerable death is one that occurs when an individual has accomplished most of what life has to offer.*

Such a biographical definition of life fails to take adequate note of the differences in the biographies of men and women. To believe that it is desirable to adopt the use of an age standard suggests that a woman's life should be viewed as completed earlier in her biological chronology than it actually is, that is, when procreation, childrearing, housekeeping, and the maintaining of conjugal relationships are complete. The argument in favor of believing that there is an appropriate time in a person's biography for claiming that her life could be considered full strikes me as advancing recognized forms of male bias: both a general *devaluation of women's concerns* and *an indifference to a woman's "life possibilities" apart from her abasement into more servile positions.* (That is not to say that I couldn't agree that one's life from a certain point forward might not be worth living or might itself be intolerable.)

Why shouldn't one believe, as James Childress (1984) has suggested, that the use of an age standard seems to symbolize a willingness on our part to abandon older female persons and exclude them from communal care?[2] Furthermore, as Childress seems to believe, the use of an age criterion for determining how to allocate health care resources seems to manifest society's perception that youth is valuable and advanced age, particularly advanced female age, has less worth. The testimony of older persons, especially older women, who profess to believe that they are willing, and maybe even morally obliged, to let a younger person (say, a child or a grandchild) live in their stead is less evidence in favor of accepting the argument than it is evidence confirming society's devaluation of older persons and advancing age. Besides, willingness on the part of some older persons to elect to forego certain resources or experiences in favor of giving them to younger persons does not imply that a standard for accomplishing that should be *imposed*. Unless Childress's claim about the use of an age criterion is true—that is, unless we really do believe that youth is more valuable—why should it be obvious that we should prefer to limit resources to older persons in favor of allocating to younger persons? Why shouldn't we believe that electing such a standard makes women's deaths premature? Why isn't it obvious that women's old age *is* full of burdens? Is it obvious that there aren't resources available to relieve them?

A biographical definition of life also seems to measure a person's life by the notion of a "range of experiences" without taking note of any qualitative measure of those experiences. This understanding of measuring one's life seems counterintuitive. It doesn't seem enough to say that the range of a person's experiences, or the range of her exposure to resources, is greater by virtue of her having lived longer. Surely the *quality* of those experiences or of those resources colors them in a way that cannot be ignored. For that reason, it seems culpable indifference to fail to count the quality of those experiences as significant. Insofar as women have historically been disadvantaged with respect to their achievements, their interests, their economic, social, and political status, and their sexuality, many would argue that the quality of their life experiences has been so low that with respect to the first criterion of what counts as a tolerable death, such a definition begs the question.

This brings me to the second part of the definition of what counts as a tolerable death:

A tolerable death is one that occurs when one has fulfilled one's obligations to all those to whom one has responsibilities.

Women are beginning to enter the paid labor force in substantial numbers, but in spite of their economic emergence, women continue to be in disadvantaged positions in the marketplace both in terms of the wages they command and the jobs open to them. As human capital, women are valued less highly than men (Bergmann 1986). This can be viewed as a natural consequence of the fact that "[i]n the past, women's place

in the economy was an assignment to sole responsibility for the care of the children, and to housework and other works that could efficiently be combined in the home with child care. Men were given sole responsibility for earning money, and exempted from taking a share in 'women's work' " (Bergmann 1986, 7). The importance assigned to earning money, among other things, helped contribute to devaluing "women's work." Reskin and Hartmann (1986) and others delineate some of the kinds of work that have been so devalued: *caring work* (child care and nursing care, for example), *consumption work* (all those tasks involved in purchasing goods and services), *kin work* (tasks involved in keeping up with family birthdays, weddings, funerals, and simply "keeping in touch"), *invisible work* (housework, cooking, sewing, washing, ironing, for example). A further indication of the lack of value attached to such work is found in the fact that government and industry have been slow to move to "industrialize" child care and housework, making it even harder for women (especially single mothers) to compete effectively in the job market (Bergmann 1986, 275–98).[3]

Because of the value attached to providing for another financially, women's responsibilities to others continue in large part to be described as consisting in caring work, kin work, consumption work and other forms of so-called invisible work. It is easy to imagine someone arguing that a woman who is single, or who outlives her spouse, or whose children are independent has outlived her usefulness and her obligations. Furthermore, because women live longer than men and have been in the work force a shorter period of time than men, and hence have contributed less to public funds and have limited provisions of their own for their old age, women could also be perceived as undeservedly requiring more in the way of others' responsibilities *to* them. As the largest and poorest population of the elderly, it is women who will make the heaviest demands on public monies for health care. It is the older woman who will have the greatest need for increased social and nonfinancial forms of support. It is she who will be society's greatest burden, and it is she for whom limits will be set.

It is this larger social and moral context to which I want to appeal in evaluating the thesis that age be a standard for rationing care. Using age as a standard for rationing is much more complex than it appears on its face. For his part, Callahan acknowledges that an age standard has "symbolic significance" when its use is colored by its context, or by the rationale articulated for its use (1987, 169). He also acknowledges that death is a tragedy and an outrage if it comes on the heels of one's having been denied what one needs through discrimination or indifference (1987, 204).

A death is tolerable when it no longer offends or engenders rage and despair.

Of course, many who advocate an upper age limit on providing health services don't necessarily desire to deal women out. If anything, their arguments are ones that I have heard many so-called senior citizens express almost as eloquently themselves. And I do agree that we have to be sensible about utilizing medical resources, especially in cases where they aren't likely to benefit the recipient or alter an inevitably bad outcome. I acknowledge that we are fast approaching a time in our history when the largest segment of our population, our largest special interest lobby, if you will, is the aging and the elderly. However, I can't agree that employing age as a standard in rationing would transform its present use into a use that "affirms" and does not denigrate old age (Callahan 1987, 170).

I want to argue that there is tremendous symbolic significance for women in adopting an age standard, a significance that derives from and is colored by women's social and moral history. Honoring a "natural life span" could mean believing that a natural life normally ends in the mid-seventies (the life expectancy for males), and in accepting that age standard, Callahan-style policy makers might adopt measures that preclude women from receiving essential services at the ends of our (longer) lives.

Among the items left over from the "old" anti-ageism agenda (Butler 1975), the widespread problem of elder abuse and neglect should generate outrage. A University of Massachusetts study suggests that there are six times as many cases of abuse of the elderly as are actually reported (Elder Abuse 1988). Abuse, neglect, and exploitation include failing to provide the ill and the fragile with minimal medical care, medication, and hospitalization. Why don't the proponents of such sweeping policy change give this problem more prominence?

Again because of their numbers, women constitute the majority of those affected by abuse and neglect. When I worry about setting limits, I worry about the attitudes engendered by promulgation of the belief that there is an age beyond which one is getting more than her fair share. I worry about the fact that so-called entitlement policies—that would focus on providing health care to "disadvantaged groups" who have been deprived of benefits available to the population as a whole—don't mention women except as their health care affects the health status of their offspring (Callahan 1990, 197).

Arguments for rationing on the basis of age seem to rest on the presumption that there is little value in providing certain health services to persons who have reached the end of full and natural lives. I protest that presumption because "natural life span" and "tolerable death" are not gender neutral. Providing health services to the very old has been devalued, in part because medical intervention can dehumanize the natural end to one's natural life span. I wonder if that absence of value is not also due in large measure to the fact that there are few male competitors for these services. Couldn't we believe that, like other items in women's social history, when men move to evaluate something that is peculiarly the province of women, it then becomes devalued?

Given this social and moral context, women's old age is not affirmed by setting limits; it is debased. Given this context, the deaths of older women *will* engender rage and despair. Given this context, appealing to an age standard will make the deaths of women premature in the fullest sense of the word. Not only will their deaths be sad, they will be a tragedy and an outrage.

NOTES

I am especially grateful to my colleague Ferdinand Schoeman for the many helpful suggestions he made about various aspects of this discussion.

1 Older women now outnumber older men three to two. This represents a dramatic increase from 1960, when the ratio of elderly men to elderly women was five to four. Furthermore, the ratio changes markedly with increased age. The 1984 census found only 40 men for every 100 women at age 85, but 81 men for every 100 women between the ages of 65 and 69. By the year 2050, the projected life expectancy for females will reach 83.6 years as contrasted with a life expectancy for males of 79.8 years. The gender ratios are important for the further reason that they indicate that more women than men will be living alone in old age. Although more than one-third of all elderly disabled men living in their communities were cared for by their wives, only one in ten elderly disabled women were cared for by their husbands (Special Committee on Aging 1985).

An obvious concern, and the concern that underlies Callahan's interest in examining medicine's goals for an aging society, is that the projected increase in the size of the older population implies correlative increases in the demand for health care resources and the provision of services to the elderly. In addition, elderly persons are more likely than other adults to be poor. However, the economic statistics are especially grim for elderly women. According to a study published in 1985 by the United States Senate's Special Committee on Aging, of those persons between the ages of 65 and 69, white males had a median income of $12,180 per year as compared to a median income of $5,599 for elderly women. Because they live longer than their male counterparts, elderly women average a longer period of retirement than elderly men and must, therefore, rely on private and public sources of income longer than elderly men. Not surprisingly, nearly three-quarters of the population of the elderly poor are women (1985, 2).

Although at present only about five percent of the elderly live in nursing homes, close to 75 percent of all nursing home residents have no spouse and are institutionalized because they have health problems that significantly limit their ability to care for themselves. Not surprisingly, a disproportionate number (74.6 percent) of nursing home patients are very old, white, female, and without spouse (Special Committee on Aging 1985). The economic implications of an aging population are obvious. If limits are not set, Callahan predicts that health care expenditures for the elderly will exceed $200 billion by the year 2000. By 2040, he predicts that pension and health programs will account for 14.5 percent of the GNP and 60.4 percent of the federal budget, respectively (1987, 228).

2 Childress does not make this argument with respect to older women in particular. He makes it with respect to all older persons.

3 Furthermore, some social changes designed to benefit women economically have actually worked to their detriment. "No-fault divorce looked like a civilized way for equal adults to deal with marital incompatibility. [Yet] its implementation has cut adrift millions of middle-aged and elderly housewives who had every right to believe they had been guaranteed a comfortable home for life. Well meaning efforts to reform welfare failed miserably to lead single mothers out of poverty" (Bergmann 1986, 300).

REFERENCES

Aging America: Trends and projections. 1983. US Senate Special Committee on Aging (in conjunction with AARP). Washington, DC.

America in transition: An aging society. 1985. US Senate Special Committee on Aging. Washington, DC. 99-B.

A profile of older Americans—1986. American Association of Retired Persons. Washington, DC.

Bergmann, Barbara. 1986. *The economic emergence of women.* New York: Basic Books.

Butler, R. N. 1975. *Why survive? Being old in America.* New York: Harper & Row.

Callahan, Daniel. 1987. *Setting limits: Medical goals in an aging society.* New York: Simon and Schuster.

Callahan, Daniel. 1990. *What kind of life: The limits of medical progress.* New York: Simon and Schuster.

Childress, James F. 1984. Ensuring care, respect, and fairness for the elderly. *The Hastings Center Report* 14(5): 27–31.

Day, Alice T. 1984. Who cares? Demographic trends challenge family care for the elderly. *Populations Trends and Public Policy.* Washington, DC: Population Reference Bureau, Inc.

Elder abuse reports are growing in SC. 1988. *The State.* Columbia, SC. June 5.

Long term care: A review of the evidence. 1986. University of Minnesota, School of Public Health: Division of Health Services.

May, William. 1982. Who cares for the elderly? *The Hastings Center Report* 12(6): 31–37.

Projections of the population of the US by age, sex and race: 1983–2080. Washington, DC: US Bureau of the Census. Series P-25, 952.

Reskin, Barbara, and H. Hartmann, eds. 1986. *Women's work, men's work.* Washington, DC: National Academy Press.

Waldo, Daniel, and H. Lazenby. 1984. Demographic characteristics and health care use and expenditures by the aged in the US: 1977–1984. *Health Care Financing Review* 6(1).

Is the Oregon Rationing Plan Fair?
Norman Daniels

Norman Daniels is professor of philosophy at Tufts University. He was a member of the White House Task Force on National Health Reform, the Advisory Ethics Working Group. Widely published in philosophy and biomedical ethics, he is the editor of *Reading Rawls* (1974) and the author of *Just Health Care* (1985) and *Am I My Parents' Keeper?: An Essay on Justice between the Young and the Old* (1988).

Daniels takes up the question of whether the Oregon rationing plan (which is discussed in the introduction to this chapter) is fair or just. In exploring this complex question, he notes ways in which particular features can be seen as fair or unfair depending on background assumptions about justice. For example, the plan may make those already eligible for Medicaid (the very poor) worse off by not funding some of the services to which they had previously been eligible; this feature counts as unjust, Daniels argues, if justice requires maximally benefiting those who are the worst off. On the other hand, the plan extends coverage to many poor persons previously uncovered by Medicaid—a feature reducing inequity between the poor and others in society. Daniels also examines the way in which (1) political judgments (e.g., regarding the feasibility of alternative strategies for implementing more egalitarian reforms) and (2) judgments about the adequacy of the public process (e.g., regarding which groups were represented at public meetings) affect our moral evaluations of the Oregon plan.

The Oregon Basic Health Services Act mandates universal access to basic care, but includes rationing services to those individuals who are Medicaid recipients. If no new resources are added, the plan may make current Medicaid recipients worse off, but still reduce inequality between the poor and the rest of society. If resources are expanded and benefits given appropriate rankings, no one may be worse off; though inequality will be reduced, alternative reforms might reduce it even further. Whether the outcome seems fair then depends on how much priority to the well-being of the poor we believe justice requires; it also depends on political judgments about the feasibility of alternative strategies for achieving more egalitarian reforms. Oregon makes rationing public and explicit, as justice requires, but it is not clear how community values influence the ranking of services; ultimately, the rationing process is fair only if we may rely on the voting power of the poor.

Reprinted with permission of the publisher from *JAMA*, vol. 265 (May 1, 1991), pp. 2232–2235. Copyright © 1991, American Medical Association.

EXCLUDING PEOPLE VS EXCLUDING SERVICES

In 1987, Oregon drew national attention when it stopped Medicaid funding of soft-tissue transplants. Officials justified the action by claiming that there are more effective ways to spend scarce public dollars than to provide high-cost benefits to relatively few people. They insisted that the estimated $1.1 million that would have been spent on such transplants in 1987 would save many more lives per dollar spent if invested in prenatal maternal care.[1] Rather than heartlessly turning its back on children in need of transplants, the state was making a "tragic choice" between two instances of rationing by ability to pay. The consequences of ignoring "invisible" pregnant women who cannot afford prenatal maternal care are much worse than are those of refusing to fund highly visible children in need of transplants.

The Oregon Basic Health Services Act boldly couples the rationing of health care with a plan to improve access.[2] It expands Medicaid eligibility to 100% for those individuals who are at the federal poverty level, creates an Oregon Health Services Commission (OHSC) to establish priorities among health services, requires cutting low-priority services rather than excluding people from coverage when reducing expenditures is necessary, mandates a high-risk insurance pool, and requires employers to provide health insurance or to contribute to a state insurance pool. Oregon must obtain a federal waiver to implement the changes in Medicaid.

Oregon explicitly rejects the rationing strategy that predominates in the United States: our rationing system excludes whole categories of the poor and near-poor from access to public insurance, denying coverage to *people,* rather than to low-priority *services.* In contrast, the Oregon plan embodies the following principles: (1) there is a social obligation to guarantee universal access to a *basic level* of health care, (2) reasonable or necessary limits on resources mean that not every beneficial service can be included in the basic level of health care, and (3) a public process, involving consideration of social values, is required to determine what services will be included in the basic level of health care.[1,3]

Though these principles are not a complete account of justice for health care, they have considerable plausibility, derive support from theoretical work on justice and health care, and are, to varying degrees, widely believed in by the US population.[4] Nevertheless, these principles permit rationing care to the poor alone, with serious implications for equality. Thus, critics attack the Oregon plan for making the poor, specifically poor women and children, "bear the burden" of providing universal access.[5]

To evaluate this criticism, we must ask three questions: (1) Does the plan make the indigent groups better off or worse off? (2) Are the inequalities the plan accepts justifiable? (3) Is the procedure for determining the basic level of health care a just or fair one? These questions raise issues of distributive justice that go beyond the principles underlying the Oregon legislation.

WHAT DOES THE OREGON PLAN DO TO THE WORSE-OFF GROUPS?

Critics of Oregon's plan appeal to widely held egalitarian concerns when they argue that it makes the poor bear the burden of this effort to close the insurance gap. The strongest sense of "bear the burden" is "being made worse off." Does the plan, as the critics charge, make the poor worse off instead of giving priority to improving their well-being?[6,7]

Consider the simplest case first, a zero sum game with resources. For example, if extrarenal transplants

are removed from coverage and no higher-priority services, unavailable before the plan, are added, then current Medicaid recipients will lose some services and the health benefits they produce. They will no doubt then make this complaint: "We bear the burden of the plan. Since we are already the most indigent group, or close to it, we should not have to give up lifesaving or other important medical services so that the currently uninsured can get basic level health care."

It is important to grasp the moral force of this complaint. Notice that *aggregate* health status for *all* the poor, including current Medicaid recipients and the uninsured, can be improved by the plan, even though current Medicaid recipients are made worse off. The loss of less important services by current recipients is more than counterbalanced by the gains of the uninsured. As a result, the plan reduces overall inequality between the poor and the rest of society, albeit at the expense of current Medicaid recipients. Therefore, the complaint cannot be that the plan makes society less equal; instead, it is that even greater reductions in inequality are possible if other groups sacrifice instead of Medicaid recipients. It is unfair for current Medicaid recipients to bear a burden that others could bear much better, especially since inequality would then be even further reduced.

How stringent is the priority owed the poorest groups when we seek to improve aggregate well-being? Three positions are possible: (1) help the poor as much as possible (*strict priority*); (2) make sure the poor get some benefit (*modified priority*); or (3) allow only modest harms to the poor in return for significant gains to others who are not well-off (*weak priority*). Critics of the Oregon plan insist that we should not settle for weak priority, especially since feasible alternatives help the poor more. The Oregon plan leaves the bulk of the health care system intact. By eliminating the inefficiencies it contains, eg, by establishing a low-overhead public insurance scheme (as in Canada), or by developing treatment protocols that eliminate unnecessary services, we might be able to avoid making current Medicaid recipients any worse off. Alternatively, by broadening rationing to cover most of society, as in Canada or Great Britain, we could avoid the criticism that only the poor are being made to bear the burden of improving access.

Proponents of the Oregon plan aim for a more complex case than a zero sum game with services, however, hoping to add either new services or new revenue sources.[1,3,8] Suppose, for example, the plan makes available "high-priority" services that are currently not adequately provided, such as prenatal maternal care, mental health, and chemical dependency services, while "low-priority" services, eg, soft-tissue transplants, are not funded. Then current Medicaid recipients will have a *higher* expected payoff from the revised benefits. Since the currently uninsured are also made better off, and no one is made worse off (except that taxes may be increased), we have what economists call a *pareto superior* outcome. Of course, those particular Medicaid recipients who need the newly rationed services will be worse off, but it is reasonable to judge the effects of the system *ex ante,* and the poor as a whole are better off despite the loss to some individuals who would require soft-tissue transplants.

Thus, with appropriate revisions of Medicaid benefits, the poor will be better off than they are now. Nevertheless, current Medicaid recipients can object, "We achieve our gain in health status by giving up beneficial services that better-off groups receive; in that sense we ' bear the burden' of the Oregon plan. The poor would improve even more if better-off groups contributed more." The complaint is that social inequality could be reduced in a way that benefits the poor even more.

One version of this complaint appeals to long-term considerations: the Oregon plan makes the poor better off in the short run but worse off than they would be in the longer run if a national health insurance scheme were introduced. This claim depends on particular political assumptions about the likelihood of alternative scenarios for reform. In reply, some proponents see the current legislation in Oregon as but the first step in a comprehensive, incremental reform; ultimately, the state would become the major insurer and most powerful purchaser by substituting its basic insurance plan for many private insurance plans as well as for Medicare and long-term care under Medicaid (Sen John Kitzhaber, verbal communication, January 1991). The debate then focuses on the means to health reform, not its ends; disagreement results from complex political, not moral, judgments.

A second complaint about reducible inequality derives from the Children's Defense Fund's charge that the Oregon plan "exempts" the elderly who are Medicaid recipients from the ranking of services.[5] Poor women and children, who constitute 75% of the Medicaid recipients, receive only 30% of the benefits in dollars. Much of the rest goes to the elderly who have "spent down" their resources in order to be eligible for long-term care, but these services—as well as all acute care for the elderly who are covered under Medicare—are

not included in the prioritization or rationing process. By not establishing priorities among health care services for the elderly, and by financing expansion of Medicaid coverage, primarily by rationing to women and children, the plan seems to suggest that any use of long-term medical services by the elderly is more important than short-term medical services for the young. This would be an irrational ranking on the face of it. If we did not know how old we were and had to allocate resources over our life span, taking our needs at each stage of life into account, we would not consider this ranking a prudent one.[9] A reasonable rationing plan would consider the importance of all health care services, short-term medical as well as long-term care, over an individual's life span, at each stage of life. To avoid what seems to be discrimination by age, rationing should include all age groups. In reply, and as noted, some Oregon proponents intend to expand the plan to cover Medicare and long-term Medicaid care.

Advocates for the Oregon plan argue that additional revenue, which would further reduce inequality, will be easier to obtain when the legislature must visibly cut beneficial services and cannot disguise rationing by raising eligibility requirements for Medicaid. This political judgment ignores evidence from the 1980s, when various states, as well as the federal government, cut important services to the poor, including prenatal maternal care and the Women, Infants, and Children's Program's distribution of food supplements to pregnant women and neighborhood mental health care services. Explicit rationing to the poor made neither politicians nor their constituents so uncomfortable that the cuts were stopped.

In short, we cannot answer the basic question about how the worse off will fare under the current legislation until we are told what they will get, that is, until the Medicaid benefit package is ranked by OHSC, is funded by the legislature, and is approved for a Medicaid waiver by the Department of Health and Human Services, sometime later in 1991. If the current Medicaid recipients are made worse off, there is a serious, though not necessarily fatal, objection to the Oregon plan. If we hold only a weak version of the requirement that we give priority to the worse off, we might still think the plan acceptable even though some of the poor bear the burden of reducing overall inequality. In any case, the Oregon planners hope that rationing will yield a result in which all the poor are better off than now. Political judgments differ about the likelihood of this preferred outcome.

ARE THE INEQUALITIES THE OREGON PLAN ACCEPTS JUSTIFIABLE?

By rationing lower-priority services to the poor, rather than excluding whole groups of the poor and near-poor from insurance, the Oregon plan reduces inequality in our society, even if current Medicaid recipients are, to some extent, worse off than they are now. Somewhat paradoxically, even under the scenario in which no one is worse off, there is still a sense in which the poor bear the burden of the plan, since the plan accepts as official policy an unjustifiable inequality in the health care system.

To see this point, contrast the kind of inequality the Oregon plan accepts with the inequality that arises in the heavily rationed British system.[10] Although about 10% of the British public buys private insurance coverage in order to procure various rationed services, the overwhelming majority abides by the consequences of rationing. This produces a more acceptable structure of inequality than would result if the bottom 20% of the Oregon population has no access to some services that are available to the great majority.[11]

To see why one structure of inequality seems worse than the other, consider how the poor would feel under both. Under the Oregon plan, the poor can complain that society as a whole is content not only to leave them economically badly off, but also to deny them medical services that would protect the range of opportunities that are open to them.[6] There is a basis here for reasonable regrets or resentment, for society as a whole seems content to shut the poor out of mainstream opportunities. They may reasonably feel that the majority is too willing to leave them behind under terms in which the benefits of social cooperation do not reflect their moral status as free and equal agents.[12,13] Alternatively, if health care protects opportunity in a way that is roughly equal for all, except that the most advantaged group has some extra advantages, then this may seem somewhat unfair, but no one group is then singled out for special disadvantages that are viewed as "acceptable" by the economically and medically advantaged majority. Consequently, no group would have a basis for the strong and reasonable regrets that the poor have under the Oregon plan, despite their improvement relative to the current situation.

Thus, even if the poor are better off under the Oregon plan than now, the plan still accepts an inequality that is not ideally just. It is more just—perhaps much more just—than what we now have, but still not what justice requires. Does this mean we should not implement it? The answer seems to depend on political judgments about the feasibility of alternatives. If one thinks that a uniform, universal plan, like Canada's, is a political impossibility in the United States, or if one thinks that introducing the Oregon plan makes further reform in the direction of a uniform plan more likely, then the Oregon plan, even if it is not ideally just, seems reasonable. But if one thinks that introducing the Oregon reform makes more radical reform of the system less likely, then one might well prefer not to make a modest improvement in the justice of the system in order to facilitate a more significant improvement later.

IS THE PUBLIC PROCESS FOR DECIDING WHAT IS 'BASIC CARE' FAIR?

The Oregon plan involves public, explicit rationing; it disavows rationing hidden by the covert workings of a market, or buried in the quiet, professional decisions of providers. Its rationing decisions are the result of a two-step process involving separate, publicly accountable bodies. First (step 1), OHSC, which is charged with taking "community values" into consideration, determines priorities among services in a possible benefit package. Second (step 2), the legislature decides how much to spend on Medicaid, given competing demands on state funds. Some lower-priority services may thus not be covered, but the resulting Medicaid benefit package must still be approved by the Department of Health and Human Services. Assessing the fairness of the rationing process requires examining both steps.

Oregon's insistence on publicity is controversial. Calabresi and Bobbit[14] argue that "tragic choices" are best made out of the public view in order to preserve important symbolic values, such as the sanctity of life. Despite the importance of such symbols, however, justice requires publicity. People who view themselves as free and equal moral agents must have available to them the grounds for all decisions that affect their lives in fundamental ways, as rationing decisions do. Only with publicity can they resolve disputes about whether the decisions conform to the more basic principles of justice that are the accepted basis of their social cooperation.[15]

Actually, going beyond a concern for publicity, Oregon calls for broad public participation in the development of priorities. Public participation is desirable because it may yield agreement about how to resolve disputes among winners and losers in a fair way. It also makes it more likely that outcomes reflect the consent of those individuals who are affected and, since there may not be one uniquely fair or just way to ration services, participation allows the shared values of a community to shape the result. Is the public participation process itself fair, and does it have a real effect on outcomes?

OHSC held public hearings on health services and asked Oregon Health Decisions to hold community meetings throughout the state "to build consensus on the values to be used to guide health resource allocation decisions."[16] At 47 meetings that were held during the early part of 1990, citizens were asked to rank the importance of various categories of treatment and were asked, "Why is this health care service *important to us*?" From these discussions, an unranked list of 13 "values" was distilled. A tally was kept of how often each value was discussed, but we cannot rank the importance of the values on that basis.

One frequent criticism of the community meeting procedure is that it did not involve a representative cross section of Oregonians. Some 50% were health professionals; too many were college educated, white, and relatively well-off. Moreover, whereas 16% of Oregonians are uninsured, only 9.4% of community meeting participants were uninsured, and Medicaid recipients, the only direct representatives of poor children, were underrepresented by half.[5,16] Even if there was no evidence of bias in the meetings, the process is still open to the charge that it consisted of the "haves" deciding what is "important" to give the "have-nots." The charge is twofold. Not only is the composition of the meetings unrepresentative of the interests of those who will be affected, but the task set for the meetings presupposes that rationing will primarily have an impact on an underrepresented minority.

It is difficult to assess the importance of either charge of bias, for we have no way to compare the outcome with an unbiased alternative. Suspicions about the effects of compositional bias would be reduced, however, if there were no bias in the task, that is, if the Oregon plan called for rationing services to the great majority rather than to the poor. We worry less about who is making a decision if it has an equal impact on everyone, including the decision makers.

The charge of bias is important only if the meetings actually influence the ranking of services (otherwise they are just window dressing). Contrary to public and media understanding, however, the community meetings do not yield a ranking of services, only a general list of community values. Moreover, the list of values cannot be used in any direct way in determining priorities among health services. Some of the "values" are really only categories of services, eg, mental health and chemical dependency, or prevention. Other values, such as equity (guaranteeing access to all) or respecting personal choice, are things we desire of the system as a whole, not of individual services. And the values relevant to ranking services, such as quality of life or cost-effectiveness or ability to function, are not themselves ranked.

OHSC is well aware of this limitation and views the list of values only as a "qualitative check" on the process of ranking services (Paige Sipes-Metzler, personal communication, June and July 1990). Thus, it believes the community concern for equity is met because the system guarantees universal access to basic care. Community concerns about mental health and chemical dependency, or prevention, are met by making sure that these services are included in the ranking process. Although no weights were assigned to values such as quality of life or cost-effectiveness, they are included as factors in the formal ranking process. The only direct community input into the first attempt at ranking services, however, came from a telephone survey aimed at finding how Oregonians ranked particular health outcomes that affect their quality of life. By combining this information with expert judgments about the likely outcomes of using particular procedures to treat certain conditions, as well as with information about the costs of treating a population with those procedures, OHSC generated a preliminary cost-benefit ranking of services. Because this ranking drew extensive criticism (*New York Times*, July 9, 1990; sect A:17) and failed to match its own expectations about priorities, OHSC modified its procedure for ranking services. As a result, the OHSC commissioners themselves ranked general categories of services according to their importance to the individual, to society, and to the health plan and "adjusted" other items.[17] It remains unclear how this process reflects community values, and until we know just how the final rankings were "adjusted," we cannot know what influence public participation has had.

The rationing process involves two decisions, not one. Suppose that we have a fair procedure and a perfect outcome at step 1: the ranking of services captures relevant facts about costs and benefits and represents community values fairly. Unfortunately, fairness at step 1 does not assure it at step 2, because the voting power of the poor is negated in a political process that generally underrepresents them, judging from past voting patterns and outcomes. Therefore, even if there is a consensus at step 1 about what the basic, minimum package should be, there may be well-founded worries that the legislature will not fund it. Indeed, the situation is somewhat worse because OHSC only ranks services, it does not decide what is basic. The funding decision of the legislature determines what basic care is provided.

Clearly, political judgments diverge on how much we can trust the legislature. The crucial issue from the point of view of process, however, is this: because the Oregon plan explicitly involves rationing primarily for the poor and near-poor, funding decisions face constant political pressure from more powerful groups who want to put public resources to other uses. In contrast, if the legislature were deciding how to fund a rationing plan that applied to themselves and to all their constituents, then we might expect a careful and honest weighing of the importance of health care against other goods. The legislature would then have stronger reasons not to concede to political pressures to divert resources, and other groups would be less likely to apply such pressure. If the plan is expanded to include other groups, then the poor may find important allies.

Worries about fairness in the Oregon rationing process thus come from the plan's being aimed at the poor rather than at the population as a whole. Concerns about fairness in the process thus converge with concerns about the kinds of inequality the system tolerates. This does not mean that the Oregon experiment should not be tried; it may produce less overall inequality in health status than we now have. But we should recognize from the start that a system that rations only to the poor is less equitable and less fair than alternative systems that ration for the great majority of people. To the extent that the inequality ends up troubling many participants in the system, including physicians who will be able to do only certain things for some children and more for others, the strains of commitment to abiding by the rationing will be greater, and rationing may get a worse name than it deserves.

Oregon's plan retains the structure of inequality that it does because states must respond to the problems imposed by a highly inequitable and inefficient national health care system. The plan contains a bizarre irony: the state's Medicaid budget is in crisis because of rapidly increasing costs, largely the result of the burden of long-term care imposed by the elderly, yet the rationing plan focuses on poor children. Oregon did not design a Medicaid system that forces the most vulnerable children and the most vulnerable elderly to compete for scarce public resources. As long as states must respond to problems created by the national system, however, their solutions will inherit its major flaws. Uncoordinated responses by states cannot solve the problems caused by the continuing rapid dissemination of technology, inefficiencies in administering a mixed system, and a growing demand for services in our aging and acquired immunodeficiency syndrome-threatened society.

Oregon offers important lessons for any national effort to address these problems. Nationally, we should embrace Oregon's commitment to provide universal access to basic care and to make rationing a subject of open, political debate, but we should not simply expand the current legislation into a national plan. That would not only reproduce on a larger scale the unjustifiable inequality that the Oregon plan permits. It would also retain at the state level competition for funds between poor children and poor elderly, and it would leave unaddressed the basic problems of inefficiency and rapidly rising costs. In contrast, rationing within a single-payer, public insurance scheme that covered all age groups would more easily address these problems. Whether such a comprehensive scheme is best introduced all at once (on the model of the Canadian system), or is phased in (building on an Oregon-style starting point), is a complex issue. In any case, we have yet to see whether the Oregon plan gives us a clear model for how community values or public participation should influence the design of a national benefit package.

ACKNOWLEDGMENTS

This work was generously supported by grant RH-20917 from the National Endowment for the Humanities and grant 1RO1LM05005 from the National Library of Medicine, Washington, DC.

Helpful information, materials, or comments were provided by Dan Brock, PhD, Arthur Caplan, PhD, Michael Garland, PhD, John Golenski, SJ, Bruce Jennings, PhD, Sen John Kitzhaber, and Paige Sipes-Metzler, DPA.

REFERENCES

1 Golenski J. *A Report on the Oregon Medicaid Priority Setting Project.* Berkeley, Calif: Bioethics Consultation Group; 1990.
2 Senate Bills 27, 534, 935. 65th Oregon Legislative Assembly; 1989 regular sess.
3 Kitzhaber J. *The Oregon Basic Health Services Act.* Salem, Ore: Office of the Senate President; 1990.
4 Blendon RJ, Leitman R, Morrison I, Donelan K.

Satisfaction with health systems in ten nations. *Health Aff.* Summer 1990:185–192.

5 *An Analysis of the Impact of the Oregon Medicaid Reduction Waiver Proposal on Women and Children.* Washington, DC: Children's Defense Fund; 1990:1–7.

6 Daniels N. *Just Health Care.* New York, NY: Cambridge University Press; 1985.

7 Rawls J. *A Theory of Justice.* Cambridge, Mass: Harvard University Press; 1971.

8 *Preliminary Report.* Salem: Oregon Health Services Commission; 1990.

9 Daniels N. *Am I My Parents' Keeper? An Essay on Justice Between the Young and the Old.* New York, NY: Oxford University Press Inc; 1988.

10 Aaron HJ, Schwartz WB. *The Painful Prescription: Rationing Health Care.* Washington, DC: The Brookings Institution; 1984.

11 Temkin L. Inequality. *Philosophy Public Aff.* 1986;15:99–121.

12 Cohen J. Democratic equality. *Ethics.* 1989;99:727–751.

13 Scanlon TM. Contractualism and utilitarianism. In: Sen AK, Williams B, eds. *Utilitarianism and Beyond.* New York, NY: Cambridge University Press; 1982:103–128.

14 Calabresi G, Bobbit P. *Tragic Choices.* New York, NY: WW Norton & Co Inc; 1978.

15 Rawls J. Kantian constructivism in moral theory: the Dewey Lectures. *J Phil.* 1980;77:515–572.

16 Hasnain R, Garland M. *Health Care in Common: Report of the Oregon Health Decisions Community Meetings Process.* Portland: Oregon Health Decisions; 1990.

17 Kitzhaber J. *Summary: The Health Services Prioritization Process.* Salem: Oregon State Senate; 1990.

Ethics and Rationing: "Whether," "How," or "How Much?"
Daniel Wikler

Daniel Wikler is professor of philosophy at the University of Wisconsin, Madison. He served on the staff of the President's Commission for the Study of Ethical Problems in Medicine and Biomedical and Behavioral Research. His articles include "Brain Death: A Durable Consensus?", "What Has Bioethics to Offer Health Policy?", and "Reflections on Research on Mentally Disabled Human Subjects."

    Wikler challenges the emerging consensus that the important question about health-care rationing is not *whether* it should occur but *how* it should be done. To clarify the issues, Wikler distinguishes three grades of rationing: (1) *trimming,* the cutting back of services that nobody needs and few people want; (2) *tailoring,* the cutting back of services that are needed but not wanted or wanted but not needed; and (3) *cutting,* or *hard rationing,* the cutting back of services that are clearly both wanted and needed. After criticizing several efforts to provide a principled framework for cutting, Wikler questions the common assumption that it is necessitated by recent massive increases in medical expenditures. He argues that we need to ask what factors are driving up costs and whether there is some way other than cutting to relieve the cost pressure. He rejects appeals to the aging of the American population and to the cost of new technology as bases for the assumption that we must accept cutting. Wikler concludes that this assumption is unfounded: "[G]iven the right kind of reforms in our health-care system, we could exchange these ethical dilemmas for the more acceptable problems which other countries face."

Reprinted with permission of the author and the publisher from *Journal of the American Geriatrics Society,* vol. 40 (April 1992), pp. 398–403.

It has become a cliche in health policy discussions that Americans no longer have the luxury of debating whether to ration health care; the only question is how this should be done. The "should" in this statement is good news for the ethics industry, the legion of consultants, contractees, scholars, and symposiasts who put "bioethics" on their business cards—for the word "should" has a moral dimension, and to ask how health care should be rationed is tantamount to calling for an ethicist to make a pronouncement. Given the inevitability of rationing, the growing sense that we can no longer resolve allocation dilemmas by spending more, we must pick and choose, which is another way of saying that we must deny. Saying "no" to people in need of health care is not easy, nor should it be easy, and if those who do say "no" are to retain a good image of themselves, they will be looking for assurances that this can be done "ethically."

In this view a sizable, even monumental, task looms ahead, one which will call for the collaborative efforts of ethicists, physicians, economists, and policymakers. We must come to some common understanding of what constitutes responsible, defensible rationing and what must instead be counted as arbitrary, capricious, unfeeling or unjust. If this shared understanding, once reached, turns out to consist of generalities and abstractions, we will then need to find a way to translate these principles into policies that could actually be used in guiding administrators, payers, and clinicians. We would have to develop a principled approach to deciding who the actual rationers should be: whether the choice among needs should be made at the bedside, in the accounting office, or far away in the state or national capital. Finally, we would need to learn how to "sell" these ideas to the American population; few people will be happy about accepting less health care than they think they need, and human nature being what it is, they may feel that when their needs are chosen by the rationers to remain unfulfilled, an injustice has been done. To the extent that the public is aware that their health care is being rationed, their willingness to put up with short rations would be enhanced if the criteria for rationing were comprehensible and consonant with moral common sense.

Here, then, is a challenge, and an opportunity, for clinicians and scientists to work with bioethicists, and economists and policy experts, too, in constructing a new ethics of health care for the leaner, and unfortunately meaner, health care system of the immediate future. It is a challenge which many of these thinkers have taken up. A steady stream of papers and reports, and now even books, throws new ideas into the hopper.

Here and there one can even see hints of an emerging consensus. The intriguing example of the state of Oregon, which is trying to set priorities among health services for some of its Medicaid beneficiaries, has drawn the attention of observers from over 40 states and several foreign countries; more than one conference has gathered experts to debate its implications. All this attention suggests that some influential people believe that Oregon's initiative may be some sort of model in this new era of ethical rationing. It is not at all surprising that one of the architects of the Oregon approach is a consulting bioethicist—a Jesuit priest, in fact.

These ideas are probably familiar to readers of this journal. In what follows, I will try to undermine most of them. Though each of the claims I mentioned builds on a kernel of truth, I will argue that in some key respects the view as a whole is confused and, ultimately, unethical. Thus my own contribution, such as it is, will not add to the growing body of literature which counsels that rationing should be done this way or that way. Instead, I will reflect on the point and function of this literature as a whole.

WHAT "RATIONING" MEANS IN THIS CONTEXT

"Rationing" is a notoriously slippery and threatening word. Politicians dislike it since it means that some who need will not get. "Rationing" means some sort of allocation short of unlimited provision, but the term itself does not specify the basis for this distribution. For example, "rationing" of commodities in wartime may involve distribution by coupon, which is an alternative to the market solution of allowing consumers to bid up the price. In this case, "rationing" means, in part, that everyone who needs some will at least get something. It specifies a minimum.

In the context of today's health care cost crisis, however, "rationing" is a different animal. It means that certain services will not be provided as an entitlement or benefit, regardless of ability to pay out of pocket. In this sense it points toward the market for distribution, not away from it. And those who urge rationing only coincidentally urge new initiatives to remove the patent inequities in distribution of health care resources that mark the American health care system as the least fair of all the industrialized nations. Though the term "rationing" in other contexts refers directly to the effort to choose fairly among claimants, the oft-heard opinion that "Americans must accept the need for rationing of

health care" is not intended to mean that we should prepare ourselves for greater fairness (along with greater
stringency). It means simply that we who now get should
learn to accept less, even when the need might be great.
In a word, "rationing" means, in this context, limitations.
For those who have faced few noticeable limitations in
the past, the more precise word is "cutbacks."

"Doing without" is rarely as threatening a prospect
as when it occurs in health care since so much is put at
risk. What, then, are Americans being asked to give up?
It will help to focus the debate by distinguishing three
grades of rationing. Because the terms in common currency are used in so many different ways, I will adopt
some new words, drawing on sartorial imagery. The
least objectionable form of rationing I will call "Trimming"; the most problematic, "Cutting." In between is
a form of rationing which we might call "Tailoring."
These correspond to what some have called "soft" and
"hard" rationing (though others use these terms to designate levels of explicitness rather than levels of denial),
with an intermediate step ("semisoft rationing"?) added.

Rationing as Trimming is cutting back on services
that few people want and no one needs. To begin, it
calls for greater efficiency in delivery where possible. It
also targets ineffective care as well as medical interventions which cost more than other, equally helpful
approaches. In this category, too, might fall certain
amenities such as pleasantness of surroundings and perhaps some convenience. Trimming is needed primarily
because America's health care system has not been
properly constrained in its spending. It is the fat which
develops from a too-rich financial diet. Though the fat
makes life easier, and difficult choices fewer, it is not
essential for good care and with some discipline can be
excised. Ethical issues are least acute for Trimming.

"Hard" rationing, here tagged Cutting, means
refusing genuinely needed and wanted care on the
grounds that the cost is "too high," ie, that payers are
balking. The most visible form of Cutting is a provider's
decision, based perhaps on a payer's refusal to reim-
burse, not to provide a non-experimental organ transplant to a medically-suited patient. But this example is
arguably not a fully perspicuous one, for if "rationing"
means "cutbacks," we would have to presume that the
patient once had, or ordinarily should have, unques-
tioned access to this procedure. This is often not the
case for organ transplants, some of which still have, or
are said to have, "experimental" status. When Americans are told that they must now get used to rationing,
the message is not only that they can no longer hope for
new entitlements, but also that they must be prepared

to give up some that they have long enjoyed. This message may not be very explicit on this point, but without
it the message makes little sense, given both its premises
and its implications.

What could "Tailoring" mean? Something intermediate, of course, between hard rationing (Cutting)
and soft (Trimming). Its particular meaning comes from
amplifying the key concepts in the two polar terms:
"soft" rationing, in the sense of Trimming, is elimination of elements in health care which are neither wanted
(very much) or needed; "hard" rationing (Cutting)
eliminates care which is both wanted and needed. In the
semi-soft, Tailoring category we might put some medical interventions which are wanted but not needed and
some others which are needed but not wanted. In particular, Tailoring eliminates care which is (1) of questionable effectiveness, even though it may be popular or
even standard, or which has marginal effectiveness relative to risk; or (2) care which prolongs conditions which
are marginally endurable, or about which patients tend
not to desire. Here the clear example is care which
might succeed in keeping a patient alive, but only with a
quality of life so poor that few patients would voluntarily accept it. It might also include some forms of care
given to individuals with severe progressive senile
dementia, in cases where the patient's wishes, expressed
beforehand, would rule out attempts to prolong life in
that condition. And it might include treatment of questionable effectiveness but significant intrusion or side-
effects. To stay within the sartorial mode: Tailoring
takes away some substantial pieces of fabric, but in a
way which still fits the customer.

Trimming, I have said, is relatively painless to
patients, however much it may discomfit those making a
living through the health care system's inefficiencies.
Cutting, once it is visible as such, needs a strenuous
sales job even to be considered. Tailoring, in which real
medical gains may be given up, sometimes goes down
fairly easily, especially if seasoned with some "medical
ethics." The value to invoke here is patient self-determination. John Wennberg, for example, has maintained
that the cost crisis can be resolved without Cutting by
leaning heavily on the innate tendency of patients to
reject burdensome care when the need or benefit for the
care is not fully documentable. Wennberg writes:

"The fear that rationing will be needed is based on
the assumption that current levels of use of expensive
treatment such as by-pass surgery or intensive care
reflect consumer demand and the pace of medical
progress. But we really don't know much about what
patients demand of the health care market, nor are we

clear about how the rates of use reflect medical progress . . . we have not had the opportunity to learn what the level of demand would be if patients were fully informed of their options and if the probabilities of the various outcomes were presented to them comprehensively . . . (C)urrent rates of use of invasive, high-technology medicine could well be higher than patients want . . . (in part because) patients will on average select less invasive strategies than physicians.[1]"

Wennberg, it must be noticed, is not denying that the treatments that would be rejected by fully-informed patients would be medically indicated, in a narrow sense of that term. But when savings are effected by catering to the preferences of informed, competent patients, this is not the kind of Cutting which we are now being told we must endure.

The kind of ethical reflection needed to respond to the prospect of health care rationing, then, varies with the kind of rationing called for. Though there is much debate over the amount of savings which could be achieved through Trimming, the arguments do not turn on any profound differences in values between the various parties—at least not values publicly subscribed to. With Tailoring, there may be real differences of opinion over the prospect of realizing large savings through patients' refusal of care their physicians believe is indicated.

But Cutting points to an entirely different set of ethical dilemmas, those which we associate with the lifeboat. If some must be denied care which is needed and wanted, who should be abandoned first? Ought we give priority to the strong, the productive, the young? Should personal responsibility for illness and injury figure in our deliberations? Once the issue of rationing is defined in hardened terms, the judgment required is Solomon-like: difficult and humbling, but necessary, lest life-determining choices be made by default.

RATIONER'S TOOLKIT

What intellectual resources, what kind of moral insight, do we draw on in answer to the demand for Cutting? Though a number of thoughtful books, by such authors as Daniel Callahan[2] and Paul Menzel,[3] have begun to provide some answers, I remain pessimistic that we can achieve the goal of setting out a principled, comprehensible rationale for justifying health care cutbacks.

I will not try to sketch the wide range of approaches to rational rationing, which is too broad a task, but I would like to make a few general remarks. The new call for Americans to accept Cutting is combined with an earnest attempt to figure out how to ration "ethically": that is, to cut back services in a way which is ethically defensible. I believe that this attempt promises more than can be delivered. I will make my argument in very general terms.

We might suppose that the first question to ask in deciding how to ration ethically is the basis on which we will decide the priority of each medical service or intervention. But this is not necessarily so. We could avoid having to decide on these criteria by leaving the choice up to the individual. If we can make these rankings a personal decision, we—and "we" can mean the society, the employer/payer, or the health policy experts—can avoid having to come up with defensible rankings.

Unfortunately, having insureds tailor their coverage to their tastes cannot be a satisfactory solution. They lack information, and their choices would unfairly reflect differences in income and wealth. Permitting insureds to pick and choose in this way would, moreover, invite adverse selection, which would undermine the insurance aspect and thus defeat the purpose of the scheme. Nor can we correct for these deficiencies by making the choice a hypothetical one—by a well-informed, average-income mythical chooser deciding on medical benefits over a lifetime—for this hypothetical choice does not represent the decision of any actual person. The hypothetical chooser approach has shown its value in pondering health-care priorities in the work of Daniels, Menzel, and others, but it should not be understood as a vehicle for individualizing the rationing decision.

Second, we could take a cue from Calabresi and Bobbit, in their celebrated essay *Tragic Choices*,[4] and avoid stating criteria not by individualizing the choice but by hiding it. The simplest way to do this is to impose a budget cut on clinicians. As with individualizing, this approach avoids the need for explicit rankings of services or patients. There is, in my view, something to be said for this approach, which is, in any case, unavoidable at some level, but we should not imagine that by hiding the rationing criteria we avoid using them. Rather, this approach substitutes recurring, on-the-fly rationing for the explicit, public, stable criteria. The choices are there, even if less visible, and we still need to decide on what basis they should be made.

If neither of these approaches solves the problem, we need explicit criteria. Indeed, one of the advertised advantages of the Oregon plan is that the basis for its rationing choices is up front, available for all to see and criticize. This is thought to conform to the so-called "publicity" requirement of some moral theorists who pose, as a test of one's moral code, that one is willing to present it to others and to defend it.

I will not dispute on this occasion that going public with rationing criteria is an ethical advantage. But this point alone does not make these criteria defensible; it depends on what basis they are drawn up. I would like to briefly sketch and challenge two alleged solutions of this problem.

The first is to earmark a certain set of medical services as "basic," the remainder being somehow "optional" or, to use a philosopher's term, supererogatory. This approach is a perennial contender, but is notoriously slippery. Using expert judgment yields little consensus beyond agreement that some appearance-enhancing plastic surgery is non-basic. Daniels, following on the theory he advanced in his influential book *Just Health Care*,[5] would protect those services which preserve equal opportunity; but few have followed his lead, and the actual import of the theory is yet unclear. The idea behind a definition of "basic" care is that this concept marks an important divide between that which cannot be rationed (the basic services) and that which can be omitted without injustice. Unless the criterion which is used to draw this line is in turn based on some nonarbitrary consideration, however, the threshold marks no such ethical divide.

The Oregon approach, as I understand it, takes a different approach to defending rationing as ethical. The threshold determining whether its Medicaid beneficiaries would get a given service moves up and down the list of priorities depending on how flush the state budget is at a given time. The Oregonians claim that their list of priorities incorporates Oregonian "values" as gleaned in public meetings held throughout the state. But the Oregon experience shows what problems can arise with this strategy. The people who attended the sessions were not the people who would be affected by the harder rationing. Few were Medicaid recipients; indeed, most were health care providers.

Moreover, it is not clear what the Oregon people meant by a "value."[6] The word means many different things, and the lists produced by these citizens' meetings are exceedingly heterogeneous. Nor did they provide any reasoned scheme for giving weight to all these apples and oranges or for incorporating them into the cost-benefit measures upon which the computer-aided list of priorities was to be based. Finally, even that list has now been rearranged by common agreement to remove apparent absurdities and incongruities, again, undercutting the claim that the priorities somehow reflect some coherent set of values of the people of the state.

The resulting list of priorities, then, has no halo over it. It may or may not match your intuitions or mine, but nothing in the process by which it was drawn up makes the proposed cutbacks inherently "ethical." Each needed service denied in hard rationing schemes presents a moral problem. The problem is not erased by simply applying the label "non-basic" or by insisting that the cutback was in keeping with the people's values.

HOW MUCH RATIONING?

While I have been argumentative, I don't think that my thesis is really controversial. I am arguing for the common-sense view that Cutting in health care is a nasty business and needs a powerful justification even when it is done well. This thesis implies another: that the important question is not only (or even primarily) how the rationing is done but how much of it needs to be done. If, to quote Robert Evans,[6] the case for Cutting trades on "illusions of necessity," there are many steps we can and should take instead of Cutting, and no manner in which the hard rationing could be carried out would be ethical.

To press this point, I want briefly to examine the case put forward by those calling on Americans to accept cutbacks in medical care. I believe that their argument is misguided. It may be well intentioned; those who press this line of reasoning almost always call for the diversion of medical funds to such pressing social needs as homelessness and education. Its backers would not call for throwing the sick off the lifeboat were it not for their belief that the lifeboat as a whole is in danger of sinking.

Nevertheless, acceptance of this view could, I think, lead to barriers to the care of many very sick and needy people. Though many of its premises are undoubtedly correct, it proceeds from them in a series of non sequiturs, unfortunately giving its conclusions the undeserved weight of its premises. In countering the moral argument for acceptance of rationing, we can refuse to enter into the selection process for throwing the helpless off the lifeboat; indeed, we can take the occasion for pondering the latent function of that kind of debate.

"Chicken Little" and the Rationing Metaphysicians

It would not be possible here to list every reason which has been given for the alleged need to accept Cutting, but this would be unnecessary in formulating a critique since the familiar arguments fall into a fairly consistent pattern. The advocate of Cutting cites data on a contemporary trend which clearly would tend to push health care costs up; it is asserted, again with justification, that this trend is inexorable and may even be increasing. And from this it is concluded that costs will be pushed past the breaking point, or at least to the point at which further spending on health care could come only at the expense of other urgent social needs such as housing for the homeless. The lesson is that in view of the nation's need to remain economically competitive, or to see to its non-medical urgent needs, we must swallow the bitter pill of Cutting and revise our conventional thinking about the moral imperative to use all the medical means we have developed to save the sick.

What is wrong with this kind of argument, in most of its manifestations, is that the relation of cause to effect tends toward the metaphysical. Not that the trends are non-existent or that they do not progress in the way they are said to do, but they are long-term, general trends and do not explain why we need rationing here and now. In particular, advocates of the acceptance of Cutting fail to show that the long-term trend explains why health care costs have taken such a big jump in recent years in the United States; and since this is the fact which is supposed to make health insurance imperative, it is the argument that must be proven.

Before turning to a review of a few of these factors, I must hedge my claim. It is pointless to deny that these factors push health care prices up. But this is not the key question, from the moral point of view, when we deliberate whether to push Americans to accept Cutting. The crucial questions, rather, are (1) what factors are pushing costs up to unacceptable levels, and (2) whether this cost pressure could not be relieved by some means which are morally preferable to Cutting. Each variant of the "metaphysical" argument for Cutting errs on one or both of these grounds.

Graying of America For example, much has been made of the increasing average age of Americans, a trend which will continue for at least the next 35 years. Old people consume much more health care than younger people, and the fastest-growing age group is the very oldest. Moreover, this increased burden of health care costs will be placed on the shoulders of fewer wage-earners as the passing wave of the postwar baby boom carries the population bulge past the age of retirement.

For some, it stands to reason that expectations must be trimmed; we would otherwise have to meet a much greater need with fewer resources. This straightforward mismatching of inputs and outputs can be averted only by a shift in attitudes whereby we learn to accept the fact that we cannot live forever and look forward to the kinds of activities which are compatible with reduced activity.[7] We must, in this view, recognize the need to allocate health care resources over the life span to maximize the goods it can bring; the present emphasis on health care spending during old age may be the result of the political clout of older voters, but it does not represent any rational allocation plan.

That the American population is getting older is undeniable; the demographic bulge of the baby boom has entered middle age and will become geriatric in less than 2 decades. Nevertheless, this fact does not support the claim it is advanced to support, which is that Cutting must be accepted now. After all, the boomers are not old yet. At the moment, those in the baby boom generation are producers, and the pyramid of production and beneficiaries tapers as it is supposed to. The graying of America is equally irrelevant to the double-digit annual inflation in health care costs that spawned the perceived crisis at the end of the 80's.

Even in respect to the future, the import of the demographic bad news is questionable. For at its peak, around the end of the first quarter of the next century, the percentage of older citizens in this country will not be much higher than it is today in such nations as Austria,[8] and Austria provides health care for all its citizens at a much lower cost: 8% of GNP in 1986 versus 11.1% in the U.S.

This comparison does not demonstrate that caring for an older population of Americans through the health care system as currently constituted would not break the bank; perhaps it would. It does, however, demonstrate that it is perfectly possible for countries of comparable wealth to provide care to a grayed population at reasonable cost. When we recall that aging has nothing to do with the current crisis, the pattern of a "metaphysical" argument is clear.

Cost of New Technology Just as common is the claim that Cutting must be accepted due to the continuing development of costly new technology. Indeed, when put persuasively, this argument almost seems self-evident. Technological advances, ranging from organ transplantation to intensive care, have certainly cost billions. New technologies just coming into use, or clearly in the pipeline, will cost billions more[9] if they are to be used for all who will benefit significantly. And Americans seem to believe that all new advances should be made generally available, not just used for millionaires.[10] This cannot continue indefinitely. As Allan Gibbard[11] has remarked, our sense of what we owe our fellow-citizens (and hence what is owed to us) must take costs into account. In an earlier, pre-industrial era, the limiting factor was the lack of wealth generally. In today's high-technology medicine, the problem could be the high cost of responding to needs. Perhaps the notion of an unlimited entitlement to all effective care was most appropriate during the interim, a period of abundance with few hugely expensive medical technologies available.

Again, the fault with this kind of argument is not that the premises are generally untrue; new technology, while bringing health benefits, usually does increase costs. And indiscriminate use of these technologies could bankrupt any health care system. But these general truths do not themselves imply that this nation's uniquely high health care costs are due to the appropriate use of this technology, nor that the prospect of further advances requires acceptance of broad-scale Cutting. If there were such a direct link between technological advancement and health care inflation, other countries with comparable health care would have experienced this inflation through the past decade.

Contrary to a widespread misimpression, however, this has not been the case. For example, in the period 1980–1986, when US health care costs increased from 9.2% to 11.1% of gross domestic product (GDP), Austria's GDP share increased only from 7.9% to 8%; Denmark's share declined from 6.8% to 6.1%, while West Germany's increased from 7.9% to 8.1%, and the Netherlands rose from 8.2% to 8.3%. Sweden's system, one of the most expensive, declined from 9.5% of GDP to 9.1%. To be sure, these comparative figures are questionable; other countries may have had higher overall growth rates, and whole sectors of health care, such as nursing homes, may be included in one country's figure and excluded in another. Still, the gap between the experience of the United States and that of the other countries—both in absolute numbers and in the direction of trends—is enormous and is unlikely to be erased by superior accounting.

While the United States is a world leader in new medical technology, the figures cited refer to countries whose health care systems are generally regarded as America's equal in overall quality. The "metaphysical" argument that blames America's crisis in health care delivery on technological advances requires us to assume that citizens of other nations are denied the benefits of these technologies.

The evidence cited in favor of these claims, however, is often misconstrued. Aaron and Schwartz's important book, *The Painful Prescription*,[12] is a case in point. Their study of allocation of resources in Britain's National Health Service documented Cutting practices, including refusal of treatment for end-stage renal disease in older patients. But their findings do not show that to keep costs down, as the British do, we must deny such care. For the British spend only a third as much as we do, per patient, per year, while providing universal access to the (generally adequate) services they do provide. If the British were willing to spend at our levels, which would entail tripling the budget of the NHS, would they have to engage in Cutting? Aaron and Schwartz, in any case, studied the most parsimonious health care system in Europe; other European countries provide much easier access to treatment for renal disease[13] and still spend less than we do.

That the new technology drives prices to unacceptable levels in the American context may say as much about the American way of delivering health as it does about the affordability of the technology. It is no advertisement for the American system that it has many more MRI scanners than Canada has if the American machines are underutilized or inappropriately utilized—a Canadian MRI scanner, for example, may be used around the clock, while the American machine is scheduled from 9 to 5.

Moreover, not all the excess in expensive care is better for patients. A case in point is coronary bypass surgery, for which waiting lines exist in Canada but not the United States. Alain Enthoven has remarked on the many hundreds of excess deaths in California due to CABG surgery done at low-volume (and hence high-risk) centers or due to inappropriate care. Have the number of excess deaths in Canada due to the waiting lists been greater?[14] The British National Health Service is less likely to treat solid tumors which Americans treat aggressively but with uneven success, while treatable cancers receive the same care in both countries.

The claim that the gradual development of new, sometimes expensive medical technology forces us to contemplate draconian Cutting, then, overlooks some important links between technological development and high health costs. The nature of the health care delivery system has an important bearing on whether the new technologies are appropriately or indiscriminately used, whether there is expensive, needless duplication, and what kinds of charges the use of the technologies will generate. International comparisons suggest that in a more efficient system, one has a choice between spending much less, with restricted access, or else spending at American levels, presumably with free access. Only in America must we accept both of the poorer alternatives.

What if good evidence turned up showing that other health care systems have avoided US-style inflation only through the sort of Cutting now being urged upon us? Such data would not, in themselves, vindicate those insisting that we accept cutbacks. To avoid comparing apples and oranges, it would need to be shown that the other systems could not have avoided these limitations even by increasing national outlays to the uniquely high American levels and even by leaving one out of seven citizens uninsured. Once again, I do not deny that new, expensive technology could someday require draconian Cutting. Just as with aging, the trend is theoretically capable of bringing about this result. My argument, instead, is that those who emulate Chicken Little in the present health care crisis are jumping from the theoretical possibility to the present-day actuality: metaphysics made into policy.

"ETHICS" AND THE RATIONING DEBATE

One loses some debates simply by joining them. As it is currently developing, the debate over the "ethics" of rationing begins in medias res: it assumes that the central question is who should be dealt out of the game, this patient in need of a transplant or that patient in need of perinatal care. By arguing in favor of one or the other, the two permitted sides of the argument, one implicitly endorses the assumption that we have to make the choice. If "ethicists" are keeping themselves occupied in debating the principles for selecting and deselecting patients, they may, in some cases unintentionally, convey the misimpression that the focus of our moral concern ought to be on whom to exclude. Though they will differ on their answers, they will each argue in favor of excluding somebody, which provides this sort of "solution" to the health care cost crisis with an undeserved ethical imprimatur.

The effort of the state of Oregon illustrates these points well. Given Oregon's need to balance its state budget, and its inability to singlehandedly reform the nation's health care delivery system, the motives and intentions of the officials proposing its rationing plan need not be impugned on moral grounds. But Oregon's program must be seen not as an exemplar in a national policy of rationing health care but for what it is: an attempt to extend the basics of care to the underserved by cutting back on the benefits to the next worse-off class, all the while preserving the inefficiencies and inequities of the world's most expensive health care system. The ethical niceties of ranking one health care service over another in the reduced package to be offered the poor lack the gravity of the larger ethical issues at stake. Whatever merit Oregon's approach may have as a solution to certain problems of state government does not extend to the currently popular idea of rationing—read cutbacks—as a national health care policy. The unusually prominent role which the Oregon government has given to "ethics" may unfortunately obscure the more significant issues of ethical concern in the national health care debate.

A growing number of health policy observers, as well as government officials, are endorsing the call for rationing. With the sense of breaking a great taboo, they ask us to accept a world of limits, both physiological and financial, and to cease reacting with moral indignation at the idea of a life deliberately not saved or a handicap intentionally not remedied. Their arguments, moreover, use the terminology of medical ethics. Whether voluntarily and wittingly or not, however, they are participating in an exercise which serves a particular ideological function. They play this role no matter how well they perform the assigned task of choosing between patients. Though the cutbacks may be explicit, and in theory more democratic, the public is being prepared to accept responsibility for choices it should not have to make. Correcting the existing flaws in the Oregon rationing procedures would not address this problem.

Well past the half-trillion dollar-per-year mark, there is no point in disputing that America's health care costs are a serious issue. The perpetually high inflation rate, resistant to all tinkering, has engendered a sense of crisis. I have argued that the pro-rationing view is not, as it is sometimes presented, a mature acceptance of the necessity of choice. International comparisons suggest that the choices that are so unwelcome are not necessary ones; given the right kind of reforms in our health care system, we could exchange these ethical dilemmas for the more acceptable problems which other countries face. If the rationing debate is, at bottom, a contest between the unjustly underserved and those who benefit from the present system's inefficiencies and inequities, ethicists ought not be on the wrong side.

REFERENCES

1 Wennberg JE. Outcomes research, cost containment, and the fear of health care rationing. N Engl J Med 1990;323:17.

2 Callahan D. What Kind of Life? New York: Simon and Schuster, 1990.

3 Menzel P. Strong Medicine. Oxford: Oxford University Press, 1990.

4 Calabresi G, Bobbit P. Tragic Choices. New York: W.W. Norton Company, 1978.

5 Daniels N. Just Health Care. Cambridge: Cambridge University Press, 1983.

6 Evans RG. Illusion of necessity: Evading responsibility for choice in health care. J Health Polit Policy Law 1985;10(3):439–468.

7 Callahan D. Setting Limits. New York: Simon and Schuster, 1987.

8 Myles JF. Conflict, Crisis, and the future of old age security. Milbank Q 1983;61(3):462–472.

9 Aaron H, Schwartz W. Rationing health care: The choice before us. Science 1990;247:418–422.

10 Thurow L. Medicine versus economics. N Engl J Med 1985;313:611–614.

11 Gibbard A. The prospective Pareto principle and its application to questions of equity of access to health care. Milbank Q 1982;60(3):399–428.

12 Aaron H, Schwartz W. The Painful Prescription. Washington: The Brookings Institution, 1984.

13 Halper T. The Suffering of Others. Cambridge: Cambridge University Press, 1989.

14 Enthoven A et al. What can Europeans Learn from the Americans? Health Care Finan Rev 1989; Annual Supplement: 49–63.

Health-Care-Delivery Systems

Universal Health Insurance through Incentives Reform

Alain C. Enthoven and Richard Kronick

Alain C. Enthoven is professor of health economics at the graduate school of business, Stanford University. Widely published in health-care economics, he is the author of "The History and Principles of Managed Competition," *Health Plan: The Only Practical Solution to the Soaring Cost of Medical Care* (1980), and *Theory and Practice of Managed Competition* (1988). Richard Kronick, who served as senior health-policy advisor in the Clinton administration, is assistant professor of family and preventive medicine, University of California, San Diego. His articles include "The Demographic Limits of Managed Competition," "Health Insurance 1979–1989: The Frayed Connection between Employment and Insurance," and "Where Should the Buck Stop?: Federal and State Responsibilities in Health Care Financing Reform."

Enthoven and Kronick defend a proposal designed to achieve universal health insurance while controlling costs by reforming the financial incentives that drive the American health-care-delivery system. The related problems of lack of access to health care and skyrocketing costs, in their view, stem from such factors as cost-unconscious demand for services in our fee-for-service system, a medical culture that favors high-technology services, market distortions, and the distribution of public funds in a way that discourages widespread coverage. The authors propose a system of policies and institutions designed to give everyone access to a choice of efficient *managed care* options (e.g., as provided by health maintenance organizations). The system would involve *managed competition*—among private-sector health-care plans—executed by large employers and the Public Sponsor in each state. Under the authors' proposal, most workers would have coverage subsidized by their employers, while others would be offered subsidized coverage by their states' Public Sponsors. Enthoven and Kronick base their contention that their proposal is workable on two claims: (1) efficient managed care already exists; and (2) people "choose value for money."

THE PARADOX OF EXCESS AND DEPRIVATION

American national health expenditures are now about 13% of the gross national product, up from 9.1% in 1980, and they are projected to reach 15% by 2000, far more than in any other country.[1-8] These expenditures are straining public finances at all levels of government. At the same time, roughly 35 million Americans have no health care coverage at all, public or private, and the number appears to be rising.[4-7] Millions more have inadequate insurance that leaves them vulnerable to large expenses, that excludes care of preexisting conditions, or that may be lost if they become seriously ill. The American health care financing and delivery system is becoming increasingly unsatisfactory and cannot be sustained. Comprehensive reform is urgently needed.

DIAGNOSIS

The etiology of this worsening paradox is extremely complex; many factors enter in. Some factors we would not change if we could (eg, advancing medical technology, people living longer). We emphasize factors that are important and correctable.

First, our health care financing and delivery system contains more incentives to spend than to not spend. It is based on *cost-unconscious demand*. Key decision makers have little or no incentive to seek value for money in health care purchases. The dominant open-ended fee-for-service (FFS) system pays providers more for doing more, whether or not more is appropriate. ("Open ended" means that no budget is set in advance within which the job must be done.) Once insured, consumers are not cost conscious. Deductibles and coinsurance at the point of service have little or no effect on most spending, which is on sick people who have exceeded their out-of-pocket spending limits. "Free choice of provider insurance" blocks cost consciousness on the demand side by depriving the insurer of bargaining power. This approach is rapidly yielding in the market-place to preferred provider insurance. In its present forms, preferred provider insurance helps to regulate price but is not yet very effective in controlling the volume of services. Medicare, Medicaid, and the subsidies to employer-provided health care coverage built into the income and payroll tax laws are all open-ended and encourage decisions in favor of more costly care. These incentives are reinforced by a medical culture that esteems use of the most advanced technology, high patient expectations, and the threat of malpractice litigation if these expectations are not met.

Contrary to a widespread impression, America has not yet tried *competition* of alternative health care financing and delivery plans, using the term in the normal economic sense, ie, *price* competition to serve cost-conscious purchasers. When there is price competition, the purchaser who chooses the more expensive product pays the full difference in price and is thus motivated to seek value for money. However, in offering health care coverage to employees, most employers provide a larger subsidy to the FFS system than to health maintenance organizations (HMOs), thereby destroying the incentive for consumers and providers to choose the economical alternative. Many employers offer no choice but FFS coverage.[8,9] Others offer choices but pay the whole premium, whichever choice the employee makes. In such a case, the HMO has no incentive to hold down its premium; it is better off to charge more and use the money to improve service. In many other cases, employers offer a choice of plan, but the employer pays 80% or 90% of the premium or all but some fixed amount, whichever plan the employee chooses. In all these cases, the effect is that the employer pays more on behalf of the more costly system and deprives the efficient alternatives of the opportunity to attract more customers by cutting cost and price.

The rational policy from an economic point of view would be for employers to structure health plan offerings to employees so that those who choose the less costly plans get to keep the full savings. Several factors discourage them from doing this. Employers became committed to paying the price of the FFS plan in the 1960s and 1970s, when costs were much lower and

HMOs were few. Now this commitment is hard to break. When an employment group considers more costly and less costly health plans, it knows that government will pay about one third of the extra cost of the more costly plan through tax remission. Labor unions see management commitment to full payment of costs of the open-ended system as a precious bargaining prize. There is a need for collective action. If one employer attempts to convert to cost-conscious employee choice while other employers remain with the employer-pay-all system, the employer will get disgruntled employees in the short run but no reformed, cost-effective health care system in the long run. For the latter to happen, most employers in a geographic area must convert to cost-conscious choice.

The second major problem is that our present health care financing and delivery system is not organized for quality and economy. One of the main drives in the present system is for each specialist to exercise his or her specialty, not to produce desired outcomes at reasonable cost. In a system designed for quality and economy, managed care organizations would attract the responsible participation of physicians who would understand that, ultimately, their patients bear the costs of care, and they would accept the need for an economical practice style. Data would be gathered on outcomes, treatments, and resource use, and providers would base clinical decisions on such data. We have few outcome data today. The FFS system often pays more to poor performers who have high rates of complications than to good performers who solve patients' medical problems quickly and economically. High-quality performers are not rewarded, because of the payment system and because employers and consumers do not have the data to identify them.

There are too many beds and too many specialists in relation to the number of primary care physicians. A high-quality cost-effective system would carefully match the numbers and types of physicians retained and other resources to the needs of the population served so that each specialist and subspecialist would be busy seeing just the type of patient she or he was trained to treat. We have a proliferation of costly specialized services that are underutilized. For example, in 1986, more than one third of the hospitals in California doing open-heart surgery performed fewer than 150 operations, the minimum annual volume recommended by the American College of Surgeons (*Los Angeles Times.* December 27, 1988:3).

The third major problem area is "market failure." The market for health insurance does not naturally pro-

duce results that are fair or efficient. It is plagued by problems of biased risk selection, market segmentation, inadequate information, "free riders," and the like.[10] Insurers profit most by avoiding coverage of those who need it most. The insurance market for small employment groups is breaking down as small employers find insurance unavailable or unaffordable, especially if a group member has a costly medical condition. Most employment groups are too small for risk spreading or economical purchase of health insurance. Systematic action by large collective purchasers is needed to manage competition to reward providers of high-quality economical care and to make affordable coverage available to individuals and small groups.

Fourth, public funds are not distributed equitably or effectively to motivate widespread coverage. The unlimited exclusion of employer health benefit contributions from the taxable incomes of employees is the second-largest federal government health care "expenditure," trailing only expenditures for the Medicare program. While providing incentives for the well-covered well-to-do to choose even more generous coverage, this provision does little or nothing for those (mainly lower-income) people without employer-provided coverage. Most of the $46 billion the federal budget lost to this tax break in 1990 went to households with above-average incomes, many of whom would have bought at least catastrophic expense protection without the tax subsidy, while little went to households with below-average incomes, people whose decisions to insure could be substantially affected by such subsidies. The system works backwards: the most powerful incentives to insure go to those in the highest income tax brackets. From a tax effectiveness point of view, it should be the reverse. Government-provided subsidies should give everyone strong incentives to purchase coverage and to choose economically.

In brief, powerful *incentives* that shape behavior in the health care system and that influence the distribution of services point the system in the wrong direction: services too costly for those who are covered, and the exclusion of millions from any coverage at all.

OUR PROPOSAL

We propose a set of public policies and institutions designed to give everyone access to a subsidized but responsible choice of efficient, managed care (HMO, preferred provider insurance plans, etc).[11,12] We propose *comprehensive reform of the economic incentives* that drive the system. We propose cost-conscious informed consumer and employer (or other sponsor) choice of managed care so that plans competing to serve such purchasers will have strong incentives to give value for money. We also propose a strategy of *managed competition* to be executed by large employers and public sponsors (explained below), designed to reward with more subscribers those health care financing and delivery plans that offer high-quality care at relatively low cost. The goal of these policies would be the gradual transformation of the health care financing and delivery system, through voluntary private action, into an array of managed care plans, each competing to attract providers and subscribers by finding ways to improve the quality of care and service while cutting costs. We propose restructuring the tax subsidies to create incentives to cover the uninsured and to encourage the insured to be cost conscious in their choice of plan. We propose the creation of public institutions to broker and market subsidized coverage for all who do not obtain it through large employers. We favor substantial public investments in outcomes and effectiveness research to improve the information base for medical practice and consumer/employer choice.

Public Sponsor Agencies

The Public Sponsor, a quasi-public agency (like the Federal Reserve) in each state, would contract with a number of private-sector health care financing and delivery plans typical of those offered to the employed population and would offer subsidized enrollment to all those who do not have employment-based coverage. Except in the case of the poor, the Public Sponsor would contribute a fixed amount equal to 80% of the cost of the average plan that just meets federal standards. The enrollee would pay the rest. (The 80% level was chosen to balance two incentives. First, we wanted the subsidy level to be low enough so that there would be room for efficient plans to compete by lowering prices and taking subscribers away from inefficient plans. Second, we wanted the subsidy to be high enough so that the purchase of health insurance would appear very attractive even to those who expect to have no medical expenses.) To the enrollee, the Public Sponsor would look like the employee benefits office.

In the case of the poor, we propose additional subsidies. People at or below the poverty line would be able to choose any health plan with a premium at or below the average and have it fully paid. For people with

incomes between 100% and 150% of the poverty line, we propose public sharing of the premium contribution on a sliding scale related to income.

Public Sponsors would also act as collective purchasing agents for small employers who wished to take advantage of economies of scale and of the ability of Public Sponsors to spread and manage risk. Small employers could obtain coverage for their groups by payment of a maximum of 8% of their payroll.

Today, a substantial part of the money required to pay for care of the uninsured comes from more or less broadly based state and local sources, including employers' payments to private hospitals for bad debt or free care and direct appropriations from state and local governments to acute-care hospitals. In our proposal, federal funds (the sources of which are described below) would be the main source of support for the Public Sponsors. These funds would be supplemented by funds from state and local sources.

Mandated Employer-Provided Health Insurance

For better or worse, we have an employment-based system of health insurance for most people under age 65 years. It can be modified gradually but not replaced overnight. Most employers and employees agree that health care will be included in the compensation package. This is responsible behavior; if one of the group gets sick, the group pays the cost. Some employers and employees do not include health care in the package. The effect is irresponsible behavior; if an employee becomes seriously ill, these employers and employees count on someone else to pay. They are taking a "free ride." It is hard to justify raising taxes on the insured to pay for coverage for the employed uninsured unless those uninsured are required to contribute their fair share.

The existence of Public Sponsors would give all employers access to large-scale efficient health care coverage arrangements. However, in the absence of corrective action, the availability of subsidized coverage for uninsured individuals would create an incentive for employers to drop coverage of their employees. This would create additional expense for the Public Sponsor without compensating revenue. To prevent this, our proposal requires employers to cover their full-time employees (employers would make a defined contribution equal to 80% of the cost of an average plan meeting federal standards and would offer a choice of health plans meeting federal standards).

Premium Contributions from All Employers and Employees

Many people who are self-employed, who have part-time or seasonal work, or who are retired and under age 65 years do not have enough attachment to one employer to justify requiring the employer to provide coverage. Thus, an employer mandate for full-time employees would leave out millions of people. Moreover, in the absence of corrective action, a requirement that employers cover full-time employees creates a powerful incentive to use part-time employees.

We propose that employers be required to pay an 8% payroll tax on the first $22,500 of the wages and salaries of part-time and seasonal employees, unless the employer covered the employee with a health insurance plan meeting federal standards. Self-employed persons, early retirees, and everyone else not covered through employment would be required to contribute through the income tax system. An 8% tax would apply to adjusted gross income up to an income ceiling related to the size of the household. The ceiling would be calculated to ensure that households with sufficient income paid for approximately the total subsidy that would be made available to them through the Public Sponsor.

The proceeds of these taxes would be paid by the federal government to the states, on a per-person-covered basis, for use by Public Sponsors in offering subsidized coverage to persons without employment-based coverage.

This tax would be at the federal level because individual states might be deterred from levying such a tax by employer threats to move to a state without the tax.

Limit on Tax-Free Employer Contributions

We propose that Congress change the income and payroll tax laws to limit the tax-free employer contribution to 80% of the average price of a comprehensive plan meeting federal standards. The average price of a qualified health plan in 1991 might be roughly $290 per family per month. As a condition of tax exemption, employer health plans would be required to use fixed-dollar defined contributions, independent of employee choice of plan, not to exceed the limit, so that people who choose more costly health care plans must do so with their *own* money, not with that of the taxpayer or employer.

The purposes of this measure are twofold. First, it would save the federal budget some $11.2 billion in 1988 dollars. This money could be used to help finance subsidies for the uninsured comparable to those received by the employed insured. Second, making people cost conscious would help enlist all employed Americans in a search for value for money in health care, would stimulate the development of cost-effective care, and would create a market for cost-effective managed care. Thus, this tax reform is defensible on grounds of both equity and efficiency.

Budget Neutrality

The Congressional Budget Office has estimated the effects of our proposal on coverage, costs, and the federal budget and has found that our proposed new revenues would equal the added outlays.[13] We have not done a state-by-state analysis, but, in the aggregate, required state and local contributions appear to approximately equal outlays for care of the uninsured.

Managed Competition

The market for health insurance does not naturally produce results that are fair or efficient. It is plagued by problems of biased risk selection, market segmentation, inadequate information, etc. In fact, the market for health insurance cannot work at the individual level. To counteract these problems, large employers and Public Sponsors must structure and manage the demand side of this market.[10] They must act as intelligent, active, collective purchasing agents and manage a process of informed cost-conscious consumer choice of "managed care" plans to reward providers of high-quality economical care. Tools of effectively managed competition include the annual open-enrollment process; full employee consciousness of premium differences; a standardized benefit package within each sponsored group; risk-adjusted sponsor contributions, so that a plan that attracts predictably sicker people is compensated; monitoring disenrollments; surveillance; ongoing quality measurement; and improved consumer information.

Outcomes Management and Effectiveness Research

As Ellwood[14] and Roper et al[15] have pointed out, there is a poverty of relevant data linking outcomes, treatments, and resource use. Although such data are costly to gather, they constitute a public good, and their production ought to be publicly mandated and supported. Combined with the incentives built into our proposal, such data could be of great value to providers and patients seeking more effective and less costly treatments. Without incentives for efficiency, such data are likely to have little impact on health care costs.

Mutually Supportive Components

Some components of our proposal have been proposed individually. However, they would be much more effective as parts of an integrated, comprehensive reform program than they would be alone. Consider, for example, a law that employers must cover their full-time employees. Alone, this law would leave out people who are not employed on a full-time basis and their dependents—12 million people. Without a payroll tax on uninsured employees, employers would have a strong incentive to escape the mandate by using part-time employees. Without Public Sponsors, the law would not address the problem of availability of affordable coverage for small employers. Without the limit on tax-free employer contributions, the law would not address the need for a cost-containment strategy.

We recognize the propensity of the American political system to seek minimal, incremental change. Some components of our proposal would be viable and helpful on their own. However, we believe that effective solution of the problems of access and cost requires a comprehensive strategy, and the merits of the combined package exceed the merits of the individual components.

WILL IT WORK?

Our confidence that a reasonably well-managed comprehensive reform plan along these lines can be made to work rests on two propositions.

First, efficiently managed care does exist. It is possible to improve economic performance substantially over the nonselective FFS, solo practice, third-party intermediary model. The best documented example was a randomized comparison of per capita resource use between Group Health Cooperative of Puget Sound and traditional third-party insurance and FFS providers in Seattle, Wash, in the Health Insurance Experiment of the RAND Corp.[16] Group Health Cooperative of Puget Sound cared for its assigned patients at a cost

about 28% lower than that in the FFS sector, resulting in essentially equal health outcomes and overall patient satisfaction about 95% as high. Satisfaction with interpersonal aspects of care and technical quality was 98% as high as in the FFS sector.[17,18] Group Health Cooperative of Puget Sound accomplished this without much cost-conscious demand and without any significant competing organized system. One wonders how much better they might have done if there had been several such organizations competing to serve cost-conscious consumers. Other nonrandomized studies have produced similar results.[19]

Many physicians and patients may prefer practice styles other than prepaid group practice. We do not have similar experimental evidence on the economic performance of independent practice associations and preferred provider insurance plans. However, we have observed wide variation in the performance of providers. For example, in Los Angeles, Calif, in 1986, one hospital performed 44 coronary artery bypass grafts with an 11.4% death rate and median charges of $59,000, while another hospital performed 770 coronary artery bypass grafts with a 3.8% death rate and median charges of $16,000 (*Los Angeles Times.* July 24, 1988:3). Some managed care plans would find ways of selecting economical providers of high quality and would channel business to them, improving quality and cutting costs substantially.

Second, people do choose value for money. Our limited experience with even attenuated price competition in employment groups such as federal employees, California state employees, and Stanford University suggests that, over time, people do migrate to cost-effective systems. A recent study of health plan choice in the Twin Cities, Minnesota, area found that employees' decisions are quite sensitive to health plan prices.[20,21] This accords with generally accepted principles of economic behavior.

We have been asked, "Why, if nonprofit HMOs are so much more efficient and desirable, have they failed to grow except very modestly?" In times past, legal and professional barriers were important, including illegal restraints of trade.[22] In recent years, the main inhibitor of the growth of HMOs has been the employer contribution policies we have discussed; that is, most employers do not structure their health plan offerings in such a way that the employee who chooses the most economical plan gets to keep the savings. Nevertheless, some nonprofit HMOs have been growing rapidly; through the 1980s, Harvard Community Health Plan averaged membership growth of more than 11% per year, and the

Kaiser-Permanente Medical Care Program averaged 5.2% growth on a much larger base. However, the success of our proposal does not depend only on nonprofit HMOs. Other forms of cost-effective managed care may do the job. What we propose is a restructured market system in which the efficient prosper and the inefficient must improve or fail.

COMPREHENSIVE REFORM THAT RELIES ON INCENTIVES IS PREFERABLE TO DIRECT GOVERNMENT CONTROLS

One alternative to the system we have proposed is a system like Canada's, in which the government is the sole payer for physician and hospital services. While Canada's system has evident strengths, there would be major difficulties in successfully adopting or implementing it in the United States. First, it would require a political sea change to adopt such a system here. A tax increase of approximately $250 billion per year would be required, the intense opposition of insurers and many provider groups would need to be overcome, and the concerns of many employers and citizens about the effects of such a system on access and quality would need to be allayed. In the era in which the Berlin wall has been torn down, one must be cautious about branding any proposal as politically infeasible, but it is difficult to imagine a politician winning election on a platform including an extremely large tax increase. Second, government regulatory processes tend to freeze industries and often penalize efficiency. The Canadian system is not as frozen as it might be because proximity to the United States exposes Canadians to our innovations. If American medical care were also entirely financed and regulated by the government, the negative effects of regulation would likely loom larger.

A second alternative would be to leave the financing of health insurance for the employed population in the private sector but to have the government regulate physician and hospital prices for all payers. It is possible to imagine a political compromise in which such a system could be adopted—in the midst of a recession, providers might agree to accept all payer price controls in exchange for an employer mandate, and employers might acquiesce to a mandate in exchange for price controls—but it is hard to imagine that such a regulatory structure could be effective over time in promoting quality or economy. Such price controls would be met by continuing provider efforts to circumvent and modify them. Providers would

lobby for adjustments and exceptions deemed to enhance equity, increasing the complexity of the regulations and the incentives for those who were not favored to seek favor. Congress would have created a rich new barrel of pork to reward electoral supporters and contributors—an especially attractive source, because price increases for private sector rates could be granted without requiring a tax increase.

Furthermore, such a system does not contain incentives to shift medical care resources from less productive to more productive uses. The current mantra in cost containment is the development of practice guidelines and the application of these guidelines to eliminate the ineffective practices that exist in our medical care system today. While we strongly support the development of better outcomes data and practice guidelines, in the absence of change in the financial incentives created by the FFS system, such guidelines will do little either to control costs or to lead to improvements in efficiency. For guideline development to succeed, medical care would have to be much more of a science and much less of an art than it is likely to be at any time in the foreseeable future.

Finally, administrative costs in the present system are high and increasing.[23] These costs arise from many causes: the multiplicity of payers, each with its own forms, processes, and data requirements; the high marketing costs associated with the coverage of individuals and small groups; the costs of determining eligibility for coverage in a system in which millions have no coverage; the costs of billing patients for covered services; the costs of payers attempting to determine whether services were actually provided and were appropriate; and others. We believe administrative costs would be greatly reduced under our proposal. After a competitive shakedown, there would be relatively few managed care organizations in each geographic area. Everyone would get coverage through large group arrangements. Eligibility determination would be simple in a system of universal coverage. Today, the best managed care organizations do not bill patients for services. Providers are paid by health plans in simplified ways using prospective payments for global units of care. In a system with relatively few managed care organizations competing to serve competent sponsors and cost-conscious consumers, payers would not have to attempt to micromanage the delivery of care because providers would be at risk. Administrative costs and the "hassle factor" would be much lower than they are today. However, the most important economies would be in the effective organization of the process of care itself.

Over time, we would expect slowed growth in the price of the average health plan and continuing improvements in efficiency comparable to those in other competitive industries.

ACKNOWLEDGMENT

The authors gratefully acknowledge support from the Robert Wood Johnson Foundation, Princeton, NJ, and the Henry J. Kaiser Family Foundation, Menlo Park, Calif.

REFERENCES

1 Office of the Actuary, Health Care Financing Administration. National health expenditures, 1986–2000. *Health Care Financ Rev.* Summer 1987;8:1–36.

2 Schieber GJ, Poullier JP. Recent trends in international health care spending. *Health Aff.* Fall 1987;6:105–112.

3 *1991 US Industrial Outlook.* Washington, DC: US Dept of Commerce; 1991.

4 Kronick R. *The Slippery Slope of Health Care Finance: Business, Hospitals, and Health Care for the Poor in Massachusetts.* Rochester, NY: University of Rochester; 1990. Thesis.

5 Wilensky GR. Filling the gaps in health insurance: impact on competition. *Health Aff.* Summer 1988;7:133–149.

6 Ries P. Health care coverage by age, sex, race, and family income: United States, 1986. In: *Advance Data From Vital and Health Statistics of the National Center for Health Statistics: No. 139.* Hyattsville, Md: Public Health Service; 1987. US Dept of Health and Human Services publication PHS 87-1250.

7 *Health Insurance and the Uninsured: Background Data and Analysis.* Washington, DC: Congressional Research Service, Library of Congress; 1988.

8 Jensen GA, Morrisey MA, Marcus JW. Cost sharing and the changing pattern of employer-sponsored health benefits. *Milbank Q.* 1987;65:521–542.

9 Foster Higgins Health Care Benefits Survey. *Managed Care Plans.* New York, NY: Foster Higgins; 1989.

10 Enthoven A. *Theory and Practice of Managed Competition in Health Care Finance.* Amsterdam, the Netherlands: Elsevier Science Publishers; 1988.

11 Enthoven A, Kronick R. A consumer choice health plan for the 1990s: universal health insurance in a system designed to promote quality and economy, I. *N Engl J Med.* 1989;320:29–37.

12 Enthoven A, Kronick R. A consumer choice health plan for the 1990s: universal health insurance in a system designed to promote quality and economy, II. *N Engl J Med.* 1989;320:94–101.

13 Long S, Rodgers J. *Enthoven-Kronick Plan for Universal Health Insurance.* Washington, DC: Congressional Budget Office; 1988.

14 Ellwood PM. Outcomes management: a technology of patient experience. *N Engl J Med.* 1988;318:1549–1556.

15 Roper WL, Winkenwerder W, Hackbarth GM, Krakauer H. Effectiveness in health care. *N Engl J Med.* 1988;319:1197–1202.

16 Manning WG, Leibowitz A, Goldberg GA, Rogers WH, Newhouse JP. A controlled trial of the effect of a prepaid group practice on use of services. *N Engl J Med.* 1984;310:1505–1510.

17 Davies AR, Ware JE, Brook RH, Peterson JR, Newhouse JP. Consumer acceptance of prepaid and fee-for-service medical care: results from a randomized controlled trial. *Health Serv Res.* 1986;23:429–452.

18 Sloss, EM, Keeler EB, Brook RH, Operskalski BH, Goldberg GA, Newhouse JP. Effect of a health maintenance organization on physiologic health. *Ann Intern Med.* 1987;106:130–138.

19 Luft HS. How do health-maintenance organizations achieve their 'savings?' rhetoric and evidence. *N Engl J Med.* 1978;298:1336–1343.

20 Feldman R, Dowd B, Finch M, Cassou S. *Employee-Based Health Insurance.* Rockville, Md: National Center for Health Services Research; 1989. US Dept of Health and Human Services publication PHS 89-3434.

21 Feldman R, Finch M, Dowd B, Cassou S. The demand for employment-based health insurance plans. *J Hum Res.* 1989;24:115–142.

22 Weller CD. 'Free choice' as a restraint of trade in American health care delivery and insurance. *Iowa Law Rev.* 1984;69:1351–1392.

23 Himmelstein DU, Woolhandler S. Cost without benefit: administrative waste in US health care. *N Engl J Med.* 1986;314:441–445.

A National Health Program: Northern Light at the End of the Tunnel
Steffie Woolhandler and David U. Himmelstein

Steffie Woolhandler and David U. Himmelstein both work for Physicians for a National Health Program and for the division of social and community medicine at Cambridge Hospital and the Harvard Medical School. Together they have authored *The National Health Program Book* (1994) and such articles as "The Deteriorating Administrative Efficiency of the U.S. Health Care System" and "Resolving the Cost/Access Conflict."

In view of 37 million uninsured Americans and dramatic increases in health-care spending, Woolhandler and Himmelstein propose a comprehensive reform of health-care financing, arguing that lesser reforms will either fuel inflation or require intrusive cost-management bureaucracies. The present American system, they argue, is burdened by the enormous bureaucratic weight of more than 1,500 different health plans, which require individual billing, patient-by-patient utilization reviews, eligibility determinations, and marketing expenses. By contrast, they contend, the key to administrative simplicity in Canada is a single-source payment system that allows Canada to spend much less per capita than does the United States, while guaranteeing universal (complete) coverage with comparable quality of care and at least comparable health indexes. The authors propose that the United States adopt a national health program (NHP) that would (1) create a single tax-funded comprehensive insurer in every state, (2) pay each hospital and nursing home a global budget to cover all expenses, and thereby (3) eliminate hospital bills, eligibility determinations, and the need to attribute charges to individual patients. To finance the system, the authors explain, Medicaid and Medicare funds would go to the NHP, employers would pay an NHP tax equal to the current average spent on health benefits, and individuals would be taxed an amount equal to current average out-of-pocket expenses. Despite the political obstacles facing such a reform, the authors conclude, nothing less sweeping is workable.

Few would dispute that our health care system is deeply troubled. Thirty-seven million Americans are uninsured, health care costs continue their exuberant growth, and bureaucracy increasingly intrudes in the examining room. Opinion on solutions is more divided.

We and many colleagues have proposed a sweeping reform of health care financing[1] because we are convinced that lesser measures will fail, as they have for the past quarter century. Expanding Medicaid,[2] mandating that employers provide health benefits,[3] setting up state risk pools, and similar piecemeal attempts to expand access either fuel inflation or install intrusive cost-management bureaucracies—usually both.[4] Providing more care to those currently uninsured must raise costs if resources are not diverted from elsewhere in the system.

Unless bureaucracy is trimmed, these resources will be siphoned from existing clinical care, a process invariably overseen by yet another layer of bureaucrats.

Medicare epitomizes the problem. It improved access for the elderly, but costs soared and diagnosis related groups resulted.[5] Moreover, cost-management bureaucracies are not only intrusive but expensive, leading to a steady fall in the care-bureaucracy ratio, which is now little better than 3:1.[6] For each dollar spent for the clinical components of care, 30 cents is spent for administrators and their tools.[6] Resources seep silently but inexorably from the clinic to the administrative suite. The shortage of bedside nurses coexists with a proliferation of Registered Nurse utilization reviewers and preadmission screeners. Few physicians now escape the pleasure of their scrutiny.

Such an enormous bureaucratic burden is a peculiarly American phenomenon. Our insurance companies take 12% of their premiums for overhead[7]; Canada's program runs for less than 3% overhead.[6] We devote more than 18% of hospital spending to administration and billing; Canada devotes 8%.[6,8] United States physicians spend 45% of gross income for professional expenses, much of it for billing; our Canadian colleagues spend 36%.[9,10] Overall, we spend 2.6% of our gross national product for health care bureaucracy, while Canada spends 1.1%.[6] Reducing our health administrative apparatus to the Canadian level would have saved about $62 billion this year.

Unfortunately, piecemeal tinkering cannot reverse bureaucratic hypertrophy. The key to administrative simplicity in Canada is the single-source system of payment[11]: in each province, virtually all bills are paid by the provincial insurance plan. Hospitals do little or no billing and need not keep track of the charges for individual patients.[12] They are paid a global annual budget to cover all costs, much as a fire department is funded in the United States. Physicians bill by checking a box on a simple insurance form and submitting it to the provincial plan. Fee schedules are negotiated annually between the provincial medical associations and governments.[12,13] All patients have the same (complete) coverage.

The fragmentation of insurance coverage in the United States (with >1500 different plans) requires the current herculean administrative efforts. Hospitals must determine eligibility, keep track of charges, and bill for each patient individually; coverage and regulations vary widely. Each insurer employs legions (6000 people work for Blue Cross of Massachusetts alone) to market their plans and minimize their costs, often by simply shifting those costs onto patients, other insurers, the government, or hospital red ink. Physicians must deal with an increasingly complex tangle of insurance forms and requirements. Our group practice pays about 10% of gross revenues to a billing service, a typical figure.[6]

The national health program (NHP) we propose would create a single tax-funded comprehensive insurer in each state, federally mandated but locally controlled.[1] Everyone would be fully insured for all medically necessary services and private insurance duplicating the NHP coverage would be proscribed, as would patient copayments and deductibles. The current byzantine insurance bureaucracy with its tangle of regulations and wasteful duplication would be dismantled. Instead, the NHP in each state would disburse all funds, and central administrative costs would be limited by law to 3% of total health spending. Cost-shifting efforts would be pointless—there would be nowhere to shift costs to. Marketing of insurance plans, health maintenance organi-

zations, and hospitals would also be eliminated, saving billions of dollars annually.

We expect that initially the NHP would cause little change in the total costs of care, with savings on administration and billing approximately offsetting the costs of expanded care.[14] The Canadian experience suggests the increase in use of care would be modest after an initial surge,[15] with most of the rise occurring among the poor and those with serious symptoms.[16,17]

Demonstration projects in one or more states might precede nationwide implementation. In these demonstrations, and during the phasing in of a nationwide system, funding would mimic existing patterns to minimize economic disruption—but all payment would be funneled through the NHP. Thus, Medicare and Medicaid monies would go to the NHP; employers would pay an NHP tax equivalent to the average now spent for health benefits; and individuals would pay a tax equivalent to the current average out-of-pocket expenditure.

The NHP would pay each hospital and nursing home a global budget to cover all operating expenses. This operating budget would be negotiated annually based on past expenditures, previous financial and clinical performance, projected changes in costs and use, and proposed new and innovative programs. Capital projects would be funded through separate appropriations from the NHP, and the use of operating funds for capital purchases or profits would be prohibited to minimize incentives for hospitals to skimp on care. Under this payment scheme, many administrative tasks would disappear. There would be no hospital bills to keep track of, no eligibility determination, and no need to attribute costs and charges to individual patients.

Physicians would enjoy a free choice of practice settings and styles. They could elect to be paid on a fee-for-service basis or receive salaries from health maintenance organizations, hospitals, or other institutional providers. The representative of the fee-for-service practitioners (perhaps the state medical society) and the state's NHP board would negotiate a simplified binding-fee schedule. Practitioners who accepted payment from the NHP could bill patients directly only for uncovered services (as is done for cosmetic surgery in Canada). The effort and expense of billing would be trivial: stamp the patient's NHP card on a billing form, check a box, send in all the bills once a week, and receive full payment for virtually all services—with an extra payment for any bill not paid within 30 days. Health maintenance organizations and group practices could elect to be paid a capitation fee to cover all services except inpatient hospitalization, which would be funded through hospitals' global budgets. Regulations on capital funding and profits would be similar to those for hospitals. Financial incentives for physicians based on the health maintenance organization's financial performance would be prohibited.

A similar system has worked well in Canada for nearly 20 years.[4,12,18] There are virtually no financial barriers to care and fewer nonfinancial barriers than in our country.[19] Health spending per capita, though 30% below the US figure, is the second highest in the world.[20] It has remained stable as a proportion of gross national product largely because bureaucracy has not hypertrophied and because the NHP, as the sole source of funds for health care, is able to set and enforce overall budgetary limits.[11] Despite disputes about the adequacy of funding for high-technology care,[21] most observers agree that quality of care has remained on a par with the United States and health status is at least as good as in our country.

Regulation of practice in Canada consists mainly of setting ceilings on aggregate physician reimbursement, hospital budgets, and capital spending and monitoring for outlandish abuses (eg, a single family physician who billed for $250,000 for urinalyses in 1 year).[11,13] Detailed oversight of the clinical encounter has proved unnecessary and clinical freedom is better preserved than in our country.[22,23] Although Canadian physicians have battled government over adequate funding, physician incomes are high and have more than kept pace with inflation.[13] Overall, 69% of Canadian physicians rate their NHP good or excellent, 61% believe it has improved health status, and the same proportion express satisfaction with their own practices.[24] Medicine remains a much sought after career, attracting nearly three times as many applicants per medical school place (and per capita) as in the United States.[25-27]

The Canadian system enjoys overwhelming support among patients.[19] Indeed, only 3% of Canadians would go back to the US-style system that predated their NHP.[19] In contrast, 61% of Americans favor a Canadian-style reform,[19] more than twice as many as support patchwork approaches like extending Medicaid.[28] United States corporations are also increasingly interested in fundamental health policy reform. Thus, Chrysler's health insurance costs ($700 per car in the United States vs $223 in Canada) have spurred Lee Iacocca to consider supporting an NHP (*Baltimore Sun.* April 16, 1989:2D).

Despite such popular and powerful support, the NHP we propose faces important political obstacles. The virtual elimination of private health insurance will meet stiff opposition from the insurance industry and necessitate a large-scale retraining program for employees of insurance companies (many might be employed as support personnel to free nurses for clinical tasks). Although business as a whole would see no rise in its health care costs, firms not now providing health benefits would face increased taxes without the offset provided by the elimination of health insurance premiums.

The long-term financial viability of the system we propose is critically dependent on achieving and maintaining administrative simplicity. The Canadian macromanagement approach to cost control—setting overall budgetary limits—is inherently less intensive administratively than the current US micromanagement approach that depends on case-by-case scrutiny of billions of individual expenditures and encounters. However, even in a Canadian-style system, vigilance and statutory limits on administrative spending will likely be needed to curb the tendency of bureaucracy to reproduce and amplify itself.

An NHP would solve the cost-vs-access conflict by slashing bureaucratic waste and improving health planning. It would reorient the way we pay for care and eliminate financial barriers to access, but preserve the physician-patient relationship. An NHP would offer patients a free choice of physicians and hospitals, and physicians a free choice of practice style and hospital affiliation. How many failed patchwork reforms, how many patients turned away from care they can't afford, how many dollars spent on bureaucracy, before we arrive at the only viable solution—a universal, comprehensive, publicly administered national health program?

NOTES

1 Himmelstein DU, Woolhandler S, the Writing Committee of the Working Group on Program Design. A national health program for the United States: a physicians' proposal. *N Engl J Med.* 1989;320:102–108.

2 Thorpe KE, Siegel JE, Dailey T. Including the poor: the fiscal impacts of Medicaid expansion. *JAMA.* 1989;261:1003–1007.

3 The National Leadership Commission on Health. *For the Health of a Nation: A Shared Responsibility.* Ann Arbor, Mich: Health Administration Press; 1989.

4 Evans RG. Finding the levers, finding the courage:

lessons from cost containment in North America. *J Health Polit Policy Law.* 1986;11:585–615.

5 Aiken LH, Bays KD. The Medicare debate: round 1. *N Engl J Med.* 1984;311:1196–1200.

6 Himmelstein DU, Woolhandler S. Cost without benefit: administrative waste in U.S. health care. *N Engl J Med.* 1986;314:441–445.

7 Levit KR, Freeland MS. National medical care spending. *Health Aff.* 1988;7(5):124–136.

8 *Administrative and Supportive Services.* Ottawa, Canada: Health Information Division, Dept of Health and Welfare; 1981.

9 Reynolds RA, Ohsfeldt RL, eds. *Socioeconomic Characteristics of Medical Practice.* Chicago, Ill: American Medical Association; 1984.

10 *Estimates of Physicians' Earnings, 1973–1982.* Ottawa, Canada: Health Information Division, Dept of National Health and Welfare; 1983.

11 Evans RG, Lomas J, Barer ML, et al. Controlling health expenditures: the Canadian reality. *N Engl J Med.* 1989;320:571–577.

12 Iglehart JK. Canada's health care system. *N Engl J Med.* 1986;315:202–208, 778–784.

13 Barer ML, Evans RG, Labelle RJ. Fee controls as cost control: tales from the frozen north. *Milbank Q.* 1988;66:1–64.

14 Himmelstein DU, Woolhandler S. Free care: a quantitative analysis of the health and cost effects of a national health program. *Int J Health Serv.* 1988;18:393–399.

15 LeClair M. The Canadian health care system. In: Andreopoulos S, ed. *National Health Insurance: Can We Learn From Canada?* New York, NY: John Wiley & Sons Inc; 1975:11–92.

16 Enterline PE, Salter V, McDonald AD, McDonald JC. The distribution of medical services before and after 'free' medical care: the Quebec experience. *N Engl J Med.* 1973;289:1174–1178.

17 Siemiatycki J, Richardson L, Pless IB. Equality in medical care under national health insurance in Montreal. *N Engl J Med.* 1980;303:10–15.

18 Taylor MG. *Health Insurance and Canadian Public Policy: The Seven Decisions That Created the Canadian Health Insurance System and Their Outcomes.* Montreal, Canada: McGill-Queens University Press; 1987.

19 Blendon RJ. Three systems: a comparative survey. *Health Manage Q.* 1989;11:1–10.

20 Scheiber GJ, Poullier J-P. Recent trends in international health care spending. *Health Aff.* 1987;6(3):105–112.

21 Task Force on the Allocation of Health Care Resources. *Health: A Need for Redirection.* Ottawa: Canadian Medical Association; 1984.

22 Hoffenberg R. *Clinical Freedom.* London, England: Nuffield Provincial Hospitals Trust; 1987.

23 Relman AS. American medicine at the crossroads: signs from Canada. *N Engl J Med.* 1989;320:590–591.

24 Stevenson HM, Williams AP, Vayda E. Medical politics and Canadian Medicare: professional response to the Canada Health Act. *Milbank Q.* 1988;66:65.

25 Jonas HS, Etzel SI. Undergraduate medical education. *JAMA.* 1988;260:1063–1071.

26 Ryten E. Medical schools in Canada. *JAMA.* 1988;260:1157–1161.

27 US Bureau of the Census. *Statistical Abstract of the United States: 1989.* Washington, DC: Government Printing Office; 1989.

28 Seaver DJ, Huske MS. *Health Care Attitude Survey Shows Surprising Results.* Cambridge, Mass: Arthur D Little; 1988.

Universal Health Care, American Style:
A Single Fund Approach to Health Care Reform
Dan E. Beauchamp

Dan E. Beauchamp is professor of health policy and management, school of public health, State University of New York at Albany. Beauchamp served as deputy commissioner of policy, planning, and resource development for the New York State Department of Health. He is the author of *Beyond Alcoholism: Alcohol and Public Health Policy* (1980) and *The Health of the Republic* (1988).

Beauchamp proposes the creation of a single fund to pay for all health care in the United States, without moving to public financing for the entire system. Health-care finance reform will require direct methods to control spending, he argues, and the only workable direct methods focus on systemwide cost controls. According to Beauchamp, the only viable options are (1) the adoption of a totally new financial structure like Canada's, and (2) restructuring our pluralistic financing system into a single-fund system while leaving a place for insurance companies. While a system like Canada's would control costs, he argues, it would create a very large public system that might be counter to American preferences. Beauchamp provides details of his proposed alternative before concluding that it is consistent with the American political tradition, much as Social Security is.

Runaway health care spending and the widespread instability in the health care system it has produced are providing the major impetus for national health care reform. The focus of attention is on directly controlling spending; all roads lead to finance reform.

In this article, I review the two major options we face in reforming our health care finance system. I focus on the option of creating a single fund for financing health care while maintaining multiple sources of public and private insurance.

INSTABILITY AND RISING COSTS

Twenty-five years of sharply rising costs have destabilized the American health care system. The middle class has joined the nation's poor in doubting its protection against unpaid medical bills. Never-ending increases in insurance costs crowd out wage increases. Employees fear changing jobs and losing their insurance while employers edgily seek to shift coverage costs to workers' shoulders. Workers strike to defend their health benefits more than for any other cause.

Reprinted with permission of the publisher from *Kennedy Institute of Ethics Journal,* vol. 2 (June 1992), pp. 125–135.

Defending against rising costs often adds more costs. Private insurers routinely require doctors and hospitals to justify their use of costly procedures, adding red tape to the system. Medicare's prospective payment system of price controls, called diagnositic-related groups, adds a new layer of administrative personnel to the nation's hospitals. Today, the United States spends well over twice what Canada does on administration (Himmelstein and Woolhandler 1986, 1991; Evans et al. 1989).

Rising costs are shredding the private insurance market. As waves of new cost increases hit every year, insurers seek ingenious ways to avoid sick people. Entire trades are "red-lined" as too costly to insure; insurance for small business is drying up.

Public programs are permanently destabilized. The urban poor, living where no doctor ever goes, crowd hospital emergency rooms and out-patient clinics. Hospitals respond with costly, often long-delayed care. Medicaid and other payers are hit with a new round of hospital increases. The increases doom legislative plans to fund more primary care for poor neighborhoods, in part to ease hospital crowding. Meanwhile, fees for physicians who accept Medicaid clients remain unacceptably low, constituting irrefutable evidence for most physicians that government cannot be trusted to oversee health care.

The worst may lie immediately ahead. In the year

2000, the United States is likely to see health care spending rise from present levels of 13 percent of the GNP to 17 percent. This growth will add $1.5 trillion extra to health care costs in the next eight years, 40 percent of which—$600 billion—will be in new taxes (Meyer, Silow-Carroll, and Sullivan 1991, p. 20). Business will spend another $600 billion to pay for increased employee health insurance costs.

At present rates of growth, Medicare and Medicaid will pass Social Security in size by the year 2000. By 2010, Medicare itself will rival Social Security in size (Advisory Council on Social Security 1991). This growth, if unchecked, will create even more pressures to ration health care for the poor or the elderly.

FOCUSING ON FINANCE

The health care system's chronic instability and sharply escalating spending will likely force action for universal health care. Public support for universal health care is at a record high. Reform will also come for two other related reasons.

First, we will act because the experts are finally recognizing that, whatever the myriad causes of sharply rising spending, directly limiting total revenues flowing to doctors, hospitals, clinics, and HMOs is the only effective remedy.

Second, the direct control of aggregate revenues cannot occur until the financing of the health care system (principally, the insurance system) shifts away from its present focus on the health care risks and health care utilization of individuals and small groups, and more toward system-wide financing and cost control. This shift can occur either under a restructuring of the public-private insurance system, or under a public sector alternative.

Prestigious voices like the General Accounting Office pinpoint broad reforms in health care financing as the path to affordable health care (Bowsher 1991). These finance reforms clearly lead to direct controls over total revenues flowing to hospitals and doctors. They include universal coverage, major insurance reform including common rules for payment, and caps on aggregate spending.

The shift to direct financial control is an admission that the chronic instability in the health care system is rooted in the radically decentralized financing arrangements for health care in the United States. Whatever other reasons attend the need for insurance reform, universal coverage, and direct limits on spending, the common theme is the struggle to move the financing of health care from an individual to an aggregate basis, controlling system-wide spending.

Insurance reforms that reinstate community rating as the norm, and that eliminate most experience rating or medical underwriting (attempts to adjust premiums to the actual sickness experience of subscribers) permit financing on a system-wide basis. Universal coverage and expenditure limits over total spending, as well as rate-setting and/or budgets for hospitals and fee schedules for doctors are an essential step in the transition to aggregate financial controls.

One critical, final step in the emerging reform agenda is still missing. This is the creation, by the method of financing, of a single fund to pay for all health care, without the necessity of shifting to public financing for the entire system. The existence of this common fund is the critical innovation to permit the use of budgets for hospitals and clinics, and to most effectively control the growth of total revenues flowing to the health care sector. I will show in subsequent sections how such a fund might be created without eliminating private sources of insurance.[1]

The shift to direct financial control is also an admission, if tacitly, that the root problem lies with what economists, political scientists, and philosophers call the assurance problem (Buchanan 1985). The assurance problem refers to the difficulty in gaining voluntary agreement to undertake common or concerted actions to alleviate a problem, especially when the resulting gains are diffuse and uncertain, and spread across society. The resolve of hospitals, doctors, or insurance companies to resist upward cost pressures is undercut because others cannot be relied upon to make the same sacrifice, or because individual efforts do not make a dent in so huge a problem. Also, as Norman Daniels (1986) argues, American physicians cannot be assured, without some overall national health plan, that the costs they save will be used to meet more pressing needs in health care, rather than in defense.

FROM UNIVERSALISM TO COST CONTROL

Most national health plans installed in Europe and Canada in the period after the Second World War either contained mechanisms of centralized financing or had other arrangements that permitted the rapid move toward more closely coordinated financial planning. All had near universal coverage, with highly uniform sets of benefits. These systems of coordinated or centralized financing and budgeting of health care also were linked to the larger political system, promoting taxpayer solidarity for controlling spending. These systems have recently been termed, aptly, single payer systems (Bodenheimer 1989), highlighting their distinctive methods of finance and payment.

At the time, however, public or coordinated financing was not installed to control aggregate spending, but was adapted to promote a politically stable solution to provision for the poor and the working classes, by offering health care to all in a common system. The solution, in its purest forms in England and Canada, was called universalism or social insurance.

At the practical political level, universalism sought to promote stable political coalitions for a wider equality—stable voting majorities composed of lower and middle income groups—forged by each citizen sharing the social good equally through a single and common system. Universalists chose to meet the problems of health care provision as a group, standing together "with their fellows," in the words of England's Beveridge Report (Beveridge 1942, p. 13). In this way they could help to keep the level of services high, and funding stable, because the middle classes would be the largest group of beneficiaries of the program. Also, universalism would be cheaper to administer, because income tests are typically avoided (Abel-Smith and Titmuss 1987, especially chap. 7).[2]

When costs began to rise in the sixties and especially the seventies, the countries with established systems of public finance, were better able to respond. This is because these systems of finance permitted budgets for hospitals, fee schedules for doctors, and controls over capital expansion—features difficult to install in a system with myriad public and private sources of financing. It was also because these systems usually had single cards and standardized levels of coverage, promoting voter and taxpayer solidarity for restraining costs, another feature almost impossible to design in a highly pluralistic financial scheme.

The decision of the United States to forego a national health program, and to opt for a combination of private and public programs like Medicare and Medicaid, offered no options for switching to such direct controls. The systems for collecting monies for payment, and for payment itself, were too focused on monitoring each patient-physician transaction to permit a more global, aggregate strategy of revenue limitation. Also, voters in the United States had no way to express disapproval of the health care system's rapid overall growth.

I will discuss in the concluding section whether the decision of the United States to forego national health insurance represented some fundamental rejection of the techniques inherent in single payer systems. For now, we should ask: What are the options for reforming finance more along the lines of a single payer system in the United States?

SINGLE PAYER SYSTEMS IN THE AMERICAN CONTEXT

Analytically, there are two options for creating a single payer system, with its unique financial structure, in the United States. We can scrap the present system, building an entirely new, tax-financed one like Canada's Medicare, finding the $250 billion in extra taxes to replace private insurance. Or we can restructure the private-public insurance system, converting a pluralistic source of financing into a "single fund" method of financing.

The option of scrapping the present system and installing a publicly-financed one would result in a very large public system. It would likely cost the U.S. citizenry less overall (as a total of public and private spending). It would also surely result in savings on the considerable administrative costs of private insurance companies. This approach would surely be effective in controlling costs (Meyer, Silow-Carroll, and Sullivan 1991). Its chief liability in the eyes of those who are fearful of public programs is that it would sharply increase the size of the public budget for health care.

Whatever the political fate of a publicly-financed single payer system, it is important to note that there is an alternative. This approach would reform private insurance, making it operate more like public insurance and, in effect, merge private and public insurance revenues into a single fund. This reform would permit the creation of a single source of financing and payment despite multiple insurance companies. In addition it would permit the addition of a single card and other stabilizing virtues of the national health plans elsewhere, such as stronger political accountability.

The New York State Department of Health takes this path with its Universal New York Health Care, or UNY-Care (Beauchamp and Rouse 1990). Under UNY-Care, health insurance would be simplified and made more uniform, stabilizing every resident's expectations about health care. First, each New York state resident would be given a UNY-Care card. The card will guarantee every citizen equal access without discrimination, standing for what each resident is entitled to, individually. Because everyone will belong to the same system, the single card will also symbolize what everyone together can afford.

Second, the rules governing payment and insurance would be made uniform. Insurance would shift to community rating principles; practices like medical underwriting and pre-existing conditions clauses would be eliminated. Health insurance would become a standard product; insurance companies would compete only on grounds of service and price (or, to a limited extent, for extra coverage).

Third, the state would set overall expenditure ceilings for doctors, hospitals, and other providers, and would reform the billing and payment system to give effect to these targets. Henceforth, all insurance companies would be required to use a new, state-wide electronics claims system. Paper claims would be rapidly phased out. Claims would be filed by physicians and hospitals through computer terminals. Patients would not file claims. Eligibility determinations would be made by the single electronics claims clearinghouse based on a state-wide file. The single payer system would pay providers. Insurers would pay the single payer system, on a lump-sum, advance basis, not on the basis of individual claims. This requirement would create a de facto, single fund for all health care in New York state. The claims system, now electronic, would be used for auditing, not payment, purposes. This simple system would eliminate vast amounts of paperwork and confusion for providers and consumers alike.

The single payer authority, managing and controlling the flow of all the money in the system, could set targets for overall growth based on negotiations with hospitals, doctors, and other providers. The payer authority could also, in time, pay hospitals and other health care settings on the basis of global budgets. The new payer authority would prepare a global state-wide budget to plan the growth for capital, as well as primary and acute care.

MEDICARE FOR THE 21ST CENTURY

There is a national variant on the New York idea, building on and expanding the Medicare program. (Many of the ideas for reforming the Medicare program discussed below were first proposed by Robert Ball (1991), the Commissioner of Social Security under the Kennedy, Johnson, and first Nixon administrations.) Medicare would become, in effect, two programs: one public, one private, operating with a single trust fund for all. The public program would cover the elderly, the unemployed, the poor, and small business employees. All business could, at its option, join the public program, paying on the basis of a payroll tax, rather than premium-based financing. Catastrophic coverage for everyone would be the responsibility of the public program, with private insurance limited to, say, $25,000 in coverage annually for each individual. In this new Medicare (perhaps renamed Med21, for Medicare for the 21st Century) the private program would contain all employees and their dependents, except for those firms that choose to enroll in the public program. Initially, premium-based financing would be used for the private program. However, it would be easy to change the basis of financing to a percentage of income, with the employer and employee paying their appropriate share. Thus, the progressivity of a tax-based system could be employed, even though the costs would be off the government's books. Medicaid would be largely abolished; the poor and near poor would be part of Med21's public program.

The key reform would have all funds of the private program deposited on a scheduled basis in a new, expanded Medicare Trust Fund. The Trust Fund, operating through state-run single or universal payer authorities, would pay all physicians, hospitals, and clinics in the United States.

(In a recent report, the Congressional Budget Office [1991] examined two alternative paths to universal coverage: a publicly financed, single payer system based on a standard Medicare benefit, and an "all-payer" system using Medicare's payment rates, but allowing private insurance companies to pay bills. The Med21 approach is different; it is a hybrid, single payer system, more accurately called a "universal payer" or "single fund" system. Again, it would be organized around a universal, Medicare-based benefit. Private insurance premiums would be deposited in the Medicare Trust Fund, on an advanced basis. The Trust Fund would oversee state-run single payer authorities.)

Everyone in the United States would use a single Med21 card. Private insurance companies would not pay bills, and all funds collected under the private and public program would be deposited with the Med21 Trust Fund. Med21 would pay hospitals and doctors on the basis of budgets and fee schedules, respectively. Everyone would carry a Med21 card.

The size of the Med21 program would be roughly one-half that of a publicly-financed system, and would require only one-fifth as many new tax dollars.

One virtue of the new Medicare is that everyone in the United States would, at one time or another, belong to the public and private program. All in the workforce would contribute to both systems, paying for their old-age system through Social Security taxes, and for their present insurance through premiums collected by employers.

The new single fund, single card system of Med21 would be part of the larger Social Security system. This approach should remind all that the United States already has a very large, successful social insurance-type system in place.

Is it necessary to make the benefits uniform in single card systems? At least in principle, the more uniform coverage, the more stable the system is likely to be overall. Uniformity facilitates voter evaluation of the functioning of the system overall. Uniformity also promotes cohesion among the middle class and the poor, among small families and large ones, and between the old and young.

In practice, however, there are no reasons why minor variations in coverage might not be permitted, based on different plans and different preferences. If airlines can arrange for special diets for passengers, hospitals and health insurance companies can surely do the same. The trick is to prevent insurance companies from using individualized coverage packages to select against risk or to divide up the hospital into a first class and a coach section.

Also, there are no administrative reasons why a single payer could not accept a range in the levels of deductibles and co-payment that insurance companies could offer; the single claims clearinghouse would find this level of detail undaunting. However, and again, insurance companies might be strongly tempted to use this device to introduce a measure of competition that might lead to selection against risk. As always, the more that financing and coverage rules becomes non-standard, the more social solidarity and taxpayer solidarity become elusive.

CONCLUSION

It is tempting to argue that the United States rejected the single fund option when it chose to expand private insurance and establish Medicare and Medicaid in 1965, and when it did not adopt national health insurance during the seventies. But, we should not overinterpret those events. The cost debate erupted in the late sixties, and rose to dominance during the seventies. However, the view that the explosion of costs left the United States with practically no option in responding, other than a universalist approach that contained single payer-style financing, is fairly recent. Even in Canada and Germany, the cost control issue, and its policy implications for directly limiting the expansion of the size of health care spending, did not become well-established until the mid- to late seventies.

Also, it is not true that our earlier rejection of national health insurance suggests that social insurance or universalism is simply not part of our political tradition. The strategy of joining the middle classes and the poor is explicit in Social Security and other broad-gauged programs like unemployment or workers' compensation.

Further, our experience with Social Security suggests that we can run big programs successfully. True, Social Security is not nearly as complex as managing the growth of the health care system. However, the pressures to push the spending on this program are very strong. Moreover, we managed to fundamentally change Social Security's finances during the early years of the Reagan administration, despite Reagan's occasional suggestions that the entire program ought to be put on a voluntary basis (Bernstein and Bernstein 1988). This suggests that, even in the United States, strong, popular social insurance programs generate a politics that is more consensual and stable, just as their advocates predicted.

NOTES

1 For a brief description of this approach for shifting to a common system, see Dan E. Beauchamp (1988, pp. 25–29).
2 For a discussion of universalism or social insurance in the American context, see Theodore Marmor, Jerry Mashaw, and Philip Harvey's *America's Misunderstood Welfare State* (1990). Thomas Edsall (1982) discusses the political bases of social insurance programs in the United States in *The New Politics of Inequality*.

REFERENCES

Abel-Smith, Brian, and Titmuss, Kay, eds. 1987. *The Philosophy of Welfare: Selected Writings of Richard M. Titmuss.* London: Allen & Unwin.

Advisory Council on Social Security. 1991. *Report on Medicare Projections by the Health Technical Panel to the*

1991 Advisory Council on Social Security. Washington, DC: U.S. Government Printing Office.

Ball, Robert. 1991. A Public/Private Partnership Providing Health Care for All: Building on What We Have. Unpublished ms., 8 April.

Beauchamp, Dan E. 1988. *The Health of the Republic: Epidemics, Medicine, and Moralism as Challenges to Democracy.* Philadelphia: Temple University Press.

Beauchamp, Dan E., and Rouse, Ronald. 1990. Universal New York Health Care: A Single Payer Strategy Linking Cost Control and Universal Access. *New England Journal of Medicine* 323: 640–44.

Bernstein, Merton C., and Bernstein, Joan Brodshaug. 1988. *Social Security: The System That Works.* New York: Basic Books.

Beveridge, Sir William. 1942. *Social Insurance and Allied Services.* London: His Majesty's Printing Office.

Bodenheimer, Thomas. 1989. Payment Mechanisms Under a National Health Program. *Medical Care Review* 46: 3–43.

Bowsher, Charles A., [Comptroller General of the United States]. 1991. U.S. Health Care Spending: Trends, Contributing Factors, and Proposals for Reform. Statement before the Committee on Ways and Means, House of Representatives, 17 April.

Buchanan, Allen. 1985. *Ethics, Efficiency, and the Market.* Totowa, NJ: Rowman & Allanheld.

Congressional Budget Office, Congress of the United States. 1991. *Universal Health Insurance Coverage Using Medicare's Payment Rates.* Washington, DC: U.S. Government Printing Office.

Daniels, Norman. 1986. Why Saying No to Patients in the United States Is So Hard. *New England Journal of Medicine* 314: 1380–83.

Edsall, Thomas. 1982. *The New Politics of Inequality.* New York: Norton.

Evans, Robert G.; Lomas, Jonathan; Barer, Morris; et al. 1989. Controlling Health Expenditures—The Canadian Reality. *New England Journal of Medicine* 320: 571–77.

Himmelstein, David U., and Woolhandler, Stefanie. 1986. Cost Without Benefit: Administrative Waste in U.S. Health Care. *New England Journal of Medicine* 314: 441–45.

———. 1991. The Deteriorating Administrative Efficiency of the U.S. Health Care System. *New England Journal of Medicine* 324: 1253–58.

Marmor, Theodore R.; Mashaw, Jerry L.; and Harvey, Philip L. 1990. *America's Misunderstood Welfare State.* New York: Basic Books.

Meyer, Jack A.; Silow-Carroll, Sharon; and Sullivan, Sean. 1991. *A National Health Plan in the United States: The Long-Term Impact on Business and the Economy.* Washington, DC: Economic and Social Research Institute.

ANNOTATED BIBLIOGRAPHY: CHAPTER 10

Callahan, Daniel: *Setting Limits: Medical Goals in an Aging Society* (New York: Simon and Schuster, 1987). This is a much expanded version of the reasoning Callahan advances in the article reprinted in this chapter.

———: "Meeting Needs and Rationing Care," *Law, Medicine, and Health Care* 16 (Winter 1988), pp. 261–266. Callahan argues that the need to provide an adequate level of health care to all and the need to control costs are in tension and necessitate rationing. He defends explicit rationing decisions as more honest and open to public debate. Callahan concludes that (1) we cannot expect to meet all needs and desires regarding human health, (2) we should shift our focus from individual need to social need, and (3) we must be prepared to set limits to what we will provide.

Childress, James F.: "Ensuring Care, Respect, and Fairness for the Elderly," *Hastings Center Report* 14 (October 1984), pp. 27–31. While granting that, under ideal conditions, some age-based rationing would be ethically defensible in principle, Childress contends that such rationing in our less-than-ideal world would be morally problematic. For the purposes of thinking creatively about allocation alternatives, he suggests replacing the military metaphor that dominates our thinking about medicine with the metaphor of nursing.

———: "Priorities in the Allocation of Health Care Resources," *Soundings* 62 (Fall 1979), pp. 258–269. Childress focuses on macroallocation decisions that require choices (1) between health care and other social goods and (2) between prevention and crisis medicine.

———: "Who Shall Live When Not All Can Live?" *Soundings* 53 (Winter 1970), pp. 339–355. Childress advocates a two-stage selection process for making decisions about the microallocation of scarce resources. The first step involves the use of medical criteria to establish a pool of medically accepted candidates. The second step is a random selection process.

Daniels, Norman: *Am I My Parents' Keeper?* (New York: Oxford University Press, 1988). Daniels seeks a principled approach to allocating health care, income support, and other types of resources to members of different age groups in society. Because we all age, he argues, each of us passes through different life stages. Thus, if we can determine how we would prudently allocate our fair share of social goods to ourselves over different life stages, we can discover what justice demands in the way of allocation among age groups.

———: "Health-Care Needs and Distributive Justice," *Philosophy and Public Affairs* 10 (Spring 1981), pp. 146–179. Daniels argues that if an acceptable theory of justice includes a principle of fair equality of opportunity, then health-care institutions should be among those governed by this principle. His article includes an account of basic needs and, in particular, health-care needs. He identifies basic needs as those important to maintaining normal species functioning, which is an important determinant of the range of opportunities open to an individual.

Dougherty, Charles J.: *American Health Care: Realities, Rights, and Reform* (New York: Oxford University Press, 1988). Dougherty provides a moral evaluation of American health care. The book divides into (1) a review of actual access to health care ("realities"), (2) a pluralistic philosophical defense of a moral right to health care ("rights"), and (3) an assertion of what reforms are needed to achieve justice ("reforms").

Fuchs, Victor R.: *The Health Economy* (Cambridge, MA: Harvard University Press, 1986). Fuchs provides a framework for thinking about the issues of cost, efficiency, access, and quality in regard to health care.

Iglehart, John K.: "The American Health Care System: Managed Care," *New England Journal of Medicine* 327 (September 3, 1992), pp. 742–747. Iglehart describes in detail the various kinds of managed care currently used in the United States and discusses general strengths and weaknesses of this type of health-care delivery. He concludes with a discussion of managed care's promise for the future as well as the challenges it faces.

President's Commission for the Study of Ethical Problems in Medicine and Biomedical and Behavioral Research: *Securing Access to Health Care,* Vol. 1: *Report* (Washington, DC: U.S. Government Printing Office, 1983). This influential report presents the commission's conclusions about (1) an ethical framework grounding a societal obligation to provide an adequate level of health care to all citizens, (2) the state of health care in America, and (3) changes in health-care delivery that can move the United States in the direction of meeting its societal obligation.

———: *Securing Access to Health Care,* Vol. 2: *Appendices: Sociocultural and Philosophical Studies.* This volume contains sociological, philosophical, and ethical studies pertaining to the issue of health-care access.

———: *Securing Access to Health Care,* Vol. 3: *Appendices: Empirical, Legal, and Conceptual Studies.* The three parts of this volume are entitled "Ethical Implications of Health Care Distribution," "Allocation in Varied Medical Settings," and "Legal Implications of Allocation Policies."

Singer, Peter A.: "How Green Is Your Grass?: A Comparative Analysis of the American and Canadian Health Care Systems," *Humane Medicine* 7 (Winter 1991), pp. 47–53. Singer provides a review of key points made in presentations at a conference sponsored by the Ontario Medical Association on comparisons between the American and Canadian health-care systems. Topics covered include malpractice and litigation, social and moral values, clinical guidelines, the consumer's perspective, and rationing.

Veatch, Robert M.: *The Foundations of Justice: Why the Retarded and the Rest of Us Have Claims to Equality* (New York: Oxford University Press, 1986). Veatch examines current conceptions of justice, equality, and social responsibility as he grapples with the question of how to allocate limited resources fairly, especially to people with inexaustible needs and little capacity for improvement.

————: "Voluntary Risks to Health: The Ethical Issues," *JAMA* 243 (January 4, 1980), pp. 50–55. Veatch explores several empirical, conceptual, and ethical issues raised by voluntary risk taking and its impact on health. He analyzes several models for approaching the issue of whether health risks are voluntary before defending a "multicausal" model. Veatch concludes that, if persons have equal opportunities for health, it is not unjust to treat those who squander their opportunities by taking voluntary risks differently from those who do not.

Wellstone, Paul D., and Ellen R. Shaffer: "The American Health Security Act: A Single-Payer Proposal," *New England Journal of Medicine* 328 (May 20, 1993), pp. 1489–1493. The authors argue for the adoption of a single-payer system of health-care delivery, citing its likely success in controlling costs while providing universal access. Their proposal permits insurance companies to offer services not covered by the public system, such as elective cosmetic surgery.

APPENDIX

Case Studies

This appendix contains a set of case studies for analysis and discussion. Some of the cases are essentially records of actual situations. Others, however, are only loosely based on actual happenings, and a few have been constructed simply for their perceived pedagogical value. Most of the cases have been developed only up to a crucial "decision point." Although retrospective case review—concerned with the appropriateness of decisions actually made in any given case—is called for in a few of the cases presented here, most of the cases ask for a prospective rather than a retrospective analysis. Thus, the more common task is to provide an analysis of what should be done within the context of a developing case rather than an analysis of what has actually been done in a case that has already run its course.

When case descriptions feature a richness of factual detail and nuance, they are sometimes characterized as "thick." By way of contrast, case studies of the type presented here may be characterized as relatively "thin," and their somewhat schematic character may cause discomfort. Individuals involved in analyzing such cases often feel that it would be desirable to have more factual details, especially clinical ones. This recurrent desire reflects the well-based axiom that good decision making must be based on "good facts." However, a perceived lack of factual detail should not be allowed to paralyze analysis and discussion. If the proper decision in a certain case is thought to be dependent on information not provided in the case description, and if it is reasonable to believe that the desired information would or could be available to those confronted with the decision, a discussion of the case can include an examination of the precise way in which the desired information is relevant to the decision.

Two final points are worth noting. First, the last paragraph of each case study identifies some questions raised by the case. These questions are not the only ones worthy of consideration, but they can be used to facilitate analysis and discussion. Second, the title of each case study is followed by a number or numbers within brackets. These numbers refer to the various chapters in this book. Thus the chapter or chapters most directly relevant to each case are identified.

CASE 1

Withholding Information about Risks [2]

Marcia W is a 40-year-old female with multiple myeloma, who upon diagnosis shows great interest in having all the information that is necessary to make a decision about further treatment. Dr. C tells her that the response rates to chemotherapy with this disease are very good and that recent research has shown that 50 percent of patients can hope for long-term survival rates, which are tantamount to cure. The other 50 percent of patients die within a year or two. What Dr. C neglects to tell her is that preliminary studies are showing that in 20 years, 10 percent of those who survive contract a form of leukemia that is highly resistant to treatment. When her treatment is discussed in a staff meeting, Dr. C says that he does not want to tell Marcia W about the 10 percent because he is afraid that it might unduly alarm her and cause her not to take treatment, thereby spoiling her chances for long-term survival. Moreover, he states (1) that the research is not conclusive enough to suit him and (2) that 10 percent is such a low figure that he is not morally required to communicate the risk. After all, he suggests, one cannot inform a patient of *every* risk.

(1) Does Marcia W have a right to the information about the possible risk of leukemia? (2) Is this 10 percent chance of contracting leukemia significant for her decision making? (3) Will this information harm her by making it impossible for her to make an autonomous decision? (4) Is the refusal to disclose justified by the low 10 percent figure and the serious consequences of refusing treatment?

CASE 2

A Patient's Request for a Possibly Useless Treatment [2]

After arriving at his doctor's office, Jeff R complains of the flu and requests an antibiotic. His description of symptoms convinces Dr. T that he has the flu. Dr. T knows that antibiotics are physiologically useless against the flu and other conditions caused by viruses (as opposed to bacteria). In dealing with patients who have the flu, she ordinarily recommends rest and fluids and sometimes recommends over-the-counter drugs. But Jeff R insists on an antibiotic, so she considers writing a prescription. On the one hand, she figures that an antibiotic will cause Jeff R no harm and might even help psychologically by making him feel that something is being done for his condition. On the other hand, she is aware that overuse of antibiotics makes it more likely that bacteria in the environment will become resistant to available antibiotics.

(1) Should Dr. T honor Jeff R's request for antibiotics? (2) Is it appropriate for physicians to offer treatments whose sole purpose is to provide psychological comfort when that comfort is based on a false belief or misunderstanding?

CASE 3

Conflict between the Interests of a Patient and His Wife [2]

An elderly man, Bill S, has been paralyzed by a stroke but apparently retains decision-making capacity. There is no significant chance that the paralysis can be reversed. The patient's physician, Dr. Z, believes the patient should enter a nursing home when he is ready to be discharged from the hospital. Bill S, however, insists on returning home, although the only available caretaker is his rather frail, elderly wife, Amy S, who has a heart ailment. Amy S knows that she is incapable of the physical demands required to care for her husband, and she also knows that he will refuse nursing care at home. She explains to her husband that if her health fails, he will have to enter a nursing home anyway and she may become bedridden or die. Amy S pleads with Dr. Z to intercede when her husband remains adamant. Because Bill S is very attached to his physician, Dr. Z believes that by threatening to withdraw from the case, he might be able to get Bill S to change his mind.

(1) How should Dr. Z deal with this situation? (2) Should the interests of family members, when they conflict with a patient's interests, have any bearing on medical decision making? (3) Is it ever appropriate for a physician to pressure a patient to do what is morally right?

CASE 4

Patient Responsibility [2]

For years Brian B has visited a public clinic that provides health care to uninsured persons. He has established a relationship with Dr. L, who always inquires about Brian's smoking habits and advises him to quit or at least curtail his smoking. Despite repeated warnings, Brian B has continued to smoke heavily, even after developing signs of emphysema in his early fifties. Now, at age 57, Brian B has a severe case of emphysema and comes frequently to the clinic—sometimes clearly for medical purposes, but sometimes apparently just to talk. The clinic, meanwhile, has been hit with budget cuts that have resulted in fewer staff to see patients. Dr. L is irritated with Brian B for ignoring all warnings and worsening his own medical condition. Dr. L tells him that, in the future, he must call before coming to the clinic and that there might not always be a staff member available to see him. Dr. L adds, "These days I am very busy with patients—patients who, by the way, follow doctor's orders—and I will be unable to see you."

(1) To what extent is Brian B responsible for his severe case of emphysema? (2) Does Dr. L have an obligation to continue to be available to Brian B? Does virtue require his continued availability?

CASE 5

Voluntary Sterilization and a Young, Unmarried Man [2]

Gregory X, who is 25 years old, unmarried, and childless, wants a vasectomy. (Vasectomy is a sterilization procedure that, until recently, had been considered irreversible but at present can sometimes be surgically reversed.) He comes to Dr. H, a urologist in a clinic in a large city hospital, because he cannot afford the surgery elsewhere. He tells Dr. H that he has decided, after several years of thought, never to be a parent. The vasectomy will now ensure that and make it unnecessary for any woman he loves to run the various risks associated with the available means of contraception. Dr. H has doubts about performing the surgery on a young, unmarried man. He asks Gregory X to consider the feelings of a possible future wife who will not have any say about the sterilization decision. Gregory X insists on the surgery.

(1) Should Dr. H accede to Gregory X's request despite his reservations, since Gregory X cannot afford the vasectomy elsewhere? (2) Is there anything morally problematic about Gregory X's request?

CASE 6

The Dentist and Patient Autonomy [2]

A 36-year-old man, Patrick M, contacts the office of an endodontist. (Endodontics is a specialized field of dentistry.) Patrick M wants to arrange for a procedure commonly called a "root canal" to be performed on each of his teeth. A root canal is a common (somewhat involved) procedure used as an alternative to extracting a diseased tooth. It consists of removing the damaged or diseased blood vessels and nerves contained within the tooth. The tooth is thus "devital" but functions normally. If this procedure is not done on a diseased tooth or if the tooth is not extracted, infection will very likely develop in the necrotic tissue and spread into the jaw bone and surrounding tissues.

The endodontist is startled by the idea of performing a root canal on all of Patrick M's teeth. Further discussion makes Patrick M's motivation clear. He is a fervent survivalist, dedicated to planning for every contingency in the expectation that some conflagration is about to destroy society. Patrick M is attempting to ensure—by having all of his teeth desensitized—that he will never suffer a toothache. Although the endodontist cannot escape a sense of amusement over what he considers a bizarre situation, Patrick M seems fully prepared both to undergo a difficult set of procedures and to pay what will be a huge overall bill. Still, the endodontist feels that it would be unethical to remove healthy tissue. He feels that he is being asked to perform a procedure that is not indicated by the existing conditions and may never be indicated, judging by the excellent overall health of the teeth.

(1) Is there any significant difference between the dentist-patient relationship and the physician-patient relationship? (2) Should the endodontist accede to Patrick M's desires?

CASE 7

A Physician's Conflicting Loyalties [2]

Dr. A, who works for a health maintenance organization (HMO), is visited by Mr. O, who suffers chronically from moderate back pain. An interview with the patient and a brief physical exam lead Dr. A to believe that Mr. O's back pain, like that of many patients, results from a combination of muscle tightness and stress. It is unrealistic to expect Mr. O to eliminate stress from his life, given his job, and he does not seem to need psychotherapy. Dr. A believes that the patient would benefit most from a combination of daily stretching exercises and, at least for the time being, massage therapy on a regular basis. But Dr. A feels constrained by the expectations within the HMO that practitioners keep costs down. More specifically, referrals for massage therapy (which is available through the HMO) are supposed to be made only for those judged to be suffering from *severe* muscle pain. Dr. A is prepared to recommend the daily exercises but wonders whether he should make a referral for massage therapy as well.

(1) Should Dr. A make the referral? (2) If Dr. A feels that his obligation to the HMO precludes a referral, should he suggest that the patient consider massage therapy outside the HMO? (3) Do physicians have an obligation to do what is in their patients' best interests, regardless of costs?

CASE 8

Hospitals, Surgeons, and Economic Incentives [2, 3]

A large, for-profit hospital chain (RASA) offers to share the profits generated by the use of its operating rooms with the staff surgeons who use them. Dr. G is one of these surgeons. Thus she benefits financially in two ways when she operates on a patient in a RASA hospital—she is paid for the operation and she receives a share of the hospital's profits. There are other, equally equipped hospitals in the community whose facilities Dr. G could use.

(1) Is Dr. G acting in a morally acceptable way by referring her patients to a RASA hospital? (2) Is RASA's profit-sharing policy morally acceptable? (3) Does RASA's policy work to the detriment of the patient?

CASE 9

The Nurse and Informed Consent [2, 3]

Michael G, who is dying of leukemia, is in a hospital where he is receiving chemotherapy. A registered nurse involved in his care, Nurse L, learns that he has never received information about alternative natural therapies. She gives Michael G the information and discusses the advantages and disadvantages of the various alternatives. After extensive reflection and consultation with his family, Michael G decides to leave the hospital and to make arrangements to try one of the alternative therapies. He informs the attending oncologist of his decision. When the oncologist learns about the source of Michael G's information, he charges Nurse L with unprofessional conduct and asks that her nursing license be revoked. Nurse L argues that the patient has the right to know about the alternatives and that a failure to inform him vitiates his "informed consent" to the chemotherapy.

(1) Was Nurse L acting in a morally correct way when she gave Michael G the information? (2) Should the physician in charge have the final word about the information a patient receives? (3) If Michael G did not know about the alternative therapies, was his assent to the chemotherapy *informed* consent?

CASE 10

The Office Nurse and Informed Consent [2, 3]

Joan R is going through menopause. Her physician, Dr. W, wants her to begin estrogen therapy. After talking with the physician, Joan R agrees to the therapy. She stops at the nurse's desk in Dr. W's office to pick up her prescription. In the course of the conversation, Nurse M realizes that Dr. W has not informed Joan R that other options are available to her and that there is wide disagreement about which option is preferable. Instead of taking only estrogen, Joan R could choose to take estrogen together with a progestin, or she could choose to take no hormones at all. Each of these options is thought to carry different potential benefits and risks.

(1) Should Nurse M provide Joan R with that information? (2) Should Nurse M suggest to Joan R that she initiate an additional discussion with Dr. W in order to obtain more information? (3) Should Nurse M express her concern in this matter to Dr. W? If so, how should she approach him?

CASE 11

An HIV-Infected Surgeon and a Duty to Disclose [2, 3]

Dr. M, a surgeon, has learned that he has been infected with the human immunodeficiency virus (HIV). A prominent study estimates that surgeons cut themselves, on average, 2.5 times for every 100 surgical procedures and that, in approximately one-third of those cases, the patient is touched with the instrument carrying the surgeon's blood. According to the study, for every 1,000 cases in which an HIV-infected surgeon's blood mixes with that of a patient, a patient will become infected in at most 3 cases. Thus there is *some* risk that a patient operated on by Dr. M will be infected.

(1) Does Dr. M have an obligation to refrain from performing surgery? (2) If not, does Dr. M have an obligation to inform those on whom he plans to operate that he is infected with the virus? (3) Suppose the positions were reversed and a patient, Dorothea L, is the one infected. Is Dorothea L obligated to inform Dr. M of her infection?

CASE 12

A Randomized Clinical Trial and a Physician's Responsibility to a Patient [2, 4]

Dr. L has agreed to request participation of his patients in a RCT designed to test a new drug whose purpose is to treat and cure a disease that is about 70 percent fatal. One of the participants in the trial, Bruce W, has been a patient of Dr. L's for 11 years. There are a total of 30 participants in the RCT. Placebos are given to 12. The other 18 are given the new drug. None of the patients are told which treatment they are receiving, although all know that they are taking part in a randomized clinical trial. After 8 of the 12 patients on placebos and 5 of those receiving the new drug die, Dr. L is asked by Bruce W whether he is one of the placebo recipients and whether there is any good reason to think that the new drug is effective. Dr. L knows that Bruce W is a placebo recipient and that the data so far support the view that the experimental drug may be effective and prevent death. Dr. L and the other physicians involved in the trial are unwilling to end the experiment because of their concern about the validity of the study if it is terminated too soon.

(1) Should the experiment be ended and the remaining patients put on the new therapy immediately? (2) Should Dr. L decline at this point to provide Bruce W with the requested information? (3) Does Dr. L have an obligation to his patient, Bruce W, which should take precedence over his concern with establishing the validity of the results of the RCT?

CASE 13

Enrolling Ineligible Patients in a Clinical Trial [2, 4]

Participation in the clinical trial of a drug intended to benefit cancer patients is contingent on the fulfillment of certain requirements. These include having only a certain type of cancer; having at least an eight-week life expectancy; having normal kidney, liver, and heart functioning; and having the ability to perform everyday functions. The validity of the trial depends on the enforcement of these requirements. The trial is being conducted by colleagues of Dr. T who have asked him to enroll eligible patients in the trial, with the latter's consent, of course. Dr. Y, who is Dr. T's patient, has exhausted the therapies available for his form of cancer. Dr. Y hears about the clinical trial. Although he knows that he cannot meet all the requirements for participation, he tells Dr. T that he wants to be enrolled and asks that Dr. T fudge the data, if necessary, since otherwise he has no chance for survival.

(1) Should Dr. T fudge the data to give Dr. Y one last chance? (2) Since Dr. Y is also a physician and understands that his participation will compromise the validity of the trial, is his insistence on participation incompatible with his professional commitment?

CASE 14

A Teenager's Consent to Participate in Research [4]

One hundred high school sophomores are asked to participate in an experimental trial of a new soap intended to prevent acne or at least to mitigate its severity. In the planned randomized clinical trial, half the students will receive the new soap while the other half will be given a facsimile without the ingredients thought to be effective against acne. No risks to the students are anticipated. The students are given consent forms to take home for their parents' signature. Lisa H's parents refuse to consent on Lisa's behalf, although Lisa wants to participate in the project.

(1) Should Lisa's consent override her parents' refusal? (2) Would the answer be different if a similar situation occurred involving children whose ages ranged from 7 to 9?

CASE 15

Baboon Colonies for Transplantable Organs [4]

Many patients who currently undergo dialysis because of end-stage renal disease could dispense with the machines and live a relatively normal life if they received a kidney transplant. The supply of cadaver kidneys, however, is severely limited. While approximately 10,000 kidney transplants are done in the United States each year, about 20,000 Americans remain on a waiting list at any given time. Concerns about the shortage of available kidneys and other organs, such as livers and hearts, lead a member of Congress to introduce a bill that would establish "baboon colonies" to support the use of xenography—the transplantation of organs from animals to humans. As yet there have been no long-term successes following xenografts. The record length of survival is 9 months, in 1963, when a man received a chimpanzee's kidney. In 1993 a man survived 71 days in a largely stuporous condition after receiving a baboon's liver—one of the most successful cases thus far. The member of Congress argues that, while xenografts have not yet been very successful, improvements in the technology in combination with the establishment of "baboon colonies" could provide a long-term solution to the organ shortage. Since baboons are not classified as an endangered species, she continues, thousands of baboons could be bred and maintained until their kidneys, livers, or hearts are needed for transplant. She adds that the baboons could be killed painlessly before their organs are taken.

Another member of Congress argues that the proposal should be rejected for several reasons. First, it is unclear that the technology is sufficiently promising. Second, there is something ethically troubling about rearing baboons for the sole purpose of using their organs. Finally, the most suitable organs for transplant—those of human cadavers—are largely wasted. We should explore options for increasing the number of transplantable organs from this "more natural" supply, he contends.

(1) Is the *likelihood* of improving xenography to the point at which recipients survive significant lengths of time with a decent quality of life crucial in a moral evaluation of the proposal? Alternatively, does *any* chance of significantly helping human patients justify the proposal? (2) If baboons raised for transplantation purposes are not made to suffer, does the second member of Congress have any reasonable grounds for ethical concern? (3) Should the United States consider ways of increasing the number of available human organs? For example, should it advertise the need for such organs? Should it adopt a "presumed consent" policy (as several European countries have), in which an adult is presumed to consent to the use of his or her organs following death unless he or she indicates otherwise?

CASE 16

Alzheimer's Disease, Memory Continuity, and Autonomy [2, 5]

Thomas P is a 78-year-old male who has cancer, with a primary site in the lung and metastases to the bone. It has been determined that nothing genuinely therapeutic can be done for the lung disease. Now he faces a decision as to whether he should have radiation to the bones to reduce the possibility of fractures. The radiation proposed has already been used once in the course of the disease, and it made the patient very ill for about six weeks. There is every reason to believe that the same morbidity will occur this time. Thomas P must now decide whether he wants to undergo a similar treatment, with its accompanying side effects, for the bone metastases. He is cared for at home by his wife, and he has five children who have genuine loving concern for him.

Thomas P's situation is complicated by the fact that he has Alzheimer's disease. His memory does not always serve him well. He remembers the side effects of the previous radiation, and he seems to be well acquainted with the disease process. However, he does not always remember what his physician tells him and then is forced to make decisions based on incomplete or unrecalled information. Furthermore, he cannot always remember what he has consented to and what he has not consented to. His locutions sometimes take the form of "Did I agree to that?" He sometimes seems to be persuaded by whomever he is discussing the matter with at the time. This ambivalence, together with the lapses in memory continuity, raises questions about his competence in making decisions.

(1) Is Thomas P sufficiently autonomous to make his own decisions? (2) How seriously

should his health-care professionals consult with him about his mode of treatment? To what extent should the family be involved?

CASE 17

Liberty and the Elderly Patient [2, 5]

Ronald X is 71 years old. A widower, he lives alone in an apartment, but he receives some assistance from a cleaning woman and a friendly neighbor. Ronald X is presently in a hospital because of a broken leg, but he is ready to be discharged. Ronald X also suffers from arteriosclerosis, a condition that results in his experiencing periods of confusion during which he sometimes wanders purposelessly around the city, running some risks to himself. Ronald X's children do not want him to return to his home. They believe that he needs the supervised care provided in a nursing home. Ronald X, when not in a confused state, repeatedly expresses his awareness of the problems he faces stemming from his arteriosclerosis and of the resultant risks he runs. Nonetheless, he would rather run those risks than be confined to institutional care. The health-care professionals and Ronald X's children decide that he will not be discharged from the hospital until an appropriate nursing home is found. At that time, he will be sent to the nursing home. When Ronald X insists on being discharged from the hospital, the medical professionals sedate him to a level sufficient to gain his compliance.

(1) Are the health-care professionals and Ronald X's children making an unjustified leap from his occasional risk-running behavior to the conclusion that he lacks sufficient competence to determine the shape of his own life? (2) Is this paternalistic limitation on Ronald X's liberty morally obligatory? morally permissible? morally reprehensible?

CASE 18

Privacy and Monitoring Systems in a Psychiatric Hospital [3, 5]

The new superintendent of the Meller Valley Psychiatric Hospital, Dr. R, has decided to install television monitoring devices in all the patients' rooms as well as in the hallways and visiting rooms of the hospital. His primary purposes are to make it easier to locate personnel when they are needed in a hurry and to help the staff, which is shorthanded, keep an eye on the doings of patients, a small number of whom are prone to violence. Patients know about the surveillance, but visitors are not informed. Some of the members of Dr. R's staff object, arguing that the system is a gross violation of the privacy of both patients and visitors.

(1) Is Dr. R morally justified in establishing the monitoring system? (2) Are patients' and visitors' rights being violated?

CASE 19

Autonomy and Mental Illness [5]

Humphrey W, a 40-year-old businessman, is committed to a psychiatric hospital at the instigation of his wife and without his consent after repeated manic episodes in public and a suicide attempt. During some of his manic episodes, he has thrown money around on street corners, harangued passersby, raged against his fellow employees, and boasted of nonexistent business deals to his boss. After commitment, Humphrey W refuses tranquilizing medication, which psychiatrists consider necessary to control his "manic flights" and strengthen his own control over his behavior.

(1) Would it be morally correct for the psychiatrists to give him the tranquilizers (e.g., by means of a syringe) against his expressed dissent? (2) Was it morally correct to commit him to the hospital without his consent?

CASE 20

A Schizophrenic Son's Refusal of Therapy [5]

William T, who is 22 years old, has a troubled history. He has been diagnosed as suffering from chronic undifferentiated schizophrenia. He has been expelled from several schools due to his severely disruptive conduct and a continuing serious deterioration in his school performance. William T has been a multiple drug abuser, he has threatened various members of his family, and his behavior has sometimes been catatonic. He has persistently refused to take any medication and has rejected all other forms of treatment. Now William T is in a state hospital after being charged with attempted armed robbery, assault, and battery. He continues to reject all treatment. William T's father, Joseph T, who has been appointed his temporary guardian, wants to consent to the administration of medication to William T. The father thinks that William T may pose a danger to others if he is discharged without treatment and thereby poses a threat of harm both to himself and others. Joseph T maintains that he is acting in the best interests of his son, who is incompetent to decide what is best for himself.

(1) Should parents in such cases be allowed to make treatment decisions that go against the expressed wishes of their children? (2) Is William T's autonomy sufficiently diminished so that his father's actions on his behalf are an example of weak, rather than strong, paternalism? (3) Is forcing medication on patients inconsistent with respecting them as persons?

CASE 21

Sterilization and the Mentally Retarded [5]

The parents of a 19-year-old, Mindy G, who has Down's syndrome and an IQ in the upper-50s range, ask her physician to implant a drug-delivery system that will serve as a relatively long-term contraceptive. The parents argue that the prevention of pregnancy will serve Mindy's long-term interests, since if she becomes pregnant she will neither fully understand her condition nor be able to care for the baby on her own. Furthermore, they are concerned about what will happen to Mindy after they die. They would like to see her settled in a group home for retarded adults and working in a sheltered workshop. They argue that continuous and dependable contraception is a prerequisite for these kinds of changes in her life.

(1) Putting aside any legal complications, would it be morally correct for the physician to implant the contraceptive device? (2) Is it plausible to see such long-term contraception as serving Mindy's long-term interests and, perhaps, as even maximizing her freedom? (3) Would surgical sterilization (tubal ligation), which would permanently prevent pregnancy, be a preferable option given Mindy G's parents' concern with her well-being after their death?

CASE 22

Depression and Autonomy [2, 5, 6]

John Q is a 56-year-old male with a wife and two grown children. He has just suffered his third heart attack in five years, and his cardiologist, Dr. Y, has told him that he must have bypass surgery if he is going to live. Dr. Y has also told him that because of the already existent damage to the heart muscles he will be a semi-invalid for the rest of his life even with the surgery. John Q had been an active businessman until his first attack, and he has resentfully had to cut back on his activity since that attack. Now the possibility of extensive surgery and living as a semi-invalid is too much for him to bear. He goes into a depressed state and refuses the surgery, saying that he is "tired of being sick" and that life holds no meaning for him any longer. He is adamant about not having the surgery. The family asks for a psychiatric consultation, and Dr. Y supports the idea because he believes that the psychiatrist might be able to talk John Q into the surgery. The psychiatrist says the depression obviously indicates that

John Q is incapable of making a rational judgment and that the family and Dr. Y should make the decision and ignore the patient's wishes.

(1) Does depression after hearing "bad news" automatically indicate that a patient is incompetent to make decisions regarding treatment? (2) Is it the consulting psychiatrist's role to try to talk the patient into doing what the attending physician wants to do? (3) How can the family serve the best interests of the patient in this situation?

CASE 23

Refusal of Life-Sustaining Treatment by a Minor [2, 6]

Jimmy T is an 11-year-old boy who suffers from lymphoma. The oncologist has indicated that without chemotherapy Jimmy is likely to die within six months. She has also indicated that chemotherapy provides an effective cure in only 20 percent of cases like Jimmy's; in most of the cases, chemotherapy produces at best an additional three-month to six-month extension of life. Jimmy is also compromised by an incurable neurological disease. This disease will eventually make it impossible for him to walk, talk, use his hands effectively, or control his excretory functions. Already his speech is slurred, and he cannot hold a pencil. Even without the lymphoma, the prognosis for him because of the neurological disease is death by the age of 18. Jimmy has been raised in a strong religious environment, and his belief in God has been an important comforting factor for him. After having the facts fully explained to him, he has accepted his situation and the inevitability of his death at a young age. He says that he does not want the chemotherapy and that he is ready to "go to God." His parents, however, cannot reconcile themselves to losing Jimmy. They override Jimmy's decision and tell the oncologist to proceed with the chemotherapy.

(1) Should minors of Jimmy's age be permitted to participate in decisions of this magnitude? (2) Whose decision, the parents' or the child's, should be decisive? (3) How should the oncologist deal with this situation?

CASE 24

Physician Disagreement Regarding a Patient's Wishes [2, 6]

John H, a 59-year-old male, has been diagnosed as having cancer, the primary site of which is the pancreas. His condition is rapidly deteriorating. John H has requested that he not be resuscitated if he should go into cardiac arrest. He has also stated that he wishes no further treatment. Dr. W, who is John H's personal physician, and Dr. R, the oncologist in the case, agree that he should not be resuscitated, and "Do not resuscitate" is written on his chart. However, when John H begins to experience severe internal bleeding, he asks his physicians if they can do something. Whether John H is competent at this point is unclear. Dr. W does not want to take measures to stop the bleeding, in keeping with John H's original request for no further treatment. Dr. R sees the request "to do something" as taking precedence over the earlier request for no additional treatment. If they do not act quickly to stop the internal bleeding, John H will die as a result of blood loss.

(1) What is the most appropriate response in this situation? (2) When a patient who is in a great deal of pain, weak, and close to death makes a request that seems at odds with a decision he made when he may have been more fully autonomous, which request should guide those caring for him?

CASE 25

Honoring the Living Will [2, 6]

Esther K, a 65-year-old woman with a long history of diabetes, has been diagnosed as having pancreatic cancer. At the time of diagnosis, she refused all aggressive therapies and later wrote a living will, in which she stated clearly that she did not want any "extraordinary means" used to prolong her life. She specified the "extraordinary means" as chemotherapy, respirators, or resuscitation efforts. Three months after diagnosis, Esther K was admitted to the hospital in a confused state with discoloration on her foot and some evidence of necrotic tissue on the top of her foot. Observation over the next couple of days revealed that the necrosis had spread, and the surgeon, Dr. P, diagnosed gangrene. Dr. P wanted to remove the foot before the gangrene spread. Esther K was still somewhat confused but nonetheless agreed to the surgery. The family was very upset with Dr. P for suggesting the surgery and for considering her competent to give consent. The family thinks that in the spirit of the living will she would not want the surgery, which would fall into the class of "extraordinary means." Furthermore, the family thinks that Esther K is too confused to give reflective consent, and this may be borne out by the fact that the patient whispered to the nurse that she consented only because she was afraid Dr. P would no longer take care of her and might order her out of the hospital.

(1) How specific must a living will be in order for it to be morally decisive? (2) Is there a danger of assuming that a consent is valid merely because it coincides with what the physician wishes to do? (3) What weight should be given to the family's judgment in this case?

CASE 26

Discriminating among Life-Sustaining Therapies [2, 6]

Shirley W is a 26-year-old female, unmarried with no dependents. She has reached the end stage of leukemia, has accepted her impending death, and has told her physician that she wishes to have no heroic measures used to preserve her life, although she also wishes to be kept comfortable. Her physician, Dr. Q, wants to honor her request but is concerned with her rapidly falling platelet count. The lower the platelet count, the greater the chance of hemorrhage. The physician does not know whether to interpret possible platelet transfusions as "heroic measures." On the one hand, a hemorrhage would cause Shirley W to die soon, and a transfusion would extend the dying process. On the other hand, if the hemorrhage occurred in the mouth, the death would be very uncomfortable because the patient would choke. If the latter were allowed to happen, Dr. Q's promise to keep the patient comfortable would be broken.

Not knowing quite how to proceed, Dr. Q consults with the staff and as a result offers the patient the following mode of treatment. If a hemorrhage were to occur in the mouth, the patient would be given platelets as a comfort-producing measure. Thus the platelets would be seen as serving a palliative function in keeping with the patient's desire to be kept comfortable and would not be seen as a heroic measure whose primary function is to prolong life. However, if the hemorrhage were to occur in some other part of the body, the priorities would be reversed; the platelets would be seen as heroic measures, and they would not be given.

(1) Is the concept of "heroic measures" a useful one for purposes of ethical analysis? If so, how should one determine "heroic measures" in general? (2) Did Dr. Q handle this situation in an appropriate manner?

CASE 27

Advance Directives and a Demented Man [5, 6]

Albert H is a 77-year-old man who lives in a nursing home. His wife is deceased, but their only child, a son, visits his father at least three times a week. Albert H began to exhibit the first signs of senility in his late sixties, and his condition rapidly deteriorated. At this point he is categorized as severely but "pleasantly" demented. Albert H needs constant supervision and assistance with basic tasks but seems undisturbed by his situation. He loves to watch TV and smoke cigars. He seldom recognizes his son but talks enthusiastically with him and anyone else who will listen. He tells the same stories over and over again; in fact, he often tells the same story to a person 4 or 5 times in a row, forgetting that he has just told the story. Almost all of his stories derive from memories of childhood; he seems to have virtually no memories of his adult life. Apart from his mental deterioration, Albert H has no notable health problems.

When Albert H was in his early sixties, he had executed a formal advance directive. Among other things, he had clearly specified that, were he to become seriously mentally impaired, he should not be given life-sustaining treatments, including antibiotics. The problem now is that Albert H has contracted pneumonia, and this disease will probably be fatal unless it is countered with an antibiotic. Although Albert H's son is aware of his father's advance directive, he nevertheless believes that an antiobiotic should be provided. He argues that his father presently has no conception of the "indignity" of his existence. Since his life, however compromised, clearly has value to him, his son contends, it is in his best interest that the antiobiotic be provided.

(1) Should Albert H's advance directive be overridden in this case? (2) Is Albert H presently the same person as the person who wrote the advance directive? If not, does that former person have the right to dictate what happens to Albert H?

CASE 28

Is Nutrition Expendable? [6]

Mildred D, a 78-year-old woman, suffers from diabetes, which has been controlled largely by diet. She has a history of heart disease and has suffered two heart attacks. She has now had a stroke, which has rendered her semicomatose and paralyzed. She must be fed through an NG (nasogastric) tube, and the sustenance that she receives in this way is the only thing that keeps her going. Mildred D has previously indicated to her family that in such a circumstance she would not want to be resuscitated. Her condition is slowly deteriorating, but it looks as though the dying process will be a long one. It seems that she will never return from the twilight zone in which she now resides. Angiography indicates that a substantial portion of the brain has been destroyed by the stroke. Her three children want to stop the tube feedings, but the physician objects that it is unethical to "starve" a patient so that she will die sooner.

(1) Is it morally legitimate to withhold nutrition in this case? (2) Does the family have the right to make such a decision for the patient? (3) Should the refusal of resuscitation be considered an indicator that the patient would also refuse nutrition?

CASE 29

Physician-Assisted Suicide in Oregon [2, 7]

In November 1994, voters in Oregon approved by a margin of 52 to 48 percent a ballot initiative known as the "Death with Dignity Act." This law (which had not gone into effect as of May 1995 because it was being challenged in federal court) permits physicians in Oregon to prescribe lethal drugs for terminally ill adult patients who want to end their own lives. In order for a patient to be eligible for such assistance, the attending physician must determine that the patient has a terminal illness and is expected to die within six months, and a consulting physician must confirm the diagnosis and prognosis. The following requirements are also stipulated: (1) The patient must make an initial oral request; reiterate the oral request after 15 days have passed; and also submit a written request, supported by two witnesses. (2) Before writing the prescription, the attending physician must wait at least 15 days after the patient's initial request and at least 48 hours after the written request. (3) The attending physician must fully inform the patient with regard to diagnosis and prognosis, as well as feasible alternatives—including comfort care, hospice care, and pain control. (4) Both the attending physician and the consulting physician must certify that the patient is "capable" (i.e., has decision-making capacity), is acting voluntarily, and has made an informed choice. (5) If either physician believes that the patient's judgment might be impaired (e.g., by depression), the patient must be referred for counseling. The Oregon law allows the attending physician and others to be present when the patient takes the lethal dose.

(1) Is the Oregon law morally sound? (2) Does it provide appropriate safeguards against possible abuse? (3) Is it necessary to have a waiting period? Is 15 days too long?

CASE 30

Death by Dehydration [6, 7]

Roberta W is a 67-year-old unmarried female. A retired teacher, she is cared for by her brother and his wife in their home. Roberta W suffers from severe emphysema and related heart problems. She also suffers from a collection of nagging medical problems, including bloatedness, hemorrhoids, and a hernia. She is largely confined to her bed. Occasionally she feels well enough to sit up for an hour or so, but eating, going to the bathroom, and personal grooming are experienced as exhausting and burdensome. Roberta W is weary of the circumstances of her life, and she regrets being a burden to her brother and his wife, although they do not seem to resent the demands placed on them by her care. Roberta W's prognosis is somewhat unclear, and she may well live for several years in her present state, but she continually says that she would rather be dead. At one point, when her hernia was especially bothersome to her, she had a conversation with her physician, Dr. R. He said that the hernia could easily be corrected by surgery, but that it was very unlikely that she would survive the surgery because of her emphysema and heart problems. She said that she wanted the surgery anyway. "If I die, fine; if I survive, at least I have one less problem." Dr. R responded that no responsible surgeon would perform an operation in such circumstances.

Roberta W now asks Dr. R to admit her to the hospital. Her plan is to stop drinking and to refuse any form of medical hydration, but she wants to be in the hospital so that any discomfort can be controlled through medication. She has read that patients who refuse all hydration will usually die within a week or so.

(1) If Roberta W refuses all hydration, is she committing suicide? (2) Should Dr. R accept Roberta W's plan and cooperate with her in executing it? Should his cooperation be understood as physician-assistance in suicide? (3) Would it have been morally justified for a surgeon to have provided the hernia surgery that she had wanted at an earlier time?

CASE 31

Anencephalic Newborns, Organ Donation, and Social Policy [6, 7]

It is estimated that 2,000 to 3,000 babies are born in the United States each year with anencephaly, the total or almost total absence of the cerebral hemispheres. Many of these infants are stillborn; the prognosis for those born alive is that they will live for only a few hours, days, or weeks. Although the organ systems of some anencephalic infants are underdeveloped, there are many cases in which organs (e.g., a heart or kidneys) could be transplanted to other infants whose lives might thereby be saved. Some parents of anencephalic infants would undoubtedly consent to organ donation as a way of creating some redeeming value out of a tragic situation. Still, numerous reservations have been expressed about the idea of transplanting the organs of anencephalic infants. In particular, for transplants to be successful, the vital organs must be taken from an anencephalic infant before it meets the criteria of (whole) brain death; thus harvesting its vital organs is tantamount to killing it. At present, there is no legal mechanism through which organ donation can be accomplished.

(1) Is it disrespectful, unfair, or otherwise immoral to transplant the organs of an anencephalic infant? (2) Should we adopt a social policy that would permit (with parental consent) harvesting the organs of an anencephalic infant? (3) If an anencephalic infant is stillborn, would it be justifiable to attempt resuscitation purely for the purpose of keeping

organs intact until they can be harvested? (4) If it is justifiable to harvest the organs of an anencephalic infant, would it be justifiable to harvest the organs of someone in a persistent vegetative state?

CASE 32

Neonatal Care and the Problem of Uncertainty [7]

Bobbie C is now six months old. He was born prematurely with a birth weight of 800 grams and had multiple problems from the beginning. Bobbie developed hyaline membrane disease due to his undeveloped lungs and the need for a respirator. He also developed rickets. A CAT scan revealed some calcium deposits in the brain that might or might not compromise his mental functions. Within the first month, Bobbie developed thrombocytopenia (low platelet count), for which he was given transfusions. He now suffers from a depression of his immunological system, perhaps related to the transfusions. He shows little interest in eating, and all attempts to bottle-feed him have failed after a couple of days. His health-care costs are being supported by Medicaid, and they are estimated to be in the neighborhood of $550,000 for his six months of hospitalization. Now the health-care staff and the attending physician are considering the possibility of a bone marrow transplant to deal with the thrombocytopenia and the immunosuppression. The chances of success in an infant this small are minimal, and the procedure is largely experimental in infants having this condition. If the transplant is successful, it will only alleviate one of his many problems.

(1) In view of the many uncertainties in this case, what is the proper treatment decision? (2) Should society be expected to shoulder such an expense for an infant who is so physiologically and, perhaps, mentally compromised? (3) Do the parents have a right to reject further aggressive therapies? to insist on them?

CASE 33

A Brain-Dead Mother Gives Birth [6, 8]

Rosa J suffered a fatal seizure while she was 23 weeks pregnant. After the seizure, Rosa J was placed on life-support systems but was declared brain-dead the next day. She was kept on life-support systems for 9 weeks, however, until she gave birth to a healthy baby girl by cesarean section. During this time the physicians used steroids to help the lungs of the fetus to mature and monitored fetal growth with ultrasound examinations. Rosa J was fed intravenously and given antibiotics for infections when necessary. After the birth, the life-support systems were disconnected. The baby was given an excellent chance to survive, although she weighed only three pounds. From the time of the seizure, all decisions about Rosa J and the fetus she was carrying were made by physicians in consultation with Rosa J's family.

(1) Should Rosa J have been kept on life-support systems for nine weeks after being declared brain-dead simply in order to give the child she was carrying a better chance to survive? (2) Was Rosa J being used merely as a means to others' ends? (3) Is someone who is brain-dead a "person" and, therefore, on a Kantian account an individual who cannot be used merely as a means to others' ends?

CASE 34

Maternal PKU and Fetal Welfare [8]

Martha J, a 23-year-old female, was born with PKU (phenylketonuria), an enzyme deficiency that prevents the metabolization of phenylalanine. Children born with PKU are ordinarily placed on a special low-phenylalanine diet for at least the first five years of their life. Although the diet is necessary to prevent severe retardation, it is very burdensome, not only because normal foods are very limited but also because the main source of protein is a bad-tasting "medical food." Because Martha J was placed on this special diet in her childhood, she does not suffer from retardation.

Martha J is four-months pregnant. Although her inability to metabolize phenylalanine is no longer a problem for her own well-being, there is a problem for the fetus she is carrying. Unless Martha J maintains the same low-phenylalanine diet throughout the course of her pregnancy, her fetus is at grave risk for severe retardation, microcephaly, congenital heart disease, and other disorders. Martha J's religious beliefs have motivated her to decide against abortion. Nevertheless, she is ambivalent about her pregnancy, because she is unmarried and depressed by the breakdown of her relationship with the child's father. She is also finding it very difficult to adhere to the same dietary restrictions that she found so oppressive in her childhood. Dr. R, the obstetrician who is caring for Martha J, has repeatedly emphasized the importance of adhering to the prescribed diet, but Martha J acknowledges that she has been inconstant in doing so.

(1) Should Dr. R encourage Martha J to reconsider the possibility of abortion? (2) If Martha J is resolved to carry her fetus to term, how should Dr. R deal with the fact that she is not maintaining the prescribed diet? (3) If all else fails, should Dr. R seek a court order that would place Martha J in a supervised setting where dietary restrictions could be enforced?

CASE 35

A Fetus with Turner's Syndrome [8, 9]

Barbara J is a 37-year-old woman who is pregnant and in her 20th week. She is married and has one child, a four-year-old girl. At the advice of her obstetrician, Barbara J has undergone amniocentesis, so that tests could be performed for chromosomal abnormalities and neural-tube defects. The tests have just come in, and Barbara J is told that the fetus has been diagnosed with a chromosomal abnormality known as Turner's syndrome.

A normal female has two X chromosomes. In Turner's syndrome, one of the two X chromosomes is missing; there is a total of only 45 chromosomes. Females who have Turner's syndrome have a characteristic appearance: short stature, webbing of the neck, sagging eyelids, low hairline on the back of the neck, and multiple moles. The syndrome is also characterized by narrowing of the aorta, the failure of menstruation and breast development, and infertility. Although many patients with Turner's syndrome have difficulty performing tasks that require spatial orientation, they can otherwise function normally in society.

(1) How serious are the appearance and developmental problems associated with Turner's syndrome? (2) Would abortion be morally justified in this case? Does it make a difference that the fetus is already at 20 weeks?

CASE 36

Prenatal Diagnosis and Sex Selection [8, 9]

A 32-year-old woman, Lisa B, comes to the prenatal diagnostic center of a major hospital. She is intent on arranging for chorionic villi sampling (CVS) in order to determine the sex of the fetus she is carrying. A genetic counselor explains to her that the center has an established policy against making prenatal diagnosis (whether CVS or amniocentesis) available for purposes of sex selection. The genetic counselor, in defending the policy, tells her that there is a collective sense at the center that abortion purely on grounds of sex selection is both morally and socially problematic.

Lisa B proceeds to explain her situation. She and her husband already have three children, all of whom are girls. They want very much to have a male child but, for economic reasons, are determined to have no more than one more child. Indeed, if they had a boy among their three children, they would not even consider having a fourth. They feel so strongly about this fourth child's being a boy that if they cannot gain assurance that it is a male they will elect abortion. Lisa B insists that it is unfair for the center to deny her access to prenatal diagnosis.

(1) Should the center consider this case an exceptional one and make CVS available? (2) Would the center be well advised to develop a different policy regarding the availability of prenatal diagnosis for purposes of sex selection?

CASE 37

Cystic Fibrosis and a Finding of Nonpaternity [9]

At the age of 19 months, Jennifer C was diagnosed with cystic fibrosis (CF), an autosomal recessive genetic disease. The characteristic pattern is that a child inherits the CF gene from both parents, each of whom is a carrier. Jennifer C's parents, who have been married about three years, are anxious to clarify their risk for having another child with this disorder. They are referred to a genetic counselor, who arranges for DNA testing to confirm their carrier status. The results from the laboratory indicate that Jennifer's mother is a carrier but her husband is not. In fact, DNA analysis shows clearly that he is not the biological father of the child. The genetic counselor is unsure how to proceed.

(1) Should the genetic counselor communicate the finding of nonpaternity to the couple, perhaps jeopardizing their young marriage? Should the genetic counselor first speak privately with the woman? (2) If the woman is willing to identify the biological father, should the genetic counselor notify him that he is almost certainly a carrier of the CF gene?

CASE 38

A Feminist Sperm Bank [9]

The Oakland (California) Feminist Women's Health Center is a sperm bank that was founded in order to make AID (artificial insemination by donor) available in a manner that is consistent with feminist ideals. Although genetic and medical screening is provided, the keynote of the center's operation is the fact that no *social* screening of applicants is done. Lesbians and unmarried women are expressly invited, along with more traditional candidates for AID, to make use of the center's services. In addition, neither standards of economics nor standards of intelligence are employed to exclude applicants, and racial matching is not done.

(1) Is the operational philosophy of this sperm bank morally sound? (2) Should a sperm bank be held accountable to society for a social screening of its applicants for AID? If so, what factors would be sufficient to disqualify an applicant?

CASE 39

IVF and a Postmenopausal Woman [9]

Emily L is a 59-year-old woman who plans to retire at the age of 60 from her job as a financial executive. She has been married for ten years to a man who also plans to retire within the next year. He is presently 64 years of age. Both Emily L and her husband are in good health and look forward to carving out a new life in retirement. In fact, they have decided that this would be a good time for them to raise a child, so they want to arrange for Emily L to become pregnant. They are aware that it is now possible for postmenopausal women to bear children by employing egg donation, in vitro fertilization (IVF), and embryo transplantation to the womb of the postmenopausal woman, who would receive hormonal treatments. The idea is that Emily L's husband would provide the sperm for IVF, making him the biological father of the child. When Emily L and her husband explain their plan to Dr. T at the Metropolitan

Fertility Clinic, Dr. T is uncertain whether the clinic should support Emily's attempt to become pregnant. Dr. T has successfully produced pregnancies in women who have experienced early menopause, but she is not comfortable with the age of the prospective parents in this particular case.

(1) Is the plan formulated by Emily L and her husband morally sound? If not, what is problematic about it? (2) Should Dr. T and the clinic support Emily L's attempt to become pregnant?

CASE 40

Justice, Mental Disability, and Public Policy [5, 10]

State representative Jeremy H has introduced a state bill that would establish homes for the care and education of children with major learning disabilities, such as severe retardation and autism. The bill would provide one home for every 12 children presently institutionalized in five state institutions for children with such disabilities. The present annual cost of maintaining the five institutions is $100 million. Providing the new form of care for the present institutionalized population of 8,000 is expected to cost about $130 million annually.

Jeremy H argues that the currently institutionalized children live in antiquated buildings lacking basic human necessities and amenities. The children frequently spend whole days in their cheerless rooms; many are not even properly clothed. Supervised by an overworked, largely untrained staff, they receive almost nothing in the way of education, entertainment, or structured activities. Jeremy H argues that justice requires removing these individuals from such subhuman conditions and offering them an opportunity for a more "normal" life.

A physician, Dr. M, is opposed to the bill and testifies at a legislative hearing. He argues that the money required to make the change could be used more efficiently to provide health care for three groups: normal children, women lacking access to gynecological and prenatal services, and working adults whose employers do not provide health insurance. He also argues that the occurrence of retardation and other mental disabilities can be greatly reduced through prenatal diagnosis.

(1) Should the proposed bill be enacted into law? (2) Do the mentally retarded have a right to lead a life as "normal" as possible, given their limitations?

CASE 41

Justice, Kidney Dialysis, and a Mentally Retarded Boy [5, 6, 10]

Joey C is a 13-year-old retarded boy living in a state-supported home for the mentally retarded. He has no relatives. Joey is suffering from uremic poisoning. Ordinarily someone in Joey's condition would be treated by dialysis three times a week. If Joey does not receive dialysis treatments, he will die. Joey is examined by four kidney experts, all of whom decide against dialysis. They give two reasons for their decision: (1) Joey will not understand the need for the therapy; he will consider the needles and the frequent confinements to the machine as torture, and, as a result, he will be unmanageable. (2) The state institution cannot provide Joey with the necessary hygienic and dietary care required for dialysis. The physicians conclude that the alternative to adopt for Joey is a slow, easy death.

Several employees of the institution protest and argue that Joey should not simply be allowed to die but should be given dialysis treatments. They offer the following reasons: (1) Retardation should not be a criterion for dialysis. (2) Any form of therapy can be perceived as a form of torture by a patient, depending on how the health professionals in charge handle the patient. (3) Other retarded children on dialysis have often been model patients. In fact, retarded young adults are sometimes perceived as overly compliant, meticulously following orders about their care.

(1) When a child has no parents or close relatives and is not competent to understand what is at issue in a life-or-death decision, who should make the decision for the child? Physicians? The courts? A guardian appointed by the courts? (2) Is severe mental retardation a morally relevant criterion when decisions are made about the use of expensive medical resources?

CASE 42

Determining the Quality of Life [6, 10]

George K is a 25-year-old male who is unmarried and has no dependents. Medicaid supports him in his health-care needs, which are considerable since he suffers from muscular dystrophy. George K is totally paralyzed and therefore confined to bed. In addition to being quadriplegic, he cannot speak, and he is respirator dependent through a tracheotomy. Ordinarily he resides in a nursing home, but periodically he must be brought to the intensive care unit of a local hospital for crisis care related to the respirator dependency. He has a woman friend who visits him occasionally as well as a mother who visits him regularly. George K communicates through smiles and raising and lowering his eyebrows. He seems to enjoy watching television and is a great fan of the Dallas Cowboys and the Detroit Tigers.

(1) What assessment should be made of George K's quality of life? (2) Should discussions be initiated with George K about withholding treatment in the case of future crises? (3) Can society afford to support, for long periods of time, individuals who constitute such a drain on health-care resources?

CASE 43

Justice and Abortion Funding [8, 10]

Sara G is a 35-year-old mother of four children whose husband deserted her about a month after she became pregnant with her fifth child. The ages of her four children range from one to six years. She knows nothing about her husband's whereabouts and is currently being supported by welfare payments including Aid to Families with Dependent Children (AFDC). Sara G is less than three months pregnant and wants an abortion. Her reasons are as follows: (1) She does not have the skills to get a job whose earnings will even come close to the welfare payments she receives. If she has to pay for child care from whatever meager wages she could earn, the money left could not support her family at even the subsistence level. So, at least until the children are older, she will be dependent on welfare and AFDC. The sums she receives are barely adequate to take care of her present family. Adding another member would mean even further deprivation for her present family. (2) Her welfare caseworker has agreed that when the four children are a bit older, Sara G will go into a job-training program that will enable her to get a job paying enough to get the family off public assistance and to give her children a better start in life. Sara G has undergone a battery of psychological tests to help determine what kind of work she should be capable of doing with the right education and training. The social worker and psychological counselor are both confident that Sara G can do the work necessary to make a good living for herself and her family. Having another child would only postpone the time when Sara G will be self-supporting, and in the meantime her family would be living at a very inadequate level.

Because Sara G is on welfare, she must get an authorization from the social work agency for any medical procedure that is not necessitated by an emergency. In cases involving abortion, the final decision is made by a social worker.

(1) Should the social worker authorize the abortion? (2) What moral justification could be advanced to support an authorization? a refusal to authorize the abortion? (3) What restrictions, if any, should there be on the Medicaid funding of abortion?

CASE 44

Justice, Age, and Personal Responsibility [10]

The intensive care unit (ICU) at a local hospital has one available bed. Two patients are in immediate and desperate need of ICU care. The first is Jeffrey O, who is 71 years old and has been severely injured in an automobile accident. Jeffrey O was in good physical shape prior to the accident and does not suffer from any debilitating condition. However, his present condition is extremely critical due to the accident. The second patient is Donald R, a 22-year-old drug addict whose present equally critical condition is the result of drug use.

(1) Which of the two should receive the ICU bed? (2) Would the answer be different if Donald R were 71 years old and Jeffrey O were 22? (3) Suppose Donald R were not a drug addict but a previously healthy 22-year-old severely injured in an automobile accident. Furthermore, suppose that Jeffrey O had been admitted to the hospital about an hour before Donald R, but the decision about putting each of them in the ICU is being made at the same time. Who should get the bed?

CASE 45

Justice, Health Care, and Poverty [10]

Amanda R is 25 years old. Although she holds both a full-time and a part-time job, she has a very low income and does not have any health-care insurance. At the same time, Amanda R's income is just high enough to prevent her from qualifying for any government-funded health care such as that provided by Medicaid. While experiencing severe chest pain and difficulty in breathing, Amanda R goes to the emergency room of a local for-profit hospital. Before she receives any care, clerical personnel in the hospital determine her financial status and the fact that she is uninsured. By the time she is examined, Amanda R's chest pains stop, and her breathing difficulties disappear. A medical staff member gives her a cursory examination, which does not include an electrocardiogram, and sends her home, suggesting that she go to her own physician the next day for a more thorough examination.

(1) If the medical staff member's decision not to give Amanda R a more thorough examination and not to admit her for further observation was based on her lack of health-care insurance, can that decision be morally justified? (2) Suppose that Amanda R's symptoms had not eased while she was in the emergency room and that the medical staff member had decided that Amanda R did need hospital admittance, observation, and testing. However, suppose that instead of admitting her to the for-profit hospital, Amanda R had been sent by ambulance to a community (not-for-profit) hospital. Would that behavior have been morally acceptable?